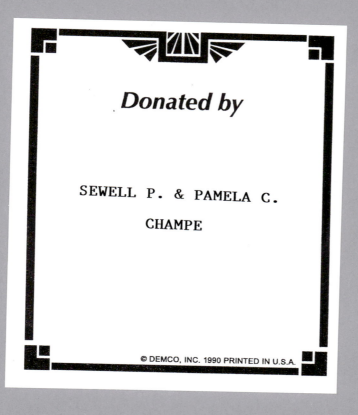

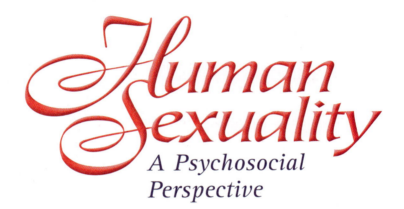

Human Sexuality

A Psychosocial Perspective

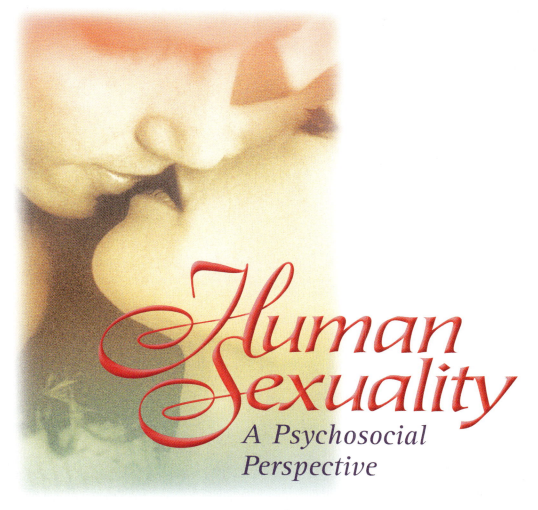

Human Sexuality

A Psychosocial Perspective

Ruth K. Westheimer
Sanford Lopater

 LIPPINCOTT WILLIAMS & WILKINS

A **Wolters Kluwer** Company

Philadelphia · Baltimore · New York · London
Buenos Aires · Hong Kong · Sydney · Tokyo

Editor: Susan B. Katz
Development Editor: Tom L. Lochhaas
Managing Editor: Matthew J. Hauber
Marketing Manager: Aimee Sirmon
Production Editor: Jennifer D. Weir
Editorial Assistants: Jennifer Pirozzoli, Loftin P. Montgomery

Art Direction: Jonathan Dimes, Jennifer Clements
Interior Design: Doug Smock
Cover Design: Armen Kojoyian
Photographers: Michal Heron, Stephen Ogilvie
Image Researcher: Barbara Feretti
Artists: Mary Anna Barratt, Jonathan Dimes, Michael Kress-Russick, David Rini

Copyright © 2002 Lippincott Williams & Wilkins

351 West Camden Street
Baltimore, MD 21201 USA

227 East Washington Square
Philadelphia, PA 19106 USA

Printed in the United States of America.

Library of Congress Cataloging-in-Publication Data

Westheimer, Ruth K. (Ruth Karola), 1928-
    Human sexuality: a psychosocial perspective / Ruth K. Westheimer, Sanford Lopater.
        p. cm.
    Includes index.
    ISBN 0-683-30138-1
    1. Sex. 2. Sex (Psychology) 3. Sexual disorders. I. Lopater, Sanford. II. Title.

HQ21 .W59 2001
306.7--dc21

00-140181

The publishers have made every effort to trace the copyright holders for borrowed material. If they have inadvertently overlooked any, they will be pleased to make the necessary arrangements at the first opportunity.

To purchase additional copies of this book, call our customer service department at **(800) 638-3030** or fax orders to **(301) 824-7390**. International customers should call **(301) 714-2324**.

Visit Lippincott Williams & Wilkins on the Internet: http://www.LWW.com. Lippincott Williams & Wilkins customer service representatives are available from 8:30 am to 6:00 pm, EST.

01 02 03 04 05
1 2 3 4 5 6 7 8 9 10

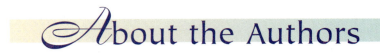

Ruth K. Westheimer, EdD Dr. Ruth Westheimer is a Psychosexual Therapist, pioneering sex educator, and long-time proponent of "sexual literacy." She received a Masters degree in Sociology and a Doctorate in Education from Columbia University. Dr. Westheimer studied human sexuality with Dr. Helen Singer Kaplan at New York Hospital-Cornell University Medical Center and is an adjunct professor at New York University and fellow of the New York Academy of Medicine. In addition, she regularly conducts seminars on adolescent sexuality for pediatric residents and interns at Brookdale Hospital, SUNY Downstate Medical Center. She is a frequent speaker at colleges and universities across the country and twice has been named "College Lecturer of the Year." Her radio program, "Sexually Speaking," which began in 1980, aired across the country, and her television show, "The Dr. Ruth Show," has been syndicated nationally and internationally.

Sanford Lopater, PhD Sanford Lopater has been a faculty member in the Department of Psychology at Christopher Newport University in Virginia since 1973. He received his Doctorate in Experimental and Physiological Psychology from the University of Virginia. Dr. Lopater has taught human sexuality courses for the past 28 years, as well as other courses in the areas of biological psychology, behavioral medicine, and health psychology, and as a two-time recipient of Fulbright awards, he has worked in the area of postsecondary teacher training in England.

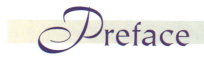

Preface

*E*very year I lecture at many college campuses across the country, and I try to keep my finger on the pulse of youthful sexual concerns and interests. While many of you have taken or plan to take a course in human sexuality, most students have not. That's a pity because college is just the place for a serious, systematic approach to the matters that concern you and have an effect on your lives. And sex is certainly one of those subjects.

One reason that some students avoid a course in human sexuality is embarrassment, and I completely appreciate that fact. It is not always easy to just start talking and reading about a topic that in the past has been a little mysterious and more than a little controversial. But a well-thought-out course in human sexuality, sensitively taught by a caring professor, can be a wonderful addition to your education.

I'm pretty sure human sexuality is one course you won't be able to forget about once the final exam is over. And I'm also convinced that a good human sexuality textbook is one you would want to make a permanent part of your personal library. The material in this book will help you to not only better understand how life is created, but also how to actually help you create life itself (or postpone doing it, if that's what you want). Sexual pleasure in the context of a mutually supportive, communicative relationship brings some of the most powerful pleasures and satisfactions you will ever experience, and I hope and believe that what you read here will help you reach this goal.

Dr. Ruth K. Westheimer

Maybe more so than in most undergraduate courses, students who enroll in a human sexuality course are highly motivated and genuinely curious, and have a number of personal questions about the area of human sexuality in general and perhaps a few specific questions in particular. Still, teaching or taking this course requires careful attention to the basic principles of learning. For this reason we have taken special care to offer a human sexuality textbook that is comprehensive, systematic, and interesting on the one hand and very easy to read and learn from on the other. Chapters are carefully ordered to introduce more basic and elementary issues at the outset and elaborate on them in depth in later sections of the book. Simply stated, more complex topics are built on more fundamental facts, concepts, and principles.

In addition to all the traditional topics of human sexuality, we have introduced a considerable amount of pertinent and interesting, nontraditional information, in part to appeal to the many different academic majors represented in most human sexuality courses. Our approach is not specific to the needs and interests of students in the social, behavioral, and biological sciences. In casting our net wide we have included novel, relevant, fascinating information from disciplines such as history, law, business administration, military science, philosophy, ethics, law enforcement, and health care administration. While no book can meet everyone's needs all the time, we have certainly tried to appeal to a broad array of student interests and academic programs.

We have worked to "nest" virtually every important topic in three domains: the personal, the interpersonal, and the societal. For every key concept, we first discuss its implications for the individual as a solitary, thinking, evaluating person. We then explore its meaning to that person in an intimate or sexual relationship. And finally, we discuss the relevance of the issue to the wider psychosocial environment. In this way, virtually every significant topic is viewed from three complementary perspectives simultaneously, offering, we hope, a more comprehensive, cohesive understanding of the material and better avenues for students to draw a personal connection.

Finally, we take great pride in offering a human sexuality textbook that is easy and enjoyable to read. Throughout, our objectives have been to educate students, to motivate them to learn more independently, and to reassure them that many of their thoughts, feelings, and fantasies are largely common and normal. We have purposely avoided an overly technical tone throughout, and we are certain that our friendly prose will be a welcome feature that will encourage reading and re-reading of the entire text.

FEATURES

Chapter Opening

Each chapter begins with a brief **Highlight** of the material to follow and a set of learning **Objectives.** The objectives state explicitly the main points the student should be able to know and understand when he or she has finished reading the chapter.

From Dr. Ruth

The introductory paragraphs, **From Dr. Ruth,** at the beginning of each chapter provide the unique, personal insight of a person who has dedicated her professional life to educating the public in issues of human sexuality.

Other Countries, Cultures, and Customs

A cross-cultural approach is explicit throughout the book. Not only is cross-cultural material integrated into the text, but also individual chapters contain a feature or features entitled **Other Countries, Cultures, and Customs,** containing a vignette, study, or story that demonstrates the application of content in the chapter to other societies and their diverse ways of life.

Research Highlights

This feature offers in-depth analysis of the nature, meaning, methods, and implications of both classical and current studies. The methodology of various studies is critiqued and their long-term value explored. By drawing on studies from different disciplines (social and behavioral sciences, law, medicine, anthropology, history), the **Research Highlights** further reinforce the multidisciplinary approach of the book, while encouraging a closer critique of research design.

Exploding Myths

Unfortunately, within the arena of human sexuality, myth often carries the authority of fact. Misinformation, misinterpretation, and over-generalization are common. In the **Exploding Myths** feature, we look at the sources of common sexual myths, their implications intellectually, emotionally, and behaviorally, and the reasons they are perpetuated.

On the Lighter Side

The **On the Lighter Side** feature will encourage students to see that we shouldn't always take ourselves too seriously. The whimsical and comical stories in this feature should do much to dilute the anxiety that might otherwise make learning human sexuality difficult or uncomfortable.

Dear Dr. Ruth

This feature shows Dr. Ruth's unique perspective from a closer angle, taking readers into the enlightening and revealing world of her role as therapist. These short "vignettes" present questions, concerns, and scenarios based on Dr. Westheimer's broad experience as both a sex therapist and an approachable, candid public personality.

ANCILLARIES

Available to instructors is a complete set of free teaching ancillaries, many located at the *Human Sexuality: A Psychosocial Perspective* companion website, **connection.lww.com/go/sexuality**:

- **Test Generator CD-ROM** containing more than 1000 questions.
- **Image Bank** of illustrations, available on CD-ROM.
- **Instructor's Manual**, including an expanded list of learning objectives for each chapter and detailed lecture outlines. Available on line and by request as a printed version.
- **Student Study Guide,** authored by Richelle Frabotta, including numerous multiple-choice, matching, short answer, and true/false questions and answers for review of the chapter material, as well as "Self-Reflection" exercises to encourage more divergent thinking. The study guide includes additional "Dear Dr. Ruth" features in most chapters for students to read and react to in a framework of personal reflection and exploration. Also included are links to relevant web sites for each chapter. Available on line and by request as a printed version.
- Customizable **PowerPoint Slide Presentation** of chapter outlines.
- **Content Updates** for each chapter, posted regularly to provide the most current information.
- **Web Resource Links**
- **Discussion Board**

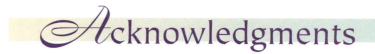

Acknowledgments

A book of this size, scope, and complexity requires the persistent, dedicated, and coordinated efforts of many people. We are especially indebted to a number of friends and colleagues, not to mention our families, who have supported and assisted us throughout every phase of the development and writing of this textbook.

Tom Lochhaas was our developmental editor, and working with him has been one of the happiest and most cooperative, productive professional relationships of our careers. Tom has a keen sense of the undergraduate readership and was adroit in encouraging ever-greater clarity of expression. He was our cheerleader, coach, and friend. This book is no less Tom's than ours. Jonathan Dimes directed the selection, evaluation, procurement, and placement of virtually every photograph, chart, table, or drawing. His personal expertise as an artist and managerial skills as a medical illustrator are apparent on every page of this textbook. We have been able to depict complex concepts, anatomical illustrations, surgical procedures, and physiological mechanisms because Jonathan was tirelessly resourceful. Our managing editor, Matt Hauber, worked hard to create and maintain a calm, focused, and astonishingly fruitful coordination of talent throughout the revision and production phases of this book. His unfailing calmness and civility were fundamental to the creation of a book of wonderful clarity and attractiveness. Tim Satterfield, the President of Lippincott, Williams & Wilkins, had faith in the entire enterprise from the outset and made generous resources available that allowed us to work unencumbered by many common constraints in the publishing industry. Tim's faith in us was an unspoken and fundamental strength throughout the development and creation of our book. Many others at Lippincott Williams & Wilkins devoted a disproportionately large share of their time and dedication to our project, and we wish to thank Aimee Sirmon, Nancy Evans, Susan Katz, Crystal Taylor, Jennifer Clements, and Jennifer Weir for their unquestioning loyalty and hard work.

Many of the more explicit photographs for our book, and the line art drawings often based on them, are of the highest available professional quality. This is due to the wonderful talent of Michal Heron and Stephen Ogilvie of New York City. With Michal, Stephen, Jonathan, and one of us (S.L.) working together, we were able to pose a score of models as we chose, refine their postures and expressions, and create the template for an art program that we feel is unsurpassed. Our thanks to them for translating many of our concepts and objectives into flawless photographs.

FROM RUTH WESTHEIMER

I'm very quick to say that I know what I know and I also know what I don't know. From the very beginning I knew that I could not write a textbook on human sexuality on my own, but from the second I laid eyes on Sandy Lopater, I also knew that he would be the perfect co-author. Undoubtedly we've both learned a great deal from working on this immense project and, as a result, the students who use this textbook will learn even more.

I first began working with Pierre Lehu in 1981 and he well deserves the title I have given him of Minister of Communications. As with every project with which I am involved, he has been of great help on this one and for that he gets my deepest gratitude.

Thanks to my family of origin, to my teachers who had the opportunity to instill in me the much cherished values of the Jewish tradition, and to the memory of my late husband, Fred, who encouraged me in all my endeavors. Thanks to my daughter, Miriam Westheimer, EdD, son-in-law Joel Einleger, MBA, their children Ari and Leora, my son Joel Westheimer, PhD, daughter-in-law Barbara Leckie, PhD, and their daughter, Michal.

Thanks to Jim Anker, Peter Bernard, MD, Mary Cuadrado, PhD, Martin Englisher, Michael Freedman, MD, David Goslin, PhD, Amos Grunebaum, MD, Allan Halpern, MD, Helen Singer Kaplan, MD, PhD, Steven Kaplan, PhD, Amy and Joel Kassiola, PhD, Robert Krasner, MD, Lou Lieberman, PhD, Vera Jelineck, PhD, Daniel Present, MD, Ira Sacker, MD, Michael Weiss, MD, and Ben Yagoda.

FROM SANFORD LOPATER

Thanks are due to the many colleagues and students at Christopher Newport University who made it possible for me to devote large blocks of uninterrupted time to work on this manuscript. I especially wish to thank President Paul Trible, Provost Robert Doane, and Dean Jouett Powell, as well as the Board of Visitors of Christopher Newport University for granting me a sabbatical to work on this project. My department Chair, Sam Bauer, arranged flexible scheduling of my course load and my administrative assistant Emilie Smith carried out an incredibly diverse number of tasks on short notice—always with my sincere thanks. Other professors in my own and other departments offered personal support and information: Robert Abdo, Tom Berry, Tim Marshall, Kelly Cartwright, Vince Rose, Joe Healey, Frank MacHovec, and Dave Dooley.

A number of students read portions of the manuscript, offering their helpful perspective and suggestions. For this I am especially grateful to Cheri Cain, Ryan Serio, and Don and Linda Mates.

Mr. John McDonald of Williamsburg, Virginia, and Ms. Elizabeth Cunningham of Hampton, Virginia, gave me dozens of books (some quite old and valuable) in the area of sexuality, and I am profoundly thankful for their generosity over the years.

Ms. Maureen Humphries and Ms. Leslie Condra worked for many years to obtain for me hundreds of inter-library loans and I am indebted to them for their industriousness and dedication to my work.

Since 1965, Ted Goble, John Russell, Gary Mull, Ron Grant, Dan Cahill, Bob Shaw, Scott Adie, and Mr. and Mrs. Bill Lewis have taken a keen, personal interest in my academic and professional success and it gives me immense pleasure to thank them here in this way.

I was fortunate to have been mentored by a number of exceptional teachers and scholars over the last forty years and here I wish to thank Bill Karasick, Donald E. Parker, PhD, John F. Hahn, PhD, Frank W. Finger, PhD, and John A. Jane, MD, PhD. Their support of my developing talents and interests has been indispensable to the initiation and continuation of a wonderful, rewarding career.

My wife Susan, and daughters Emily, Erin, and Robye have been there for me throughout the last 5 years. Susan read and commented on virtually every word of the manuscript and the kids so much enjoyed telling me all that I *really* needed to know about sex.

No list of acknowledgments would be complete without attributing my thanks to my parents, Harold Jack Lopater and Shirley H. Lopater. They both taught me to work hard and to enjoy it.

Finally, I wish to offer my sincerest thanks to Ruth Westheimer. Ruth and I have worked on this project for more than 5 years and throughout that entire time she was there to offer assistance, share her clinical experience, and explore the best ways of blending my didactic classroom experience with her enormously diverse and interesting clinical experience.

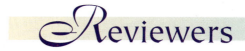

Thomas Billimek, MA, LPA
Department of Psychology
San Antonio College
San Antonio, Texas

Sandra L. Caron, PhD
University of Maine
Orono, Maine

Bart Cilento, MD
Department of Urology
Children's Hospital
Boston, Massachusetts

Rita J. Clark, MS
Department of Behavioral, Social and Economic Sciences
Aims Community College
Loveland, Colorado

John Collins, PhD
Department of Psychology
North Dakota State University
North Fargo, North Dakota

Lorry Cology, PhD
Department of Social and Behavioral Sciences
Owens Community College
Toledo, Ohio

Linda Costanzo, PhD
Department of Physiology
MCV
Richmond, Virginia

Connie Edlund, MA
Chair, Wellness
Kalamazoo Valley Community College
Kalamazoo, Michigan

Richard Ellsworth, PhD
Assistant Professor of Psychology
Chapman University
Palmdale, California

Richelle Frabotta, MSEd, CSE
Miami University
Middletown, Ohio

Sue Frantz, MA
Assistant Professor of Psychology
New Mexico State University-Alamogordo
Alamogordo, New Mexico

David A. Gershaw, PhD
Professor of Psychology, Emeritus
Arizona Western College
Yuma, Arizona

Matthew Hogben, PhD
Behavioral Interventions & Disease Research Branch, DSTDP
Center for Disease Control and Prevention
Atlanta, Georgia

David Johnson, PhD
Department of Sociology and Anthropology
University of South Alabama
Mobile, Alabama

Julie Johnson-Pynn, PhD
Assistant Professor of Psychology
Berry College
Mount Berry, Georgia

Dawn Larsen, PhD, CHES
Department of Health Science
Minnesota State University
Mankato, Minnesota

Frank Ling, MD
Chair, Department of Obstetrics & Gynecology
University of Tennessee, Memphis
Memphis, Tennessee

Andrew R. McGarva, PhD
Assistant Professor of Psychology
Dickinson State University
Dickinson, North Dakota

Stephanie McGowan, PhD
Department of Psychology
University of Albany, SUNY
Albany, New York

Chris Moyers, PhD
Department Chair, Sociology and Anthropology
Mission College
Felton, CA

Maureen O'Brien, PhD
Northwest Iowa Community College
Le Mars, Iowa

Michael Perry, MD
Professor of Internal Medicine
Nellie B. Smith Chair of Oncology
Director, Division of Hematology/Oncology
University of Missouri/Ellis Fischel Cancer Center
Columbia, Missouri

Rusty Pippin, PhD, CHES
Professor and Division Director, Health Division, HHPR
Baylor University
Waco, Texas

Sherman Sowby, PhD, CHES
Health Science Department
California State University—Fresno
Fresno, California

Mary Wyandt, MEd, CHES
University Health Center
University of Arkansas
Fayettesvillle, Arkansas

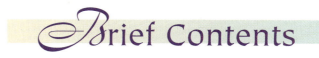

Brief Contents

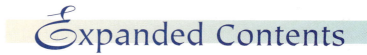

Expanded Contents

Hence a man leaves his father and his mother and clings to his wife, so that they become one flesh.

Genesis 2:24

The two of them were naked, the man and his wife, yet they felt no shame.

Genesis 2:25

The Place of Sexuality in Our Lives

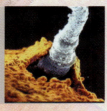

OBJECTIVES

When you finish reading and reviewing this chapter, you should be able to:

1. Describe some common assumptions students have about a course in human sexuality.

2. Describe your own expectations and assumptions about a course in human sexuality.

3. List several sciences and professions related to the study of human sexuality.

4. Discuss how sexual topics are included in the subject matter of different sciences.

5. Describe what is meant by "levels of analysis" and give examples of macro and micro levels of analysis of sexual topics.

6. Discuss the prevalence of sexual concerns to people with different lifestyles and levels of personal development.

7. Suggest additional sexual issues affecting our lifestyles that have not been introduced in this chapter.

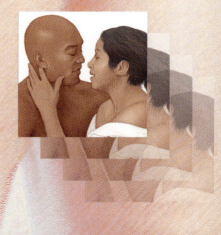

From Dr. Ruth

What an opportunity! How exciting to be in a course that can inform, motivate, and reassure you about one of the most fundamental, fascinating, and pervasive aspects of human nature. Not every course can help you better understand yourself, other people, and society all at the same time. But we must tell you from the beginning that this subject is sometimes quite complex; that it is a *serious* academic discipline with its own traditions, methods, and controversies. Some of the things you will read you may already know about, other things may surprise you, and still others really may astonish you. The discipline of human sexuality can improve the quality of your life and, in some cases, even the length of your life.

Sexuality surrounds us every day because in one way or another we encounter sexual "concerns," "issues," and "questions." But you most likely have not had the chance to study these topics in much depth. This is your chance to do just that. Although we have written this book to teach you about human sexuality, we want to encourage you to use this information to learn still more and to critically assess what you read and hear in the media and from your friends. You can think of this as a "life skills" course.

ASSUMPTIONS ABOUT A COURSE IN SEXUALITY

Because our assumptions guide our perceptions, an understanding of our own beliefs helps us better comprehend events in the world around us. This is a good time to examine some common beliefs about this course you are taking. The following common assumptions are not a complete list, but they are a good starting point. We want to encourage you to think about your expectations for this subject matter and for this book.

ASSUMPTION 1: Human sexuality is a single, integrated subject in which facts, concepts, and principles are all clearly related to each other. This assumption cannot be fully supported. Just browsing through this book will reveal an enormous variety of topics. For example, one chapter includes complicated descriptions of the action of sex hormones on reproductive behaviors and fertility, while other chapters discuss social perspectives on issues such as homosexuality and sexual assault. This diversity of topics presents an interesting challenge for the course but can also stimulate curiosity about relationships among facts that, at first, might seem unrelated.

Just as human sexuality includes diverse topics, so too are the methods sex researchers use to discover trends, facts, and generalities. As medical scientists use sophisticated physiological and biochemical techniques to make discoveries, social and behavioral scientists use many other methodologies, such as observational techniques, carefully controlled experiments, and survey and questionnaire investigations. Consider, however, that this research always takes place within the context of a cultural value system, and different cultures sometimes have very different perspectives on sexual issues.

ASSUMPTION 2: Most students already have learned a lot about human sexuality in elementary school, high school, their homes, or their church groups. We wish this were true, but it is unusual for undergraduates to have learned much yet about many of the topics in this course. Now you have the opportunity to enrich your life by exploring this most interesting aspect of human nature. Much may be new to you, but you'll experience the excitement of discovery. You have already heard much about some aspects of human sexuality, but some of this is likely not based on careful study. The material in this book, however, is *organized* and *authoritative* to help make your learning *thorough* and *systematic*. Instruction in human sexuality may have changed in recent years, but the serious, organized, and factual quality of the discipline has not (Fig. 1-1).

Some of what students know or think about sex may involve feelings of guilt or anxiety. Accurate, useful information, however, can be a powerful antidote to such feelings. This is just one of the benefits of a course like this: to gain a new understanding in a nonjudgmental, safe, academic setting.

ASSUMPTION 3: Students will think critically about what they learn and will apply it in their interpersonal relationships and preprofessional studies. We're counting on this. Our experience has shown that knowledge of human sexuality can change lives, almost always for the better. Still, there is sometimes a gap between learning something and incorporating it into one's life. Feelings of nervousness about sex do not suddenly disappear when one learns new information. Accurate information is only the first step in developing a personal sense of "sexual literacy."

We urge you not to take a simplistic "take it home and put it to work" approach to sexual information. Most sexual expression takes place in an interpersonal context, and that means someone else is involved in your sexual discovery and development. Be cautious about sharing what you learn without clear communication first.

One of our most important goals in this book is to provide enough information for you to make intelligent sexual decisions and enhance your reproductive and sexual health. This involves much more than erections and secretions. We urge an active personal commitment to maintaining personal health through such things as testicular or breast self-examination, regular mammograms if appropriate, responsible consideration and use of contraception, and sensitivity to the risks of sexually transmitted diseases.

Finally, you will find this information indispensable in many different professions. Those majoring in nursing, social work, psychology, physical therapy, occupational therapy, health education, physical education, premedicine, prelaw, or gerontology, to name only a few, will gain pertinent and interesting information for your life's work. More obviously, this knowledge is essential and important for parenting skills.

ASSUMPTION 4: Human sexuality has central importance in the liberal arts and sciences. We think so. If liberal learning implies that exposure to the arts, sciences, and social sciences enhances our lives and prepares us for an ever-changing world, then certainly this course is part of this tradition. But you should know that others may react differently when they learn you are taking this course. Some of your friends and fellow students may find something slightly suspect about this course. Although everyone accepts that metabolism, digestion, and neural functioning are "natural" aspects of humanity to study, unfortunately some do not include human sexuality as a "natural" function. Some may even feel the topic or the course involves erotic, titillating, exhibitionistic, or obscene elements. With an understanding of the breadth and depth of this subject, however, you can easily legitimize its place in the curriculum.

ASSUMPTION 5: Students always see the relationship between physical aspects of sexuality and the importance of communication, intimacy, and individuation. This assumption involves an interesting challenge. Many people mistakenly believe that if they just knew more about touching and lovemaking techniques, then their sexual selves would be complete and satisfied. But of course, tactile stimulation and sexual intercourse without communication and commitment are usually less than fully rewarding experiences. A thorough familiarity with anatomical, physiological, and hormonal aspects of human sexuality in no way insures a person can communicate with another openly about sensitive issues. Shared intimacy exists in an interpersonal relationship, of which sexuality is just one dimension.

A genuine capacity for intimacy often depends on a climate of psychological safety and a couple's willingness to share their vulnerabilities. Real mutuality involves accepting the other without expecting the other to change to please you. These relationship dimensions do not automatically flow from one's knowledge of the physical aspects of sexual interaction.

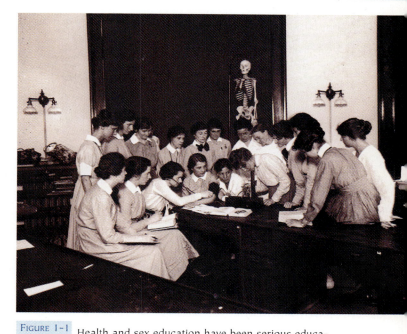

FIGURE 1-1 Health and sex education have been serious educational priorities in many countries throughout the world for the past half-century.

Yet there are reciprocal influences of the physical and emotional aspects of sexual expression that you will come to better understand.

We started out with the observation that our assumptions often guide our perceptions. The assumptions we discussed may not match your own, but we urge you to examine carefully your beliefs and values related to sexuality and how they may affect your expectations for this course.

A MULTIDISCIPLINARY APPROACH TO SEXUALITY

Perhaps nowhere more so than in the study of human sexuality do so many arenas of human inquiry come together. Each discipline has its own rules and traditions for what constitutes a "fact," the generalizing of findings, research methods, and the application of knowledge to help people. Many academic specialties engage in the discovery, analysis, and application of sexual information. Of the following disciplines considered throughout this text, listed here in arbitrary order, no one is more important than others.

Sociology

Sociology is a branch of the social and behavioral sciences concerned with the nature of social and cultural norms and problems. Sociologists are generally interested in the trends and traditions of groups of people, as well as the impact of their behavior on society. Sociology is a "big picture" discipline, giving less attention to individuals. For example, a sociologist might study why certain sexually transmitted diseases are more prevalent in certain socioeconomic groups or geographic areas.

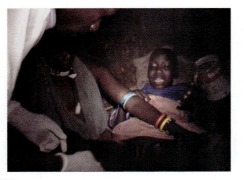

FIGURE 1-2 Female circumcision is often performed under unhygienic conditions and remains a subject of much debate among women's advocacy groups.

Social workers, on the other hand, might apply the findings of sociologists when helping individuals.

Anthropology

While sociology deals primarily with social issues and problems in a single society, cultural anthropology takes a cross-cultural approach. Multicultural similarities and differences in human sexual behavior are a recurring focus of this book. Sex is a fundamental human drive affected by society and other factors; different societies have different ways of giving form and direction to sexuality. Sexual behaviors and traditions that seem barbaric or abhorrent in one culture may seem normal and acceptable in another. For example, human rights and women's organizations throughout most of the world have condemned the practice of female circumcision in some societies and criticized its brutal physical impact on women and their potential to enjoy sexual intercourse or any pleasurable genital sensations at all. On the other hand, one anthropological perspective claims it is inappropriate to judge this custom in some cultures by the standards and norms of other cultures, even if it seems cruel and painful. Figure 1-2 is an illustration of female circumcision.

Psychology

Psychology is a variegated and diverse discipline difficult to describe with a single definition. Basically, psychologists study individual organisms (both human and nonhuman) to figure out what behavior is normal and predictable. "Behavior" is broadly defined and refers to observable actions as well as subtle, invisible cognitive, neural, or endocrine activities. Organism-environment interactions are a primary focus for psychologists. There are several different kinds of psychologists, many of which study various aspects of human sexual thinking, feeling, and behaving. For example, biopsychologists are primarily interested in the relationship between behavior and neuroendocrine activity. Clinical psychologists study the development and manifestations of emotional and behavioral problems as well as their diagnosis and treatment. Some clinical psychologists, social workers, and other professionals specialize in *sex therapy*—the assessment, counseling, and treatment of sexual dysfunctions. *Developmental psychologists* examine behavioral changes that occur over time as we age, some focusing on children and others on adolescents, young adults, or aging and elderly individuals. *Personality psychologists* study consistency and predictability in human behavior, usually over long periods of time. *Social psychologists* explore how our complex interpersonal environment affects our thoughts, feelings, and actions. Figure 1-3 shows two psychologists working in very different settings, yet both strive to understand the relationship between environmental stimuli and human behaviors and feelings.

■ ■ ■

These three broad disciplines—sociology, anthropology, and psychology—share the concept that human growth, development, and behavior should be viewed as an interactive process: private, psychological, and societal factors work together to influence the many manifestations of our emotional, cognitive, and physical functioning. This psychosocial approach is important for an understanding of how people's sexual learning and behaving begin to emerge. Psychosocial influ-

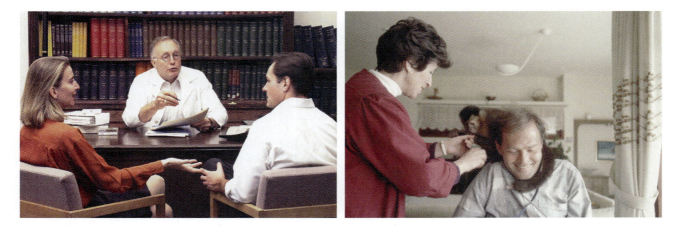

FIGURE 1-3 Psychologists work in many different arenas to better understand an enormous variety of behavioral, cognitive, emotional, and physiological issues.

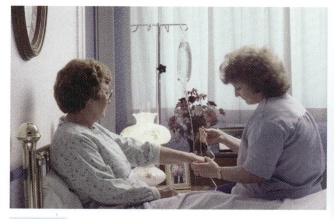

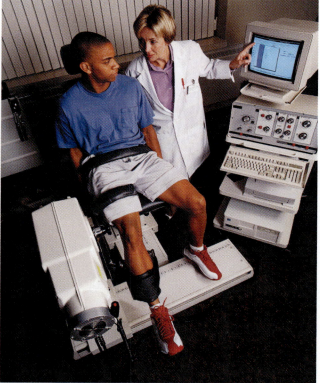

FIGURE 1-4 Health care specialists use a variety of clinical methods and technological tools to better understand illness and effective therapies.

ences also powerfully affect a person's adult sexual self-concept. Throughout this book we will frequently return to this psychosocial approach because it is very important to our understanding of eroticism and intimacy.

Medicine and Allied Health Sciences

Many health care specialists are concerned with human sexuality in wellness and disease: nurses, physicians, midwives, and physical therapists to name just a few. Several physician subspecialties focus on sexual, reproductive, and interpersonal difficulties. For example, *urologists* specialize in conditions of the genitourinary system and *gynecologists* specialize in wellness and diseases of the female reproductive system and breasts. *Andrologists* focus on issues of fertility in men, as well as their sexual functioning. *Surgeons* correct anatomical abnormalities, such as those affecting fertility, and, along with *oncologists* (cancer specialists), remove growths and tumors. *Psychiatrists* diagnose and treat mental disorders using counseling techniques and medications. When sexual problems result from psychological trauma or abuse, psychiatrists may use long-term psychotherapy with clients.

Health care specialists generally act from a set of implicit assumptions often called the medical model. In this model, sexual abnormalities are considered diseases with specific symptoms and suggested medical treatments. Biological factors are considered more important than psychosocial influences in the development of sexual problems. Although the medical model is appropriate in many health care settings (hospitals, doctors' offices, etc.), the psychosocial perspective embraces a much broader set of influences. Figure 1-4 illustrates different kinds of activities in health care related to physical ailments.

Law and Business

All societies develop and elaborate codes of conduct to protect people and their property—this is the basic function of law. In-

terestingly, this profession that addresses such broad societal concerns also has a profound impact on so intimate an area of human behavior as sexuality. Virtually every culture has a complex system of laws, norms, and mores to regulate, encourage, or punish different aspects of human intimate expression. Laws dealing with human sexuality are not always developed, revised, or eliminated as promptly as changes in social custom occur, however. We have all heard of unusual, outdated statutes that stipulate the "illegality" of behaviors that have become common. For example, oral-genital stimulation, homosexual behaviors, and male-female intercourse in postures other than the traditional "missionary" position are felonies in some states, theoretically punishable by fines or imprisonment. Such laws often remain on the books, even though they no longer reflect society's views and are seldom enforced, perhaps because no one (especially elected officials) wants to conspicuously work for more "liberal" sexual laws now when there is so much dialog about morality and ethics in the society as a whole.

Although outdated frivolous statutes stipulate various "normal" human sexual behaviors, the law does offer everyone essential basic protections against abuse, exploitation, coercion, and assault. The law defines the boundaries of acceptable sexual expression and punishes departures from norms involving our safety and the very dignity of our personhood. Just as the basic function of law in all cultures involves protecting people and their property, the basic objective of laws related to sexual expression generally have in common the protection of the private nature of sexual behavior and the inappropriateness of force, intimidation, or coercion (Fig. 1-5). Legal tradition upholds the fundamentally *consensual* nature of erotic and reproductive behaviors.

Theology and Religious Traditions

In one way or another, our notions of right and wrong are often powerfully influenced by the religious traditions in which we are raised or those we adopt. How most people think about ethics and appropriate conduct toward one another is also affected by these influences. Some people prefer a concrete code of "Thou shalt" or "Thou shalt not," and are uncomfortable with ambiguity or flexibility in personal or societal morality. Others let the nature of the situation influence the moral judgments made. Still others recognize that their personal view of right and wrong results from a long socialization process everyone goes through when growing up and that it is really our personal history that affects our definitions of good and evil. Yet almost everyone accepts that religious and ethical issues are a fundamental part of how we begin to think and feel about sexual experience and expression. Spiritual leaders, therefore, have a powerful impact on how many people think and feel about their sexuality (Fig. 1-6). There is some debate about the extent to which one can ever *unlearn* the religious perspective about sexuality with which one was raised. Just as many people have trouble talking openly about sex, talking about sex and religion is even more difficult.

Our modern conceptions of rectitude are rooted in ancient Greek and Roman traditions, especially the writings of Plato (427–347 BC) and Aristotle (384–322 BC). Plato's *Re-*

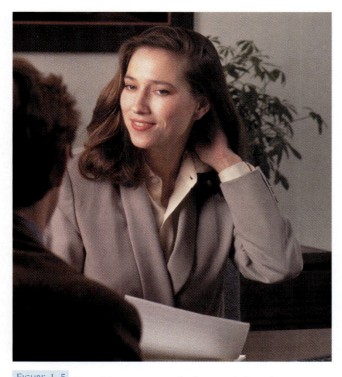

FIGURE 1-5 Sexual harassment, whether carried out by men or women, involves sexual attention or overtures that are both unwanted and unwelcome.

public introduces us to the role of popular beliefs about goodness and righteousness in the governance of an entire society—a concern that still occupies our attention. Virtues, vices, and the importance of moderation were explicated in Aristotle's *Ethics,* which teaches that in each sphere of human action, favorable and unfavorable feelings and behaviors exist on a continuum. Aristotle thought that our notions of "good" and "bad" are somewhat relative, a view at odds with some religious perspectives based on moral absolutes.

LEVELS OF ANALYSIS

The study of human sexuality has "big picture" and "little picture" dimensions. On the one hand, broad societal and cultural issues definitely affect our perceptions, thoughts, and feelings about sexual matters. The civilization in which we are born and develop plays a major role in telling and showing us what to view as normal, necessary, important, or unusual. At the same time, individuals grow up in a family (defined in various ways), or maybe an extended kinship group or an ethnic or racial subculture. How we think about sex is affected by each of these nested social environments. Different disciplines view these issues at different levels. For example, sociology and anthropology typically explore sexual issues in large cultural groups or the entire culture, while the medical sciences frequently focus on individuals.

At a middle level of analysis is the human body, observable without sophisticated equipment. We are concerned with the appearance and condition of our physical selves in both normal and unusual states. Our body's appearance is such an important part of our self-concept that it can be difficult to examine it or think about it apart from our feelings about the "attractiveness" of what we see. We may think about the details of our appearance in relation to our desire to be considered appealing or alluring. Try this: ask some close friends which part of their bodies they are most pleased with and which they are most displeased with. You might be surprised to find out how quickly and specifically they will answer you, as most people have already thought about it. Not surprisingly, the most common elective surgeries in the United States are performed by plastic surgeons to change some aspect of physical appearance.

At the smallest level of analysis are anatomical, physiological, and hormonal issues. Microscopic structures and individual cells in the pituitary gland, testes, and ovaries are involved in the production of hormones, sperm, and eggs. Cells in the ovaries and testes produce hormones that affect the body in many ways. Other endocrine glands also produce hormones that affect fertility, physical appearance, and sexual functioning.

In all, we have to use lenses of different power to examine the wide range of topics important in this course. Macro or "big picture" levels of analysis are important for large social concerns and demographic aspects. At the other extreme, the micro or "little picture" level of analysis is needed for hormonal, anatomical, neurological, and physiological matters.

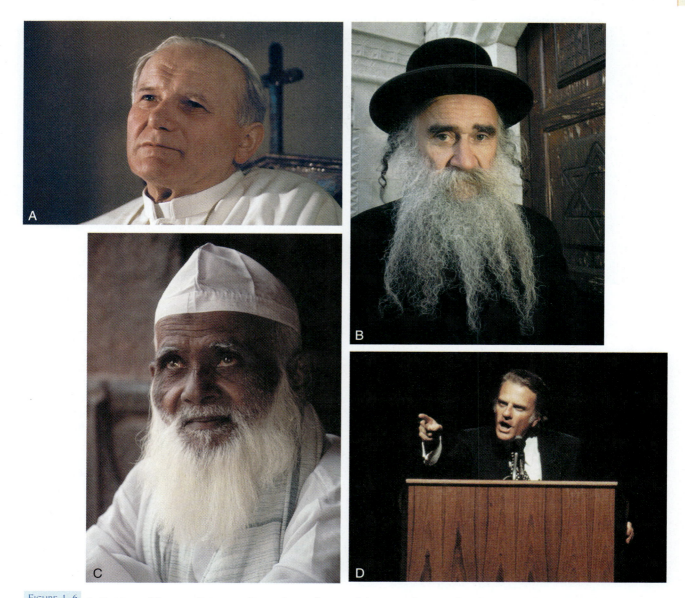

Figure 1-6 A–D. Many different religious traditions have all created doctrines, laws, and traditions regarding acceptable and unacceptable sexual behaviors.

The intimate, interpersonal nature of sexual relationships is generally between these two extremes. Figure 1-7 contrasts examples of a macro perspective on one sexual issue and a micro perspective on a different issue.

WE ARE SURROUNDED BY SEXUALITY

The following sections in this chapter present a number of everyday vignettes that illustrate sexual issues. Each of these realistic little stories involves an issue that will be examined in later chapters. None of these anecdotes has a definite ending, but by the time you have finished this course you will understand their likely outcomes.

Hector

Hector lived in a quiet suburban community in Virginia, a tidy and conservative place by most standards. Hector and his wife Maria both thought it was a great place to raise kids. The schools were good, and there were many parks and swimming pools. Most families belonged to a church or synagogue and attended regularly. All in all, Hector and Maria felt they had a high quality of life. Their two children, Mike, age 4, and Ellen, age 3, were well assimilated in their preschool and peer groups. But then something very disturbing happened in their town, and Hector and Maria didn't know what to make of it, but they felt very angry and vulnerable for the first time in such a pleasant place.

The local newspaper was running stories about a 19-year-old man charged with sexually molesting children between the

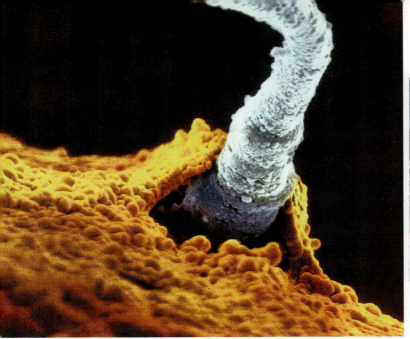

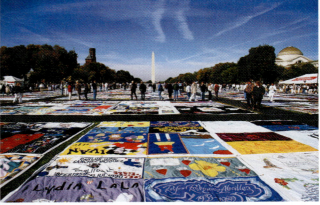

FIGURE 1-7 A sperm penetrating an egg is an example of the micro perspective (**left**), while social and cultural awareness of the AIDS epidemic represents the macro perspective (**right**).

ages of 4 and 7 while working at a local church preschool. The photographs of him in the newspaper showed a clean-cut kid, neatly dressed, in handcuffs. His family was devastated. People were talking about what kind of home he must have come from. The parents of the children who were molested were outraged and retained attorneys. Their quiet community was now full of reporters with cameras and satellite gear. Hector wondered if the town itself seemed suspect in public opinion. Were people in faraway cities wondering, "*What kind of people are they?*"

How ironic. The preschool was in an old and distinguished church, founded during colonial times, the spiritual home to generations of citizens of this community. It was such a strange site for the horrible victimization and abuse of trust-

ing youngsters and their families. Wasn't there any way for church authorities to have screened this young man? Didn't they ask for references? Hector and Maria worried about the long-term consequences of this experience for the children and their families. They also wondered in private whether the reports of children that young were reliable and accurate and how they would respond to questioning by attorneys, psychologists, and judges. Was there a chance none of this ever really happened? And if not, what would happen to the accused young man?

Hector and Maria are not unique. What parent wouldn't have these questions and concerns about their preschool? Scenes such as the one shown in Figure 1-8 have unfortunately become common in the news. Do they reveal some terrible flaw in our society? Do we really understand the people who commit these crimes? Is it true that someone abused as a child is more likely to repeat the pattern of victimization—and is it really just that simple? These questions will be addressed in Chapter 19.

Moira

"Growing up really sucks!" Moira just couldn't understand it at all. Here she was, a proud and popular sixth-grader and all of a sudden, people were *really* looking at her in a strange new way. She used to think it only got better as you got older, but now that seemed a big mistake. She was getting taller, but so were her girlfriends. Why in the world weren't the boys getting taller too? They were so much smaller, and now they were staring at her.

Having all those giggling little guys acting pop-eyed around her was really unnerving. Her mom and dad seemed to take it all in stride, but their friends always acted surprised when they hadn't seen her in a while: "*No! This isn't our little Moira. My goodness, have you ever changed, sweetie! I'll bet there are lots of boys sniffing around here these days.*" If only they understood how immature and vulgar those boys were.

Everything seemed to be changing. When Moira's breasts began to develop, she felt so conspicuous. All those boys she

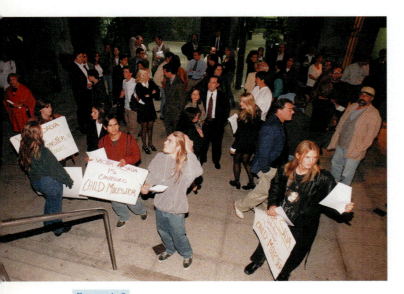

FIGURE 1-8 Communities often react with anger and outrage when child sexual abuse is discovered.

Research Highlight

THE CASE STUDY METHOD

Much of this chapter is devoted to vignettes that describe real-life circumstances of people dealing with different sexual issues. These are fairly common situations in our society, even though only a few of them might seem relevant to you personally. We can learn much about general topics by examining individual life histories; this is the basis of an interesting research method called the *case study,* which has been used by many sexuality investigators.

Most research in the social and behavioral sciences seeks to establish general laws about human nature by studying a large number of people to determine what they have in common. However, some scientists believe the individual cannot be fully understood by examining large groups because the individual's unique attributes are lost as data from many individuals are averaged.

A case study is an intensive description and analysis of an individual. By carefully examining single cases we often can better understand common, or classic, phenomena, perhaps some syndrome or disorder. Although the focus is only on a single case, the full color and detail of that human reality are often better revealed. What scientists lose in not being able to make broad generalizations from a single case, they gain in interesting and often telling details. The case study method has other advantages too. An unusual event can be analyzed in a single case, whereas a large number of such cases would take a long time to collect. Thus, interesting and potentially telling phenomena can more easily be shared with the scientific community.

Case studies also can present stark exceptions to "common knowledge" and widely accepted ways of thinking about a subject (Kazdin, 1980). Exceptions to the rule cannot always be dismissed as bizarre, once-in-a-lifetime events, for often they reveal significant information and contribute to our fuller understanding. For example, this chapter includes a story about a newly married young man experiencing premature ejaculation. This is a common sexual problem in which a man is unable to delay ejaculation until his partner has reached a level of sexual enjoyment. This vignette conveys some of the frustration of this dysfunction. Here the case study method reveals the personal impact of such a problem on both the person experiencing it and his partner. A more rare condition is the case of women who have orgasms as soon as they are entered and then quickly become uninterested in continuing sexual intercourse (W.H. Masters, personal communication, November, 1978). This is the exception that becomes a focus of interesting speculation and study.

Although case studies are engaging and have real immediacy, they are not a true experimental design. Actually, they are more like demonstrations (Bordens & Abbott, 1996). Variables cannot be manipulated, and the general causes and consequences of behavior cannot be determined based on single cases. Still, when many case studies are collected, summarized, and reported (as we will see in the next chapter in the work of Alfred Kinsey), the investigator can make stronger generalizations.

A final potential drawback to case studies is known as observer bias. Scientists too can have preconceptions, expectations, and prejudices, and these might possibly distort the recording and reporting of individual case studies.

The stories described in this chapter are not from the scientific literature, but they have the color and personal details of case studies. They are short, simple examples of how case studies reveal information about sexuality. They might even validate some of your own experiences or observations.

swam with this past summer were now talking about her, and sometimes she heard the less-than-polite things they said. Her girlfriends weren't getting this treatment; they were *lucky,* their breasts weren't growing as big as hers. Not only that, but now Moira was beginning to develop a real "figure," with a waist and hips and everything!

This puberty thing was getting out of hand. A few weeks ago Moira was at a slumber party with a bunch of her girlfriends, and they had a *fantastic* pillow fight. It got loud and unruly very fast. Then her so-called friend Beth sneaked up behind her and pulled her pajama bottoms clean down to her ankles! Oh, my God, *everyone* saw her pubic hair—and she just knew she was the only one it had happened to. She just screamed in embarrassment.

Then, of all times, Christmas morning! Moira and her mother were close and could talk to each other about almost anything. Her mother had told her about menstruation, so she knew what was coming. But with all these other things happening and the hustle and bustle of the holiday, this was just too much. Everyone was downstairs opening presents and here was Moira, crying upstairs in the bathroom while her mother tried to show her how to put on a pad.

All these changes were happening too fast, she thought. No, growing up wasn't easy. Now, as if she didn't already have enough on her mind, there was this problem of pads or tampons, and how was she supposed to keep them hidden in her purse? Did all women have to go through this?

Adolescence can be a hard time. Not all teenagers develop at the same rate (Fig. 1-9). At puberty, the secondary sexual characteristics appear, and getting used to them can be a challenge. Our bodies change, and other people react to us differently. The impact of puberty on our bodies and self-concept will be discussed in Chapter 12. How was your puberty compared to Moira's? Did you feel as self-conscious as she? Did you have acne too?

An issue not mentioned in this story about Moira is the fact that many adolescents are using contraceptives, as they need to be.

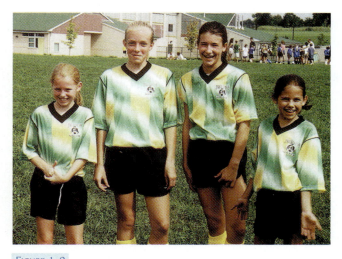

Figure 1-9 Physical development in puberty can be highly variable. All of these youngsters are within 12 months of each other in age.

This is another important aspect about growing up that people have to learn to cope with, and it will be discussed in Chapter 12.

Congressman Frank

Early in the summer of 1996, an unusual thing happened during a debate on the floor of the United States Congress. An openly gay congressman, Barney Frank, was arguing for the right of homosexuals to legally marry one another. One of his colleagues was attacking him bitterly and personally. Congressman Frank's lifestyle, gender orientation, significant other, legal opinions, and priorities were brutally attacked—on television. It was by no means a civil debate. Congressman Frank was being victimized by gay slurs from another congressman, Dick Armey, who called him "Barney Fag." C-SPAN showed the whole episode about the extremely controversial subject, including arguments about the marital bond and the nature of commitment between lifetime partners. Even though the debate reached no answers, viewers came away with a number of important questions. Discussing this subject in Congress would have been unimaginable a generation ago.

Should government recognize such unions? The debate is ongoing elsewhere, as well as in the United States. For example, as of this writing, a court case is pending in Hawaii that could recognize the legality of same-sex marriages. Some believe that the Supreme Court of Hawaii will give gay couples the right to marry (Shumate, 1995). Some see the issue as an intrusion of government into the private lives of citizens, when many have viewed marriage as a matter of religion and private interpersonal relationships. Indeed, one writer notes the issue of gay marriage "will make the battle of gays in the military look like a Sunday school picnic" (Shumate, 1995). Note that the issue of gay marriage is different from the issue of laws that prohibit sexual behaviors among homosexuals.

What Congressman Frank and others argue for would change historical and contemporary standards. For example, gay couples could file joint tax returns and could include each other in health insurance program benefits. Inheritance rights and joint property ownership would be allowed. Congressman Barney Frank (Fig. 1-10) was making a lucid, civil attempt to sensitize other legislators and the public to controversial but important gay rights issues.

It is sometimes hard for people to view homosexuality from a perspective of lifestyle issues and the psychosocial environment. We too often focus on their erotic interests and behaviors and don't consider the issues of companionship, bonding, love, and mutuality in their relationships. The debate described above will not end soon or quietly. Chapter 9 examines gay relationships and the emerging dialogue about gay marriage and gay rights. How do you feel about a law sanctioning gay marriages?

Sandra

Sandra was a single mom and had been since her son Kyle was 4 years old; he was now 9 and a real handful. Sandra came from a rural community and married Kyle's dad, Joe, when she was 16—she felt she had to since she was pregnant. It was a

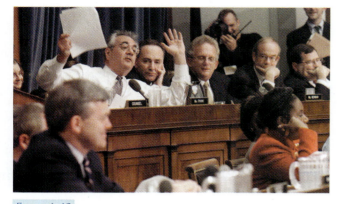

FIGURE 1-10 Congressman Barney Frank is an advocate of the legal recognition of homosexual bonds.

confusing time in her life. She had been dating him about a year, and they had a pretty good relationship. But she didn't feel very ready for or informed about sex. She was lonely, and her mother and father didn't spend much time with her. They never talked to her about school, dating, or the future. They *never* talked about sex. When Sandra had her first period she didn't know what was happening to her, and she thought she was dying. Joe was different, though—he knew about sex. But she noticed that he used a condom only some of the times they had sex. He kept telling her not to worry, but then she became pregnant.

At first their parents were angry. There was a lot of screaming and finger pointing. After a while, they got used to the idea and were more supportive. Sandra and Joe got married. Sandra dropped out of high school to have the baby. Their marriage lasted 4 years. They discovered they were very different people and had different ideas about the future. Sandra found a job and put Kyle in a day-care center. From the start, she distinguished herself as a good employee. She advanced quickly and after 5 years was earning a good salary, enough for her and Kyle to be comfortable.

Sandra made herself a promise. Kyle would *never* be ignorant about sex. She would see to it. She kept an eye on him and was sensitive to those teachable moments when a parent can ask a question or say a few words about sexual matters, such as when the neighbor's cat had kittens. Sandra was pleased that the state legislature just passed a comprehensive Family Life Education Act. She believed this would be a good way for Kyle to fill in any gaps in his knowledge. The local newspaper described the program as an excellent introduction to a wide range of sexual, relationship, family, and health concerns. The legislators felt that their work would enhance the quality of life of citizens and that children and adolescents would receive timely, useful information. Then Sandra read on.

The Act had a provision that every local school board in the state had the right to choose which aspects of the program to teach in its jurisdiction, and it could prohibit other parts. The more Sandra thought about it, the less optimistic she felt.

She knew the people on the local school board, and she suspected they would destroy this effective program just to satisfy a few vocal citizens in the community. She read that in the next county the school board disallowed any instruction about contraception, homosexuality, sexual assault and abuse, and other topics. What was left?

Kyle was now 9. Because they had a good relationship and could talk, she knew he had already heard some bizarre things from his friends, and she had to gently correct these incorrect notions. Was she going to have to do this whole job alone? And what about all those other kids whose parents wouldn't do the job well? Sandra had the unhappy feeling that these kids were growing up in an environment no different than the one where she had—and look at what happened to her because of a lack of information about sex. Maybe, she thought, she should talk to the school board . . .

Sexuality involves not only personal and relationship issues, but also political and legislative ones. Everyone has a voice in a democracy, and often those voices do not agree about important matters affecting the health and well-being of the community. Chapter 12 describes how youngsters who receive effective sex education in elementary school begin sexual behavior at a later age and more responsibly. Youngsters who receive little sex education begin their sexual explorations earlier and much less carefully.

Ellen

It wasn't easy being a 49-year-old accountant, wife, mother, and homemaker. Ellen, however, was proud of her accomplishments. After raising two children (both in college now), Ellen finished her BA degree in business administration and became a certified public accountant. She found that many companies liked to hire mature women because they were efficient, rarely missed work, and had good time-management skills. With the kids away and her career going well, Ellen and her husband Jack had more time to spend with each other. Things seemed to be going very well.

Then Ellen began to notice some gradual changes. At first they were so slight that she didn't think very much of them. But gradually they became more noticeable and a little troubling. She occasionally missed a period, and when she did have one it had a very light or very heavy flow. Sometimes she noticed clotting in her menstrual discharge. Her skin seemed dry. It used to be a bit oily, but now she needed to use hand cream at times and found that facial moisturizers helped. She was also feeling mood swings. Some days she felt fine and in an "up" mood, but on other days she felt distracted and forgetful. She was surprised how quickly she became irritated by minor frustrations and how long she brooded over them.

She felt tired a lot, and this surprised her because she had always been a sound sleeper and got all the rest she needed. Some days she was exhausted by 3:00 in the afternoon. She had gained a few pounds, and this bothered her too. She had always eaten wisely, walked regularly, and had been proud of her figure. Her muscles were losing their youthful tone.

Ellen also noticed that intercourse with Jack was becoming a bit uncomfortable for her because her vaginal membranes were drier. Also, she would flush, blush, and sweat quite suddenly and unpredictably from time to time. She woke sometimes to find herself completely soaked. How long would all this go on? She knew about menopause, of course, but hadn't imagined it would be like this. Couldn't anything be done about any of this?

And she wished Jack would be more sympathetic. He didn't seem to have much idea what she was going through, and she was a little angry with him for not understanding. Why didn't *he* try to be more sensitive and helpful? He was going on with his life as if nothing at all had changed.

Contrary to common belief, menopause causes no significant changes in a woman's personality. In addition to the physical and emotional issues shown in this story are other important changes of menopause: the higher risk of cardiovascular disease and osteoporosis. Ellen's story is not an unusual menopause experience, but it should make us realize how important it is to establish an open relationship with a primary care physician in order to maintain good sexual and reproductive health. Had Ellen had a yearly physical and gynecologic examination, many of her symptoms would not have worried her because she would have been prepared for them. Figure 1-11 illustrates Premarin, *an estrogen replacement agent commonly used by some women going through menopause;* K-Y Jelly, *used for lubrication to make intercourse more comfortable; and* Replens, *a vaginal moisturizing cream. Chapter 13 examines the physical and emotional aspects of menopause. This process can be challenging. Indeed, it is a kind of developmental milestone in a woman's life. Some positive aspects of menopause not mentioned yet might surprise you.*

Keisha and Ernest: Ironing Out the Kinks in a New Marriage

Where did the time go? It seemed just yesterday they were eating wedding cake. It's been a whole year, already, and my goodness have they had to make adjustments! Keisha and Ernest knew they wanted to spend the rest of their lives together, but their busy work schedules, a tiny apartment, little money, and subtle hints from their families about them starting a family made for some real stress. People dropping by unannounced at all hours didn't help things either. They didn't know if living so close to their families was a good thing or not. It didn't seem fair. Before they got married they had to go to extremes to enjoy private times with each other, but they didn't mind. They hadn't particularly liked having to keep watch while making out in Ernest's car, but where else could they go for a little privacy? They knew that some day they'd have a place of their own.

Keisha and Ernest enjoyed sharing their lives. They never argued, and they saw eye-to-eye on most things. They were both proud of being sensitive to each other's wants and needs. They were developing a real sense of mutuality while still maintaining their own independence. This mature intimacy was very different from their earlier infatuation; yet they had an extremely frustrating problem that neither of them knew quite what to do about.

Whenever they made love, Ernest ejaculated very soon after entering Keisha. Maybe old habits were tough to break. All those times in Ernest's car they'd felt anxious about being discovered, and they'd rushed things. They never really had a

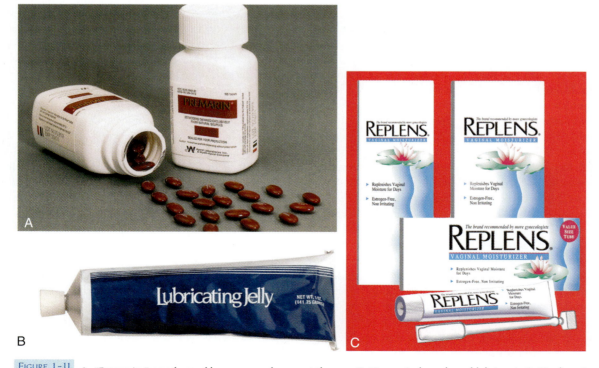

FIGURE 1-11   **A.** "Premarin," one form of hormone replacement therapy. **B.** Non-petroleum based lubricant. **C.** "Replens," a vaginal moisturizing cream. All may help women continue to enjoy sexual expression during menopause.

chance to explore each another in a relaxed, private place. But it seemed this frustration just wouldn't go away, no matter how slowly they went or how relaxed they were together. Keisha didn't want to hurt Ernest's feelings by saying anything about it, since he already felt bad enough; but she just didn't feel like a "full partner" in their lovemaking.

Neither of them knew what to say or even how to raise the subject. Ernest wondered if there was something wrong with him, and Keisha hoped he wasn't just trying to get the whole thing over with as soon as possible. People had told them lots of things about marriage, but nothing like this. Was it a physical problem or something psychological? Whatever it was, it was causing some tension. Keisha had noticed that now Ernest was initiating sex less frequently than he used to. To make things worse, Keisha felt nervous whenever Ernest started to approach her sexually. She didn't know if he really wanted to or just felt that he had to. How did things get so complicated? What could they do about this? Where do you go for help with something like this? Keisha could never talk to her mother about sex. Maybe her doctor....

Premature ejaculation is the most common sexual dysfunction—and also the easiest to remedy with counseling and behavioral treatment. But that doesn't make it any less frustrating to experience. Chapters 14 and 15 discuss some of the causes of this difficulty and its treatment. With some help Keisha and Ernest should be able to solve this problem without too much trouble.

Jane: "I Can't Believe This Is Happening to Me!"

Jane was frantic, hurt, frightened, and just plain mad. He'd given her a disease! She felt stupid and vulnerable as well as naive. How could it have happened?

Mid-America USA, a tiny college town in the Midwest, Saturday night and not much to do. Jane and her three suitemates, all freshmen, shared two bedrooms and a bathroom in a college dorm. None had a steady boyfriend, and they constantly teased each other about that. But it was now February and Jane and her roommates still felt like high school girls, not college women. The nerds went to the dances and the drunks went to the bars. Wasn't there anything in between?

A new club had just opened in town, and people said the food and the bands were both great. So Jane and her roommates decided to give it a try and see if they'd meet some men. They were nervous when they first walked in, but after a few beers they felt more relaxed. It was Ladies' Night, so their drinks were half price, and they took full advantage of the bargain. After a while, they were all dancing. A guy named Dennis had taken an immediate liking to Jane, and she enjoyed his attention.

Dennis was a senior, tall, good-looking, and well-dressed. They really hit it off. When Jane talked to him, he listened as if he really cared for her. All too soon it was 1:00 in the morning and the club was closing. Dennis politely asked if she'd like to stop at his apartment for a nightcap on the way home. She liked the idea. So she told her roommates goodbye and left with Dennis.

Dennis' place was cozy and quiet. They had a few more beers. One thing seemed to lead to another, and before she knew exactly what was happening, they were in bed together having sex. She'd had so much to drink that she didn't really feel much of anything.

The next day she felt really strange about it, however, and was wondering what she should say to him when he called. She wasn't sure how much she really liked him, it had all happened so suddenly. After all, this was her first time. Shouldn't they have used a condom or something? After everything she'd heard about "safe sex" and "knowing your partner," she was surprised she hadn't thought about it last night.

But he didn't call. Not at all. Not a word, as if the whole thing had never even happened. Until today—2 weeks later. Dennis sounded aloof and casual on the phone. He said that he'd had some symptoms and had gone to the campus health center. The doctor said he had chlamydia, a common sexually transmitted disease. Then he mumbled something about how she better "get yourself checked" and abruptly hung up. The way he talked so matter-of-factly about the whole catastrophe really angered Jane.

She didn't have any symptoms, however, so she wondered if she had gotten the infection from Dennis. Could she have it without even knowing it? Suddenly she realized she could get other sexually transmitted diseases without knowing it too. Didn't people get AIDS that way? Now she really felt frightened, and embarrassed, and dirty too. Why didn't they teach her about this in high school?

Chapter 17 discusses many different sexually transmitted infections and related problems. Sometimes very frightening things happen to good, but sometimes careless people. Specific diseases are discussed, as well as their symptoms and treatments. The emphasis is on prevention. The most important factor for avoiding sexually transmitted disease is knowing your partner very well. We will also sensitize you to your rights to capable, confidential, nonjudgmental medical treatment. As you can see in Figure 1-12, local health departments are one setting that provides care for health problems, such as sexually transmitted diseases.

Cindy and Phil: A Whole New Way of Thinking About the Rest of Your Life

Cindy and Phil were depressed and devastated. Nothing in their lives had prepared them for this. What they thought about marriage, adulthood, and the rest of their lives had been turned upside down. They were numb and didn't know what to say to each other, and they didn't want to talk to anyone else about it. They felt they were losing a life they hadn't had a chance to experience. For two 26-year-olds, it was beyond belief. Whose "fault" was this?

After a year of their trying to conceive, Cindy's gynecologist recommended she have a complete fertility assessment. She and Phil had been having intercourse two or three times a week without using contraception for over a year, and it seemed they might be an infertile couple.

They had known each other for 4 years and got married 2 years ago. They were really happy. They both came from

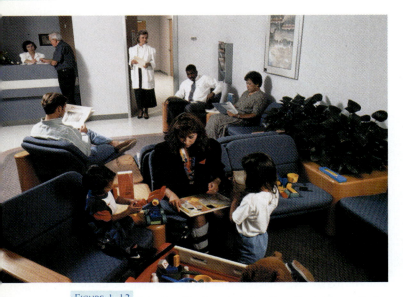

Figure 1-12 Local health departments offer affordable medical care for a variety of problems, including sexually transmitted diseases.

large families and wanted the same for themselves. Cindy had three siblings and Phil had four. The hustle and bustle of a large family was something they cherished. Even if there wasn't always much money to go around, there was always lots of love. After dating for a few months they talked easily about their dreams of a big house with lots of little "rug rats" running around. Their plan was simple: finish school and get married, both work for a year and save some money, and then start their family. Their energy, optimism, and love convinced them it was a workable plan.

But now what? She'd never be able to get pregnant and have babies? She couldn't imagine going through life without children. She felt stupid and angry. Was this common? Her doctor said they couldn't know what the problem was without the tests. He also said, depending on the results of her fertility work-up, Ron might need to be evaluated also. Just now they didn't know where the "problem" lay.

Cindy and Phil were learning a lot of things they never knew, lots of terms like "ovulation," "fertilization," "implantation," "sperm count," "sperm motility." But they couldn't pay much attention to all this technical information when their anxiety level was through the roof. How would they tell their parents? Sooner or later they would have to. What would life hold for them if they couldn't have children? Would it just be the two of them forever?

Phil didn't quite know where he stood in this whole situation. He realized that rearing children was part of traditional female socialization and empathized with Cindy's fears and feelings of inadequacy. But he had some very real anxieties himself. Phil saw himself as a "daddy" taking his kids to swim meets, museums, the zoo, and the first day of school. He saw himself cleaning up cuts and scrapes and putting on Band-Aids. What would there be now besides going to work every day, coming home, eating dinner, and falling asleep on the couch? What would he do if their fertility problem was his "fault?"

Fertility problems are far more common than in the past, and we know only some of the reasons why. Infertility is a major stressor in a relationship, and resolving it one way or another takes time, patience, and sometimes considerable money. Chapter 10 discusses issues related to fertility and infertility and the modern, highly technical treatments for infertility. Although most couples do not have to face this problem, there is value in understanding and being prepared for it. A national organization named Resolve (Fig. 1-13) helps people cope with infertility and work through the alternatives in trying to conceive.

The Neighborhood

The neighbors had had enough of it. As often happened in inner-city neighborhoods, a number of pressing problems had created fear in the people living there. The pride that people once took in the appearance of their homes was almost gone. Now it seemed more important to "look out for one another." Poor people who had no air conditioning stayed in their apartments with windows locked to defend themselves from break-ins, robberies, assaults, and drive-by shootings. People selling and using drugs on the street and in abandoned homes had created a very dangerous environment. And now there was a new problem that was making some residents angry.

A lot of unfamiliar cars parked in the neighborhood in the evening. Men from outside the neighborhood went into row houses where prostitution seemed to be thriving. Sometimes it was obvious they were drunk or high on something. They were noisy and boisterous, and their presence further

The mission of RESOLVE, a nonprofit organization founded in 1974 by Barbara Eck Menning, is to provide timely, compassionate support and information to people who are experiencing infertility and to increase awareness of infertility issues through public education and advocacy. Infertility is a disease or condition that results in the abnormal functioning of the male or female reproductive system. It includes difficulty conceiving and the inability to carry a pregnancy that results in a live birth (miscarriage). RESOLVE supports family-building through a variety of methods, including appropriate medical treatment, adoption, surrogacy, and the choice of child-free living.

Figure 1-13 RESOLVE is an organization that serves as a support group and information resource for couples dealing with infertility.

changed the character of the neighborhood. With drugs, guns, violence, and now prostitution spreading through the neighborhood, long-time residents wondered if they could ever reclaim their neighborhood. And now the problem was occurring throughout the daylight hours too.

The police were unable to do anything, so finally some of the residents decided to act. They started walking the streets late and recording the license plate numbers of the "patrons'" cars. It was a scary job, but a lot of the residents joined in. Actually, it was almost comical: men looking for prostitutes were slinking around, followed by neighbors slinking right after them writing down their license plate numbers.

The neighbors visited their local newspaper offices, hoping to get some help. The editor of the paper couldn't believe her ears. "You want me to do *what*?" she demanded. "I'm not sure that's even legal!" She held her ground and refused to publish the license numbers of the men visiting prostitutes.

But the citizens in the neighborhood wanted the Johns out *now*. They started putting a poster of "Johns of the Week" on telephone poles. They listed the names and addresses of men arrested for soliciting prostitutes in their neighborhood. They put a warning on the posters: "Johns! Stay out of this neighborhood or your name will be here next week." And the posters worked. Prostitution moved out of the neighborhood. Other big-city newspapers ran stories about it, leading to similar citizen activism elsewhere. What was most important, however, was that people felt they could improve their quality of life and their neighborhood. As you can see in Figure 1-14, residents are not always polite in how they preserve the safety and integrity of their neighborhoods.

Prostitution is a complicated issue. This story should encourage you to think about the nature of what is sometimes called a "victimless crime." Sex-for-money is always complicated and involves legal and public health risks, and it affects people far beyond its immediate sphere of influence. The motives for becoming a prostitute, the reasons for buying time with one, and the societal impact of prostitution are considered in Chapter 19. Perhaps nowhere else is there such a connection among self-esteem, body image, economics, and basic biological drives. Do you think prostitutes are "bad" people? What do you know about the different kinds of prostitutes?

Peggy

The judge was furious. Standing before her was Peggy, 20 years old, who had three young children and a long history of cocaine abuse. She was in court on charges that she had repeatedly neglected and otherwise physically abused her children during the last 18 months. In cases like Peggy's there were no "extenuating circumstances." What could be done for her or about her? Should anything be done *to* her? Now the state, the defendant, the attorneys, and representatives for the defendant's children stood before the judge. Peggy had been here before, charged with the same offenses. She had been warned. But she was back.

Peggy was a single parent and head of the household with virtually no financial resources. She had never been married and did not live with her parents or anyone else who might offer some stability or support to her life. She did not work and

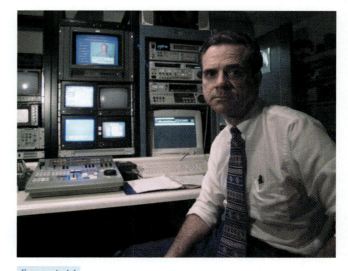

FIGURE 1-14   Bill Frohmberg is a videographer who produces a program called "John TV" in Kansas City, MO. The show presents the pictures and names of people arrested on charges involving prostitution and is thought to be related to a significant drop in the number of arrests for prostitution in that city.

depended totally on public assistance for her and her children's survival. She was also pregnant again and was asking for additional funds to have an abortion. The judge was sympathetic to Peggy's request but knew she had a long history of negligence with contraceptives and used cocaine, known to be horribly harmful to unborn embryos and fetuses. The two lawyers, the state, the judge, and Peggy were in a terrible predicament.

Cases like Peggy's are, unfortunately, not at all unusual, although modern contraceptive technology may provide an alternative that was unavailable not long ago. What choices does the judge have in this case?

The judge was considering mandating that Peggy receive a contraceptive called "Norplant" instead of sentencing her for drug abuse and child neglect and as a condition for public funding for an abortion. With this type of contraception, six little capsules are surgically inserted under the skin of her upper arm. These capsules contain female hormones like those in birth control pills, but these are time-released over several years. Essentially, this is effective, no-fuss contraception. Norplant is very reliable and is effective almost immediately, although some women who use it have side effects that can be uncomfortable and persist for months. If the court could not improve Peggy's life situation immediately, at least with Norplant it could ensure that she would have no more children to care for until she got on her feet. The judge was also offering Peggy one-on-one counseling with a therapist at the Community Services Board. While these measures seemed a comprehensive "package" to help this young woman, there were some ethical considerations the judge had to think about.

For example, can a court intervene in any woman's reproductive choices and curtail her fertility, even temporarily? How is this ethically different from permanent sterilization of people who do not conform to society's expectations regarding their sexual and child-bearing choices? Should all women who abuse their children have their fertility temporarily taken away? Who would monitor Peggy to be sure that she didn't have the capsules removed by a doctor—and what would be the penalty if she did? What if Peggy had a terrible reaction to Norplant? What if, for religious reasons, Peggy refused to use *any* contraceptives? Her situation involved issues of reproductive freedom, public policy, contraceptive technology, and moral and ethical aspects of a terrible family situation.

Chapter 11 discusses contraception. Understanding the different methods and their relative effectiveness and possible side effects is not difficult. The broader psychosocial issues involved in the various methods of birth control, as well as some of the reasons why people are negligent in using them, are more complex. We will explore the immediate and broader cultural environment in which contraceptive choices are considered and made, and understand why the availability of contraceptives does not ensure they are used.

David

David just turned 18 and was in the middle of his senior year of high school. More than ever before, he felt overwhelmed by issues he was facing. Something inside him didn't have the strength to deal with it all, but he knew he couldn't stop the calendar or fail to acknowledge what is in his head and his heart. He was having a problem understanding himself.

For several months he had been thinking a lot about college. He had done very well on his SATs and was getting letters asking him to apply to some of the best colleges. Virtually all offered him some scholarship assistance. His grades were extremely strong. Being a great football player didn't hurt either, and he had some good athletic scholarship offers to consider too.

His dad had moved away, but his mom had been attentive and helpful to his education and athletics ever since he was 10 years old. She was very proud of him and optimistic about his future. It was his dream to become an art critic, and he wanted to study art history and museum studies. He knew these interests didn't fit the typical profile of an All-American high school running back, and there were other things that didn't fit either.

David's junior prom had been a real mess, and he was already feeling uptight about his senior prom. He'd known Danielle since he was in the sixth grade, and they were very good friends. They talked easily and trusted each other completely. In most ways he was very comfortable with her. They had dated steadily for over 2 years, and they'd never really talked about going to the prom, it was just understood that they would. The dress, the tuxedo, the corsage, the dance—it all overwhelmed him. He told himself it was just that he was a very simple person. But when his friends wanted to get rooms at a local motel, buy some booze, and spend the night with their dates, David felt uncomfortable. Danielle wanted to go, however, and they had an argument. He seemed to have so many things on his mind . . .

David was also worrying about leaving his mother alone when he went away to college. For almost 8 years now, he knew she had built her life around him, savoring his every achievement and award. He felt protective of her and didn't know what she would do if he went to school far away.

In addition to all this, he had more pressing thoughts that formed a constant, disturbing emotional background for his entire life. David was pretty sure he was gay. He had never actually had an "encounter" with another male, but he wasn't averse to the idea. When masturbating he usually had fantasies of having sex with other boys or men. His awareness of being gay had developed slowly, though for the past year he had felt an almost painful self-consciousness. How could he be sure about this, when he knew how scorned and reviled gays were in society? How was he supposed to handle his public self as an amazing athlete while he was attracted to other men at the same time? He just didn't feel he fit in, either way. He was keenly aware of how abusive people can be to gays, and he didn't think he had the gumption to handle it himself.

So David kept his secret to himself. There was no one he could talk to—no one. Not his mom, not Danielle, not his coach, certainly not any of his friends. He didn't go to church. For a while he thought about going to talk to a school counselor, but he worried someone would see him and people would start asking questions. He knew about the quiet network of gays at school, but he wasn't friends with any of them and didn't know how to approach any of them. How had life suddenly gotten so complicated? How was he going to make it through the year with all these problems?

Homosexuality is an issue relevant to many chapters in this book, but we will take a systematic, comprehensive look at this topic in Chapter 9. The issue of gender orientation is not an either/or designation, and the expression of one's sexuality should be viewed within different contexts: one's social situation, how one thinks of oneself, and one's feelings of emotional affiliation. "Coming out" is rarely an easy decision. We will explore how society facilitates or inhibits the decision to self-identify as gay. We will recognize the basic worth and humanity of individuals of all gender orientations and the normality of their lives, drives, and desires.

Tara and Jason: A "Hands-On" Learning Experience

Tara was 3 years old, and Jason was her best friend. They lived across the street from each other. They did everything together, like having Pop-tarts after pre-school, watching TV side-by-side on the floor, and going to the neighborhood swimming pool in the afternoon. Jason had a big sandbox in his back yard, and Tara came over often with her toy trucks and earth movers. They were great friends.

One Saturday afternoon Jason's mom came home from a yard sale with an old canvas army pup tent. They set it up in the back yard, and Jason and Tara loved it. It was a magical place; it felt like there was nothing outside the tent and the closeness within was safe and quiet. Later that week, Jason and Tara were playing alone inside the tent. Jason was so engrossed in his Legos that he ignored the need to urinate until it was almost too late, so he went to the tree beside the tent to relieve himself. Tara came out and watched him intently. She told

Jason that *she* certainly didn't have anything like that, and she wanted another peek.

This was new to Jason. He was surprised she didn't have one too. So he tugged his shorts down so she could have another look. Then Tara did the same to show him that she didn't have one. For just a few minutes they just inspected each other. Neither knew what to say, and after a few minutes they yanked their shorts back up and went back to their Legos.

That evening, just after Jason's mother had read him a story and was about to turn off his light, he asked her why he and Tara looked so different "down here," and he pointed to himself. His mother's eyes opened wide; she was clearly surprised. She asked him what he meant and Jason comfortably told her what had happened that afternoon. Then she told him those are "very private places" you shouldn't show to others until you got much older. She said that what he and Tara did was okay, that it wasn't any big deal this time, but that there were better ways to play with his friends. Then she told Jason that if anyone ever made him show himself to them, he was to tell her right away. As she left his room she told him that he could come to her with questions like that one whenever he wanted to. As she went back downstairs, she was thinking that parenting was getting more interesting every day.

Sexual curiosity in childhood is very common and normal. Figure 1-15 shows how utterly unselfconscious young children are with respect to their nudity and curiosity. We are all sexual beings from birth to death—this is a fundamental aspect of our shared humanity. This story is a good example of what sex educators call a "teachable moment," an occasion when a parent or caretaker can take the opportunity to teach and reassure a youngster about some sexual, intimate, or reproductive issue. Chapter 12 discusses a number of issues related to the emergence of sexuality in childhood. Think back to your own childhood. Can you recall incidents like the one in this story? How did your parent(s) react? How did you react to the discovery of sexual curiosity in your own children? How do you think you will in the future if you become a parent? Events like this are upsetting to some parents, while to others it is perfectly normal and expectable behavior.

Donna

Finally, Donna had landed a really good job! After working in fast-food restaurants and as a maid at a motel, she was hired at the new computer chip facility in her small community in upstate New York. She was 19 and ready for a challenge. She knew she had superlative manual dexterity, and this intricate work felt perfect for her. She got along with her co-workers. Management found her productive and cooperative. The pay was excellent, and the health care benefits were very good.

She was also meeting lots of new people from all over the region. She had gone out a few times already with Danny, a quiet, polite guy who worked with computers in the accounting department. She was impressed with his poise and self-confidence. He never tried to be someone he wasn't. He was only a few years older than Donna, and they formed a comfortable friendship. They went to the company picnic together, and everyone assumed they were now a couple in a relationship.

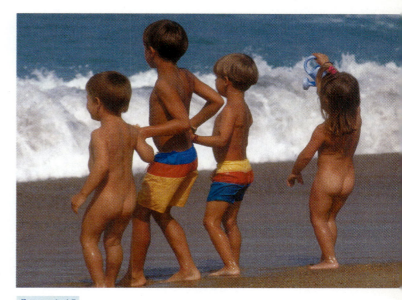

FIGURE 1-15 While sexual curiosity among young children is common and normal, they are also quite unselfconscious about their nudity.

Very early one Saturday morning (much too early for her tastes), Donna found herself in Danny's pick-up truck on the way to his favorite fishing spot. She had made sandwiches, and Danny brought a big cooler of drinks. He was driving with an open beer between his legs. It seemed pretty early in the day for a beer, Donna thought. He turned off the two-lane highway and drove a long way over dusty, unpaved roads full of bumps and ruts. Finally, they got to a beautiful blue lake. There was no one else around.

They fished all morning. The sun got higher and it got hot. Danny drank beer all morning; Donna had iced tea. For lunch they ate the sandwiches she'd packed. Having gotten up so early, the heat and food now made Donna very drowsy. Danny had become pretty animated, though, and Donna was surprised how different he acted after drinking beer all morning. She told him that she was going to take a short nap in the truck and left him to his fishing. Almost as soon as she lay down across the seat she went to sleep.

Donna awoke to find Danny naked beside her in the truck. He had a strange look on his face and was rubbing her legs. She was frightened—this didn't seem like the Danny she knew. "What are you doing?" she demanded. He said nothing; he didn't smile or look her in the eye. Then in an instant he was on top of her. Loudly and firmly Donna said, "No, Danny. No. Stop now. Now!" He didn't stop. He acted belligerently. He didn't listen to her. Soon he'd pulled her blouse and bra off and jerked her jeans open. She was paralyzed with fear but kept yelling "No. Don't. Stop. Please get away from me!" She couldn't believe this was happening to her. He took her brutally, painfully, abusively. She was terrified, and for a while all she felt was fear and disgust. Then her sense of shame and loss of control were overwhelming.

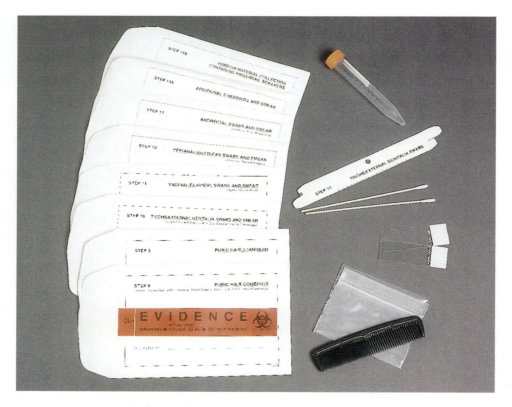

FIGURE 1-16 A rape investigation. Many kinds of evidence are all helpful in arresting and prosecuting men who rape.

Figure 1-16 shows a rape investigation kit used by medical and law enforcement personnel to collect evidence about a sexual assault.

Date rape is common. Unfortunately, all forms of rape are common. Chapter 19 explores the motives for rape and assesses its consequences—psychological, legal, and emotional. Donna's story is not unusual. Danny sexually assaulted her. His sexual advances were unwanted and unwelcome. He failed to comply with her demand to be left alone. He ignored her "No." Donna may wonder forever if she did or said something to encourage Danny, but she should never wonder about the appropriateness of his behavior. It was wrong, and it was illegal.

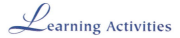

SEXUAL EXPRESSION AND SEXUAL EXPERIENCE SURROUND US

We share these stories with you because the emotional texture of sexual expression and experience cannot be conveyed simply through a summary of the primary literature in the key disciplines. These vignettes show many of the ways that sexuality touches human experiences. Our lifestyles, our development, our biology, and our wider psychosocial environment are all deeply influenced by our sexuality.

We also think that the issues dealt with in these vignettes may relate in one way or another to your own experience or the experiences of someone close to you. In a sense, we want to validate the realities of sexuality in your own life, and in

some cases perhaps reassure you of their normalcy. Thinking about certain experiences can help us be prepared for them if and when they happen to us or those close to us.

By the time you finish reading this book, we hope sexuality still holds much of its magic and mystery for you, while at the same time you are more knowledgeable, comfortable, and tolerant about it. This is indeed a subject that can enhance the quality of your lives. So hang on! It's going to be a *very* interesting ride.

Learning Activities

Following are activities to help you review what you have learned in this chapter. Your instructor might ask you to think through these questions or write down your answers.

1. At the beginning of this chapter we discussed several assumptions related to a course in human sexuality. Now let's take a different look at this issue of "assumptions."
   a. By this time, some of your friends and perhaps family members know you are taking this course. Describe *their* reactions to your taking a class with this title.
   b. When you tell others that you are taking calculus, they usually don't ask to see your calculus text. Has anyone picked up or asked to see your human sexuality book? Can you tell if they are looking for anything in particular? Do they quickly skim the book

or pause to study parts more closely? Has anyone asked to borrow the book? Have you noticed that anyone else, such as a roommate or family member, has been reading this book?

2. If you work very hard on this course throughout the term but don't get what you consider a good grade, would that affect how you feel about your own sexuality? Can you think of any situations in which what you *knew* and how you *acted* seemed inconsistent?

3. In the section on the multidisciplinary nature of human sexuality, this chapter introduced you to a number of areas that overlap in their study of this subject. Have other disciplines been omitted? Do you feel that this course can be taught successfully by only one instructor? Can it be taught successfully from within only one department? Do you think female and male instructors would bring different perspectives to this course?

4. Discuss some sexual issues you think could be most productively studied with a macro perspective. What methods would be best to answer these questions?

5. Discuss some sexual issues you think could be most productively studied with a micro perspective. What methods would be best to answer these questions?

6. What image do you have about the type of person who would sexually molest children in a day-care center? Describe their gender, age, and background.

7. In your own adolescent development, what was the most difficult challenge you faced as your body began to change?

8. In which grade should sex education in schools begin? Why? If you feel that sex education should *not* be taught in the schools, *where* should this information be offered and *how* should those responsible for it prepare themselves?

9. Without looking ahead in this book, describe the symptoms of one sexually transmitted disease. How long does it take for these symptoms to appear after the exposure to the bacteria or virus?

10. If you had always planned to have children and found out that you couldn't, how would you feel and what would you do?

11. Should the courts have the power to restrict a woman's fertility? If so, what actions should receive this penalty? If a male rapist requests surgical castration instead of prison, should a court honor this request?

12. At what age do you think people become aware that they are gay? How do people deal with pressures to stay "in the closet" or "come out?" Is there a best way to "come out?"

13. With condoms so readily available, why don't all people use them conscientiously and consistently?

14. How should women resist sexual assault?

*K*ey Concepts

- In a climate of psychological safety, two people feel unconditional acceptance for one another, shared mutuality, nonjudgmental communication, and a sense of security about revealing their vulnerabilities.
- A multidisciplinary approach uses facts, concepts, principles, and methods from a number of different sciences and/or academic disciplines to explain a particular phenomenon under study.
- Cultural anthropology is concerned with a cross-cultural analysis of the customs, norms, and mores of different societies, often with regard to conventions serving similar objectives of the cultures under study.
- Clinical psychologists specialize in the study of the development and manifestations of emotional and behavioral problems, as well as the diagnosis and treatment of these difficulties. Some clinical psychologists, social workers, and other professionals specialize in sex therapy.
- In the study of human sexuality, the macro or "big picture" level of analysis deals with larger social concerns and demographic aspects of an issue, while the micro or "little picture" level of analysis focuses on hormonal, anatomical, neurological, and physiological matters.
- The case study method is an intensive study, description, and analysis of a single individual and the life circumstances surrounding that person.
- Biopsychology researches and applies information about the biological foundations of human and animal behavior, which may involve the anatomical, physiological, and endocrine basis of thought, emotion, and action.
- The psychosocial approach analyzes and explains human behavior in a context of the broader social environment in which it occurs, dealing with the reciprocal influences between people's actions and the surroundings in which they operate.
- The medical model views abnormal or unusual behaviors as symptoms of an underlying disease state that can be diagnosed and appropriately treated.

2

Historical and Current Traditions and Perspectives in Human Sexuality

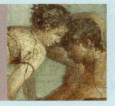

OBJECTIVES

When you finish reading and reviewing this chapter, you should be able to:

1. Differentiate among various meanings of the term *sexuality*.

2. Differentiate among various meanings of the terms, *sex, gender role,* and *gender identity*.

3. Describe the four major theoretical perspectives in the study of human sexuality: psychobiological, psychosocial, clinical, and cross-cultural.

4. Discuss the influence of ancient Jewish beliefs on modern traditions in terms of male dominance, intercourse within the marriage bond, and sexual pleasure in marital intimacy.

5. Explain the long-lasting impact of the writings of St. Augustine and St. Thomas Aquinas on attempts to understand and systematize thinking about human sexual inclinations.

6. Describe the impact of the Protestant Reformation on ideas about sexual feeling and behavior in the context of marriage.

7. Describe the elements of Victorian sexuality and note their impact on contemporary thinking about male and female gender roles.

8. Describe the contributions of Richard von Krafft-Ebing and Havelock Ellis and their relationship to the Victorian influences of the 19th century.

9. Summarize Freud's thinking on the distinction between "sexuality" and "sensuality," and describe the following concepts in his psychoanalytic theory: determinism, libido, erogenous zones, pleasure principle, and reality principle.

10. Describe the methods employed by Alfred Kinsey and his colleagues and the importance of their findings.

11. Summarize the methodologies and findings of William Masters and Virginia Johnson and explain their contributions to sexuality research.

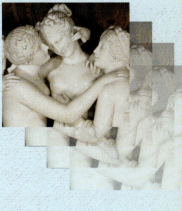

From Dr. Ruth

As you read this chapter, which includes the history of Western sexual tradition, note an important point: those who wrote the cultural records were typically men, and the generalizations they made about their own culture and those preceding them often reflected a male perspective. This is not to say that women have not held an important place in the history of sexuality as we know it today. Although women do not have to enjoy sex in order to further procreation, they are all born with sexual feelings and the capacity to have orgasms, and their sex drive most definitely affects their behavior, as well as the behavior of the men around them.

If you believed cartoonists, sexual relationships between men and women in prehistoric times happened only after the cave man had clubbed the woman senseless and dragged her off into the bushes. But is that really how early humans had sex? I doubt it, and one proof comes from our studies of some modern, undeveloped, geographically isolated societies. For example, missionaries who went to preach in the South Pacific were shocked at the variety of sexual positions they found the natives using. They engaged in many different sexual activities that pleased both men and women. It was no accident that the so-called "missionary" (male superior) position advocated by those visiting men of the cloth happens to offer women the least freedom to control the angle, rate, and depth of penile penetration.

But even much later, women were often not full partners in sex. I like to quote the Victorian mother who told her soon-to-be-married daughter that sex is not something to be enjoyed but instead she should "lie back and think of England." Still, throughout history, despite the often deadly consequences of being branded an adulteress, women have strayed from the marital bed in search of intimate pleasures their husbands weren't giving them.

In the Ancient Jewish tradition, sexual satisfaction is part of the wedding contract for both men and women. Celibacy is not a virtue—orgasms are. And certainly the Greeks and Romans celebrated their sexuality, perhaps to excess, which is what instigated the sexual reserve inherent in Christian teaching for the last 2000 years or so. Sexual satisfaction, particularly for women, was pushed into the background. As you read this chapter, you'll see that women today seek their own sexual self-determination, and that more than ever before they are true partners in all aspects of their relationships with men. But it hasn't been easy to reach this point, and the story is a long and interesting one.

Because the words we use color the way we think, we should examine the term *sexuality* and explore both its obvious meanings and its less obvious connotations at the outset. From a young age you may have recognized that whenever the word "sex" was used, it provoked an assortment of reactions, some positive, others negative, and still others aversive. Words with different shades of meaning carry quite different implications and inferences. So just exactly what does the term **sexuality** mean?

Let's begin with an objective definition. Biologists typically use the term "sexual" to refer to the type of reproduction in which a cell from a male of the species is joined with a cell from a female to produce a *new* member of the species. If our thinking about sexuality focused just on trading DNA, however, this book wouldn't need to be very long at all. Sexuality involves other terms with other sexual implications or connotations. For example, the word **carnal** typically implies "crude" sexual pleasures—an "appetite" or hedonistic motivation; it is used more often in legal and historical/theological contexts. **Erotic**, another word referring to sexual thinking and behaving, is commonly used to describe something that arouses sexual desire or love with a powerful sexual component. Instead of "carnal," we will use *erotic* in this book to convey some of the subtle emotional texture surrounding that which we find sexual.

Later on, this chapter will introduce Sigmund Freud's theory of psychosexual development. His term **libido** describes a basic, primitive "force" in the personality that seeks sexual or aggressive expression. Freud coined the term to convey the idea that what human beings find "lustful" is based on a deep biopsychological drive that may not be completely sexual in nature. How Freud used the term indicates that he thought sexual feelings derive from strongly felt pleasures, regardless of where they come from in the body. Such pleasures need not be entirely genital in origin.

Another word commonly used in reference to sexual matters is *passionate*. This conveys the spirit of intense, ecstatic feelings surrounding sexual arousal and expression. It connotes a loss of reasoning and total absorption in the object of one's desires. This word is also used to refer to other desires as well, such as when someone says that they "feel passionately about human rights." Finally, the word **sensual** is often used to describe pleasures of many kinds, one of which is sexual. For example, although a person's back and thighs are not as sensitive as their genitals, a slow, warm massage is for most individuals a highly sensual experience.

All these terms have different nonjudgmental connotations. As you know, however, some other terms for sexual matters are not nearly so wholesome. Since language reveals thoughts and judgments, negative terms convey a different perspective about intimacy and sexual enjoyment. For example, words such as "infatuation," "lustful," "horny," and "dissipated" have sexual overtones, and none conveys an unambiguously favorable picture of sexual motives or behaviors. The point here is simple: language helps shape thought. The terminology used says much about the individual using the words. As we will see in Chapter 12, when children are taught cute terms for their sexual anatomy, this often implies a lack of cleanliness and self-respect. One of the most important objectives of this book is to give you an appropriate and accurate sexual vocabulary.

HISTORICAL CHANGES IN PERSPECTIVES ON SEXUALITY

Today an enormous amount of information is available about virtually all aspects of human sexuality. Although there are pockets of sexual repression in our society, the number of accurate publications and audiovisual resources available is truly enormous. Our culture has become progressively more comfortable with sexuality. It hasn't come easy, however, and the times weren't always as progressive. Throughout history, attitudes about sexuality have swung like a pendulum from the comfortable and open to the restrictive and restrained. How and why has this happened?

More than 2300 years ago Aristotle wrote about the importance of moderation in the pursuit of human appetites (Fig. 2-1). "All things in moderation" is clearly an Aristotelian notion, characteristic of his view of human nature. In *The Nicomachean Ethics* he writes:

The temperate man holds a mean position with regard to pleasures. He enjoys neither the things that the li-

centious man enjoys most (he positively objects to them) nor wrong pleasures in general, nor does he enjoy any pleasure violently; he is not distressed by the absence of pleasures, nor does he desire them—or if he does, he desires them in moderation, and not more than is right, or at the wrong time, or in general with any other qualification.

—*THE NICOMACHEAN ETHICS,* BOOK III, CHAPTER XI

Later he is more specific: "Now you can have an excess of bodily goods; and it is the pursuit of this excess, not that of the necessary pleasures, that make a man bad; because everyone enjoys tasty food and wine and sex in some degree, but not everyone to the right degree." (Book VII, Chapter xiv). But what is "moderation" in sex? The following historical review shows that with a few exceptions the rule of thumb, through much of Western history has been: "The less, the better." Nonetheless we are dealing with one of the most powerful human motives, which demands expression, more or less publicly.

Between 400 BC and 400 AD relationships between women and men in the Greco-Roman world were characterized by an enormous asymmetry in power. Men were dominant and women were submissive. Most women were exploited sexually by the men who owned or controlled them–slaves, former slaves, wives, servants, and women captured in war (Boswell, 1994). This manipulation and abuse was common and questioned by few. Uninhibited historical descriptions of such sexual encounters show that many sexual unions took place with-

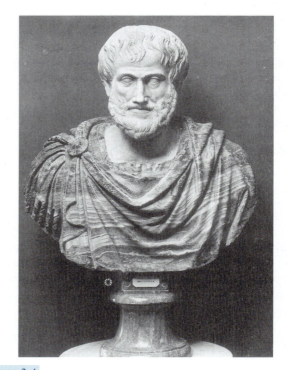

FIGURE 2-1 The Greek philosopher Aristotle taught the basic importance of moderation in all things, including sexual expression.

out affection, respect, or comforts and protections. Marriage, which was not a romantic institution, involved the exchange and sharing of property, land, and financial assets as a link between kinship groups. Sexual attraction was less important to the ancients as a motive for marriage.

This sexual inequality persisted well into the Middle Ages, with one interesting development. The wealthy upper class was more influenced by the Church's demands for a circumspect sexual code (at least publicly). The peasantry, however, had sexual freedom and felt few qualms about pursuing erotic adventures with or without the knowledge or consent of anyone else.

The private and public aspects of human sexual expression have always been two sides of the issue, and writings ranging from the secretive to the scientific characterize the history of the study of human sexuality.

While historical and religious influences have shaped thinking and behaving about sex, philosophical and scientific factors have also had an enormous impact. **Epicureanism**, an important Roman philosophy, held that the highest good is the unrestrained pursuit of pleasure, including sexual adventures. In contrast, **Stoicism** believed that women and men should conduct themselves with intelligence, restraint, and dignity. The Epicurean view is still a popular approach to life, emphasized by advertising slogans such as "You only go 'round once in life." Here is the contrast between the repressive, secretive, exploitative aspects of human sexuality on the one hand, and the public pursuit of pleasures on the other. Now add to this mix the influences of science and things become more complicated. Long before the industrial revolution of the 1840s, the Church was gradually replaced by the spirit of scientific inquiry as the sole and final authority on morality and public conduct; we will explore this later in the section on the Victorian Era. As well, ethics began to emerge as a freestanding branch of philosophy, divorced from theological tradition and based more on pragmatic, situational factors. Today we are left with the remnants of these conflicting historical, philosophical, religious, and scientific influences.

"SEX," "GENDER ROLE," AND "GENDER IDENTITY"

These three terms are often used interchangeably, although they have different meanings. Their definitions should be clear, because they will appear often in this book. The word *"sex"* is often used to refer to the biological designation of being either male or female. In this respect, *sex* is the clearest and least ambiguous of these terms. Still, *sex* refers to both the individual's genetic and anatomical composition, and these are not always in perfect agreement.

Gender role is more complex. It refers to a wide assortment of expectable or "appropriate" thoughts, feelings, and behaviors of males and females. Keep in mind, however, that "expectable" and "appropriate" are specific to one's sociocultural environment. Feeling that you are required or expected to behave in a particular way because you are a man or woman oc-

curs because gender role involves what is socially acceptable. Even without knowing it we may be influenced by these expectations. Our ideas of **masculinity** and **femininity** are based on gender roles. Those terms can be complicated because they often represent a distillation of everything it means to be a "real man" or a "real woman." Our clothing, social demeanor, and even grooming habits may be affected by traditional or contemporary notions of masculinity and femininity.

Finally, **gender identity** refers to our self-awareness of our maleness or femaleness. This may involve the degree to which our biological characteristics and our gender role are commensurate. For many of us there is no confusion or "mismatch," although some feel a distressing bewilderment. For example, the next chapter discusses **transsexuality**, a condition in which a person feels "trapped" in the body of the opposite sex. Gender identity develops gradually in a social and familial context. As all of us have some traditionally "feminine" attributes, as well as traditionally "masculine" ones; forming a comfortable gender identity is not always straightforward.

These three terms, *sex, gender role,* and *gender identity,* encourage us to ask three questions of ourselves: "What do I look like?" "How should I think, feel, and behave as a man or a woman?" "How do I feel about the 'fit' of my sexuality and my gender role?" We may not think often about these concerns, but occasionally they emerge as questions. Because popular conceptions of masculinity and femininity change, it is normal to have such questions. They involve male/female differences and how we express such differences in our demeanor, dress, and behavior.

THEORETICAL PERSPECTIVES

The previous chapter discussed some of the disciplines involved in the study of human sexuality. Here we will explore in more depth four broad approaches. Virtually everything in this book can be understood within these (sometimes overlapping) contexts. Each is a kind of lens through which we look at topics with sexual meaning.

Psychobiological Perspective

Since the time of the Greek physician Hippocrates (c. 400 BC), thinkers have wondered about the precise relationship between the brain and our feelings and behavior. Aristotle popularized the notion that what we experience through our senses ultimately becomes our emotional and cognitive picture of reality (c. 300 BC). Scientific thinkers did not have a good understanding of the brain's structure until the Belgian anatomist Vesalius (1514–1564) created wood-cuts illustrating the surface and structure of the brain in accurate detail. In the mid-1600s the French philosopher/mathematician René Descartes (Fig. 2-2) introduced a **mechanistic** view of the brain. He approached the brain like a machine, thinking that if we wanted to understand how the machine worked we had to learn about its parts and how they interacted. Descartes introduced the interesting philosophical dilemma that came to be called "dualism." Dualism addressed this question: "How

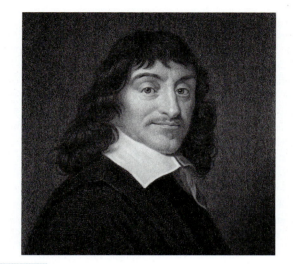

FIGURE 2-2 The French philosopher and mathematician René Descartes wrote about the relationship between the mind and the body, and maintained that the body could be studied as if it were a machine.

can the spiritual, substanceless, incorporeal 'mind' control and direct the physical reality that is the human body?" A clear answer to that question has not yet emerged, even following "The Decade of the Brain" (the 1990s), even with other great advances in the neurosciences.

This mechanistic approach to brain-behavior relationships, which have become the cornerstone of contemporary psychobiological studies, suffers from the problem of **reductionism,** which literally means "nothing but." For example, as you'll read later on, in reference to deeply emotional, sexual feelings that are processed in certain brain centers, some analysts claim that sexual feelings are "nothing but" neural activity in certain parts of the brain. The full emotionality, meaning, and importance of sexual feelings is difficult to reduce simply to sequences of nerve impulses in brain tissue, even though some scientists are comfortable with this approach.

Still, despite the attractions of reductionism, the psychobiological approach offers much to the study of human sexuality. This approach is also concerned with the impact of hormones on behavior and human drives. Indeed, the endocrine glands and hormones are basic to any understanding of human sexuality. Brain activity stimulates hormonal secretion, and hormonal secretion stimulates brain activity.

This is a simplistic but basically accurate description of the **psychobiological approach.** Psychobiologists are interested in the neural basis of thinking, emotions, and behaviors, yet generally they try to avoid being reductionistic. These investigators also call themselves "physiological psychologists" or "behavioral neuroscientists." The study of sexual behavior in both animals and humans is a large part of their research.

Psychosocial Perspective

We briefly described the psychosocial perspective previously in terms of the *reciprocal* relationship between the behaviors of

human beings and the social and cultural environments they inhabit. This perspective pays much less attention to the neurological and biochemical approach of the psychobiological view. The focus is on broader (*macro*) psychological and sociological influences. Our rich inner cognitive and emotional lives are important. Further, the social and cultural environment help shape our perceptions and motivations related to sexuality. The influences are numerous and diverse. Powerful psychosocial influences come from our national, regional, and local geographic localities. National, ethnic, and racial traditions influence our personal development of sexual norms and mores. Finally, religious, economic, and even scientific and technological influences color our development of a personal sexual ideology.

The psychosocial perspective can help interpret the development of an individual throughout the life span, or understand a person at a single, discrete point in life. It can be developmental or situational, or both. Students studying social work learn about "psychosocial assessments," in which personal or family difficulties are examined and documented in order to formulate a plan for helping the client. The aim of such an assessment is to document psychological and social influences that led to personal, interpersonal, or legal problems.

A few important points must be made about the psychosocial approach. First, we are not all equally influenced by society's expectations. While most people are keenly attuned to what they're "supposed to do," others are less so, and some are utterly indifferent. Differences in interpreting social norms contribute to both sexual variations and deviations in many people's lifestyles. Second, human beings do not have to *experience* the consequences of a behavior in order to *learn* the consequences of a behavior. We learn a lot from our psychosocial environment by observing *other people* when they engage in specific behaviors. This capacity for **vicarious learning** is wonderfully adaptive, and you will see later how it affects our learning about our sexuality. By observing others we learn what the probable outcomes of our own actions will be. When we see others avoid contracting sexually transmitted diseases or prevent an unanticipated pregnancy by using condoms, we learn the utility of that behavior by observing it, not by making mistakes ourselves. Finally, a psychosocial approach is highly *synergistic:* our private psychological characteristics interact with the public attributes of the social environment to create powerful, *mutually reinforcing* influences on behavior. Just as we affect our environment, our environment assuredly affects us too.

Clinical Perspective

The word **clinical** refers to various settings and research approaches beyond medical uses of the term. For example, in the social and behavioral sciences, *clinical* typically means the investigator is using controlled observation along with an in-depth interview. After having scrutinized some record of human behavior, the investigator asks the subject about certain actions under study. This leads to a personal recollection of the person's behaviors, thoughts, emotions, and motivations. The combination of the behavioral record and subjective assess-

ment often reveals interesting things about how humans behave. The period of observation helps render a highly **naturalistic** picture of behavior.

Have you ever been told that you flirt a lot? Did you
know it? Did you deny it? What if we showed you a videotape
of you having coffee with other students that revealed you as a
shameless flirt? In an interview we might learn how much you
are aware of your behaviors. We would then be able to learn
about your intentions, feelings, and possible motives for your
flirting. Observing human behavior with a follow-up discussion provides a fuller understanding of the behavior dynamics
being studied.

The clinical approach also involves an objective, analytical
type of investigation. The investigator's biases, expectations,
hopes, and speculations should play no role in planning the
study, carrying it out, or analyzing the data. The individuals being studied are told enough about the project to give their informed consent, although telling *too much* about the hypotheses and anticipated results would bias the subjects' responses. To
avoid this ticklish problem, a **double blind** study is used—neither the person administering the study nor the person participating in it knows the true nature of the study. Thus, the
thoughts and emotions of the experimenter and the subject are
much less likely to lead to inaccurate or prejudiced data.

The term "clinical" also involves a distinction between
basic science and applied science. Basic science involves investigations undertaken purely to gain knowledge; no immediate
use of the collected data is intended. In contrast, applied science is concerned with real-life human problems and their solutions. The clinical approach is one manifestation of this. In
medicine, for example, the basic sciences include **anatomy,
physiology,** and **embryology.** Information in these areas has
no immediate or direct usefulness in the treatment of illnesses.
However, when knowledge of anatomy, physiology, or embryology is used to develop a better treatment for a disorder, then
we have entered the realm of therapeutics, the applied science
of treating disease.

In summary, the term "clinical" involves a diversified approach with several important, subtle distinctions. In common
use, "clinical" is usually synonymous with scientific, experimental, or methodological rigor and care in the development,
execution, and analysis of thorough, well-controlled studies.

Cross-Cultural Perspective

In the previous chapter we introduced several disciplines that
study human sexuality; one of these is cultural anthropology. It
is a rich and fascinating approach to the unique characteristics
of different cultures and environments and their distinctive customs. Words like "different" and "distinctive" refer to something
strange, but strange in comparison with what? The answer is
simple: strange in comparison with our culture, as if ours should
be the standard by which others are judged. What a high-and-
mighty way to look at the world! We must understand that "different" means just that—different, not better or worse. The
word **ethnocentrism** refers to the attitude that one's own group
or culture is superior to others and that others can be judged in
reference to one's own society. Ethnocentrism shows an utter
lack of objectivity about cross-cultural differences, and we
should always be sensitive to its biases and influences.

Many of the interpersonal and sexual customs of other
cultures might seem unusual, but they give a fascinating
glimpse of the lives of people in distant and sometimes exotic
places. The same is true of some subcultures in our own society. For example, historically, some Native American tribes believed there are three genders. In addition to male and female
were *diconidique* or *diconidiniin,* thought to be remarkable
types of women and men corresponding to our contemporary
designation of lesbian or gay (Day, 1995). Within the tribe's
social structure lesbian or gay people were highly spiritual individuals who named newborn infants, acted as tribal healers,
and created art. This shows the importance of standing outside
of the traditions and standards of one's own culture in order to
understand others. A cross-cultural approach emphasizes our
shared humanity, despite major differences among cultures.

Table 2-1 summarizes the four perspectives described
above.

Many aspects of human sexuality take different forms in
other cultures. **Circumcision** of males or females, arranged marriages, expressions of childhood and adolescent sexual interest,
and attitudes about extramarital sexual relationships vary in distinct ways in different cultures. Much can be learned from a
cross-cultural analysis of such differences. Throughout this book
are examples of cross-cultural sexual differences, although the
ways in which we are different from one another are perhaps not
as interesting as the ways in which we are similar. Interestingly,

---

TABLE 2-1

Four Theoretical Perspectives in the Study of Human Sexuality

Psychobiological Perspective	Psychosocial Perspective	Clinical Perspective	Cross-Cultural Perspective
Mechanistic approach to mind-body interaction	Reciprocal relationship be-tween human behavior and the social environment	Controlled observation and in-depth interview	Description and comparison of different cultures and their customs
Reductionistic approach	Vicarious leaning may play an important role	Naturalistic descriptions of human behavior	Emphasis on shared human values and traditions
Brain-behavior relationships		Applied science orientation to human problems and their solutions	

Other Countries, Cultures, and Customs

THE SAMBIA OF NEW GUINEA

Semen conservation theory, explored later in this chapter in connection with Victorian sexual norms and mores, emphasizes sexual restraint and the inappropriateness of "wasting" semen through masturbation and too-frequent intercourse. This has been an influential idea in one guise or another in the Western world. An interesting custom in contrast to semen conservation theory has been called "semen investment theory" (Money, 1992).

The anthropologist Gilbert Herdt did a field study of the Sambia, an aboriginal tribe in eastern New Guinea. Notable were his descriptions of customs related to the development of masculinity and male sexual behavior during childhood and early adulthood. The Sambia believe that semen has powerful properties and that to embark on the path to manhood young boys must drink the semen of young men in their village. These homosexual interactions are brief and do not involve relationships of any permanence.

Sambian boys are taught the growth-promoting qualities of semen through a ritual teaching process:

Now we teach you our customary story . . . . And soon you must ingest semen in the culthouse. Now there are many men here; you must sleep with them. Soon they will return to their homes. Now they are here, and you ought to drink their semen. In your own hamlets, there are only a few men. When you sleep with men, you should not be afraid of sucking their penises. You will soon enjoy them . . . . If you try it [semen], it is just like the milk of your mother's breast. You can swallow it all the time and grow quickly. If you do not start to drink it now, you will not ingest much of it. Only occasionally . . . . And later when you are grown you will stop. If you drink a little semen now, you will not like the penis much. So you must start now and swallow semen. When you are bigger your own penis will become bigger, and you will not want to sleep with older men. You will then want to inseminate younger boys yourself. So you should sleep with men now.

—HERDT, 1987, 150

Both semen conservation and semen investment theories attribute powerful qualities to semen. This Sambian custom is thought to be independent of heterosexual interests, which begin in later adolescence and develop slowly and tentatively. Indeed, young Sambian men are truly bisexual. Very rarely do adult Sambian males adopt a homosexual orientation; the pressures to establish and provide for a family are keenly felt (Herdt, 1987).

virtually all cultures establish norms and laws to recognize and regulate the appropriate expression of sexual behavior.

BRIEF HISTORY OF HUMAN SEXUALITY

It is hard to imagine experiencing the sexual norms of another era, as it is difficult to generalize about changes over time in how people experience sexual feelings and express their sexual tastes. Yet to gain a fuller appreciation of sexuality in the present, historical precedents and traditions must be understood. Following is a condensed, chronological view of sexuality based on historical artifacts, manuscripts, and illustrations. It is noteworthy that no matter how liberal or repressive any his-

torical era was, sexual interest was expressed consistently and graphically in the arts. It seems humankind has always had a sense of wonder, mystery, curiosity, and respect for sexuality.

Early Historical Records

Before ancient Egypt recorded its technological achievements and intellectual accomplishments, early European and Middle-Eastern cultures had already created artifacts revealing an interest in sexual feelings and a sensitivity to sexual attractiveness, produced as early as 4500 BC. Stone Age statues illustrate themes of fertility and masculine sexual potency. Female figurines have large breasts and explicit feminine body configurations, and statues with prominent penises seem to celebrate male sexual arousal. The people who created them may have had a poor understanding of the cyclic nature of human fertility. Tannahill (1980) suggests that as prehistoric women and men watched their livestock, they became aware that intercourse leads to procreation. Anatomical exaggeration in this statuary may illustrate emotionally invested human curiosity about bodies, sexual excitement, intercourse, and fertility. Every age communicates with the symbols at its disposal. The carvings left by civilizations more than 11,000 years ago demonstrate that preliterate bands of people wished to preserve or celebrate some of the deepest feelings and awarenesses they had—a universal characteristic of art. Figure 2-3 shows some erotic art that reveals that people in various historical periods were attuned to pleasures from stimulating the body's most sensitive areas.

Some of the earliest signs of sexual restrictiveness emerged in Egyptian civilization. Most notable are incest and its permissible and impermissible variations (Tannahill, 1980), although these sanctions applied only to the pharaohs and their families. This custom dates back at least to the Eighteenth Egyptian Dynasty (1570–1320 BC). This is important because, for the first time, sexual mores were being created. Prohibitions regarding incest evolved in the psychosocial environment, not from the existing theological climate of the day. So far, sex was an entirely secular matter.

Ancient Hebrew Influences

Many ancient Jewish beliefs about sexuality have come through history remarkably unchanged. These traditions originated as long ago as 3000 BC. Sexual norms and behaviors that consolidated the integrity of the nuclear family were esteemed, while those detracting from the solidarity of marriage in the community were condemned. Religiously sanctioned monogamous marriage was the only appropriate arena for sexual intercourse. Yet, within this private relationship, sex was considered a blessing to be enjoyed uninhibitedly as a mutually pleasurable reflection of the all-important bond between a man and a woman, who were part of the wider religious and civic community.

The Talmud, an ancient Jewish holy book, is a commentary of authoritative tradition, as well as exposition and debate among great Rabbis on the Old Testament. It exhorted women and men to marry and have children and enjoy their mutual sexuality within God's plan for the prosperity of the Jewish people. Those who remained single or married without having children were considered somewhat unusual, but received the community's compassion. Sexual intercourse was to be practiced primarily for procreation. Today's traditions of male dominance and sex-for-procreation originated partly in these Jewish traditions. Among the ancient Jews, men were the undisputed masters of their homes and enjoyed the leadership roles in the community. Moses, who lived in the thirteenth and early twelfth century BC (Fig. 2-4), is one of the well-

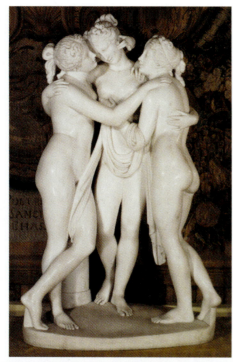

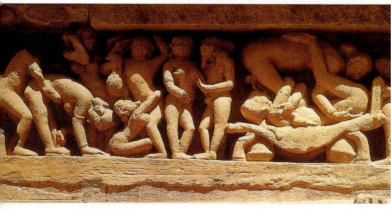

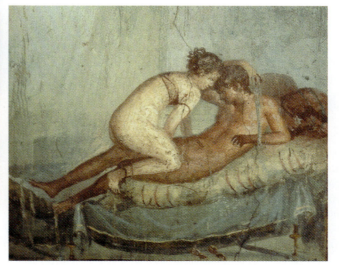

FIGURE 2-3   Throughout history, erotic themes have been a popular artistic focus in virtually all of the world's cultures.

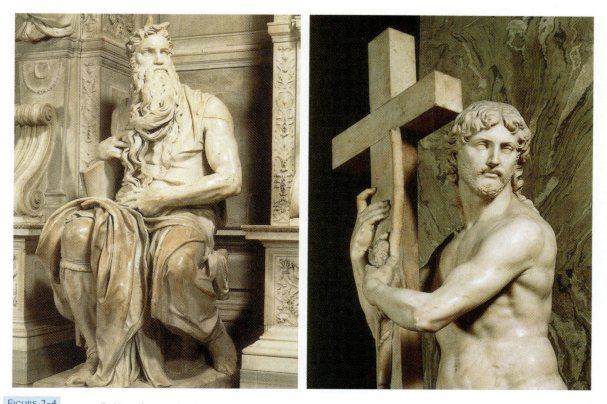

FIGURE 2-4   Moses **(left)** and Jesus **(right)**. Ancient Jewish and Christian traditions have had a powerful impact on contemporary Western perspectives on human sexuality.

known ancient Jews whose traditions and customs still influence our thinking about human sexuality.

Greek and Roman Traditions

Ancient ideas about the beauty of the human body are related to early notions of sexuality in relation to marriage and the social environment. Between 500 BC and Aristotle's time (384–322 BC), sexual attraction was an important theme in art, philosophy, and literature. The role of sexuality in human affairs can be understood through the early Greek distinction between eros and philia. "Eros" was the Greek god of erotic love. Erotic love involved the uninhibited expression of sexual desire and full enjoyment of passionate pleasures. Eros was not associated with a thoughtful, deliberate consideration of a relationship. "Philia," on the other hand, refers to devoted, compatible friendship. It is a less subjective, but more "elevated" notion of the attachment between two people; its ascetic qualities clearly contrast the erotic feelings. Sometimes eros and philia were two parts of the same sexual relationship. Figure 2-5 reveals that the ancient Greeks were comfortable with a variety of sexual behaviors and depicted them in their art.

Pederasty, for example, refers to the love of boys, usually involving sexual behavior, typically anal intercourse. Among the ancient Greeks, men commonly initiated a sexual relationship with adolescent boys who were their pupils. These liaisons combined eros and philia and were considered special teacher/student attachments with physical, spiritual, and intel-

lectual aspects. Sexual exploitation of boys younger than this was forbidden. These behaviors were not considered homosexual. The older man typically was married and had established a large kinship group. Similarly, the young man usually went on to heterosexual marriage and made his primary sexual affiliation in that relationship. Neither man's gender role prohibited this arrangement; in fact, being chosen by an important older man enhanced the young man's esteem and popularity.

Homosexuality in general was an acceptable lifestyle in ancient Greece. It carried no stigma such as sometimes occurs in our own society. Same-sex unions were often thought to involve a "purer" or "higher" form of human attachment. In *Same-Sex Unions in Premodern Europe,* historian John Boswell reminds us that in Plato's Symposium, "heterosexual relationships and feelings are characterized as 'vulgar,' and their same-sex equivalents as 'heavenly'" (Boswell, 1994, p. 74). This attitude involves gender inequality because although male homosexual relationships and friendship were thought to represent the highest form of love and friendship, women were not thought to possess the intelligence or moral integrity needed for such friendship (Boswell, 1994).

Same-sex marriages in ancient Greece often involved an older male and a younger one, similar to common age differences in marriages of men and women. In the *Politics,* Aristotle tells of two male lovers who lived together in one dwelling throughout the course of their whole adult lives and were buried together. These "marriages" were not unusual. It

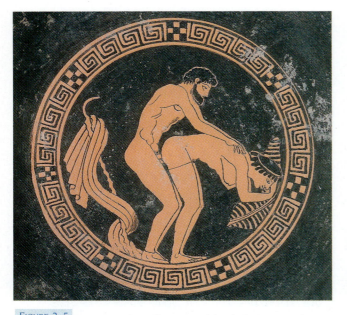

FIGURE 2-5   Many Greek artifacts reveal frank depictions of a wide variety of sexual behaviors.

was a hallowed tradition for Greek warriors who had fought side-by-side to pledge their love and devotion to one another and live together for decades (Boswell, 1994). Further, an older male Greek citizen commonly "adopted" a younger man as his "brother," thereby establishing a long-term same-sex union in which the adoptee inherited an enhanced social standing, as well as joint property. These relationships were enjoyed openly. Boswell (1994) describes elaborate wedding ceremonies in which oaths were exchanged and pledges made.

Just as same-sex unions in Greco-Roman times might strike today's reader as unusual, heterosexual marriages too were not much like contemporary marriages. As noted above, women in the ancient Mediterranean were often seen as property of their husbands; they had virtually no sexual choices. While women and men from affluent families saw marriage as an opportunity to consolidate land holdings and wealth, these bonds had little romantic or sexual motivation. Among poorer couples, however, emotional affinity and sexual attraction had a greater role in creating and maintaining marriages. A wealthy Greek or Roman might have a wife to help consolidate his line of inheritance and another woman for his sexual pleasures and companionship. "Concubines" were women kept by wealthy men for their sexual fulfillment. They might be maintained in the family household or a separate dwelling. Many unmarried men had concubines too (Boswell, 1994). Yet even though relationships with spouses and concubines were public and comfortable for all parties, extramarital sexual relations were still common. As Boswell notes, marriage in Greek society was "a union of 'spirits' or harmony of minds—but not erotic satisfaction, sexual fidelity, or romantic fulfillment." (1994, p. 47).

As Greek power diminished in premodern Europe and

Roman influence grew, sexual norms changed little in this part of the world. Yet one important development did begin—with far-reaching consequences. Instead of marriage being primarily for property reasons, personal choice, affection, and attraction emerged as key factors in marriage. According to Tannahill (1980), many of these changes did not become apparent until about 1800. Marriage became less of an economic institution and more of a romantic partnership (Boswell, 1994). Yet this change did not occur throughout the Roman Empire. Emperors such as Julius Caesar and Caligula were renowned for their fluid gender preferences and uninhibited sexual orgies. Sexual intercourse was not necessary in Roman conceptions of marriage, nor was marriage expected to result in children. A wedding was more of a ceremony celebrating partnership and compatibility than sexual interest and fidelity (Boswell, 1994).

Greek and Roman writers give us insight into their beliefs about different aspects of human sexuality. The Greek physician Hippocrates (460–377 BC), perhaps the most influential doctor of ancient times (Fig. 2-6), described his perceptions of female orgasm:

During intercourse, once a woman's genitals are vigorously rubbed and her womb titillated, a lustfulness [an itch] overwhelms her down there, and the feeling of pleasure and warmth pools out through the rest of her body. A woman also has an ejaculation, furnished by her body, occurring at the same time inside the womb, which has become wet, as well as on the outside, because the womb is now gaping wide open.

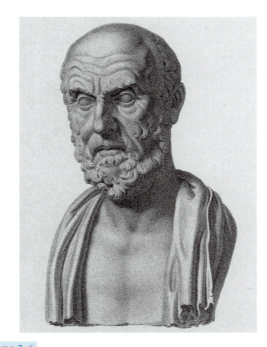

FIGURE 2-6   The famous Greek physician Hippocrates left us an interesting description of female orgasm.

A woman feels pleasure right from the start of intercourse, through the entire time of it, right up until the moment when the man pulls out; if she feels an orgasm coming on, she ejaculates with him, and then she no longer feels pleasure. But if she feels no oncoming orgasm, her pleasure stops when his does. It's like when one throws cold water onto boiling water, the boiling ceases immediately. The same with the man's sperm falling into the womb, it extinguishes the warmth and pleasure of the woman.

Her pleasure and warmth, though, surge the moment the sperm descends in the womb, then it fades. Just as when wine is poured on a flame, it gives a spurt before it goes out for good.

—ZACKS, 1994, 9–10

While Hippocrates is not physiologically accurate by contemporary standards, his remarks communicate his insights into a shared sexual experience.

Long after Hippocrates, the Roman philosopher Lucretius (c. 96–55 BC) had some interesting and clear ideas about the appropriate positions for women to assume during intercourse:

The sexual position is also important. For wives who imitate the manner of wild beasts and quadrupeds— that is, breast down, haunches up—are generally thought to conceive better, since the semen can more easily reach the proper place. . .

For a woman prevents and battles pregnancy if in her joy, she answers the man's lovemaking with her buttocks, and her soft breasts billow forward and back; for she diverts the ploughshare out of the furrow and makes the seed miss its mark. Whores practice such movements for their own reasons, to avoid conception and pregnancy, and also to make the lovemaking more enjoyable for men, which obviously isn't necessary for our wives.

—ZACKS, 1994, 17–18

The Roman Stoic philosopher and statesman, Seneca (4 BC–65 AD), was a keen observer of human nature and society. His comments on the clothing of some women are similar to the thoughts of some in our own society:

I see silk clothes, if these qualify as 'clothes,' which do nothing to hide the body, not even the genitals . . . These clothes are imported from far-off countries and cost a fortune, and the end result? Our women have nothing left to show their lovers in the bedroom that they haven't already revealed on the street.

—ZACKS, 1994, 16

Finally, Zacks (1994) relates an early tale of highly creative advertising: "A pair of sandals owned by a Greek prostitute have survived, and embossed on the soles in raised letters,

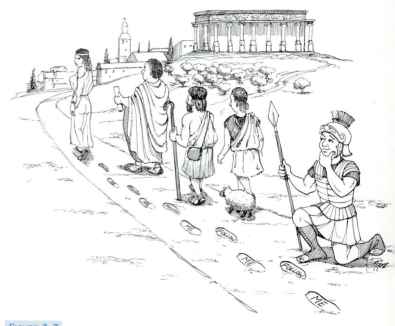

FIGURE 2-7 Roman prostitutes were very innovative in finding ways to advertise their services.

which would leave an impression wherever she walked, were two words: 'Follow me!'." It's hard to imagine more frank sexual advertising (Fig. 2-7).

We include these passages here to emphasize the timeless nature of some observations and concerns regarding human sexuality.

Early Christian Teachings

Just as the ancient Hebrews encouraged conformity with a religiously based code of sexual conduct, the early Christian thinkers and theologians did the same. While the Jews seemed more accepting and comfortable with sexuality in life generally and marriage specifically, early Christians created more negative injunctions for human sexuality. The reasons for this are not hard to understand. In the first century AD, Christian thinking concerning sexuality was based on the teaching of St. Paul. At this time, the sexual excesses of the Roman Empire were everywhere and obvious, and adultery and orgies were often carried out in public. These excesses had a profound effect on early church doctrines.

Jesus of Nazareth, who was celibate throughout his life, saw marriage as the only appropriate arena for sexual expression. Christ said virtually nothing about homosexuality and taught tolerance for sexual indiscretions, seen in the biblical description of his encounter with a woman accused of adultery. Still, Paul believed that the highest spiritual state derived from a celibate lifestyle. He felt the most profound inner tranquility could only be found apart from the excesses of the flesh. To remain without sin, however, it was preferable to marry than to go to hell. Paul apparently considered celibacy a personal victory over worldly temptations. Indeed, many early Christian writings painted a lucid picture of conflicts between desires and religious beliefs— conflicts that are still a part of the human condition.

Many of Paul's beliefs were elaborated and revised by St. Augustine (354–430 AD). Augustine's teachings were as strict as Paul's, and he passionately sought to eradicate sexual excess from the human psyche. (Augustine, it is interesting to note, abandoned his mistress and their son after having a vision of God.) Because of Augustine's writings, the Church took a firm position against sexual intercourse outside marriage. Further, the Church denounced sexual intercourse unless procreation was intended, and any sexual behavior in which procreation would not or could not result became sinful. This included homosexual behavior, masturbation, and oral-genital stimulation.

The Church's positions on sexual concerns gained clearer focus in the writing of St. Thomas Aquinas (1225–1274 AD), who reinforced the notion that sexual behaviors, especially those not resulting in procreation, were inherently sinful. For example, Aquinas believed that masturbation was worse than rape because it could not result in conception, the fundamental objective of sexual activity. In his book, *Summa Theologica,* Aquinas wrote about virtually every aspect of human sexuality, including the nature and content of sexual fantasies, the "aberrant" nature of homosexual behaviors, and the vice of fornication. While little he wrote was new, his work was a lucid, organized, comprehensive commentary on a wide diversity of sexual inclinations and

behaviors. Perhaps more than anyone else, St. Paul, St. Augustine, and St. Thomas Aquinas (Fig. 2-8) were responsible for a church philosophy that has lasted well over 1000 years.

Despite the highly negative injunctions of the church against homosexuality, same-sex unions have been widely documented in Europe during the Middle Ages, as they were in Greco-Roman times. Indeed, some of these homosexual marriages took place within the church itself and involved its senior functionaries. For example, the older Roman tradition of forming a same-sex bond by proclaiming him a "brother" continued well into the Middle Ages. Boswell (1994) notes that "Basil I (867–886), the founder of the Macedonian dynasty that ruled the Byzantine Empire from 867 to 1156, was reported to have been twice involved in ceremonial unions with other men" (p. 231). Indeed, in one of these relationships Basil was named "companion of the bedchamber" to the Emperor Michael III (Boswell, 1994, p. 237).

Some people now consider these early Christian teachings and traditions as a part of past history, but the reader should remember that some of these old ideas are still part of our socioreligious landscape today. For example, in 1995 the University of Texas at Austin offered workshops to students on the topic of sexual abstinence; conservative student groups applauded giving this sexual lifestyle choice a greater voice on campus. Apparently many of these students felt the Student Health Center was "devoting too much attention to birth control and homosexuality and not enough to abstinence." The campus chapter of the Young Conservatives of Texas complained when the Health Center offered workshops addressing gay, lesbian, and bisexual issues (The Chronicle of Higher Education, October 6, 1995, p. A44).

Similarly, the *US Catholic* (April, 1996) published an article titled "Ten Consequences of Premature Sexual Involvement." Here are those "consequences":

1. "worry about pregnancy and AIDS
2. regret and self-recrimination
3. guilt
4. loss of self-respect and self-esteem
5. the corruption of character and the debasement of sex
6. shaken trust and fear of commitment
7. rage over betrayal
8. depression and suicide
9. ruined relationships
10. stunting personal development"

Clearly, many of the beliefs and attitudes of Paul, Augustine, and Aquinas remain with us in a contemporary guise and continue to reinforce one perspective toward sexuality.

A final example of a contemporary theology regards homosexuality and the church's view of its ultimate origins and resolution. Seitz (1995) writes that "the Old Testament considers humanity in two categories: one fallen and outside God's special relationship with Israel, the other fallen but marked with the potential for knowing the will of God, a knowledge that sadly cannot preclude disobedience" (p. 239).

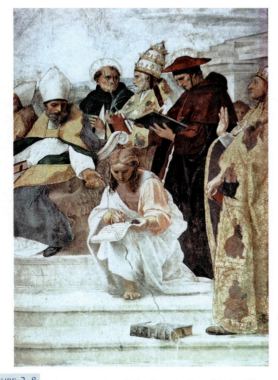

FIGURE 2-8   Saint Augustine (left, dictating) and Saint Thomas Aquinas (in black) were among the most influential early churchmen to address the role of sexuality in Christian life.

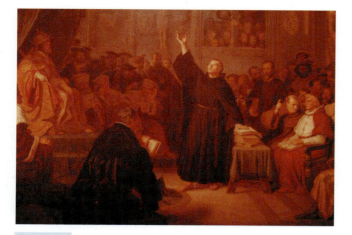

FIGURE 2-9   Martin Luther, a powerful, charismatic preacher, held a more permissive, practical perspective on sexual expression than did his Roman Catholic contemporaries.

The author then goes on to note that aberrant expressions of sexual desire (homosexuality) defy Scripture's "lone voice" of benign reason.

European Developments in the 16th, 17th, and 18th Centuries

The Protestant Reformation was a widespread, passionate challenge to the irrefutable authority of the Roman Catholic Church. It was led by Martin Luther (1483–1546). Luther was an angry, rebellious young man who struggled with his own sexuality and its involuntary, guilt-provoking attributes (erection, nocturnal emission). He was certain that celibacy was unnatural and that the Roman Catholic Church was wrong about it. He concluded that sexual desire is a natural aspect of being human and is not sinful, though its only appropriate arena is marriage. Luther was acutely aware that sexual motivations, once aroused, can be quite distracting (Erikson, 1962). He left the priesthood, married a nun, and had 6 children with her. Luther did not believe priests should not marry or have children. Perhaps most remarkably, Luther did not believe that the only rationale for sexual intercourse was to conceive. Much of the force of Luther's thinking was based on his charismatic, powerful style of preaching (Fig. 2-9).

Following is a passage Luther wrote in 1531; it summarizes his thoughts on marriage and sexuality:

I find there's nothing but godliness in marriage. To be sure, when I consider marriage, only the flesh seems to be there. Yet my father must have slept with my mother and made love to her and they were nevertheless godly people. All the patriarchs and prophets did likewise. The longing of a man for a woman is God's creation— that is to say when nature's sound, not when it is corrupted as it is among the Italians and Turks. [Luther is here referring to the practice of homosexuality among these peoples.]

—ZACKS, 1994, 148

Within this emerging tradition of self-awareness and defiance, Protestant sects began to emerge as alternatives to Catholicism. Similar ideologies emerged in the thinking of another important 16th-century theologian, John Calvin (1509–1564), who believed in the powerful benefits of sexual expression for diminishing daily pressures. Indeed, Calvin felt that the marital bond could only be enhanced through the renewing intimacy of sexual intercourse. Still, premarital and extramarital sexual expression threatened the integrity of the family and were viewed harshly by Protestant churches, as we will see shortly with the Puritans. Calvin (Fig. 2-10) was a connection between the spirit of the reformation in Europe and the emergence of Puritan traditions in North America.

So far we have looked only at changes in the perception of the appropriateness of sexual inclination in marriage. Its enjoyments apart from procreation were now acknowledged. Elsewhere on the continent other developments were occurring and being written about with candor. In France there was a significant, abrupt drop in the birth rate in women over the age of 20. The rural birthrate declined from 7.2 children in 1760–1769 to 6.4 children in 1780–1789 (Van De Walle & Muhsam, 1995). Limiting family size became a popular idea. The statistics did not vary much across the social classes. In a country where procreation and large families (and church communities) were so esteemed, what led to this sudden decline? Although infant mortality declined during this era, contraception was also becoming more popular in France. Interestingly, although the declining birthrate primarily involved married women, the developing means of contraception first gained popularity in the contexts of premarital and extramarital intercourse.

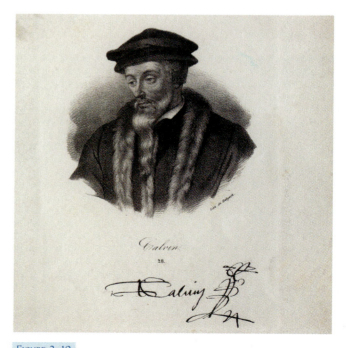

FIGURE 2-10   John Calvin believed in the importance of sexual expression in marriage as a vehicle of intimate bonding and relief from the pressures of daily life.

Any contraceptive measure at the time was thought to involve "homicide," and contraceptive information was often referred to as "fatal secrets"—secrets because such information was not considered appropriate for people of nobility and good taste (although many were its most avid practitioners!). Anything that might lower the birthrate was seen as a threat to the integrity and growth of the French nation. Yet whatever the French were doing, it was working! What is important here is that public discourse on contraceptive techniques was entirely new in that society, as well as most of Europe, and discussed for the first time with an intention to change behavior and offer reproductive choices where few had existed before. These contraceptives included early versions of the condom, inserting small pieces of sponge into the vagina (sometimes first dipped in brandy), and other agents introduced into the vagina in suppositories, douches, and pessaries. Withdrawal became more common, along with other nonintercourse avenues of physical intimacy such as oral and anal intercourse, mutual masturbation, and fondling to orgasm. The falling birthrate could also partly be attributed to the growing popularity of abortion, which then was not commonly performed by physicians. A number of popular pamphlets were available that disseminated contraceptive information. Further, condoms became known also for preventing the transmission of sexually transmitted diseases and had become more popular.

Of the contraceptive tactics then available, the one that was most obviously seen as "cheating nature" of its procreative imperative was **coitus interruptus,** or withdrawal before ejaculation. Pornographic literature of the late 1500s offered explicit descriptions:

> [T]o put inside and take their fun to their heart's content, as long as [the women] do not receive any of their

> seed . . . 'Move around as much as you want . . . but on your life, have care not to spill anything in there . . .' So that the other had to be careful and to watch for the time of the tidal wave when it was coming . . .

> —BRANTOME, 1666, AS CITED IN
> VAN DE WALLE & MUHSAM, 1995

Puritan Tradition in North America

The sexual ideology of Luther and Calvin was the legacy upon which the Puritans created their notions of sexual morality in North America. The creation and maintenance of the nuclear family within the church-affiliated community was of central importance for this early Protestant sect. Their general view of human nature was pessimistic. People were thought to have inherited sin from the Fall. The Reverend Thomas Shepard preached that the human heart:

> . . . is a foul sink of all atheism, sodomy, blasphemy, murder, whoredom, adultery, witchcraft, buggery; so that if thou hast any good think in thee it is but a drop of rose water in a bowl of poison.

> —TANNAHILL, 1980

Tannahill (1980, p. 329) reminds us that "13 of the 18 wives [on the Mayflower] died during the first winter," and that the shortage of women created a setting for the displaced expression of sexual expression. Fornication and adultery were punished harshly and publicly with floggings and the stocks. Bestiality was punished by execution, as in the case of Thomas Granger who had ". . . carnally abused a mare, a cow, two goats, five sheep, two calves, and a turkey" (Tannahill, 1980, p. 329). Interestingly, Puritan society was apparently somewhat open minded, if not entirely silent, about homosexuality—perhaps not unusual in a culture with such clearly defined roles of masculine dominance. Because many immigrants to America in the 1700s were also members of Protestant sects, Puritan perspectives on sexuality and the nuclear family would become an important feature of the emerging codes of sexuality in the New World. The social cohesiveness of the family and village were extraordinarily important to the Puritans (Fig. 2-11). In fact, attitudes regarding premarital intercourse became more relaxed because a higher birth rate meant more farm workers were available. The Puritans had an interesting custom called *bundling,* in which a potential suitor from a distant village would stay the night at the home of a young lady in whom he was interested. The two often shared a bed, although the woman would be enclosed in a large sack closed at the neck or a wooden divider separated the couple in bed. This was *not* what we now call a "barrier method" of contraception, of course, and these measures were rarely effective in preventing intercourse before marriage. But once a conception took place, the marriage was inevitable and the growth of the community aided.

Every society discussed here so far built on inherited notions about sexual morality and behavior while at the same

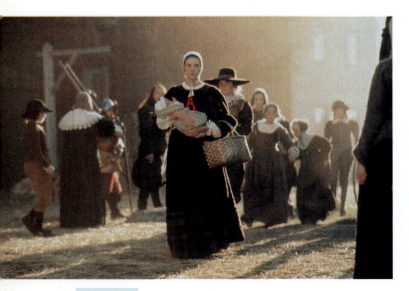

FIGURE 2-11   The novel *The Scarlet Letter* described the powerful Puritan condemnation of adultery. At the same time, the Puritans were surprisingly permissive about other forms of sexual expression, such as premarital intercourse.

Dear Dr. Ruth

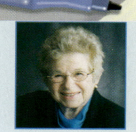

Question:

There's a girl in one of my classes who is "working" her way through college by turning tricks. She always has plenty of money and seems very happy. She offered to help me learn the trade, but I've always refused. But once in a while I start to think differently about it, especially when I'm really strapped for cash. Is it really that bad to be paid for having sex? My friend says that sometimes she even enjoys it.

Answer:

It's not called the world's oldest profession for nothing, and I doubt it will ever disappear. In fact, I'm for legalizing prostitution so that health authorities can maintain the highest standards of hygiene. I've personally visited the Mustang Ranch in Nevada.

Having said that, my advice is not to follow the path of that girl. First of all, prostitution is not legal outside some parts of Nevada, so if you get caught, there goes any chance of ever getting a good job. You'll have put all that effort into getting a degree, which will then be almost worthless. And illegal prostitution bears many other risks. If you read the papers, you know that prostitutes are often injured or even killed by the strangers they meet. And there's the chance too of a very long lasting psychological impact. You might later on find that sex with a lover or spouse doesn't bring the pleasure it might have if you had not sold yourself to other men.

How we interpret the religious and moral codes with which we have been raised often helps us formulate the values we live by. Listen to your conscience; it's a better guide for behavior than your financial needs.

time finding ways to bend the rules. While their expectations seemed rigid, the Puritans were also highly pragmatic. Their religious and social mechanisms intended to strengthen the nuclear family probably had some flexibility, as we have seen in other cultures. While the Puritans could in no way be described as permissive, it is likely that minor infractions that did not threaten the family or community would have been quietly tolerated.

Early Medical and Pseudoscientific Disciplines

The development and dissemination of sexual knowledge in Britain and Europe was strongly influenced by medical practitioners. A history of this trend by Porter & Hall (1995) reveals an interesting intertwining of medical, ancient philosophical, and moralistic influences in popular literature beginning in the mid-1600s. Although these publications often had little accuracy and legitimacy, anyone who *could* read seemed to be reading them.

An early tract titled Aristotle's *Master-Piece* was one of the best-known volumes about sex and procreation before the Vic-

torian era. It first appeared in English in 1684. It was written not by Aristotle but by compilers and medical popularizers of the day. Several different versions enjoyed long publication lives concurrently, and in one form or another it stayed in print for over 200 years. An interesting aspect is that this book divorces sexuality from its psychological and emotional aspects; it takes a clinical, objective approach to its subject. This book (Fig. 2-12) contributed significantly to the gradual loss of the church's authority over sexual information and is an early example of how to many, scientific information (even when inaccurate) seemed more believable than church teachings. Aristotle's *Master-Piece* contained folk wisdom about intercourse during menstruation, a practice which had been thought to contribute to the birth of defective, malformed children. Early urine pregnancy tests were described, and there was commentary about some emotional aspects of infertility. This colorful book combined inaccurate drawings and misinformation with support of pronatalism in marriage. It was aimed at simple people with little education but a sincere curiosity about reproduction. Another well-known sex manual of this day, called *Tableau de l'amour conjugal,* was written by Nicolas Venette, a

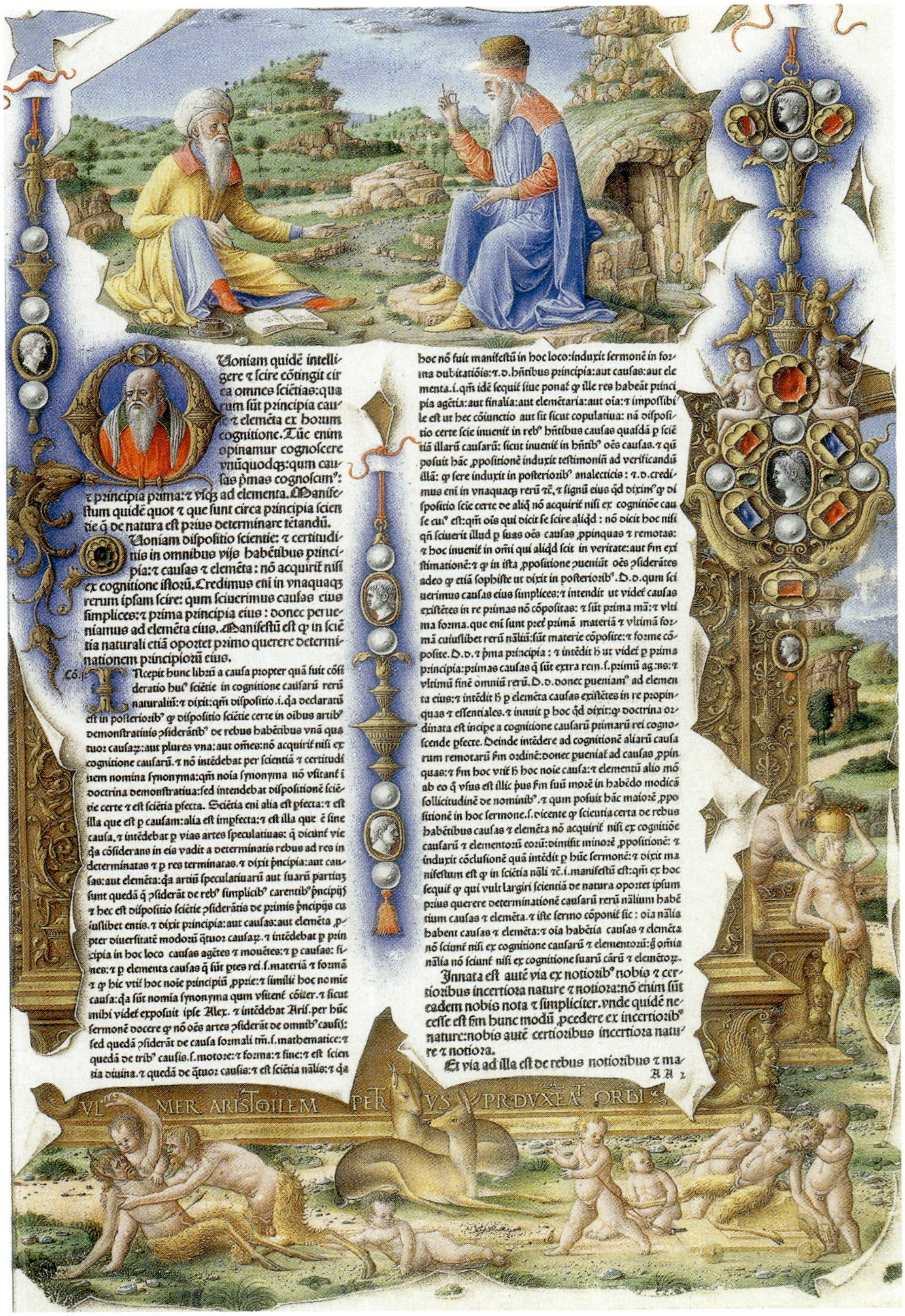

FIGURE 2-12   Aristotle's *Master-Piece* (actually written by numerous anonymous popularizers of medical fact and myth) was among the first books to examine sexual expression from an objective, non-religious perspective.

physician of some repute. Like Aristotle's *Master-Piece,* this book was reworked and revised by countless anonymous contributors. It contained more than 400 pages and appealed to a more erudite audience; it had been translated into Dutch in 1687, German in 1698, and English by 1703. This was an anatomy and physiology book with an important twist. The

psychological and physiological aspects of sexual intercourse were seen as equal, complementary elements of one experience.

Venette believed that people's sex drive was an overall indicator of their general physical and psychological health. Still, he cautioned the reader to avoid excessive indulgence, noting, like Aristotle (the real one), that moderation in eroticism is the ideal (Porter & Hall, 1995). Impotence and fertility received much attention, as did aphrodisiacs, and he wondered aloud about exactly where conception occurred. He also proclaimed that a pregnant woman's thoughts cannot affect her fetus in any obvious way; this was (and even today remains) one of the more interesting superstitions about pregnancy. Venette saw this as an example of how misinformation about sex persists without any proof at all.

After 1660 there was a notable increase in sexual tracts intended for a popular readership. The two recurrent themes in the bulk of this folk literature were the horrible consequences of sexually transmitted diseases and the sins of "excessive" masturbation. One author, John Martin, believed that it was his duty to provide information to increase the quality and length of life by informing readers of the "facts" about "diseases venereal" so that they could take foresightful measures to avoid them. In his book, *Treatise of All the Symptoms of the Venereal Diseases in Both Sexes* (1708), he notes "that no Persons therefore for the future may be drove to the Necessity of Ship-wrecking their Bodies, Purses, and Reputations upon those Rocks of Destruction, (I mean those wretched Ignoramus's QUACKS, MOUNTEBANKS, and ASTROLOGERS that swarm in every Corner, imposing on the too credulous World their peddling insignificant Remedies)." (Marten, 1708, cited in Porter & Hall, 1995, p. 93).

Yet the anxiety surrounding masturbation garnered more of the reader's attention. By the time Tissot published *Onanism* in 1760, there was practically an epidemic of apprehension about "self-abuse." *Onania,* published anonymously in 1710, was a precursor of things to come in the almost explosive growth of this literature. Current opinion taught that masturbation led to the loss of rationality, innocence, and the wastage of valuable human seed. Guilt surrounded both purposeful self-stimulation and nocturnal emissions.

Much quackery was involved in this publicity movement. Georgian society in England had come to associate sexual expression with "health, happiness, beauty and fertility" (Porter & Hall, 1995, p. 107), and medical quackery made every effort to elevate these objectives. A conspicuous public posting advertised "An Herculean Antidote Against the POX," while another promised "A Most Infallible, and Sure Cheap Secret Safe and Speedy Cure for a Clap" (Porter & Hall, 1995, p. 107). The best known of these colorful figures selling sex advice and remedies was James Graham, who advertised his "Celestial Bed," a 9 x 12 foot creation of glass, magnets, and elegant carved figurines of cupid and psyche. Its down was packed with spices, and a music box created orchestral sounds while messages painted in ornate calligraphic style exhorted to "be fruitful, multiply, and replenish the earth" (Porter & Hall, 1995, p. 109). Yet behind such pseudoscientific ventures, the repressive spirit against masturbation and too frequent intercourse was to remain for at least another 150 years.

By the early 1800s, the stage had been set for the Victorian Era. One thing was beyond doubt: the public had developed a great appetite for sexual information, both frivolous and factual, just at the time when the spirit of science was beginning to supersede the influence of the Church in human affairs. The rational spirit of objective investigation had made its way to one of the most private of all human enterprises.

Victorian Era

From our contemporary vantage point, if ever there was a time when a population was known for its sexual phobias and straight-laced attitudes toward sexuality, the reign of Queen Victoria was most certainly that time. It was a time of repression and self-control, and the very nature of the relationship between women and men was scrutinized and revised. These were not merely quaint, old-fashioned customs. Much of the sexual morality of the United States in the first half of the twentieth century originated in Victorian attitudes. Queen Victoria was crowned in 1837, and the sexual climate of the remainder of the 19th century was profoundly influenced by the customs she condoned. The Victorian Era intervened between the outlandish characters described above and the twentieth century's serious and intellectual approach to human sexuality. The influence of Queen Victoria (Fig. 2-13) was in large measure due to her extremely long reign (1837–1901).

The impact of this era on sexual connotations in common language was enormous. Pianos didn't have "legs," they had "limbs," and these were discretely hidden in cloth adornments (Mason, 1995) in case the symbolism became overwhelming. At the traditional Sunday dinner one didn't ask for the "breast" of roast chicken but rather the "white meat."

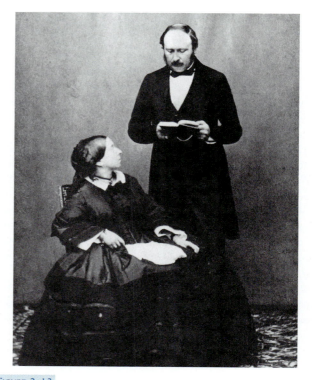

FIGURE 2-13 Queen Victoria and Prince Albert, her husband. Victoria's reign saw an interesting conflict between the public's keen interest in sexual matters and a more aloof, proper public perspective.

Women weren't "seduced" but "betrayed." These were not playful manipulations of words; rather they reveal how language was a vehicle for an entirely different way of thinking about the physical aspects of sex.

This spirit of sexual repression made its way to North America, where a clergyman in New York City preached enthusiastically against the dangerous effects of "excessive" sexual activity. Sylvester Graham believed that men younger than 30 were not fit enough to have sexual intercourse without exhausting physical consequences and that married couples should avoid having sex more than once every 3 years (Francoeur, 1991). Graham believed that certain foods unduly stimulated the digestive tract and led to sexual arousal. If cheeses, milk, and eggs were eliminated, along with meats and spicy foods, and replaced with bland grain crackers (which incidentally became known as "Graham crackers"), then women and men would regain control over their sexual urges. Interestingly, Dr. John Kellogg (founder of Kellogg's cereals) developed corn flakes as an alternative to Graham crackers. These are just examples of how the ideological climate in England had a profound impact on sexual thinking in the United States as well.

Not all English social classes felt the repressive Victorian spirit equally; in fact, the British aristocracy of the day was somewhat permissive of adultery, although this was not the case among rural landowners. In many instances servants and maids upheld a more stringent moral code than the lords and ladies they worked for. Young girls in wealthy homes often enjoyed a lack of supervision as they courted young men and were comfortably uninhibited in their references to sexuality (Mason, 1995). Despite the tone of sexual restraint prevalent in the culture, there was little hesitation to use, and talk about using, contraception. Coitus interruptus was common, and in the second half of the 19th century a condom cost only a halfpenny (Annan, 1995). Mason (1995) notes that abstinence was plainly unpopular with British wives. Victorian society involved interesting and enigmatic paradoxes: sexual restraint versus sexual liberality, open sensuality versus a repressive social environment, and anxiety about too frequent intercourse versus the availability of inexpensive condoms. Perhaps most interesting of all, an enormous number of prostitutes were engaging in a thriving trade in England's large cities. Mason (1995) notes that citizens of London, who were asked to estimate the number of prostitutes working in London, reported half a million! This was in contrast to the more conservative police estimate of "only" 30,000. While one standard of public morality was being upheld at home, another was being pursued extramurally—not the first time this has occurred in history. In public, the Victorians were very concerned with formal appearances and proper behavior (Fig. 2-14).

As every period in history has sexual excesses, as well as some conservatism, the same is true of Victorian England. A notable example of Victorian excess is found in the diary of "Walter," who described explicitly his sexual adventures beginning in the 1830s and spanning a period of 50 years. He described sexual encounters with over 1500 women. Walter was

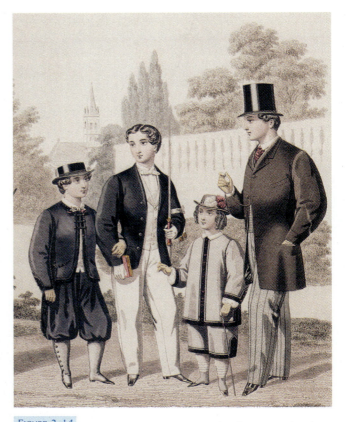

FIGURE 2-14   Victorian men were expected to be unemotional, poised, and controlled, and children were dressed and treated much like little adults.

an affluent Englishman with a penchant for lower-class women; many were prostitutes. He believed that any woman beneath his social station had no right to decline his advances. When the book was first published in 1869, its publisher was sentenced to 2 years in jail and fined 20,000 pounds for obscenity (Koenig, 1995). This aggressive and exploitative memoir is a telling supplement to the "marriage manuals" of Victorian times, described below. The sexist and classist traditions that sanctioned Walter's encounters are perhaps the saddest and most thought-provoking aspect of his dairies. The contempt for poor girls and society's quiet acquiescence are traditions that have not entirely disappeared.

As noted above, scientific standards of inquiry began to replace sacred standards of faith in Victorian England. An interesting manifestation of this trend is the appearance of a large number of "marriage manuals" that appeared in shops everywhere in cities in the United Kingdom. Most were a collection of simple biology, elementary sketches and drawings, speculation regarding conception, and advice about intercourse, sexually transmitted diseases, and the sins of "excessive" masturbation. These books themselves are not as noteworthy as the fact that most everyone was reading them. There was an enormous private curiosity about virtually all aspects of human sexuality, and the new legitimacy of objective science gave further impetus to this interest.

One of the better-selling marriage manuals is titled *Elements of Social Science or Physical, Sexual and Natural Religion*, 100,000 copies of which had been purchased by 1900. It was written by George Drysdale (Korn, 1995), although the authorship was anonymous for 50 years. This long book (more than 600 pages) discussed the importance of regular sexual activity for maintaining good mental health, the normality of happiness, and the significance of coming to terms with one's sexual inclinations. The author disapproved of condoms ("dulls the enjoyment and frequently produces impotence in the man and disgust in both parties" [Korn, 1995]). He favored the sponge, primarily because he felt that contraception was fundamentally a woman's job: "Any preventive means, to be satisfactory, must be used by the woman, as it spoils the passion and impulsiveness of the venereal act if the men have to think of them." (Korn, 1995). Like others of his time, Drysdale believed that masturbation was a misdirected erotic desire.

Semen conservation theory, mentioned earlier, was an important folk belief that influenced Victorian thinking about masturbation, homosexuality, and frequent intercourse. Semen has an almost legendary meaning in history, going back to China and India more than 2500 years ago (Money, 1991). It was seen as the most visible symbol of procreative potential, and semen conservation theory suggested not only that it must never be wasted, but also that a man's character would be enhanced through his cautious dispensing of it. Any waste was a sin, and horrible consequences were promised those who indulged in its nonprocreative dissipation. Physical and mental infirmity were the consequences of masturbation, according to Ellen White, the founder of the Seventh Day Adventists during the mid-1840s (Tannahill, 1980).

While most Victorian sexuality traditions are associated with England, an analysis of Irish women sheds some light on similar concerns in that country (McLoughlin, 1994). As in England, a global perception of cultural prudery is inaccurate. Economic and class factors also played a major role in sexual relationships. "Respectable" Irish women had three primary attributes. They wanted to marry, remain faithful, and establish a subservience to their husbands. Parenting and homemaking were their central priorities. Finally, female sexuality was expressed only inside the marital bond. Expectations of male sexual expression were far more flexible, and this discrepancy led to a number of interesting situations.

A sexual relationship between a gentleman and a lady provided her with his "lifelong interest and protection" even if they did not marry (McLoughlin, 1994, p. 271). A dwelling was provided for her and any children, and she held some rights of inheritance. Such relationships might be brief or last many years. "Overall there was a kind of grudging admiration of this woman's economic astuteness, and her ability to take care of herself and her own interests" (p. 272). Again, regardless of prudish Victorian traditions, "alternative" sexual lifestyles often had a pragmatic quality. A different fate awaited poor women who had a child (or children) without benefit of marriage, however. These women were openly scorned, especially in cities where their circumstances were more apparent.

If an unmarried young woman became pregnant and the man responsible refused marriage, she had only one opportunity to avoid public censure: an enormous dowry offered by her father to lessen her shame and help rebuild her standing in the community. By 1880, this option was seen as far less desirable than remaining virginal.

One final aspect of Victorian sexual traditions deserves discussion: the impact of these conventions on the gender roles of women and men. The inequalities we have discussed grew from very different expectations of behavior for the sexes, which affected gender roles in North America well into the 20th century. Victorian women were expected to be passive, chaste, and focused on their children and husbands. "Independent woman" was a contradiction in terms. In contrast, men were to show emotional restraint and a cold, objective rationality in their work and marriage. They were to be in control without looking like they were trying very hard. Emotional spontaneity was unusual among both women and men. Note, however, that this century ended on a very different note with the writings and slowly growing popularity of Havelock Ellis and Sigmund Freud (Annan, 1995), who introduced a decidedly more liberal intellectual climate with respect to sexual matters.

Late 19th and Early 20th Century

The following sections review the contributions of several pioneers of the objective, applied study of human sexuality. Here we find a big change from the Victorian era. The study of sexuality became respected, if not entirely acceptable. No longer was there a focus on the "dark power" of sexuality and its titillating or bizarre aspects. The approach became systematic and quantitative. In the infancy of any science, investigators must first determine what phenomena fall into the new discipline, and then classify them according to various criteria, and that is what these early thinkers did. Richard Krafft-Ebing, Havelock Ellis, Sigmund Freud, Magnus Hirschfeld, Alfred Kinsey, and William Masters and Virginia Johnson all had certain personality attributes in common: courage, competence, curiosity, thoroughness, and keen social insight. They were interested in not only the diverse and fascinating manifestations of human sexual motivation, but also, more basically, the place of sex in a person's life and its impact on the quality of life.

Richard Krafft-Ebing and Havelock Ellis

Richard von Krafft-Ebing's (1840–1902) *Psychopathia Sexualis* (1886) and Havelock Ellis's (1859–1939) *Studies in the Psychology of Sex* (1900) are milestones in the scientific study of human sexuality. Krafft-Ebing denounced masturbation for its potentially harmful psychological effects. He believed that masturbation blocked the development of normal erotic inclinations and made a young man impotent in early heterosexual relations; this, in turn, would lead to homosexuality in adulthood. In contrast, Ellis found no harm in masturbation, but believed its capacity to reduce tension had a beneficial effect. Both writers believed that homosexuality was a psychopathology, although Ellis believed that a person was born homosexual and did not become that way. His perspective on the origin of homosexuality is similar to some contemporary views, as we will see in Chapter 9. Although mental health professionals no longer believe that homosexuality is a psychological disorder, that notion affected thinking and writing about homosexuality until the early 1970s. Nonetheless, Krafft-Ebing and Ellis (Fig. 2-15), both trained as medical doctors, were pioneers in the scientific study of human sexuality.

One of Krafft-Ebing's contributions is the first clinical description of **masochism**, which refers to erotic pleasures from being physically hurt in certain controlled circumstances. (The counterpart concept is called **sadism**, which involves sexual arousal from inflicting such pain.) Additionally, he described a number of fetishes, which involve inanimate objects used in masturbatory rituals or intercourse itself. Krafft-Ebing's approach to sexual variations and deviations was systematic; he was a physician who worked for the police in Austria. Eventually, the

works of both Krafft-Ebing and Ellis were banned, despite their serious psychological intent and scholarly quality. While these two authors were writing, Sigmund Freud had not yet undertaken his explorations regarding the nature of sexual motives.

SIGMUND FREUD

No figure in the history of sexuality in the late 19th and early 20th centuries was more productive and controversial than Freud (1856–1939). Freud's theories are often criticized because of the emphasis on sex. Yet one seldom hears this criticism from anyone who has read Freud's works in his own words. Common views of the term "sexuality" often focus on the genitals and the feelings we have when they are stimulated erotically; however, Freud did not hold such a narrow definition. He believed that sexuality was less concerned with "genitality" than with sensuality generally. According to Freud, sexual feelings could come from stimulation of many parts of the body, not just the genitals. He called these **erogenous zones**, which include the mouth and anus, as well as the genitals. These Freud called the primary erogenous zones. (Chapter 12 explores in greater depth Freud's psychosexual theory of development.) Freud also assumed the existence of secondary erogenous zones, which, through our personal experiences, come to be associated with sensual pleasure when they are stimulated. Many people find a massage sexually stimulating because many secondary erogenous zones are being touched and rubbed, such as the buttocks, back, thighs, breasts, or chest.

Freud pioneered the study of how infantile and childhood indulgences and frustrations are incorporated into our personalities. His controversial theories are based on his clinical practice, and disagreements and alternative explanations have certainly emerged. At the heart of Freudian theory is the concept of **determinism**. This implies that virtually all adult

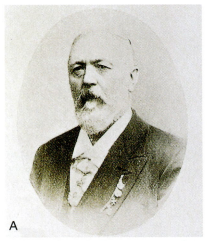
A

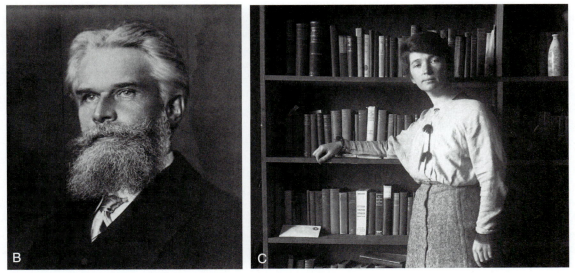

FIGURE 2-15   **A.** Richard Krafft-Ebing, 19th century writer who explored the relationship between sexual expression and psychological disorders. **B.** Havelock Ellis, author of *Studies in the Psychology of Sex.* **C.** Margaret Sanger (1883–1966), a contemporary of both Krafft-Ebing and Ellis, was a pioneer advocate for women's reproductive and contraceptive rights, and about whom we will learn more in Chapter 11.

thoughts, feelings, and behaviors have been determined in the personality by about age 6 and that after that time our personalities are formed and cannot be changed. There is little contemporary support for this idea, although it has historical significance. In his theory, adult sexuality has its roots in childhood experiences of pain, pleasure, and interpersonal control. Freud's beliefs were so unusual that he was often harshly criticized. During the Hamburg Psychiatric Congress in 1910, someone in the audience stood up and mentioned Freud's theories, and the chairman of the session, William Weygandt, ". . . stopped him, saying: 'That is no subject for a scientific congress; it is a matter for the police'" (cited in Lewinsohn, 1958, p. 365). Throughout most of his professional life, Freud (Fig. 2-16) was criticized for his work on the development and manifestations of erotic motives and behaviors.

Earlier we introduced you to Freud's term *libido*, which refers to a primitive motivational force in the personality that expresses itself sexually and aggressively. Freud believed that the libido operated on the basis of the **pleasure principle**, the desire to seek pleasures (mostly physical pleasures) and to avoid pain. Further, the pleasure principle cannot accept delayed gratification; if it could speak, it would say, "I want what I want when I want it!" The pleasure principle has neither patience nor foresight. There is a characteristic of the more "mature" personality called the **reality principle**. The reality principle "negotiates" human motives for pleasure to act within the laws, morals, and norms of the society at large. Basic to Freud's approach to sexuality is the ever-present conflict between these two internal "voices."

Freud's theoretical system, called **psychoanalysis**, involves a theory of personality, a theory of human growth and development, and a method of **psychotherapy**. The psychoanalytic approach studies the development of emotional states and their impact on adult feeling and behaving. Freud believed that virtually all aspects of adult sexuality are rooted in a person's infancy and childhood. Therefore, to understand sexual difficulties of an adult, it is necessary to go through therapy to discover what historical events might have led to the problem. In Freud's view, the problem cannot be helped until its antecedents in the person's past are understood. Although this was once a popular view, many sex researchers and therapists today no longer accept this rigid deterministic perspective. Even the most dedicated Freudians say (tongue in cheek) that although therapy won't necessarily make you feel better, it will help you understand why you're miserable!

In Freud's long career (he lived from 1856 to 1939), he worked intensively with only about 130 patients, and despite his theories about child development, he never psychoanalyzed a child. Yet he pioneered the early attempts to understand the power of the unconscious mind on adult emotional and behavioral states virtually by himself. He did not perform controlled experiments, but that was never his intention as a practicing psychiatrist. Further, he was not willing to accept the normality of female sexual feelings or homosexuality. Despite these outdated perspectives, his writings continue to have a powerful effect on our conceptions of human eroticism and sexual motivations. His ideas about unconscious motivations,

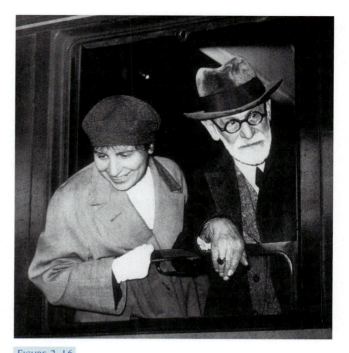

Figure 2-16 Sigmund Freud, here with his daughter Anna. Freud was responsible for exploring the nature of erotic motivations and feelings and the impact of sexuality on normal and abnormal psychological functioning.

early sensual pleasures, the importance of dreams in psychotherapy, and "slips of the tongue" are still important concepts for psychotherapists using different approaches.

Magnus Hirschfeld

Another noteworthy figure was Magnus Hirschfeld (1868–1935), a Berlin physician who founded the Institute for Sex Research. Hirschfeld was a homosexual whose professional productivity was remarkable; he became one of the best known figures in Germany. He organized psychological and medical associations, arranged international meetings on a variety of sexual topics, and generally promoted the scholarly examination of human sexual concerns. He fought to gain acceptance of homosexuality in the wider society. One of his most important contributions was the enormous (over 1000 pages) *Homosexuality in Men and Women* (1918–1920). Here, Hirschfeld suggested that over 90% of the German people would vote to repeal laws punishing homosexuality if they only knew the medical and psychological truth about it (Plant, 1986). His confidence had little foundation in reality, however, given the emerging Nazi regime. Like other pioneers in the study of sexuality, Magnus Hirschfeld (Fig. 2-17) was harshly criticized for his scientific findings and beliefs, especially his assertion that homosexuals should not be persecuted.

Hirschfeld's scholarly writings were encyclopedic. His books, pamphlets, and arguments amounted to over 200 publications. In addition to his famous book on homosexuality, he also wrote *Natural Laws of Love* (1912), *Sexual Pathology* in

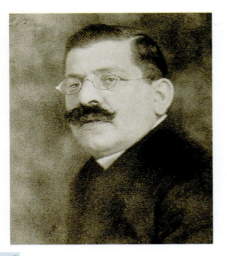

FIGURE 2-17 Magnus Hirschfeld was one of the first scientific investigators to seriously and systematically examine homosexuality and urge public acceptance of this gender preference.

three volumes (1920), *The Science of Sexology* (1920), and *Sexual Knowledge* in five volumes (1926–1930). He founded the *Yearbook for Intersexual Variants,* serving as editor until 1923 (Plant, 1986). Until 1910, Hirschfeld believed that homosexuals comprised a third sex, a biologically separate gender. In 1898 he published *What People Should Know About the Third Sex,* but there was little support for his theory. The ultimate scientific and political lot of Hirschfeld's life's work is described in Richard Plant's *The Pink Triangle* (1986):

> *On May 6, 1933, a gang of "outraged students" stormed the famous Institute for Sex Research, directed by Magnus Hirschfeld, the father of the new science of sexology. For three decades Hirschfeld and his team of legal and medical associates had assembled an invaluable collection of documents, photographs, treatises, and statistics about sex. For the Nazis, Hirschfeld—a Jewish physician, a homosexual, and a liberal propagandist—was an ideal target. The fascist press had denounced him with lavish insults for many years. The eager fascist students rummaged through the building, throwing books, photos, paintings, and files into the yard; around the growing fire they sang patriotic songs about Germany's awakening. Four days later they returned and put the ransacked building to the flame, and with it the bust of their patron-Satan, Dr. Hirschfeld. Out of the country on a lecture tour, Hirschfeld never returned to Germany.*

> —PLANT, 1986, 16–17

While Magnus Hirschfeld is not often considered a major figure in histories of human sexuality, his professional output, his involvement in the professional societies of his day, his courageous claim that homosexuality is not a psychological disorder, and his courage in a brutally repressive fascist political climate all reveal a personality who pioneered

an unpopular aspect of sexual expression with professional integrity.

ALFRED KINSEY

Alfred Kinsey (1894–1956) became a professor of zoology at Indiana University in 1929 after earning his doctorate at Harvard. He spent the early part of his career in entomology, until an interesting thing happened to him in 1938. Because he was such a congenial teacher, several of his students approached him with questions about marriage and the place of sex in marriage. He was impressed by their naiveté and at first said nothing because he felt that he was not enough of an authority on these topics. He resolved to try to find answers for them and carefully read through the existing literature on the subject. He was surprised and disappointed at the poor quality of existing research and its lack of depth and quantity. Several of his students then appealed to the university to offer a course on sexuality and marriage.

What began as a matter of intellectual curiosity became Kinsey's preoccupation for the rest of his life. With seven other instructors, he coordinated a scholarly course on a topic not previously considered a legitimate academic interest in the United States. His wife told her friends, "I hardly see him at night any more since he took up sex." (Halberstam, 1993). Kinsey began by interviewing his students about their sexual experiences; these interviews were confidential and their substance not associated with the students' names. His course became more popular; eventually 400 students took it each time (Halberstam, 1993). Soon he was traveling on weekends to find more people to interview. He was preoccupied with categorizing and analyzing data. In 1940, the president of Indiana University, Herman Wells, asked Kinsey to his office for a chat. Local ministers had complained about Kinsey's marriage and sexuality course, and the University was feeling the heat of the community's opinion about the inappropriateness of this subject. Wells gave Kinsey a choice: he could surrender the course or give up his research, but he could not continue to do both. Kinsey gave up the course and devoted his time to research on human sexuality (Halberstam, 1993). Beginning that year, he received financial support from the National Research Council, the Rockefeller Foundation, and the University. In a country still affected by Puritan traditions, Alfred Kinsey (Fig. 2-18) succeeded in helping to make the study of sex legitimate and respected.

From the beginning, Kinsey was struck by the enormous gap between public morality and private behaviors. This insight was tantalizing. His first book, *Sexual Behavior in the Human Male,* was published in 1948. It was based on 5300 case histories collected by Kinsey and his collaborators, the psychologist Wardell Pomeroy and statistician C. E. Martin. The text was over 800 pages in length and written for a scientific audience. Some of the findings presented in the book were surprising even to informed readers. For example, Kinsey noted that approximately 95% of males in this country were sexually active by the age of 15, that the "average" single male experienced 3 or 4 orgasms each week, that 70% of his sample subjects said they had had sex with a prostitute by age 35, that 37% ac-

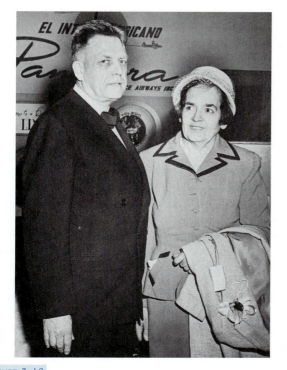

FIGURE 2-18 Dr. and Mrs. Albert Kinsey. Research carried out by Kinsey at Indiana University candidly revealed the nature and diversity of sexual behavior among American men and women in the 1940s and 1950s.

knowledged that they had had homosexual experiences by age 21, and that about half the married men in the sample disclosed that they had had extramarital sex by age 40 (cited in Francoeur, 1991). The book shot up the bestseller list and eventually sold 275,000 copies by 1954. Almost everyone who read a newspaper knew about the book and was talking about it. (Remember the popularity of the Victorian marriage manuals and why people read them.) His work was both praised and criticized. Some of the disapproval came from powerful, conservative segments of American society, and soon the Rockefeller Foundation doubted the wisdom of continuing its support. Kinsey was hurt by some of this criticism but maintained a professional, objective attitude. University President Wells asked Kinsey to publish nothing more while the state legislature was in session for fear of reduced funding levels for the university.

In 1953, Kinsey and his colleagues braced for an anticipated even harsher round of criticism. When *Sexual Behavior in the Human Female* was published, the reaction was much stronger because "he was, after all, discussing wives, mothers, and daughters" (Halberstam, 1993, p. 42). This book would sell more than 250,000 copies, and again the reviews were mixed. The Rockefeller Foundation withdrew its funding in 1953.

In this study Kinsey found an enormous range of sexual appetites and behaviors in a number of dimensions: frequency of orgasm, preferred sexual behaviors, duration of sexual intercourse, number of sexual partners, and frequency of intercourse in marriage according to the duration of the marriage

all revealed tremendous variability. Kinsey found that higher levels of education were associated with more open attitudes toward sexual behaviors, such as oral-genital sex. Further, Kinsey revealed that many people had had a sexual encounter with another person of their gender (50% of the males and 28% of the females in his sample). Masturbation did not cause psychological problems but indeed helped many people learn about their sexual responsiveness. Extramarital sexuality was far more common for both women and men than society acknowledged. Good sex was an important factor for building and maintaining a good marriage.

Although much of this may seem obvious now, in the late 1940s and early 1950s many people felt that Kinsey had taken something highly personal and subjected it to cold, objective scrutiny. His work has been criticized for focusing on measurable behaviors while neglecting the psychological domain. Kinsey's samples had inherent biases as well. Virtually all racial minorities were excluded, and a disproportionately large percentage had high levels of education. Aging and elderly people and those in rural areas were similarly underrepresented. Still, Kinsey's research was tremendously important in the study of human sexuality. It is amazing to look back at that little discussion between Kinsey and his students in 1938 and realize what came from it.

How present sexuality researchers formulate questionnaires and interviews is based on Kinsey's thorough methodical model. Similarly, our current concerns with confidentiality and the ethical conduct of sex research owe much to Kinsey's personality, as well as his professional standards. Even though his work was not based on a representative sample of Americans at this time, this inadequacy motivated later researchers to study sample groups that mirror our population as a whole as closely as possible.

WILLIAM MASTERS AND VIRGINIA JOHNSON

After Kinsey, serious interest in human sexuality grew in medical and academic circles. By far the most significant sex researchers since the mid-century have been William Masters and Virginia Johnson (Fig. 2-19). They have been dedicated to the scientific examination of the physiology of sexual responsiveness, therapy for sexual dysfunctions, and other basic aspects of the discipline, including the study of homosexuality and the development and refinement of sex research. Their names have become synonymous with rigor and reputability in the arena of human sexuality, although all of their publications have not been viewed as balanced and authoritative.

William Masters was born in Cleveland, Ohio, in 1915. While in college he became interested in research and entered medical school at the University of Rochester in 1938. Masters was more interested in a laboratory research program in the physiology of sexual responsiveness than a career in clinical medicine. At this time, the physiology of sexuality was one of the last unexplored areas of sexology. His mentor, Dr. George Washington Corner, told him that because of the highly controversial nature of the subject, certain qualifications would be essential for a career in this arena: "that he be a man of mature age, about forty years old, to reduce suspicion of prurient interest; that he first establish a reputation in a different area of

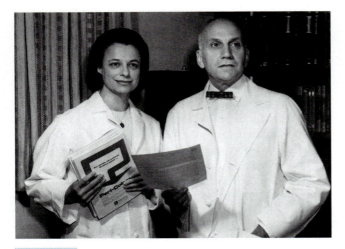

FIGURE 2-19   William Masters and Virginia Johnson. Masters and Johnson were the first to carry out exhaustive laboratory investigations of human sexual response and later wrote comprehensively about sexual dysfunctions and sex therapy.

research; and that he secure the backing of a university" (Current Biography, 1968, p. 247). Kinsey's career had set the example for these suggestions.

Over the next decade Masters trained in obstetrics and gynecology, pathology, and internal medicine, and in 1947 he joined the faculty of the medical school at Washington University in St. Louis. He had already established his reputation as a researcher in gynecology. By 1954 he was ready to undertake his research agenda, beginning where Kinsey had finished. Kinsey's work was based on interviews and case studies without direct observation of sexual behavior or responses. Masters thought the time was right to explore this unexamined territory with the aid of modern medical instrumentation. He asked the most basic question: how does the body respond physiologically to erotic stimulation? In 1964, he founded the Reproductive Biology Research Foundation in St. Louis to gain the funding necessary to expand his research. It is today known as the Masters and Johnson Institute.

His study of the physiology of sex began with prostitutes, but Masters soon found out that they were an unusual sample of subjects, and he was able to recruit subjects from the university community. He hired Virginia E. Johnson in 1956 because he thought that as a woman and as a person deeply interested in working with people, she was the research assistant he was seeking. Since that time she has been his partner and collaborator on virtually all important research projects. They were married to each other for a time but are now divorced. Their collaboration resulted in the Institute's most important research publications, which rival Kinsey's for thoroughness and breaking new ground. Masters and Johnson had decided that they would publish nothing until they had studied it systematically for a minimum of 10 years (Personal Communication, 1978).

Their first two books, *Human Sexual Response* (1966) and *Human Sexual Inadequacy* (1970), were each based on 11 years of research. Their *Homosexuality in Perspective* (1979) was based on 14 years of research. Through these books the public and scientific community gained accurate information about how women's and men's bodies respond to erotic stimulation in the **sexual response cycle**, how **sexual dysfunctions** develop and why they do not necessarily indicate a psychological disorder, strategies for treatment of sexual dysfunctions, and much about homosexual lifestyles and patterns of sexual expression. These books were a long time in development. Masters and Johnson began their program of sex therapy for husbands and wives with sexual problems in 1959, at first charging no fees because they thought their methods were too experimental (Personal Communication, 1978).

Basic to Masters and Johnson's approach to sex therapy is a behavioral perspective on the development of sexual dysfunctions. At the time, Freud's deterministic perspective was the most powerful approach. Behavioral theories, however, are theories of learning. Masters and Johnson discovered that sexual dysfunctions frequently resulted from maladaptive learning and could be "unlearned" in a relatively brief time compared to long-term psychoanalysis. Indeed, if sexual dysfunctions were generally the result of emotional traumas in the distant past, as the Freudians believed, then it would be unlikely that they could be cured in the 2- to 3-week therapeutic program used at the Masters and Johnson Institute. Masters and Johnson believe that the persistence of sexual difficulties means these problems continue to be reinforced in some way. If this reinforcement is discontinued and new behaviors and reinforcements are substituted, then the former maladaptive behavior will eventually be extinguished. This does not deny the usefulness of the Freudian approach with some types of sexual problems, however. Chapter 15 discusses in depth the nature and success of their program.

Masters and Johnson have contributed enormously to the professionalization of the study of human sexuality. Their efforts led to high ethical standards in sex research (see below) and authoritative standards of proficiency for becoming a sex therapist. Despite facing outrage and criticism as Kinsey had, Masters and Johnson firmly established a legacy of information, methodologies, and standards of proper conduct for sex research.

RESEARCH METHODS IN THE STUDY OF HUMAN SEXUALITY

For facts in any discipline to be useful and generalizable, they must be collected over a long period of time in a careful way. This is true also in the scientific study of human sexuality. Throughout this book you will read about many facts, concepts, and principles, and you need to understand how this information was collected, tested, replicated, and shared with others. This section, therefore, introduces some of the techniques researchers have used to discover useful and valid facts about all aspects of human sexuality.

First, one must understand that scientific research progresses in a cautious, conservative, step-by-step manner. Useful facts and theories in reality accumulate slowly over a long time,

Research Highlight

HISTORICAL RESEARCH

A lucid introduction to the methods of historical research can be found in the work of Shafer and his colleagues (1980). Their techniques and concerns remind one of the standards of proof required to be used by attorneys when reconstructing the past. The first step in any historical analysis of an issue is a thorough bibliographic survey of the subject and its major historical personalities, with an exhaustive analysis of critical essays on both. Although this can take a long time, it is the essential foundation for valid, reliable statements about events and people in the past. When researching more contemporary topics, this step may be simpler, and current sources are likely to be more complete.

The historian next confronts matters of conclusive proof and speculative probability. In some cases there is extensive documentation and corroborative evidence, whereas in other instances little survives other than the writings of generations of scholars, some of whom may have introduced personal interpretations or translations. For example, although Aristotle's thinking on the importance of moderation in all things seems a clear notion, the manuscripts that record his thoughts were damaged, revised, translated, and interpreted by many different people over literally thousands of years. In contrast, we have authoritative information about Alfred Kinsey, William Masters, and Virginia Johnson because modern scholars and journalists asked them questions, recorded their answers, corroborated their substance and meaning, and printed them for the wider public. Although we are forced to rely somewhat on speculation in the case of Aristotle, we have widely authenticated and confirmed sources in the latter.

When examining the historical record, criteria for different kinds of historical evidence must be considered. The raw materials of historical methods thus come under scrutiny. Ideally, both physical and oral historical records exist to support the interpretations of the modern historian; however, these data do not always exist, and when they do, they may not allow an unambiguous analysis of the past. The personal values and professionalism of the historian are therefore highly relevant, indeed fundamental, to a sound retrospective perspective. How the modern historian categorizes and analyzes notable records and reminiscences affects how the research is summarized, interpreted, and shared. Exhaustive data from the laboratory research of Masters and Johnson still exist, whereas virtually no early drafts of Victorian marriage manuals can still be found and analyzed.

Historians distinguish between external and internal criticism. External criticism involves the noted documents and data themselves, whereas internal criticism is concerned with the meaning of those sources from a current perspective. Finally, historical scholars both analyze and synthesize their research. Both are exhaustive, systematic attempts to put all the pieces together; skill, perceptiveness, and critical acumen are obviously important here. The historian's working hypotheses should be clear. At this point, the historian judges the adequacy and reliability of the sources and reports on any biases in the interpretations of others. The researcher also supports and defends her or his assessment of the relevance of the sources used, as well as the rationale for selecting them. Interpretations and generalizations are tentatively offered, accounting for the possibility of additional undiscovered information.

Different disciplines create and maintain diverse methodologies for discovering and assessing data and presenting it to professional and lay audiences. Historical research is no less rigorous or exacting than research in other areas of intellectual exploration.

in contrast to the common *misconception* that scientific break-throughs happen often and critical studies frequently provide important, widely applicable data. Such breakthroughs happen very, very rarely. Most scientists are patient women and men who are comfortable with data collection that can take many years. As mentioned earlier, Masters and Johnson followed their rule to "publish nothing unless you have studied it and collected empirical evidence for a minimum of *10 years."*

Second, scientific research is very different from personal observation and common sense. While many of us trust our own eyes and the value of our own experience, we must remember that compared with potentially thousands of subjects in a research study, our observations reflect the perspective of only *one* person. We, therefore, must acknowledge that our experience is highly personal and likely to be somewhat biased. These biases probably color what we see, how we interpret it, and how we apply that information. The value of scientific research is based on the fact that data collected from many subjects over a long period of time are likely to lead to a truer understanding of what applies to most of the people most of the time.

Many philosophers of science and historians attribute the early development of the scientific method to Sir Francis Bacon (1561–1626), the famous English essayist and philosopher. Bacon wanted to create a new system of knowledge that would replace Aristotle's, and his writings about how scientific investigations should proceed were a step in this direction. Bacon believed that philosophical inquiry could progress objectively only when unencumbered by religious dogma, and he sought to create criteria for truth that did not depend on spiritual explanations. Bacon believed that science would advance on the basis of *inductive reasoning.* In other words, useful and generalizable laws could be formulated only by determining what was common in many observations. Laws were built based on what was discovered from numerous individual cases. The more observations you make, the stronger the law you create.

For Bacon, the scientific method was simple. You begin with a *hypothesis* or some hunch about how the world works. A hypothesis is like an educated guess about the way things work or a question we ask ourselves often: "I wonder what would happen if. . . ." When you have formulated your hypothesis, the second step is to make as many objective, unemotional, rational observations as you can—the more the better. The third step is to analyze the observations (data) you have collected to see how they differ and what they have in common. Ask yourself what might have contributed to their variability or consistency. Finally, you return to your original hypothesis and ask whether the data show your hunch was correct or incorrect or whether more data are needed to decide. Because an infinite number of observations cannot be made, the original hypothesis is accepted only on the condition that still more observations in other circumstances will support it. Some statistical tools can tell us how sure of our results to be.

Bacon was also a keen observer of human nature and understood that many factors might prejudice one's inductive search for facts. He described a number of "impediments" to unbiased induction. These included the usual personal biases we all have, including loyalty to religious or racial doctrines, a lack of clarity or care in how we define our terms, and blind beliefs in historical traditions or political authority. These ideas, first introduced in about 1620, are still basic to training in the sciences today.

IMPORTANT PRINCIPLES IN RESEARCH METHODOLOGY

Before any scientific study begins, several decisions have to be made about the nature and scope of the investigation. Basic issues have to be decided. What sample of subjects are to be studied, where will they be found, and how are they to be paid for participation? What methods will be used to make the observations? How will observations be recorded? How are the findings to be categorized and statistically analyzed? (The statistics to be used are decided *before* your results are collected, not afterwards). How are the results to be shared with fellow professionals or the public? How will subjects be assured that they will be treated ethically?

Sampling Procedures

Scientists think in terms of two groups of subjects: the *population,* which includes every person from whom you could conceivably collect data (e.g., all college students in the United States), and the *sample,* a much smaller group of subjects (e.g., a few hundred students at your community college, college, or university) who you think will give you enough information to make inferences about the entire population. Sampling involves a huge risk. Scientists do not want their claims about a population to turn out half-baked because they weren't careful to select a sample that was as large, feasible, randomly selected, and as representative of the population as possible. Scientists in all disciplines undergo training in inferential statistics so that their analysis can be as strong as possible. But scientists do not always have access to the exact type of sample they would most like to study. For example, Alfred Kinsey's sample of subjects did not represent minorities or less well-educated individuals, and Masters and Johnson's subjects were often college or medical students. Certainly, such individuals do not represent the entire population of Americans or human beings in general. When we report studies in this book, we will point out any shortcomings that might detract from the usefulness and generalizability of the results.

Variables

A variable is any characteristic of a subject or quantity that can change. A variable can be an attribute of an individual, the magnitude of a stimulus presented to an individual, or the nature, magnitude, or latency of an individual's response to a stimulus. Describing, defining, and measuring variables is central to how researchers think about their studies. In the social and behavioral sciences, investigators typically define their research in terms of three different variables: independent, dependent, and intervening variables. An independent variable is some *stimulus or characteristic of the subject.* It is called "independent" because it can be selected or varied *independently* of a subject's response to it. Dependent variables are the subject's responses to the independent variable. Scientists are interested only in independent and dependent variables that can be *measured.* Measurement and quantification are the hallmarks of scientific investigations. Yet human beings are much more than mere responders to stimuli. Something happens within us—within our sense organs, brain, and endocrine glands—between the moment we receive a stimulus and our response to it. These invisible but inferred events are called "intervening" variables. Intervening variables, by definition, cannot be observed and measured, but we presume they are present because of changes in the subject's behaviors.

As you read about the many research studies summarized in this book, identify the independent and dependent variables being examined and consider the private and psychological events taking place inside the subjects. No single study can exemplify "typical" or "standard" variables, but as you think critically about research studies you will gain a good grasp of such variables.

Correlational Methods

Independent variables do not always *cause* changes in the dependent variable. An entirely different approach to research design explores relationships between two variables without assuming that changes in one cause changes in the other. Although some scientists think correlational studies are less rigorous than experimental laboratory studies, there is often much to be learned from them. A correlation *coefficient* is a measurement of the strength of the relationship between two variables. With a positive correlation coefficient, an increase in the magnitude of one variable is associated with an increased magnitude of the other. For example, as an adolescent's age increases from 13 to 19, there is also an increased likelihood that they have had sexual intercourse. But age in itself does not *cause* this increased likelihood, because many other psychosocial factors enter the picture. An example of a negative correlation you will read about later is that the more serious sex education children and teenagers have, the less likely they are to be involved in an unanticipated pregnancy. But again, education by itself may not cause a decline in teen pregnancy, because many other things are happening in these individuals' lives. Even though correlations do not indicate cause-and-effect relationships, they can guide further research studies in which causal relationships may be discovered.

TYPES OF RESEARCH METHODS

Sex researchers have gained much information through many different research methods. No one method is better than the others, as the type of question being explored determines the appropriate method. Various research methods have different strengths and weaknesses that affect how useful or generalizable the data may be.

Laboratory Investigations

With laboratory methods and controlled direct observations of sexual behaviors, scientists have considerable *control* over the quantification and presentation of stimuli and *precision* for measuring and recording subjects' responses. Independent and dependent variables are ideally both observable and measurable, and laboratory investigations make this feasible. Laboratory methods, therefore, usually allow scientists to make strong cause-and-effect statements about the effects of independent variables on dependent variables. As noted earlier, subjects selected to participate in laboratory investigations must be selected randomly from the population and their characteristics must be representative of that population.

William Masters and Virginia Johnson began their pioneering laboratory and direct observational analysis of human sexual response in 1954. For the first time, scientists, therapists, and the public could learn from studies that measured sexual arousal and orgasm in controlled conditions. Masters and Johnson electronically measured indicators of sexual excitement and orgasm while observing their subjects masturbate or have sexual intercourse. Important consistencies and differences between sexual response in women and men were thereby discovered, and these data could be generalized to most healthy people.

Although control and precision are a major strength of these methods, they have some drawbacks too. Laboratories are highly *artificial environments and people do not always behave normally and naturally in them.* While much is gained in control and precision, something is lost because one cannot be certain people respond sexually in the lab the same as they do at home or elsewhere.

Before carrying out an experimental laboratory design, the investigator must also decide either to randomly assign different groups of subjects to different levels of the independent variable or to present different levels of the independent variable to only a single group of subjects. The former is referred to as a *between-subjects design,* and the latter a *within-subjects design.* Generally, data from within-subjects designs have much less variability and are often thought more valid. Collecting data from many subjects receiving different levels of the independent variable can introduce more variability and, thus, diminish the generalizability of the results.

Longitudinal and Cross-Sectional Studies

In addition to defining the independent and dependent variables in a study, the investigator also decides whether to study the same subjects over a long period of time or only briefly. *Longitudinal studies* require the careful, frequent collection of data from the same individuals over a prolonged period of time. Longitudinal studies can last for several months or, in some cases, up to several decades. These studies reveal how time, age, and various life and cultural events affect the dependent variable being measured. We will see later on, for example, how the normal human aging process affects sexual expression, arousal, and responsiveness; often longitudinal studies are well-suited for such analysis. Longitudinal studies are complex and expensive, however. It takes considerable work and funds to follow people over long periods of time.

Subjects may disappear or die, and then the researcher loses valuable data. But these types of studies are well-suited for assessing the impact of time, age, and major sociocultural phenomena, for example, the impact of the Great Depression on the availability of contraceptives and subsequent changes in the birth rate. Another drawback to longitudinal studies, especially those that take place over many years, is that although the study may have started with a large, randomly selected sample representative of the population, as subjects drop out, the likelihood that the remaining subjects are similarly representative of the population decreases. In fact, the final subjects could be quite different.

When a researcher is interested in studying a group of similar subjects at a specific point in time, these studies are called *cross-sectional.* They involve the investigation of a cross section of the population in just one period of analysis. For example, a cross-sectional study would be well suited to examine whether women and men at mid-life really have some kind of "crisis" and change partners, families, and sexual habits during this supposedly tumultuous time. Cross-sectional investigations require less time, research assistance, and money, but there is no way of knowing what happens to the research subjects after the study is over or how their thoughts, feelings, and behaviors change. In a sense, a longitudinal study is like a movie while a cross-sectional study is like a snapshot.

Surveys, Questionnaires, and Interviews

A basic premise in research in the social and behavioral sciences is that if you want to learn something about people, just ask them! Surveys and questionnaires are not the same, however. A survey is a research strategy in which the researcher asks a large number of subjects questions about their thoughts, feelings, and behaviors that have occurred in the past, are occurring now, or are likely to occur in the future. The subjects' answers reveal to the researcher information about what variables might underlie behaviors. The paper-and-pencil *instrument* used to carry out a survey is called a *questionnaire,* a collection of questions intended to elicit the information the scientist is seeking. Designing good questionnaires is a real art, however, and must be carried out in a careful and unbiased manner. Questions must be phrased in ways that do not influence the responses, with alternatives unambiguously different from each other. Surveys are used in both longitudinal and cross-sectional studies. In a longitudinal study, for example, a subject's response to a question about their feelings toward premarital intercourse is likely to differ when they are 18 compared to a later time, say when they have an 18-year-old child. In a cross-sectional study, responses from different samples at the same point in time will likely reveal differences about how different groups think and behave concerning sexual issues.

Interviews have long been used to learn about human sexual behaviors and how people feel about their sexuality. Not everyone is comfortable answering intimate questions about such personal issues, however, and there is always the chance that subjects' responses might not be open and honest. Often interviewees need time to "warm up" to this conversational format, and some are never completely at ease, while others who are itching to tell you about their sexual thoughts and activities may not be representative of the population. This research stumbling block is called *volunteer bias,* and it can lead researchers to conclusions that do not accurately describe the larger population. Many of the sex surveys commonly published in magazines, for example, may suffer from this bias, because readers who take the time to fill out a questionnaire may not be "normal" readers or representative of society as a whole.

There is still another concern for scientists who use sex surveys. They can never be certain that their subjects are telling them the truth. Some subjects might not want the interviewer to think they have engaged in "bad" sexual behaviors and, therefore, might not be forthcoming about their actual sexual history. Also, the gender, personality, race, or age of the interviewer may make some subjects more or less comfortable about disclosing details of their sex lives.

Another way to learn details about a subject's behaviors uses the case study method, which describes how an individual has developed, behaved, or reacted to various circumstances. This method was described in Chapter 1. It is important and useful in many respects.

Field Studies

Sometimes it is most informative to study people's behavior in their own home and work environment. Because most people act naturally in familiar places, researchers believe that our "real" selves can often be studied better this way. Field studies are also carried out in other countries or cultures. This book will share many interesting and sometimes unusual sexual practices from other countries, often resulting from methodical field observations. One of the most interesting challenges for social scientists is viewing the sexual behaviors of other cultures without using their own as the standard for "normality." It can be difficult to view apparently odd sexual customs from the perspective of the culture in which they occur rather than from one's own culture, but this is important for unbiased objectivity and a scientific approach.

In 1951, Ford and Beech published *Patterns of Sexual Behavior,* which employed field study methods to study sexual behaviors and customs in dozens of world cultures. Their findings surprised many in the United States. For example, they found that homosexual behaviors are acceptable in many cultures throughout the world, including many Native American Indian tribes during religious ceremonies. Field studies show us that the sex drive is given form and direction by culture. Much of what we know about certain sexual habits, variations, and preferences such as voyeurism and sadomasochistic behavior has been learned through field studies.

Participant-Observer Research

In some cases, researchers decide that the best way to study something is to get into the situation and see for themselves. For example, to learn about "pick-up lines" people use when they meet in bars and clubs, you might decide to go there yourself and listen to what people say to each another to signal their interest or sexual receptivity. Participant-observer research offers the researcher an authentic glimpse into an issue.

HOW TO INTERPRET DATA COLLECTED BY SEX RESEARCHERS

An inspection of your local bookstore will reveal that human sexuality is an active area of publication. Many excellent (and not so excellent) books teach about human sexuality in general, and others focus on problems in intimate relations or sexual arousal or responsiveness. Most of this information and that published in popular magazines, however, is quite different from that found in scientific journals. Even in scientific journals, only when a study's findings are replicated by other research can one be confident of their validity. Information presented to the public is often simplified, and such writers seldom admit any doubts about the validity or reliability of what they report. Readers can therefore be given a false sense of certainty about what is "right" or "wrong" in such sexual information. An important function of a textbook such as this, therefore, is to summarize and explain complex findings published in the scientific literature, as well as to encourage you to read this "primary literature" yourself. Yet even then it is often difficult to evaluate original research reports.

As hard as researchers try, it is extremely difficult to ensure that the sample subjects truly represent the population as a whole. A sampling error may occur so that the sample differs in subtle but important ways from the population. This problem, of course, makes it risky to generalize broadly about the study's findings. Subjects in sex research studies often have different levels of knowledge about sex and different sexual experiences. These factors must be examined when considering whether a study's findings relate to society as a whole.

How the findings can be applied is another challenge in interpreting research. To what extent can one put this information to work in one's own life?. In many instances the application is clear, but in other cases application requires assistance from medical, psychological, or psychiatric professionals in human sexuality, who have highly specialized knowledge. Finally, although having new information does not always change how a person behaves sexually, it can have tremendous reassurance value for people who are doubtful, uninformed, or fearful about some sexual issue.

ETHICAL CONSIDERATIONS IN SEX RESEARCH

Before Alfred Kinsey undertook his studies of male and female sexuality, the ethical conduct of research in this private arena did not receive much attention. Indeed, before Kinsey, most knowledge about sexuality came from medical or clinical settings. By the late 1940s, however, the social and behavioral sciences were studying sexuality, and ethical considerations and

protections became part of sex research and therapy. As the discipline grew, more than a simple understanding of confidentiality became necessary.

In 1953, the American Psychological Association first published Ethical Standards for Psychologists, which, through subsequent editions, has defined the ethical issues for social scientists. These guidelines insure that research subjects enjoy basic care and security. Following are the most important protections:

1. Informed Consent. Any research study involving human beings must begin by first acquiring the subject's permission; this usually involves obtaining a signed statement describing the nature of the study and the subject's awareness of what she or he will do as a participant. Deceiving the subject as to the nature of the study should be avoided in every way possible. In those instances in which deception is used, it must be ". . . justified by the scientific, educational, or applied value of the research and that alternatives to deception are not feasible" (APA, 1992, Sections 5 and 6).

2. Confidentiality. Researchers must make every effort to keep confidential all data collected. Further, a subject's data must not be associated immediately and obviously with their name or any other identifier. Ideally, coded identifiers should be used. In this way, both confidentiality and anonymity will be assured.

3. Discontinuance. Experimental subjects must be given every assurance that they are free to discontinue their participation at any time without being required or expected to offer any explanation.

4. Debriefing. At the conclusion of the investigation, the experimenter is required to offer his or her participants a full and thorough debriefing as to the scope, substance, and outcomes of the study. However, subjects can only be offered generalized group data and must not be told how their personal responses compared with the group data.

This list touches only on key points in the most basic ethical standards for research with human beings. These basics are all relevant in sex research and any inquiry soliciting personal information. As the scope of sex research expands, new ethical considerations confront the researcher. For example, research on high-risk behaviors associated with acquiring sexually transmitted diseases and AIDS should be undertaken with great sensitivity to privacy and confidentiality. Similar ethical challenges would be involved with research on factors that predispose adolescents to pregnancy or research on extramarital sexuality,

An example of the sensitive nature of such ethical concerns is found in the work of Korn et al (1992), who asked male and female undergraduates to evaluate the ethical acceptability of two published studies on the use of guided imagery in recreating rape circumstances. Guided imagery is a technique, sometimes used in counseling, in which a person imagines a specific situation, usually one that provokes significant fear or anxiety, while being "talked through" the scene in order to diminish the fear or anxiety through the supportive, relaxed situation. Korn and his colleagues asked their female subjects to evaluate the ethics of an experiment that asked women to imagine themselves as rape victims; the male subjects were told to imagine themselves as rapists. Both women and men said that the research question was important, but they found its ethics less than fully acceptable. The guided imagery of a sexual assault was particularly stressful for the women, none of whom said they would have chosen to participate in the evaluated studies, and none thought the research was at all ethical.

In addition to the American Psychological Association, the Council for International Organizations of Medical Sciences (CIOMS), a branch of the World Health Organization, has as its primary mission considering the ethics of human research. According to CIOMS, four ethical principles govern all research with human subjects:

1. Respect for persons, which includes both autonomy, or the respect for the self-determination of those who are capable of deliberating about their personal goals, and protection of persons with impaired or diminished autonomy;
2. Beneficence, which is the ethical obligation to maximize benefits and minimize harms or wrongs;
3. Non-maleficence, which means 'do no harm"; and
4. Justice, which requires that subjects in studies are treated equally, and studies are designed so that the subjects of study are also the beneficiaries of the study (although clearly they may not be the only beneficiaries).

The general ethical standards are clear, but how are they implemented in research settings? Were you asked to participate in an experiment, as students often are, you would want to know.

Whether research is carried out in medical or academic settings, the researchers cannot begin without permission from the Institutional Review Board (IRB). This is true with both human and animal research. Every organization has an IRB that evaluates the ethics of research proposals. The IRB usually consists of people from different disciplines who read and discuss every proposal before voting to grant or withhold permission to proceed. Regardless of who is funding the research or how "important" they are, the local IRB has total control over this determination.

CHANGING PERSPECTIVES ON HUMAN SEXUALITY

This chapter has introduced many changes in societal, historical, and cultural perspectives on human sexual thinking, feeling, and behaving. Sexual attitudes that were once considered prurient or that provoked guilt have become issues about which the public is more comfortable thinking and talking. Anxieties about masturbation or "too frequent" sexual intercourse once concerned a lot of people. Sexual feeling and expression are now meaningfully discussed among people who are close to each other. Quacks and pseudoscientific sources of information about sex have been replaced by professionals with extensive training. When Masters and Johnson began collecting data on sexual arousal and orgasm, they opened a new era of human inquiry. *Human Sexual Response* (1966) brought empirical legitimacy in the scientific examination of sexuality, in which objective evidence is gathered under controlled conditions and evaluated with robust statistical tools.

Learning Activities

1. Before starting this course, you may have thought about sex mostly in terms of genitalia and erotic feelings. What other meanings did the term "sex" have for you? How would you now describe your general emotions about this topic?
2. Try to describe specific ways in which our society sends messages about how women and men should behave. At what age do you think that girls and boys begin to notice these messages? What can happen when someone does not act in conformity with these expectations?
3. Can you describe a sexual custom in another society that would be utterly inappropriate in our culture?
4. How do you think that historical beliefs about male dominance still affect ways in which women and men interact sexually?
5. You have been introduced to several contemporary and historical perspectives on same-sex marriage. In your opinion, will federal, state, or local laws ever sanction such unions? Why do you think this concept is so controversial?
6. This chapter presents 10 consequences of "premature sexual involvement" published in *US Catholic* (1996). Describe your reactions to these and explain why you feel as you do.
7. The study of human sexuality began as a "pseudoscientific discipline." Do you know any contemporary, less-than-legitimate approaches to the study of sexuality? To whom do these seem to appeal?
8. Do you recognize the remnants of any Victorian sexual beliefs in society now? What, specifically? Why do you think that modern movies about the Victorian period (e.g., *Sense and Sensibility, Howard's End, The Return of the Native*) have been so popular?
9. Why do you think that Sigmund Freud has been criticized for his work on the development of sexuality? Can you think of any other historical or contemporary figure conspicuously identified with sexuality?
10. While at Indiana University, Alfred Kinsey was asked not to publish his research during times when the state legislature was in session. How does this mesh with the concept of academic freedom? Do you think such a thing would or could happen today?
11. Can you think of special ethical challenges sex researchers might face when investigating controversial is-

sues (e.g., child sexual abuse, extramarital affairs, making condoms available to high school students)?

Key Concepts

- Epicureanism was a Roman philosophy that sought the highest good through the pursuit of intellectual pleasure.
- Stoicism, another Roman philosophy, held that the central challenge of existence was to live in harmony with nature and conduct ourselves with dignity, intelligence, and compassion.
- The term *sex*, strictly defined, refers to reproduction in which reproductive cells from males of a species join with reproductive cells of females to produce offspring.
- *Gender role* refers to society's expectations for "appropriate" thoughts, feelings, and behaviors of people based on their sex.
- Our self-awareness of our maleness or femaleness is our *gender identity.*
- The psychobiological perspective views all cognition, emotion, and behavior as resulting from activity of the nervous system. Neurophysiological and neurochemical foundations of behavior are of primary interest.
- Many psychobiologists take a mechanistic approach to behavior. The brain is considered a machine, with its functions understood by learning about the parts of the machine and their interactions.
- The psychosocial perspective accounts for diverse human behavior in terms of the reciprocal relationship between individuals and their social and cultural environments.
- Investigators attempting to understand the dynamics of human behavior through a combination of observation and in-depth interview take a clinical perspective.
- The cross-cultural approach examines characteristics of different cultures and explores similarities and differences to understand how people achieve similar social and behavioral ends in their own environments.
- For centuries, the reproductive potential of semen has been recognized. Semen conservation theory maintains that men must never waste their semen through masturbation or intercourse not intended for conception. It was once thought that a man's character was enhanced by abstaining from such "nonproductive" ejaculation.
- In Sigmund Freud's psychosexual theory, libido is the primitive motivational force in the personality, expressed through sexual and aggressive behaviors.
- The libido functions on the basis of the pleasure principle, the desire to seek pleasures and avoid pain and deprivation.
- According to Freud, as one matures, the personality acknowledges that pleasure seeking must be achieved within the context of society's laws, morals, and norms. The personality thus functions on the reality principle.
- Freud said that the libido is invested in the erogenous zones—areas of the body that when stimulated yield sexual pleasure.
- In Freud's theory, all adult thinking, emotion, and behaviors are determined in infancy and early childhood.
- Psychoanalysis refers to a theory of normal human growth and development, a theory of personality, and a method of psychotherapy.
- Research involving human beings requires informed consent, meaning that potential subjects know the nature of the investigation, what they will do as participants, and that they will be protected from harm.
- Sex researchers use the scientific method and rigorous methods to collect data. They are cautious in making generalizations about the population based on information from the sample subjects.
- The history of human sexuality helps us understand the origins of our thoughts, feelings, and behaviors in relation to this complex aspect of human nature.

Glossary Terms

anatomy	gender identity	psychotherapy
carnal	gender role	reality principle
circumcision	libido	reductionism
clinical	masculinity	sadism
coitus interruptus	masochism	sensual
determinism	mechanistic	sexual response
double blind	naturalistic	cycle
embryology	pederasty	sexual
Epicureanism	physiology	dysfunctions
erogenous zones	pleasure principle	sexuality
erotic	psychoanalysis	Stoicism
ethnocentrism	psychobiological	transsexuality
femininity	approach	vicarious learning

Suggested Readings

Halberstam, D. (1993, May/June). Discovering sex. American Heritage, 39–58.
Kinsey, A., Pomeroy, W., & Martin, C. (1948). Sexual behavior in the human male. Philadelphia: Saunders.
Kinsey, A., Pomeroy, W., Martin, C., & Gebhard, P. (1953). Sexual behavior in the human female. Philadelphia: Saunders.
Masters, W., & Johnson, V. (1966). Human sexual response. Boston: Little, Brown.
Masters, W., & Johnson, V. (1970). Human sexual inadequacy. Boston: Little, Brown.
Plant, R. (1986). The pink triangle. New York: Henry Holt and Company.

3

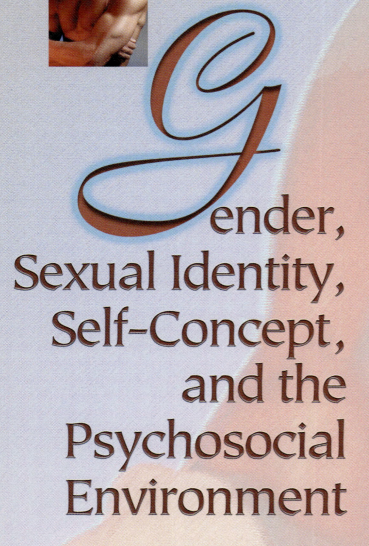

Gender, Sexual Identity, Self-Concept, and the Psychosocial Environment

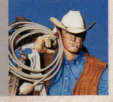

OBJECTIVES

When you finish reading and reviewing this chapter, you should be able to:

1. Explain how the concept of gender can be considered from three different but related perspectives: biological, psychological, and social.

2. Explain *attribution theory,* discuss the distinction between internal and external attributions, and describe the fundamental attributional error.

3. Describe the role of sex chromosomes and genes in influencing the sex of human offspring.

4. Define what a *hormone* is, and discuss hormones that affect male and female prenatal sexual differentiation.

5. Describe the internal and external male and female sexual differentiation in the human embryo and fetus.

6. Summarize the relationship among sex hormones, sexual feelings, and sex drive in women and men.

7. Describe the psychosocial aspects of how children learn traditional gender roles, and discuss the impact of this learning on self-concept and self-esteem.

8. Describe androgynous ways of thinking, feeling, and behaving.

9. Define *transsexuality* and *transgenderism,* and explain the general medical and psychosocial approaches to the treatment of *gender dysphoria.*

10. Summarize some male responses to feminism and reasons for these reactions.

11. Describe how gender differences influence male/female relationships and sexual communication between men and women.

12. Summarize the relationship between sexuality and advertising, and describe societal responses to such advertising.

13. Explain how children, adolescents, and adults interpret and evaluate sexual messages in the media.

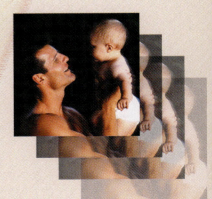

From Dr. Ruth

I'm sure you've heard the phrase "the battle of the sexes." Not that long ago I co-hosted a comedy special with George Hamilton with just that title. In it, we poked fun at American stereotypes of differences between the sexes. But as we enter the new millennium, that battle has de-escalated into just minor skirmishes for many couples. As more women have entered business, industry, medicine, law, and education, men and women haven't had the time or energy to fight, but have pooled their abilities and resources to survive these stress-filled times.

Of course, this change has occurred mostly in Western cultures. Many other parts of the world haven't even reached the "battle of the sexes" stage because women are so completely dominated by men that they don't dare disobey. I know what one kind of that discrimination is like: when I was a young girl in an orphanage in Switzerland, only the boys were allowed to study academic subjects. The only training girls got was how to be a housekeeper. (Thanks to my boyfriend at the time, I got some schooling from reading his books at night.) Of course, many men and women in the United States today still have not been fully enlightened. I believe that the pace of rapprochement is speeding up, however, so it won't be long before some of the prime battlefields of old will have been totally forgotten.

Still, differences between the sexes do exist, and one of the aims of this chapter is to describe them and how and why they develop as they do. Although there are obvious biological differences between men and women, those don't explain very much about the stereotypes of being a man or being a woman. Our goal in discussing gender differences is not to see them as good or bad, but only different and certainly interesting.

The last chapter introduced some terms that are important for a wide variety of sexual issues. We'll briefly review them here because of their relevance in this chapter. Note that although they are often used interchangeably, these terms do have essential differences in their meanings.

The term **sex** is usually used to describe the biological or genetic designation of maleness or femaleness. In most cases, this designation is clear, based primarily on chromosomal, anatomical, physiological, and endocrine considerations. This is perhaps the most basic and obvious way that most of us began learning and thinking about sexual matters and questions, but this is only part of the story. The term **gender role** is a more complicated notion. This term refers to a variety of societal expectations about "appropriate" or "expected" ways we are supposed to behave as females or males. In addition to overt behaviors, gender roles concern how we think and feel about being women or men. Not everyone in our culture, or people throughout the world in diverse cultures, thinks of gender roles in exactly the same ways. Our perceptions influence how sensitive we are to such psychosocial "demands" in the environments in which we live. For example, sometimes we do not even notice the traditional role expectations for masculin-

ity and femininity, but at other times we might genuinely feel stifled by a perceived need to act in a way expected because of our maleness or femaleness. Finally, **gender identity** refers to how comfortable we are in our gender roles. Gender identity is influenced by society's expectations. Sometimes we are attuned to the congruence of our biological attributes as women and men with our interpretations of our gender roles. At other times we are entirely unselfconscious about this subtle internal comparison.

Although you may not have thought in these terms before, you have probably thought about things related to these concepts. For example, if you've ever looked in a mirror and wondered whether you were an attractive man or woman, then you have been analyzing the implications of biologically based conceptions of sexuality for you personally. Similarly, if you have wondered whether you think like a "typical" or "real" man or woman, you are wondering about your own gender identity. The question concerns the fit between your biological sex and how you think you are supposed to think, feel, or act as a woman or a man. Behind these private personal questions lies another important question: "Which is more important for my physical and psychological sexuality—my own opinions or those of others or society as a whole?" Much of this chapter deals with this question.

A NOTE ON CHAPTER ORGANIZATION

As you have already noted, gender issues can be quite complex. We believe that they are best approached from three complementary perspectives: biological, psychological, and social. We begin by viewing gender as a *biological construct.* An incredible number of complex hormonal events trigger the differentiation of male and female internal and external sexual anatomy before birth. Sometimes this process does not go smoothly, and "mismatches" occur between a developing embryo's genetic sex and the appearance of the body. Another issue concerns the impact of sex hormones on feelings of well-being and on what is sometimes called the "sex drive." We will explore whether stereotypical differences between women and men are indeed based on real hormonal differences.

Our approach then switches to consider gender as a *psychological construct,* including what happens inside our own minds in relation to gender issues. We will explore why and how and to what extent we are comfortable with our masculinity or femininity. We will examine how gender roles develop throughout childhood and adolescence in a process some scientists call "gender-role typing." Learning to be a boy or girl is by no means a simple or brief process but one that takes many years and involves many kinds of messages from the family and the social environment. We will also look at some noteworthy racial differences in gender-role typing in this country.

Last, we will examine gender as a *social construct.* This approach concerns *interpersonal* aspects of gender, behavior, and the wider social setting. Gender and role expectations are related to where and how we grow up and live our lives, as well as our thinking about maleness and femaleness. Sometimes these concerns are not easy to predict or understand. For example, many men have highly negative reactions to militant feminism and express their feelings freely. There are also scientific data to support some of the aspects of the old sexual stereotypes about men and women. Another important issue involves the media. Sex sells. Television has an immense influence on many people, especially the young. Finally, there is something to be learned from other societies and how they view their women and men and their respective roles.

ATTRIBUTION THEORY

Psychologists use the term **attribution** for how people try to explain what they see in the behavior of other people. As we observe women and men in our day-to-day activities, we can ask whether observed behaviors are due to gender-based attributes or the circumstances. For example, let's say that someone of unspecified gender has a flat tire on an isolated road late at night. If a male stopped to help, it is likely that we would make an attribution based on the particular situation. After all, in circumstances involving cars, flat tires, lonely roads, and the need for help, we would expect a man to stop and offer aid. If

you think that this attribution is based on a stereotype about men, you are correct. Consider, however, a lone woman stopping and offering help in the same situation. This is not something women usually do, and it may take an unusual woman to do it. Here, the attribution is based on the individual's strong altruistic tendencies. In all, stereotypes, personality, and situation should all be considered when we try to understand reasons for what we observe. We are introducing attribution theory early in this chapter because it helps sort out how gender, stereotypes, unique personalities, and the social setting all interact to influence how we explain a variety of behaviors we observe every day.

An important aspect of attribution theory is *the fundamental attribution error.* This refers to the bias in how we try to explain behaviors we observe: generally, we tend to attribute too much importance to personality factors and discount social factors. For example, Dave has promised his wife Nan that he will clean out the garage Sunday afternoon. But when Sunday arrives, Dave backs out of his promise. The fundamental attribution error might lead some to say: "Isn't that just like a man!" when actually Dave has obtained a rare ticket to a Rembrandt exhibit. The error is to de-emphasize the personal qualities that led Dave to break his promise and dwell on a stereotype of how men behave when faced with an unpleasant domestic task. This theory can be useful for explaining the behaviors of women and men based on gender stereotypes (Fig. 3-1). Wouldn't it be nice if we just saw people as they are rather than as what we expect them to be as women or men?

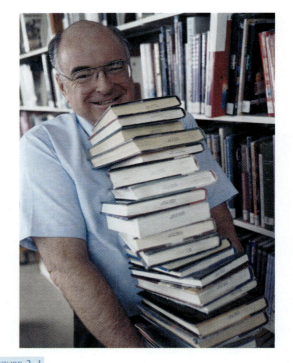

FIGURE 3-1   Historically, most librarians were women, but today this profession has many men working at all levels of responsibility. The stereotype of the "spinster" librarian is no longer supported by our common observations.

GENDER AS A BIOLOGICAL CONSTRUCT

Genes and Chromosomes

Beginning at conception, there is a complex sequence of events involving chromosomes and the genes on them. These formulate the directions for normal female or male development to begin. Later, the embryo's early sex glands and the tiny amounts of hormones they produce become very important.

Sex cells are called **gametes**. Female gametes are called ova (singular, ovum) or sometimes "eggs"; male gametes are sperm. Other body cells are called **somatic cells**. Somatic cells have 46 chromosomes grouped in 23 pairs (Fig. 3-2). Twenty-two of these are matched pairs, meaning that both chromosomes of the pair are similar. Each matched set is called an **autosome**. Autosomes are the same for genetic males and females and have little to do with the creation of maleness or femaleness. The twenty-third pair has two chromosomes that are different in males and females; these are called **sex chromosomes**. Females have two of the same sex chromosomes, both called X chromosomes, giving genetic females an XX sex chromosome designation. In contrast, males have one X and one Y sex chromosome, or an XY sex chromosome designation.

Gametes are not like somatic cells; they do not have twenty-three *pairs* of chromosomes, but twenty-three chromosomes, period. Twenty-two are autosomes, and one is a sex chromosome. An ovum has 22 autosomes and an X sex chromosome, and a sperm has 22 autosomes and an X or Y sex chromosome. At the moment of fertilization, 22 of the mother's autosomes are joined with 22 of the father's autosomes. The ovum contributes an X sex chromosome and the sperm contributes either an X sex chromosome or a Y sex chromosome. If the fertilized ovum has an XX sex chromosome composition, the embryo and later the fetus will be female. If the fertilized ovum has an XY sex chromosome composition, it will be male. These sex chromosomes guide the development of the internal, external, and hormonal characteristics of the offspring.

The process of sexual differentiation in the developing fetus is quite complicated. Let's begin with the **gonads** (the sex glands)—ovaries in females and testes in males. A gene on the Y sex chromosome directs the formation of the male's testes; if there is no Y sex chromosome, there are no instructions for the creation of testes, and ovaries will instead develop. There is apparently also a gene, or perhaps several, on the X chromosome with a role in the development of ovaries (Eicher, 1994; Bardoni et al., 1994).

Hormones

Until 6 weeks after conception, the gonadal sex of the embryo is not apparent; *sexual differentiation* has not yet occurred. In the genital region of this early embryo there is virtually no difference between genetic males and genetic females. As soon as the gonads become functional, however, this situation changes dramatically and quickly. **Hormonal sex** now becomes obvious. A **hormone** is a chemical substance produced in one of the body's **endocrine glands** secreted directly into the blood stream. (There are many different endocrine glands, e.g., pituitary, thyroid, thymus, pancreas, adrenal, testes, ovaries, etc.) Sex hormones are examples of a larger family of chemical compounds called **steroids**. Once in the circulatory system, hormones travel to their destination (usually another endocrine gland) and affect the activity of that "target organ." As the ovaries of a genetic female begin to develop, they secrete hormones called **estrogens** and a hormone called **progesterone**. There is actually no single hormone called "estrogen;" this term refers to a family of eight different hormones that differ in chemical structure and potency. The testes of a genetic male begin to secrete **androgens**; the best known of these is **testosterone**. While these hormones have several functions in the developing and mature individual after birth, their prenatal action contributes to normal sexual differentiation. In tiny amounts, these agents direct the development of internal and external sexual anatomical structures in women and men. Our biological sexual characteristics thus begin only a few weeks after conception.

Internal Sexual Anatomy

The internal and external sexual anatomy of the embryo begins to develop very early. At 7 or 8 weeks after fertilization, one of two different internal systems of ducts and tubes begins to develop, depending on the genetic sex. Both were present before differentiation began. In genetic males, the *Wolffian ducts* begin to develop; in genetic females, the *Müllerian ducts* mature. These in turn will further differentiate into all of the internal male and female sexual anatomical structures. In genetic males, androgens stimulate the Wolffian ducts to differentiate into many internal anatomical structures: epididymis, the seminal vesicles, the vas deferens, and the ejaculatory ducts. In addition to androgens, the embryonic testes also secrete a substance called *Müllerian-inhibiting substance,* which acts to cause the

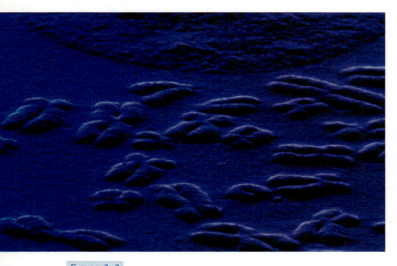

FIGURE 3-2   A scanning electron micrograph of human chromosomes.

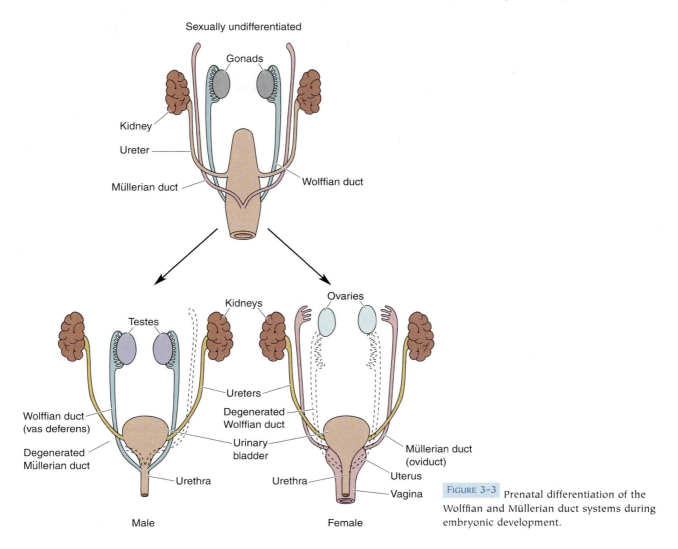

Sexually undifferentiated

Gonads

Kidney

Ureter

Müllerian duct

Wolffian duct

Kidneys

Ovaries

Testes

Ureters

Wolffian duct
(vas deferens)

Degenerated
Wolffian duct

Degenerated
Müllerian duct

Urinary
bladder

Urethra

Urethra

Vagina

Müllerian duct
(oviduct)

Uterus

Male

Female

FIGURE 3-3 Prenatal differentiation of the Wolffian and Müllerian duct systems during embryonic development.

Müllerian ducts to regress and disappear. A 1994 study (Hack et al.) demonstrated that a gene on the Y chromosome is responsible for the secretion of Müllerian-inhibiting substance. The male hormone that directs this remodeling process, testosterone, is converted into dihydrotestosterone (DHT), which stimulates the development of the prostate gland.

Because no androgens are present in the female, the fetus begins to develop female internal and external sexual structures. The Müllerian ducts develop into fallopian tubes, the uterus, and the upper part of the vagina, while the Wolffian duct system regresses and disappears. This occurs mainly because the fetus' ovaries do not secrete testosterone or Müllerian-inhibiting substance, which leads to sexual differentiation in genetic males. While these changes are occurring internally, sex-specific external anatomical structures are also developing (Fig. 3-3).

External Sexual Anatomy of the Fetus

Many of the external sexual anatomical structures are *homologous,* meaning that they are similar in position and structure, though not necessarily in function, in females and males.

Hormones have a major role in directing the development of external sexual anatomy. If DHT is not present, as in genetic females, the genital tubercle (Fig. 3-4) develops into the clitoris and the genital folds become the labia minora and outer por-

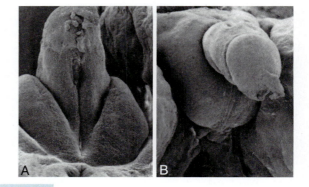

A   B

FIGURE 3-4 Embryonic appearance of external female genitalia **(left)** and external male genitalia **(right).**

tion of the vagina. The labioscrotal swelling, in turn, differentiates into the labia majora. If DHT is present, however, as in genetic males, the genital tubercle develops into the tip of the penis (glans) and the genital folds become the shaft of the penis. The labioscrotal swelling differentiates into the scrotum, although at this prenatal stage of development the scrotum does not yet contain the testes (Eicher, 1994). The development of internal and external sexual anatomy is complete by the end of the third month of pregnancy. Table 3-1 lists some homologous sexual structures in males and female.

Although most people know the anatomical differences between women and men, not everyone is aware of the significant similarities. Often people are surprised to learn how much alike the two sexes really are. As in other aspects of sexuality discussed elsewhere in this text, the similarities between women and men are more interesting than the differences.

Anomalies in Sexual Differentiation

Sometimes development, as described previously, does not go smoothly, resulting in some very unusual outcomes. Examples of abnormal sexual differentiation are described here not to shock you with bizarre tales of genetic and hormonal mishaps but in order to clarify some basic concepts. First, anything unusual in early embryonic sexual differentiation will have effects that accumulate and are magnified as tissues develop and the organism matures. Second, sometimes discrepancies occur that are not always apparent in physical appearances; in many cases these abnormalities cannot be detected by only looking. Although the conditions described here involve biological aspects of gender, how individuals cope with them and the gender identity challenges they pose involve psychological and social issues as well.

CONGENITAL ADRENOGENITAL SYNDROME

In some cases, female embryos are inadvertently exposed to male hormone (androgen). This can happen in a number of ways. For example, if the adrenal glands of the developing female embryo produce too much androgen, this has the effect of masculinizing the female embryo's genitalia. (Male and female adrenal glands secrete both estrogens and androgens in both sexes). An excessive amount of androgen causes the con-

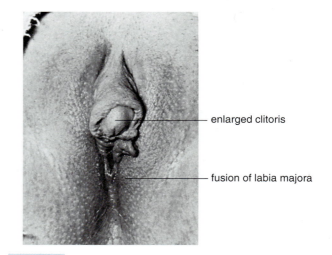

FIGURE 3-5 In congenital virilizing adrenal hyperplasia, masculinized genitalia are common. The labia majora are fused. Here, a highly enlarged clitoris is obvious.

genital adrenogenital syndrome, sometimes referred to as **congenital virilizing adrenal hyperplasia** (Fig. 3-5). "Virilizing" means to make masculine or male-like (virile); "hyperplasia" refers to an abnormal or unusual increase in the number of cells comprising the adrenal gland.

Normal genetic female embryos have been exposed to excessive androgen in another way as well. From the late 1940s into the late 1950s, some obstetricians used androgen as a **progestational drug**—an agent intended to reduce the risk of miscarriage. Androgen was an effective progestational agent; however, androgen also masculinizes female embryos. While having an XX sex chromosome designation, these female infants are born with an enlarged clitoris that looks very much like a penis. The labia are joined together in such a way that they look almost exactly like a male infant's scrotum. In some instances, a tiny vaginal opening is apparent. Despite these external masculine traits, the internal sexual anatomy is clearly female: ovaries, fallopian tubes, a uterus, and a vagina are present.

Careful diagnostic assessment typically reveals this abnormality. Plastic surgery is usually performed and/or hormones administered so that genital appearance conforms with the female's genetic sex. This individual has normal fertility in later life. Obviously it is important to diagnose this problem as early as possible and correct the situation so there is a match of chromosomal and genital sexual attributes through normal childhood development.

CONGENITAL INSENSITIVITY TO ANDROGEN SYNDROME

An inherited X-sex chromosome-linked trait called **androgen insensitivity syndrome** or "testicular feminization" occurs rarely. A genetic male with appropriate X and Y sex chromosomes has a body in which somatic cells are not sensitive to and do not respond to androgens. In androgen insensitivity syndrome the gonads (testes) and internal sexual ducts are male though they have not descended, as the testes usually do,

---

TABLE 3-1

Homologous Sexual Structures in Males and Females

Male	Female
Testes	Ovaries
Prostate gland	Skene's glands
Cowper's glands	Bartholin's glands
Shaft of penis	Labia minora
Scrotal sac	Labia majora
Foreskin of penis	Hood of clitoris
Glans of penis	Clitoris

by birth. There is no scrotum for them to descend into. The external genitalia are female, with the vagina ending in a kind of dead-end pouch. The internal sexual anatomy, however, is not female, because the testes of the fetus secreted the Müllerian-inhibiting substance causing the lack of a uterus or fallopian tubes; the individual is therefore sterile. By the appearance of the external genitalia, the new baby seems a female and is therefore raised as a girl. Often nothing seems unusual until adolescence, when the young "woman" and perhaps her parent(s) become concerned that she has not started having periods. Interestingly, breast development progresses "normally" as the process is normally affected by the secretion of estrogens. Adjustment to traditional female gender role expectations is generally uncomplicated in these individuals.

DHT Deficiency

As described above, dihydrotestosterone (DHT) is one of the metabolic by-products of testosterone. Testosterone passes easily through the cell membranes of genetic males and is then converted to DHT. DHT is far more potent than testosterone itself. A rare abnormality of prenatal sexual differentiation involves a mutant gene that inhibits the conversion of testosterone into DHT. The testes do not descend into the scrotum before birth, and the external genitalia have an ambiguous, somewhat female appearance. Internal sexual anatomy is male.

The first clinical assessment of DHT deficiency was reported in the Dominican Republic in the 1970s (Imperato-McGinley, 1976; Money, 1976). Reports revealed that 38 villagers had a most unusual puberty. Because of their apparently female external genitalia, these youngsters were raised as girls. As commonly occurs with other problems of prenatal sexual differentiation, development seemed to proceed normally until puberty, when the expected appearance of secondary sexual characteristics does not happen. Yet in the case of DHT deficiency, these adolescent "girls" began to develop male secondary sexual characteristics. Their clitorises enlarged significantly and turned into penises. This condition was referred to in the Dominican Republic as *guevedoce*, which literally means "penis at 12." They were also referred to as *machi-hembra*, "first woman, then man." Apparently at puberty the increased secretion of testosterone from the newly descended testes is sufficient to trigger an external masculine appearance. An interesting aspect of this study is that these individuals reported that they had never felt fully comfortable with their "assigned" feminine sex and had experienced ambivalence about the female gender roles in which they were raised.

A Case of Genital Mutilation in Infancy

Some highly convincing data support the idea that one can learn a gender identity different from one's biological sex and that in some cases the adjustment is very successful. An interesting example of this occurred in 1965.

Money and Tucker (1975) relate the story of a couple who took their healthy seven-month-old twin sons to their doctor to be circumcised, resulting in an unfortunate accident:

The physician elected to use an electric cauterizing needle instead of a scalpel to remove the foreskin of the twin who chanced to be brought to the operating room first. When the baby's foreskin didn't give on the first try, or on the second, the doctor stepped up the current. On the third try, the surge of heat from the electricity literally cooked the baby's penis. Unable to heal, the penis dried up, and in a few days sloughed off completely, like the stub of an umbilical cord. (91-92)

The parents were, of course, devastated. A local plastic surgeon referred them to the Johns Hopkins University Medical Center at about the same time that the couple saw a television program about transsexuality (a topic considered later) and the counseling and surgery for such a gender transition at Johns Hopkins. By the time of their initial consultation, the infant was already 15 months old. Was it too late for this baby to begin anew as a girl? The medical psychologist involved, Dr. John Money, thought it definitely was not too late and said that the parents had until the child was 30 months old to make this difficult decision.

The mother and father decided to proceed. Several operations were required. The boy's testicles were removed, his urethra repositioned, and his scrotum was fashioned into an anatomical structure resembling a vagina. Female external genitalia could be created surgically, and later hormone supplements would feminize "her" body into a feminine form. Of course, conception and pregnancy were out of the question, but she could become a fully adequate and supportive mother to an adopted child.

In 1997 (Colapinto, 1997) the case was reported thoroughly. It became known as the case of "John/Joan," and it turned out that this individual *never* felt comfortable in the feminine role he was given for the first 15 years of his life. Colapinto depicts Dr. Money as an assertive and somewhat dogmatic researcher who was not always kind, open, and honest with John and his family. Apparently, John knew from his earliest memories that he was not a girl, and he did not have any of the traditional interests of girls. He felt odd and was abusively taunted by his male playmates while growing up.

As puberty approached, a decision had to be made about giving John estrogen supplements and surgery to create a vaginal "pouch" inside his "vagina." John took the estrogen pills (irregularly) and developed small, rudimentary breasts, but he and his parents refused the genital surgery. At the age of 14, "Joan" stopped living as a girl and began to dress like a boy. In 1980 "Joan" had her slightly developed breasts removed, and plastic surgeons fashioned a penis; since that time "Joan" has been "John." But the terrible psychological problems of his past continue to haunt him well into adulthood.

We share this story with you to demonstrate that while chromosomal, anatomical, and physiological aspects of sex and gender identity are powerful factors in how we grow up as boys and girls, the process also strongly depends on the psychosocial environment and the nature of support or reinforcement one receives for gender-related behaviors. "John/Joan's" story is a compelling example of the importance of an interaction among biological, psychological, and social ways of thinking about gender.

KLINEFELTER'S SYNDROME AND TURNER'S SYNDROME

So far we have examined instances of abnormal sexual differentiation and some of the problems associated with having physical characteristics that do not correspond to XX and XY sex chromosomal designations. In other types of chromosomal disorders a different problem occurs. In Klinefelter's syndrome, a genetic male has an extra X sex chromosome, creating 47 chromosomes instead of 46, with an XXY sex chromosome configuration. Its prevalence is approximately 1 in every 500 live male births, but this condition is typically not diagnosed until adulthood. This male has testes and all normal internal and external sexual anatomy. However, testosterone production is significantly reduced and the testes produce no sperm; the man is sterile and often impotent. Testosterone injections can often increase sexual interest and restore potency (Kolodny, Masters, & Johnson, 1979).

In Turner's syndrome, the Y sex chromosome is missing; the affected individual has 45 chromosomes and only one sex chromosome (the X). This female's ovaries do not form properly, but her external genitalia are normal. She has a uterus and fallopian tubes. A characteristic constellation of signs accompany Turner's syndrome: infertility, absence of menstruation, shortness of stature, unusual facial appearance, and heart and kidney anomalies. Often the condition is not diagnosed until adolescence when the girl does not start to menstruate or experience the normal adolescence growth spurt. Turner's syndrome has an incidence of 1 in 2500 live female births.

HERMAPHRODITISM AND PSEUDOHERMAPHRODITISM

Hermaphrodites are extraordinarily rare; the exact prevalence of this highly unusual abnormality in sexual differentiation is not known. They are born with both ovarian and testicular tissue (Fig. 3-6). Some have one gonad of each type, and others

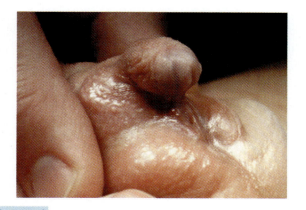

FIGURE 3-6   Hermaphroditism. Both internal and external sexual and reproductive structures of women and men are present to some degree. External genitalia are an anatomical "blend" of female and male structures.

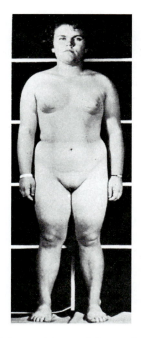

FIGURE 3-7   Female born with pseudohermaphroditism.

have gonads that combine the two types of tissues. The internal sexual anatomy of hermaphrodites is confused: most have a uterus, and some have a fallopian tube on one side of the body with a vas deferens and/or epididymis on the other side. In some instances male and female internal anatomical structures develop on both sides (Parker, 1998).

Pseudohermaphroditism, an abnormality in sexual differentiation, refers to a mismatch between an individual's genetic sex and the development and appearance of external genitalia, such as in the fetally androgenized female discussed above. The prevalence of this anomaly is estimated to be one in every 1000 live births (Green & Green, 1965) (Fig. 3-7).

Differences in Male and Female Human Brains

In recent years much research has investigated whether the brains of women and men are identical or perhaps different in some ways. This can be a complicated subject. If there are differences, are they consistent and significant? If there are consistent, significant anatomical differences, are they reflected functionally in the ways men and women think, emote, or behave? Another crucial issue would be the meaning of any observed anatomical and/or physiological differences in male and female brains. Such information would have to be assessed within the context of the psychosocial environments in which brains function. According to Kolb and Whishaw (1996), there are important sex-related differences in how the cerebral cortex is organized in women and men.

Since the 19th century we have been aware of consistent, measurable differences in the size and weight of the brains of adult human men and women. But when we correct for differences in body size, the sex differences are much less obvious (Peters, 1991; Ankney, 1992) or not even worth mentioning (Gould, 1981). Brain size differences have not been found to be very large or important.

Neuroanatomists have examined several specific areas in the brain to look for any measurable, consistent differences between men and women. They have examined the cerebral hemispheres, the hypothalamus (whose importance is explained in the next two chapters), and the corpus callosum (the thick band of nerve fibers connecting the left and right cerebral hemispheres). No large, consistent differences have been found in the gross anatomical structures of the brains of women and men. It remains to be seen whether there are functional differences in these areas, however. For example, verbal abilities seem to be localized primarily in the left hemisphere, and women tend to perform better on tests of these skills. Spatial abilities seem to be localized primarily in the right hemisphere, and men tend to perform better on tests of these abilities. While such performance differences might seem clear, any anatomical differences are not. Kolb and Whishaw suggest that six possible factors account for sex differences in neurological functioning: "(1) differential brain organization, (2) hormonal effects on cerebral function, (3) genetic sex-linkage, (4) maturation rate, (5) environment, and (6) preferred cognitive mode" (p. 227). Clearly it's risky to attribute behavioral differences between women and men to differences in brain structure.

Sex Hormones, Sexual Feelings, and Sex Drive

A final issue of gender as a biological construct concerns the extent to which sex drive, sexual inclinations, and sexual feelings are associated with sex hormone levels in women and men. This question directly confronts stereotyped differences in sex drive between women and men. One stereotype regards men as "ever-ready" sexually—that men are always thinking about sex, exploring sexual opportunities, enjoying sexual interactions, and planning the next encounter. This stereotype may be entirely inaccurate, but one should ask if there is anything behind it.

In contrast, the stereotypes about the sex drive of women are different. Folk beliefs suggest women are not as erotically motivated, nor are their world views supposed to be quite so geared toward frequent intercourse and orgasm. Different attitudes are present at different times, however, such as the Victorian notion that women were a threat to a man's self-control, as we saw in the last chapter. Whether these stereotypes have any truth behind them cannot be determined conclusively. The estrogen levels in a woman's bloodstream and the testosterone levels in a man's bloodstream clearly are important. Still, are sex drive and the desire for sexual intercourse and orgasm tightly tied to the nature and amount of sex hormones in women and men? Is it that straightforward?

While we recognize the importance of biological and hormonal factors, we must at the same time remember that even as biological beings we function in a psychosocial environment. Does the presence of testosterone in men create a "predisposition" to perceive sexually "eroticized" environments, while psychosocial factors influence whether such perceptions actually occur? Although there are no simple answers to these questions, we do know much about the impact of sex hormones in men and women. Note, however, that much of this research was done with animals. Indeed, virtually every biological aspect of human sexuality has been explored in other species as well, and what we have learned shows there is a common heritage among many animals in the evolutionary process.

Sexual desire in men is clearly related to levels of testosterone, but, interestingly, arousal is not (Wallen, 1995). For example, males with very low levels of testosterone become sexually aroused promptly when shown erotic materials (Kwan et al., 1976; Bancroft et al., 1974). These men do not say that their erections are especially enjoyable, however, nor do they seem motivated after arousal to pursue sexual activity (masturbatory or with someone else). In other words, arousal seems unrelated to hormone levels, while motivation is. The same phenomenon occurs in women. Sexual arousal in women is independent of the amount of circulating estrogen in the bloodstream, and the capacity to become sexually aroused seems unrelated to where a woman is in her menstrual cycle (Slob, Erneste, & van der Werff ten Bosch, 1990). Nonetheless, a woman's desire to *act* on her sexual feelings clearly fluctuates throughout the menstrual cycle. Becoming sexually aroused and desiring to act on that arousal are not the same thing.

In other words, there is a very real and important difference in the cyclicity with which sex hormones are secreted in women and men, and this difference has a measurable effect on what is commonly called "sex drive" (Fig. 3-8). That term is usually used to refer to a person's inclinations to behave in a sexual way. Males have a fairly constant level of testosterone that leads to a fairly constant sensitivity to erotic cues and desire to act on them. The words "compulsive" and "driven" are

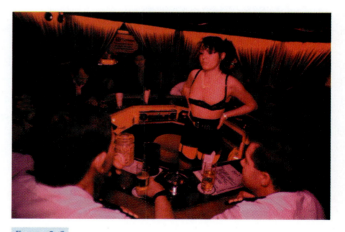

Figure 3-8 Erotic stimuli are reliably effective in increasing sexual motivation among men. In women, however, fluctuating hormone levels are more clearly related to feelings of sexual interest and inclination.

Research Highlight

ANATOMICAL AND GENETIC CORRELATES OF HOMOSEXUALITY

Because one's sex has a clear genetic foundation, many people wonder whether differences in gender roles and gender identity also have a biological basis. Homosexuality is a controversial case in point. The causes of homosexuality have been investigated for a long time. Many years ago Dr. Cornelia Wilbur (1964) suggested that a homosexual orientation in adulthood derives from the psychosocial characteristics of the family in which one is raised, particularly one's relationship with parents. Fathers of children who eventually self-identified as homosexuals were supposedly passive, hostile, indifferent, weak men, apparently seen as ineffectual compared to their wives. Since Wilbur's original speculations, research has not supported her claims, and today research is more biological in its focus.

Recent publications on possible biological causes of homosexuality have raised public and scientific debate. This research offers a good opportunity to evaluate the validity and reliability of different investigative approaches to this subject. As clear as the claims of these research studies might seem to some, there are some serious problems in accepting them without question and in widely generalizing their findings.

In 1991, Dr. Simon LeVay, a neuroanatomist at the Salk Institute, examined a tiny part of the brain called the hypothalamus, far below the surface of the cerebral hemispheres. The hypothalamus is near the center of the brain and has long been known to be involved in many individual- and species-supporting behaviors, such as eating, drinking, aggressive behavior, and sexual motivation and behavior. It is the size of your smallest fingernail and is composed of many separate clumps of nerve cells called *nuclei*. Dr. LeVay was examining a structure referred to as INAH3 (the third interstitial nucleus of the anterior hypothalamus). The exact functions of this tiny clump of nerve cells are not clearly understood.

Dr. LeVay inspected this area in 19 gay men and one bisexual man who had all died of AIDS. He examined the same area in 16 heterosexual men, six of whom had died of AIDS, and in six women who identified themselves as heterosexual. Dr. LeVay discovered that this specific area of the hypothalamus was two to three times larger in heterosexual men than in homosexual men. The difference was large and consistent in this sample of subjects. However, LeVay pointed out that it was extremely difficult to find the borders of this tiny nucleus of nerve cells and that in many cases it was a poorly defined scattering of neurons whose size was difficult to accurately determine (LeVay, 1991). These data became the focus of much controversy and discussion about the scientific and societal implications. Many people in the gay community claimed that these findings "proved" that people are born gay or heterosexual, and that one's sexual orientation is not a purposeful choice.

Some basic issues must be considered before LeVay's results and interpretations can be accepted as consistent and convincing. According to Dr. William Byne, director of the neuroanatomy laboratory of neuropsychiatric disease at New York's Mount Sinai Medical Center, "A general problem with this work is that there have been dozens and dozens of reports of sex differences in the human brain since the middle of the last century. But not a single one of these has been corroborated, except for the one that men tend to have slightly larger brains than women." Byne notes that there are sex differences in virtually every organ of the body, but it is very difficult to be specific about what these differences mean (cited in Finn, 1996).

In addition, LeVay's data might possibly have been affected by the fact that many of his subjects had AIDS. As well, the differences LeVay reported may have been attributable to some other, still unexamined factor. For example, Byne notes that many men who die of AIDS experience some shrinkage of their testicles before they die. Animal experiments have shown that hormones from gonads can affect the size of several different nuclei in the hypothalamus, but the possible effects of diminished testosterone were not examined in this research.

Our goal here is to consider the validity of LeVay's controversial findings and the possibility of other explanations for the observed differences between heterosexual and homosexual men. Any research findings should be interpreted with caution, as one should think critically about the nature of scientific research. There has been no large-scale attempt to replicate LeVay's research, and the small sample size should encourage caution about the validity of his findings.

Similarly debatable data were published in 1993 by the National Institutes of Health (NIH) about a possible genetic basis of male homosexuality. The NIH research indicated a "correlation" between a particular region of the X sex chromosome and male homosexual gender orientation. Again, we must be cautious interpreting these data. For example, this report does not identify a specific gene on the X chromosome that supposedly determines gender orientation or indicate that this chromosome region accounts for all instances of male homosexuality.

These studies and others demonstrate the recent interest in exploring the biological foundations of sexuality, which likely has a role together with psychosocial influences.

often used for this aspect of male endocrine function (Wallen, 1995, p. 75). Something very different happens in women, whose cycles of fluctuating estrogen levels relate to a changing sex drive. In general for women, through less of their cycle does the idea of having sex seem especially pleasurable, and they may, therefore, seek intercourse less often. Wallen (1995) makes this point clearly: ". . . peak sexual desire does not differ between men and women; what differs is how consistently they experience intense sexual desire" (Wallen, 1995, p. 75).

This important difference probably affects how women and men daily look at the world. Because women do not generally desire sexual intercourse or other sexual expression as constantly as men, they are thought to more carefully evaluate mating opportunities and the assets of someone with whom they might have intercourse and conceive a child. In other words, women might be more aware of mating alternatives and their potential outcomes. Chapter 7 discusses this subject in terms of developmental issues of adults. Men, in contrast, experience relatively constant levels of testosterone with an accompanying higher level of sexual interest and sensitivity to erotic cues. This basic biological/hormonal difference between men and women is thought to significantly affect gender roles and behaviors.

Understanding gender as a biological construct, the focus of this section, is essential for a clear understanding of the psychological and social aspects of maleness and femaleness, the focus of the next section: gender as a *psychological construct.*

GENDER AS A PSYCHOLOGICAL CONSTRUCT

Just as basic to our maleness and femaleness as our anatomy is how we interpret the meaning of our sex in the psychosocial arena. What does it mean to be a man or a woman? How do we learn gender roles? Who or what reinforces our behavior for

acting in a "gender appropriate" manner? How and why are we stigmatized for not acting in a "gender appropriate" manner? All of these psychological issues are affected by our social environment, as we will see later on. These psychological questions involve our self-concept and the feelings of adequacy and self-esteem that arise from our self-concept. This complicated process, often called **gender role typing,** is the developmental process of how we come to think about ourselves as one sex or the other and the congruence or incongruity we feel between our biological sex and our gender identity.

How and When Do Children Learn Gender Roles?

Children begin to learn gender roles between the ages of 3 and 6 years of age. The process is gradual and involves becoming aware of how the social environment regards the actions of men and women. Generally, the more intelligent the child, the more rapid the gender role learning (Papalia & Olds, 1995). It can be surprising to see how quickly and uncritically children at this age make conventional generalizations about what men and women are "supposed" to act like. According to Haugh, Hoffman, & Cowan (1980), 3-year-old children used the words "big," "mad," and "strong" to describe boy babies and "little," "scared," and "weak" to describe girl babies. Unfortunately, gender stereotypes can foster beliefs about the restricted aptitudes and abilities of boys and girls. Bem (1976) emphasizes that the process of learning gender roles in early childhood may foster the development of adults who are unsure of themselves in tasks supposedly done better by the other gender. The effects of early gender-role learning can be far-reaching.

The educational environment seems especially important in gender role learning. Fagot et al. (1992), Fagot & Hagen (1991), and Huston (1983) reported that even in preschool (typically ages 3 to 5), children are rewarded for behaving in a way congruent with their sex and may be punished for behaving in ways associated with the opposite sex. The same is often true in daily interactions between parents and their children.

With pressures like these on children this young, not to mention those in elementary and middle school, one can see the educational arena is especially important in gender-role learning. Rewards and punishments powerfully affect the gender-role learning process, even though some behaviors are also affected by biology (e.g., boys tend to behave more aggressively than girls at this age, apparently a result of the actions of testosterone).

The family and psychosocial environment are apparently more important than biological factors in the development of gender roles (Fig. 3-9). Even though our society now supposedly is more flexible in its expectations of males and females than in the past, old stereotypes die hard. Lytton and Romney (1991) analyzed almost 200 studies of the socialization of boys and girls between 1952 and 1987. Their findings are surprising to some. Most parents still try to influence their sons to act in independent, assertive ways, while they encourage their daughters very differently, though girls are not observed or monitored as closely as their brothers. Parents didn't seem as concerned about who their daughters played with, the games they played, or their clothing. Aggressive behavior was viewed as more appropriate for boys, and expressions of warmth were more acceptable for girls. This leads us to wonder whether the personal, educational, and occupational gains women have made in the last generation are reflected in child-rearing practices. Has there been any diluting of the old stereotypes?

Bronstein (1988) found clear differences in how fathers related to their sons and daughters. Their interactions with their daughters had more "social" flavor; they were also more encouraging, loving, and accepting. In contrast, fathers' interactions with their sons involved more regulating and supervising of their behavior; fathers focused more on their sons' intellectual achievements than on their daughters' cognitive abilities.

One American family in four now is a single-parent female-headed household, and researchers have studied how this affects the learning of gender roles. Katz (1987) found that these children are far less influenced by conventional gender stereotypes than children reared in two-parent households, presumably because a single female parent often tries to act as both mother and father. Children modeling this maternal behavior, therefore, are less likely to associate specific tasks, achievements, or emotional styles with either men or women, and their behavior and feelings reflect both traditional masculine and feminine traits. The term **androgyny** refers to this compatible blend of male and female traits, a topic we consider later on.

With more single-parent families and more two-paycheck families today, children are more likely than children only a generation ago to see their parent(s) doing more and different things in maintaining the home and caring for the family. Older ways of thinking about what men and women do and how they participate in child rearing are changing, but only very slowly. Children of both genders see parents of both genders doing many tasks which would probably puzzle their grandparents. Men cook and clean and nurture little boys with scraped knees. Mothers shout at soccer matches and lubricate the chain on the trail bike. Generally, by adolescence most children have been exposed to traditional gender roles, as well as unique family circumstances and expectations.

As children grow up, they observe same- and other-sex adults behaving in ways that often confirm traditional gender-role expectations. These observations happen constantly and exert powerful influence as children begin to behave in ways they interpret as expected of them. This process of observational learning (Bandura, 1965) seems to play a major role in the process of learning to think of ourselves, behave, and monitor our behavior in accordance with what we think our society expects. In other words, we learn not only by doing but also by watching as well.

Observing adult men and women and seeing the consequences of their behaviors provides developing children with consistent models of maleness and femaleness. This social learning process is a key part of the psychosocial approach to developing gender identity. Simply stated, adults are important models in gender-role typing. According to Albert Bandura, the developer of **social learning theory,** much of children learning about behaving in social situations is vicarious. Much of gender-role learning thus takes place quietly and covertly, based on long-term observations in many different social settings.

There is one other interesting aspect of male gender role development in traditional nuclear families. Although, as Bandura suggests, little boys are aware of and sensitive to the behaviors of their fathers or other men, often the father is away from the home a great deal and the mother or other women do most of the childrearing in the child's early years. In this scenario, is there enough time and meaningful contact between the young boy and his father and other males for male roles to be learned vicariously (Craib, 1987)? Even more interesting is, in terms of social learning theory, what is the impact of a long-term, close, constant contact with only the mother? These questions may be tangential to sexuality issues, but they are

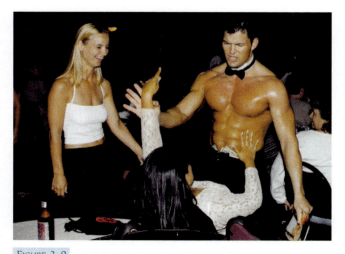

FIGURE 3-9   Until the last few decades, female gender roles did not generally allow or condone observing sexually provocative male dancing.

significant for human growth and development issues. The family situation described above tends to create another distinction between traditional masculine and feminine roles, so that even young children may gradually come to think the man's life and work are outside of the home, while the woman's life and world are inside of the home. Even though more women work full-time outside the home now than at any time in history, most housekeeping and child rearing is still done by women.

Gender Roles, Self-Concept, and Self-Esteem

Gender and self-concept are closely related. Just as we gradually develop a sense of maleness and femaleness, part of this development affects how we think of ourselves more globally. The sum of all our thoughts and feelings about ourselves is called our **self-concept.** When a person thinks of "I" or "me," he or she is actually referring to his or her self-concept, and gender is a large part of this. Because we have observed role models and become sensitive to how society expects us to act as males and females, our self-evaluations in these terms are an important part of the self-concept. This situation can become rather complicated. For example, our self-concept is in some ways based on a personal comparison between the person we are and the person we would like to see ourselves becoming. Our most honest, here-and-now view of ourselves, including both abilities and inabilities, is called the **perceived self;** it is our personal awareness of all that we are physically, intellectually, socially, and, perhaps, spiritually. On the other hand, most of us also have a private mental picture of who we would like to be when we are older, more mature, more developed, or perhaps more at peace with ourselves—in other words, our future best self. This is usually called the **ideal self.** When we feel we are making progress from the perceived self toward the ideal self, we usually experience feelings of self-esteem or self-respect. Sometimes, however, we do not see ourselves making progress towards our ideal selves, and this may lower our self-esteem. In summary, there are two key points here. First, our gender identity is often an important part of our self-concept. Second, as we grow and develop and begin to feel more at home in our gender roles, this has an important and positive impact on our self-esteem.

How we conduct ourselves in social situations depends to some degree on our gender identity, self-concept, and self-esteem. In other words, our social behaviors are related to our thoughts about ourselves as women and men, and we "regulate" our actions accordingly. We believe there is also a "sexual self-esteem," which involves feeling comfortable with our gender identity (whatever it might be) and being honest and open with others about those feelings. It can take a long time to reach this point in one's development, but we feel it is an important personal goal worth working hard to attain.

In addition to Bandura's social learning theory, there are other ways of thinking about how children learn gender roles. For example, **cognitive-developmental theory** asserts that as children grow up and interact with their peers, they receive af-

firmation of their roles as little girls or little boys after having come to understand their gender at about 4 years of age. These self-reinforcing contacts with other children help create a mental "model" of maleness and femaleness, and the child then consciously behaves in a way congruent with her or his gender. At the same time, in Freud's theory, children at this age identify with their same-sex parent. This identification and the selective validation of the peer group are at the heart of cognitive-developmental theory.

Still another theoretical approach to how children learn to behave as males or females is called **gender-schema theory.** The word "schema" refers to a set of beliefs about something that is generally accepted in a society. Gender schemas are common, sometimes stereotypical ways of thinking about the characteristics, abilities, and interests of women and men. A gender schema acts like a lens through which children observe and interpret how women and men behave and interact. In this way, children monitor the degree to which their own actions fit with what they observe and perhaps change their behaviors to become more in line with what they have learned is common and "normal."

The Emergence of Masculine Roles

Because biological, psychological, and social factors all interact as little boys learn about maleness and traditional ideas of masculinity, their development has many influences, many of which center on gender stereotypes. One of the more persistent of these concerns supposed differences between males and females with respect to interest and excellence in sports. Sports are commonly considered a metaphor or model for life in general—a way of thinking about our daily activities according to the rules of games. The development of male roles has been explored within the context of organized sports activities, although it is now incorrect to say that only boys engage in highly physical, competitive sports.

For many, masculine identity is profoundly affected by participation in organized athletics in childhood and adolescence. Why does this experience seem to perpetuate the physical, competitive aspects of developing male identity? First, family influences often "push" young boys in the direction of organized athletics, while they give girls less encouragement to participate in sports. Traditional male stereotypes seem to foster the belief that a young boy's opinion of himself can be helped or hurt by success or failure in early sports activities. They can have good or bad effects. On the one hand, it might seem that sport isn't the best way to establish enduring self-worth. On the other hand, it seems beneficial that more females now can participate in the same games that fostered the masculine stereotype in the past: soccer, baseball, and even football (Messner, 1990) (Fig. 3-10). Note too that only a minority of youngsters in high school participate on organized athletic teams. An interesting unanswered question involves what the consequences are for a developing sense of masculinity for boys if they compete with girls in sports and lose to them. But of course, our understanding of masculinity involves much more than can be found in the games boys and men play.

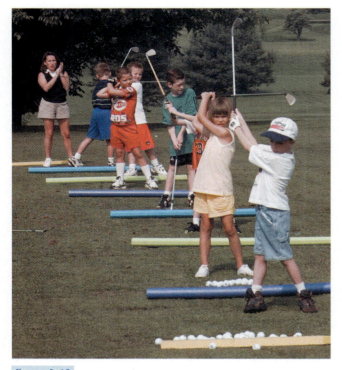

FIGURE 3-10   Sex roles for little girls and boys are more likely today to involve participation in a variety of competitive athletic activities. In the past, girls were rarely encouraged to participate in sports.

Another aspect of masculinity and the development of masculine roles is not discussed often: the relationship among self-esteem, masculinity, and body image in men. Interestingly, much attention has been given the equivalent subject in women, by both scholars and the popular press, but little has been written about the supposed physical manifestations of masculinity. Mishkind, Rodin, Silberstein, and Striegel-Moore (1986), who studied how body image may be related to self-esteem and a sense of masculinity in men, report that 95% of the college men they surveyed expressed explicit feelings of dissatisfaction with some part of their bodies; most often they were dissatisfied with their chests, waists, and overall weight. Many men surveyed said that they thought a well-defined musculature was attractive and desirable (Tucker, 1982). This type of physique is sometimes called "mesomorphic." While women express ambivalence about the attractiveness of this body type, both women and men tend to describe muscular males in positive terms and to use negative terms for skinny or overweight men (Wells & Siegel, 1961).

Traditionally masculinity is characterized as "strong," "powerful," or "effective." Other terms sometimes used are "aggressive," "independent," "dominant," "self-confident," and "unemotional" (Rosenkrantz, Vogel, Bee, Broverman, & Broverman, 1968). Such traditional notions are thus based on common stereotypes of physical appearance and behavior. The significant correlation between men's self-esteem and the way they evaluate their bodies has been known for years (Lerner,

Karabenick, & Stuart, 1973). Men generally focus on two aspects of physical appearance when considering their attractiveness: the face and the general muscular physique (Franzoi & Shields, 1984). The desire to become more attractive, therefore, involves a range of different strategies. A man can change his haircut, grow or remove facial hair, choose different eyeglass frames or change to contact lenses, or even undergo plastic surgery. Changes in general physique usually involve exercise and dieting or both. Note that most of the research on masculinity has used college-age subjects, and it is not as well known how older and perhaps more mature men think about these issues.

Another issue involved in masculinity is varying ways in which different subcultures perceive the appearance of a man's body. Kleinberg (1980, cited in Mishkind, Rodin, Silberstein, & Striegel-Moore, 1986) notes that the gay male subculture puts a premium on a highly attractive physical appearance that includes physique, clothing, grooming and hygiene, and specific facial features that are considered attractive. Miskind, Rodin, Siberstein, & Striegel-Moore (1986) found that this population of men, because of this premium, were more likely to report dissatisfaction with their bodies. The gay men in their sample of collegiate respondents reported significantly more dissatisfaction with their general body build, waist, biceps, arms, and stomach (p. 555). Gay men also reported a greater gap than the heterosexual men in this sample between their actual body shape and their ideal body shape.

With so many subcultural and racial groups in our society and throughout the world, researchers have wondered whether the development of masculine traits is similar or different in different groups. An important example of a different conceptualization of masculinity in American society occurs among many African American young men. Harris (1995) believes that European American masculine norms emphasize the roles of provider, protector, and disciplinarian (p. 279). African American males who feel such roles are less relevant in their circumstances may develop a different set of masculine values and roles. For example, in some cases where limited educational opportunities have blocked full enfranchisement in a professional workforce, other ways of developing a sense of manhood are commonly pursued (Harris, 1995). A low-income, alienated social status often fosters a concept of masculinity emphasizing sexual promiscuity, toughness, thrill seeking, and violent interactions and confrontations with others (Harris, 1995, p. 280). Psychological attributes of this concept of masculinity include suppressing the expression of emotions, a suspicion of organized bureaucracies and authority figures, a need for peer acceptance, disrespect for feminine traits, overcompensatory masculinity, and the false belief that one is invulnerable.

Other problems occur with traditional masculine roles. For example, about half as many male college students as females seek counseling for personal problems, a relative difference about the same as in the adult population (Wills & DePaulo, 1991). Eisler & Blalock (1991) point out that the personal qualities necessary to seek help are incompatible with

On the Lighter Side

The stereotypes about traditional masculine values and behaviors have given rise to much modern humor and irony. In 1996, *Psychology Today* published a little piece called "Great Moments in American Masculinity," excerpted from Michael Kimmel's book, *Manhood in America: A Cultural History* (1996). Here are some selections (pp. 12-15):

1820: Henpecked husband Rip Van Winkle awakes from a 20-year nap and learns his wife has died. "When he found out," notes Kimmel, "a smile creeps across his face and he lives happily ever after, hanging out in front of the saloon."

1832: Henry Clay's declaration that "we are a nation of self-made men."

1840: During the presidential election campaign, challenger William Henry Harrison plays the "wimp card," portraying himself as a manly man—born in a log cabin and fond of hard cider—while casting aspersions on incumbent Martin Van Buren for his ruffled shirts and for installing indoor plumbing in the White House. Harrison wins but in an ironic coda catches pneumonia on the day of his inauguration when he manfully braves the weather sans overcoat despite record cold temperatures. He dies a month later.

1845: Henry David Thoreau ventures into Walden Woods and does his own Robert Bly initiation ceremonies. Thoreau dunks himself in Walden pond and barely contains his urge to devour a raw woodchuck. "If he could have," Kimmel quips, "he would have gone to the sweat lodge."

1860: The Civil War, with a manly metaphor—"brother fighting brother." The message: Events are experienced through masculinity. Shortly before the war's end, Confederate leader Jefferson Davis allegedly escapes from Richmond, which is surrounded by Union troops, by dressing as a woman.

1910: The Boy Scouts is founded "to rescue boys from the feminizing clutches of mothers and Sunday School teachers, and to get them out into the woods to learn how to be men."

1905—1915: Fed up with wimpy ministers and a bland Savior, the Muscular Christian movement reinvents Jesus as "a kind of religious Rambo." The movement emphasizes the Son of God's carpentry background and such macho Bible tales as Jesus kicking the money changer out of the temple.

1930: A Hollywood producer recommends that a budding actor named Marion Michael Morrison change his name to something less feminine. Morrison later becomes an icon under a macho, monosyllabic moniker: "John Wayne."

1936: Legendary social psychologist Lewis Terman invents the "M-F" scale, a behavioral checklist that alerts parents if their boys aren't turning out okay (i.e., heterosexual). Among the "danger" signs: boys who keep a diary or like to take baths.

1965: President Lyndon Johnson opts not to withdraw the American troops that JFK had sent to Vietnam, lest he be thought "less of a man than Kennedy."

1967: The hippie movement rejects the traditional view of masculinity, embracing long, flowing hair and clothing. Hit song: "Are You a Boy or Are You a Girl?"

1982: *Real Men Don't Eat Quiche* hits the best-seller list. Some men don't get the joke and mistake the book for a manifesto.

1991: Robert Bly's *Iron John* inspires thousands of men to head into the woods rediscovering their wild, "warrior selves."

1992: Bill Clinton becomes the first president with a dual-career marriage—and is promptly wimp-baited for having a successful, ambitious wife.

traditional notions of masculinity: being able to acknowledge having a personal problem and the desire to do something about it, a desire to "open up" to someone else, being able to admit personal vulnerabilities, and sensitivity to one's feelings and an ability to express them. Many men, however, do not have problems doing these things. These men, interestingly enough, often have a different difficulty: **gender role conflict.** This term refers to conflicting feelings about behaving in a way that does not conform to traditional gender stereotypes. This is a "damned if you do, damned if you don't" situation: there are problems with males not being able to ask for help, but a gender role conflict can occur for those who do. Indeed, Good & Mintz (1990) demonstrated that men who experience high levels of male gender role conflict are more likely to feel depressed and less likely to seek counseling services.

Some social observers claim there is a subtle, persistent desire among men to more clearly define their masculinity. Books have been published that address this uncertainty and ambivalence (i.e., Bly, 1990), and an almost adversarial dialog has emerged between contemporary feminists and men who feel they have been occupationally displaced by women. Lashmar (1996) notes that in Britain there are more women than men in the work force, and that in many areas women are surpassing the academic achievements of men. Inequality in pay between women and men in Britain and the United States is diminishing, and many of the traditional roles that once solidified a man's sense of himself are now often shared with women or undertaken exclusively by them: breadwinner, craftsman, parent, and soldier (p. 33). Plainly, the concept of masculinity is a more complex and fluid one now, more than in the history of Western societies.

Sociologists use the term **sociality** to refer to interpersonal attraction of a nonsexual nature, and this concept helps clarify other ways of thinking about masculinity. Developmentally, little boys usually first think about maleness as simply not being female, and they often actively suppress female qualities when more traditional male roles begin to emerge. Bird (1996) has shown that in same-sex interactions, men see emotional detachment as not only desirable but necessary, and reinforce one another accordingly. Even the most personal, meaningful, and emotional subjects are explored without much overt feeling. Although contemporary attitudes often tout more emotional men and suggest that modern women welcome this change, powerful peer pressures still influence men to maintain a traditional emotional reserve among themselves. Another male "virtue" prized by many men is competitiveness, and as emotional detachment is discouraged, competitiveness is encouraged and rewarded. The male respondents in Bird's (1996) interview study stated that a competitive outlook on work and play is a basic part of "non-femaleness." A final traditional masculine value according to Bird is **sexual objectification**, which refers to how men brag about gaining women's affections, usually sexual. Men often refer to women with words like "them," "other," or "girls" (Bird, 1996, p. 128)—like sex objects. Men also exhibit their competitiveness when seeking the attention or sexual favors of women who meet their peer group's notions of attrac-

tiveness. According to Connell (1992), these two male values comprise the basic attributes of maleness in our society today, at least among the college students who are usually the subjects in this research.

What happens if a man doesn't go along with his buddies in emotional detachment, competitiveness, or sexual objectification? Bird (1996) believes that he will be "pecked" to a lower status among his male friends. She maintains that most men comply with peer pressures to avoid this loss of masculine esteem. One of the respondents in Bird's study explained clearly:

> *there's always an assessment going on in the group. Always ... some guys will go along but wouldn't make a degrading comment about women themselves. But when some guy says something, because you want to be a member of the group, it becomes "Yeah." You follow the lead.*

—BIRD, 1996, 130

Because the men in this investigation were between 23 and 50 years of age and most in an academic community, these findings may not generalize fully to other segments of society.

As there are negative sanctions against men departing from those norms described above, males may also be viewed negatively for engaging in nurturant behaviors toward children, especially holding and caressing. Rane and Draper (1995) studied a large sample of mostly unmarried male and female undergraduates who were read stories depicting women and men engaging in loving, nurturant touching of young children. Interestingly, both male and female respondents rated males behaving in this way negatively and as unmasculine, while the women in the stories behaving in this way were rated very highly in terms of "goodness" and "social acceptance." Interestingly, at a time when men are trying to get more comfortable with their feelings, a large random sample of young people still viewed nurturant touching of young children by males as something they find uncomfortable (Fig. 3-11).

The Emergence of Feminine Roles

Feminine roles develop according to different rules involving very different variables. Remember that one of the interesting things about learning male roles is that young boys typically spend much of their time with women and therefore have limited time to observe male models and identify with them. The same generally cannot be said about young girls. Because they spend much time at home and school with primarily female role models, their gender-role typing is easier to understand. Carol Gilligan (1982) analyzes this situation and points out an important difference between males and females. Because boys begin to achieve a male identity through separation from their mothers, they are often intimidated by intimacy. In contrast, because girls begin to develop their female sex role through attachment to their mothers, they come to feel threatened by separation from those they love.

The psychosocial environment influences females just as it does males. We mentioned earlier that as children grow up,

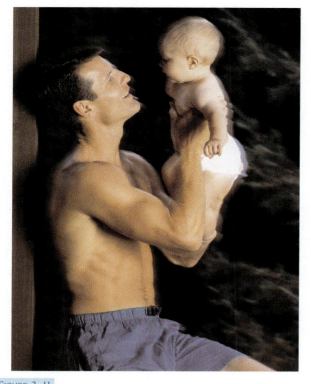

FIGURE 3-11   Many men today find it comfortable and enjoyable to spontaneously express their love and nurturance, although traditional masculine emotional control is still seen by many as very important.

The message of the research of Rosenzweig and Dailey (1991) is that women might experience special stresses when they perceive a need to behave in a traditional feminine gender role but don't feel inclined to do so. Indeed, anyone who feels compelled to behave inconsistently with conventional sex role stereotypes might feel uncomfortable about the need to conform to the norm. For example, we explored above how many men feel a need to be emotionally detached. It might therefore be stressful for a man to feel he should comfort an upset male friend. This situation would probably not be as troubling for a woman because nurturance is commonly attributed to femininity.

Gillespie and Eisler (1992) developed a "Feminine Gender Role Stress scale" to quantify and better understand those stresses women feel. This paper-and-pencil test assesses how women appraise the magnitude of various stressful situations, some of which conform to gender stereotypical expectations of women. These investigators identified five areas of stress in the responses to the questionnaire. Each is a focus of stress for women as they experience their female roles in their daily lives, and each can lead to feelings incompatible with what it stereotypically means to "be a woman" (Fig. 3-12):

1. fear of being involved in unemotional (unrewarding) relationships
2. fear of being/feeling physically unattractive
3. fear of victimization (personal safety)
4. fear of behaving assertively
5. fear of not being nurturant

they often see the "outside world" as a male arena and the "inside [the home] world" as a feminine arena, although this way of looking at things has changed much in recent years. When women explore (and excel in) the outside world, this involvement and success can involve some ambivalence.

Rosenzweig and Dailey (1991), who have studied women's gender roles outside and inside the home, report that it doesn't make much difference whether a woman sees herself as a masculine, a feminine, or an androgynous individual; the social contexts of work and home exert powerful pressures to conform to a traditional picture of femininity. Women in different jobs at a large Midwestern university answered a questionnaire that assessed their conformity with traditional gender role stereotypes for women. This sample scored relatively high in the masculine index (traits related to autonomy, assertiveness, and competitiveness), which was not surprising since these traits are often helpful for succeeding in employment outside of the home. At the same time these women felt keen pressures from their male counterparts to "behave like women" in occupational, social, and sexual situations despite their apparent masculine traits. This study serves to remind us that, despite an unambiguous female sexual identity, the psychosocial environment still exerts its expectations clearly. Yet this investigation does *not* tell us whether the felt need to conform to traditional female gender-role behaviors actually becomes manifest in the daily behaviors of these women.

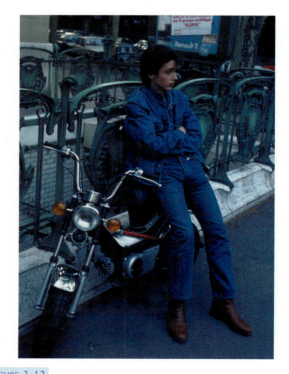

FIGURE 3-12   The traditional feminine gender role does not usually include such activities as motorcycle riding, and some women find it difficult to enjoy participating in such activities.

Although this list does not include all potential stressors in a woman's life, it shows common arenas of distress causing feelings of anxiety, fear, or inadequacy. In addition, there were significant differences in how women and men sized up these fears. These writers conclude, "For women who strongly adhere to feminine gender role imperatives, situations that signify interpersonal inadequacy may be particularly relevant to the self-concept and threatening to self-esteem" (Gillespie & Eisler, 1992, p. 435).

Women who appraise situations as threatening to their traditional feminine gender role frequently experience considerable stress, which can impact their health. Martz, Handley, and Eisler (1995) demonstrated that women with eating disorders report much more stress about conforming to conventional feminine gender roles than other women who do not, as measured on the Feminine Gender Role Stress scale. Such studies help clarify the relationship between common cultural values about femininity and body form and the development of eating disorders.

For women, feelings of psychological well-being and participation in full-time employment may interact in ways that lead to feelings of role overload. Many women who both work outside the home while still doing most of the domestic work in the home simply have too much to do, and sometimes they feel they cannot be both "good" mothers and wives. Recent research (Dennerstein, 1995) shows that there are positive effects for women who work outside the home while still feeling effective in their many different family roles. The drawbacks in this situation, however, may diminish the positive outcomes. If a woman's husband or significant other does not emotionally support her work outside the home and does not take his fair share of child care and home responsibilities, the woman is much less likely to feel a sense of personal adequacy and enjoyment in her work outside the home. It might be simplistic to say that this situation alone causes feelings of inadequacy or depression, but certainly women in this situation frequently experience role conflicts.

We will conclude this section by noting some interesting differences in how white men and African American men view traditional female roles, especially related to work outside the home. Blee and Tickamyer (1995) analyzed with a sociological perspective the longitudinal data collected between 1967 and 1981 in the National Longitudinal Surveys. Their analysis reveals clear differences between white and African American men in attitudes about women's traditional gender roles. Interestingly, there is no evidence that differences in the behaviors of these men's mothers might have led to these differences; they note, "While African American young men clearly grow up in different home environments than white young men, there is little in our analysis to suggest that these differences influence adult role attitudes" (Blee & Tickamyer, 1995, p. 29). They note that African American men are much more liberal in their thinking about working wives, possibly because they are more likely to have grown up in a household with a working wife/mother and, therefore, may better understand the practical nature of this situation. In contrast, young white men were more traditional in wanting their wives to stay home engaged in domestic tasks. This may explain only one reason for these different attitudes about women's gender roles; other factors remain to be explored. We raise the issue only because it is a good example of how an important psychosocial factor has effects that can be seen throughout society.

Androgyny

Our discussion of gender as a psychological construct has so far dwelt primarily on *differences* between women and men and how they experience their gender roles. Some people, however, seem to possess a blend of traditional masculine and feminine traits called "androgyny"—a word referring to both "male and female." Is it really possible to have the conventional traits of both sexes? What are the emotional, cognitive, and behavioral manifestations of androgyny? What do supposedly androgynous people say about it? Finally, can a person try to be or become androgynous, is it something that develops over time, or is it just there?

Sandra Bem (1974, 1976) believes that the healthiest adult personalities hold in equilibrium the best traditional gender traits of both women and men. Someone like this would be independent, in control, and assertive, while at the same time nurturant, empathetic, and caring. Bem suggests that androgynous individuals can evaluate their day-to-day social situations and interactions based on the fundamental attributes of those circumstances, instead of being bound by their masculine or feminine socialization experiences or the expectations of others because they are women and men. Several different concepts about androgyny have been explored. For example, Bem (1975) believes that androgynous individuals can evaluate some situations from a masculine perspective and other situations from a feminine perspective; this is called *situational flexibility.* Another approach to androgyny emphasizes the individual's ability to combine masculine and feminine perspectives in social situations; the term *integration* is used to describe this approach (Sedney, 1989). Finally, androgyny can also be thought of as a *transcendence* of the requirements and expectations of male and female gender roles (Sedney, 1989).

A validity test of these three ways of thinking about androgyny was undertaken by Vonk & Ashmore (1993). These investigators used questionnaires to examine whether subjects identified as androgynous would describe themselves in ways that supported one of these ways of conceptualizing androgyny. They found support only for the first view, that of situational flexibility. According to Vonk and Ashmore, integration and/or transcendence were not very apparent in the self-descriptive statements of these subjects. Perhaps, these writers suggest, androgyny is a more general capacity for role flexibility in daily life that many people possess in varying degrees (Fig. 3-13).

Writers have suggested that androgyny is a desirable personality attribute because androgynous people do not feel confined by a need to "act like men" or "act like women." Although this gender role flexibility may seem highly desirable, androgyny may not be an attainable or desirable attribute in all

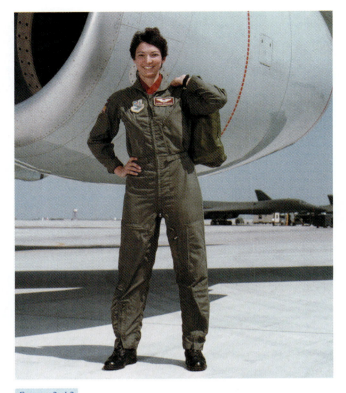

FIGURE 3-13 Androgynous individuals enjoy a happy blend of both traditional feminine and masculine characteristics and interests.

cultures. It is difficult to generalize about how androgynous individuals fit in our culture. Bem (1984) has softened her earlier enthusiasm for androgyny, suggesting that a fuller understanding of how gender differences might affect perceptions of the world is more important. For example, in societies with rigidly defined male and female roles (Saudi Arabia, Turkey, India, and parts of the United Kingdom), androgynous individuals might have problems "fitting in" with conventions for male and female behavior. Assertive, emotionally detached, independent women do not receive as much social support in a culture such as Iran. Similarly, emotional, empathetic, and submissive men do not meet expectations of male gender roles in a country like Jordan.

Transsexuality

> I was three or perhaps four years old when I realized that I had been born
> into the wrong body, and should really be a girl. I remember the moment
> well, and it is the earliest memory of my life.
>
> —JAN MORRIS, *CONUNDRUM,* 1974, 15

Jan Morris was born James Humphry Morris, who at an early age became aware that, in his case, traditional male and female biological, psychological, and social attributes had somehow become confused. As we grow up, we all try to find out "who we are," but an awareness like Morris's is unusual. Because much of our socialization is based on learning to recognize our gender roles, circumstances like this would be problematic for someone like James Morris. Eventually, Morris had a "sex change operation," more accurately termed sex reassignment surgery.

Morris was not the first to feel a major mismatch between physical sex and psychological awareness of gender. Tennis player Renee Richards, who competed first as a man and later, following sex reassignment surgery, as a woman is perhaps more widely known (Fig. 3-14). However, Morris was among the first to write with candor and self-awareness about what is called **transsexuality.** Just as conventional gender-role typing takes place early in life and rarely changes thereafter, the same is true of transsexuality. Once an individual is certain of a fundamental incompatibility between his or her gender identity and biological sex, the feeling won't go away. No one knows exactly how transsexuality develops or even when it develops, although Morris's story suggests that it takes place early in life.

Transsexuals want sex change operations and usually desire intimate sexual behavior. People do not *become* transsexuals by having gender reassignment surgery. Long before surgery or living as a member of the other sex, the individual is certain about how he or she feels and wants to look. Such individuals are constantly aware that their external sexual anatomy and physical appearance are not congruent with how they think of themselves and how they experience their psychosocial environment. Transsexual individuals do not think of themselves as homosexuals.

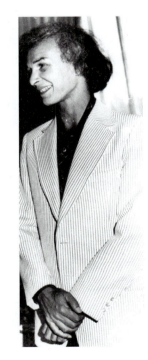

FIGURE 3-14 Dr. Richard Raskin at a dinner party in 1975. Dr. Raskin later became Dr. Renee Richards.

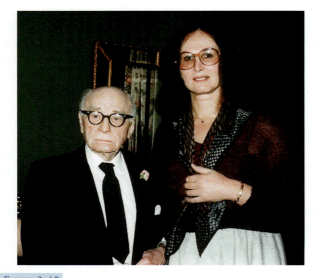

FIGURE 3-15   Dr. Harry Benjamin on his 80th birthday with Dr. Renee Richards.

Transsexuality is also called "gender dysphoria," which means something like "having bad feelings about one's gender." Usually, transsexuals go through a long period of counseling before gender reassignment surgery, which is irreversible. This medical treatment may last several years (Cole, Emory, Huang, & Meyer, 1994), during which time psychological and psychiatric assessments are made and "real life" simulations take place and are evaluated. Hormone therapy helps create some of the desired secondary sexual characteristics. Finally, surgery is done after this period of usually mandatory evaluation.

To aid individuals in gender reassignment counseling and surgery, a document was drafted at the Sixth International Gender Dysphoria Symposium in 1979, which has been revised since. Because many people are considering this surgery, a statement was formalized for professional standards of care for those seeking hormonal and surgical treatment. In 1979 it was estimated that 3000 to 6000 people had been hormonally and surgically sex-reassigned and that as many as 30,000 to 60,000 American citizens thought of themselves as candidates for the procedure.

HISTORY OF THE STUDY OF TRANSSEXUALISM

The physician Harry Benjamin, one of the six founding members of The Society for the Scientific Study of Sex (Fig. 3-15), made significant contributions in this area of study. Benjamin is best known for his pioneering studies on gender dysphoria, which initiated the careful study of transsexuality. He studied his first ten cases between 1938 and 1953 (Schaefer & Wheeler, 1995). Benjamin's patients used the same words to describe themselves as transsexuals use today, speaking of being "trapped" in a body of the other gender. Virtually all of his transsexuals came to him self-diagnosed; in the 1930s and 1940s virtually nothing had been written about this subject,

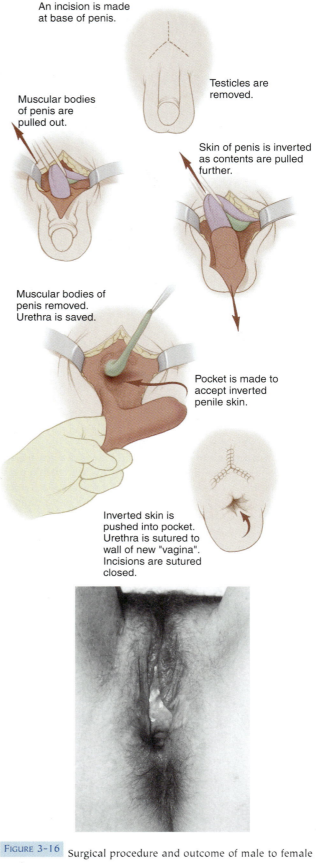

An incision is made at base of penis.

Testicles are removed.

Muscular bodies of penis are pulled out.

Skin of penis is inverted as contents are pulled further.

Muscular bodies of penis removed. Urethra is saved.

Pocket is made to accept inverted penile skin.

Inverted skin is pushed into pocket. Urethra is sutured to wall of new "vagina". Incisions are sutured closed.

FIGURE 3-16   Surgical procedure and outcome of male to female gender reassignment surgery.

and these patients couldn't have read descriptions matching their own feelings and inclinations. Alfred Kinsey referred three individuals he had interviewed to Benjamin in the late 1940s; he had never encountered anything like what they had told him and was truly perplexed. Benjamin was among the first to administer hormonal treatments and make referrals for surgery, which was not performed in the United States early in his career. Benjamin was a perceptive, sensitive, caring physician (Schaefer & Wheeler, 1995).

SEX REASSIGNMENT SURGERY

Sex reassignment surgery is complicated and requires a highly experienced medical team. Historically, more men than women sought this surgery, but in recent years the numbers of women and men having it have become more equal. The male-to-female procedure is usually a one-stage operation, while the female-to-male procedure requires at least two surgeries.

In the male-to-female operation (Fig. 3-16), the penis and testes are removed. The tissues of the penis are used to construct a vaginal canal, and the scrotal tissue is fashioned into labia. Sensory nerves from the penis are moved inside the new vagina, and many transsexuals report that they experience sexual arousal and orgasm. Removing the testes eliminates the primary source of male hormones, aiding in the eventual development of a more female body when estrogen is also given.

In the female-to-male operation (Fig. 3-17), the internal female reproductive organs are removed, including the ovaries, uterus, and fallopian tubes. Breast reduction surgery may be necessary. Because the woman has already been using male hormones, the clitoris is enlarged; the urethra is now channeled through it. With tissues from the lower abdomen and the labia, a penis-like organ and scrotum are created. This new penis has no nerve or blood supply and therefore cannot become erect; penile implants are used, and sometimes artificial testicles are placed in the new scrotum. Tissue from the clitoris is moved to the base of the new penis, allowing feelings of arousal and in some cases orgasm. Most transsexuals who have had the surgery feel gratified that finally their biology matches their feelings and perceptions of their "real" gender.

What happens to transsexuals who have had sex change operations? Abramowitz (1986) notes that about two-thirds of those who undergo the surgery are either improved or highly satisfied. Some estimates are as high as about 75% (Pauly, 1981). Most transsexuals think the tremendous changes brought about by this program of diagnosis, evaluation, counseling, hormone therapy, and surgery were "worth it." Still, some individuals had negative results. Abramowitz reports that 7% of those polled reported "unsatisfactory" or even "tragic" outcomes; many of these patients requested a surgical reversal of the sex change operation, had serious psychotic episodes, were hospitalized for psychiatric reasons, or even committed suicide. The long period of evaluation and counseling obviously seems warranted, although there may not be an accurate way to predict who is likely to have an adverse psychological result.

Snaith, Tarsh, and Reid (1993) reported that based on the subjective assessments of 36 female-to-male and 105 male-to-

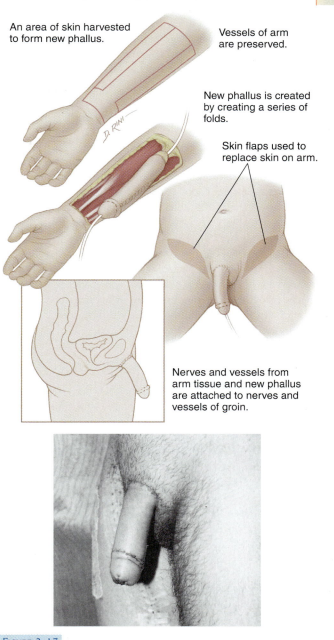

An area of skin harvested to form new phallus.

Vessels of arm are preserved.

New phallus is created by creating a series of folds.

Skin flaps used to replace skin on arm.

Nerves and vessels from arm tissue and new phallus are attached to nerves and vessels of groin.

FIGURE 3-17   Surgical procedure and outcome of female to male gender reassignment surgery.

female transsexuals who had sex reassignment surgery in the Netherlands, the course of treatment and surgery had highly therapeutic effects on these subjects. Both groups had comparably beneficial outcomes, and the combination of psychosocial and medical components of the treatment program was considered essential for the favorable outcomes. Another study in the Netherlands (Hage, 1995) addressed the adequacy of the traditional course of counseling and treatment and found that it is especially important to inform transsexuals fully about the surgical procedures used.

Kockott & Fahrner (1987) studied what happens to transsexuals who do not undergo sex reassignment surgery even when it has been offered to them. Patients who considered the surgery but declined it were often older and usually married; they frequently had children and had lived for many years with a spouse of the opposite sex. These patients who decided not to have the operation continued to have the adjustment problems and social difficulties as when they were first evaluated by the medical/psychological team.

POSSIBLE CAUSES OF TRANSSEXUALISM

A variety of explanations have been offered about the causes of transsexualism, although none is entirely satisfactory. Some believe that exposure of an embryo or fetus to excessive amounts of hormones that differ from those of its genetic sex may later contribute to the emergence of transsexualism (Pauly, 1974). Other investigators believe that social learning theory is involved (Green, 1974). For example, if a child is selectively and consistently reinforced for behaving in a way congruent with stereotypes of the other sex, it could be a challenge to develop a gender identity congruent with his or her genetic sex. At this time the factors and conditions likely to lead to a transsexual orientation are unknown.

GENDER AS A SOCIAL CONSTRUCT

The final part of this chapter will examine still another way of considering gender. In addition to biological and psychological approaches, the social construct approach examines how we function in our social and cultural environment. This environment exerts subtle and obvious pressures on us to behave in accordance with our biological sex, regardless of our psychological characteristics. Obviously there are important differences between women and men. But how much should we make of those differences and what adjustments, if any, should be made for them? Should women or men be given special consideration in certain arenas because of their differences? Can society legislate gender equality if there are authentic distinctions between the sexes? How do men feel about women being given special treatment? How do women feel about men being given special treatment? How do women feel about having been discriminated against for so long? These are just some of the issues addressed in this section.

Analysis of Gender Differences

The scientific study of gender differences advanced with the publication of *The Psychology of Sex Differences* in 1974 by Maccoby and Jacklin. Many social and behavioral scientists have explored differences between women and men without being judgmental. There are very important political implications to the study of gender differences (Eagly, 1995). If there are significant, measurable differences between women and men, would this information be used to open opportunities for some people and to limit opportunities to others? For example, many studies have revealed a male advantage in quantitative problem-solving by late adolescence or early adulthood (e.g., Benbow, 1988). Other investigations have

shown a clear female advantage in tests of verbal fluency and word and sentence meaning (e.g., Maccoby & Jacklin, 1974). Recognizing and measuring sex differences and acting on their basis are two very different issues, however. As well, because studies on gender differences have not been conducted in many different countries and cultures, we cannot know that differences observed result from genetic/biological influences or social/cultural forces. Although many social and behavioral scientists take a perspective between these two extremes (sometimes called an "interactionist" perspective), convincing data supporting either extreme are not found consistently.

The study of sex differences was greatly influenced by the feminist movement. If it could be scientifically proven that there were no significant differences between women and men, then it would be inappropriate to limit opportunities for women based on stereotyped beliefs about their abilities. Many feminists didn't want to find or acknowledge any significant differences between the sexes for this very reason. Gilligan (1982), however, believes that moral reasoning develops along different lines in males and females, that females are more likely to develop a caring perspective and males to develop a more rational, rule-oriented perspective. Women are also thought more likely to develop relationship skills and a desire for close interpersonal bonds because of the close relationship they often had with consistent female parenting figures (Chodorow, 1978). These are two examples of consequences of the different social/familial worlds of little girls and little boys. These examples also conform to the common stereotype that females are more nurturant and caring than males. In other words, rigorous studies of gender differences are often seen to *confirm gender stereotypes we have about male and females.* Our everyday experiences and inferences thus have an element of truth in them and perhaps are not merely stereotypes after all. Nonetheless, when it comes to judging a man or a woman for a job or other position, what's important isn't the degree to which a person conforms to gender stereotypes or gender differences but rather their ability and promise to meet the requirements of the position.

Differences Between Females and Males
1. Girls tend to have greater verbal ability than boys, a difference that is obvious by high school.
2. Males tend to perform better on tasks requiring visual-spatial ability, such as to recall and detect shapes, engage in mental rotation tasks, solve problems in geometry, learn mazes, and read maps.
3. Boys tend to have greater skill in mathematics than girls, a difference that widens by early adolescence.
4. Boys tend to be more aggressive physically than females, a difference already apparent by the age of 2 or 3.

—FROM KOLB & WHISHAW, 1996, 221–223

This chapter began with an overview of attribution theory, in which we asked whether we perceive and relate to people based on their real qualities or instead on qualities we at-

Dear Dr. Ruth

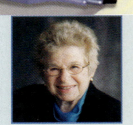

Question:

I've been married a little over a year now. However, my husband and I have been having the same problem ever since our wedding—and even before. He does not like to have intercourse very often. He accuses me of being "obsessed" with it. I attribute this to several things: 1) he has not had a lot of sexual experiences, 2) his previous girlfriend cheated on him, and 3) I had a lot of male companions (before we met). We've talked about this, but he just says that I'm obsessed and he doesn't like to do it too much. I sometimes wonder if maybe it's me and maybe I'm not much of a turn-on for him. But when we do have sex, he says he enjoys it very much. I'm becoming pretty confused and frustrated. We both think it's important for our good relationship to make love, and I know it shouldn't take precedence over everything else we share, but what am I doing wrong? I just can't understand why he doesn't want to make love to his new wife who is faithful and loving.

Answer:

I'm fond of saying that husbands and wives are not Siamese twins, and it is very common that one desires more sex than the other. It's a common misconception that it's always the man who complains about not getting enough sex. While more men do voice this concern, there are many women in your situation.

If you were interested in sex more than he was, even before you got married, you should not be surprised that nothing has changed since you walked down the aisle together. First of all, forget about whose "fault" it is. Having different sexual appetites is not a fault any more than one person being a "morning person" and the other a "night owl." Sex drive varies between people, as well as within one person from time to time. He did want to marry you, so stop thinking that he's not attracted to you. I have always believed that one of the most important aspects of a relationship is finding ways to appreciate your similarities and negotiate your differences. Whether you are a man or a woman, and no matter how you feel about how men and women "should" behave, this is an important part of any good relationship.

But you two need to communicate better. You told me what you think the reasons are for his lack of interest, but you didn't tell me what he says about this. Just as men are supposed to always be "ready" for sex, men are also supposed to have problems talking about their feelings, so this might be the best place to start. Talk about what each of you thinks you are "supposed" to do, and maybe then you can communicate better about what each of you wants to do, and when, and how often, and why, or why not.

tribute to them. The study of sex differences has been stimulated in part by a sincere interest in proving the unacceptability of sex discrimination. As Eagly (1995) has written, "The common description of empirical research as showing that sex-related differences are small, usually unstable across studies, very often artifactual, and inconsistent with gender stereotypes arose in part from a feminist commitment to gender similarity as a route to political equality" (p. 155). This study is an excellent example of how social and behavioral scientists have the obligation not only to tell the truth as they see it, but also to consider very carefully how their research results might be used. If differences between women and men were clear and unambiguous, then they wouldn't be such an interesting topic for study and debate.

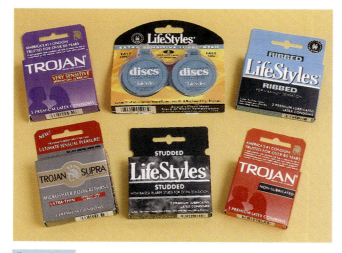

FIGURE 3-18 Condoms are commonly colorfully packaged and frequently appeal to both women and men when they're making a decision to purchase them and act intelligently about safer sex.

Gender Differences in Negotiating Safe Sex

So far we have been discussing aspects of gender as a social construct related to understanding the dynamics of male/female relationships. Certain aspects of this subject can have applied value as well, such as how women and men negotiate the use of condoms. Public safe sex information campaigns are generally aimed at women because it is often the female who agrees to a sexual encounter. Without her assent, sex doesn't happen except in cases of assault. What happens when men decline to use condoms? Can women learn to exercise tactful assertiveness to direct their partner to use a condom? Keep in mind gender-role differences: assertiveness is not a common feminine virtue, and some men frankly dislike it. Appealing to women to assume responsibility for safe sex may be ineffective because of traditional gender roles. Lever (1995) points out that women's insistence that their partners use protection can evoke men's resistance because it may seem the woman is "taking control"—something many men *won't* let happen. Lever notes that this power struggle alone can make men be irresponsible about using condoms. Understanding traditional gender roles and expectations, however, may help one anticipate this struggle and perhaps resolve it.

When condom manufacturers direct their sales messages to women *and* men (Figs. 3-18 and 3-19), they may not account for the fact that many young men are not used to taking directions from young women. A woman acting independently, intelligently, and assertively can be a "turn off" for some men, especially young men. Lever (1995) notes that young women when role playing or recollecting sexual encounters often *lower their voices* when asking, "Did you bring any protection?" (Lever found that most women were uncomfortable even using the word "condom.") In other words, they tried to seem less demanding or independent at this important and ticklish moment. Interestingly, most men who use condoms do so without saying much about it.

Sexuality, Sales, and the Media

In 1957, Vance Packard published *The Hidden Persuaders,* a psychological and sociological analysis of how advertising techniques influence people to buy things. Among other factors, he discovered that sexual reassurance was a very influential factor. Women and men wanted some assurance that they were undeniably feminine or masculine, and advertisements appealing to this need were especially eye-catching. While everyone likes to feel attractive, this trend of reassurance seemed to be something new in the American psyche. Its causes and consequences both are complicated. Traditional gender roles of the 1940s and 1950s had perhaps become so comfortable and unselfconscious that Americans began to look for some "extra-special" attention. The publication of Kinsey's studies perhaps stimulated questions about what men and women want sexually. For whatever reason, advertisers soon understood that "sex sells." Whether it was a hem line or a novel scent, Americans seemed to be asking for attention. Even steel, chrome, and glass automobiles were being referred to as "sexy." Since that time, our culture has not outgrown the need for sexual reassurance. Perhaps by buying certain products and creating a particular "look," people gain the sexual reassurance Packard thought people wanted. Many advertisements, whether for a deodorant or mouthwash, appeal to viewers because of the supposed attractiveness and attention they will get if they use that product. But isn't just dressing up our appearance a superficial way to get others to notice us? Yes, but that doesn't seem to bother many consumers. Sex gets people's attention, and anything that gets people's attention is a useful tool of the advertising industry (Fig. 3-20).

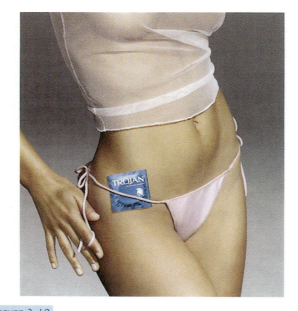

Trojan® latex condoms. What everyone will be wearing this year.

FIGURE 3-19 Advertisements frequently encourage women to behave foresightfully and responsibly with respect to avoiding pregnancy and sexually transmitted diseases.

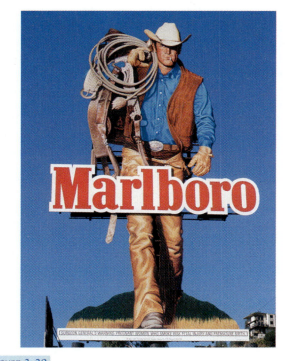

From early toddlerhood, children are exposed to media messages and images that reinforce or sometimes criticize traditional views of maleness and femaleness. Television is, of course, the most powerful and pervasive medium in this respect. Decades ago Sternglanz and Serbin (1974) revealed that females on television were not portrayed as competent as males were and that 70% of the characters on prime-time television were men. These men were usually depicted in the workplace, while women were shown in domestic roles. Children watching television in this era saw men in high-status, high-income professions, acting in assertive, effective ways. Women were shown in loving and sensitive roles. In the last two decades this situation has changed dramatically. Divorced families, single moms with children, single dads with children, and cohabitation arrangements are all common today on prime-time television. Children and adolescents today are more frequently exposed to depictions of role flexibility.

Judy Kuriansky, a clinical psychologist and host of the "Love Phones" radio show, wrote about these issues in *Advertising Age* magazine in 1995. She quotes the President-CEO of Candies, Inc., a large shoe manufacturer, on television advertising: "In 30 seconds, to keep people from going to the refrigerator, you have to astound them—and sex does" (p. 49). Consider the sexually obvious advertisements on television of the past quarter century. Kuriansky cites a number of powerful examples. Several female office workers take a break at precisely 11:30 a.m. to all rush to the window to watch a classic hunk construction worker take his shirt off, expose his well-muscled torso, and down a Diet Coke. This simple message appeals to the stereotype of masculine muscle-men being attractive to women, even though we have already seen that this traditional belief is fading. Yet this is what little girls are seeing on TV as they begin to think about females and males and their differences. The same is certainly true of the "Marlboro Man."

A second example is more subtle but no less powerful. Kuriansky points out that by 1970, the indirect erotic message of advertisements that "Virginia is for Lovers" led to an immediate, dramatic increase in tourism in one of the most conservative states in the country. Kuriansky notes that not all "successful" sexual advertising is as blatant as the Diet Coke Man or the 1960s Noxema shaving cream commercial in which an attractive blond with a Swedish accent fingers the foam while cooing, "Take it off. Take it *all* off." There is a more subtle trend today, possibly due to the influence of the women's movement. Now the "family man" is sexy, with his polite, monogamous, family-oriented approach to products ranging from Folger's Coffee to the American Express Card (p. 49). Men who take women seriously also sell products successfully. Kuriansky notes that how women and men were portrayed in commercials between 1971 and 1988 changed remarkably. Although sexual stereotyping is still common, women are increasingly the central characters in these newer commercials, and men are more likely to be portrayed as spouses and fathers. Considering that a typical 30-minute television show contains *twelve 30-second commercials,* the influence of these images of women and men is indeed very powerful.

Advertising using sexual imagery has recently led to a consumer backlash, however (Elash, 1995). In the 1990s, Calvin Klein's advertisements, for example, were called provocative and pornographic by different segments of the population (Fig. 3-21). *Very* young adolescents were shown in Klein's underwear ads. Although for the most part teens were not upset by this, many adults were. The FBI investigated the ad campaign to determine whether child pornography laws were violated, and Klein himself came under fire for what many consider poor taste and sexual exploitation of children. At a time when much attention is being given to child sexual abuse, this was not the best publicity for Calvin Klein. Suzanne Keeler of the Canadian Advertising Foundation noted, "I think there is a more conservative attitude in our society . . . Ten years ago, sexuality was not nearly the issue it is now" (Elash, 1995, p. 36).

Still, some advertising depicts women in passive, submissive poses (Fig. 3-22). While passivity and submissiveness were once part of a traditional female gender role, today these traits are not viewed so wholesomely. An advertisement for the French perfume "Jaipur" showed a naked woman with wrists bound behind her back by a bracelet-shaped perfume bottle. When the ad ran in Canada, many women contacted the retail clothing merchant who ran it and strongly complained. The merchant immediately bought space in newspapers to apologize for any unhappiness or "distress" the advertisement caused. These examples of consumer activism demonstrate the influence we consumers can have on both electronic and print media. If you believe that sexism exploits consumers, make your feelings known.

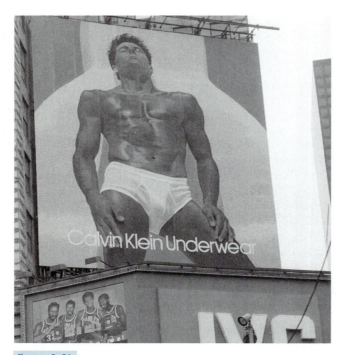

FIGURE 3-21   Some advertising with sexual imagery has been criticized as inappropriately provocative.

Another interesting example of possible sexism and the exploitation of traditional gender roles might enter your home in a different way—you might buy it for your children! Thirty-seven years ago Mattel introduced the "Barbie" doll, which has been an icon for two generations of girls and an interesting introduction to the feminine form. Is that what we want little girls to think they should grow up to look like?

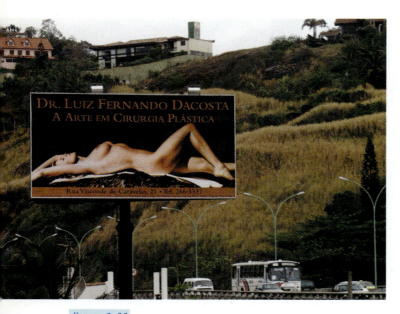

FIGURE 3-22   Advertisements frequently depict women as passive and sexually receptive. Of course, such stereotypes are frequently perceived as inaccurate and offensive.

Erica Rand's *Barbie's Queer Accessories* (1994) is an insightful exercise in cultural criticism, revealing Barbie as an interesting vehicle for looking at social conceptions of the "ideal" female form, heterosexual feminine attractiveness, and a belated nod to multiculturalism—belated because versions of Barbie other than white, blond girls were late to arrive in the long list of Barbie dolls. More recently, Mattel developed a line of software products with Barbie as star. "Fashion Designer," "Barbie Storymaker," and "Barbie Print 'n Play" are an attempt to appeal to girls in the software market. This line of toys has a subtle and important aspect perhaps not immediately apparent. The president of Mattel, Jill Barad points out that if girls do not play with and learn to excel at computer toys early in life, they may be at a disadvantage compared to boys. Barad says that whatever it takes to get girls on the computer will have big payoffs later when they use other software for educational and occupational purposes (*Time*, November 11, 1996). Of course, there are many other software packages available for both boys and girls that do not exploit sexual stereotypes.

Television, Cinema, and the Family

Social and behavioral scientists have been interested in how television influences children for decades. While many studies focused on depictions of aggression, more recently, studies have examined the impact of sexual themes. The power of television to create gender images and expectations of "appropriate" gender behaviors is enormous; this really isn't even debatable. Still, we need to learn more about the *specific* influences of television on how boys and girls learn to think about sex, men, and women. Ward (1995) analyzed 12 prime-time programs for their sexual themes. Table 3-2 lists the programs she assessed, the network presenting them, and their scheduled time slots.

Ward found that discussions about sexual issues were extremely common in these shows, accounting for an average 29% of character interactions and as much as 50% in some episodes. More interactions concerned the male sexual role

TABLE 3-2

Programs Analyzed for Sexual Themes[a]

Program	Network	Viewing Time
The Fresh Prince of Bel-Air	NBC	8:00
Blossom	NBC	8:30
Roseanne	ABC	9:00
Martin	FOX	8:30
The Simpsons	FOX	8:00
Beverly Hills, 90210	FOX	8:00
In Living Color (the first season)	FOX	9:00
Full House	ABC	8:00
Hangin' with Mr. Cooper	ABC	8:30
Home Improvement	ABC	8:30
Step by Step	ABC	8:30
Family Matters	ABC	8:00

[a]After Ward (1995).

than the female sexual role. More discussions dealt with sex in a recreational rather than a procreational context. The most common sexual statements concerned competitive aspects of sexual relationships; males commented openly on the appearance and desirability of women's bodies and physical attractiveness. These programs presented a conception equating masculinity with being sexually "successful" with attractive female characters. The most consistent theme in these programs was that physical attractiveness is a "key asset" for masculinity and femininity (Ward, 1995, p. 595). With messages like these contributing to the socialization for children and adolescents, it is no wonder that people have difficulty escaping the old stereotypes about what women and men are supposed to look and act like.

Rock music videos have a powerful, pervasive influence on how children and adolescents think about gender roles, although more research is still needed about their impact. Still, we have learned much, such as from a recent analysis of the influence of rock music videos on premarital sexual attitudes. Strouse, Buerkel-Rothfuss, and Long (1995) explored how gender and family influences affect adolescents' interpretation of sexual themes in rock music videos. Exposure to videos was generally associated with more permissive sexual attitudes, particularly among females. Perhaps females watch more rock music videos than males and spend more time listening to popular music. This impact was even greater in young women in inadequate family environments. These authors do not suggest a cause-and-effect relationship between frequent exposure to rock music videos and more permissive premarital sexual attitudes. Rather, they believe that because a female's sexual attitudes are more influenced by psychosocial factors, and a male's sexual attitudes more by biological factors, young women may be more vulnerable to such influences. More research into the impact of music and music videos is needed. In the meantime, since music videos are an art form in their own right, we believe it would be premature and inappropriate to condemn them because of a *suspected* influence. This study is important in part because its approach to just one aspect of the issue is cautious and illustrates a small but important part of the issue without leaping to more grandiose conclusions.

In both prime-time television and rock music videos, children and adolescents are being influenced regarding traditional gender roles. An interesting question arises: what about the influence of roles that do not conform to these traditional images? An excellent example is a series of roles played by the actress Jodie Foster (Fig. 3-23). Movies often depict "larger than life" men and women who are indisputably masculine and feminine and who are often presented as symbols of what "real" men and women are like. For example, actors like Arnold Schwarzenegger typically portray determined, assertive, and emotionally detached characters, and actresses like Emma Thompson have played obviously feminine characters who defer to men and are passive, submissive, quiet, and the object of affections. Some have suggested that Jodi Foster, in contrast, has cultivated a film persona that is either sexually ambiguous or plainly androgynous (Lane, 1995), although this issue evokes some debate. Foster clearly excels in roles

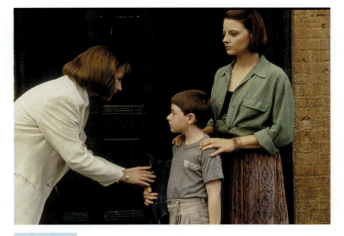

FIGURE 3-23 In the movie *Little Man Tate*, Jodie Foster plays the part of a single mother who is an independent, strong, and encouraging figure in her intellectually gifted son's life.

requiring a delicate amalgam of feminine fragility and masculine independence and assertiveness. In *Taxi Driver* she played the role of a tough yet sensitive prostitute. In *The Accused* she played the victim of a horrible gang rape who nonetheless had tremendous strength and self-respect. In *The Silence of the Lambs* she played the role of Starling, an FBI agent who pursues an inhuman and ruthless serial killer and reveals her own private doubts and demons related to an emotionally isolated childhood. She both directed and starred in *Little Man Tate* as a character with strength and persistence as a single mother raising a gifted boy, yet still vulnerable and nurturant with her son. Great artistry and sensitivity are required to play such characters convincingly, and these depictions of feminine strength no doubt have some influence as well on our views of gender.

Cross-Cultural and Sub-Cultural Conceptions of Gender Roles

We conclude this chapter by looking at how other cultures conceptualize male and female roles. Of all the differences among societies, gender-based behaviors and expectations are perhaps the most intriguing. Some differences are just interesting, while others might make you angry. These differences often involve deep and enduring social, cultural, and religious mandates about what women and men are supposed to be like for a society's *status quo* to be maintained. Although we might be tempted to judge societies different from our own, we should beware of **ethnocentrism**, an attitude stemming from the belief that one's own culture is the only "right" one and that others are "wrong." Sometimes differences are only that: differences.

In many societies throughout the world, women's status is low and every effort seems to be made to keep it that way. Gender identity and roles are powerfully affected by cultural traditions. For example, women have low-to-no social or legal status in Turkey. Despite legislative reforms intended to enhance women's status, no substantive progress has been made. The disadvantages of being a woman in Turkey are profound.

Other Countries, Cultures, and Customs

MASCULINITY AND MALE BONDING AMONG JAPANESE BUSINESSMEN

Anne Allison's fascinating sociological study of Japanese "hostess bars" (1994) describes establishments where Japanese businessmen go after work to engage in a corporate male bonding and reaffirm their masculinity in a way necessary for business success. The author worked in one for 4 months as part of her scholarly study of this institution. The Japanese *sarariiman* is like the American conception of a "workaholic." The word itself is actually based on the English "salary man." He usually lives simply and frugally in a small apartment, and he spends an enormous amount of his day at his job and often much of the evening.. His job is his whole life, and only through his dedication to it will his loyalty and industry be rewarded with security, seniority, and good salary.

There is a clear etiquette about who goes to hostess bars and what happens there. The experience is closer to work than relaxation; thus the title of Allison's book: *Nightwork: Sexuality, Pleasure, and Corporate Masculinity in a Tokyo Hostess Bar* (1994). Hostess bars are expensive. Most professionals cannot afford to go to them, although there are other places where drink and female companionship can be had. Businessmen always go in groups headed by one obviously senior member. The clubs are sumptuously appointed and immaculately clean. Business expense accounts cover the costs of drinks and companionship, which seldom involves anything more than flirting and never includes sex. The men often make rude jokes as they become drunk and may sing along with electronic karaoke music. From the outside there may seem little value to the experience: everything is expensive, the female companionship involves only implied intimacy and no meaningful conversation or interaction, and everyone is exhausted the next day. Yet the tradition continues because hostess bars are an arena of corporate male bonding and trust building. Men develop lifelong business contacts in these clubs, explore commercial opportunities and plans, and demonstrate their company loyalty. Hostess clubs reveal masculine values somewhat different from those seen elsewhere and are an interesting reminder that such values need occasional reinforcement.

Geisha houses are another venue in which Japanese women entertain men. These women, however, wear more formal, ceremonial attire and are rigorously trained to play musical instruments and engage in conversation with their clients (Fig. 3-24).

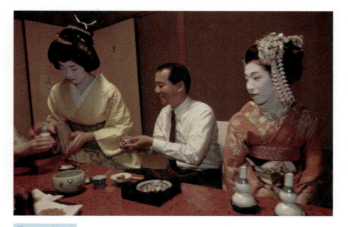

FIGURE 3-24   In Geisha houses, Japanese men are attended to deferentially by women trained for years to entertain them and offer them relaxation. Sexual contact is not customarily part of a Geisha's interactions with her clients.

Turkish women have no right to dissent. According to Turkish law, the man is "the head of the family" and in family disputes only his views are valid. The man decides where to live without consulting his wife or family members. The man represents the family in all matters outside of the home and makes all business arrangements that affect the family. Turkish women cannot own property, and in a divorce the man is awarded all tangible "immovable" property; women may lawfully be thrown out on the street with their children, utterly destitute (Chittister, 1995).

Adultery is a crime for both women and men in Turkey, but the law has a gender bias. For women, a single act of infidelity legally constitutes adultery. Men, however, can be charged with adultery only after living with another woman for at least 6 months or having had sexual intercourse with her in his own family's home. Although public education is compulsory and free, one-third of Turkish women are illiterate because their fathers refuse to allow them to attend school, with the support of local legal officials. The 1995 World Conference on Women revealed circumstances such as these, but this situation is not likely to change much or quickly.

We have seen significant differences in male and female gender roles in Japan and Turkey—but what about within our own? A common American stereotype is that Southerners have rigid male and female gender roles (Fig. 3-25). Rice and Coates (1995) investigated this stereotype and found that Southern attitudes about gender roles have changed substantially in recent years. With 1972–92 data from the National Opinion Research Center, they analyzed how Southerners feel about a variety of gender role issues, especially those dealing with women. They assessed attitudes toward working mothers, employed women, and women in politics. The results are interesting. Southerners are much more conservative in their attitudes about these gender role issues than subjects polled in the Northeast, Midwest, and West, with African Americans giving the most conservative responses. Through the 2 decades of study, a more egalitarian climate of opinion emerged, although Southerners continue to have very conservative opinions about the inappropriateness of women in politics and moderately conservative opinions about women working outside the home.

A recent study (Quadagno, Sly, Harrison, Eberstein, & Soler, 1998) explored differences in sexual behavior among 438 women 18 to 45 years old in African American, Hispanic, and white samples. They found some interesting differences among

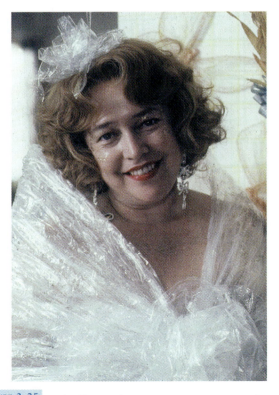

Figure 3-25 In the film *Fried Green Tomatoes*, actress Kathy Bates plays the role of a traditional Southern wife who tries to spice things up in her marriage by greeting her husband at the door dressed in clear wrap.

these groups. Whites and Hispanics reported participation in oral sex twice as frequently as African American women, and Hispanic women reported engaging in anal sex almost three times as often as African Americans and whites. These women's ages were unrelated to the reported frequency of vaginal, oral, or anal sex, although women with more education reported more frequent oral sex. It is noteworthy that measurable differences such as these occur in a large sample of American women, and that ethnicity may influence a woman's sexual behaviors.

Another example of cultural differences in gender roles is somewhat unusual. Only rarely can one examine the impact of relatively quickly occurring social and technological changes on gender and family roles. One interesting case is found in northernmost Norway where people of the Sami society have lived a rural existence for centuries. The men hunted reindeer and farmed, and women stayed at home and raised children. Over the last 30 to 40 years, Norway's government has attempted to integrate these people more completely in their nation state with all the rights and benefits of full social enfranchisement. The impact of this "modernization" program has not always been positive, however, especially for Sami youngsters born in the late 1940s and early 1950s. These individuals most keenly felt the conflicts between their culture's ancient traditions and the contemporary social agenda. Many of this generation's women were discouraged from exploring occupational opportunities outside their homes and villages because these aspirations were "inappropriate" for women (Stordahl, 1995). Some women were encouraged to resign from teaching positions as soon as they married in order to become part of their husband's "ground crew." In the past, women had helped with hunting and skinning reindeer, but as the industry became more mechanized, their contribution was no longer as needed for the family's economic survival. Husbands felt that part-time teaching was sufficient for them and became suspicious when women expressed interest in local and, later, national political positions. Apparently, full-time teaching and political positions were incompatible with traditional Sami feminine gender roles.

When a new public education system was implemented in the 1960s and 1970s, the changing opportunities for women led to problems for Sami families. Many Sami men felt displaced by the increased participation of women throughout Sami society. Stordahl (1995) reports that today social workers, teachers, and physicians point to problems Sami men and boys have had to deal with as a result of these changes. Sami boys and men have a far higher incidence than Sami girls and women of alcohol dependency, drug abuse, suicide, dropping out of school, difficulty in keeping a job, and difficulty maintaining interpersonal relationships. Far more Sami girls than boys are in the educational system at all levels, including university. We should not assume a simple cause-effect relationship about the changed gender roles and family functioning with the increased incidence of these problems, but Norwegian physicians and social scientists believe that the two are clearly related.

In a more positive example, gender equality has recently received much attention in the African nation of Kenya.

Wainaina (1997) suggests that gender equality is central to that country's desire to implement a more democratic form of government. This writer calls for Kenyan men to work on eliminating domestic violence, emphasizing that such behavior is an "affront to manhood" (p. 38). When women are fully enfranchised in Kenyan society, a greater prosperity for all and increased value of life are hoped-for benefits for both women and men. In conclusion, Wainaina proclaims that "power shared is power increased" (p. 38).

CONCLUSION

This chapter has introduced different ways of thinking about "sex," "gender roles," and "gender identity." Gender as a biological construct includes genetic and chromosomal aspects, normal and abnormal sex differentiation, and the hormonal mechanisms of genital development, as well as the relationship between sex hormones and gender stereotyped behaviors and sexual inclination.

Examining gender as a psychological construct includes exploring the meanings of "masculinity," "femininity," and "androgyny," along with the development of sex roles, the variables influencing this long process, and important gender similarities and differences. Transsexuality and gender dysmorphic disorders were discussed along with some of the psychological, medical, and surgical aspects of these issues. The social construct of gender includes exploring the impact of television, advertising, music videos, and movies. Cross-cultural and sub-cultural examples also illustrate the impact of social influences on gender roles.

Now that you have been introduced to the place of sexuality in our everyday lives, the history of the study of human sexuality, and important concepts of sex, gender roles, and gender identity, we will turn to "hardware" issues: the anatomy, physiology, and endocrinology of female and male sexuality.

Learning Activities

1. Imagine that you are a female physician in a local urgent care facility. A man is brought in with a severe laceration on his forehead from falling out of his recliner during the Superbowl. You start to evaluate his injury when he turns to you and says, "I don't want a silly nurse taking care of me—go get me a doctor, honey!" Explain the nature of the attribution he is making and fully describe your response to him.

2. You have read about the effects of sex hormones on the pre- and postnatal development of male and female bodies, including rare anomalies. Having read about such conditions, how do you assess the relative importance of biological versus psychosocial factors in the development of gender identity? When a "mismatch" occurs between physical appearance and genetic sex, which do you think is more important in establishing a sense of identity?

3. Genetic counselors often use the results of prenatal tests (such as amniocentesis) to inform prospective parents about potential problems of a fetus long before it is born. If *you* were a genetic counselor and knew of an abnormality of sexual differentiation in a couple's fetus, for example Klinefelter's Syndrome or Turner's Syndrome, what would you tell them? Ethically speaking, you can advise them about a specific course of action.

4. Here is a true story. A man tells his son whose wife is pregnant, "Your mother and I saved your electric train. If you and Mary have a son, we'll send it to you so that he can play with it when he gets older." The son says, "Dad, are you telling me that if we have a girl you won't send it for her to play with?" His father replies, "Why would you want to screw up a little girl's development?" Comment.

5. In your own experience, how do children at a young age respond to early observations that male and female external genitalia are different? What do you think about how they respond?

6. Describe different ways adults behave toward male and female newborn babies.

7. Men are sometimes stereotyped as being "ever ready" for a sexual encounter, and women as more "choosy" about when and with whom they will have intercourse. Based on what you have learned about male and female hormones and how they change or don't change cyclically over time, do you think these stereotypical differences are more biological or psychosocial in origin? Or could they be both?

8. Is it "good" to be androgynous? Does being androgynous "dilute" a person's masculinity or femininity?

9. An episode on a popular television series described how a man became a woman through sex reassignment surgery and then enjoyed a successful career as a model. A routine physical examination revealed her genetic maleness, and the model was subsequently fired. Do you think this woman was unjustifiably deprived of her livelihood? Why or why not?

10. In your opinion, how often are gender-neutral selling techniques used in television commercials? What types of products would likely sell best using gender-neutral appeals?

11. The 1948 Combat Exclusion Act disallows women from combat assignments in the Navy, Air Force, and Marine Corps. The Army has a similar policy. These restrictions are based on traditional and perhaps outdated ideas about how wars are fought. By modern legal standards, these statutes may be discriminatory. Since 1948, other countries, notably Israel, have used women in armed combat roles, and Israeli women have fought effectively. Yet their deaths, often gruesome in war, were profoundly demoralizing to male soldiers. Do you think women and men should fight side-by-side? Why or why not?

12. Dr. Matina Horner (1970, 1972), a social psychologist, studied whether women would feel that occupational success, especially in competition with men, had negative consequences for them. She discovered that many

women believe they will be viewed as less feminine, would endure negative job consequences, and would worry about being rejected by both female and male coworkers if they were conspicuously more competent than male co-workers. They also worried about being perceived as less desirable marriage partners. These concerns were seen in girls as young as those in junior high school. Even more surprising, a motive to avoid success was seen in women who had *already succeeded* in business, government, industry, and education. Do you believe that there is really a motive for women to avoid success in their work when they compete with men?

Key Concepts

■ The term sex is usually used to describe the biological or genetic determination of maleness or femaleness. Gender role refers to societal expectations about what is expected of our behavior as males or females. Gender identity refers to the degree to which we feel comfortable in our social roles as men and women.

■ Psychologists and other behavioral scientists use the concept of attribution to explain how we try to explain other peoples' behavior. If the behavior we observe seems attributable to another person's personality or personal qualities, we are making an internal attribution. If the behavior seems attributable to the circumstances, we are making an external attribution.

■ Differences in sex based on different sex chromosomes are referred to as chromosomal sex, and differences based on differing sex glands is referred to as gonadal sex. Hormones secreted by the gonads create differing male and female body forms. This difference is called hormonal sex.

■ A hormone is a chemical substance secreted by an endocrine gland into the blood stream, where it travels to other organs or glands and changes their activity in some way, such as increasing or decreasing that activity.

■ Gender role typing is the developmental learning process of how we come to think of ourselves as a member of one sex or the other.

■ The concept of androgyny denotes a compatible blend of traditional female and male psychological traits in the same person.

■ In the course of growing up, children observe same and other-sex adults behaving in ways that confirm or disconfirm traditional gender-role expectations. This observational learning is the central feature of social learning theory, which posits that the behavior of others gradually becomes a model for our own as we learn vicariously by watching the actions of others.

■ The sum of all our thoughts and feelings about ourselves is called our self-concept. It combines our here-and-now,

most honest thoughts about ourselves (our perceived self) and our vision of ourselves in the future when we have become the man or woman we would like to be (our ideal self). When the person we are seems to be developing into the person we would like to be, this enhances our self-esteem.

■ A gender-role conflict is any feeling of restriction that accompanies the desire to behave in a way that does not conform to traditional gender stereotypes.

Glossary Terms

androgen insensitivity syndrome (testicular feminization)	endocrine glands	progestational drug
	estrogens	progesterone
	ethnocentrism	self-concept
	gametes	sex
androgens	gender identity	sex chromosomes
androgyny	gender role	sexual objectification
attribution	gender role conflict	sociality
autosome	gender role typing	social learning theory
cognitive-development theory	gender-schema theory	somatic cells
congenital virilizing adrenal hyperplasia	gonads	steroids
	hormonal sex	testosterone
	hormone	transsexuality
	ideal self	
	perceived self	

Suggested Readings

Allison, A. (1994). Nightwork: Sexuality, pleasure, and corporate masculinity in a Tokyo hostess club. Chicago: University of Chicago Press.

Bem, S. L. (1976). Probing the promise of androgyny. In A. G. Kaplan & J. P. Bean (Eds.), Beyond sex-role stereotypes: Readings toward a psychology of androgyny. Boston: Little, Brown.

Eagly, A. H. (1995). The science and politics of comparing women and men. American Psychologist, 50, 145–158.

Gilligan, C. (1982). In a different voice: Psychological theory and women's development. Cambridge: MA: Harvard University Press.

Harris, S. M. (1995). Psychosocial development and black male masculinity. Implications for counseling economically disadvantaged African American male adolescents. Journal of Counseling and Development, 73, 279–287.

Martz, D. M., Handley, K. B., & Eisler, R. M. (1995). The relationship between feminine gender role stress, body image, and eating disorders. Psychology of Women Quarterly, 19, 493–508.

Morris, J. (1974). Conundrum. New York: Harcourt Brace Jovanovich, Inc.

Rosenzweig, J. M., & Dailey, D. M. (1991). Women's sex roles in their public and private lives. Journal of Sex Education and Therapy, 17, 75–85.

Ward, M. (1995). Talking about sex: Common themes about sexuality in the prime-time television programs children and adolescents view most. Journal of Youth and Adolescence, 24, 595–615.

4

Female and Male Genital and Reproductive Anatomy, Physiology, and Endocrinology

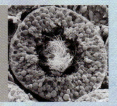

OBJECTIVES

When you finish reading this chapter, you should be able to:

1. Describe the differences between "anatomy" and "physiology," including the hormonal aspects of physiological processes.

2. If you are a woman, recall and describe the anatomical structures seen in your genital self-examination, including color and texture, and state your thoughts about privacy in relation to physical examinations, particularly regarding the use of a chaperon during your examination by a physician.

3. Describe the three layers of tissue in the vagina, their structure and functions, and the functions of this organ at different times. Explain why the vagina can comfortably stretch to accommodate a penis of almost any size.

4. Summarize the arguments and the data supporting and refuting the presence of a G spot in the vagina, along with your personal opinion.

5. Review the location, structure, and functions of the fallopian tubes. Describe their role in facilitating conception and the implantation of a fertilized ovum.

6. Describe the location and function of the hypothalamus and the pituitary gland. Define "negative feedback mechanism" and give some examples involving the hypothalamus and the pituitary gland.

7. Describe the events in the hypothalamus and pituitary that initiate ovulation. Describe what happens in the ovaries during the follicular, ovulatory, luteal, and menstrual phases.

8. Describe the events in the uterus during the menstrual, proliferative, and secretory phases.

9. Describe the external appearance of the scrotum and the structures inside it. What are the functions of the scrotum, and how are these carried out?

10. Define "meiosis" and discuss spermatogenesis as an example. Where and how does it occur?

11. Discuss in anatomical order the structures sperm pass through on their way out of a man's body. Describe the contributions of each structure to semen and its functions. List the substances that make up semen.

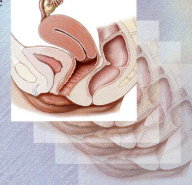

12. Describe similarities in the female and male sexual and reproductive systems.

From Dr. Ruth

In some aboriginal tribes, nudity is the norm. In Europe, seeing a topless woman on the beach is no big deal since this is so common. Even in staid old London, one of the most popular newspapers features a picture of a topless woman every day. In the U.S., however, human anatomy is still covered up.

Having lived in many different cultures, I have learned to accept their norms, and so the puritanism that permeates our culture doesn't bother me very much. What does bother me is that this sense of shame also keeps us from learning how our bodies work. If people want to hide themselves head to toe from others, fine, but for them to hide from their own bodies is a ridiculous and even dangerous attitude.

In this chapter we cover, or maybe I should say uncover, the reproductive organs, including the male and female genitalia. Although these are the parts of the human body that come closest together, actually inserting one into the other, far too few people understand how their own or their partner's sexual equipment really functions.

Now, I am famous for saying that the most important piece of sexual paraphernalia lies not between your legs but between your ears—that is, your brain. But your brain cannot function without information, and it needs—you need—to know as much as possible about penises and vaginas and other organs. To maximize good sexual functioning you need to examine your own and to understand your partner's. I don't care if you want to make love with every light on surrounded by mirrors or in the dark under the sheets. If you feel uncomfortable parading around in the nude, you don't have to. But for your own health and pleasure you need to become familiar with human sexual anatomy.

Before you start any exploration, you need a road map. You need to know what you are looking at and how it functions, and that's what you'll get in this chapter. Read it carefully and remember it in your travels. Begin with your own body. Women especially need to make an effort to see their genitals. At some point you can broaden your studies with a partner. Your knowledge will not only contribute to a good grade but will help guarantee improved sexual functioning, and let me tell you, that's important.

This chapter focuses on our bodies: how they're built and how they work. Much is visible and can be easily observed, and much can be understood only at a microscopic or molecular level. **Anatomy** concerns the physical structure of our bodies and the design of organ systems (e.g., the circulatory, respiratory, nervous, genito-urinary, and reproductive systems). **Physiology** concerns the *functions* of these parts and organs—how they work. **Endocrinology** is the study of the glands that make and secrete hormones into the circulatory system. We defined and discussed some sex hormones in the previous chapter. This chapter will discuss the anatomy of human sexual and reproductive organs, how those structures function, and the role of hormones in regulating fertility and sex drive. Understanding the following chapters depends on first understanding the anatomy, physiology, and endocrinology of sexuality.

Studying the body is one thing, but understanding how we *feel* about our bodies is quite another. One of the themes throughout this book is that the relationship between self-esteem and body-image is an important part of one's sexuality. Someone who thoroughly understands how their body is built and how it works is much less likely to have inaccurate beliefs about their sexuality. Someone who knows their own body well and the basic anatomy of their sexual partner is in a better position to talk about intimate sexual feelings and concerns.

Thus the biological and physical aspects of human sexuality are prerequisite knowledge for understanding other interesting and complex issues. For example, a clear grasp of sexual arousal and orgasm depends on understanding external and internal female and male anatomy and the changes that accompany erection in men and vaginal lubrication in women. Similarly, understanding sexually transmitted infections involves knowing basic anatomy and physiology. Understanding the biology of sexuality is a necessary first step for understanding many issues in human sexuality.

This chapter necessarily uses many technical terms. We hope you will take the time to learn these words. Your instructor also is an important guide as you learn an appropriate sexual vocabulary. Remember the old saying: "style is the mirror of the mind." If you use sexual language carefully and correctly, your thoughts and actions will be similarly sophisticated. Often some practice is necessary. You already know that sexual words and terms often carry powerful meanings. Your instructor may use "desensitization exercises" to help you become more comfortable with some of this emotional language.

A WOMAN'S BODY

Ladies first! We're going to explore female anatomy, physiology, and hormonal mechanisms before we discuss the same dimensions in men. But let's begin with the common observation that for many people, the sight of the genitalia and a woman's breasts evokes strong emotions. Many societies throughout the world have developed clothing customs and even legal statutes for "decency" to regulate what body parts are shown in public. The explanation for such multicultural traditions is probably simple. Humans have evolved to be sensitive to cues that motivate the perpetuation of the species. The evocative appearance of female and male genitalia helps assure sexual interactions that may result in conception, gestation, and the birth of a child.

Diversity Is Normality

One overriding principle should guide any discussion of female and male external genitalia: *diversity is normality.* Whether dressed or undressed, no two of us look exactly alike, and this is true of our genitalia and breasts as well. There is a wide range of variation in virtually all anatomical structures. Teenagers undressing together in a changing room in the school gym or community pool are acutely aware of different rates of pubertal development and differences in the appearance of their genitals. Most adults, however, forget there is a wide variation also in adult genital appearance. Because such differences are normal, no one should be concerned about their own differences (Fig. 4-1).

Self-Examination of the External Female Genitalia

Many writers have emphasized the mysteries of humankind with sayings such as "We are infinitely mysterious to ourselves," or "What becomes too familiar becomes practically invisible." These phrases have meaning too for how many of us think about our bodies. Because of the powerful feelings associated with our genitals, many parents do not take enough time, care, and attention to teach children exactly about their sexual anatomy and the appropriate names for those parts. This is a very common problem. There is value, however, in coming to understand your own anatomy through careful self-examination.

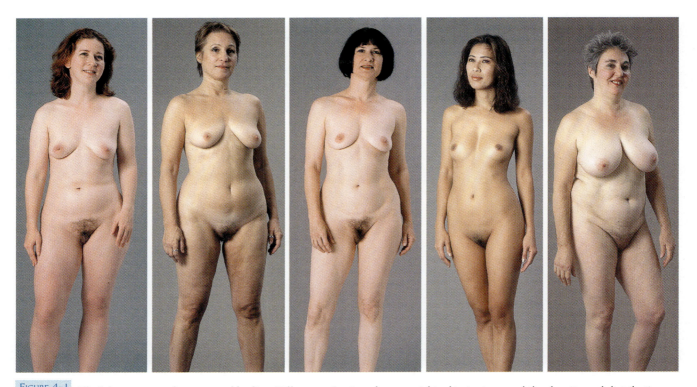

FIGURE 4-1   All of these women have normal bodies. Differences in size, shape, weight, skin texture, and the density and distribution of pubic hair are all obvious but at the same time certainly "average" or "typical."

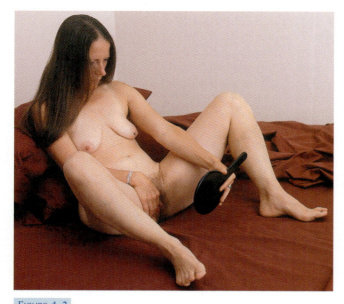

FIGURE 4-2 A genital self-examination allows women to learn the location, coloration, and texture of the structures which comprise the external genitalia.

When alone and assured of privacy, take the time to examine your own genitalia. Use a hand mirror or position yourself before a full-length mirror in such a way that you can see your external genital anatomy and vaginal opening. A flashlight might also be helpful. Slowly look carefully at yourself, using your fingers to open and make more visible your genitals. Don't hurry. When touching different parts of your genitalia, you will notice significant differences in their sensitivity, as well as their relative size and color shadings. If you experience some excitement or arousal, that's o.k.

There are two good reasons for self-examination. First, self-awareness is the first step to self-knowledge and self-

understanding. As well, taking personal responsibility for one's sexual and reproductive health is an important objective of this course. Knowing what you look and feel like when you are not experiencing any problems provides a "baseline" for later comparison if you suspect any problem. This self-knowledge will also help you communicate accurately with health care providers. Again, take your time. You might keep this book handy and use the sketches and photographs to learn the correct anatomical terms as you examine your own genital structures (Figs. 4-2 and 4-3).

THE VULVA

The **vulva** is the collective term for everything seen in an examination of the external female genitalia. These structures are sensitive to the touch, and most become wet or moist during sexual arousal. The vulva includes the mons veneris, labia majora, labia minora, clitoris, vestibule, urethral opening, introitus and hymen, and perineum (Fig. 4-4).

The Mons Veneris

About 3 or 4 inches (8–10 centimeters) below the navel, right on top of the pubic bone, is a small, dense cushion of fat called the **mons veneris,** which in Latin means "mountain of Venus," the ancient Roman goddess of love. The technical name for the pubic bone is the **pubic symphysis.** Most women have discovered that pressing on the mons produces sexual pleasure, the result of being richly endowed with nerve endings, and many women press on the mons when they masturbate to heighten the pleasure of clitoral stimulation. The mons is covered by a moderate to dense distribution of pubic hair, which appears in early adolescence. Sex hormones determine the specific patterns of pubic hair found in women and men. The amount of pubic hair varies considerably from woman to woman, depending also on the woman's age. The prominence of the mons is also somewhat variable.

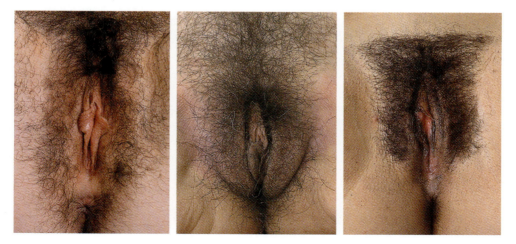

FIGURE 4-3   Despite differences in the prominence of the structures of the external genitalia, all of these photographs are of normal women.

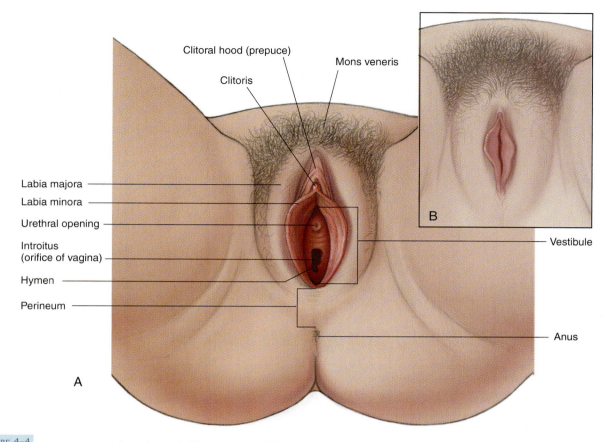

Clitoral hood (prepuce)

Mons veneris

Clitoris

Labia majora

Labia minora

Urethral opening

Introitus
(orifice of vagina)

Hymen

Perineum

B

Vestibule

Anus

A

FIGURE 4-4   A. Structures of the vulva with labia major and labia minora parted to allow observation of the vestibule. B. Structures of the vulva in a woman who is not sexually aroused.

The Labia Majora

In Latin, **labia majora** means "large lips." These are one of two sets of skin folds flanking the vestibule. On their outer surfaces facing the thighs is more pubic hair, while the inner surfaces adjacent to the labia minora have no pubic hair. These soft folds often have more skin pigmentation (coloring) than adjacent tissues and have many free nerve endings, making them extremely sensitive to touch.

The Labia Minora

The **labia minora** are the "small lips" that bound the vestibule. These delicate folds of skin have no pubic hair and vary greatly in appearance and prominence among women. They are extremely sensitive to touch. When women are pregnant and after a vaginal birth, the labia minora are darker in pigmentation than in nonpregnant women and women who have not given birth vaginally. These folds of skin are joined at the **clitoral prepuce,** or hood. They extend from the clitoris past the **external urethral meatus,** or urethral opening, and the vagina. The two vestibular bulbs extend under the labia minora. When a penis, fingers, or a dildo penetrates a woman's vagina, the side-to-side stretching of the labia minora causes the clitoral hood to rub against the clitoris, which is usually perceived as erotically exciting.

The Clitoris

The last chapter explained that the **clitoris** is a homologue of the penis, but of course it has no urinary functions in women as a penis does in men. Like the penis, during arousal the clitoris becomes turgid and sends the nervous system information about tactile stimulation, which is usually interpreted as erotic. The anatomy of the clitoris is nearly identical to that of the penis. It is a small cylindrical structure with a small shaft and a tip, called the **glans.** Unless you manually part the labia minora and pull the tissue slightly back, you cannot see the shaft of the clitoris, although the glans is usually visible without this maneuver. Inside the crura and body of the clitoris are two **cavernous bodies,** which become engorged with blood during sexual arousal, giving the clitoris a somewhat turgid, stiff feeling and appearance. The shaft of the clitoris lying deep within the mons is keenly sensitive to touch, but most women report that the glans is too tender for direct manual or penile stimulation, especially immediately after orgasm. Actually, the clitoral prepuce covers the glans until orgasm, which is one reason many women report that direct touching of the clitoris after intercourse is a little uncomfortable.

It has been estimated that the glans of the clitoris has approximately as many free nerve endings as the glans (tip) of a man's penis, an area of skin substantially larger—this

THE IMPORTANCE OF PRIVACY AND MEDICAL CHAPERONES

*G*ynecology is the medical specialty concerned with the health of a woman's genital and reproductive organs. Women are generally encouraged to have a yearly gynecologic examination including pelvic and breast exams and usually a rectal exam. A yearly gynecological examination is recommended for women after the age of 18 or who have started having sexual intercourse or using birth control pills. Few women claim to enjoy these exams. Although these diagnostic exams are not completely comfortable physically, they are not really painful either. Also, many women feel shy and reserved about exposing the most private parts of their bodies to a medical professional they see only once a year. More women today are also aware of the medical, legal, and privacy issues involved in an examination of their genitalia by a physician who they might not know very well. After all, one visit a year does not offer much opportunity for establishing a good rapport. For all these reasons, a medical chaperone is often a good idea. A medical chaperone is usually a nurse or member of the doctor's office staff who is present during gynecological examinations or other office procedures to ensure the legitimacy of what happens in the examination room.

Unhappily, reports of sexual misconduct are becoming more common in all arenas. Many physicians and patients therefore believe that having a third person in the examining room offers both parties important legal protections. Doctors want to feel assured that their appropriate examination is witnessed by a third party and that they will not be accused of improper behavior. Similarly, patients often feel that a chaperone's presence eliminates the risk of impropriety. But there are some drawbacks as well. For example, a woman who feels uncomfortable about revealing her genitalia and breasts to one professional person might feel even more reserved with two professionals there (Greider, 1995).

Many doctors speak to their patients alone and privately, generally either before or after the pelvic, breast, or rectal exam. Sexual and reproductive privacy is extremely important to most people.

Every woman needs to decide on her own about using a medical chaperone and should talk to her doctor about her expectations and wishes. In health care, as in any other business or industry, being an informed consumer is very important and often necessary to be satisfied with the services received.

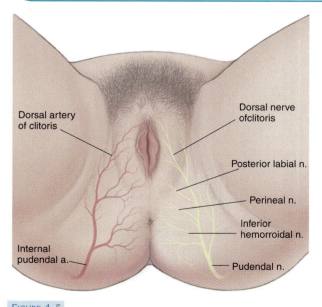

Dorsal artery of clitoris

Internal pudendal a.

Dorsal nerve ofclitoris

Posterior labial n.

Perineal n.

Inferior hemorrhoidal n.

Pudendal n.

FIGURE 4-5 Blood and nerve supply of the female external genitalia. Given the extreme sensitivity of these structures, the rich network of blood vessels and nerve endings in this region would be expected.

helps explain why this structure is so sensitive. Verkauf, Von Thron, and O'Brien (1992) reported that in a large sample (200 women) of subjects receiving routine gynecologic examinations, the average diameter of the glans was 3.4 +/− 1.0 mm. The total length of the glans was 5.1 +/− 1.4 mm, and the total length of the exposed portion of the clitoris, including the glans, was 16.0 +/− 4.3 mm. Clitoral dimensions were unrelated to the woman's age, height, weight, or current use of oral contraceptives. Generally, women who had had children had a slightly larger clitoris than women who hadn't. If there is any meaning or relevance to these variations in size, it remains obscure. We know of no data that show that larger or smaller clitorises or penises are any more or less sensitive (Fig. 4-5).

Because of the dense nerve endings in the clitoris, it is not surprising that manual stimulation of the clitoris is the most common method of female masturbation. Rarely is an object inserted into the vagina during masturbation; rather, the shaft of the clitoris is stimulated, sometimes while rubbing and pressing the mons veneris at the same time. The clitoris is also especially sensitive to vibratory stimulation. Chapter 8 discusses female masturbation in more detail.

Other Countries, Cultures, and Customs

RITUAL FEMALE GENITAL SURGERY IS NOT THE SAME EVERYWHERE

All cultures have customs, and many customs vary among different cultures. Rituals involving the surgical alteration of female genitalia differ in severity and extent in Asia and Africa. In some societies these are a rite of passage for females entering adolescence, and they do not resist or challenge these practices. The procedure typically causes significant scar tissue, which leads to painful menstruation and childbirth complications. When the woman begins having intercourse, it takes months for the vaginal opening to become wide enough for comfortable penile penetration. Not all societies that practice female circumcision do so in the same way, however. An informative example are the Bedouin in Israel, who are caught between two different cultures in the Middle East.

Asali et al. (1995) studied Bedouin women living in Israel using controlled observation and in-depth interviews. A female social worker with a background in human sexuality interviewed 21 Bedouin Arab women, who were also examined by an experienced gynecologist. The authors knew that ritual female genital surgery is commonly carried out in different societies and sought to determine the nature and extent of the procedure in these women. For example, in the most radical surgical procedure, called the "Pharaonic" operation or "infibulation," ". . . the clitoris is removed along with the labia minora and at least two-thirds of the labia majora . . ." (Asali et al., 1995, p. 572). A somewhat less invasive surgery known as the "Sunni" type removes the clitoral prepuce. Geographically and culturally, these two procedures are not entirely separate, and many groups practice both forms (Hosken, 1978). Asali et al. (1995) sought to learn whether one or both of these techniques were common among Bedouin women in Israel.

Extensive interviews were conducted. Five or six women spoke with the interviewer at one time because of the cultural inappropriateness of outsiders talking to Bedouin women alone. After some trust was established, one-on-one interviews were conducted. Surprisingly, *none* of these women could describe which part(s) of their genital anatomy had been altered in their ritual procedure. There was significant social pressure for young girls to undergo these rituals. The tribes believed that girls who had the ritual circumcision were more "clean." In most instances, the girl's mother pressured her daughter to undergo the procedure. Razors were typically used without anesthesia.

The physical examinations of these women were somewhat surprising. None of these women had a clitoridectomy or removal of the labia minora or labia majora. However, virtually all had small scars on the clitoral prepuce or the portion of the labia minora closest to the clitoris. Some women had a single scar, whereas others had multiple vertical and horizontal scars on the clitoris and labia minora, ranging in length from 0.5 to 1 cm (0.2 to 0.4 inch). Virtually all of these subjects remembered bleeding and discomfort, and three recalled needing medical attention.

The Bedouin women in Israel demonstrate the diversity of ritual female genital surgery. Although explicit clitoridectomy and infibulation are performed in other parts of the world, other less radical variations are performed also. Yet behind all of these customs is the folk belief that women will become cleaner and more attractive because of this ritual. Genital mutilation is also often practiced to ensure that the young woman is a virgin, a matter of great pride for her family. Asali et al. (1995) also note that these women reported that they had received somewhat contradictory messages: they would experience enhanced fertility and also diminished sex drive (Fig. 4-6).

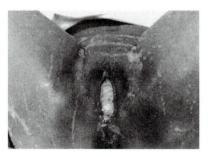

FIGURE 4-6 Scarring from ritual genital surgery. Different cultural traditions involve various patterns of skin markings after these wounds have healed.

Sometimes there is an accumulation of dead skin cells and dried urine with a white to yellowish color just underneath the hood of the clitoris. This pasty substance is called **smegma.** It can be removed using a cotton swab and warm, soapy water. A significant accumulation of smegma can cause discomfort during intercourse. While small amounts of smegma do not usually indicate poor hygiene, a woman should check carefully just under the clitoral hood during the self-examination.

Many African and Mideastern cultures practice a "coming of age" ritual involving a form of genital mutilation in pubescent girls. Clitoridectomy is the surgical removal of the clitoris and labia, often done with appallingly inadequate hygiene that results in infections that often leave the woman deformed for life. This procedure is usually referred to as **female circumcision,** although it is not an exact counterpart to male circumcision, which removes the foreskin covering the glans of the penis. Removing a woman's clitoris deprives her of a primary source of sexual pleasure, and clitoridectomy is often viewed as another way in which men impose their control over women. Women in these societies often see this ritual as an essential cultural requirement that enhances their appeal and acceptability to young men looking for a wife, and therefore they may hesitate to resist. As painful as this custom seems from the perspective of our own society, many well-meaning social scientists, including cultural anthropologists, have defended the right of other societies to perpetuate traditions and customs they have evolved over thousands of years. In the case of female circumcision, however, few informed Westerners would condone or defend this practice.

The Vestibule

The smooth tissue inside of the labia minora surrounding the opening to the vagina and urethral opening is called the **vestibule,** a term referring to an entranceway. While not very large, it is very sensitive and becomes slippery during vaginal lubrication. Figures 4-3 and 4-4 can help you locate the vestibule; pulling back the labia majora and labia minora in the self-examination may slightly distort how this area looks.

The External Urethral Meatus

The **urethra** is the tube that carries urine from the bladder to outside the body. It usually is located just below the clitoris and above the opening to the vagina. Because its location varies somewhat, it may be difficult to see unless you know what you're looking for. The tissues of the vestibule and external urethral meatus are very delicate and may become irritated for a variety of reasons discussed in the next chapter.

The Hymen

The entry to the vagina, the **introitus,** is surrounded with a thin membrane called the **hymen,** which in most women partially covers the vaginal opening. The hymen has been the focus of much attention because of the common belief that its appearance signifies whether a female has had her first intercourse. Because of its location, some tearing of the hymen and bleeding are common during first intercourse, but not in all cases. In fact, often the hymen isn't torn until a woman has a vaginal birth. The appearance of the hymen also varies considerably, as shown in Figure 4-7. Although most young women have a small opening in the hymen before intercourse, in some cases the membrane is completely closed and obstructs the passage of

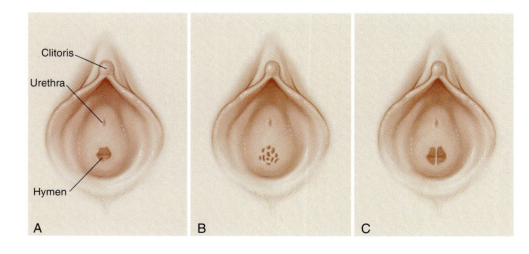

FIGURE 4-7 The appearance of annular (A), cribriform (B), and septate (C) hymens. Variations in the appearance of the hymen are common.

menstrual discharge. In such cases a doctor usually makes a small hole in the hymen to allow normal menstruation.

The tearing of the hymen with first intercourse does not produce substantial discomfort for most women (Weis, 1985). In a study of over 300 undergraduates, only 28.3% of the women reported that their first intercourse was physically satisfying. Most of the others said that they were a little uncomfortable physically, and many reported that a lack of emotional satisfaction and feelings of inexperience contributed to a lack of physical enjoyment and responsiveness (Darling, Davidson, & Passarello, 1992). Women's feelings about their first intercourse and the tearing of the hymen depend on many factors, not just physical discomfort. For example, these authors reported that whether the first intercourse was planned, involved contraception, and involved a partner who was loved in a relationship of some length all affected both the psychological and physiological aspects of this important sexual encounter.

Many women in many cultures believe it is important and desirable to be virginal before marriage. Some cultures even have a ceremony in which the bed sheets of the newlyweds are publically displayed to prove that the bride was a virgin on her wedding night. As well, many females define their virginity in personal ways, and some teenage females may engage in a variety of sexual behaviors, such as heavy petting, mutual masturbation, oral sex, and anal intercourse, but still not have penis-in-the-vagina intercourse. Such women may consider themselves virgins, and perhaps technically they are.

In any case, remember that the absence of a hymen does not necessarily mean that a woman has had penis-in-the-vagina intercourse, and the presence of a hymen does not necessarily mean that she has not. A girl's hymen may be torn through a variety of physical activities and mishaps that can occur in childhood and adolescence.

LOSING ONE'S VIRGINITY

Personal decisions about having sexual intercourse for the first time are complicated and are difficult to study. Langer, Zimmerman, and Katz (1995) collected data from over 1300 tenth-graders in Miami, Florida. Questions were asked about how virgins and nonvirgins felt about themselves in regard to sexual intercourse. The way nonvirgins felt after having had sex was not as positive as they had anticipated. The nonvirgins who anticipated having good feelings about having sex were likely to be male, not interested in postponing sex, influenced strongly by friends, and African-American. Those who said that they felt very good about having lost their virginity were likely to be male and to have had more sex partners. These data hold meaning for those who advise youngsters who are thinking about having sex for the first time. Encouraging caution about unanticipated pregnancy, sexually transmitted diseases, and AIDS, these writers emphasize that "feeling good" about yourself after having sex is by no means as important as carefully considering the unwanted consequences.

The previous chapter introduced attribution theory as a way people explain human behavior. This theory suggests that how people look at the world as either actors or observers affects how they explain their behaviors. Schechterman and Hutchinson (1991) use this theory to explore how different "virginity statuses" affect sexual perceptions and behavior. They defined four virginity statuses. *Adamant virgins* have not had sexual intercourse and are unlikely to before marriage. *Potential nonvirgins* have not yet had intercourse but are likely to with the appropriate person in certain circumstances. *Nonvirgins* have had intercourse and anticipate continuing to do so. *Regretful nonvirgins* have had intercourse but do not plan to continue to do so in the foreseeable future. This study suggests that virginity status affects how people feel about making personal sexual choices. For example, female adamant virgins were reportedly *less likely* to have a lot of control over sexual decisions; apparently, female adamant virgins might actually be more easily persuaded to be physically intimate. Perhaps adamant virgins are therefore less likely to enter situations in which their beliefs might be tested. Interestingly, female potential nonvirgins saw their sexual decisions as externally based while male potential nonvirgins saw their sexual decisions as internally based. The overriding conclusion of this study is important: how people approach sexual decisions depends heavily on their perceptions of the psychosocial environment and their place in that environment as women and men.

The Perineum

The **perineum** is the small area of smooth skin between the vaginal opening and the anus. It is very sensitive to touch and temperature. Many women find manual stimulation of this area, such as during foreplay, highly pleasurable. Because of its location, perineal tissue often tears when the newborn's head passes through the birth canal. Some obstetricians surgically cut the perineum, using a procedure called an episiotomy before the passage of the baby's head to prevent this tearing. Other obstetricians do not routinely make such an incision.

INTERNAL SEXUAL AND REPRODUCTIVE ANATOMY

In addition to the ovaries, fallopian tubes, uterus, and vagina (Fig. 4-8) there are other underlying internal structures not visible with self-examination.

The Crura

These spongy bodies composed of corpora cavernosa are the root of the clitoris. They attach the clitoris to the pubic bone, and like the clitoris, become engorged with blood and slightly rigid during sexual arousal. Women who manipulate the clitoris during masturbation often feel this stimulation much deeper in the pelvis, not only within the clitoris itself.

The Vestibular Bulbs

The **vestibular bulbs** are located deep under the labia minora, alongside the vestibule. They too become engorged with blood during sexual arousal. Their swelling can be perceived by women and men during penile penetration of the vagina, contributing to the feeling of "penile containment"—the feeling men have of being "held" during intercourse. As the vestibular bulbs swell, both women and men report feeling more genital pleasure. Anatomical research has documented that the erectile tissue in the vestibular bulbs extends into the clitoris and terminates in the glans. Thus there seems a continuity in many of the structures that become engorged with blood during sexual arousal (van Turnhout, Hage, & van Diest, 1995).

Bartholin's Glands

Before Masters and Johnson's first book, *Human Sexual Response,* was published in 1966, many believed that **Bartholin's glands** secreted much of the liquid that acts as a lubricant during sexual intercourse. These two small glands, about the size of small beans, are located on both sides of the opening to the vagina. Although they may produce very small amounts of liquid during arousal and orgasm, this is almost insubstantial. Most of the lubrication that eases penile insertion during intercourse comes from inside of the vagina. Some writers have suggested that this slight secretion may contribute to a woman's genital scent. In reality, no one knows for certain what important functions Bartholin's glands might serve.

Muscles Underlying the Vulva

Beneath the external genitalia is a complex network of muscles that support the vagina, give some tone to the opening to the vagina, and provide elasticity to accommodate the passage of a

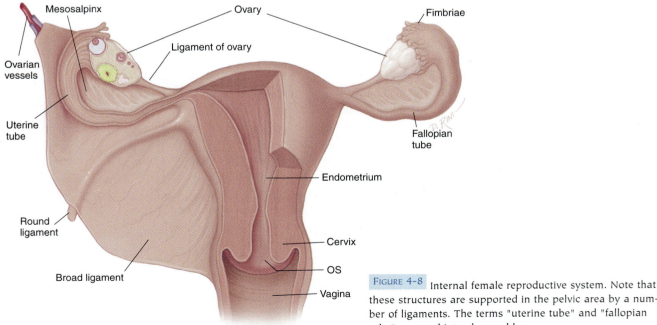

FIGURE 4-8   Internal female reproductive system. Note that these structures are supported in the pelvic area by a number of ligaments. The terms "uterine tube" and "fallopian tube" are used interchangeably.

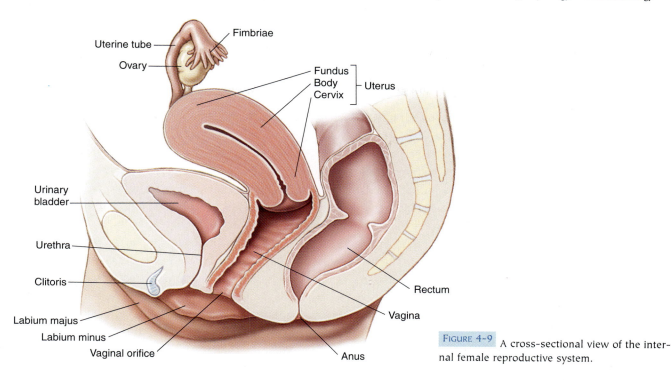

Figure 4-9 A cross-sectional view of the internal female reproductive system.

baby's head through the birth canal during childbirth. They are collectively called the pelvic floor muscles and they surround the urethral opening, the vagina, and the anal opening. The configuration and position of these muscles allows them to act as a "sling" to support a woman's internal organs during pregnancy. Good tone in these muscles gives good urinary control and helps provide the feeling of tightness men experience during intercourse. During a woman's orgasm, the rhythmic contractions of these muscles are sometimes quite strong, along with contractions of the muscular tissues surrounding the clitoris, vagina, and anus. An important pelvic floor muscle is the pubococcygeal muscle, which surrounds the vaginal opening. During childbirth, it may become stretched and temporarily lose its tone.

In 1952 Dr. Arnold Kegel discovered that exercising the pelvic floor muscles could improve vaginal tone, enhance pleasure during intercourse, and improve urinary continence, which diminishes with normal aging. **Kegel exercises** are short, rhythmic contractions and relaxations of the muscles along the pelvic floor; many gynecologists believe these exercises should be lifelong personal health habits for all women. These exercises may also benefit pregnant women because the fetus's head may press on the bladder, making urinary control difficult. The best way to learn Kegel exercises is to release urine in small amounts while sitting on the toilet, using a "start-stop" technique until the bladder is empty. After mastering this, it is recommended that women tighten and relax the same muscles during various "exercise periods" throughout the day when not urinating. Women should do 10–20 contractions at a time, working up to 60–80 contractions a day. Ideally, one should be able to sustain a contraction for 10 seconds without interruption.

The Vagina

The **vagina** is a collapsed sleeve of three different layers of tissue. Masters and Johnson referred to it as a "potential space" because it can stretch significantly, allowing most women to comfortably accommodate a penis of almost any size. The word "vagina" in Latin means "sheath" or "scabbard," referring to a sheath for a sword. Its posterior surface is a little longer than its anterior surface (Fig. 4-9). In most women who have not had a vaginal birth the vagina is about 3 inches (7.5 cm) long, and it is about 1 inch (2.5 cm) longer in women who have. Projecting from the roof of the back of the vagina is the cervix, the opening to the uterus. The vagina has four important functions. It is the female organ for sexual intercourse, although women and men, as well as women and women, enjoy many forms of physical intimacy other than penis-in-the-vagina intercourse. It is the passageway to the uterus for sperm, and the route through which menstrual flow leaves a woman's body. Finally, it is the birth canal through which babies are born (with the obvious exception of Cesarean section births). It has a highly adaptive structure for these functions.

The innermost layer of the vagina is a mucous membrane. This is the tissue you can feel inside the vagina with your finger. The secretions of this membrane increase during sexual arousal, providing lubrication that make penile penetration more comfortable. As well, this mucus helps keep the interior of the vagina clean and maintain an acid-alkaline balance. Tiny droplets of mucus are constantly produced within this layer. A number of ridges in this inner membrane give the vagina a furrowed texture that allows for expansion. The next layer of the vagina is muscular, which offers firmness to the otherwise soft

IS THERE SUCH A THING AS A G SPOT?

*I*n recent years there has been controversy about a supposed "super-sensitive" area inside the vagina that, when stimulated, is believed to precipitate an orgasm and even ejaculation through the external urethral meatus. This is still controversial, in part, because only a generation ago did women begin to feel sufficiently comfortable with themselves and their sexuality. Research has occurred only in recent decades.

In 1950 Dr. Ernest Grafenberg published a paper on the role of urethral stimulation in female orgasm. Dr. Grafenberg described an area located toward the front of the vagina along the anterior wall about 1 inch (2.5 cm) inside the vaginal opening. This area has no specific, consistent appearance or texture in unaroused women but becomes larger and has more clearly defined boundaries during arousal. It is about the size of a coin—smaller than a dime in unaroused women and becoming larger than a quarter as women become more excited. Many gynecologists claim not to have palpated the G spot (named for Grafenberg), perhaps because in most cases, women undergoing pelvic examinations are not sexually aroused. When this area is touched during arousal, many women first report a sudden urge to urinate but then quickly discriminate the feeling as erotic. When a woman needs to urinate, the bladder is distended, and gently touching the inside of the vagina at this time may help a woman localize this area.

Davidson, Darling, and Conway-Welch (1989) reported that stimulation of the G-spot independent of clitoral stimulation will lead to an orgasm that is qualitatively different from that attained through clitoral stimulation. Responses from almost 1300 questionnaires showed that 84.3% of the respondents believed in a sensitive focal area inside the vagina and that highly pleasurable feelings result from its stimulation; 72.6% reported experiencing an orgasm from stimulation of this area. Many respondents also reported a small fluid spurt from the urethral meatus associated with orgasm, although some noted it was difficult to discriminate between normal vaginal lubrication and this apparent ejaculation. However, Ladas, Whipple, and Perry (1982) write that female ejaculation is reported by approximately 10% of women.

What is there about stimulating this specific area that elicits a spurt of fluid from the urethral meatus? A number of tiny glands called Skene's glands surround the urethra just inside the urethral opening. These glands come from the same embryological tissues that give rise to the prostate gland in males. Presumably, stimulating the Grafenberg area causes the secretions of Skene's glands to enter the urethra and to be expelled during ejaculation. The data are inconsistent regarding the composition of the female ejaculate itself. While some researchers report finding an enzyme found in a male prostatic fluid (prostatic acid phosphatase), it is actually a somewhat altered form of the enzyme. Other researchers report the presence of urea, a basic component of urine. As of this writing, it is not known where female ejaculate is stored or the specific relationship between the Grafenberg area and ejaculation in women.

We should note that some investigators (Hoch, 1986) have failed to find a localized area in the vagina that changes in shape and prominence during erotic stimulation. However, virtually all of the anterior wall of the vagina was found to be especially erotically sensitive, whereas the remainder of the interior of the vagina was decidedly less so or even entirely insensitive.

Regardless of whether there is or is not a G spot, we are concerned that a belief in it may motivate some people to try to find it and neglect many other aspects of intimate sharing. Research has found no "magic method" in lovemaking that regularly and reliably causes a woman to have long and strong orgasms. Seeking such a technique while ignoring the wide variety of other pleasurable forms of stimulation is short-sighted. We discourage an overly mechanistic, routine, and invariable approach to sex, even when some suppose it to have immediate and wonderful results (Fig. 4-10).

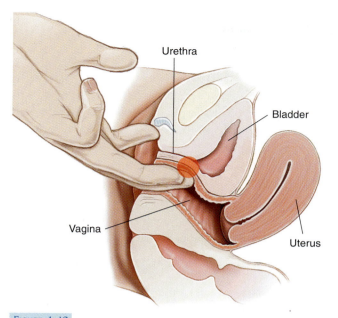

FIGURE 4-10   A cross-sectional view of the vagina, bladder, and uterus. A red dot marks the location of the Grafenberg area—usually referred to as the "G spot." Manual stimulation of this area, shown here, is thought to precipitate orgasm.

tissue. The outermost layer is composed of elastic connective tissue, giving the vagina much flexibility. Together these layers of tissue create an optimal organ for its functions.

When a woman is not sexually aroused or having sexual intercourse, the inner walls of the vagina contact each other. While the opening to the vagina is very sensitive to tactile stimuli, most of the interior of the vagina is not very well endowed with nerves; the inner two-thirds of the interior of the vagina has very little sensitivity. Occasionally women report feelings of discomfort while having intercourse, especially rapid, deep pelvic thrusting by their partner; in such instances it is not the interior of the vagina that causes these feelings, but rather the stretching of ligaments that support the uterus.

The normal secretions of the vagina facilitate penile penetration and also at other times signal periods of peak fertility in the menstrual cycle. Mucous membranes inside the vagina and cervical tissues produce liquid secretions that vary in color, viscosity, smell, and taste throughout the monthly cycle, as well as during sexual arousal. These secretions are more or less obvious in different women. For example, younger women generally experience more vaginal lubrication during sexual arousal than older women. Even in the same woman, the amount of such liquid varies over time. Generally speaking, the more sexual stimulation the woman experiences before penile penetration, the more vaginal lubrication occurs.

At the time of ovulation, a woman might notice a clear-to-yellowish, odorless vaginal secretion. When a potentially fertilizable egg has been released by the ovaries, the cervical mucus has a decreased viscosity thought to be a biological

adaptation to increase the chances of conception. The texture of this secretion helps sperm swim more easily through the cervix, into the uterus, and on to the fallopian tubes. It is also somewhat alkaline and offsets the normally acidic environment of the vagina, enhancing sperm motility. These issues are discussed in greater depth in Chapter 10 in terms of factors affecting fertility and conception.

The Uterus and Cervix

When a woman is not pregnant, her **uterus** is about the size and shape of a pear. It is a multilayered, hollow, muscular organ located between the bladder and the rectum and, like the vagina, it has multiple roles. The uterus is often called the "womb"—a more comfortable term for many people. It is a complex structure despite its simple appearance (Fig. 4-11). The size of the uterus varies significantly through a woman's life span. When a female baby is born, her **cervix** is relatively large, primarily because of the influence of the large amount of estrogens in the mother's blood stream. The uterus and cervix are fairly small during the childhood years. The uterus grows significantly during pregnancy. In adult, non-pregnant women it is about 3 inches (7.5 cm) long and about 2 inches (5 cm) wide. The uterus is made up of three layers: the perimetrium, the myometrium, and the endometrium.

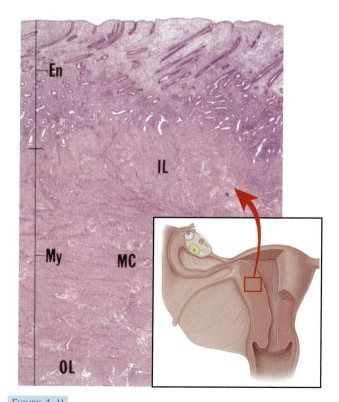

FIGURE 4-11   A microscopic section of the uterus illustrating the various muscular layers. "En" denotes the endometrium and "My" denotes the myometrium. IL, inner longitudinal muscle; MC, middle circular muscle; OL, outer longitudinal muscle.

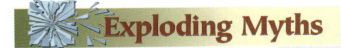

Exploding Myths

The Media, Women's Bodies, and Feminine Health and Hygiene Products

Even a quick glance through many "women's magazines" reveals something that might seem a little odd: dozens of advertisements for feminine hygiene products imply that women's vaginas smell bad. For example, advertisements for aerosol "feminine deodorants" imply such products are necessary if a woman wants to feel "really fresh and clean." In fact there is no good reason for healthy women to use these products. Both women and men have a "genital scent" from normal perspiration and oil gland secretions of the external genitalia and the secretions of Bartholin's glands in women. This is a normal odor, however, and aerosol fragrances used on the external genitalia are both unnecessary and potentially highly irritating. Another, perhaps more important problem is that such ads associating something unpleasant with the normal appearance and functioning of the vagina may cause some women to feel there is something bad or unclean about themselves. The normal secretions of the vagina's mucous membranes have a self-cleaning function, and women should be encouraged to trust their body's capacity to keep itself sanitary.

Some sanitary napkins and tampons are also scented—for no good hygienic reason. Although menstrual discharge does have a slight odor, it's seldom significant. Again, regular bathing is more than adequate to keep a woman feeling fresh and clean during her period.

The most controversy involves douching, the introduction of various types of fluids into the vagina under low pressure, usually with a hand-held squeeze bottle. An estimated 67 million American women have douched, (Rosenberg, Phillips, & Holmes, 1991), with approximately 20 million douching regularly (Rosenberg & Phillips, 1992). Since 1974, the sale of over-the-counter douching products has tripled (Chow et al., 1985). In the study by Rosenberg et al. of 618 women, three characteristics were associated with douching: lower socioeconomic status, increased risk of acquiring a sexually transmitted disease, and symptoms that might indicate a vaginal infection. These three attributes were most clearly associated with women who douched frequently. These data suggest that many women douche if they suspect they might have a sexually transmitted disease or vaginal infection instead of going to a doctor, and this behavior could lead to a delay in being treated.

A study by Wolner-Hanssen et al. (1990) demonstrated a strong correlation between frequent douching and pelvic inflammatory disease (PID). Acute PID affects the lining of the fallopian tubes and may impair later fertility. The more often one douches, the greater the probability of developing PID. These researchers suggest that douching may flush the vagina of healthy microorganisms that resist the bacteria that cause PID, or it may force those dangerous bacteria into the uterus from which they then spread to the fallopian tubes. Recent data support the connection between frequent douching and reduced fertility (Baird, Weinberg, Voigt, & Daling, 1996) in women who are trying to become pregnant. As well, Chow, Daling, Weiss, More, and Soderstrom (1985) report that women who douched at least weekly were twice as likely to have an ectopic tubal pregnancy as woman who did not douche at all. On the other hand, in couples being treated for infertility, Everhardt, Dony, Jansen, Lemmons, and Doesburg (1990) showed that douching with a dilute sodium bicarbonate solution significantly reduced the viscosity of cervical mucus, theoretically improving the chances of conception.

A final aspect of feminine hygiene products concerns how they are commonly displayed in stores. Because douches and feminine deodorants (also sold in suppository form) are often located next to condoms and spermicidal jellies, foams, and suppositories, some women without much sexual awareness believe all these items are contraceptives, when of course they are not.

The outermost layer is the perimetrium, sometimes called the serous layer, which includes most of the uterus except the cervical canal. The primary layer of the uterus is called the myometrium. The muscular fibers of the myometrium are arranged in various directions and are interspersed with blood vessels, lymphatic vessels, and nerves. These muscles are quite powerful in order to push the newborn out of the birth canal during childbirth. Each individual labor contraction is a synchronized action of all the muscle fibers in the myometrium. The innermost layer of the uterus, the endometrium, adheres to the inside of the myometrium. It has many blood vessels, mucous membranes, and connective tissues. The endometrium thickens in each menstrual cycle because hormones have prepared it to receive a fertilized egg. At the end of the menstrual cycle in which fertilization has not occurred, it is sloughed off. This is discussed in more detail in a later section on the menstrual cycle.

A number of ligaments in the pelvic area support the uterus. The position of the uterus in the body varies. In most women the vagina and uterus are at about a 90-degree angle to each other, affected somewhat by how full the bladder is. The uterus in some women is tilted back toward the lower spine; this is called a retroverted uterus. The uterus has three parts. The top is called the fundus, its narrowing middle section is the isthmus, and its opening is the cervix.

The opening to the cervix is called the os. The cervical canal running through the middle of the cervix is flattened, with tissue ridges running along its length. The mucus within it has the consistency of a gel. Cervical mucus varies in viscosity through the menstrual cycle; this substance comes from a number of small glands inside the cervix. Estrogen thins the mucus, and progesterone thickens it. The thickness of cervical mucus affects how easily sperm can swim through the cervix into the uterus. When cervical mucus is clear and stringy, sperm readily swim through it. Thickening is caused by long molecules that form a tangled network in the mucus (Carlstedt & Sheehan, 1989). Later chapters discuss cervical cancer and the role of the cervix in fertility.

The Fallopian Tubes

The famous Italian anatomist Gabriel Fallopius in the mid-1500s first described the appearance of what later came to be called the **fallopian tubes.** These two passageways connect the uterus with the area around the ovaries; they are 3 to 5 inches (7.5 to 12.5 cm) in length and very narrow and fragile. The opening of each fallopian tube adjacent to each ovary is surrounded by fimbria, which resemble the petals of a flower. These "funnel" the egg released at ovulation into the upper portion of the fallopian tube, where fertilization may occur. The fallopian tubes are also called "oviducts" or "uterine tubes." Sperm deposited in the vagina during intercourse swim through the cervix, up the uterus, and through the fallopian tubes toward the ovaries. A fertilized ovum travels back down the fallopian tube to the uterus where it is implanted in the uterine wall.

The lining of the fallopian tubes is a mucus membrane that is continuous with the mucus membrane inside the uterus. It is covered with tiny, hair-like cells called cilia that "sweep" the fertilized ovum down to the uterus with the currents they set up. The lining of the fallopian tubes is covered with delicate folds of tissue that nourish the fragile fertilized egg (Fig. 4-12). Very small muscle fibers in the walls of the fallopian tubes, thought to be stimulated by the ovary's release of a mature egg, create a gentle suction that draws the egg into the fimbria of the fallopian tubes. Tiny glands in the walls of the fallopian tubes produce nutrients that sustain the fertilized egg on its trip toward the uterus. All adaptations work together to help ensure the implantation of a fertilized egg in the lining of the uterus. It generally takes 3–7 days for a fertilized egg to reach the uterus.

Sometimes the fertilized egg gets stuck in the fallopian tube and begins to develop there. This is called an ectopic pregnancy. The term "ectopic" actually refers to the development of a fertilized egg anywhere other than in the uterus, which may also include the pelvic cavity. Such a pregnancy cannot proceed to birth. Significant discomfort usually occurs, and surgical treatment is required; the fallopian tube and developing fertilized embryo must be removed. Without surgery, the fallopian tube would burst and cause life-threatening internal bleeding. One of the negative consequences of delayed treatment for sexually transmitted diseases is pelvic inflammatory disease, which often involves scarring inside the fallopian tubes. Such scarring increases the risk of a fertilized egg lodging in the fallopian tube and causing an ectopic pregnancy. Since some common STDs (gonorrhea and chlamydia) frequently do not cause any early symptoms in women, tissue damage may occur before medical assistance is sought.

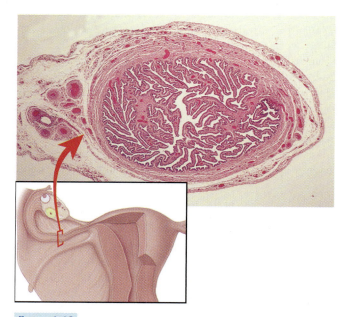

FIGURE 4-12 A cross-sectional photograph of a fallopian tube. Note the many delicate membranes within it. Not simply a "hollow tube," the fallopian tubes are elegant in their complexity.

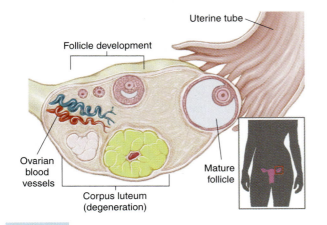

FIGURE 4-13 An ovary, showing stages in the development of a primary follicle. Note that the ovary is well-supplied with blood vessels. These carry a number of hormones, especially from the pituitary gland, to the ovary where they stimulate the ovary to produce its own hormones.

The Ovaries

The **ovaries** are a woman's gonads, the sex-cell–producing glands. The two ovaries are located on both sides of the pelvis (Fig. 4-13). In younger women they are almond-shaped, smooth, and white. With aging they become puckered, shriveled, and gray, the result of scars (corpus albicans) left by each egg that leaves the ovary. The ovaries are attached to one of the ligaments that supports the uterus.

Within each ovary are many primary follicles, each of which can mature into a fertilizable egg. At birth, a female infant has an estimated 200,000 to 400,000 primary follicles in each ovary; most of these deteriorate before the onset of menstruation, when only a few hundred are left. The ovaries have two functions: to produce eggs and to produce hormones, including the estrogens and progesterone. These hormones regulate ovulation and the menstrual cycle and are basic to a woman's fertility. Ovulation refers to the production of a mature, fertilizable egg from an ovary. A woman usually ovulates from one of the ovaries each month, sometimes from both— but not necessarily at the same time. At puberty, increased estrogen secretion by the ovaries initiates the appearance of secondary sexual characteristics. Very small amounts of these hormones have powerful effects on fertility and body configuration. The many roles and effects of these hormones will be discussed at various times through this text.

THE MENSTRUAL CYCLE

While the term **menstruation** refers to the regular sloughing off of the endometrium and the accompanying vaginal bleeding, this is only the most obvious sign of the cyclic, monthly variation in a woman's reproductive system. Although many women find menstruation a painful or disagreeable time of the month, many others do not experience much inconvenience or discomfort at all and may even feel affirmed in their femininity by this sign of their capacity to conceive and bear a child. The psychological and

social aspects of menstruation are interesting and complex. But before we discuss these, we need to understand the complex hormonal mechanisms responsible for the menstrual cycle.

The menstrual cycle involves the preparation of the endometrium for the implantation of an embryo after an ovum is fertilized high in the fallopian tubes and makes its way down to the uterus. For implantation to be successful, the endometrium must become thick, spongy, moist, and well supplied with blood vessels carrying oxygen. This is an ideal environment for the beginning of life: soft, wet, rich in oxygen, dark, quiet, and very still. Anything that compromises this environment may impair or stop implantation, even though fertilization has occurred. Conception does not always lead to implantation and pregnancy. If conception does not occur, the endometrium gradually separates from the wall of the uterus and is expelled through the cervix over a number of days as menstrual discharge.

Many girls and women do not know how long their menstrual cycle lasts, how long their periods last, or when during their menstrual cycle they are most fertile. We recommend that women keep a written record of the beginning and end of their menstrual cycles and how long their menstrual discharge lasts. This information can be very helpful if a menstrual problem requires a visit to one's gynecologist. For those using oral contraceptives this is a moot point, because the length of the cycle and the number of days of menstrual discharge are determined by the synthetic hormones in these pills. This discussion of menstruation concerns cycles unregulated by oral contraceptives.

The menstrual cycle begins on the first day of the period and ends the day before the next menstrual discharge begins. The length of a woman's menstrual cycle can vary from as short as 21 days to as long as 41 days in rare cases. The menstrual discharge can last from 2 to 6 days. Stress, fatigue, illness, regular strenuous exercise, and eating disorders can all affect the length and regularity of a woman's menstrual cycle. With a reasonably regular lifestyle, however, the menstrual cycle is generally very regular.

The Brain, Endocrine System, and Hormones

The last chapter defined hormones as chemical substances which are produced by endocrine glands and secreted directly into the bloodstream. Once there, they travel to various parts of the body and affect the activity of those "target" organs. The most important endocrine gland is the pituitary gland (Fig. 4-14). The **pituitary gland,** the size of a lima bean, is located in the middle of the head, just beneath the brain, to which it is connected through a network of blood vessels and nerve fibers. The hypothalamus is the part of the brain that communicates with the pituitary gland. The pituitary is composed of three lobes and is encased in a hard, bony capsule. It can be seen in x-rays of the head. The pituitary is called the master gland because it tells the other endocrine glands what to do and when. It sends hormonal messages that cause them to start and stop their own secretion of hormones. Female sex hormones are secreted by the ovaries in response to the pituitary

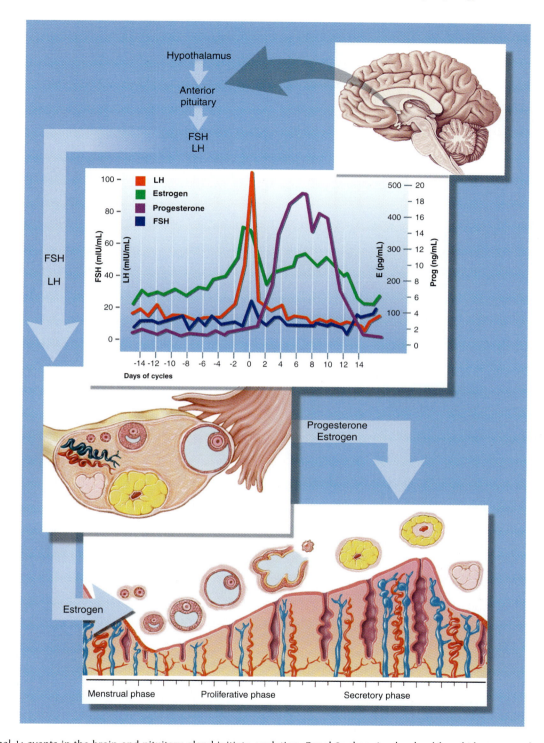

FIGURE 4-14   Panel 1: events in the brain and pituitary gland initiate ovulation. Panel 2: changing levels of female hormones throughout the menstrual cycle. Day "0" represents the occurrence of ovulation, day -2 is two days before ovulation, etc. Panel 3: the ovary. Panel 4: various stages of the development of the primary follicle, and (below) changes in the lining of the uterus and phases of the uterine cycle.

gland's instructions. In addition to affecting reproduction, hormones from the ovaries affect breast development, the development in puberty of an "hour glass" feminine shape, and the density and distribution of pubic hair. Chapter 12 dis-

cusses this in greater detail in the context of adolescent sexuality and puberty.

If the pituitary gland "senses" that another endocrine gland needs to begin or increase the secretion of its own hormones, it will send its own hormonal instructions to that gland. When the target gland follows these directions and increases the secretion of its hormones, the pituitary gland recognizes this and stops the stimulating message. This process is just like the thermostat in your home, which senses cool air and sends a message to the furnace to increase its production of heat. The room temperature rises, and the thermostat detects this and sends another message to the furnace to shut off. This is called a negative feedback mechanism. The menstrual cycle depends on such negative feedback mechanisms involving the hypothalamus, the pituitary gland, the ovaries, and the endometrium.

The Follicular Phase

The follicular phase begins on the first day of a woman's menstrual cycle when a chemical messenger secreted by the hypothalamus, gonadotropin-releasing hormone (GnRH), travels to the pituitary gland. The term "gonadotropin" means a hormone that stimulates the gonads, in this case the ovaries. GnRH stimulates the pituitary gland to secrete two of its own hormones, follicle-stimulating hormone (FSH) and luteinizing hormone (LH). Working together, these two hormones cause a number of immature ova in the ovaries to begin to mature and to secrete estrogen. Of the several ova that begin to develop, usually one matures more than the others and expands toward the surface of the ovary. This well-developed ovarian follicle, sometimes called the Graafian follicle, becomes an obvious swelling on the surface of the ovary.

The Ovulatory Phase

The ovulatory phase begins on about the eleventh day of the menstrual cycle. As the Graafian follicle gets progressively larger, a nipple-like protuberance forms on its surface called the stigma. Then an increased pituitary secretion of LH from the pituitary gland causes the follicle to rupture. The ovum within it is released along with fluid from inside the Graafian follicle. This is called ovulation, and it typically occurs on the 14th day of the menstrual cycle. The fluid escapes into the pelvic cavity and sometimes causes discomfort, which can allow the woman to feel that she has ovulated. This discomfort is referred to as Mittelschmerz, German for "middle pain"—referring to pain in the middle of a woman's body. It can cause mild discomfort or, in rare cases, enough pain to mimic appendicitis.

The Luteal Phase

After the Graafian follicle releases the ovum, the cells remaining in the follicle become a temporary endocrine gland called the corpus luteum ("yellow body," named for its appearance). The corpus luteum secretes progesterone and some estrogen, and the body's level of progesterone rises substantially during this phase. Progesterone sends a chemical message back to the pituitary to stop further secretion of FSH and LH. In essence, the corpus luteum is telling the pituitary that in case fertilization has occurred, it should not secrete any more FSH and LH or start another menstrual cycle. If fertilization and implanta-

tion have not taken place, the corpus luteum disintegrates, forming a small scar (corpus albicans) on the surface of the ovary. However, if a pregnancy has begun, a hormone from the developing embryo called human chorionic gonadotropin (HCG) signals the corpus luteum to continue producing hormones. This continues until the placenta forms and produces estrogen and progesterone on its own; then the corpus luteum deteriorates.

The Menstrual Phase

If conception and implantation have not occurred, the final events in the ovaries during the menstrual cycle lead to the shedding of the endometrium. The rapid drop in secretion of estrogen and progesterone from the corpus luteum sets into play the gradual separation of the endometrium from the myometrium and its slow disintegration. As this occurs, there is a gradual increase in the pituitary gland's secretion of FSH to begin a new cycle with the growth of more immature primary follicles.

The Uterine Cycle

So far we have looked at what is happening in the ovaries and in the hormonal communication between them and the hypothalamus and pituitary gland. Now let's look at the changes in the uterus correlated to the ovarian cycle just described. While most women are somewhat aware of their feelings associated with changing hormone levels, virtually all women feel the sensations accompanying changes in the uterus during their menstrual cycle.

THE MENSTRUAL PHASE

Like other events inside the uterus in the menstrual cycle, the sloughing off of the endometrium is under hormonal control. The decreased secretion of estrogen and progesterone sets the following events into action. As soon as estrogen and progesterone levels fall, the cells of the endometrium begin to shrink substantially, by some estimates to as little as 65% of their premenstrual size. Following this, a day or two before the menstrual flow begins, the blood vessels supplying the endometrium are closed off, causing these cells to begin dying. The death of endometrial cells causes the endometrium to separate from the myometrium. This tissue, along with blood in the hollow center of the uterus, stimulates uterine contractions that gradually force the menstrual discharge through the cervix into the vagina. These contractions are what are commonly called menstrual cramps. Blood, water, tissue fluid, and tissue debris are expelled. If the ovum was not fertilized, it is not expelled during menstruation but gradually disintegrates on its own. Menstruation typically lasts 3 to 5 days.

THE PROLIFERATIVE PHASE

After menstruation, the growth of primary follicles and the Graafian follicle during the follicular phase in the ovary cause secretion of estrogen. This hormone stimulates the cells of the endometrium, which thickens and becomes richly supplied with

DOES MENSTRUAL SYNCHRONY REALLY EXIST?

*W*hen women live together and interact frequently, they sometimes develop similar menstrual cycles; this is called "menstrual synchrony." It is not known how this happens. Although the sense of smell is often mentioned as a factor involved in menstrual synchrony, its role is not yet known. The data regarding menstrual synchrony are often inconsistent and inconclusive.

Weller, Weller, and Avinir (1995) studied menstrual synchrony among college roommates in dormitories in Israel. These data were collected prospectively: subjects recorded their menstruation as it happened rather than relying on memory to report how their periods gradually reached more or less similar beginning and ending times. Data were collected for an entire academic year among young women who were not using oral contraceptives. Menstrual synchrony was found to occur among women who were close friends and who had social interactions. Women who were not close friends did not show menstrual synchrony. Weller and Weller (1993) also reported menstrual synchrony among mothers and daughters living together in the same house, college roommates living together in private homes, and college roommates living in dormitories. As clear as their results were, other studies failed to recognize menstrual synchrony under similar circumstances. Why menstrual synchrony occurs or does not occur is still unknown.

Trevathan, Burleson, and Gregory (1993) studied the existence of menstrual synchrony in lesbians living together. Subjects kept careful records of their menstrual starting dates, intimate interactions, and sexual behavior. None of these subjects reported having any sexual contact with men during the study. Interestingly, there was no indication at all of menstrual synchrony. Wilson, Kiefhaber, and Gravel (1991) studied menstrual synchrony among sorority members and roommates, as well as a sample of 24 women living in cooperative student housing. No indication of menstrual synchrony was found in either study.

The data seem to both support and refute the existence of menstrual synchrony. It remains an interesting and enigmatic phenomenon.

---

blood vessels. This estrogen secretion also causes the cervical mucus to become thinner and easier for sperm to swim through. The proliferative phase ends at the moment of ovulation.

THE SECRETORY PHASE

As long as the corpus luteum exists in the ovary, the progesterone it is secreting stimulates tiny glands in the endometrium. The endometrium produces a form of sugar to nourish an implanted fertilized egg. Progesterone, unlike estrogen, causes the cervical mucus to become extremely thick, forming a little "plug" in the cervix (Carlstedt & Sheehan, 1989). If fertilization has not occurred, the menstrual phase described earlier begins again. These events are all summarized in Figure 4-14.

Awareness of Ovulation

Because fertility depends on producing fertilizable eggs, women often wonder when or whether they are ovulating normally. In fact, a woman can get a good idea about ovulation from certain body changes. The first has already been mentioned. Mittelschmerz, or lower abdominal discomfort, sometimes accompanies the release of a mature ovum from the ovary because the ovarian fluid may irritate the peritoneum. Women who report mittelschmerz on one side of the pelvis 1 month often report a similar feeling on the other side the next month. Another clue

to ovulation involves the cervical mucus, which becomes very thin due to the action of estrogen. Many women notice a clear-to-yellowish, odorless vaginal discharge in their underwear around the time of ovulation. Chapter 10 discusses how a woman can test the viscosity of her cervical mucus to determine her peak period of fertility during her menstrual cycle.

On waking in the morning, the body temperature is the lowest of the day. This is called the basal body temperature (BBT). Because changes in basal body temperature signal the approach and onset of ovulation, BBT charts can show a woman when she is approaching the peak period of fertility during her menstrual cycle (see Chapter 10 for an example of a BBT chart). A special basal thermometer is needed that registers lower body temperatures with high accuracy. Following are guidelines:

1. Before going to bed, shake down the thermometer and place it within easy reach. On waking, without getting out of bed and moving as little as possible, put the thermometer under the tongue for 5 minutes while holding perfectly still.
2. Read and then record the temperature on a BBT chart (see Chapter 10). Woman will see the basal body temperature fluctuate within a relatively narrow range for about the first 12 days of the cycle.

3. When the temperature has dropped by one half to a degree or more, this means the woman is getting ready to ovulate and that she is fertile at this time.

4. The next morning the woman will notice that the temperature has increased by at least one degree or more. This means that she has ovulated and that the corpus luteum has formed and begun to secrete progesterone. Progesterone reliably causes an increase in body temperature. As long as the temperature remains elevated (usually 3 or 4 days), the woman is fertile. When it begins to decline, menstruation will occur in a few days. The ovum that has been released from the ovary is fertilizable for about 24 hours, although recent data indicate that intercourse occurring before ovulation is most likely to lead to conception. Like cervical mucus tests, the BBT chart can be used to time intercourse to maximize or minimize the probability of conception.

The factors that affect the length of the menstrual cycle also can cause irregularities in the timing of ovulation: stress, fatigue, illness, strenuous exercise, and eating disorders. Chapter 10 shows an idealized BBT chart. In reality, wide variations in body temperature often occur for no apparent reason. A woman can make a BBT chart to learn more about her menstrual cycle and the interesting interplay between the pituitary gland and the ovaries.

Intercourse During Menstruation

Unlike many other animals, humans are not predisposed to have intercourse only when fertilization is likely. Humans are influenced by biological, social, and interpersonal stimuli to have sex even when conception is unlikely (such as during menstruation) or very unlikely (such as when using contraceptives appropriately). Some couples wonder or worry about having intercourse during menstruation, when things can get a little messy. Of course, there is no reason not to. Many women report that they desire to have intercourse during their periods, and some say that orgasms help relieve feelings of pelvic fullness that sometimes accompany menstruation. As with all sexual interactions, the couple should talk and share their feelings openly to validate and affirm their desires. Still, many people prefer to avoid sexual intercourse during menstruation.

A study involving 287 women and 206 men in Chile found that 70% of the women and 72% of the men made a point of not having intercourse during menstruation (Barnhart, Furman, & Devoto, 1995). This was a large urban sample, and there is little reason to think this culture is unique in this aversion. Women with higher education were less likely to avoid intercourse during menstruation than women with only an elementary or secondary education (57% versus 73%); the same was found among the men.

One aspect of intercourse during menstruation deserves mention in this context. Endometriosis is a condition in which endometrial tissue is discharged into the pelvic cavity through the top of the fallopian tubes during menstruation rather than

out through the cervix. It can cause discomfort and infertility. A study of almost 500 women found a strong statistical association between having intercourse frequently during menstruation and the development of endometriosis (Filer & Wu, 1989). We are careful to say that frequent intercourse during menstruation does not *cause* endometriosis—only that they may be related. One's personal physician can give the best advice on this issue. Recent studies also suggest a relationship between vaginal yeast infections, called candidiasis, and intercourse during menstruation (Hellberg, Zdolsek, Nilsson, & Mardh, 1995), but again, this is only a statistical association, not a clear cause-and-effect relationship.

The decision to have intercourse during menstruation usually involves the couple's wishes and desires, and sometimes health-related concerns. Nonetheless, some societies have powerful beliefs about menstruation (see the box Other Countries, Cultures, and Customs).

A WOMAN'S BREASTS

Because of where they are, how they are shaped, and what they do, a woman's breasts are well suited to nurture and provide warmth to the newborn, as well as help the mother and baby bond. In addition to the milk of breast feeding, the act involves eye contact between the mother and newborn, olfactory cues to mother's uniqueness, and intimate cuddling that adds to the relationship. Breasts may differ significantly in size and shape (Fig. 4-15).

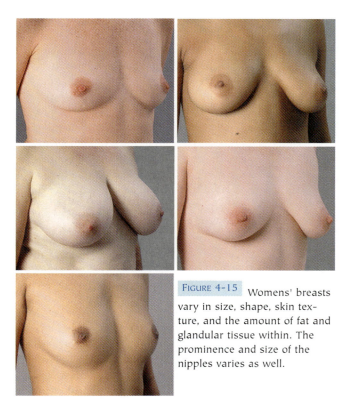

FIGURE 4-15 Womens' breasts vary in size, shape, skin texture, and the amount of fat and glandular tissue within. The prominence and size of the nipples varies as well.

Other Countries, Cultures, and Customs

WOMEN, MENSTRUATION, AND THE SLAUGHTER OF PIGS IN RURAL PORTUGAL

Buckley and Gottlieb's 1988 book about the anthropology of menstruation, *Blood Magic,* describes many interesting studies and anecdotes about customs related to menstruation. An interesting chapter by Denise L. Lawrence describes the sexual politics of menstruation in rural Portugal. Lawrence shows how menstruation is embedded in the wider factional relations between women and men in this culture. Sometimes, for example, women play upon male-perceived menstrual-related taboos in order to achieve their own needs in their society.

Most families in rural southern Portugal raise pigs. The meat is used to make sausages for the family's diet and for gifts to other villagers in return for their help throughout the year. Each year at a ceremony called the "matanca," families with the help of friends and neighbors slaughter a pig and make the sausages. This is a very important family and village ritual. It is thought that if menstruating women even gaze upon the butchered pork, it will be polluted and turn blue and rot. Even a casual glance is thought to have this power, but the "fixed gaze" of a menstruating woman is most destructive . Every precaution is taken to ensure that menstruating women do not come near a butchered pig. Furthermore, if a menstruating woman has intercourse with her husband at this time, he is thought to be "cross-polluted," that his presence also will cause the pork to spoil. Of course, this is very serious because if the family cannot make sausages, then they must find alternative sources of protein and cannot repay friends and neighbors for their help.

Because no one family alone can do the butchering and make the sausages, they seek the help of a few special friends. This important job is the wife's responsibility, and through her careful choice of helpers, the family's alliances in the village are reinforced. The wife thus "screens" potential helpers for the job, including asking about the menstrual status of women. She accepts help only from women who swear that they are not menstruating, and she must disqualify herself if she is menstruating.

Although this custom might seem mythical and magical, it is unique and interesting in one respect. Most rituals about menstruation center on *men's* fears and phobias about menstruating women, but in this case menstruation becomes a point of leverage that *women* use at a crucial time to solidify political and friendship patterns in the community.

The pituitary gland secretes hormones that stimulate milk production and ejection in **mammary glands** throughout the breast tissue. The mammary glands are surrounded by fat and connective tissue, which give breasts, especially in younger women, their softness. With age, connective tissues gradually lose their elasticity, contributing to the sagging usually seen in women's breasts as they get older. Younger women with large breasts who often do not use the support of a bra may experience stretching of the ligaments that support the breasts and have an earlier loss of firm breast appearance (Fig. 4-16).

A woman's nipples may be raised, flat, or even inverted; all are common. As a woman becomes sexually aroused, the nipples generally become more erect, but this varies much among women. The area of the breast surrounding the nipple, called the **areola,** varies much in size and pigmentation among women. Just as "diversity is normality" in genitalia, the same is true regarding breasts (Fig. 4-15). Reynolds and Wines (1948) analyzed a very large sample of young women, photographed frontally and in profile, and concluded there are three general

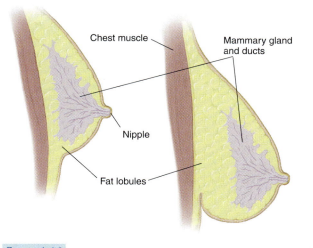

Chest muscle

Mammary gland and ducts

Nipple

Fat lobules

FIGURE 4-16   Cross-sectional drawing of two breasts that differ notably in overall size. Note that despite differences in breast size, the amount of milk-producing tissue is usually quite similar.

ONE OF THE MOST COMMON ELECTIVE SURGERIES IN AMERICA

*M*ost elective surgery involves procedures people don't really need, such as plastic surgery. Breast augmentation is one of the most common elective surgeries in this country, usually involving breast implants. (Far fewer women have breast *reduction* surgery.) Implants are usually filled with silicone gel or saline solution (Fig. 4-17). Women seek breast augmentation surgery for two very different reasons. The first is cosmetic: some women desire to have a bustline that they perceive is more attractive. The second is breast reconstruction after a mastectomy, usually for a cancerous tumor.

How common is breast augmentation surgery? Manufacturing numbers along with survey data suggest that about 8 in 1000 women in the United States have had breast implants (Cook & Perkins, 1996). About 60% of these procedures were undertaken for cosmetic reasons, and about 95% were performed in Caucasian women. Younger women had more implants for cosmetic reasons, while older women had more reconstruction surgery due to mastectomies. Most of the women were between the ages of 45 and 54 years. These researchers estimated that by 1989, over 815,000 American women had received breast augmentation.

In recent years, anxiety and controversy have occurred over the use of silicone gel breast implants. Some writers suggested that silicone has a chronic, nonspecific activating effect on the immune system (Jenkins, Friedman, & von Recum, 1996), but a clear causal relationship has not been demonstrated. Concerns about the risks of silicon have apparently affected how satisfied women who have had breast augmentation are with their implants. In a survey of 174 women with implants, 43% reported that they were completely satisfied with their outcomes (Fee-Fulkerson, Conaway, Winer, Fulkerson, Rimer, & Georgiade, 1996). Only 3% said that they were "not at all" satisfied. These data were collected after news stories had alerted the public to medical concerns about silicone. Women with implants reported that they were very pleased with how their clothes fit and said they felt they looked more "normal." Thinner, healthier women generally were the most satisfied with their implants. More than a third of these women (34%), however, said that if given the choice now, they would probably not choose to have silicone implants.

Because of concerns that silicone breast implants may be somehow associated with breast cancer, immune system disorders, and connective tissue disease, these implants have been banned since 1992. Implantable silicone has also been banned in Australia as liability claims mounted (Renwick, 1996). Medical researchers have been analyzing the risks of silicone implants for many years. Handel, Jensen, Black, Waisman, and Silverstein (1995) calculated the rate of implant ruptures as 1 per 760 implant-years, and the prevalence of implant-related connective tissue disorders as 1 per 3801 implant-years. Sanchez-Guerrero et al. (1995), at Harvard Medical School, assessed the long-term health consequences of silicone- and saline-filled breast implants in a large study. In a sample of almost 1200 women, they found no statistical association between silicone gel breast implants and connective tissue disease.

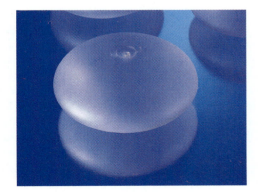

FIGURE 4-17   A breast implant.

Dear Dr. Ruth

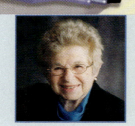

Question:

I am very self-conscious about my breasts because they are much smaller than my friends' and I am wondering whether they will ever get any larger. I am 21 years old. Will they grow more?

Answer:

Some teenagers have late growth spurts, so there is a possibility your breasts will grow some more, but there is no way of knowing whether or not that will happen. At 21 years of age, I would say the likelihood isn't very high that they will. If you are really concerned, you might take this question to your doctor.

Are small breasts some sort of death sentence? You may think so, but it really isn't. Yes, some boys are attracted to more visible breasts, but for more mature men choosing a mate, the size of her breasts ranks somewhere along with the length of her eyelashes—not very high. Your personality is really much more important, so give your attention to traits that you can control, like having a good sense of humor, being a good conversationalist or a good listener. These are the real keys to finding the man of your dreams, and isn't that wonderful?

---

categories of breast shape—conical, round, and flat—and that breasts can also be classed as small, medium, and large. In their sample, 72% were in the small and medium categories.

We have often commented on the important relationship between self-esteem and body image. For some reason, in American culture some men equate "bustiness with lustiness," as if women with large breasts were more interested in sex or more easily aroused. This is a myth, however; no systematically collected data suggest there is any relationship among breast size, shape, or sensitivity and erotic interest in women. Breast sensitivity may be affected by experience. If a woman has learned to associate erotic arousal with breast stimulation, she will probably continue to do so.

Although breasts vary much, size is mostly due to fat and not mammary glandular tissue. Therefore, women with small breasts can breast feed an infant with no difficulty at all. Health issues concerning a woman's breasts are discussed in the next chapter.

A MAN'S BODY

The structures, functions, and hormones involved in the male reproductive system are similar to what you have just read about women. Think of these as "variations on a theme." Although a woman's external genitalia are not as visible as a man's, an important truth about women's external genitalia is no less true for men: *diversity is normality* (Fig. 4-18). The penis and scrotum vary considerably among different men at the same or different ages. The same "selective perception" that makes peo-

ple so attentive to women's genitalia is also relevant to men's external genitalia. Nudity usually gets our attention—as it's supposed to. Such perceptions involve powerful imperatives that lead to attraction and intimate interest. In Chapter 12, we will discuss how to make the most with your child (or grandchild) of "teachable moments" involving the human body.

The female form has been adored and celebrated throughout the history of art, and the erotic appeal of a man's body is no less compelling or diversified. Historically, there has been little shyness about depicting male external genitalia, often in almost comically exaggerated form (Fig. 4-19). Artistic depictions of the penis—or "phallic symbols" ("phallus" means "erect penis")—typically celebrate male generativity. Although the phallic symbols depicted in Figure 4-19 might seem bizarre or humorous, in a sense they celebrate masculine power, procreativity, and even political influence. Chapter 2 discussed some of the roots of contemporary traditions of male dominance in social, commercial, and family arenas. These phallic symbols religiously or ritualistically affirm these traditions. Most interpretations of such historical artifacts suggest that an especially prominent penis symbolizes male-dominant attributes. Later in this chapter we examine myths of "sexual superiority" related to large penises and consider just exactly what "large" means in this context.

Self-Examination of the External Male Genitalia

As we discussed with women, genital self-examination for men is just as important. As is the case among women, men's self-esteem is often based in part on their body image, and a can-

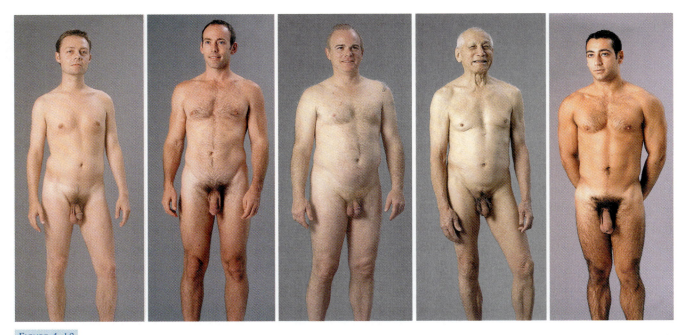

FIGURE 4-18   All of these men have normal bodies. Differences in size, shape, weight, skin texture, and the density and distribution of pubic hair are all obvious but at the same time certainly "average" or "typical."

did self-examination helps assure us of our normality (see Fig. 5-17). A mirror may be helpful but is not necessary, and examination is easier when the genitalia are warm, such as after a warm bath or shower when the weather is cool. Consulting the illustrations in this chapter will be helpful for learning the names of the different parts of the genitalia, which is important for communicating accurately with health care professionals when needed.

Take your time to note the softness of the tip of the penis (the **glans**). Men who have not been circumcised need to retract the foreskin a little to see all of the glans. Note the appearance of blood vessels along the shaft of the penis (Fig. 4-20) and the little "notch," called the coronal ridge, that separates the shaft from the glans. The **external urethral meatus,** as in the female, is the little hole through which urine leaves the male's body. Note the very smooth mucous membrane just inside this opening. The underside of the glans, called the **frenum,** is one of the most sensitive parts of the penis. Take a moment to feel the oval shape of your testicles inside the scrotum; note the soft, fibrous tissues and how sensitive to touch the testicles are.

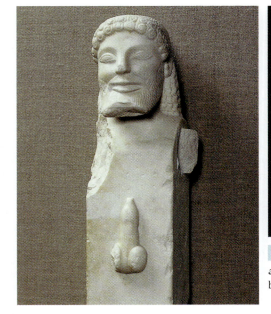

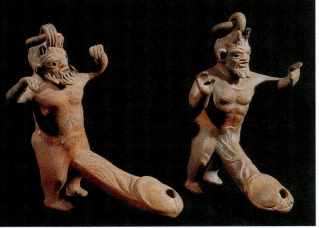

FIGURE 4-19   Historical artifacts frequently represent penises in an unusual or exaggerated form. The penis is sometimes a symbol of dominance, power, or authority in works of art.

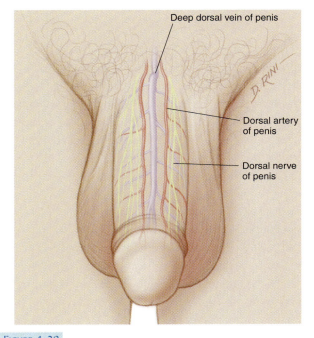

FIGURE 4-20   Blood and nerve supply of the penis.

The next chapter describes testicular self-examination as a screening test for testicular cancer in more detail.

As gynecology is the medical specialty dealing with a woman's sexual and reproductive health, urology is the specialty for men's sexual and reproductive health. **Urologists** also diagnose and treat disorders of the urinary system in both women and men. Some urologists specialize in **andrology**, which focuses on men's fertility problems. Your primary care physician can refer you to such a specialist.

Men in our society are more likely to see one another nude, in keeping with the general (though incorrect) assumption that men do not need or desire as much privacy as women. For example, in high school, males are likely to use an open group shower room after physical education or athletic activities, while females often have individual shower stalls. Males are therefore more likely to observe differences in the shape and size of the penis and scrotum, as well as the different rates of development through puberty. As we begin to discuss in detail the male's anatomy, remember that diversity is normality.

EXTERNAL SEXUAL AND REPRODUCTIVE ANATOMY

The Penis
Although the **penis** looks simple at first glance, its interior is actually complex. The penis is composed of three, independent "cylinders" of tissue bound together by connective membranes. The cross-sectional view of the penis shows these three elongated structures (Fig. 4-21). The most prominent are the paired **corpora cavernosa.** Like the spongy tissue within the clitoris, these fill with blood during sexual arousal; this swelling is called **tumescence,** which is obvious in both the shaft and glans of the penis. The third cylinder is called the **corpus spongiosum;** within it is the urethra, which carries both urine and semen out of the body. The corpora spongiosum extends into the glans as the tip of the penis. The glans is keenly sensitive to touch and, as we noted above, the underside of the glans is especially responsive. The frenum (sometimes called **frenulum**) connects the ventral portion of the glans with the foreskin on the underside of the shaft. The **coronal ridge,** which divides the glans from the shaft, has the highest concentration of nerve endings in the male body. The base of the penis, called the root, connects the penis with the pelvic bony structures. While pubic hair surrounds the base of the penis, there is virtually no hair growth on the penis beyond this point.

As the penis becomes larger during sexual arousal, it may also shrink somewhat when the man is very cold or immersed in cold water, such as at the pool or beach.

In males who have not been circumcised, a small length of the skin of the shaft covers some of the glans; this loose fold of skin is called the **foreskin** and as in women is also called the *prepuce.* Just as smegma may accumulate beneath a woman's clitoral prepuce, it may also gather under a man's foreskin. Pulling back the foreskin regularly and washing beneath it helps keep this area clean. **Circumcision** is the surgical removal of the foreskin. Circumcision is common generally only in North America and Israel. Although this procedure was once thought to enhance male genital hygiene, regular washing under the foreskin is more than adequate to ensure cleanliness. The tradition of circumcision

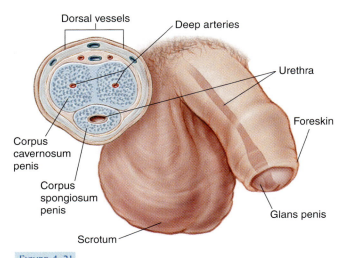

FIGURE 4-21   Illustration of the penis (uncircumcised) and scrotum. A cross-sectional illustration of the penis reveals the three independent cylinders of tissue within.

THE DEBATE OVER CIRCUMCISION

*B*etween 1875 and 1950 there was little public disagreement about the desirability of circumcision in the United States, even though during this time period no other country or culture (with the exception of Jews) embraced circumcision as a routine procedure for male newborns. Muslims and Africans sometimes practiced it at adolescence. Despite its acceptance in the United States, there was little scientific rationale for circumcision. In 1971 and again in 1975 the American Academy of Pediatrics issued a policy statement announcing there were no convincing medical data for routine circumcision. In 1978 the American College of Obstetrics and Gynecology endorsed this position as well. In 1983 both of these professional organizations reasserted their policies. All these pronouncements did not, however, lead to a notable decrease in the number of circumcisions performed in the United States. Circumcision continues to be common in the United States because of confusion and misinformation concerning pain, sexually transmitted diseases, cancer, and personal hygiene (Wallerstein, 1985). In addition, very often young boys are sensitive about the different appearances of circumcised and uncircumcised penises and wonder what a penis is "supposed" to look like. Adult men too often wonder whether circumcised men experience more pleasure during intercourse than uncircumcised men because the glans of the penis is exposed.

For some reason, folk myths have associated circumcision with sexually transmitted diseases. There are virtually no good systematic studies that show conclusively that circumcised males are any more or less likely to acquire a sexually transmitted disease of any type if they are not wearing a condom.

It was also once thought that circumcision prevented penile cancer, but this has been shown incorrect. While cancer of the penis is rare (about 1000 cases are diagnosed in the United States each year [Rosenberg, 1992]), cases do occur in circumcised men. The American Cancer Society has flatly stated, "Circumcision is not of value in preventing cancer of the penis." Penile cancer occurs primarily in older men and seems related to such factors as cigarette smoking, genital warts, and having had 30 or more sexual partners, more than to whether a man has been circumcised (Cold, Storms, & Van Howe, 1997). Another study of men with cancer of the penis found that of the 110 subjects, 32 had been circumcised at birth and 19 later in life (Maden, C. et al., 1993). These data seem to show clearly that circumcision offers no consistent protections against this rare disease. Additionally, current data do not support any relationship between lack of circumcision and prostate cancer in uncircumcised men or cervical cancer in their female sexual partners.

Wallerstein notes that mothers who agree to or request their son's circumcision say that they are mostly concerned with hygiene. Because the foreskin does not separate from the glans of the penis until a few months or even years after birth, mothers are advised not to try to retract the foreskin during bathing. In adolescence and adulthood, the foreskin is easily retracted for cleaning the glans beneath it in a matter of seconds. While some have suggested that uncircumcised babies are more likely to develop urinary tract infections in infancy, no clear causal relationship has yet been found, and more research is needed to determine if such a connection exists (Altschul, on-line).

Although the debate over circumcision might seem just another "great big issue over a little bit of tissue," a new facet has emerged with the HIV epidemic in Africa. In 1996 Caldwell and Caldwell published an article in *Scientific American* titled "The African AIDS Epidemic" in which they discussed a positive correlation between lack of circumcision and the transmission of HIV in heterosexual intercourse, implying the lack of circumcision may be a causative factor in the spread of AIDS in some parts of Africa. However, Falk (1996) argued with this assertion and points out that existing published data fail to demonstrate a statistically significant increase in HIV among uncircumcised men (de Vicenzi & Mertens, 1994). Nonetheless, the belief that lack of circumcision might play a role in the transmission of HIV alarmed many men in Africa. The Caldwells note that in Tanzania men, often with their sons, are coming to hospitals asking to be circumcised. Additionally, private medical facilities specializing in adult circumcision began appearing and advertising in Tanzanian newspapers.

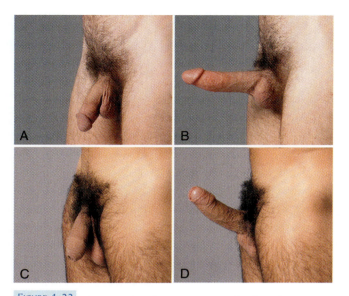

FIGURE 4-22 Photographs of two penises in the flaccid, or nonerect, state at left (A and C), and in the erect state at right (B and D). Note the angle of the erection with reference to the body, as well as the slight upward retraction of the glans.

among the ancient Jews began as a symbol of God's "special relationship" with the peoples of the tribes of Israel. Much controversy surrounds circumcision and whether it is advantageous in any way to men and their sexual partners (Fig. 4-22).

The Scrotum

The **scrotum** is composed of thin, delicate skin well endowed with hair follicles and sweat glands. The scrotum's functions are to contain the testes and help regulate their temperature. "Scrotum" comes from the Latin "scutum," meaning "shield," although the scrotum is so delicate that it doesn't shield the testes very well from injury. Much of its surface is covered with pubic hair in an amount that varies significantly among men; it becomes more sparse in middle and older age. The size of the scrotum also varies among men. Beneath the soft skin of the outside of the scrotum is a second layer of smooth muscle fibers and connective tissue, called the tunica dartos (Fig. 4-23). One of the functions of the dartos is to raise the testes toward the body when it is cold and to allow the testes to hang further away from the body at warmer temperatures—this is to maintain the testes at the ideal temperature for their functioning. When immersed in cold water, for example, the testes are pulled up toward the body as the scrotum becomes hard and puckered. The same thing happens to the scrotum during sexual arousal.

Early in prenatal development, around 7 or 8 weeks after conception, the **testes** begin to form in the embryo's abdominal cavity, near the kidneys. Through prenatal development they gradually descend through two inguinal canals, which eventually close, leaving them in the scrotum. In a condition called cryptorchidism one or both testes may not fully descend before birth. In many instances this condition corrects itself

shortly after birth; if not, then surgery is performed to put the testes in their appropriate place.

The position of the testes is important because they produce sperm at an optimal rate only if they are about 6 degrees (Fahrenheit) cooler than the core body temperature. Anything that causes a consistent warming of the testes may temporarily reduce a man's fertility—but this is not an immediate or dependable effect that can be used for contraception! For example, frequent long hot baths can have this effect, and a man who has had a prolonged high fever may have reduced sperm production for a few months. Men who have sedentary jobs in which they are literally "sitting on their testes," such as long-distance truck drivers, cab drivers, or even many sedentary office workers, may have measurable reductions in sperm count. When steel workers work close to blast furnaces for prolonged periods they often have somewhat diminished fertility. When a couple is experiencing a fertility problem, the urologist may recommend that the man switch from "jockey" shorts to looser fitting underwear to allow his testes to hang more freely rather than more warmly against the body.

Prolonged, severe stress also influences sperm production. In World War II, airmen flying nighttime bombing mis-

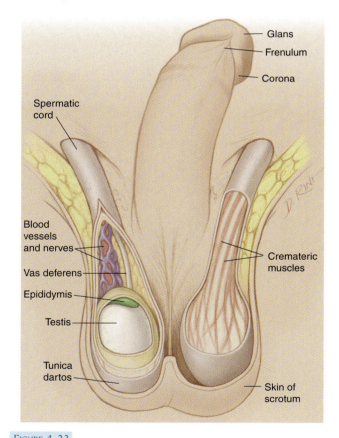

FIGURE 4-23 The structures within the scrotum. Structures adjacent to the testes are illustrated: the epididymis and vas deferens. The tunica dartos is a layer of smooth muscle and connective tissue. Cremasteric muscles retract the testes.

Other Countries, Cultures, and Customs

MEN'S ANXIETIES ABOUT THEIR PENIS

How men feel about their bodies—and their penises—is influenced by their psychosocial environment. This is well illustrated by an unusual psychological disorder that has been documented in Asia. Koro is an emotional problem that has been recognized for hundreds of years in Asian cultures but known to Westerners only since 1895. Investigators have debated whether to include this disorder in the DSM (Diagnostic and Statistical Manual of Mental Disorders). This book is important because it identifies accepted psychological problems, their distinguishing symptoms, and their prevalence in the general population and in at-risk groups. Cases of koro have been reported in Southeast Asia, India, the Caribbean, China, and North America. Koro is a condition in which the man believes his penis is shrinking and will disappear, resulting in his death. In fact, his penis is not shrinking—he only believes it is (Fig. 4-24).

Early reports of koro from Malaysia included, in addition to men's perceptions of penile shrinkage, women's perceptions of labial and breast shrinkage. An epidemic of koro was described in 1963, and more than 1000 cases were reported in Thailand just after the Vietnam War. Some men afflicted with koro said they saw ghosts of the dead without penises, who were conspiring to steal penises from the living. Because koro tends to appear in epidemics, psychosocial factors would seem important as possible causes. Men suffering from koro usually experience panic as they believe their penis is retracting into the abdomen. They often fear imminent death and have a constant desire to hold the penis to prevent its retraction. There is, however, no physical disorder that results in penile retraction. Koro can be treated successfully with the drug haloperidol, a powerful anti-psychotic agent.

---

sions over central Europe for months became infertile, and this condition reversed itself when their flights ended. As well, prolonged exposure to high altitudes may also impair male fertility. Peruvian shepherds who spend months with their flocks high in the Andes Mountains often are not fertile until they have been back at sea level for a few months. Finally, exposure to high doses of radiation may inhibit or completely stop the production of sperm, although such exposures are very unusual.

The Testes

The testicles produce male sex hormones and sperm. They are suspended in the scrotum by two tubular membranes called spermatic cords, which contain the vas deferens along with blood vessels, nerve fibers, and cremasteric muscles. The size of the testes varies much among men, but they are between the size of a hazelnut and a walnut. A man's sex drive and fertility have little to do with the size of his testes in most cases. The testes have a dense nerve and blood supply. As a woman's ovaries produce her sex cells (ova), a man's testes produce his (sperm). Similarly, as meiosis is the type of cell division that creates the ova, it is similarly involved in the creation of sperm. The most important structures for sperm and hormone production are the **seminiferous tubules** (Fig. 4-25). Sperm are produced in more than 800 sections of these tubules, which, if they were uncoiled, would combine to a length over a mile. These tubules are very narrow, with a diameter of 0.12 to 0.3

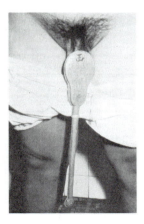

FIGURE 4-24   Koro is a psychological disorder in which a man believes his penis is shrinking into his body. This man has attached a long jeweler's clip in an effort to prevent this retraction. Of course, the penis is not actually shrinking.

millimeters. Interstitial cells of Leydig between the tubules manufacture testosterone, perhaps the most important male sex hormone. The male sex hormones are collectively known as androgens.

Testosterone and Other Male Sex Hormones

As in women, negative feedback mechanisms in men involving the hypothalamus, the pituitary gland, and the testes maintain adequate levels of the sex hormones needed for sperm production. Levels of **testosterone** and other hormones in a man's bloodstream are strongly related to his "sex drive." Although in women the relationship between sex hormones and sexual motivation is powerfully affected by psychosocial variables, the relationship in men is more direct and depends less on psychosocial factors. Interestingly, the testosterone levels of a male newborn are similar to those in teenage boys, but in infancy these levels fall rapidly and remain low until puberty. Once these adolescent changes begin, there is much hormonal communication among the testes, adrenal glands (two adrenal glands in all people), and the pituitary and hypothalamus. Testosterone has many functions beyond those of sexual interest and performance; it is involved in other so-called masculine attributes, such as aggressiveness, general body configuration, bulk and weight, hair pattern and hair loss, and the gradual build-up of abdominal fat. In most but not all men, testosterone levels decline as they get older (Flieger, 1995). Even normal levels of testosterone seem associated with some health risks, such as prostate enlargement. (The next chapter discusses this further.)

Because of the connection between testosterone levels and sex drive, some men have tried to enhance their performance by using synthetic testosterone obtained illicitly. The supposedly powerful effects of testosterone were first described in what today seems a bizarre experiment. The respected French physiologist Charles Edouard Brown-Sequard was 72 in 1889 when he reported to his scientific colleagues that he had injected himself with a liquid derived from the testicles of dogs and guinea pigs. He reported enhanced mental alertness, physical strength, and improved urinary force but said little about enhanced sexual arousal. In another unusual experiment in 1918, Dr. Leo Stanley, a physician at San Quentin prison, removed the testicles from executed inmates and transplanted them into prisoners who were suffering from various maladies, including impotence. His patients noted an increased sex drive and had erections more frequently. When testicles from executed inmates were unavailable, Stanley used the testes of deer and boars and claimed to observe similar effects. Investigators today attribute these findings to a placebo effect (Karlen, 1996).

In 1939, Adolf F. J. Butenandt from Germany was a co-recipient of the Nobel prize in chemistry for his work in synthesizing sex hormones. For the first time testosterone could be manufactured from chemicals, and scientists no longer had to rely on a meager supply from agricultural sources. Af-

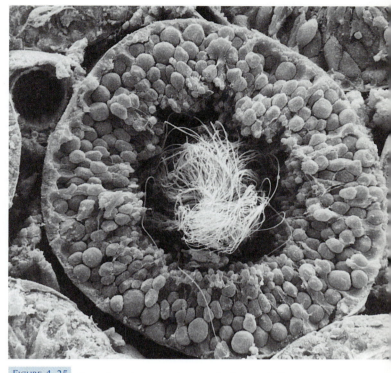

FIGURE 4-25   Scanning electron micrograph of a seminiferous tubule. Immature sperm forms begin their development at the periphery of the tubule, while mature sperm forms (with tails) are adjacent to the hollow center of the tubule.

ter synthetic testosterone became widely available, some of its abuses began. Testosterone is an especially potent *anabolic,* or "tissue building" steroid. Athletes in many sports learned of the muscle building properties of synthetic testosterone, and abuses became common. As well, aggressiveness and endurance were apparently enhanced. An enormous black market grew up around these practices, so that now athletic competitions routinely screen competitors for performance-enhancing agents. Serious side-effects often accompany medically unsupervised consumption of high doses of anabolic steroids, including a significant shrinkage of the testes, loss of libido, loss of sperm production, dizziness, muscular pain, and liver tumors and damage. Male breast enlargement, clotting abnormalities, anxiety, depression, and elevated cholesterol levels are also common. Anabolic steroids shut down the normal functioning of the male reproductive system and change the body's metabolism in often dangerous ways. Although some athletes have said such effects might be worth it for their career, we disagree completely. Overdosing with testosterone is a form of substance abuse.

Sometimes there are, however, medically appropriate reasons for using testosterone to treat certain problems in men. Testosterone enhances fertility in men whose pituitary gland has stopped stimulating their testes or whose testes do not produce testosterone. Finally, in aging or elderly men testosterone

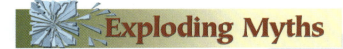

Exploding Myths

Why Do Some People Make Such a Big Deal About Penis Size?

Almost everyone has heard some interesting ideas about the supposed importance of penis size. Because this is a serious textbook about human sexuality, it's appropriate to address this issue and correct misconceptions. There are several false beliefs people have about penis size. During the 1950s and 1960s, a cigarette brand was advertised with the slogan "It's not how long you make it, it's how you make it long." That advertising raised some eyebrows and led to a lot of jokes. Much could be said about psychosocial elements in that message, but there is a significant message there too. It isn't penis size alone that determines the pleasure of a sexual experience, but the whole physical interaction of the couple, as well as the caring and sharing and communication involved in their relationship. In addition, a focus on penis size implies that penis-in-the-vagina intercourse is the only way to make love, and this is certainly not the case. Many kinds of erotic touching are keenly arousing and for many are more enjoyable than intercourse.

One common myth is that penis size is related to masculinity. In the last chapter you learned that masculinity is a multifaceted and complicated concept that cannot possibly be based on a simple measurement figure. Masculinity involves many aspects of a man's personality and psychological attributes. Different people describe masculinity in various ways. Some say it has to do with self-assurance and competence. Others claim that it involves the ability to stay "cool" under pressure. Some are sure it is a matter of body hair and muscular bulk. Still others refer to the idea of "quiet strength." No one trait, especially one physical measurement, could adequately characterize this complicated quality called masculinity.

As well, one should note that the size of a man's penis when it is flaccid (not erect) is not an accurate predictor of its size when erect. When a man's penis is small when flaccid, it usually increases in size substantially when he becomes aroused and erect. Similarly, when a man's penis is large when flaccid, it does not increase much more when erect. In other words, when aroused, men's penis size does not vary all that much. Virtually all biological structures vary along a normal distribution, or "bell curve." Although a few cases can be found at the two extremes of the distribution, the vast majority are fairly close to the mean or average. This is no less true of the length of a man's penis than of the length of his torso or his nose.

Finally, remember that the inner two-thirds of the vagina have virtually no nerve supply and that only the outer one-third has much sensitivity. For this reason, during full penile penetration or containment, most of the length of the penis is not accurately perceived or related to felt stimulation by the woman.

is sometimes used to treat decreased sex drive and sexual functioning, although other drugs are more frequently used for this problem today.

The same pituitary hormones that contribute to the production of ova in women stimulate the testes of men to produce sperm. FSH regulates sperm production, and LH stimulates the interstitial cells of Leydig's cells, increasing testosterone secretion. Also, as in women, the pituitary is directed by the hypothalamus, which monitors testosterone levels in the bloodstream. Low levels of testosterone stimulate the

hypothalamus to stimulate the pituitary, which, in turn, increases its output of interstitial-cell-stimulating-hormone that causes testosterone increase.

Spermatogenesis

As shown in Figure 4-26, each testicle has several compartments, or **septa**, that contain the seminiferous tubules. **Spermatogenesis** is the production of sperm through meiosis. This process begins in boys by about the age of 12, and by 13 or 14 most boys have mature sperm in their ejaculate (the

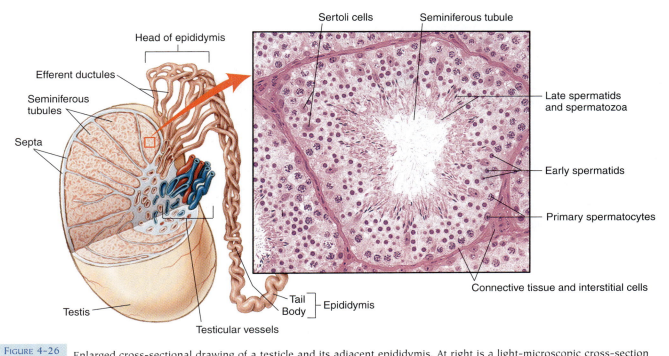

term for everything that leaves the penis during ejaculation). The production of mature sperm takes about 72 days, occurring in the linings of the seminiferous tubules. The process occurs along the length of the seminiferous tubules and is unaffected by behavioral variables or the frequency of sexual intercourse. Early sperm cells begin their maturation at the outer periphery of the tubules, and as they grow they slowly migrate inward toward the hollow center of the tubule, from which they may then begin the journey out of the body. Figure 4-26 shows relatively mature sperm as they approach the interior of the seminiferous tubules. Although sperm production is initiated by FSH, testosterone is also involved in their maturation. Spermatogenesis is a constant process, different from how a woman's body produces ova in 28-day cycles.

Developing sperm go through several meiotic stages as they mature in the linings of the seminiferous tubules. The earliest form is the **spermatogonium,** which begins in the outer wall of the tubules. It grows into a **primary spermatocyte,** which eventually divides into two **secondary spermatocytes.** Each secondary spermatocyte divides into two **spermatids.** The spermatids develop a highly compact head, and each of these spermatids finally becomes a **spermatozoon.** Thus, each spermatogonium eventually becomes four mature sperm. Cells lining the seminiferous tubules, called sustentacular cells, or Sertoli cells, provide nutrition for the developing sperm. Each sperm contains 23 chromosomes. Half of the sperm have the X sex chromosome and the other half have the Y sex chromosome. Figure 4-27 shows a sperm and its most conspicuous parts.

A sperm has a head, neck, body, and tail. The head contains a dense accumulation of genetic material that enters an ovum during fertilization; the whole sperm does not. The surrounding cellular membrane compacts the head into an efficient vehicle for the man's genetic contribution. On top of the head of a sperm is a small capsule called an **acrosome** within which is hyaluronidase and other protein-dissolving enzymes.

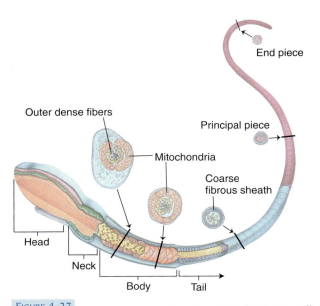

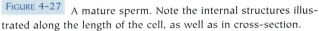

FIGURE 4-27   A mature sperm. Note the internal structures illustrated along the length of the cell, as well as in cross-section.

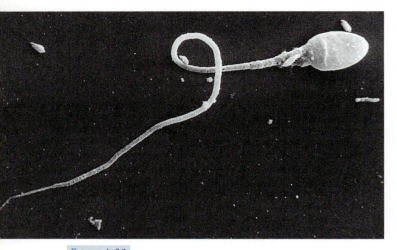

These substances help gradually break down the egg's surrounding substances and membranes so that the head of the sperm can enter. The body of the sperm is well supplied with mitochondria, the subcellular organelles that provide energy for the sperm's swimming.

Sperm swim with side-to-side lashing movements of their tails (Fig. 4-28). They travel in a fairly straight path at the rate of 1–4 millimeters per minute (Guyton, 1992). Considering how tiny sperm actually are (1/5000 of an inch in length, or about 1/200 of a mm.) and how far they have to swim through the vagina, through the cervix, up the uterus, and then to the ends of the fallopian tubes (a trip of 6 to 8 inches), this is a long journey. Not surprisingly, most sperm die somewhere along the way. Even before sperm leave a man's body, they have already made a long and complex journey involving stops along the way that better prepare them for the trip through a woman's reproductive system.

After their production in the testes, sperm pass into the **epididymis,** a comma-shaped structure on the posterior surface of each testicle (Fig. 4-29). The upper end of the epididymis surrounds the top of each testicle, and its tail extends toward the lower portion. A small amount of sperm is stored here. The epididymis is important for the further maturation of sperm. When sperm pass out of the seminiferous tubules they are not yet motile (cannot yet swim). Sperm begin to develop the potential for swimming after being in the epididymis about 24 hours, but the surrounding fluid inhibits movement. Sperm are not fully capable of swimming until ejaculation (Guyton, 1992), but the amount of time they spend in the epididymis is essential for maturation.

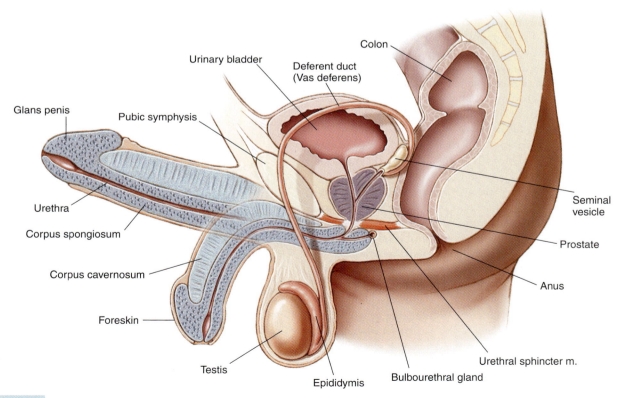

FIGURE 4-29   A cross-sectional view of the male reproductive system.

The Vas Deferens

The **vas deferens** is a long passageway (18 inches, or about 45 cm) that emerges from the tail of each epididymis. Sperm can be stored here for at least a month without loss of function, although with regular sexual activity they keep moving through the system. Sperm that do not leave the body during ejaculation are reabsorbed back into the body through the walls of the vas deferens or epididymis. The vas deferens from each testicle exits the scrotum and follows a twisting pathway behind the bladder where it joins with the seminal vesicles. Cutting or tying off the vas deferens in the surgical procedure called a **vasectomy** ends this passage of sperm and renders the man sterile. This common contraceptive surgery is performed on an out-patient basis, as discussed more in Chapter 10. Interestingly, one vasectomy in 800 spontaneously reverses itself when the two ends of the severed vas deferens reconnect, and the man regains fertility without knowing it.

Vasectomy does not affect a man's sexual arousal or response. Of the teaspoon of semen that leaves the penis during ejaculation, only about 1% is made up of sperm cells. There is no significant decrease in the amount of ejaculate from men who have had vasectomies.

The Seminal Vesicles

The **seminal vesicles** are two pouches of glandular tissue about 2 inches (5 cm) long. They do not hold sperm but produce important secretions essential for sperm's motility, including significant amounts of the simple sugar fructose. Additionally, the seminal vesicles secrete prostaglandins, which are essential for normal male fertility. Fructose provides energy for swimming sperm, and prostaglandins make the cervical mucus easier for sperm to swim through. Prostaglandins are also believed to stimulate a gentle, rhythmic sequence of muscle contractions that "nudge" swimming sperm up the uterus and fallopian tubes more quickly than their own swimming could get them there. The base of the seminal vesicles joins the vas deferens at the ejaculatory ducts, where sperm and the secretions that support the sperm are mixed together. These ejaculatory ducts pass through the prostate gland, where more secretions are added.

The Prostate Gland

The **prostate gland** (not "prostrate" gland) is located below the bladder and surrounds the urethra. It is about 1.5 inches (4 cm) by 0.75 inches (2 cm) and is composed of muscle fibers and glandular tissues that make prostatic fluid. Prostatic fluid is white, viscous, and alkaline and contains citric acid and calcium. The inside of the vagina normally is acidic and, therefore, potentially very hostile to the delicate sperm. The alkalinity of prostatic fluid neutralizes some of the vagina's acidity and, therefore, enhances the motility and survival of sperm deposited there.

The prostate gland is the place where sperm and secretions enter the urethra to be conveyed out of the body through the penis. Semen is held in the prostate, seminal vesicles, and

upper portion of the vas deferens just before ejaculation. Twelve to 20 prostatic ducts empty their secretions into the urethra. Prostate health issues are described in the next chapter on sexual and reproductive health.

Cowper's Glands or Bulbourethral Glands

Cowper's glands or **bulbourethral glands** are two tiny glands located beneath the prostate gland and that secrete directly into the urethra. When the penis becomes erect during arousal, a clear droplet of liquid is usually released through the urethral meatus. Although this liquid isn't as milky as semen, there may be substantial numbers of sperm in it. Although the man may not feel that ejaculation is about to occur soon, as long as he is penetrating his partner, significant numbers of sperm are being released. Withdrawing the penis before ejaculation, therefore, is not a foolproof means of contraception, as we'll discuss further in Chapter 11 on contraception. While the precise functions of the secretions from the Cowper's glands are not fully understood, they likely help lubricate the inside of a man's urethra for a smooth passage of sperm during ejaculation.

Virtually every structure sperm pass through from the testes where they are produced to their release into the urethra contributes something to help these tiny, fragile cells survive and reach their destination (Fig. 4-29). The intricate adaptations of all these organs in the male and female reproductive systems are astonishing and beautiful in their complexity.

Semen

Earlier we noted that everything that leaves the penis during ejaculation is called the **ejaculate**. In addition to sperm are the secretions of the epididymis, seminal vesicles, prostate gland, and Cowper's glands (see Fig. 6-12). Of the total volume of ejaculate, about 1% is sperm. Several characteristics of the ejaculate significantly affect a man's fertility. Most urologists can perform a fairly straightforward semen analysis that provides significant information related to fertility.

An important characteristic of semen is its volume. Ejaculate normally contains 3–5 cc of fluid. **Sperm count** is a second crucial characteristic. Normally, there are 40–100 million sperm per cc of ejaculate, meaning that up to 500 million sperm may be deposited in the vagina through intercourse. If the sperm count is below 20 million sperm per cc of ejaculate, the man's fertility is seriously compromised. A third important characteristic is **sperm motility.** Ideally, all the sperm are swimming and moving in the same direction. If substantial numbers of sperm are nonmotile, fertility is diminished. Finally, **sperm form** affects fertility. There is some normal variation in the size and shape of sperm; for example, sperm carrying the female chromosome are smaller and swim more quickly than those carrying the male chromosome. If many grossly abnormal sperm forms are present, however, the progress of normal sperm may be blocked. Chapter 10 will discuss these factors in relation to techniques to improve a man's fertility.

Dear Dr. Ruth

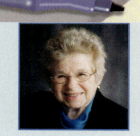

Question:

I have a question about ejaculation. When ejaculating, should my sperm shoot out of my penis? I mean, how far? It does come out but does not shoot any distance. It more or less just flows out. Is this a problem—can I still fertilize the egg if it does not shoot out? What should I do?

Answer:

Don't confuse your penis with a gun. Sperm are not bullets that fly up into the woman, but instead they swim up through the cervix. Since your penis penetrates into the vagina, the speed at which the sperm are deposited doesn't matter because they're in the right place to get where they have to go. It is true that some men can't produce babies if they don't make enough sperm, but that has nothing to do with how vigorously the semen comes out.

SIMILARITIES IN FEMALE AND MALE ANATOMY

Because all too often people see the two sexes as very different, it is helpful and interesting to review the similarities between the female and male sexual and reproductive systems.

Common Genetic Issues

Gametes in both women and men are very small cells, and like virtually all animal and plant forms, we produce far more than needed to reproduce and perpetuate the species. Another basic similarity is that both eggs and sperm each have 23 chromosomes, not 23 *pairs* of chromosomes, as in all other human somatic cells. As well, eggs and sperm are the only body cells that divide through meiosis rather than mitosis.

Common Embryological Developmental Issues

Both males and females begin embryological development with an undifferentiated "bipotential" gonad, a sex gland that can take on female or male form and function depending on the genetic instructions. Not until 7–8 weeks after conception do these ambiguous early genitalia begin to differentiate, with different internal male or female duct systems then beginning to develop: the Mullerian duct system in genetic females and the Wolffian duct system in genetic males. As Chapter 3 described, many internal and external sexual and genital structures are homologous. For example, a woman's clitoris is the counterpart of the man's penis; the prepuce or hood of the clitoris is the parallel to the foreskin of the penis. Further, the female labia majora

correspond to the male scrotum, and the labia minora and vestibular bulbs are the counterpart to the corpus spongiosum of the penis. The corpora cavernosa, as well as the glans of the penis and clitoris, are comparable as well.

Common Steroid Biochemistry of Sex Hormones

As shown in Figure 4-30, molecules of steroid hormones have a similar common "core." Shown are the molecular structural diagrams for the three most common estrogens along with two

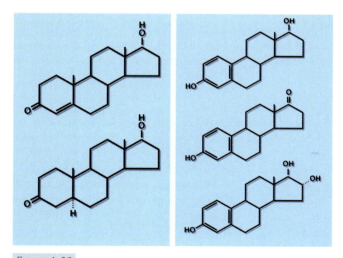

FIGURE 4-30   Note the common steroid core to both male (left) and female (right) sex hormones. At left are the hormones testosterone (top) and dyhydrotestosterone (bottom). At right are estradiol-17β (top), estrone (middle), and estriol (bottom).

forms of testosterone. While there are important differences in some of the side chains of these molecules, there is an obvious uniformity at the core of these molecules.

Another significant hormonal similarity between women and men is that the adrenal glands in both women and men secrete both androgens and estrogens. We all have the sex hormones of both sexes in our bodies, albeit in very different amounts. One of the factors thought to contribute strongly to a woman's sex drive is the amount of androgens her adrenal glands are secreting. Chapter 13 discusses this more in terms of hormone replacement therapy for women in later adulthood.

Common Genital and Internal Adaptations for Conception

Because both eggs and sperm are incredibly delicate cells easily killed by even tiny adverse changes in their chemical environments, special protections for these special cells have evolved. Small changes in moisture, temperature, acidity or alkalinity, and even light affect the reproductive system, and, therefore, both women and men have evolved internal and external genital structures to protect gametes from these potential threats.

For example, one of the reasons for the shape of the penis is that it facilitates inserting semen far into the woman's body. Similarly, the vagina's depth helps isolate sperm well away from the outside environment's potential hazards. Although the interior of the vagina is acidic, secretions from the prostate gland neutralize this acidity without impairing sperm motility. Secretions from the cervix, uterus, fallopian tubes, prostate gland, seminal vesicles, and Cowper's glands all act to preserve the viability of eggs and sperm and to facilitate their getting together. Despite obvious differences, both women's and men's bodies are well suited to manufacture and nurture gametes and ensure that they eventually get together.

Common Hormonal and Behavioral Adaptations

Women and men have many of the same sex hormones, particularly those secreted by the pituitary. The pituitary gland in both sexes secretes FSH and LH. Although these are chemically the same in both sexes, their actions on the ovaries and testes are very different. In other words, the production of eggs in women and spermatogenesis in men are both stimulated and regulated by the same pituitary hormones. In both sexes, the hypothalamus secretes the same substance, gonadotrophic releasing hormone (GnRH), which stimulates the pituitary.

Finally, the combined actions of pituitary and sex hormones on the behavior of women and men involve activities that serve to prepare for, provide for, and protect the newborn. For example, in females, several hormones regulate pregnancy precisely, stimulate milk production at the right time, and foster the mother-baby bonding that is so important for the survival of the infant and the development of a nurturing relationship. Similarly, in men, androgens that build body bulk and increase aggressiveness had an important historical role for hunting, gathering, and defending behaviors that helped ensure the survival of the newborn and the mother. Although these structures look different, their basic developmental and biological similarities are important. They are variations on a theme rather than entirely different melodies.

CONCLUSION

This chapter emphasizes the important relationship between a healthy self-concept and a healthy body image. We feel the most successful sexual communication can take place only when people understand the structures and functions of their bodies and appreciate that diverse sexual anatomy is the rule. Despite many people's idealized notions about physical attractiveness, the human body has many different forms and configurations, and one needs to be comfortable with this fact. Genital self-examination is a simple exercise in self-discovery. The more you know about yourself and the more of yourself you have seen, the more comfortable you will feel.

Although the anatomical issues in this chapter are fairly straightforward, one gains a real sense of the beauty and wonder of the human body from close examination. While women have always been aware of some of the ways their bodies change through the menstrual cycle, learning about the intricate communication among the hypothalamus, pituitary gland, ovaries, and uterus often inspires a new sense of wonder. Similarly, while most men know the appearance of their ejaculate, a fuller understanding often leads to an appreciation of just how many things have to go right for mature, motile sperm to arrive in the penis and then to reach the ovum.

This chapter focuses on the "normal" state of affairs in healthy individuals in adolescence, young adulthood, and adulthood. We have not yet looked at many of the predictable changes that accompany the aging process or any of the problems that can occur in sexual or reproductive health or wellness. These are topics for the next chapter. The next chapter deals with some illnesses that may, from time to time, afflict some of us, and later chapters examine sexually transmitted diseases and sexual dysfunctions. These later chapters, along with this chapter, will help make you more aware of your own body so that any problems that may occur can be treated promptly and appropriately.

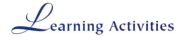

Learning Activities

1. Describe when an adolescent female should have her first gynecologic examination. Do you think a chaperone should be present during this examination? In some states, the person paying for medical services is entitled to learn the outcome of the medical examination or laboratory tests—do you think such laws are fair and appropriate?

2. Advertisements often depict menstruation as inconvenient, painful, or unclean, sometimes also implying temporary personality changes. Women with normal, menstruation-related mood changes are offered many over-the-counter products of questionable effectiveness. Consider that the word "medicine" itself implies the person has some sickness and potential incapacity. Do you think these medications and products are necessary? If you have ever used one, does it work?

3. Speculate why in our society females generally have more privacy than males in situations of nudity.

4. Many people have deeply felt beliefs about circumcision—either for or against. What factors might be related to a person's perspective? Do you think aesthetic concerns contribute to this perspective?

5. This chapter discusses the anxieties of some men about penis size and myths of how size relates to masculinity and female responsiveness during intercourse. Some "men's magazines" have advertisements of products that supposedly address these concerns. These magazines, while depicting nude women in provocative poses, advertise various sex "aids" and devices. The claimed benefits are stated clearly, but the validity of these claims is highly dubious. For example, here is an advertisement for an elaborate suction pump that is applied over the penis:

   > Have you ever wanted an 8-inch penis? Or even 10 or 12 inches? Let's face it, all men are not created equal. If you have ever been jealous of men with a huge, thick penis, the MONGO is the answer for the man with a small penis. The MONGO prosthesis design must add a minimum of 4 inches to your penis and add 30 percent to the diameter of your penis or your money will be refunded.

   a. Consider whether this product might be potentially harmful or painful.

   b. Speculate on a woman's reaction to being involved in a sexual interaction using this device.

   c. Describe the emotional and intellectual characteristics of a man who would purchase this device.

6. Many feminine hygiene products, including genital deodorants, are marketed for women. Why do you suppose similar products have not been developed and marketed for men?

7. Why do you think men might be embarrassed to purchase tampons or pads for their partners when needed?

8. We have discussed the important relationship between self-esteem and body image, such as it is related to female self-esteem and breast development and appearance. What aspects of a *man's* body are considered "masculine"? Is there a stereotypical ideal male body? What does it look like?

*K*ey Concepts

- Anatomy is the study of the physical structures of the body and organ systems. Physiology deals with the functions of these parts and organs. Endocrinology is the study of the body's ductless glands that manufacture hormones and secrete them into our circulatory system.

- Self-esteem and body image affect each other throughout the life span.

- Hormones usually work on the basis of negative feedback systems, in which shortages or excesses of hormones in the blood stimulate the secretion of more or less of that hormone.

- Cultural and subcultural customs and rituals often influence the meaning of menstruation within a society.

- It is important for both women and men to be thoroughly familiar with the structures and functions of their bodies. A genital self-examination can teach a person much about his or her genital anatomy and allows both women and men to become more "at home" with their bodies.

- Common or sometimes unusual anxieties surround the importance of penis size. Most of these concerns are unnecessary and without foundation.

- The female and male sexual and reproductive systems have several interesting and important similarities. There are common genetic, embryological, biochemical, anatomical, and hormonal aspects of these two systems. These commonalities reveal that women and men are more alike than many people realize.

- The female and male sexual and reproductive systems both function in intricate ways to ensure the best conditions for the development of ova and sperm and their union for reproduction.

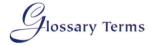 lossary Terms

acrosome	coronal ridge	female	menstruation	secondary	spermatids
anatomy	corpora	circumcision	mons veneris	spermatocytes	spermatogenesis
andrology	cavernosa	foreskin	penis	seminal vesicles	spermatogonium
areola	corpus	frenulum	physiology	seminiferous	spermatozoon
bulbourethral	spongiosum	frenum	pituitary gland	tubules	testes
glands	Cowper's glands	glans	primary	septa	testosterone
cavernous bodies	endocrinology	gynecology	spermatocyte	smegma	tumescence
circumcision	epididymis	labia majora	prostate gland	sperm count	urologist
clitoral prepuce	external urethral	labia minora	pubic symphysis	sperm form	vasectomy
clitoris	meatus	mammary glands	scrotum	sperm motility	vulva

5

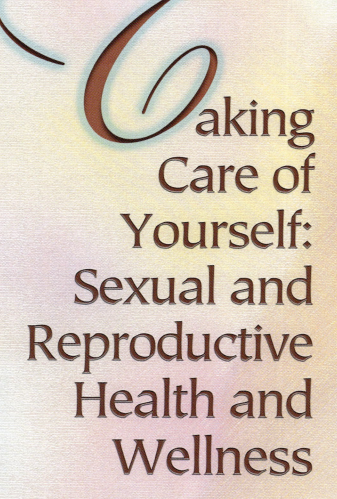

Taking Care of Yourself: Sexual and Reproductive Health and Wellness

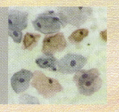

OBJECTIVES

When you finish reading and reviewing this chapter, you should be able to:

1. Describe a routine gynecological examination and the information the doctor gains through regular examinations.

2. Describe different ways to do a breast self-examination, and explain why different postures and positions are important for doing it.

3. Describe a mammogram and explain why it is useful for diagnosing breast disease.

4. Describe a Pap smear and how it can detect early signs of cervical cancer.

5. Note and explain the distinguishing symptoms of dysmenorrhea, amenorrhea, and premenstrual syndrome. Summarize the controversy about PMS as a clinical disorder.

6. List the most common vaginal infections and the microorganisms responsible for each one. Describe the distinguishing symptoms of each and their treatments.

7. Describe the causes, symptoms, and treatments for each of the following disorders: endometriosis, pelvic inflammatory disease (PID), cystitis, and toxic shock syndrome.

8. Describe how to do a testicular self-examination, and describe the signs of testicular cancer. Note the high-risk age group for testicular cancer.

9. Describe the causes, symptoms, and treatments for each of the following disorders: epididymitis, cryptorchidism, balanitis, varicocele, priapism, and phimosis. Indicate the consequences of delayed treatment for each.

10. Describe the location and function of the prostate gland. Summarize the symptoms of prostate cancer and benign prostatic hyperplasia, their treatments, and their prognosis.

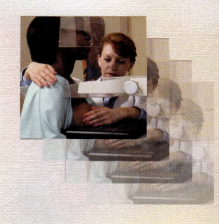

From Dr. Ruth

Through the years, I've always said that it's worth sounding like a broken record about contraception and using condoms if I helped save even one person from an unintended pregnancy or prevented one case of AIDS. Since I started my crusade back in 1981, hopefully more than one person took this advice, but I can't know that for sure. Hundreds of people have thanked me for helping them improve their sex lives, but when it comes to preventing an unintended pregnancy or case of AIDS, there is no way of knowing—because the good news is that "nothing" actually happened.

When a team of experts helped me put together *Dr. Ruth's Encyclopedia of Sex*, even I learned a few new things, one of which was the importance of the male testicular examination. I learned that most cases of testicular cancer occur in fairly young men, and that self-examination could potentially save many lives. I tried then to pass on that nugget of information whenever I was interviewed in the media. Over and over again I tried to spread the word to men that they should regularly examine their testicles and that if they ever felt anything irregular, they should immediately go to a doctor.

A few years ago in a restaurant, one of the waiters pulled me aside. People often do that, to ask me some question about their sex life or relationship difficulties, and unless I'm in a rush, I don't mind. This time I was very glad that I stopped to listen. The young man told me that he had heard me talk about the testicular examination, and then he examined his testicles and found something irregular. He went to a doctor and found out it was cancer, but because he had caught it in time, he was going to be OK and he wanted to thank me.

It made me feel really good. But the most important part of this story is not how I felt, but that this young man had acted and caught the problem in time. Modern medicine is full of unbelievable miracles, but they do no good if doctors don't have the opportunity to put them to work before it's too late. In this chapter you're going to read about many different health problems affecting our sexual and reproductive organs. It may not be a very agreeable subject, but you should study this chapter carefully because the information it contains could save your life. So read on and, just as importantly, check yourself out. Examine your body as described here. If you feel anything is not quite right, even a little thing, get it checked by your physician. People often think that they are invincible, but they're not, so do yourself a favor and think about this and take a good look at yourself.

Most of us take good health for granted. Only when we have a problem or when our good health is gone do we sometimes reflect on this effortless well-being and lack of anxiety. We need to think more about our health, however, because our actions when we are healthy often determine or affect whether we remain healthy. This chapter discusses many common health problems that can affect one's sexual and reproductive health. But before we get started, it is important to make our perspective on this subject clear. We want you to keep in mind some general principles as you read this chapter. This chapter can sensitize you to key information you need to avoid or minimize the seriousness of many health problems.

Three basic premises summarize our approach to sexual and reproductive health:

1. Your health is *your* responsibility.
2. Preventing a condition is always better than trying to treat it if it does occur.
3. Seeking treatment early in a condition is always better than delaying until later.

The previous chapter described human anatomy, physiology, and endocrinology in health. This chapter builds on that information to better understand the nature of illness. While some of these issues can be frightening, such as breast cancer or prostate cancer, others are much less serious or even more of an annoyance than a concern. Knowing about these problems helps one understand why medical counsel should be sought promptly when signs and symptoms occur, and also helps one communicate more clearly with health care providers. Using your sexual vocabulary developed from this text, you can converse intelligently with health care providers about issues that can improve the quality and even the length of your life. Overall, this chapter can help you to develop skills in personal responsibility and intelligent self care.

Not all health problems related to sexuality are discussed in this chapter. Sexually transmitted diseases, including AIDS, are discussed in Chapter 17; only a few communicable conditions are described in this chapter. How many other medical conditions affect sexuality is discussed in Chapter 16. For women, the focus of this chapter is primarily breast cancer and other types of breast disease, cancers of the female reproductive system, menstrual problems, endometriosis, and vaginal infections. For men, we will look at testicular cancer, prostate cancer, and benign prostatic hyperplasia. Although you yourself are probably in good health at this time, you know or will know someone with many of the conditions described in this chapter.

As noted above, we believe it is crucial to take responsibility for one's own health and to recognize the importance of prevention and early diagnosis and treatment. People often delay seeking treatment even though they know they should act more promptly and assertively. It has been estimated that one in nine American women will at some time in their life be diagnosed with breast cancer and that one in eleven American men will be diagnosed with prostate cancer. Yet as many studies reveal, many women still don't do regular breast self-examinations, don't seek mammograms as recommended, or procrastinate about their yearly appointment with their gynecologist. Similarly, many men avoid regular examinations that include a digital rectal examination, which is an important early screening for prostate problems.

Health care is changing rapidly in the United States. In the past, people commonly believed that their health was their *doctor's* responsibility. This is no longer a common attitude. Physicians and other health care professionals increasingly tell us that they are our partners in *our* efforts to take care of ourselves. This is an important change in focus on health and wellness. Doctors today are more willing to teach us about how to avoid ailments or minimize the seriousness of conditions we already have. The next time you visit your physician, ask any specific questions you have about your health concerns. Look for leaflets and health information sheets as well. Remember, your doctor is your partner. The better you understand health issues, the better a partner *you* will be.

Minimizing the risk of disease often requires changes in lifestyle—and these changes are examples of what we mean by *taking care of yourself*. For example, some gynecologists ask their patients to record information about their menstrual cycles on a chart, such as the day their period starts, the day it ends, any mid-cycle bleeding, bloating, or mood changes, and when they occur. Even a simple task like this can help the doctor offer specific and effective treatment for a number of menstrual problems.

The study of health problems can be complex. To ease this process we'll use a standardized approach with the wide variety of conditions. We begin each by discussing the general nature of the disorder, followed by its distinguishing symptoms and signs and an explanation of how it is diagnosed. Next, we consider who may be at greatest risk for the illness. Finally, we discuss the treatments for the problem, its long-term consequences for the individual, and how the ailment can be managed if there is no cure.

THE IMPORTANCE OF PERSONAL RESPONSIBILITY AND PREVENTIVE MEASURES

Adherence to Medical Recommendations

Health psychologists report that about two-thirds of all people do not follow their doctor's directions for long-term illnesses, and fully half do not carefully follow the doctor's advice for short-term ailments. Why? The answers involve complex human issues. Basically, when following health recommendations helps people feel better and diminishes discomfort, most people will follow them. Of all the medications that people are to take exactly as prescribed, for example, pain killers are taken most conscientiously. Yet many signs and symptoms of illness do not seem serious to the person with the problem. For example, high blood cholesterol levels do not cause any discomfort, and people can have high blood pressure and not know it. The earliest stages of some serious cancers also do not involve any discomfort. Because people don't feel bad with these conditions, they are not motivated to seek care. Nonetheless, it is a good idea to have regular check-ups to ensure one stays healthy. Regular check-ups give you and your doctor a "baseline" to which later changes in your health can be compared. Some of the disorders described in this chapter cause symptoms that get a person's attention very quickly, such as vaginal yeast infections. Other conditions advance slowly and painlessly, such as prostate cancer. Therefore, it is a good idea to work with your health care provider regardless of how well you feel at the time.

Throughout this chapter we will talk about screening tests and the value of participating in preventive testing—and who does or does not participate. Bostick, Sprafka, Virnig, & Potter (1994) noted that women with higher incomes were more likely to have mammograms, for example, and that higher education might be associated with a greater willingness to have regular cancer screening tests. In one Australian study of 72 women aged 18 to 63 (Barling & Moore, 1996), 85% indicated that they intended to have a Pap smear (a diagnostic test for cervical cancer), but only 39% actually did so regularly. Another study (Funke & Nicholson, 1993) reported that whether a woman had regular Pap smears was *not* statistically associated with her current health status, age, ethnicity, relationship status, education, or the presence of physical symptoms of an STD. Even when psychological tests showed that a subject felt "in control of her life," this attitude was not associated with having a regular Pap smear.

True, receiving the news from the doctor's office that the Pap smear had a few abnormal cells in it provokes a lot of anxiety (Bell, Porter, Kitchener, & Fraser, 1995). But wouldn't a woman rather get this news early in the progression of a disease when it can be treated effectively than later on, when treatment may not be as successful, because she had been a little negligent in taking care of herself? If people hesitate to have such an easy and convenient test for cancer, what kind of co-operation do you think typically occurs with mammograms or prostate examinations, which can be a little uncomfortable?

Breast self-examination is another example in which a brief and relatively painless procedure may be ignored by young women at a time in their lives when it is a good idea to begin developing good health care habits. Cromer, Frankel, Hayes, and Brown (1992) used a confidential questionnaire to learn whether high school students who had been taught how to do breast self-examinations actually did them 3 and 8 months later. The results are both troubling and surprising. At 3 months, 40% reported they had done a self-examination at some time since the initial session. At 8 months, however, only *2%* had continued to practice breast self-examinations since the 3-month follow-up.

A study like this one raises questions about how common breast self-examinations are among women at a higher risk of developing breast disease. Dunbar-Jacob, Begg, Yasko, & Belle (1991) found that of almost 500 women at high risk for the development of breast cancer and over 50 years old, 30% did breast self-examinations every month, 26% more often than that, and 26% less often. Astonishingly, 19% did no breast self-examinations at all. Almost 90% of these subjects indicated that they had visited their doctors during the previous two years and that their physicians had played an important role in teaching them how to do the examinations and in motivating them to do so regularly. Yet even when doctors take time to instruct women about the different positions appropriate for breast self-examinations, less than half of women studied actually use even one of these (Stevens, Hatcher, & Bruce, 1994).

When one goes to the doctor, he or she makes notes in the person's chart about the reason for the appointment and the nature of the health complaints or questions. These chart notes do not have much of an impact on the patient's self-care behaviors. Yarnall, Michener, Broadhead, and Tse (1993) asked women to fill out a health assessment form (HAF) instead of using the patient's chart notes. Forms such as these allow patients to describe fully their health-enhancing behaviors. This simple idea had a big impact on the number of women who followed up on their doctors' recommendation for regular mammograms. These investigators found that when a chart note was made recommending that the patient receive a mammogram, only 7.2% of the women followed up on this advice. However, when patients took the time to fill out the health assessment form, fully 32% actually had a mammogram done.

When the women in this study had a record of their regular check-ups, their compliance rate with the recommendation for a mammogram rose to over 65%. This study showed that when patients took time to report and record information about themselves and established a record of regular check-ups, they were more likely to practice intelligent self-care. Whether these data generalize to other studies and other health risks needs more research. Another study suggested that women living in rural locations who must travel appreciable distances to visit their doctors and have mammograms were not dissuaded by the travel time alone, as several other factors which were shown to be associated with a patient's desire to comply with a doctor's recommendations (Kreher, Hickner, Ruffin, & Lin, 1995). These investigators reported that education, family or personal income, and having medical insurance all influenced a woman's decision to have regular breast cancer screening tests. Gaston and Moody (1995) have reported that even among women at a higher risk of dying of breast cancer (African-Americans), simple improvements in patient interviews and medical office procedures can increase the percentage of these women who eventually have mammograms. Overall, these diverse investigations reveal it is difficult to predict which patients follow their doctor's recommendations.

Acting Foresightfully to Take Care of Yourself

The last chapter discussed "normal" male and female sexual and reproductive anatomy, physiology, and endocrinology. This chapter introduces "abnormal" health conditions. But just what do these two terms actually mean? Does "normal" equate with "good" and "abnormal" with "bad?" The situation is seldom that simple. Scientists in different disciplines have argued about the meaning of the term "normal" for a long time. In the context of health, these terms have different meanings depending on one's age and health history. Normal and abnormal are not two mutually exclusive categories in which a person falls into either one or the other. Normality and abnormality are actually on a continuum, with many shades of normality and abnormality between the extremes.

Another issue related to self-care is the fact that the absence of pain and other symptoms does not always indicate the absence of disease. For example, usually there is no discomfort associated with early prostate or breast cancer. Because many urologic and gynecologic conditions do not cause discomfort, this criterion cannot be used as an index of wellness. People certainly don't want to have illnesses, but that desire sometimes lulls people into feeling they are invulnerable if they feel no symptoms. Since careful and health-conscious people can still develop serious health problems, however, it is important to detect these problems early, act on them promptly, obtain the best available medical counsel, and often enjoy a full and thorough recovery.

The Impact of Illness on Our Lives

When people are sick, they don't act like their usual selves. They usually experience subjective, inner turmoil. They are frequently anxious or depressed and may be reevaluating their body image and self-concept as a "sick" person. These concerns are important in a discussion of sexual and reproductive illnesses. Diseases can affect our functioning in our families, our jobs, and relationships outside of these contexts. This is true when we think something might be wrong, when we are pretty sure that something is wrong, and when we're certain of it. Illnesses occur in stages, as do their effects on human function. What should be emphasized, again, is the fact that the earlier one finds out about an ailment, the better are the chances of getting rid of it and recovering fully.

Sick people need support. **Support systems** become particularly important to people experiencing illness and its special challenges. Someone in your support system offers you unconditional positive regard—they will be there for you no matter what. A support system can also offer an emotional challenge; these people can motivate us to ask ourselves how to become the best people we can be in our circumstances. They also express a sense of emotional appreciation. This means that they can understand, without judging, human emotion and its expression. Sickness affects more people than just the sick person; a sickness affects a whole network of people (Aronson, Pines, & Kafry, 1981). The better and more adept the support system, the better the sick person's chances of coping and dealing with the symptoms, manifestations, and treatments.

People react to being sick in slightly different ways, but there are a few commonalities in the adjustment process. Scientists who study the effects of stress on psychological and social functioning distinguish between coping with stressors and dealing with them (Lazarus & Folkman, 1984). To cope with a stressor means the person has found a way to live with it and get along with it—but not to get rid of it. Some stressors are a permanent part of the human condition, of course, and learning to cope with them successfully is a real achievement. Dealing with stressors, however, is very different. To deal with a stressor means that the person has found a way to eliminate it. The experience of being sick can involve both coping and dealing. Consider for a moment: are girls raised to be copers or dealers? Are boys raised to be copers or dealers? Is the illness experience fundamentally different for women and men? How do one's perceptions of an illness experience affect how promptly one seeks medical care?

Chapter 1 relates the story of "Dave," who was experiencing urinary symptoms at midlife. At first he didn't know what to make of them, but then he understood that confronting these symptoms was a problem-solving issue and that he needed the counsel of his doctor to figure things out. Dave's story is a common one with important, long-range consequences. It is also a symptom that is similar to the way in which a woman often deals with any unusual feelings and textures she might feel during breast self-examinations.

Taking Personal Responsibility for One's Health

A person's willingness to be foresightful and conscientious about taking care of himself or herself seems to be related to a number of personality characteristics. A fundamental aspect is

self-esteem, the image everyone has of himself or herself. If people feel that they appear and behave in a way that matches the picture of themselves they like to hold, then their self-esteem is pretty good. Similarly, when people's appearance, thoughts, and behaviors do not seem congruent with how they like to see themselves, then their self-esteem suffers and is said to be poor or "low." This personality dimension is clearly related to people's images of their bodies and the activities they engage in with their bodies. People who know a lot about their bodies and who are comfortable with their physical selves are less hesitant to notice unusual or troubling symptoms and report them to their doctor. But many people are not as knowledgeable and comfortable with their bodies, and low self-esteem is often associated with extreme shyness or dissatisfaction with one's body. This outlook may contribute to procrastination in taking care of oneself or taking action when a problem occurs. Self-esteem is not improved overnight, however. Self-esteem develops through years of childhood, adolescence, and young adulthood and is a complicated process involving many family and social influences all working together. This subject is outside of the scope of this book, but reading further about self-esteem can help one learn more about himself or herself.

Another personality trait related to one's willingness to engage in health maintenance behaviors is called **locus of control.** This idea was first introduced in 1966 by the clinical psychologist Dr. Julien B. Rotter. Basically, locus of control involves the answer to the question "Who's in charge of your life?" Rotter developed a test to determine whether one has an "internal locus of control" or an "external locus of control." With the former, *you* feel in charge of your life: *you* make the important decisions, and *you* take responsibility for making choices, taking chances, and exploring challenges. With an external locus of control, however, you believe that factors and forces outside yourself control your life and determine the quality and nature of your existence. Although most people do not generally always behave one way or the other all the time, people may tend toward either internal or external control and, therefore, have different attitudes about the relationship between behaviors and the rewards one ultimately enjoys or does not receive.

People with an internal locus of control generally believe that their health results from their actions and their health-promoting and maintaining behaviors. These are the people who believe that they are taking care of themselves because they expect their efforts to enhance the quality and length of their lives. Even if they face a high risk of developing a health problem because of their family history, they refuse to do nothing and wait for the problem to appear. They understand that lifestyle modifications, regular medical counsel, dietary changes, and perhaps medical care can substantially reduce their risk.

People who have an external locus of control act very differently. They generally believe their health is outside their control and that there isn't much they can do to minimize their risks of developing health problems or to reduce the severity of illness. They believe they must wait for the "inevitable."

Women with an external locus of control are far less likely to perform regular breast self-examinations or have regular mammograms or Pap smears. They may feel hopeless when experiencing menstrual problems that cause discomfort and disrupt their social and occupational functioning. The issue here is not whether one type of locus of control is "good" or "bad" but that people who understand this personality characteristic may be able to behave more independently and effectively when it comes to taking care of themselves. Like self-esteem, locus of control emerges during one's growth and development.

Social and behavioral scientists who study personality have discovered another personality dimension related to health care behaviors, known as **self-monitoring**. This is the degree to which a person is aware of where she or he is, whom she or he is with, what she or he is saying, how her or his utterances are being received, and the general impact of her or his presence on the immediate social environment. People high in self-monitoring have a keen sense of what is going on both inside and outside themselves. They always feel "on stage." Indeed, people high in self-monitoring often experience an almost painful self-consciousness. In contrast, people who are low in self-monitoring are less aware of what is happening around them. Generally, they have less self-consciousness and are less aware of the impact of their behavior on others or their social circumstances. Although they might seem very relaxed, they do not fully attend to relevant and sometimes important environmental cues. What they feel happening inside and outside of them lacks detail and clear reference in place and time. Self-monitoring is clearly related to one's behavior concerning health care. People who are more attuned to their surroundings and themselves are more likely to pay attention to anything unusual happening in their bodies. People low in self-monitoring might not attend to such information as promptly and may delay seeking medical counsel for anything unusual.

Overall, these personality factors influence how proactive people are in their health care behaviors. Certainly, more studies are needed. These issues relate to both women's and men's sexual and reproductive health care issues. It boils down to one basic issue: *taking personal responsibility.*

WOMEN'S SEXUAL AND REPRODUCTIVE HEALTH CONCERNS

Routine Gynecological Examination

Women often experience some anxiety about having a pelvic examination. Younger women may feel this more acutely, but the examination still causes some unease for women of all ages. The anxiety accompanying pelvic examinations has received much attention in medical education (Frye & Weisberg, 1994), and doctors now are trained in techniques to minimize this anxiety.

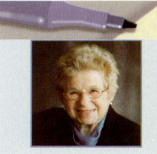

Dear Dr. Ruth

Question:

My doctor always seems in such a hurry during my yearly GYN examination. What can I do to get him to take more time with me and answer my questions more thoroughly?

Answer:

In the days before HMOs, it was easier to spend more time with a doctor. Now many people complain their doctor's office is like a factory line as the doctor moves from one patient to the next. Still, there is certainly no harm in trying to get more personal attention.

First of all, go to your next visit with a written list of questions to be sure you don't forget any. Let the doctor see that you have a list, so that he or she knows you took the time to think about your questions. Then the doctor should be more willing to respond in greater depth.

If your doctor refuses to cooperate, check out other doctors, even if you are limited to those approved by an HMO. If you let another doctor know why you are wanting to switch, he or she might be a little more cooperative. And unless you might be having a child in the near future, try going to a GYN who doesn't deliver babies. Such a doctor won't have a schedule constantly interrupted by births and won't be so tired from spending days in a delivery room.

Most physicians recommend that a woman have her first pelvic examination when she turns 18, as soon as she becomes sexually active, or when she wants to begin taking birth control pills. Women have different circumstances, however, and these are only general recommendations.

An important part of the gynecological examination is a health history. The doctor is in a better position to evaluate potential health problems with the information gained from asking various health-related questions. These include questions about one's overall health and specific questions about menstruation. The doctor may ask about breast tenderness during the menstrual cycle and the type of bra worn during exercise. Many doctors now also ask about caffeine intake because this may be related to breast tenderness or other problems.

One's past medical history is also relevant: surgeries, menstrual history, pregnancies, and breastfeeding. A family history of breast cancer, other reproductive system cancers, and other breast diseases are investigated. The doctor may ask about whether and how often a woman douches and what kinds of contraception she has used in the past. Routine questions are asked about any problems a woman might be experiencing sexually, including the age at first intercourse, how often she has intercourse, what type of contraception or protection against STDs is used, and sexual orientation. The doctor will ask about any medications being taken, as well as tobacco and alcohol habits. The doctor will also ask about one's specific reason for the visit if that is not already clear.

The examination usually follows the history. Much of the following description of this examination is based on the excellent book by Edge and Miller (1994). After emptying her bladder and undressing, the woman is draped and every effort is made to preserve her privacy. She is positioned as needed for the doctor to examine her, beginning with visual inspection of the external genitalia. The physician should tell her what he or she is going to do before doing it. The doctor will palpate (feel) the labia majora and labia minora, as well as the lymph nodes in the groin area, and will then put a finger into the vagina and feel its anterior surface (the front of the vagina). Skene's glands surrounding the urethra are palpated. The doctor may ask her to "bear down" in order to determine the tone of the muscles and ligaments that support the pelvic organs. Doctors often ask their patients to try to tighten the muscles at the opening of the vagina to assess the general muscular tone of the introitus (Fig. 5-1).

A **speculum**, a metal or plastic instrument that allows the doctor to see inside the vagina, is used for the examination of internal structures (Fig. 5-2). When inserting the speculum, the doctor encourages the woman to breathe slowly and regularly through the mouth. The doctor visually examines the inside of the vagina and the cervix and usually takes a Pap smear sample. If other tests requiring vaginal or cervical smears are necessary (such as those for sexually transmitted diseases), they also are taken at this time.

A **bimanual pelvic examination** comes next ("bimanual" literally means "two-handed"). While this might be a little un-

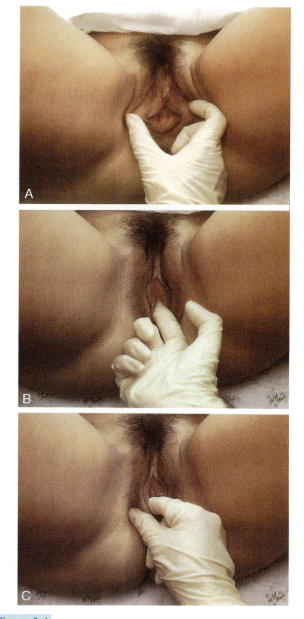

FIGURE 5-1 Examination of the external female genitalia during a pelvic examination. (A) Palpation of the labia. (B) Palpation of the immediate interior of the vagina. (C) Palpation of Bartholin's glands.

comfortable, it is a brief, relatively painless, necessary part of a thorough gynecological examination. Wearing sterile, lubricated, latex-free (some people are highly allergic to latex) gloves, the doctor places a finger from one hand into the vagina and the other hand on top of the abdomen. Internal sexual structures can now be palpated between the doctor's hands. By moving one hand and then the other, she or he can feel the cervix and the ligaments which support the uterus, ovaries, and fallopian tubes (Fig. 5-3). This examination provides the doctor with important information.

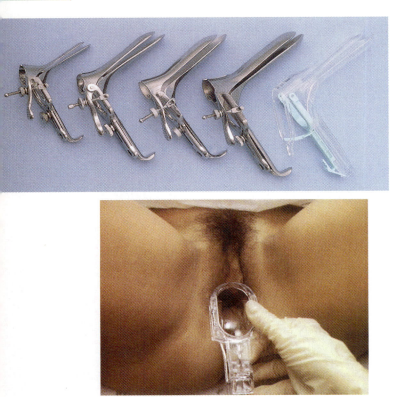

FIGURE 5-2   (Top) Various sizes of specula, both stainless steel and plastic. (Bottom) Plastic speculum inserted into the vagina allowing visualization of its interior.

As described in the previous chapter, the back of the vagina is adjacent to the front of the rectum, and the standard gynecological examination usually also includes a rectal examination. Wearing fresh gloves, the doctor inserts one finger into the vagina and another into the rectum to assess the tone of the muscles that hold and release urine. The doctor can also feel the back of the uterus.

That usually concludes the examination—15 to 20 minutes of slight discomfort each year for the assurance of good sexual and reproductive health or to find any problem early, while it is most treatable. The Pap smear is sent to the laboratory, along with any other tests, and in a few weeks the results are sent back to the doctor. The woman should call the office a few weeks after the examination in case the office hasn't yet called her to say that everything is fine or that the doctor wants to talk to her again about something.

Women often think of their gynecologist as their primary care physician and do not regularly visit a family practitioner or specialist in internal medicine. Therefore the gynecologist sometimes runs tests not directly related to sexual and reproductive health, such as blood sugar and cholesterol levels. Remember that you and your doctor are *partners* in your health maintenance and care. One of the most important things the doctor can teach a woman is the importance of breast self-examination and how to do it.

Breast Cancer

BREAST SELF-EXAMINATION

Despite some conflicting data, breast self-examinations can be extremely important for women to recognize breast changes that may signal various problems, including cancer. Women who discover lumps in their self-examinations understand the importance of seeking medical care. Women having periods should do the examination about halfway between periods. Postmenopausal women should choose a day during the month that is easy to remember. The procedure for a breast self-examination, as described by Edge and Miller (1994, p. 294), is shown in Figure 5-4.

Remember that not all lumps are cancerous. Many different conditions can cause breast lumps or bumps as symptoms, as we will discuss soon. Although the steps outlined

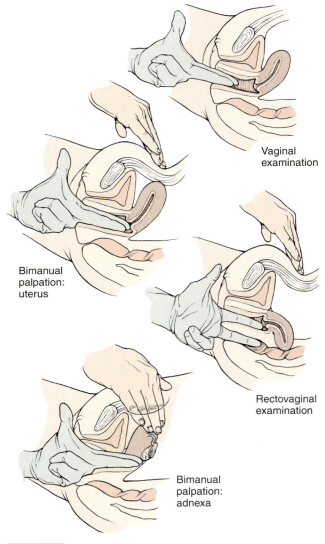

Vaginal examination

Bimanual palpation: uterus

Rectovaginal examination

Bimanual palpation: adnexa

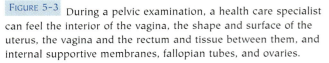

FIGURE 5-3   During a pelvic examination, a health care specialist can feel the interior of the vagina, the shape and surface of the uterus, the vagina and the rectum and tissue between them, and internal supportive membranes, fallopian tubes, and ovaries.

above take only a few minutes, women commonly are some-what careless about doing regular breast self-examinations. Health educators have wondered about how best to motivate women to do the self-examination regularly. Their studies show that the more involved women are when being taught about breast self-examinations, the more consistently they will do them in the future. To compare three different teaching techniques, women were divided into three groups. The first

group only received information about how to do breast self-examinations. The second group received the same informa-tion, but also practiced using a model of a breast that had lumps of various size in it. The final group received the same information but were guided through an examination of their own breasts. More women in this last group later continued to do regular self-examinations (Alcoe, Gilbey, McDermot, & Wallace, 1995). Other data (Stevens, Hatcher, & Bruce, 1994)

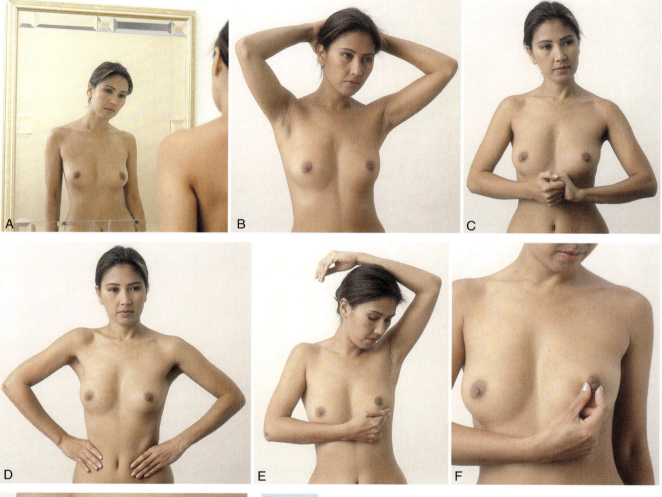

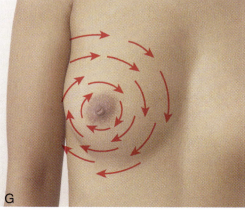

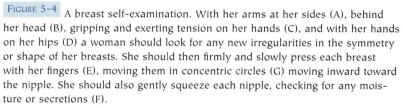

FIGURE 5-4   A breast self-examination. With her arms at her sides (A), behind her head (B), gripping and exerting tension on her hands (C), and with her hands on her hips (D) a woman should look for any new irregularities in the symmetry or shape of her breasts. She should then firmly and slowly press each breast with her fingers (E), moving them in concentric circles (G) moving inward toward the nipple. She should also gently squeeze each nipple, checking for any mois-ture or secretions (F).

indicate that when women are taught a number of postures and positions for breast self-examination, only 40% of the women used three different positions each month. In this study, 42% of the women employed only one position (lying on her back), but other studies have shown that women who use more than one method of breast self-examination are more consistent and conscientious about doing so regularly and are more successful in identifying lumps in silicone models of breasts (Atkins, Solomon, Worden, & Foster, 1991).

Another study of over 200 women aged 22 to 67 working in a large southern university revealed that only 31% practiced regular breast self-examinations, and the women who had been patiently taught how to do it by their doctors were much more likely to do so regularly (Hailey & Bradford, 1991). Generally, both younger and older women did fairly well in detecting lumps in silicone breast models, but older women were less likely to be as accurate in detecting *all* the lumps in test models (Rutledge, 1992). These data are interesting. Although one might have thought that there was a "practice effect" in breast self-exams, that the more a woman does it the better she gets at it, this is apparently not the case. Perhaps over years of practice some women become more hurried or less focused during their breast self-exams? This question deserves more research in health education.

Although finding a breast lump does not necessarily signal cancer, it should be checked by the doctor promptly. Women react to finding a breast lump in different ways, depending in part on their experience with friends and family members who might have had problems. Studies show, however, a problematic situation when it comes to women reporting and acting on breast lumps they find. Redman, Henrikus, Clover, and Sanson-Fisher (1993) found that fully 29% of their sample of 745 women had symptoms of potential breast cancer but *never contacted their doctors at all!* Another 21% of this sample didn't make an appointment for more than 2 weeks after finding a lump. Given that this is a symptom potentially of a very serious disease, these results are surprising and disheartening.

DIFFERENT TYPES OF BREAST LUMPS

Many factors can contribute to the development of benign (noncancerous) breast lumps. Sometimes changes occur during a woman's menstrual cycle, during a pregnancy, or with aging. Of all breast lumps suspicious enough that a doctor recommends a biopsy, 80% are noncancerous. (A biopsy involves the surgical removal of a small amount of the tissue in the lump, usually under local anesthesia, which is then microscopically assessed.) Because breast tissue is composed of lobes of milk-producing glands, the ducts connecting them, and fat with a muscular layer beneath, there are many tissues and textures that sometimes feel lumpy. Women with small breasts and especially thin women are more likely to notice breast changes and lumps. Because the breasts respond to changing levels of hormones during normal menstruation, it is not unusual for women to notice lumps at various times during their menstrual cycle. In most cases, such changes disappear by the

end of a woman's period, and they seldom occur at all after menopause. The National Cancer Institute estimates that about half of all women will at some time experience a breast lump, breast tenderness and pain, or nipple discharge.

A discharge from the nipple is not unusual and may not indicate a disease or disorder. Breast discharge is common in women who use birth control pills or some sedatives and tranquilizers (CancerNet, 1995). This discharge may be clear or whitish. A woman who notices a breast discharge, however, should still mention it to her doctor. Even if the discharge is caused by a breast disease, that disease is most likely benign. The doctor may prescribe an antibiotic if the discharge is caused by an infection.

Some women may be more likely to develop benign breast lumps, although the evidence is still tentative. Women who have never had children, who have irregular menstrual cycles, or who have a family history of breast cancer are more likely to develop benign breast lumps (CancerNet, 1995). Benign lumps are *less likely* in women who use oral contraceptives and those who are overweight. Because of the action of female hormones on breast tissue, benign breast lumps are more common in women of child-bearing age.

Fibrocystic disease is a condition of generalized breast lumpiness. Women with this condition performing self-examinations generally feel lumps having a knotty, ropy, or granular texture. These are most frequently felt in the area around the nipple and in the upper and most lateral parts of the breast. Women with fibrocystic disease typically notice breast changes about a week before their period begins, and they report that the nodules are round and generally regular in shape. Some women report soft lumps, others firmer lumps. Most say they feel tender or a little painful. These symptoms diminish markedly about a week after the period is over. A woman who thinks she may have fibrocystic changes in her breasts should see her doctor to rule out more serious conditions and learn more about this common disorder. Some physicians believe women who consume high levels of caffeine may feel more severe discomfort from fibrocystic breast disease.

A wide variety of benign breast lumps are often referred to collectively as **fibroadenomas**, which are the second most common type of noncancerous breast lumps. They are usually ½ to 1 inch (1.25 to 2.5 cm) in diameter and are made up of developing cells and fibrous tissue (Beckmann et al., 1998). The woman feels a single well-defined, painless lump that does not seem near or connected to other lumps. These lumps frequently have a soft texture and can be moved within the breast easily. Of all the types of breast lumps detected by women in their late teens and early twenties, fibroadenomas are the most common. The National Cancer Institute notes that fibroadenomas are twice as common in African-American women than in other American women (CancerNet, 1995). Fibroadenomas do not become cancerous but may become larger during pregnancy and breast feeding. A doctor who suspects a fibroadenoma may recommend a mammogram, which can distinguish between fibroadenomas and malignant tumors, although many surgeons believe that only by removing the mass can a definitive diagnosis be made. Sometimes other diagnostic tests may be ordered to rule out an infection.

One of the best and most authoritative sources of information on benign breast lumps is the National Cancer Institute. It and other health agencies provide information about medical conditions people may confuse with cancer and therefore experience unnecessary anxiety. Only in the most rare and unusual situations might a benign breast condition evolve into a malignancy.

Breast cancer is, of course, more serious. As noted earlier, some health experts estimate as many as one in nine American woman will develop this disease. The causes of breast cancer can be very complicated. Physicians and health educators often employ the **diathesis stress theory** to emphasize the many factors that may contribute to the development of cancer. This theory describes how genes or combinations of genes may predispose a woman to develop breast cancer, especially in concert with environmental factors, including diet and/or alcohol consumption. Early detection and treatment is essential for successfully treating breast cancer. For this reason elementary and high school health classes teach that one of the seven "early warning signs of cancer," is "a lump or thickening in the breast or elsewhere." Because the breasts are accessible for a thorough tactile examination and mammography, every woman should make a conscientious effort to perform self-examinations and have regular check-ups.

Who is most likely to develop breast cancer? In relation to the following risk factors, remember that these are not the *causes* of breast cancer but rather are *statistically associated* with the development of breast malignancies. Few oncologists (cancer specialists) would definitely state what causes breast cancer, although in some instances genetic factors seem to play an unusually powerful effect. Generally, women who develop breast cancer are over 40 years of age and have a family history of the disease. The closer the relationship between a woman and a relative with breast cancer, the higher the risk. Early menarche and/or late menopause may be associated with the development of breast cancer, but the words "early" and "late" are relative and imprecise terms. Women who have their first child after the age of 30 may also be at increased risk.

Women who have had some types of cancer previously are also at an increased risk for breast cancer. Having already had breast cancer places a woman at an increased risk for its reappearance. Women who have had colon, ovarian, endometrial, or thyroid gland cancer also are at a greater risk for breast cancer. Excessive alcohol and fat consumption may be risk factors as well, but these roles are still controversial. Although these factors are thought to increase a woman's risk of breast cancer, they are present in only 25% to 30% of all cases, and approximately 70% of women diagnosed with the disease do not consume alcohol excessively or eat a diet particularly high in fat (Edge & Miller, 1994).

Breast cancer is thought to develop primarily in three breast tissues: the milk ducts, the breast lobes, and the nipple. Tumors in these areas may be either clearly defined and well-localized or invasive, meaning that they are capable of spreading. The word **metastasis** refers to the spread of any cancer. The most common sites to which breast cancer spreads are the lymph nodes in the lungs, liver, and bones. It is generally believed that even well-localized tumors will eventually spread if not treated. Health educators point out that pain and tenderness do *not* usually occur in the earlier stages of breast cancer.

The breast region is often defined in quadrants (Fig. 5-5). The upper outer quadrant is closest to the arm pit and shoulder, and the upper inner quadrant is closest to the neck and breastbone. The lower outer quadrant is nearest to the lower rib cage, and the lower inner quadrant is adjacent to the upper abdomen. According to Belcher (1992), 50% of cancerous tumors occur in the upper outer quadrant, 15% in the upper inner quadrant, 11% in the lower outer quadrant, and 6% in the lower inner quadrant. These data should not encourage more or less careful examination of certain parts of the breasts, however. Because it is difficult to predict how fast a tumor will grow or whether it will spread, a biopsy of suspicious breast lumps should be prompt or it should be removed and examined.

A lump that is surgically removed from a woman's breast is examined carefully in a surgical pathology laboratory, where it is quick-frozen and slices mounted on a microscope slide, or mounted in paraffin and sliced. Stain applied to the tissue is selectively absorbed by different cells in the specimen, making it possible to examine and identify specific types of cells in the lump. Breast cancer can involve several different types of abnormal cellular growth, and the appropriate form of surgery and/or treatment depends on the exact type of tumor. Other tests of the tissue may take a few days. Generally, if the microscopic examination reveals cancer, the surgeon often elects also to remove a number of lymph nodes from the woman's arm pit. If cancerous cells are found here, the cancer may have begun to metastasize.

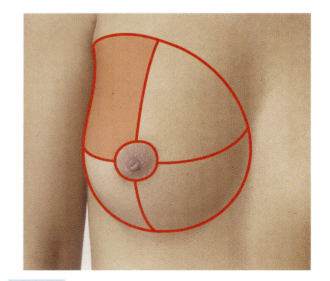

FIGURE 5-5 Four quadrants of a woman's breast. The upper outer quadrant (shaded) is where 50% of cancerous breast tumors are found.

Several medical specialists are usually involved in the diagnosis and treatment of breast cancer. The primary care physician may be a family practice specialist, internist, or gynecologist. A surgeon removes the lump, a pathologist examines it microscopically, and an oncologist makes recommendations about further treatment.

MAMMOGRAMS

In addition to breast self-exams, mammography is an important diagnostic tool for learning about breast lumps. We described benign and malignant breast disease first because mammography generally makes better sense once those issues are clear. A **mammogram,** an x-ray of the breast, is sensitive enough to reveal tumors so small that they would not be detected for another 1 to 2 years through breast self-examination (Fig. 5-6). An extremely small amount of radiation is used in a mammogram. It is a quick, inexpensive test that offers women a good way to take care of themselves and minimize any anxieties they may have about breast changes.

The procedure is fairly straightforward. The woman sits or stands, resting one breast on a cassette containing x-ray film. A transparent glass or plexiglass panel then compresses the breast, flattening it to enhance the image of the tissues within it. Because the breast is compressed significantly, this is somewhat uncomfortable (Fig. 5-7). Two films are taken of each breast, one frontally and one laterally. The procedure is repeated on the other breast, and the woman is usually asked to wait a few minutes while the films are developed to be sure that

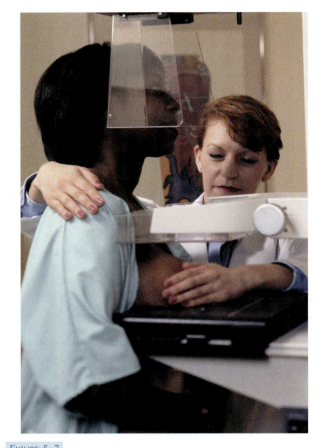

FIGURE 5-7 A woman having a mammogram. Brief compression of the breast is somewhat uncomfortable, but most women tolerate this procedure very well.

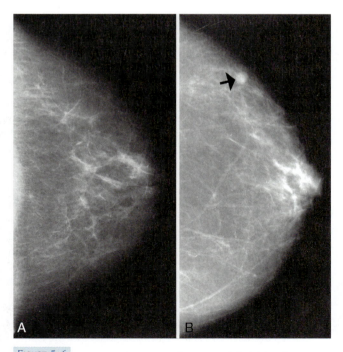

FIGURE 5-6 Two mammograms. The one at left (A) is of a normal breast. The one at right (B) reveals a benign (non-cancerous) breast mass. Learning to interpret mammograms requires significant medical training.

the image quality is good enough for the radiologist's examination. A mammogram can help a doctor discriminate among different breast diseases and between benign and malignant breast disorders, although the mammogram alone cannot make absolute distinctions.

Some women are uncomfortable disrobing and displaying their breasts for a mammogram. Women are entitled to a cotton gown covering the rest of their body, as well as usual office privacy. At the time of the test, the technician may ask the woman about her breast self-examination practices and may offer help or information about this important health care measure. This is also a good opportunity for her to ask questions about breast self-examination.

In addition to doctors' offices and breast diagnostic centers, this test is now commonly done in mobile mammography vans that offer this screening to women who otherwise might not have it. Newspapers often report the location of these mobile vans, which, like breast diagnostic clinics, often offer mammograms at low cost. Depending on a woman's age and health history, her doctor often recommends a first "baseline" mammogram around age 40 and then yearly after age 50. As described in the Research Highlight, there is much controversy about the age at which women should begin having regular

Research Highlight

BREAST CANCER SCREENING FOR WOMEN BETWEEN THE AGES OF 40 AND 49

Because mammography is such a powerful tool for the early detection of breast cancer, why don't all women after age 40 have one every year? What could be simpler? This question has generated much controversy, however, about the necessity and importance of mammography in women in their 40s. In 1997 a large number of oncologists, statisticians, epidemiologists, and radiologists were convened by the National Institutes of Health (NIH) to determine the necessity and/or desirability of mammograms for women in their 40s. The outcome of their deliberations surprised many people.

NIH noted that a 40-year-old woman has a 2% chance of developing breast cancer before age 50 but only a 0.3% risk of dying from the disease during this time. With this incidence of malignancy, are the costs and benefits of mammography enough to merit a blanket recommendation that all women in their 40s should have regular mammograms? This question is also important because there may also be *risks* associated with mammograms. Women can be harmed if their mammograms are interpreted as negative when they actually are positive, or vice versa. In fact, among women between 40 and 49, up to one-fourth of invasive cancers are not picked up on mammograms, compared to one-tenth for women between 50 and 59. There are also more false-positive mammograms among younger women, in which the radiologist believes that something on the film is suspicious when actually there is no problem. The anxiety caused by false-positive readings often dissuades women from continuing to have regular mammograms. Such factors detract from the unquestioned reliability many women attribute to their mammograms. As well, no data have proved that beginning regular mammograms at age 40 increases or decreases adherence with screening recommendations later in life.

This NIH study produced no data on the effect of early breast cancer screening on high-risk women. Before the benefits of early breast cancer screening can be fully assessed, its impact on women at highest risk for developing malignancies requires extensive study.

The most controversial aspect of the NIH consensus report was that "the available data do not warrant a single recommendation for mammography for all women in their 40s. Each woman should decide for herself whether to undergo mammography" (Draft Report, National Institutes of Health, Consensus Development Statement, "Breast Cancer Screening For Women Ages 40–49). In other words, women in their 40s are encouraged to discuss their personal situations with their primary health care providers and together come to an agreement about the desirability and frequency of mammograms. Interestingly, we see in this investigation that a scientific study cannot always lead to a clear health care directive. The more data that are collected, however, the clearer will be the appropriate medical recommendation.

The NIH recommendations were made public in January 1997, but only 2 months later, in March 1997, The American Cancer Society recommended that women should begin to have annual mammograms at the age of 40 (*New York Times*, March 23, 1997). Although we would all prefer the issue to be simple and the answer to be clear-cut, medical scientists and physicians view mammography, especially for younger women, in somewhat different ways, and differences in medical opinion naturally result. Despite this controversy, we recommend that all women have a baseline mammogram at age 40 and discuss with their doctors the frequency of mammograms thereafter.

mammograms and how often thereafter. But remember that regular doctor visits, regular breast self-examinations, and regular (when recommended) mammograms all offer a tremendous benefit for early detection of any breast diseases. One large study of almost 5000 men and women between the ages of 25 and 74 (Bostick, Sprafka, Virnig, & Potter, 1993) revealed that 80% of this sample believed that cancer was preventable, but their understanding of cancer's warning signs was poor. In this sample, 95% of the women had a Pap smear, visited a doctor for a breast exam, or had carried out breast self-examinations themselves. Almost two-thirds of the women between the ages of 50 and 65 had had a mammogram. While **adherence** to medical recommendations is still far from ideal, signs like this that women are taking better care of themselves are heartening.

Treatment of Breast Cancer

When breast cancer occurs, several treatment options can be considered by the patient and her physicians. The earlier the diagnosis is made, the smaller the malignancy, the less invasive the tumor, the better the prognosis. The type of tumor may determine what therapeutic options are recommended. If the tumor is very small, removing it and the area of normal tissue surrounding it may be adequate—a procedure called a **lumpectomy**. This is often combined with removing the lymph nodes in the armpit and radiation therapy. For larger, more aggressively growing breast disease, a **partial mastectomy** involves the removal of the tumor and a large amount of surrounding tissue. In some instances, a **mastectomy** (Fig. 5-8A) is the treatment of choice. There are several types of mastectomy, generally all involving the removal of all breast tissue and lymph nodes in the armpit. In only some instances are underlying chest muscles also removed. Many women choose to have plastic surgery to rebuild the breast after a mastectomy, and a number of options are available (Fig. 5-8B).

Drug therapy may also be used. **Chemotherapy** is the administration of drugs that selectively find and kill malignant cells. Several treatments are necessary, and the woman often experiences nausea, hair loss, and a low red blood cell count while undergoing treatment. Not all women have the same side effects or the same severity of effects. Premenopausal women who undergo chemotherapy typically stop menstruating during and after treatment. **Hormone therapy** is another type of drug therapy for breast cancer. Hormones or agents that block the actions of hormones may be prescribed. Hormone therapies may involve long-term treatment, such as with the drug *tamoxifen,* which some women take for several years.

Finally, **radiation therapy** is another treatment alternative. In some cases, small pellets of radioactive material are implanted directly into the breast, while in others an external radiation beam is directed through the breast.

A number of variables affect the doctor's treatment recommendation for any individual woman's breast cancer. Her age and pre- or postmenopausal status are important, as are the size, type, and location of the tumor(s) removed. Whether the lymph nodes show the disease spreading is a very important factor. Each treatment modality also has potential risks and complications. In some cases one treatment may be used, while in others multiple or even all treatment modalities may be employed. We began this chapter by emphasizing that everyone is a partner with their doctor in health care. Decisions how to treat a breast malignancy should result from an open collaboration between patient and physician, and the patient always has the right to express her preferences and concerns.

IF YOU FIND A LUMP IN YOUR BREAST

As noted earlier, about 90% of the time a woman finds a lump in her breast it isn't cancerous. Still, this can be an unsettling or frightening experience. If women know what to expect from the health care system if they find a lump, then they are better able to handle the stresses of medical testing procedures and examinations.

Finding a lump should lead to a call to the primary care physician. An appointment will be scheduled very soon, and the doctor will do a thorough breast examination in the office. Because of the anxiety of finding a lump, women often press or squeeze the suspected area repeatedly to learn more about it, but this can lead to soreness that only makes the woman more nervous. Instead, the woman should try to avoid manipulation of the suspicious area.

A mammogram will likely be performed next. This imaging technique allows the doctor to make a reasonably good diagnosis about the nature of the lump, although this technique has limitations. The only sure way to determine what kind of cells are in the lump is to do a biopsy. This involves surgically removing the lump or inserting a needle into it to draw out cells and fluid to be examined microscopically. The doctor also may recommend a biopsy if the nipple is irritated and inflamed, encrusted with discharge, or has scaly sores that are not healing well. For women who have not gone through menopause and who lack any other indications of a malignancy, the doctor may delay the biopsy about a month to be sure that the lump isn't caused by hormonal changes related to the menstrual cycle.

For women who have had breast cysts in the past, however, or if there are other indications of the possibility of cancer, the doctor may perform a fine needle aspiration in the office (The PDR Family Guide to Women's Health and Prescription Drugs, 1994). This procedure takes only seconds, causes little discomfort, and can determine if the lump is a cyst. The doctor washes the breast with an antiseptic, inserts a thin needle into the lump, and withdraws some fluid. In some cases local anesthesia may be used. The fluid sample is then examined under a microscope for signs of cancer.

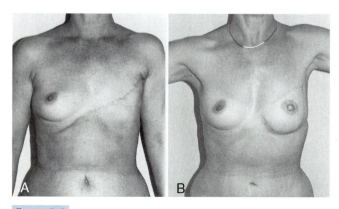

FIGURE 5-8 Post surgical appearance of a mastectomy (A), and after plastic surgery to reconstruct a new breast (B).

Breast cysts are hollow, fluid-filled sacs, whereas tumors are solid. The physician learns much from how much resistance the needle encounters as it is advanced into the lump. Hard lumps are a greater cause for concern. When a breast cyst is penetrated by the needle it collapses and the lump disappears. In such cases a follow-up mammogram may be performed in a few weeks to be sure that the lump was really a cyst. If the lump does not return, cancer can usually be ruled out. However, if in the fine needle aspiration the doctor cannot draw off any fluid, if the fluid is tinged with blood, if the mass does not go away, or if the lump returns after repeated aspiration procedures, then a surgical biopsy is usually recommended. In other words, if the needle biopsy does not produce clear results, another way of examining the lump is needed.

Breast biopsies are usually performed on an outpatient basis, and the patient goes home afterwards. Breast biopsy techniques have changed much over recent years. Most surgeons now use a two-step procedure. The lump is removed, the tiny incision is closed, and the woman is taken to the recovery room. If the lump is cancerous, a second procedure is necessary, but all further medical treatment decisions are made after the patient and doctors discuss the benefits and drawbacks of treatment options. In the past, women justifiably feared that if they went into surgery to have a lump removed and it proved to be malignant, they might wake up without a breast. It has been demonstrated, however, that a short wait between the two surgeries does not affect the woman's chances for full recovery. This delay also gives the doctor a chance to carry out more tests if needed, the results of which may influence the treatment options.

Ultrasound is another diagnostic test sometimes used with breast lumps. An image is formed by sound waves bouncing off breast tissues. Ultrasound can be especially useful for learning more about lumps deep in the breasts of younger women, which are often hard to feel and difficult to reach with a needle. Younger women have denser breast tissue than older women, and mammograms are often less accurate in finding lumps in them.

Cervical Cancer

Chapter 4 described the structure, function, and location of the cervix. It is the opening to the uterus, and the tiny aperture in it (the os) is the passageway for arriving sperm and the channel through which menstrual discharge leaves the uterus. Cervical cancer usually begins as a tiny growth between the outer surface and the layer of cells lining the cervical canal. Because it is usually a slow-growing cancer, if it is found with early diagnostic screening, this disease is curable for many women. Although the exact causes of cervical cancer are not fully understood, studies have shown an important association between a common sexually transmitted disease, the human papillomaviruses (HPV), and cervical cancer. There are over 60 varieties of the human papillomavirus, but only a few have been shown to cause cellular changes in the cervix that may progress to cancer. There are other risk factors as well. Women who began having sex in their early teens have a higher risk, and the

risk is doubled in women who smoke cigarettes. Women who have had many male sex partners are also at an increased risk for cervical cancer. Generally, as women age, their risk of developing cervical cancer increases; this is compounded by the fact that cervical cancer detected in older women often is more advanced. Finally, African-American women are twice as likely to develop cervical cancer than American women of other races. Although family history clearly plays a role in a woman's predisposition to develop breast cancer, the link is not clear with cervical cancer. Cervical cancer accounts for an estimated 15% of all cancers in women. The American Cancer Society estimates that 12,800 women will be diagnosed annually with cervical cancer, 4800 of whom are expected to die as a result.

There is no usual clinical profile of signs and symptoms for cervical cancer, although some signs are often associated with its appearance. A blood-tinged discharge that becomes progressively darker may indicate cancerous lesions on the cervix. Edge and Miller (1994) note that prolonged menstrual periods, more frequent periods, and bleeding after intercourse all may indicate potential cancer. Because early cellular changes in the cervix are not usually accompanied by clinically obvious symptoms, screening and early detection are especially important. Fortunately, a simple, painless, inexpensive, and accurate diagnostic test,—the Pap smear—is very effective.

THE PAP SMEAR

The **Pap smear** is a highly accurate diagnostic test for cervical cancer. It was developed by Dr. Georges Papanicolaou (Fig. 5-9) who discovered that cells on the surface of the cervix begin their development deep within the tissues of this structure. As they grow and develop, cells migrate outward to the outside layers of the cervix (Fig. 5-10). Therefore, if a cell on the surface of the cervix is unusual, the problem likely lies deeper in the tissue. Abnormal cervical cells show when there is something wrong under the surface requiring further testing. A Pap

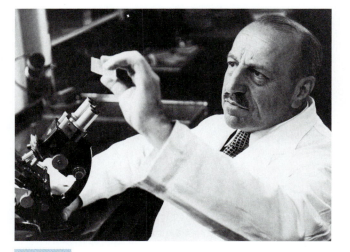

FIGURE 5-9 Dr. Georges Papanicolaou, developer of the "Pap" smear.

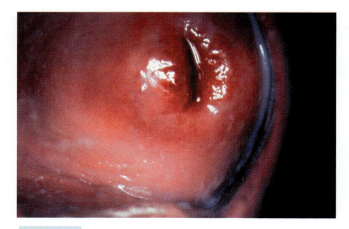

FIGURE 5-10   Appearance of a normal cervix.

smear is taken during the pelvic examination, when a small wooden spatula or nylon brush is brushed across the cervix (Fig. 5-11) to collect cells from the cervix and, possibly, the cervical canal.

The cells are placed on a microscope slide and examined by a cytopathologist, a specialist trained to identify changes in body cells that may reveal illness. The laboratory report is sent to the doctor describing the presence or absence of abnormal cells and the extent of any signs of disease suspected. Women should contact their doctor's office a few weeks after a Pap smear to learn the outcome of the test. Generally, women should start having Pap smears when they turn 18, become sexually active, or want to begin using birth control pills, whichever occurs first. Because of the association between sexually transmitted diseases and cervical cancer, regular Pap smears are particularly important.

The results of the Pap smear may reveal normal cervical cells (Fig. 5-12); mild, moderate, or severe **dysplasia**; or carcinoma *in situ* (localized cancer). The term *dysplasia* means that cells are developing abnormally, which might reveal a precancerous condition. Abnormal cervical cells may also indicate a noncancerous ailment. The most common cause of an abnor-

mal Pap smear result is infection, such as a yeast infection (discussed later). A woman with a yeast or bacterial infection is treated with antibiotics or other medication, and a follow-up Pap smear is usually performed a month or two later. Some studies suggest that up to one-fifth of all Pap smear results may be inaccurate, usually indicating an abnormality when none exists.

Follow-Up on Abnormal Pap Smear Results

If a Pap smear reveals abnormal cervical cells, the doctor may decide to take tissue samples for further analysis. Abnormal cervical cells do not necessarily mean that a cancerous tumor is growing. As noted above, many abnormal Pap tests result from infections that can readily be cured. If the cause is not an infection, however, a cervical biopsy may be needed for the diagnosis. A number of different procedures are used. Most common is **colposcopy**, in which a special microscope called a colposcope is positioned at the opening to the vagina for a magnified view of potentially abnormal areas of the cervix. A solution is applied to the cervix that causes abnormal cells to turn white or yellow. The doctor then knows exactly which areas of the cervix to biopsy. Only a small pinch of tissue is taken, causing very little discomfort. Colposcopy is carried out in the doctor's office and takes only a few minutes.

While the colposcope is in place, other tests may also be done. **Endocervical curettage** (ECC) involves removing cells from the cervical canal. When the outer boundary of the cervix is normal, there still may be problems within this passageway. This test is highly effective in detecting a type of cervical cancer that is common in younger women and grows relatively quickly. This test, combined with colposcopy, provides much important information to help the woman and her doctor plan treatment. In other diagnostic procedures, **loop electrocautery**

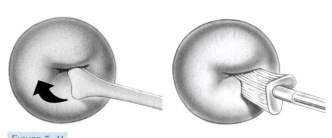

FIGURE 5-11   In taking a Pap smear, a wooden probe (left) is rubbed on the surface of the cervix to collect cells, while a small nylon brush (right) can gather cells from within the cervical canal.

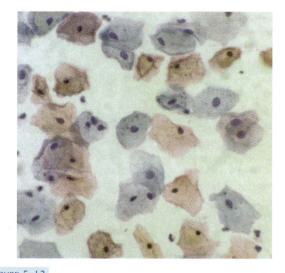

FIGURE 5-12   Normal cervical cells.

Research Highlight

CERVICAL CANCER SCREENING AND FOLLOW-UP

In the late 1980s and early 1990s in North Carolina a long-term study was conducted regarding the high prevalence of cervical cancer in African-American women. The "Forsyth County Cervical Cancer Prevention Project," a 5-year program funded by the National Cancer Institute, offered public health education through a variety of media, including the mass media and workshops. Information about cervical cancer detection and treatment was given to local health care providers. Dignan, Michielutte, Wells, & Bahnson (1994) reported a significant increase in overall awareness of cervical cancer and the importance of Pap smears for detecting a malignancy early. However, while *awareness* of these issues increased because of these educational interventions, knowledge, attitudes, and behaviors did *not* change substantially, with one exception. Women at the highest risk for cervical cancer had greater participation in cervical cancer screening for the 6 months following the study. Although 6 months might not sound like a long time for an effect to last, what can be learned during this period may be crucial to a woman's continued good health or getting treatment that may increase the length and quality of her life. When women in the study were informed of abnormal Pap smear results, they had greater compliance with follow-up care while the community education program was going on, but after it ended, women were less likely to follow-up on abnormal Pap results (Michielutte, Dignan, Bahnson, & Wells, 1994).

Earlier we discussed the importance of compliance with health care recommendations and how difficult it is to predict who will assume responsibility for their own health. This issue is especially important with cervical cancer screening, as with breast cancer screening. It has been demonstrated that women with an internal locus of control were *not* more likely to get follow-up medical treatment when diagnosed with the human papillomavirus that had become clinically obvious during routine Pap testing (Funke & Nicholson, 1993). To learn more about compliance with recommendations for follow-up treatment after abnormal Pap smears, Funke and Nicholson (1993) examined the relationship between beliefs about one's health and locus of control in women with human papillomavirus. In their analysis of 272 women, only 29 indicated that they had failed to comply with their doctor's suggestions for follow-up care. However, a few questions on this questionnaire were especially revealing. For example, subjects who agreed with the statement, "The uncertainty about my Pap test makes me nervous," were *four times as likely* to adhere to medical recommendations as the women who disagreed with this statement. Further, women who agreed with the statement, "I have not been able to cope with my abnormal Pap test," were three times as likely to fail to adhere to medical suggestions as the women who disagreed with this statement. While many women get very apprehensive about abnormal Pap results, not all of them do anything about it.

Another interesting study examined psychological issues in women who had just had a Pap smear. When the results indicated mild or moderate dysplasia or led to a recommendation for colposcopy, women experienced high levels of distress; they reported and revealed more depression and anxiety, as well as problems in social adjustment. Women encouraged to have colposcopy had the highest levels of anxiety among the 225 British women in this investigation (Bell, Porter, Kitchener, Fraser, et al., 1995).

excision procedure (LEEP) and conization, abnormal tissue is cut out using a sharp wire loop, and then the area is cauterized. Cauterization uses electrical current to burn out suspicious tissue. **Conization** is cutting out a cone-shaped area of the cervix with a scalpel or laser to examine the cells microscopically. These more aggressive treatments are often performed on an outpatient basis in the hospital as well. Many physicians believe that loop electrocautery excision and conization should be used when invasive cancer is believed present and other diagnostic procedures suggest this probability. Finally, **cryotherapy** involves freezing a well-localized lesion on the surface of the cervix. Ice crystals form in cells that might be abnormal, destroying them (Beckmann et al., 1998). The earlier that all of these procedures are begun, the less tissue is involved and the better the woman's prognosis. Which procedures are used depends on the unique circumstances for each woman.

Although some of these procedures can be used for treatment, as well as diagnosis of early signs of cervical cancer, when clear abnormalities are found in cervical cells, other approaches are necessary for the best prognosis. Since mild dysplasia is not cancer, many doctors take a "wait and see" approach. For moderate or severe dysplasia, however, generally more immediate and assertive therapeutic strategies are advised. Depending on the type of cellular abnormality, surgical, chemotherapeutic, and radiation therapies may be used alone or in combination.

Menstrual Problems

The issues described so far are those most commonly discussed in routine gynecological examinations. Menstruation problems are another source of dismay or discomfort that lead many women to visit health care professionals. The last chapter described hormonal and physiological aspects of menstruation, but here we will examine menstrual abnormalities, their symptoms, and women's reactions to them. Although not every possible variation is covered here, common menstrual problems are discussed.

Some women wonder whether *all* women have problems with their periods. The answer is yes, at one time or another, if "problem" means anything from puzzling irregularities to debilitating discomfort. In an important *American Journal of Public Health* article entitled, "Chronic Gynecological Conditions Reported by US Women: Findings from the National Health Interview Survey, 1984 to 1992," we learn that about 97 out of every 1000 American women reported gynecological problems of one kind or another. Menstrual problems are the most common disorders reported, with an annual prevalence of 53 per 1000 American women. When we add in women experiencing irregular and/or very uncomfortable menstruation early in adolescence, the similarly unpredictable periods seen early in menopause, and the common mood changes that often accompany menstruation, women who never have menstrual problems may be rare. The following sections describe the most common difficulties.

DYSMENORRHEA

Dysmenorrhea means "menstrual pain." One form, characterized as primary dysmenorrhea, is menstrual discomfort resulting from the increased secretion of **prostaglandins** in the endometrium and uterine wall. These chemicals increase the strength of uterine contractions before and during menstruation, causing significant discomfort. Secondary dysmenorrhea is caused by physical problems outside the uterus (e.g., endometriosis), in the wall of the uterus (e.g., endometrial implants in the uterine wall), or inside the uterus (e.g., infections). Dysmenorrhea causes severe menstrual cramping, and about 10% of the women who have it miss school or work at times because of it. Primary dysmenorrhea can be especially debilitating in teenage girls. In addition to cramping, dysmenorrhea may be accompanied by nausea and vomiting, extreme fatigue, diarrhea, lower back pain, and headaches. Having all of these symptoms occurring each month can significantly disrupt one's lifestyle and interpersonal relationships.

While primary dysmenorrhea often begins 1 or 2 years after menarche, secondary dysmenorrhea can begin suddenly after years of normal menstruation. The discomfort of these disorders may last from hours up to 2 days. Women may also report feelings of bloating associated with their discomfort. If menstrual discomfort disrupts a woman's lifestyle, she should consult her primary care physician, who typically does a pelvic examination and may order a Pap smear and blood tests. In some instances, an ultrasound examination of the uterus is performed and other procedures are considered, such as a biopsy of the endometrium. It is important to understand that persistent, severe menstrual pain is not normal and requires medical evaluation.

The management of dysmenorrhea may take various approaches. Many doctors recommend over-the-counter nonsteroidal anti-inflammatory drugs, such as aspirin, ibuprofen, or naproxen. For many women these are effective and convenient to take. Some investigators believe that the most important cause of secondary dysmenorrhea is an excess of *prostaglandins*. These naturally occurring hormones play a role in initiating contractions of the myometrium. Nonsteroidal anti-inflammatory drugs help block the action of prostaglandins and therefore can help reduce menstrual discomfort. Additionally, hormone therapy is often effective in treating dysmenorrhea. As many as 4 out of 5 women with this disorder are helped by taking birth control pills, especially among younger women with primary dysmenorrhea. Home remedies may also be effective, such as hot baths, heating pads, and regular aerobic exercise, which all minimize the discomfort that accompanies dysmenorrhea.

It is not easy to predict who is most likely to suffer from dysmenorrhea. In a large study of the types of problems that primary care physicians encounter, 90% of the 701 18- to 45-year-old women in the sample had visited their physicians for menstrual pain at one time or another (Jamieson & Steege, 1996). Factors such as age, having had children, marital status, race, income, and education were not correlated with the presence or absence of dysmenorrhea. Another study evaluated a large number of young women (aged 17 to 19) entering college to assess factors that might contribute to dysmenorrhea at this age. Harlow and Park (1996) found that women who had started having periods earlier in adolescence were likely to experience more severe menstrual discomfort that also occurred more frequently and lasted longer. Additionally, women who smoked cigarettes had cramps that lasted longer during their cycles. Overweight women had twice the risk of having long episodes of discomfort each month. Interestingly, women who often drank alcohol were less likely to have severe cramping, but the women who drank and did have menstrual pain had pain that lasted longer and was more severe than among women who did not drink as much. Therefore, although it is difficult to precisely characterize women as high risk for dysmenorrhea, a number of controllable lifestyle factors apparently play a role in the occurrence, duration, and intensity of menstrual pain, and altering these may help diminish these menstrual complaints.

Finally, it should be noted that women have highly diverse socialization experiences involving menstruation, especially their earlier periods. If a young girl gets the message that menstruation is debilitating and uncomfortable, she may be more likely to report discomfort and distracting mood swings associated with her periods. Such psychological factors can be as important as the physical causes noted above.

AMENORRHEA

When a woman's previously normal periods suddenly stop for 3 or more months, this condition is called **amenorrhea**, which literally means "no menstruation." (Some physicians use a criterion of 6 or more months without menstruation.) Technically, this is secondary amenorrhea. If a woman reaches the age of 16 without starting to menstruate, the condition is called primary amenorrhea. Amenorrhea is very different from a period being late or menstruating in a 5- or 6-week cycle.

Numerous studies show that severe physical or emotional problems can significantly disrupt the menstrual cycle, as can high levels of stress (even a woman's stress of worrying about whether she is pregnant if her period is late!). As we will see later, significant weight loss can lead to the cessation of menstruation.

Amenorrhea is related to abnormalities in the secretion of hormones that regulate the menstrual cycle. As described in the previous chapter, there is a very delicate interplay among the glands that secrete the hormones responsible for regular, cyclic periods. In addition to the pituitary gland and the ovaries, a woman's adrenal glands and thyroid also play subtle, but significant, roles. Any delay, interruption, or cessation in the secretion of hormones from these glands may cause an abrupt cessation of menstruation. Additionally, after stopping birth control pills, it often takes a long time to resume normal menstruation, sometimes as long as 6 months. In some cases of secondary amenorrhea, the ovaries do not respond properly to the pituitary's secretion of FSH and LH and do not ovulate. Because this delicate interplay of hormones is essential for normal menstruation, a number of factors that disrupt the balance of these chemicals can disrupt menstruation. For example, demanding physical exercise (as in athletic training) may cause menstruation to stop, especially if the woman has very little body fat. Additionally, obesity, inadequate nutrition, diabetes, chronic nonalcohol-related liver disease, tuberculosis, and various medications (such as oral contraceptives, narcotics, tranquilizers, and chemotherapy) may all cause the cessation of regular periods (PDR Family Guide to Women's Health and Prescription Drugs, 1994). A woman who has been having regular periods and suddenly stops doing so should consult her primary care physician. Often addressing the suspected cause of the amenorrhea eventually leads to returning to a regular menstrual cycle. In some cases it may take longer to find the specific cause of the amenorrhea, but generally not having periods is not problematic during this period of medical evaluation.

Finally, it is important to note that amenorrhea is common among women with the eating disorders **anorexia nervosa** and **anorexia athletica** (Yates, Leehey, & Shisslak, 1983). The former is systematic self-starvation with no accompanying organic illness, and the latter is a restriction of caloric intake while undergoing arduous athletic training. When women eat too little during prolonged athletic training, it is not at all uncommon for them to stop menstruating. The exact reason for this is not clear but is thought to involve the body leanness resulting from long-lasting athletic training. In both types of anorexia, an appetite is present but the person does not consume adequate nutrition. When women lose a significant percentage of normal body fat, an important trigger for normal menstruation is lacking, and amenorrhea results. Although the precise limit is not known, when a woman's percentage of body fat falls into the 11% to 14% range, her periods are likely to become irregular or stop altogether. Regaining weight to a normal level restores regular menstruation, usually after a few months.

PREMENSTRUAL SYNDROME

Whether there is an authentic clinical entity called **premenstrual syndrome** (PMS) is a highly controversial issue. Although almost everyone agrees that women experience menstrual-related mood changes, there is substantial disagreement about the degree to which such changes affect women's intellectual, emotional, and behavioral characteristics (Table 5-1). Further, there is significant disagreement over just when such effects begin before menstruation. Despite these unknowns, the treatment of PMS has become something of an industry. Over-the-counter medications claim to minimize or eliminate physical and emotional aspects of PMS, and some counselors and psychotherapists now specialize in PMS treatment.

Most investigators who study PMS believe that the physical and psychological complaints begin at about the time the corpus luteum is formed during a woman's menstrual cycle. Many women report symptoms beginning 5 to 10 days before their periods begin. This distress usually starts in a woman's late twenties and may increase in severity until she reaches menopause. It is estimated that about half of all women at one time or another experience PMS, and 9 to 12 million women in

---

TABLE 5-1

Symptoms Often Seen in Premenstrual Syndrome

Irritability
Depression
Mood swings
Changes in sleep patterns
Loss of energy
Breast tenderness
Headaches
Distractibility
Weight gain
Cravings for certain foods
Loss of enjoyment in activities which in the past offered relaxation and fun

the United States (6% to 9% of American women) are affected regularly. While no single physical cause of the complaints of PMS has been found, a number of biological factors are thought to play a role. Changes in estrogen and progesterone levels (especially after a fall) and a lack of certain vitamins (especially vitamin B_6) have been suggested. Women who suffer from PMS frequently report significant fluid retention, irritability, depression, and mood swings. The actions of hormones and vitamin B_6 are thought to affect certain neurotransmitters in the brain (especially dopamine and serotonin) that can have a direct impact on the experience and expression of emotion. The troubling symptoms typically go away a day or two after menstruation begins. The signs and symptoms of PMS are numerous and diverse, making it difficult to identify a specific syndrome.

Until fairly recently, the treatment for PMS included diverse and sometimes unusual treatments for which health insurance companies often would not pay. Today, however, there is more uniformity in treatment, and many health insurance companies are more willing to pay a share of the counseling that often helps women deal with PMS. The *Diagnostic and Statistical Manual of Mental Disorders* (fourth edition) now includes a category called "Premenstrual Dysphoric Disorder."

The word *dysphoric* refers to feelings of being physically ill or unhappy. The inclusion of this diagnosis in the DSM-IV is important because it standardizes the language for distinguishing symptoms of different psychological disorders and because a diagnostic category is necessary for most insurance reimbursements. Still, psychologists and psychiatrists do not all agree that premenstrual dysphoric disorder is a standard diagnosis, and there is still controversy about how much of the problem is psychological and how much is physical in origin. In addition to the symptoms previously described, the DSM-IV also includes emotional liability (e.g., "feeling suddenly sad or tearful or increased sensitivity to rejection."), decreased interest in usual activities, difficulty concentrating, lethargy, fatigability or marked lack of energy, marked change in appetite (overeating or specific food cravings), excessive sleep or insomnia, a subjective sense of being overwhelmed or out of control, and often other physical symptoms such as breast tenderness or swelling, headaches, joint or muscle pain, and weight gain (DSM-IV, 1994, p. 717).

The treatments for PMS include lifestyle changes such as a reduction in salt intake, animal fats, caffeine, sugar, alcohol, and mood-altering drugs. Women are encouraged to consume more unrefined carbohydrates (e.g., pasta, potatoes, whole-

---

IS THERE A "MENSTRUAL ETIQUETTE?"

Because of the discomfort and other symptoms that sometimes accompany menstruation, women may ask themselves, "How am I supposed to act when I'm having my period and feeling terrible?". Sometimes it takes real effort to maintain control of one's emotions, especially when feeling upset or unwell for one reason or another. Yet mothers, when teaching their daughters about menstruation, seldom mention that although a period may cause some moodiness and discomfort, *the show must go on!* Grief and Ulman (1982) noted that adolescent girls approach their first period not as a rite of passage but more as a turning point in personal hygiene. They are less likely to feel enfranchised in adult feminine society but instead become concerned about being clean and staying fresh. Still, a young woman who has been well prepared for her first period is far more likely to develop a more positive attitude about her body and her fertility and to deal well with the discomfort and annoyance that sometimes accompany menstruation (Koff, Rierdan, & Sheingold, 1982).

Various over-the-counter preparations promise to relieve the discomfort, cramps, and bloating that may occur with menstruation. There is a powerful and persistent message that menstruation is somehow unclean-isn't it interesting how the word *sanitary* is used to describe these products? Delaney, Lupton, and Toth (1988) note that advertisements for these products have traditionally employed a revealing vocabulary:

"... menstruation is still usually discussed with euphemisms: "those special days," "those difficult days," "that time of the month." "Special' is double-edged, used to imply both "noteworthy" and "problematic." Equally covert is the treatment of what to do with used menstrual paraphernalia. "Now-one more thing not to worry about ... that little discussed disposal problem. Now-neat, discreet, disposal bags come in each box of new Scott Confidets." Menstruating women should be embarrassed, say advertisers. (p. 132)

Interestingly, while terms like "secure," "confident," and "free," are most often included in these ads, the word "absorbent" is used much less frequently (Delaney, Lupton, & Toth, 1988).

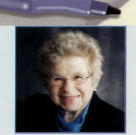

Dear Dr. Ruth

Question:

I've noticed that I often feel really aroused when I have my period, though my husband and I don't have sex for those 4 or 5 days. Is it because it's a "forbidden" activity that makes me feel this way? Or is it hormonal, or what?

Answer:

You're not alone in this, and the answer probably has to do with extra blood flowing in the area, making your genitals slightly engorged so that you feel aroused.

You should know that there's no good reason not to have sex with your husband during your period. Old Biblical taboos against it probably originated in the fact that you can't make a baby during that time, but there's no medical reason to avoid sex. It will be a little messy, but just put a towel underneath you and have some tissues nearby. If you don't want to have intercourse, you can always masturbate each other.

grain breads, and rice), protein, and fiber. Regular aerobic exercise and stress management strategies are encouraged. Several drugs may also help manage PMS, such as those that suppress ovulation, progesterone, antiprostaglandin agents (to lessen cramping and diarrhea), minor tranquilizers, antidepressants, vitamins B_6 and E, and magnesium.

Overall, PMS is a broadly defined disorder in which women suffer varying degrees of discomfort and debility. Many health care professionals are skeptical of patients who aggressively demand treatment for alleviation of their PMS symptoms. Although physicians and nurses are trained intellectually and temperamentally to deal with many kinds of ill people, they often become impatient with what they say are unusually pushy and persistent demands for help from women diagnosed with PMS. Often physicians who were trained to think of illness as physiological in origin use the phrase "just psychological" as if psychological problems were somehow less authentic. A woman who suffers from PMS, however, is likely to feel very different about this.

Part of the problem involves the nature of the syndrome. The word itself refers to a combination of symptoms, most or all of which indicate the presence of a specific disease or abnormal condition. Abplanalp (1983) suggested that the wide diversity of symptoms thought to comprise PMS is so broad, and the symptoms' degree of severity so wide, that the term *syndrome* may not be appropriate. As well, for many women the

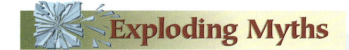

Exploding Myths

Having Your Period Doesn't Mean That You Are Not Pregnant

While a missed period is often a sign of pregnancy, that's not always true. The reverse situation is also not true: having a period does not necessarily mean a woman is not pregnant. About 20% of women have one or two periods after they become pregnant, without any harm to the pregnancy. A woman who has had unprotected intercourse and is worried about being pregnant should therefore not be too quick to breathe a sigh of relief when her period starts. As well, some pregnant women experience cycles of light vaginal bleeding throughout their pregnancy. Generally speaking, if a woman's basal body temperature stays elevated for 21 days after the date of suspected ovulation, she may be pregnant. Even though progesterone levels may be elevated, some shedding of the endometrium may still occur, which does not necessarily mean the pregnancy is at risk. A woman seeking the truth should take a pregnancy test.

symptoms are not consistent from month to month. Another argument involves the "P" in PMS. The timing of symptoms connected with menstruation may vary significantly month to month—thus "pre-" can refer to the onset of symptoms at varying times during the latter half of a woman's cycle. The validity and reliability of PMS studies into this factor are difficult to interpret because data are often collected retrospectively, which introduces bias. PMS has been related to emotional and behavioral difficulties during the last 3 to 14 days before the beginning of a period. This range seems unacceptably wide for the term "pre-" to have much predictive meaning.

In all, more studies are needed. Obviously there are a number of menstrual cycle-related mood changes, but research still needs to explore whether this is a genuine syndrome and how its timing can be understood. As more is learned about the psychological and physical aspects of PMS, its distinguish-

ing symptoms should become clearer, giving rise to better treatments.

Common Vaginal Infections

A number of other sexual and reproductive problems are common among women that often may involve substantial discomfort and annoyance or more serious health issues. There are a number of different types of vaginal infections, described in the following sections.

VAGINAL INFECTIONS

The most common gynecological problem in the United States is **vulvovaginitis**, usually called vaginitis. It causes irritation, inflammation, and itching at the opening to the vagina and the delicate mucous membranes inside the vagina (Table 5-2). Pain is common during intercourse. With vaginitis, the normal clear,

---

TABLE 5-2

Vaginitis

	Trichomonas Vaginitis	Candida Vaginitis (Monilia)	Bacterial Vaginosis[a]	Atrophic Vaginitis
Cause	*Trichomonas vaginalis,* a protozoa. Often but not always acquired sexually	*Candida albicans,* a yeast (a normal vaginal inhabitant). Many factors predispose	Unknown; probably anaerobic bacteria. May be transmitted sexually	Decreased estrogen production after menopause
Discharge	Yellowish green or gray, possibly frothy; often profuse and pooled in the vaginal fornix; may be malodorous	White and curdy; may be thin but typically thick; not as profuse as in *Trichomonas* infection; not malodorous	Gray or white, thin, homogeneous, malodorous; coats the vaginal walls. Usually not profuse, may be minimal	Variable in color, consistency, and amount; may be blood-tinged; rarely profuse
Other Symptoms	Pruritus (though not usually as severe as with *Candida* infection), pain on urination from skin inflammation or possibly urethritis, and dyspareunia	Pruritus, vaginal soreness, pain on urination (from skin inflammation), and dyspareunia	Unpleasant fishy or musty genital odor	Pruritus, vaginal soreness, or burning and dyspareunia
Vulva	The vestibule and labia minora may be reddened	The vulva and even the surrounding skin are often inflamed and sometimes swollen to a variable extent	Usually normal	Atrophic
Vaginal Mucosa	May be diffusely reddened, with small red granular spots or petechiae in the posterior fornix. In mild cases, the mucosa looks normal	Often reddened, with white, often tenacious patches of discharge. The mucosa may bleed when these patches are scraped off. In mild cases, the mucosa looks normal	Usually normal	Atrophic, dry, pale; may be red, petechial, or ecchymotic; bleeds easily; may show erosions or filmy adhesions
Laboratory Evaluation	Scan saline wet mount for trichomonads	Scan potassium hydroxide (KOH) preparation for branching hyphae of *Candida*	Scan saline wet mount for clue cells (epithelial cells with stippled borders); sniff for fishy odor after applying KOH ("whiff test")	

[a]Previously termed *Gardnerella* vaginitis.
From Bickley: Bates' Guide to Physical Examination, 7th edition, p. 427.

nonodorous vaginal discharge may be discolored (gray, green, yellow, or white) and is likely to have a bad smell. An estimated 10 million visits are made to gynecologists each year for this infection, not counting the many women who treat themselves with over-the-counter medications. While vaginitis is uncomfortable, it is a relatively harmless health problem and is easy to cure.

Vaginal infections can often be prevented. As described in the previous chapter, the inside of the vagina is somewhat acidic, but various factors can disrupt the acid-base balance. The microorganisms that cause some sexually transmitted diseases can do this, as can pregnancy, menopause, some medications (certain antibiotics), long-term illnesses, excessive douching, severe emotional stress, and types of clothing that hold heat and moisture close to the vaginal opening. Women are advised to wear undergarments made of cotton rather than synthetic material. Diet may also be an important influence (PDR Guide to Women's Health and Prescription Drugs, 1994). The use of condoms and spermicide is important to avoid sexually transmitted diseases. Generally, a healthy diet, regular exercise, and good stress management have many health benefits in addition to helping prevent vaginal infections. Bacteria live in the area of the vulva, and daily washing with a fragrance-free soap is usually sufficient to keep this area clean. Women who exercise frequently, wear pantyhose, or are overweight may need to wash more frequently. Sometimes a woman might forget to remove her diaphragm or forget that she has a tampon inside her—this will be noticed eventually. If so, the object should be removed, and the woman should douche *once* with plain water and vinegar; consulting a doctor is usually unnecessary.

Anytime the symptoms of infection persist or worsen, a woman should see her doctor. The doctor might ask about many factors, such as a new sex partner, when the symptoms began, and anything that is different or unusual, even new sexual practices. A smear can be taken in the office and often a diagnosis made immediately in order to begin effective treatment as soon as possible (Reed & Eyler, 1993). Treatment may include oral medications, as well as vaginal creams and suppositories.

MONILIAL VAGINITIS

This disorder is usually referred to as a fungal, yeast, or candidal infection; it is caused by an organism called ***Candida albicans.*** Doctors often use the term yeast infection. Women who are obese, diabetic, pregnant, or who use oral contraceptives are more likely to develop this infection. An estimated 3 of every 4 women will have a yeast infection at some time in their lives. Not all women with yeast infections have obvious symptoms, however. *Candida albicans* is one of the microorganisms that normally lives in the vagina, but when some factor changes the acidity in the vagina, its growth may become unchecked and cause symptoms.

Yeast infections usually cause a thick, cheesy malodorous white discharge. Genital itching and burning may be severe. Oral yeast infections (called *thrush*) may develop if the microorganisms spread through oral-genital contact. A number of over-the-counter preparations are effective, inexpensive treatments for yeast infections, such as miconazole nitrate vaginal suppositories. Women often can diagnose this disorder themselves and begin treatment without having to consult a

THE PROS AND CONS OF USING OVER-THE-COUNTER MEDICATIONS FOR VAGINAL INFECTIONS

*A*t least one type of common vaginal infection can be treated effectively with over-the-counter medication without a doctor's prescription. This option involves risks as well as benefits, however.

If a woman who has never had any type of vaginal infection before begins to experience one or more of the symptoms described here, it is a good idea for her to see her primary care physician or gynecologist. This visit affords an opportunity for patient education and reassurance, as well as appropriate treatment. During the office visit, the doctor will ask about the symptoms and take a vaginal smear that can immediately be examined under the microscope. Other tests may also be ordered. The woman therefore should not douche or use spermicidal jellies or foams for at least a day before the appointment. Some medications should not be used in the first trimester of pregnancy. In many instances the doctor will advise the woman to purchase the necessary nonprescription medication.

Even though nonprescription medications are available, often the symptoms of a simple infection are very similar to those of more serious types that will not respond to a nonprescription medication, so a woman would be prudent to call her doctor or other health care professional and discuss her symptoms. A woman who uses an over-the-counter product should read the instructions very carefully and use the medication exactly as stated. A woman who has reason to suspect that she has acquired a sexually transmitted disease shouldn't even think of self-medication but should contact her doctor promptly.

doctor, although a phone call to one's health care provider can be a good idea.

TRICHOMONIASIS

Trichomoniasis (often called "trick") is an inflammation of the labia and vulva that occurs most frequently in women between the ages of 16 and 35 (Edge & Miller, 1994). It is more prevalent in pregnant women. Trichomoniasis is caused by a single-celled protozoan, *Trichomonas vaginalis,* which has a long, whip-like tail. The infection is usually transmitted sexually but may also be contracted by swimming in water infested by these organisms, using a contaminated hot tub, or using towels that have been used by an infected person. After exposure to this microorganism, a woman may have symptoms starting in 3 to 28 days later. Symptoms are obvious, including a heavy, greenish-gray discharge that may foam and bubble, and itching that can be extremely distracting. This discharge is distinctly unpleasant. The external genitalia are highly irritated and may be swollen. Fortunately, this disorder can be inexpensively treated with metronidazole, an oral medication. If the woman had intercourse around the time the symptoms appeared, her partner may be treated as well, and intercourse during therapy should involve the use of a condom until a follow-up test shows the infection is over. This drug is not recommended for women in the first trimester of pregnancy.

BACTERIAL VAGINOSIS, OR "GARDNERELLA VAGINALIS"

Bacterial vaginosis is an umbrella term that refers to vaginitis of unknown or unclear origin. The term *Gardnerella vaginalis* refers to the symptoms of nonspecific vaginitis, which may involve one or more of several different microorganisms (Weaver & Mengel, 1988). The incidence of Gardnerella is higher among women who use hormonal contraceptives (i.e., birth control pills, Norplant, or Depo-Provera). The bacteria that cause this infection are normally present in the vagina, but a change in vaginal acidity leads to increased numbers. Women with bacterial vaginosis notice a watery, grayish or yellow discharge usually with an unpleasant odor. This odor is often more obvious after intercourse. Burning and itching are usually not intense, and inflammation or irritation of the external genitalia is not common. Metronidazole is an effective treatment for Gardnerella (ACOG Patient Education Pamphlet, APO28, February 1994).

The vaginal infections discussed so far may all be sexually transmitted but are not necessarily so, and accordingly they are described here rather than in the later chapter on STDs, which concerns those infections that are only transmitted through sexual contact.

ATROPHIC VAGINITIS

The vaginal infections described thus far result from generally well-known microorganisms. Atrophic vaginitis, on the other hand, is a vaginal inflammation due to a significant decline in estrogen levels. This usually happens at menopause but may also occur after childbirth, irradiation or chemotherapy, or surgical removal of the ovaries. With low estrogen levels, women often experience vaginal dryness, irritation, and burning, which result from a lack of lubrication (Beard, 1992). Intercourse is often uncomfortable, and women frequently feel sexually inadequate or unappealing. The inflammation is often markedly improved by hormone replacement therapy. Vaginal lubricants and moisturizing creams often provide immediate relief, with effects lasting up to 72 hours. This is not an infection but an uncomfortable irritation that requires medical attention or appropriate self-medication before microorganisms normally present in the vagina cause a more painful ailment.

ENDOMETRIOSIS

Any woman who is having periods could develop **endometriosis.** Its main distinguishing characteristic is the presence of endometrial tissue outside its normal location in the uterus. When the uterine muscles contract during menstrual cramps, the sloughed off endometrium may not always be expelled into the vagina through the cervix; bits of it may lodge in the fallopian tubes. Endometrial tissue may then begin to grow in the fallopian tubes, on one or both ovaries, on the outside of the

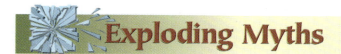

Exploding Myths

That Burning Sensation Could Be an Allergy to Semen

If a woman feels a burning sensation after intercourse, she shouldn't assume that her partner gave her a disease. Some women are allergic to semen, and unless they are trying to become pregnant, they should ask their partners to use a condom. Skin allergy to semen is rare but is troubling and uncomfortable when it occurs. Some women and men are allergic to condoms as well. They may be allergic to latex or a spermicidal agent on the condom, such as nonoxynol-9. These allergies can be diagnosed with certainty only by an allergist, who carefully monitors how the person's skin reacts to a tiny amount of the substance. Because of allergies to latex, vinyl condoms are being tested for effectiveness as contraceptives and for the prevention of vaginal infections and STDs.

uterus, on the large intestine, or in other areas of the pelvic cavity. Some gynecologists estimate that 20–25% of all women will have endometriosis at some time in their lives. This disorder affects the woman's reproductive system and may impair her fertility. It often is painful but in some instances may have no obvious symptoms at all. When the endometrium inside the uterus begins to thicken and grow due to the action of hormones during the menstrual cycle, endometrial tissues *outside* of the uterus will too. At the end of the menstrual cycle, when the endometrium inside the uterus begins to disintegrate and bleed, the same thing happens to endometrial tissues outside the uterus. Since the endometrial tissue outside the uterus cannot leave the body, inflammation surrounds it, causing pain and swelling. Scar tissue then surrounds it. In some cases, scar tissue surrounds a bit of endometrial tissue and cuts off its blood supply, making the tissue unresponsive to hormonal fluctuations. In other instances, the little clumps of endometrium may break apart during menstruation and further spread through the woman's pelvic cavity. For this reason, endometriosis may become progressively worse over time (ACOG Patient Education Leaflet, APO13, March 1991).

Most women with endometriosis experience secondary dysmenorrhea, unusual uterine bleeding, and pain during intercourse, yet many women do not promptly seek medical care with the onset of symptoms (Hadfield, Mardon, Barlow, & Kennedy, 1996). In very rare cases (less than 1%), a malignancy may occur in the endometrium outside the uterus. To accurately diagnose endometriosis, the doctor may do pelvic examinations at different times during the menstrual cycle to compare any changes in the pelvic area. The most accurate diagnostic procedure is **laparoscopy,** which involves inserting a thin microscope and light into the abdominal cavity through a small incision in the lower abdomen. This allows the doctor to view the inside of the pelvic cavity and check for endometrial

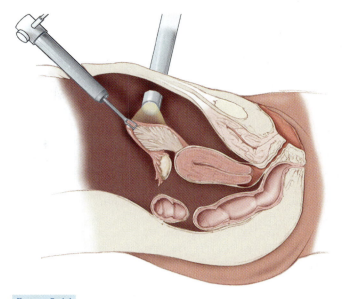

FIGURE 5-14 Illustration of the use of laparoscopy in the treatment of endometriosis. Small patches of endometrial tissue can be identified and removed through the use of this procedure without having to make a large abdominal incision.

tissue (Fig. 5-13). Because 30–60% of infertile women are diagnosed with endometriosis, laparoscopy is often included in an infertility work-up. Endometrial tissue inside the fallopian tubes can block sperm, the movement of the ovum, or the progress of a fertilized egg toward the uterus. Although surgical removal of endometrial deposits in mild forms of this disease may not automatically improve the woman's chances for pregnancy, it does provide a marked reduction in pelvic pain (Falcone, Goldberg, & Miller, 1996).

There are a variety of treatments for endometriosis. In many cases, oral contraceptives effectively minimize or eliminate the discomfort associated with endometriosis. Other hormonal therapies too work well but also suppress ovulation, so women cannot get pregnant while using these medications. Surgery is often effective as well. Electrocautery, laser treatment, or dissection can remove small patches of endometrial tissue (Fig. 5-14). These procedures generally leave the ovaries, fallopian tubes, and uterus in place, removing only deposits of endometrial tissue. In more severe cases, removal of the uterus, fallopian tubes, and/or ovaries may be necessary. For additional information, contact the Endometriosis Association at the address listed at the end of this chapter.

PELVIC INFLAMMATORY DISEASE

Pelvic inflammatory disease (PID) is an infection of the female reproductive tract that ascends from the vagina, through the uterus, and then up the fallopian tubes, spreading to the pelvic cavity. Its manifestations vary in seriousness, but it can be a quite destructive illness that impairs a woman's fertility by scarring the fallopian tubes. Often there are no symptoms, but sometimes the woman feels extreme abdominal pain. A number of different microorganisms

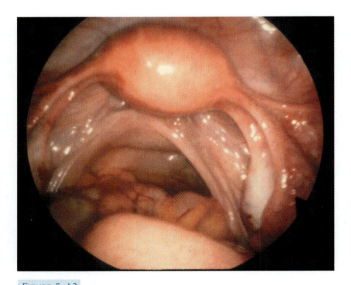

FIGURE 5-13 Surgeon's-eye-view of a woman's lower pelvic area through a laparoscope. Note the oval-shaped top of the uterus and the two fallopian tubes attached to its two sides.

cause PID, including some that cause sexually transmitted diseases. *Any person* feeling serious abdominal pain should seek medical attention.

The bacteria that cause PID are not always easy to identify. Approximately one American woman in ten will have PID at some time during her reproductive years. PID often has serious consequences, such as infertility, ectopic pregnancy, and chronic pelvic pain (Newkirk, 1996). Diagnosis can be difficult because no single symptom strongly points toward this disease. Often, an open, thorough, and comprehensive discussion with the woman helps the doctor begin to suspect PID. Doctors often start patients with suspected PID on broad-spectrum antibiotics even before laboratory tests confirm the diagnosis. Doctors today are more likely to hospitalize a woman with PID when conventional antibiotic treatment doesn't work promptly.

The risk factors for PID are not completely clear, although some factors have been shown to put a woman at a higher risk of developing this disease. Jossens, Eskenazi, Schacter, and Sweet (1996) studied 234 women with PID and found that women who had more than one sexual partner during the past 30 days, who had sexual intercourse during their most recent menstrual cycle, and who did not use contraceptives reliably or regularly were at greater risk for PID. Certainly, having intercourse during menstruation is not likely to cause PID, but this factor, along with one or more of the other risk factors, can be a problem. Investigators also have reported a relationship between bacterial vaginosis and PID (Sweet, 1995). Because of the connection between PID and both STDs and bacterial vaginosis, doctors often use broad-spectrum antibiotics (effective against many different bacteria), such as doxycycline, for PID. However, it has been demonstrated that women diagnosed with PID in the emergency room of a large, urban teaching hospital are not very conscientious about taking their medication, even though it is effective and inexpensive (Brookoff, 1994). This large sample of 386 women were surveyed by telephone to determine how well they adhered to their follow-up antibiotic treatment, which took 10 days. Fewer than one-third of the subjects (31%) reported they fully complied with the course of treatment. Unbelievably, 28% reported that they did not even fill their prescription for the medication, saying that the cost was too high (highly unlikely), they seemed to be feeling better, and it was *inconvenient* to go to the pharmacy! Also surprisingly, another 41% of the subjects stopped taking their pills early and failed to complete the course of treatment. When women do not follow their doctor's directions for treating a serious, fertility-threatening, painful disease that can be quickly, effectively, and inexpensively treated by oral medications, it is not surprising that compliance is such an important issue in medicine.

CYSTITIS

Cystitis, a bladder infection, is the most common type of urinary tract infection in women. Bacteria in the urethra may cause a local infection or spread upward to the bladder and/or kidneys. Urinary tract infections are usually caused by bacteria from the skin near the rectum and vagina that reach the urethra (ACOG Patient Education Leaflet APO50, 1992). Other causes of urinary tract infections include sexual intercourse. Because the external urethral meatus is located close to the opening of the vagina, during intercourse the movement of the penis can rub some of the bacteria normally found in the vagina into the urethra. Bladder infections are also common in women who significantly increase their frequency of intercourse. A woman should urinate before and after intercourse because this helps keep the urethra flushed clean of harmful bacteria that may cause a bladder infection.

The most obvious and compelling symptom of a bladder infection is an urgent need to urinate. Intense pain and burning in the urethra occur when urination begins, and usually very little urine is voided; the urine may be discolored with blood. Often only a few minutes later, the woman again feels the need to urinate. Despite the discomfort of urination, it is important for a woman who suspects that she has a bladder infection to drink a lot of water. In addition to these symptoms, pain in the lower abdomen, lower back, and along the sides of the body can be very uncomfortable. The need to urinate frequently at night is also a symptom of a bladder infection or diabetes.

To aid in the diagnosis, the doctor examines a urine sample and counts the bacteria and white blood cells. A pelvic examination is often performed. Several different antibiotics are effective for bladder infections, with a course of treatment from 7 to 10 days; in some cases only one dose of an antibiotic is needed. The doctor may schedule a follow-up urine test about a week after the course of antibiotics.

TOXIC SHOCK SYNDROME

Toxic shock syndrome is a systemic, acute infection by the *Staphylococcus aureus* bacteria. An estimated one in every 20,000 women will develop toxic shock syndrome (TSS). Although usually associated with menstruation and the use of "superabsorbent" tampons, TSS can also occur when bandages and dressings are used after surgery in other body areas. TSS was identified in 1978, although its symptoms were reported as early as 1942 (Hanrahan, 1994; Arrow & Wood, 1942). As of this writing, no single test can diagnose the presence of TSS, there is no vaccine to prevent it, and no antitoxin is available to treat it (Hanrahan, 1994).

TSS affects several different organ systems and causes many diverse symptoms. A sudden high fever is usually the first sign, typically over 102° F. A rash develops, and vomiting and diarrhea commonly occur. The skin on the palms and soles begins to peel, and blood pressure may drop substantially; dizziness and fainting are common. Muscular aches and pains may occur, and the kidneys and liver are affected as seen through blood tests. A woman with TSS is very sick. Antibiotics such as erythromycin are generally effective for treating this disorder.

In the early 1980s, studies discovered an association between the use of certain types of tampons and TSS (Davis et al., 1980). Accumulating data revealed that women who used tampons were ten times as likely to develop TSS as those who did not. Other lifestyle factors were unrelated to TSS (e.g., type of birth control used, having intercourse during menstruation, method of tampon insertion, wearing pantyhose, swimming, etc.) (Hanrahan, 1994). By the late 1980s it was clear that TSS was related to the chemical composition of tampons and their level of absorbency. Tampons made of synthetics such as rayon, polyester, and carboxymethylcellulose were far more likely to be associated with TSS than those made of cotton, and most scientific evidence pointed to synthetic materials that were especially absorbent. Because highly absorbent tampons do not need to be changed as frequently, it was thought that leaving a synthetic tampon in the vagina for a long period of time had a definite role in TSS. This was demonstrated in *in vitro* bacterial cultivation studies in laboratory settings (Parsonnet, Modern, & Giacobbe, 1995).

Reports of TSS naturally had a big impact on the American public and the tampon products industry. Tampons were first manufactured in 1933 (Delaney, Lupton, & Toth, 1976). Because tampons are **nonsterile** and absorbent and can cause tiny tears in the mucous membranes of the vagina, they may play a role in a gradual break-down of this tissue (Jimerson & Becker, 1980). As a result of public attention to TSS, women changed the type of tampons they used and how they used them. Women today are more aware of TSS and understand it is important to change their tampons as frequently as recommended in the product information inserts. Women are encouraged to purchase the least absorbent tampon that is effective for them personally. The disease still occurs, however, and is conclusively related to menstruation. It is extremely important, particularly for adolescents, that women using tampons receive clear, simple information about TSS and how to avoid it.

Less Common Cancers of the Female Reproductive System

Breast and cervical cancer were discussed earlier in this chapter; both are common, and women would do well to take steps to detect their earliest signs. Cancer can also affect other parts of a woman's reproductive system, however, including ovarian, endometrial, and uterine malignancies. Tests for these disorders are not always as reliable as mammograms, breast examinations, and Pap smears for detecting breast and cervical cancer. These other cancers often go undetected until it is too late to treat them with any confidence of a cure.

OVARIAN CANCER

According to Edge and Miller (1994), **ovarian cancer** is the sixth most common kind of cancer in women and the fourth leading cause of death due to cancer (p. 121). No one knows exactly what causes ovarian cancer, but it occurs most frequently in industrialized nations in the West, particularly in Caucasians of Northern European descent over the age of 50. It is especially difficult to treat this tumor effectively because it is usually not detected before it reaches an advanced stage of growth and metastasizes (spreads), usually within the pelvis and associated lymph nodes. It may cause vague feelings of abdominal discomfort, indigestion, and bloating, but there are no early, reliably specific symptoms of ovarian cancer. Even though its exact cause is unknown, some risk factors seem clearer. One theory suggests that the more a woman ovulates

during her reproductive years, the higher is her probability of developing ovarian cancer. Therefore, risk factors include having ovulated for more than 40 years, never having been pregnant or having one's first pregnancy after the age of 30, and entering menopause relatively late.

A doctor who during a pelvic examination feels any mass that indicates an enlarged ovary generally recommends an ultrasound examination of the entire pelvic area. The procedure is usually carried out in the doctor's office. A single small mass is more likely to be an ovarian cyst rather than malignant tumor. The doctor may also order a blood test called the CA-125, which measures amounts of substances related to cancerous ovarian tumors. False-positive or false-negative results may occur, however. If the ultrasound examination and blood test both suggest the possibility of cancer, a laparoscopy is usually recommended to visualize the area or tumor and allow an accurate diagnosis to be made. In this procedure, a tiny amount of tissue will be removed and examined under a microscope.

The treatment of ovarian cancer includes the same options used for other cancers depending on how early they are detected. Surgery is common to remove the ovaries and fallopian tubes, and sometimes the uterus too. Chemotherapy and radiation therapy may also be used, or some combination of all three.

Social workers often help women understand the importance of ovarian cancer screening programs, especially for those at a higher risk for the disease. It can be a challenge to improve the access to and use of health care for all women. Smith and Schwartz (1993) describe a comprehensive screening program for women at high risk of ovarian cancer. Questionnaires and interviews were used to assess each woman's risk, as well as her adaptations to her family, school, work, and other social groups—her entire psychosocial environment was evaluated. The woman's perceptions of her risk, particularly when it has occurred in a first-degree relative (usually her mother), are evaluated and her functioning at her current developmental stage is studied. Considering these psychological and social issues helps these women deal with their feelings of vulnerability and become more proactive in taking care of themselves.

ENDOMETRIAL CANCER

Cancer of the endometrium (lining of the uterus) is the most common cancer in women's reproductive organs (Von Gruenigen, & Karlen, 1995). The cure rate is very high (almost 90%) because these tumors are well-localized and grow very slowly. Women 55 to 60 years old have the highest risk for endometrial cancer. As with many other forms of cancer, the exact causes of **endometrial cancer** are not known. An abnormal growth of the cells of the endometrium occurs commonly among women approaching menopause. In most cases these growths are not malignant, but sometimes they may become so. The term *cancer* refers to an uncontrolled growth of cells, and endometrial cancer actually involves several different forms of abnormal growth and development of cells. There is no sure way to be certain about what kind of cells are growing in the endometrium without removing tissue and examining it microscopically. Although unusual cellular growth is common in

Research Highlight

WOMEN AT INCREASED RISK FOR OVARIAN CANCER

Schwartz, Lerman, Miller, Daly, and Masny (1995) examined factors likely to lead to psychological distress in women at greater risk for developing ovarian cancer. Women with a first-degree relative with ovarian cancer are three to four times more likely to develop the disease. Although many people with a hereditary predisposition to an illness often try to avoid thinking about it, this was not the case among the women in this study.

Some very strong stresses accompany living with this risk and/or living with a close relative who is battling the disease. One of the reasons these scientists were studying how women at risk cope with their distress is that some studies have shown women at elevated risk for breast cancer are *less likely* to get regular screening for that disease (Kash et al., 1992; Lerman et al., 1993). Could the stress of knowing you are at a high risk for a disease be so debilitating that you could not act in a way that helped ensure early detection and, thereby, lead to a better prognosis if the disease did develop?

One of the factors apparently relevant to this question is attentional style. Some women at higher risk are especially attentive to cues and information related to the threat of ovarian cancer, while others are less so. For example, when young and middle-aged women learned that Gilda Radner and Madeline Kahn died of ovarian cancer, some may have felt vulnerable themselves simply because they too were young and seemingly healthy, as were these two well-known actresses (Fig. 5-15). Generally, someone who is attentive to threatening information experiences more distress. Schwartz and co-workers found that the subjects in their study monitored their environments carefully for distressing information and that among younger women such distressing information was highly distracting. Women who experience high levels of stress because of their perceived risk of developing ovarian cancer would benefit from supportive interventions tailored to help them put the risk in perspective and not overreact to it.

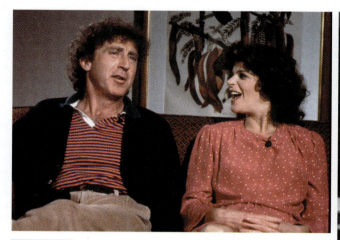
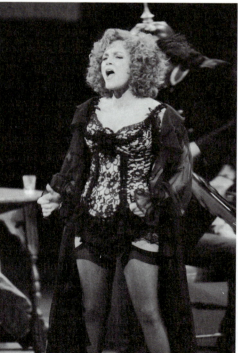

FIGURE 5-15   (Left) Actress Gilda Radner and her husband, actor Gene Wilder. (Right) Actress Madeline Kahn. Both of these talented young women died of ovarian cancer.

women before menopause, the most common type of endometrial cancer usually is not diagnosed before age 60. Women at the highest risk of endometrial cancer generally began their periods early, went through menopause relatively late, are decidedly overweight, and never had a child (PDR Family Guide to Women's Health and Prescription Drugs, 1994). Women with high blood pressure or diabetes are also at a higher risk (Von Gruenigen & Karlen, 1995). The most common early symptom of endometrial cancer is uterine bleeding after menopause.

Although a Pap smear is an excellent diagnostic tool for detecting early signs of cervical cancer, it is not as useful for detecting early endometrial cancer. Only about 50 out of every 1000 women with endometrial cancer are estimated to have an abnormal Pap smear (Berek & Hacker, 1989). **Diagnostic hysteroscopy** uses a very thin fiberoptic telescope inserted through the cervix into the uterus to biopsy selected areas for evaluation. This is an outpatient procedure performed under local anesthetic.

The treatment for endometrial cancer is generally clear-cut: a complete abdominal hysterectomy is performed, and the fallopian tubes and ovaries are removed. Radiation therapy is often recommended after surgery. Chemotherapy is generally not as effective with this disease. Hormonal therapy may also help shrink cancerous endometrial tumors (Berek & Hacker, 1989). As hormone replacement therapy using only estrogen is thought to perhaps increase the risk of endometrial cancer, many doctors recommend a combination of estrogen and progestogens to minimize this potential problem.

Most important for early diagnosis and treatment is that a woman at mid-life or beyond should act promptly if abnormal uterine bleeding occurs.

MEN'S SEXUAL AND REPRODUCTIVE HEALTH CONCERNS

So far in this chapter we have discussed sexual health and wellness issues concerning women, but men also experience problems in this area. The situation is only slightly simpler for men, as there are fewer structures affected by infections and malignancies. Although women experience physical and psychological changes in their monthly menstrual cycle, men do experience similar changes and, therefore, are not as frequently reminded of changes or issues related to sexuality and reproduction. Men do not typically have regular physical examinations that focus on their genitalia and reproductive functioning, nor do they require regular diagnostic tests, such as mammograms and Pap smears (although at mid-life prostate examinations become very important). As with women's health issues, the most important men's health issue is taking responsibility for one's own health and developing a conscientious, thoughtful approach to taking care of oneself.

Earlier, we discussed three personality attributes related to a person's willingness to take preventive health measures. Self-esteem, internal locus of control, and attentive self-monitoring are all related to a person's comfort with physiological functions and readiness to act autonomously to seek medical counsel when necessary. These considerations are just as important for men as for women. These traits are also related to who is likely to follow a doctor's recommendations and treatment instructions. Men, however, are often thought to have a "macho" mentality and to be more likely to "tough it

Research Highlight

ARE MEN OR WOMEN MORE LIKELY TO FOLLOW A DOCTOR'S ADVICE?

Earlier, this chapter discussed the degree to which women follow their doctor's recommendations for breast self-exams, Pap smears, and regular gynecological check-ups, but less is known about how men attend to their sexual and reproductive health. For example, little is known about how concerned men are about having prostate examinations or doing testicular self-exams. Studies have shown, however, some interesting similarities and differences between women and men in following the counsel of their doctors. For example, Ward and Morgan (1984) reported that women and men are about equally likely to begin an exercise program and are equally likely to drop out. Laforge, Green, and Prochaska (1994) noted, however, that women stick to a healthier diet far better than men, eating a minimum of two servings of fruits and vegetables each day when their doctors encourage them to do so. Women are also more likely to follow their doctor's recommendation for taking medication for psychological disorders than men (Sellwood & Tarrier, 1994).

While women and men differ in some respects regarding taking care of themselves, we know of no large scale studies that demonstrate that either gender is more conscientious about preventive or therapeutic care for sexual or reproductive health.

out" than ask for help. Are men in fact at a higher risk for a disease because they are slower to act on its early symptoms? The accompanying Research Highlight considers this interesting question.

Chapter 4 discusses the importance of regular genital self-examinations for both women and men and describes techniques to help you learn more about your body. This self-examination is simpler for men because the external genitalia are visually and manually accessible. Still, before one can recognize anything unusual, it is important to be familiar with the normal appearance and feeling of one's genitals, and that is an important reason for both men and women to do a genital self-exam. Men, like women, have some anxiety about the possibility of developing a problem involving sexual health. Men worry about prostate cancer and, to a lesser extent, testicular cancer. As women are concerned about the possibility of a mastectomy, men too are concerned about surgery that may result in impotence or incontinence.

The one fundamental difference between female and male urogenital anatomy and physiology is that in men the urethra in the penis has both urinary and sexual functions, while women have two separate, adjacent openings for these functions.

Testicular and Penis Problems

All men should examine their testicles regularly, especially those under the age of 35 (Fig. 5-16). Testicular cancer is not as common as other cancers, but in men younger than 35 it is one of the most common types. Therefore, it is especially important that younger men learn this simple diagnostic measure and practice it regularly. No one wants to think of the possibility of cancer, but everyone should be aware of the risks and take intelligent precautionary measures. The earliest stages

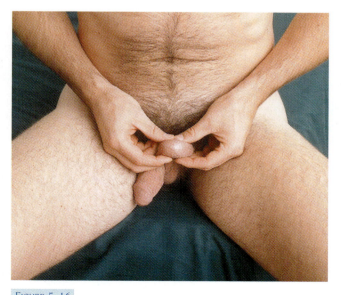

FIGURE 5-16   Testicular self-examination (see text for explanation).

of testicular cancer are painless, and without doing self-examinations a man may not notice any irregularities in the shape, size, or texture of his testes. The American Cancer Society's leaflet "How to Examine Your Testes" includes the following instructions. Copies are available at the local chapter, and more pressing questions can be directed to the American Cancer Society Helpline at 1-800-227-2345 or one's primary care physician.

- Examine the testes when the body is warm, usually during a hot shower or after a warm bath. At this time the scrotum is very soft and hangs away from the body and allows keen tactile sensitivity when feeling the testes within.
- Try to determine if there is anything new or unusual in the texture, symmetry, or size of each testicle. Lumps, bumps, and granular surfaces, especially along the front of each testicle, are not supposed to be there.
- Gently push each testicle against the surrounding scrotum and roll it between the thumbs and fingers of one's hands in order to feel all sides of it. The testes should feel firm but not hard. They should be smooth.
- Feel the epididymis of each testicle. Even though this structure is very sensitive, feel it thoroughly in order to find out if it is tender to the touch.
- Feel the spermatic cord leading away from each testicle; it should be firm and smooth.

This examination should be done once each month. Choose the same date each month (such as the 1st) or another date easy to remember (such as the day of one's birthday). Although testicular cancer occurs primarily in young men, it is increasingly common in men over 50, and all men should get into the habit of examining their testes regularly. The European Health Behavior Survey, an international project that assessed health beliefs and health behaviors of over 16,000 university students, revealed that of the 7304 men questioned, 87% reported that they had never done a testicular self-examination. Only 3% of this sample did self-examinations regularly, and 10% did so occasionally. Wardle et al. (1994) note that these data suggest that European young men do not consider testicular cancer an important health risk.

TESTICULAR CANCER

An estimated 2500 cases of **testicular cancer** are diagnosed each year, with about 60% of new cases found in men between 25 and 44. In about one-third of the cases, the cancer has already spread from the testicle at the time they are diagnosed (McConnell & Zimmerman, 1983). There are 2 to 3 cases of testicular cancer per 100,000 men, with a somewhat lower incidence in African-American males. Only in very rare cases are both testicles affected. While the specific cause or causes of testicular cancer are unknown, there is a strong relationship between failure of the testes to descend before and after birth and the later development of this disease. While family history may play a role, this statistical association has not been conclusively proven.

The earliest stage of testicular cancer is characterized by a small nodule or a change in the texture and/or consistency of the testicle. In rare cases, patients report a dull ache in the lower pelvic area, scrotum, or groin. These changes strongly suggest testicular cancer. In such a case, the doctor will thoroughly examine the affected testicle, comparing it to the unaffected one. A chest x-ray may be taken to check for any signs of the tumor's spread. Just as blood tests can help detect signs of breast cancer, similar tests can reveal telltale signs of testicular cancer. When the tumor is detected in its earliest stages before metastasis occurs, the American Cancer Society estimates a cure rate of about 90%. As with other cancers, early detection is the key to effective treatment and cure.

The treatment for testicular cancer is surgery, possibly along with chemotherapy and/or radiation if there is a chance the tumor has spread. Surgical removal of the testicle is the first step, which allows the doctor to determine the exact kind of tumor and how advanced its growth is. In some cases, a gel-filled testicle prosthesis is placed inside the scrotum to create a normal appearance. Even when a testicle is removed, along with lymph nodes to check for metastasis, the vast majority of men will continue to be able to attain and maintain an erection and ejaculate. As well, men with a single testicle are still fertile and usually can impregnate their partner. Overall, if diagnosed early, testicular cancer has a very optimistic prognosis, and therefore testicular self-examination should be a part of all men's personal health and hygiene routine.

OTHER DISORDERS OF THE TESTES AND PENIS

Although other problems of the testes and penis are less common than testicular cancer, they can provoke anxiety, and men should seek medical attention if they feel they have related symptoms.

Epididymitis

As described in Chapter 4, the epididymis is a crescent-shaped structure at the top of each testicle that serves as a temporary holding area for sperm progressing to the vas deferens. Epididymitis is a localized infection of this structure. It usually affects only adults and is rare before puberty. It is commonly associated with chronic urinary tract infections, particularly in men over the age of 35 (McConnell & Zimmerman, 1983). In some cases, an undiagnosed sexually transmitted disease (particularly gonorrhea and chlamydia) may be the cause. It is also a rare complication of the surgical removal of the prostate gland. A large American study revealed a strong statistical association between epididymitis and having had a vasectomy or prostate infections (Walrath, Fayerweather, & Spreen, 1992). Epididymitis is diagnosed by identifying certain bacteria in a urine sample. Epididymitis is discussed further in Chapter 17.

Men with epididymitis usually spend a few days in bed when the discomfort from the infection is at its worst, and an antibiotic is usually prescribed. If the man delays seeking treatment, an abscess can form on the epididymis that can spread

to the rest of the testicle. In some cases, the vas deferens may accumulate scar tissue that may cause infertility. For all these reasons, a man should act promptly on the earliest signs of this disease.

Cryptorchidism

Chapter 4 mentioned that in some cases, a male infant's testicles have not descended into the scrotum when he is born. This condition, called **cryptorchidism,** occurs in a small percentage of full-term births and is usually self-correcting shortly after birth. In some instances surgery or hormonal therapy may be necessary to relocate the testicles appropriately in the scrotum. Berkowitz et al. (1993) studied almost 7000 male infants, of which 3.7% had both testicles undescended at birth. Because the testicles can produce a normal number of sperm only if they are a few degrees cooler than the rest of the body, a man's fertility would therefore be impaired if the testicles remained in the warmer abdominal cavity. Lee, O'Leary, Songer, and Coughlin (1996) studied whether the probability of becoming a father is decreased in men who had a testicle surgically removed to correct cryptorchidism. They found fertility was indeed compromised in this circumstance.

Balanitis

Various factors can cause localized irritations of the foreskin and glans of the penis, a condition called **balanitis.** Because many different infectious agents can cause balanitis, visual examination usually cannot determine the precise cause. Some microorganisms that cause this disorder also cause vaginal yeast infections, such as *Candida albicans* and *Gardnerella* (Edwards, 1996). Simple skin irritation (dermatitis) resulting from frequent showering and washing of the genitalia can also cause balanitis. Less frequent washing and the use of skin softening creams proved highly effective in reducing the frequency of episodes of irritation and the discomfort in men with recurrent balanitis (Birley et al., 1993). Balanitis is most common during the preschool years and before toilet training (Escala & Rickwood, 1989). A foreskin that is completely or partially non-retractable is often associated with the problem.

Varicocele

The vein that supplies the testicles with blood sometimes becomes enlarged, causing a condition called **varicocele.** It usually affects the left spermatic vein. This problem occurs in about 10% of men and may play a role in male infertility. The doctor can often detect this problem through manual examination of the testicles; radiologic imaging techniques may also help make the diagnosis (Kurgan, Nunnelee, & Zilberman, 1994). Some men with this condition have fewer sperm in the ejaculate, more immature sperm, and fewer sperm with good motility (Lund & Nielsen, 1996). If there are a large number of dilated veins close to the testicle, the body's warmth affects the number and motility of the sperm produced. Surgery can correct this condition by tying off some of these extra blood vessels. Many doctors screen adolescent males to detect and correct the problem before fertility is compromised at an early age (Kurgan, Nunnelee, & Zilberman, 1994). The symptoms of varicocele include a dull discomfort or a feeling of tugging inside the scrotum.

Priapism

Priapism is a condition producing a long-lasting, very uncomfortable erection unrelated to erotic stimulation. Only the corpora cavernosa becomes engorged with blood and remains that way; the glans penis does not, nor does the corpus spongiosum (McConnell & Zimmerman, 1983). Priapism can be an effect of various serious diseases, such as leukemia, sickle cell anemia, or some malignancies. An injury to the penis involving the tearing of some of the internal membranes may also cause this condition. A distorted appearance and discoloration are not unusual, along with difficulties urinating. Priapism requires immediate medical attention because prolonged erection may damage tissues inside the penis. Treatment usually involves surgery. In some instances, drugs that lower blood pressure are beneficial.

Phimosis

Phimosis is a condition in which the foreskin of an uncircumcised penis is too tight to retract, making hygiene very difficult (Fig. 5-17). Men with phimosis often report that they experience itching beneath the foreskin that can be very distracting. Infections may develop under the foreskin. The prolonged irritation caused by the tight foreskin may cause changes in the tissues beneath. The treatment involves antibiotics and sometimes minor surgery to relieve the pressure. Men who suspect they might have this problem should contact a urologist.

Prostate Problems

The prostate gland is made up of both glandular and muscular tissue. It is located at the base of the bladder and surrounds the urethra. Secretions from the prostate gland include fructose, a source of fuel for sperm, and other

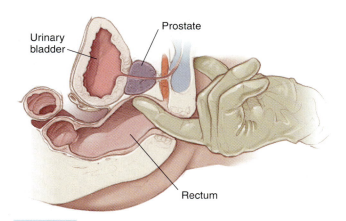

FIGURE 5-18   Digital rectal examination involving palpation of the prostate gland. A doctor can easily determine the size, smoothness, and symmetry of the gland in this way.

substances that increase the alkalinity of semen, which help neutralize the acidic environment of the vagina. Because of its location, changes in the size of the prostate gland often cause urinary symptoms. Three main disorders affecting the prostate gland are prostate cancer, benign prostatic hyperplasia, and prostatitis.

Just as many women are not very conscientious about visiting their gynecologist yearly, many men are not very conscientious about having an annual physical examination that includes checking their prostate gland, particularly after age 40. The most common screening test for prostate problems is a digital rectal examination. The doctor uses a non-latex glove with sterile lubricant jelly and inserts one finger through the anus into the rectum (Fig. 5-18). Along the front (anterior) wall of the rectum, 2 to 3 inches (5 to 8 cm) beyond the anus, the doctor can feel the prostate gland through the wall of the rectum. In younger men, the prostate usually feels small, smooth, and symmetrical. By gently pressing on the prostate gland, the doctor can force a small amount of prostatic fluid into the urethra, which may then be collected on a microscope slide for visual examination and laboratory analysis. An enlarged, asymmetrical prostate gland with lumps or bumps does not always indicate a malignant tumor.

This examination takes only a few seconds, is not uncomfortable, and is an excellent screening for prostate and rectal cancer (Fig. 5-19). Yet many men delay in having it or fail to have it regularly. Men may exaggerate the slight discomfort of the examination or feel embarrassed about digital rectal penetration. As well, because no one wants to learn something potentially serious is wrong with them, this too may help explain why people fail to seek preventive screenings for illnesses such as prostate cancer.

PROSTATE CANCER

After lung cancer, **prostate cancer** is the second most common kind of cancer in men, and the risk increases with age,

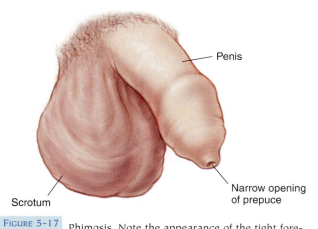

FIGURE 5-17   Phimosis. Note the appearance of the tight foreskin.

Research Highlight

PROSTATE CANCER SCREENING IN AFRICAN-AMERICAN MEN

Research has sought to learn why African-American men have a higher death rate for prostate cancer. Price, Colvin, and Smith (1993) assessed the knowledge of 290 black men about the development and symptoms of this disease. Many subjects did not know that urinary difficulties, such as problems in beginning to urinate, pain during urination, or blood in the urine could be important warning signs of prostate cancer. About 60% did not know that black men had a greater risk for this disease, and three-fourths thought that prostate cancer was always fatal. Most reported that they had no particular problems with having their prostate checked, some said they thought it was too expensive. Generally, black men with more education and higher income were more likely to have prostate exams.

Boehm, Coleman-Burns, Schlenk, Funnell et al. (1995) recognized the central role of the church in the lives of many African-Americans and studied subjects within this context. In all, 123 subjects from 174 churches participated, ranging in age from early 30s to late 70s. Black men who had been previously diagnosed with prostate cancer served as role models for the men in the study. With the encouragement and support of these models, subjects demonstrated increased knowledge about prostate cancer and had higher self-efficacy scores at the end of the study. In other words, these men felt more in charge of their own health with respect to this disease and understood it better as well. This study showed that encouragement is critical to helping these men become more aware of the risk of prostate cancer and understand the importance of regular screening. Such encouragement should be equally effective for men of other racial groups.

particularly after age 50. Almost all very old men have some cellular indications of prostate cancer found after they die of any cause, regardless of whether they had clinical signs of the disease. About 1 in 11 American men will be diagnosed with prostate cancer. The disease is twice as prevalent in African-American men as in Caucasian men, for unknown reasons.

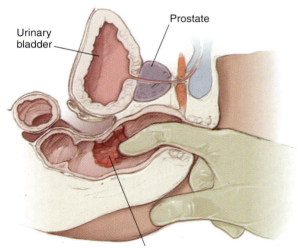

Urinary bladder

Prostate

Rectal mass in lower rectum

FIGURE 5-19   A digital rectal examination can also detect rectal cancer.

The mortality rate is very high in African Americans, perhaps due in part to discovering the disease late because of less regular screening. Japanese men have the lowest death rate for prostate cancer.

Usually no pelvic discomfort is associated with prostate cancer, although urinary symptoms may become obvious as the cancer progresses. Painful urination, difficulty in starting to urinate, frequent urination, and complete urinary retention may occur, and rarely, there will be traces of blood in the urine. Digital examination may reveal an extremely hard prostate texture. In many cases the disease is not diagnosed until it is somewhat advanced. Digital prostate examination is estimated to be 50% to 70% accurate for diagnosing this disease. Because there are usually no early warning signs, doctors recommend a yearly digital examination for men after age 40.

Another diagnostic test for prostate cancer is the blood test for **prostatic specific antigen (PSA)**, which screens for malignancies in the prostate gland. Prostatic specific antigen is a substance found in the blood that was once thought clearly associated with prostate cancer. It was found, however, that PSA levels normally fluctuate with increasing age and prostate enlargement that isn't cancerous (Pfeiffer, 1995). Because of problems with this test's reliability, many health insurance companies were hesitant to pay for this test, especially in younger men. However, the refined blood test now being used has apparently more accurate results, assessing not just the total amount of PSA but levels of free antigens, which more accurately indicate prostate cancer. Doctors are confident that the newer test will significantly reduce the number of unnecessary biopsies previously performed when cancer was suspected based on PSA levels (Tamkins, 1995).

Ultrasound is another important diagnostic tool for prostate cancer. When an ultrasound transducer is placed in the rectum, a sonographic image of the prostate gland can be made. This technique can locate a tumor in the prostate gland long before it could be felt in a digital examination (Fig. 5-20). Ultrasound is also used to guide surgical instruments to remove small tissue samples for biopsy.

Because prostate cancer often grows slowly, its treatment is controversial. Surgical removal of the prostate gland is called a *prostatectomy.* Impotence and urinary incontinence are potential side effects of the surgery, although recent innovations in prostate surgery have made these less common. One technique selectively freezes portions of the prostate while bathing surrounding tissues in warm water to preserve them and spare the nerves to allow for normal erection and urination (*Health Industry Today,* June 1996). Most doctors now believe that if the tumor is slow-growing and confined to the prostate, and if there are few clinical signs of disease, more conservative therapy may result in a normal life expectancy without surgery and its side effects. A biopsy can determine if the tumor is likely to spread and how quickly it will grow. If there is no immediate threat, an approach called "watchful waiting" is used instead of surgery. In some cases, hormone and radiation therapies may be used. The age and general health of the man also influence the treatment options considered.

BENIGN PROSTATIC HYPERPLASIA (BPH)

Benign means "nonmalignant," and *hyperplasia* refers to an unusual growth of cells—in this case, in the prostate gland.

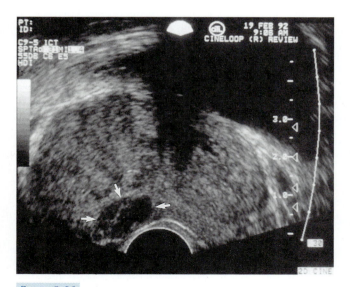

FIGURE 5-20   Ultrasound image of the prostate gland. The dark area within three white arrows is a small tumor. Only microscopic examination of the tumor can determine whether it is cancerous or benign.

BPH normally occurs with aging in men and causes enlargement of the gland, often resulting in the same urinary symptoms as occur in prostate cancer. BPH often stimulates men to get up several times a night to urinate, leaving them very tired the next day. Prostate cancer and BPH may coexist at the same time, and treating one does not necessarily minimize the symptoms of the other. The incidence of BPH increases with age: it is estimated that BPH occurs in more than half of men over the age of 50 and in more than 80% of those over 70 (Mayo Clinic Health Letter, May 1996). BPH is diagnosed through digital rectal examination, as well as urinalysis and blood tests that may be used to rule out urinary tract infections and prostate cancer. When BPH is not treated, it will improve by itself in 40% of cases, remain unchanged in 45%, and worsen in 15%. A number of medications are currently used to treat BPH. In cases in which BPH is unresponsive to medication and worsens, surgery may remove a portion of the gland (Benign Prostatic Hypertrophy Guideline Panel, 1994). About 6 million men in America had this disorder in 1995, a number expected to double by 2002 due to the progressive aging of the population (Jacobsen, Girman, Guess, Oesterling, & Lieber, 1995).

PROSTATITIS

Prostatitis may cause enlargement, inflammation, or infection of the prostate gland. Some cases are caused by bacteria, others by other factors. Symptoms include a dull ache in the lower pelvis, lower back pain, and, sometimes, difficult urination. In some cases, urethral discharge may occur. Sexual functioning may be affected: painful erections and uncomfortable intercourse are not unusual. Different bacteria have been found to cause prostatitis, including the bacteria that cause gonorrhea. The diagnosis of prostatitis may require a digital rectal examination and tests to determine the kind of bacteria causing it. A bacterial infection may appear suddenly or develop more slowly and persist for some time. Treating prostatitis with antibiotics generally eliminates the symptoms, but determining the best drug for the particular bacteria can be difficult. Often a 4- to 6-week treatment with a sulfa drug is highly effective, but strict patient compliance with the medication regimen is essential. In some cases, prostatitis is not a bacterial infection but a chronic inflammation of the gland itself, which may be caused by a change in frequency of ejaculation (either much more or much less than previous frequency for the man). In these instances antibiotics have no effect. Medications that reduce the spasms of muscular tissue within the prostate often provide some relief, as do alpha-blocker drugs. Prostatitis can be a prolonged, uncomfortable ailment, and men should consult their physicians promptly whenever they develop any type of genitourinary symptom. Prostatitis is the most common cause of urinary tract infections in men, which seem to recur frequently. Many doctors believe that regular sexual intercourse along with a high consumption of liquids may help to relieve this problem.

COPING WITH SEXUAL AND REPRODUCTIVE ILLNESSES

In several different contexts this book has discussed the relationship between self-esteem and body image. Serious and life-threatening illnesses can severely disrupt this connection. People with serious ailments often feel very alone, and sometimes even stigmatized, as if there were something fundamentally wrong with them as people. Feelings of physical and emotional intimacy are often distorted. Women and men may not feel much like sexual beings. Loneliness often is a powerful aspect of being sick and believing you might get even sicker. All the ailments discussed in this chapter have a very good chance of being cured, however, if they are detected early enough. As well, people with serious illnesses are often helped much by the social support of others. Data indicate that **support groups** can help people live longer after being diagnosed with a life-threatening illness.

Students preparing for a career in the health sciences, social work, or behavioral sciences may already know that support groups can help an individual adjust to illness. Sick people who can share their fears and anxieties with others similarly afflicted often feel much better and less isolated or unusual. Data indicate that women being treated for breast cancer who attend support groups live longer, sometimes much longer, than those who don't. Women with advanced breast cancer who participated in weekly support groups enjoyed better emotional health and survived the disease by an average year and a half longer than similar women who did not attend support groups (Evans, 1994). People who are members of support groups also experience less anxiety, depression, and pain than those who do not (O'Brien, 1994). Similarly, people who don't have a spouse or significant other are much more likely to die from heart attacks (Kukula, 1996). By sharing their concerns and worries, as well as their optimism for a good prognosis, people lower the inevitable stresses that accompany serious illness. Lower levels of stress improve the functioning of the immune sys-

Other Countries, Cultures, and Customs

"TALKING CIRCLES" AMONG NATIVE AMERICAN WOMEN

People's attitudes toward revealing private information about themselves are in many ways conditioned by their culture. Although others in the group, including the leader, are strangers, people often disclose very personal feelings about their disease and mortality. Different cultures have different attitudes about personal privacy, of course, particularly in relation to disease. This is true not only for illness itself but also for screening and detection of illness.

Native American women have higher mortality rates and lower survival rates for cervical cancer than other ethnic groups in the United States. Perhaps less access to medical care makes it difficult for them to get regular Pap smears. Because of the high risk of this cancer and the importance of early detection and treatment, a way had to be found within their cultural norms and mores to teach Native American women about cervical cancer and encourage them to be more proactive in taking care of their health. Hodge, Fredericks, and Rodriguez (1996) accomplished that in both urban and rural Native American health clinics in California.

Researchers developed a cervical cancer screening program for this population of women, using focus discussion groups. A "focus group" was already a somewhat different cultural tradition among these Native Americans, who called these groups "Talking Circles." The investigators adapted this tradition, including ancestral Native American stories, as a way of introducing information about cancer and encouraging screening for cervical cancer. Two hundred Native American women over the age of 18 participated in this study at eight different health clinics.

In the study, the women responded very well to this culturally tailored message. They attended closely to this health information framed within their cultural traditions and acted on it. For the Native American women in this sample, the Talking Circle was an efficient way to learn about their health risks and be encouraged to have regular screening for the early detection of cervical cancer. Apparently the same messages conveyed through traditional Native American communication channels were not as effective in promoting these health behaviors.

tem and thereby improve the recovery process. A support group is not necessarily a formal gathering of people with a similar ailment. Many people's own support system often can provide the validation, understanding, and empathy found in support groups led by trained facilitators. The most important element in a support system is honest, unguarded communication about one's personal fears and apprehensions, as well as the joys of improvement. In addition, support group leaders have skills for moderating the behavior of aggressive or domineering participants. When women in a support group are of similar ages and stage of disease, the group is especially effective (Evans, 1994).

Stressors not only can delay the recovery from serious illness but also seem correlated with the recurrence of cancer. (Remember that correlation does not imply a cause-and-effect relationship.). One study found that a major life stressor, such as bereavement, was correlated with a five-fold increase in the recurrence of breast cancer after surgery (Chollar, 1994). On the other hand, participants in support groups have an increased number of immune system cells that attack cancer cells (O'Brien, 1994). Support groups supplement medical treatments; they do not substitute for them. Most support groups are free or accept voluntary contributions; some may have a small membership fee. Support groups that charge high fees may be suspect and should be avoided. The American Cancer Society program for women recovering from breast cancer, "Reach to Recovery," has proved an excellent arena for sharing emotional fears and concerns, as well as practical advice on health issues after treatment (Williams, O'Sullivan, Snodgrass, & Love, 1995).

Some support groups offer participants pragmatic approaches for dealing with their health problems. For example, Goodale, Domar, and Benson (1990) taught women with premenstrual syndrome a structured relaxation technique called the relaxation response. Their ability to cope with symptoms was shown to be better than that of women who were not given this instruction. This is a simple, free, effective intervention worth examining by women experiencing PMS.

CONCLUSION

Although some of the material in this chapter is not very cheerful, there is much room for optimism for those who have these health problems, particularly when detected early. This is why people need to understand that their sexual and reproductive health and wellness require *informed vigilance.* The more one knows about health risks and the early symptoms of health problems, the more promptly one is likely to be to seek medical assistance. People need to be *proactive* in preventive measures. A person's relationship with his or her doctor also is extremely important because it affects one's willingness to ask questions and seek assistance when needed.

This chapter closes with the names, addresses, and telephone numbers of several important health care and support organizations; local agencies too may respond promptly to

one's questions and concerns. These agencies can provide more extensive and specific information regarding sexual health and wellness.

Hotline of the American Cancer Association
1 - 800 - 562 - 2623

American Cancer Society Helpline
1 - 800 - 227 - 2345

Department of Health and Human Services (HHS)
Hubert H. Humphrey Building
200 Independence Avenue, SW
Washington, DC 20201
202 - 619 - 0257

The Endometriosis Association
8585 North 76th Place
Milwaukee, WI 53223

National Center for Health Information
Office of Disease Prevention and Health Promotion (ODPHP)
PO Box 1133
Washington, DC 20013-1133
1 - 800 - 336 - 4797 or 301 - 565 - 4167

National Women's Health Network
1325 G Street, NW
Washington, DC 20005
202 - 347 - 1140

Learning Activities

1. Many women are so anxious about breast cancer that they avoid measures that would lead to early detection. What type of appeal would help motivate fearful women to follow medical advice for screening? Who might be especially influential in encouraging a woman to have a mammogram?

2. Linda is a 27-year-old virgin. She believes it is very important for her to be married before having sexual intercourse. Therefore, she doesn't take birth control pills because she feels there really is no reason to do so. She is attractive, healthy, and comfortable with her values. However, Linda has never had a gynecological examination and can't see the need for one. If you were Linda's friend, what could you say to persuade her to be proactive in her sexual and reproductive health?

3. Is it appropriate to "eroticize" personal sexual and reproductive health care examinations? For example, should men participate in their female partner's breast self-examinations, and should women take part in their male partner's testicular self-examinations?

4. Men whose wives and partners have had mastectomies are generally very supportive and helpful during recovery from surgery. They frequently express their devotion and try to minimize their partner's anxieties about feeling unattractive or unfeminine. What can men (or women in lesbian relationships) do to help their partners deal with recovery from this kind of surgery?

5. There is an estimated 10 to 15% false negative rate in mammogram results; that is, in 10 to 15% of cases the radiologist says there is no sign of a suspicious lump or mass when really there is one. Can you think of ways in which women can use this information?

6. Many nuns who are celibate believe that having a regular Pap smear is unnecessary, since problems revealed by Pap smear results are often associated with sexual intercourse early in adolescence, having many sexual partners, and some sexually transmitted diseases. Yet, reportedly, cervical cancer in nuns is about as common as in the general female population. What measures might be taken to encourage nuns to have regular yearly Pap smears and who could best encourage this simple screening test?

7. Let's say that you are a mid-level manager in a large company. One woman who works under your supervision is a bright, competent 30-year-old who recently has had problems being punctual, productive, and cooperative. In a private discussion with her you learn she has PMS. What do you do?

8. Many doctors see patients who genuinely believe that they are ill but really are not. A patient may make many appointments, miss much time at work, and run up a high bill because of many diverse, although often nonspecific, complaints. Gynecologists often see such patients. Many women, for example, overreact to minor changes in the appearance or feeling of their vaginas. If you were a gynecologist, how would you reassure such a patient when you know they are normal and their concerns are only minor?

9. Testicular cancer occurs primarily in younger men who also happen not to be conscientious about testicular self-examinations. What might be an effective way to persuade young men of the importance of this simple self-exam?

*K*ey Concepts

- Health is not just the absence of illness. It includes positive striving for wellness and taking personal responsibility for the early detection of potential problems and their treatment.

- Adherence is the degree to which a person follows the instructions of a health care professional for reducing the risk of disease, minimizing its severity, or hastening recovery, often involving medication and lifestyle.

- In reference to sexual health and wellness, "normal" generally implies an absence of disease and physiological functioning that is good for a person's age and circumstances.

- Everyone needs a support system in order to feel connected to others. Members of a support system share each other's lives and offer unconditional positive regard, emotional challenge, and emotional appreciation.

- Coping with a problem involves finding ways of living with it or getting along with it, and the problem remains unsolved. Dealing with a problem, on the other hand, means solving it and making it go away. While we can learn to cope with many problems and stressors, we cannot always deal with all of them decisively.

- The relationship between self-esteem and body image is involved in how we monitor our health and act promptly on signs of illness.

- Locus of control and self-monitoring are two personality attributes involved in the degree to which we feel in charge of our lives and are aware of what is going on both inside and outside of ourselves.

- In a routine gynecological examination, the health care professional examines a woman's external genitalia, the interior of her vagina, and the inside of her rectum.

- A breast self-examination can help a woman recognize normal conditions, as well as unusual changes in her breasts that may require medical attention. Breast self-examination by itself cannot allow either the woman or her doctor to diagnose conclusively the nature of any unusual lumps. In about 90% of cases, breast lumps are not cancerous.

- Breast cancer will be diagnosed in about 1 in 8 American women at some time in their lives. It may develop in the milk ducts, the breast lobes, or the nipple. This is the most common kind of cancer in women. No one knows exactly what causes breast cancer. Mammograms are special x-rays for detecting and diagnosing different kinds of breast lumps. Women over the age of 40 should have a mammogram every year. Ultrasound may also be used to examine the breasts. Breast cancer is treated with surgery, chemotherapy, hormone therapy, radiation therapy, or some combination of these, depending on a range of different factors.

- Cervical cancer is a slow-growing, easy-to-diagnose malignancy that is more prevalent as women get older. To screen for it, a Pap smear is given, which involves scraping a few cells from the surface and interior of the cervix and examining them microscopically. A Pap smear is painless. Many effective therapeutic options are available when abnormal cells are discovered.

- Dysmenorrhea is menstrual discomfort with psychological and/or physical causes. Amenorrhea is the cessation of menstruation, usually due to abnormalities in hormonal levels related to the menstrual cycle.

- Premenstrual syndrome involves a number of psychological and physical symptoms that often precede menstruation.

There is much disagreement about the specific symptoms of this disorder and its timing in relation to a woman's period. Its manifestations range from mildly annoying to severely debilitating symptoms.

- Vaginal infections are caused by various microorganisms and are common. While sexually transmitted diseases cause some types of vaginal infections, other vaginal infections are unrelated to these disorders. Yeast infections, trichomoniasis, and bacterial vaginosis are common vaginal infections.
- Endometrial tissue that usually lines the uterus sometimes grows outside the uterus in a condition called endometriosis, which may involve the fallopian tubes and pelvic cavity. It is causes discomfort and may impair a woman's fertility.
- Pelvic inflammatory disease (PID) is an infection of the female reproductive tract that ascends from the vagina, through the uterus, and up the fallopian tubes, spreading to the pelvic cavity.
- Cystitis is a bladder infection, the most common type of urinary tract infection in women.
- Toxic shock syndrome is a systemic, acute bacterial infection by *Staphylococcus aureus*. It is often associated with menstruation and the use of some types of highly absorbent tampons, especially those with synthetic fibers.
- Ovarian cancer is difficult to diagnose early and therefore more difficult to treat. Its symptoms include vague feelings of abdominal discomfort, indigestion, and bloating; it is more common in women over the age of 50. Endometrial cancer is the most common kind of cancer of the female reproductive tract. Its earliest symptoms include abnormal uterine bleeding; with early detection, this cancer has a cure rate of 90%.
- Testicular cancer occurs primarily in men under the age of 35. Lumps, bumps, and granular surfaces can be felt on the affected testicle during a testicular self-examination, which all men should do monthly.
- Epididymitis is a localized infection of the epididymis often associated with chronic urinary tract infections and undiagnosed sexually transmitted diseases.
- Cryptorchidism is a condition of undescended testes that occurs in a small percentage of full-term babies but is more common in infants born prematurely. It sometimes corrects itself spontaneously, but often surgery is required to relocate the testicle in the scrotum.
- Balanitis is a localized irritation of the foreskin and glans of the penis.
- The vein to the testicles sometimes becomes enlarged, leading to a varicocele. This condition occurs in about 10% of men and may play a role in infertility.
- Priapism is a long-lasting, very uncomfortable erection that is unrelated to sexual stimulation.

- Phimosis is a condition in which the foreskin of an uncircumcised penis is too tight to retract, making hygiene very difficult.
- Prostate cancer is the second most common kind of cancer in men. In its earliest stages there may be no symptoms. In more advanced cases, urinary symptoms often occur. Screening for prostate cancer involves a digital rectal examination. There are a number of effective treatments for prostate cancer.
- All men as they age have some signs of a noncancerous prostate enlargement. Benign prostatic hyperplasia often causes urinary symptoms. Drugs are often effective in reducing the enlargement.
- Prostatitis may involve enlargement, inflammation, or infection of the prostate gland. Only in some instances is it caused by a bacterial infection. Antibiotics are often effective in treating bacterial prostatitis.
- Support groups often help people with serious or life-threatening illnesses express their feelings about being sick and the isolation they sometimes experience. Scientific investigations show that those who participate in support groups often live longer than those who do not.

Glossary Terms

adherence	endometriosis	phimosis
amenorrhea	epididymitis	premenstrual
anorexia athletica	fibroadenoma	syndrome
anorexia nervosa	fibrocystic	(PMS)
balanitis	disease	priapism
bimanual pelvic	hormone therapy	prostaglandins
examination	laparoscopy	prostate cancer
breast cancer	locus of control	prostatic specific
Candida albicans	loop	antigen (PSA)
chemotherapy	electrocautery	prostatitis
colposcopy	excision	radiation therapy
conization	procedure	self-esteem
cryotherapy	(LEEP)	self-monitoring
cryptorchidism	lumpectomy	speculum
cystitis	mammogram	support groups
diagnostic	mastectomy	support systems
hysteroscopy	metastasis	testicular cancer
diathesis stress	nonsterile	toxic shock
theory	ovarian cancer	syndrome
dysmenorrhea	Pap smear	trichomoniasis
dysplasia	partial	variocele
endocervical	mastectomy	vulvovaginitis
curettage	pelvic	(vaginitis)
endometrial	inflammatory	
cancer	disease (PID)	

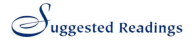

Suggested Readings

Bechtel, S., & Stains, L. R. (1996). Sex. A man's guide. Emmaus, PA: Rodale Press.

Boston Women's Health Book Collective. (1992). The new our bodies, ourselves: Updated and expanded for the 90s. New York: Simon & Schuster.

Carlson, K. J., Eisenstat, S. A., & Ziporyn, T. (1996). The Harvard guide to women's health. Cambridge, MA: Harvard University Press.

Edge, V., & Miller, M. (1994). Women's health care. St. Louis: Mosby.

The PDR Family Guide to Woman's Health and Prescription Drugs. (1994). Montvale, NJ: Medical Economics.

6

Sexual Arousal and Responsiveness: Personal and Social Perspectives on Pleasure and Sharing

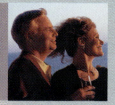

OBJECTIVES

When you finish reading and reviewing this chapter, you should be able to:

1. Relate interpersonal sexual communication factors in arousal and response to anatomical and physiological aspects of human sexual response.

2. Describe the diverse aspects of eroticism and the many manifestations of learning, thinking, and feeling underlying human sexual motives, desires, and preferences.

3. Discuss individual differences in the ways in which we receive, evaluate, and act on sexual cues in our environment.

4. Describe the structures in the central and peripheral nervous systems involved in our sexual responses.

5. Describe the most important sex hormones in women and men and their functions.

6. Discuss the four stages of Masters and Johnson's sexual response cycle in women and men, emphasizing the anatomical and physiological changes in each.

7. Discuss the three stages in Kaplan's model of sexual arousal and response, including psychological issues in the first stage and anatomical and physiological changes in all stages.

8. Summarize the perceptual and cognitive aspects of sexual arousal and response in the approaches of Reed and Palace.

9. Discuss the notion of a "climate of psychological safety."

10. Summarize biological factors affecting sexual arousal and response, including issues such as cyclic hormone changes in women, the use of oral contraceptives, and pregnancy.

11. Evaluate the effects of various substances thought to have an aphrodisiac effect and those that inhibit sexual arousal and response.

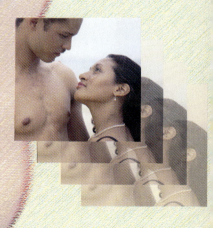

From Dr. Ruth

My field, sex therapy, would no doubt not exist if it weren't for Masters and Johnson, who studied thousands of sexual episodes to learn how sexual functioning really occurs. Because of them we have scientifically validated information that we sex therapists use to help people have better sex lives.

When you think about these scientists watching people having sex, some of you might think, "What a great job!" And, yes, at the beginning they may have been "turned on" by seeing all this sexual activity. But I'm certain that after a few thousand observed episodes, their watching people have sex ended up much more routine and scientific.

Some of you in fact may be turned off at the thought of watching even one couple have sex. That's part of what this chapter is all about-the different things people find arousing or not. Because sex is so personal, many people don't know or care much about other people's sexual desires. In relationships where one partner wants sex once a week and the other ten times a week, however, the two may criticize each other, calling each other "pervert" or "prude." And people who have unusual sexual desires, like fetishists, are often scorned. Thanks to Masters and Johnson and others who have followed, we now know a lot about eroticism and what turns people on. Although it is natural to seek out your own sexual self in this chapter, make sure you keep in mind the differences among all of us.

If there is one word that crops up more than any other in questions people ask me, it is not penis or vagina or orgasm, but "normal." Many people are concerned with whether or not their body or their sexual response is like everyone else's. Since these topics don't ordinarily crop up in conversation ("Did you and your husband have sex last night? What exactly did you do?"), it's understandable that people might want a yardstick by which to judge themselves. You can see how tall the people around you are and judge normal height, and you can pay attention at work or school to judge what performance there is "normal." But you rarely see other people's genitals and even more rarely get a peek at them having sex. The research of Masters and Johnson provides some of those yardsticks, however. And the one conclusion we can reach from their work is that the norm does not fall within a small range but rather extends broadly to include most of us.

Finally, while you may be tempted to look for yourself in this chapter to compare yourself to the "norm," please keep in mind the differences in sexual functioning among people. For you see, sex, at its very core, is the sharing of pleasure between two people. For you to limit your horizons to only your own sexual arousal is really to miss the boat. Yes, you want to receive pleasure from sex, but to get the most out of it you should also want to give pleasure. You can do that successfully only if you accept and understand the needs and desires of your partner, as well as your own.

BASIC CONCEPTS OF AROUSAL AND RESPONSE

We all know that sexual excitement changes us. Our thoughts change, our bodies change, and our thoughts about our bodies change. Since we are usually not taught this while we are growing up, we often learn about it on our own; then we usually wonder if we are "normal." People find arousing and respond to a large number of interesting and diverse erotic stimuli, but what one person finds erotic may not interest another person.

Despite the fact that our bodies respond in fairly similar ways to sexual stimulation, the different stimuli that elicit those responses can be quite varied. Interestingly, many people believe that if you study this subject too objectively or too scientifically, you take the "magic" out of it and are left only with "cold, hard facts." We don't believe this. As you have read in other chapters, accurate and complete sexual information only enhances the quality (and perhaps even the quantity) of a person's life.

One of the more interesting aspects of sexual excitement is the many different changes that accompany arousal. For example, there are many physiological and hormonal changes. Not all are easy to observe and measure, but all certainly play a role in erection, vaginal lubrication, orgasm, and ejaculation. Many physical changes take place in the same time interval, making it hard to focus on any one aspect at a time. These *physical* changes also affect what we pay attention to, think are erotic, and respond to. This is extremely important: our psychological perceptions of sexual interaction affect how we interpret the physical aspects of arousal and response. Therefore, it only makes sense when studying arousal and response to, at the same time, ask what is going on in the minds of the people involved and in their social environment.

The Interpersonal Context

Most books about human sexuality present extensive, detailed information about what happens in our bodies during the stages of arousal and response, and this chapter also will include that information. It is based on extensive, thorough, controlled laboratory observations. In 1954 William Masters began the first systematic, empirical study of human sexual response. Scientific research came late to this study of human physiology, perhaps because the personal and fundamentally private nature of our sexuality created a sense of "specialness" about erotic arousal and response. As Masters discovered, the ways we become sexually excited and respond to erotic stimulation follow a fairly predictable sequence of events.

This objective and straightforward discussion of human sexual response leaves something out, however, and, therefore, we will explore human sexual response within the *psychosocial and communication context* of two people being intimate with each other. Of course, this doesn't mean that physical changes accompanying masturbation aren't "normal." Rather, the environment in which we live, what we have learned to think of as erotic, and how we communicate with each other in sexual settings are important topics not to be divorced from what is happening in our bodies. In other words, the "big picture" is generally more informative than just what the physiologist's "microscope" shows us. Our approach to arousal and response is, therefore, more "macro" than the traditional "micro" perspective, as we introduced these terms in Chapter 1.

Eroticism: The Driving Force Behind Sexual Arousal and Response

Our environment is full of sexual signs, symbols, and stimuli, and our interpretation of this information has a major role in sexual interest, arousal, or responsiveness. Everyone has his or her own **sexual value system,** which is the sum of all those stimuli that have erotic meaning for the person individually (Masters & Johnson, 1978, personal communication). What some think is sexy, others may think is stupid. This very personal perspective on what we think are sexy colors, what we pay attention to, and how we respond. These underlying beliefs about what is attractive or exciting is a necessary part of the study of the physiology of sexual arousal and orgasm.

Because what we perceive is so basic to what we think is sexual, our study must also include the importance of our senses in receiving and interpreting information. Eroticism involves sensory experiences that focus our attention on personally relevant sexual stimuli.

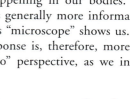

Consider the little things we do when we are trying to make a good impression on someone we find sexually attractive. We try to present that person with a number of cues they will like and associate with us. We dress attractively, even sometimes provocatively. We style and color our hair. We try to speak in soft and inviting tones. We use soap, perfume, deodorant, toothpaste, and mouthwash. We may reach across the table for a tender touch or caress. When all of this sensory information is perceived by the other as enjoyable and even a little novel or exciting, the moment becomes special and perhaps sensual and exciting. This is a big part of "eroticism." Other people may be less attentive to these stimuli and, instead, focus on factors such as personality, intelligence, wit, sense of humor, self-confidence, or nurturance and caring. We are all different with respect to what we think is erotic and how we respond accordingly (Fig. 6-1).

Psychologists and other social and medical scientists know that when the ex-

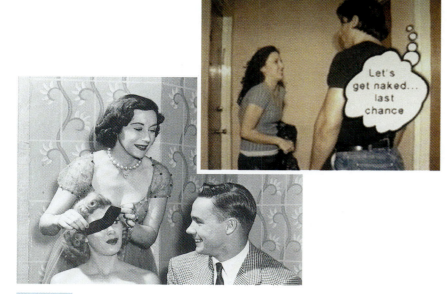

FIGURE 6-1 Television shows depict society's ideas about what is erotically interesting; as society changes, so too do these portrayals. At left is a scene from the show "Blind Date," which aired between 1949 and 1952. At right is a scene from a current program.

perience of a stimulus is pleasurable, a person is attentive to the possibility of experiencing that stimulus again. This association is a powerful factor for learning a relationship between environmental elements and sexual feelings. This process begins early in life and in some ways forms the foundation on which further sexual learning takes place. By adolescence, most people feel that sexuality has meanings that are *strong and special.* Images of sexual attractiveness in art, literature, and the media often become part of one's sexual value system. Yet as long as we live, we have the capacity for growth, change, and choice. What is erotic at one time in our lives may not be at another time.

Despite the fact that erection, vaginal lubrication, orgasm, and/or ejaculation are obvious signs of erotic arousal, they are by no means the whole story. Generally, as long as people are aware of their sexual desires, they have a better understanding of the stimuli to which they are most responsive. But sexual desire has to be refreshed and maintained. Affectionate, sensual, and sexual stimulation is the cornerstone to understanding desire and one's own sexual value system, and ideally still is an important part of any couple's intimate behaviors (McCarthy, 1995).

An interesting and informative approach to sexual desire and the problems that sometimes surround it is that of Barry W. McCarthy (1987, 1995). His approaches emphasize that our personal eroticism is enhanced if we *take time to think about it,* and this is one important objective of this chapter. An important part of the arousal accompanying sexual anticipation is *spontaneous sexual expression.*

Another aspect of sexual desire and eroticism, according to McCarthy, is taking personal responsibility for one's own sexuality. This means that a person feels comfortable making their sexual preferences and standards known to their partner without fear of being evaluated or judged. When one has learned communication skills to enhance sexual sharing, McCarthy believes the next main aspect of desire is feeling *deserving* of the enjoyment of sexual pleasure. In other words, regardless of our life circumstances, we are all worthy of the special enjoyments from that intimate sharing. A person who thinks that sexual arousal and responsiveness are only for the young, thin, rich, or "well-adjusted" has made a fundamental error about human nature. The next important aspect of sexual desire involves recognizing how broad and diversified sexual responsiveness actually is. It is often said that there is more to sex than orgasm, and more to orgasm than sex. Powerful and poignant enjoyments come from sexual sharing of many kinds, and orgasm is only one part of sexual pleasure. Finally, McCarthy emphasizes emotional intimacy as a building block for healthy sexual desire. This means that a couple feels comfortable sharing their vulnerabilities and knows the other person would never exploit this information to hurt him or her. Intimacy is a reciprocal sharing of thoughts and feelings and frequently promotes a loyal bonding. When one's partner feels free and uninhibited sexually because they feel valued and worthy, their responsiveness is easily communicated and becomes very exciting.

Because eroticism is so personal and specific to one's own tastes and experiences, it is not easy to compare one person's sexual interest with another's. One's own feelings of intimate attraction to someone may be very different from that person's. Does this mean there is no common ground for what we do and think when attracted to someone else? Not at all. Everyone knows what flirting is; most people have done it and most have had someone else flirt with them. Flirting is interesting because it is conditioned by the psychosocial environment, and its expression reveals much about what facilitates sexual arousal.

Abrahams (1994) carried out an analysis of what is conveyed during flirting and found that both women and men have the same general ideas about what flirting communicates. For example, both women and men in this study recognized flirting as an expression of *sexual assertiveness.* In other words, flirting is a proactive behavior that states one's interest in someone; it says "I'm interested in you and am taking the initiative to tell you." As well, flirting is *overt,* with little about it that is subtle because flirting is meant to be noticed. Flirting is also an *invitation* and reveals an open, welcoming attitude toward the other person. Like other invitations, the person flirting wants to find out if it is accepted or declined.

Another characteristic of flirting described by Abrahams is its *playfulness;* in other words, flirting isn't deadly serious, and the person just wants to find out if the other will notice them and is safely exploring their desirability in a social setting. Perhaps the playfulness of flirting is an easy way to explore someone's interest without them beginning to think about a "relationship." Another aspect is that flirting can be *nonverbal,* which does not imply that verbal flirting does not convey much information. The human face can reveal an astonishing array of subtle expressions that communicate a wide variety of interests, feelings, and judgments (Fig. 6-2). On the other hand, it may be that the lack of thorough and accurate

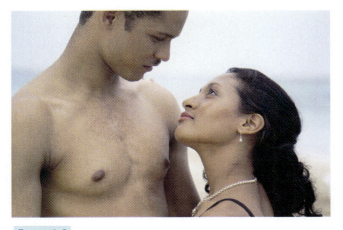

FIGURE 6-2 Facial expressions convey a lot of information about feelings of attraction. Here these two people demonstrate focused gaze, an enigmatic smile, and an inviting, friendly expression.

Dear Dr. Ruth

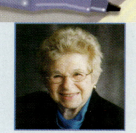

Question:

My girlfriend always wants the same "routine" when we make love and has no spontaneity or variation in her behavior. Is this normal? I'd like it if we had more variety.

Answer:

It's not uncommon for people to fix on a certain pattern and then use it over and over again. This doesn't apply just to sex. For example, some people always eat their meat first, then the potato, and then the vegetable. They enjoy the pattern and, in some cases, may feel safer because of it.

I don't know how easy it will be for you to motivate her to change, but perhaps you can work out a compromise that will help her try something new. Ask her if she wouldn't mind having sex once in a while with some variation in style just for your satisfaction. Let her know in advance what variation you'd like to try, so that she won't worry that it might be something that she abhors. Perhaps she'll get into it and enjoy the experience, and perhaps she won't, but at least you'll have had the pleasure of trying.

---

disclosure of intention makes flirting so provocative and interesting. A wag once commented that flirting is like a bathing suit: what it reveals is often very interesting, but what it conceals is vital! Finally, Abrahams demonstrated that women and men respond to the *unconventionality* of flirting communication. How a person flirts says a lot about their uniqueness and personal characteristics. Little nuances in traditional flirting "scripts" may have a powerful attention-getting appeal. While the way we dress and hold ourselves can sometimes be provocative, unusual and unconventional ways of communicating personal interest introduce creativity into the social rituals with which we attempt to get to know other people. This study probably confirms what many of us already suspected about the nature of flirtation.

Psychological Aspects of Sexual Arousal

Many psychological factors affect sexual arousal. Our awareness of our genitals and our thoughts certainly are linked. Since Masters and Johnson's work was first published, investigators have seen that human sexual arousal and response can be subjects for empirical investigation, adding to information from anecdotes and case histories that do not tell the whole story about how people become aroused and have orgasms. An interesting place to begin is the hypothesized existence of a basic, primal "sexual energy" that leads to sexual behaviors (Bancroft, 1983). Although clearly most people are motivated to act on their feelings of sexual interest and/or arousal, no convincing data support the existence of a specific sexual energy that can be observed and measured with existing scien-

tific instruments. As discussed in Chapter 3, Sigmund Freud believed in a basic motivational energy in the personality he called the libido, but this idea was more a hypothetical construct than an observable or verifiable force. Note that different scientists define the terms "arousal" and "response" in different ways. Some make no significant distinction between these words, while others (including we authors) see sexual arousal as leading to sexual response. It is too simplistic, however, to say that sexual response *is* orgasm, because sexual response involves a number of feelings and physiological changes.

If erotic stimuli can have such powerful effects, what is the role of romantic feelings in fostering sexual arousal? In a number of different controlled laboratory experiments, physiological measures of sexual arousal were made while subjects were presented with erotic audio tapes (Heiman, 1977) or erotic films (Fisher & Byrne, 1978) or asked to participate in sexual fantasies (Mosher & White, 1980). In these experiments, the content of the tapes, films, and fantasies either were explicitly sexual or emphasized the committed, romantic nature of the encounter being depicted. These investigations all revealed that sexual arousal as measured physiologically was most pronounced when the content of the message was frankly sexual; arousal was significantly lower when themes of attachment, love, and romance were presented to the subjects. Apparently, arousal is stronger with specific erotic stimuli that come to be associated with arousal close together in space or time.

Another important aspect of sexual arousal involves the degree of assertiveness or dominance that a person exercises during the intimate interaction. This refers not to unwanted aggressiveness but rather to a more positive and confident interpersonal demeanor. When measuring physiological responses to the presentation of erotic audio tapes, Heiman (1977) explored the impact of tapes in which the man or the woman took a more assertive, independent role in eliciting and furthering the sexual action. Among the female subjects in this study, greater genital response was noted when the female in the tapes took the initiative rather than in other tapes in which the male was the sexual initiator. Maybe these women identified with the women they were listening to in the tapes and felt a greater sympathy with a more independent, assertive feminine sexual style. In another experiment, Garcia et al. (1984) asked female and male subjects to read erotic stories in which women or men were more active in initiating and guiding a sexual encounter. Here again, women were more aroused as measured genitally by reading stories about dominant women, and men were more aroused as measured genitally by reading stories about dominant men. Together, these studies suggest a lot. Perhaps feeling "in control" or "in charge" is an important determinant of sexual arousal (Fig. 6-3). Of course, these data were collected under highly controlled laboratory conditions,

and whether these conclusions apply in the real world is a question to be approached with appropriate, rigorous scientific methods.

Only a few psychological determinants of sexual arousal have been discussed here, but you can see that the results of some laboratory studies do not always support one's "common sense" view of things, while other results may confirm hunches we all have about how women and men interact sexually. Remember that simple fact discovered more than a century ago: the more frequently a stimulus is paired with pleasurable consequences, the more readily does one attribute pleasurable properties to that stimulus. This is true with stimuli such as a soft caress, a particular perfume, or the proverbial candlelight dinner.

"Normal" Sexual Arousal

A later section in this chapter discusses the biological changes that occur when people experience sexual arousal and response. We go through different stages, or a sequence of changes, that are obvious anatomically and physiologically. Yet we all do not go through this cycle of sexual arousal and response in exactly the same way. Arousal does *not* imply an invariant, perfectly predictable sequence of changes and stages, but instead involves normal variations from person to person, and from time to time as well.

Because "normal" sexual arousal may change from time to time, personal issues play a big part in our receptivity to the intimate overtures of another person. A pattern of consistent, enjoyable sexual excitement is often hard to maintain, even within a comfortable, monogamous relationship. Sometimes it is important to explore variety during intimacy in order to renew the "spark."

It should be obvious by now that "normality" isn't always easy to describe or define unambiguously. In sexual arousal there are no simple "normal" and "abnormal" feelings and physical changes. These are not two discrete categories but rather two ends of a wide continuum. Remember that often women and men feel tired, frustrated, angry, depressed, or anxious, and such feelings may affect whether and when a person becomes sexually aroused or how responsive they might be. But the fact that arousal is delayed or diminished does not mean that anything abnormal is happening.

"Natural" Conceptions of Sexual Arousal and Response

Masters and Johnson revealed or rediscovered some very important although obvious truths. For example, people often find it difficult to accept sexuality as a "natural" function, as we might, for example, the circulation of the blood or the activity of the nervous system (personal communication, 1978). Think about this for a moment. During a visit to your physician, you probably find nothing at all odd or anxiety provoking about having your temperature taken, your blood pressure taken, or your throat examined. But as soon as you begin to anticipate a pelvic examination, breast exam, or prostate exam, things change in your mind. Suddenly this isn't just clinical, its *really personal.*

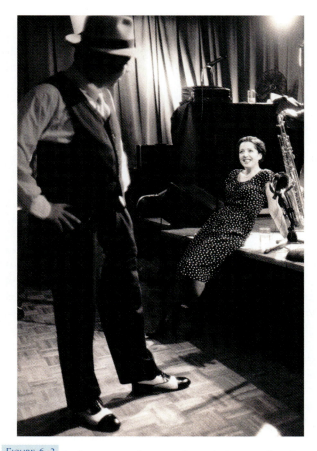

FIGURE 6-3 Body posture often reveals erotic interest, but this type of sexual assertiveness in a woman may make some men uncomfortable.

Research Highlight

MEASURING SEXUAL AROUSAL IN THE LABORATORY

A critical characteristic of scientific investigation is that it deals with *observable and measurable* phenomena. If something cannot be seen either directly or indirectly and cannot be described quantitatively, then scientists cannot study it scientifically. In addition, most scientists believe it imperative to describe the conditions in which a phenomenon occurs and that it occurs regularly and reliably in those conditions. Many interesting aspects of human nature, however, cannot be studied in this way. For example, "will power" is an interesting concept, but scientists can *not* define with any certainty the independent variables that foster it. This issue, although interesting, is not readily open to scientific investigation, and, therefore, it is extremely difficult to make statements about will power that are widely generalizable. Similarly, statements about sexual arousal and response must be based on observable, quantifiable data.

As described in Chapter 2, Masters and Johnson were the first investigators to study human sexual response in the laboratory. Earlier writers and scientists had certainly explored many aspects of human sexual interest and behavior, but they had not carried out laboratory investigations of observable, measurable aspects of sexual arousal and response. Masters and Johnson used not only observational methods but also a more informative research method called the *clinical study method,* which combines direct observation and in-depth interviews. After observing their subjects in a variety of circumstances that led to arousal and orgasm, they questioned them about the feelings, perceptions, and emotions that accompanied these physiological events. The verbal records of these interviews are at least as important as the data collected with sophisticated electrophysiological instruments. Masters and Johnson studied the associated physiological and psychological aspects of human sexual response. Masters and Johnson measured the physical manifestations of arousal and response both inside and outside the body. Films were taken and the tension in the body's musculature recorded. Breathing rate, heart rate, blood pressure, and perspiration were also measured quantitatively. The presence of a "skin flush" was recorded photographically. Breast changes accompanying arousal and response were measured and photographed. The physiological and anatomical changes of the penis and inside the vagina were measured with two special instruments. The **penile strain gauge** (Fig. 6-4A), which looks like a narrow rubber or stainless steel noose, fits around the base of the penis. Inside this little loop is a thin filament of mercury through which a tiny electrical current passes. During erection, the circumference of the penis increases, causing a change in the amount of current passing through the mercury filament as it is stretched. This minute electrical change is measured to show changes in penis circumference, which are shown on an oscilloscope or polygraph.

To observe and record changes in the vagina that accompany sexual arousal, a **vaginal photoplethysmograph** (Fig. 6-4B) is used. This device is smaller than most tampons and is inserted directly into the vagina. Just as a man's penis engorges with blood during erection, a woman's vagina also swells slightly due to the engorgement of blood vessels. The increased blood circulating in the vagina is measured by the photoplethysmograph. A tiny bulb inside it emits light that is reflected back from surrounding tissue. The amount of light reflected back is measured. Sexual arousal and vaginal engorgement are correlated with less light being reflected back from the interior of the vagina. As with the penile strain gauge, this physiological measure is observed on an oscilloscope or a printed polygraph record.

A wide variety of people volunteered as subjects in Masters and Johnson's experiments. In all, 382 subjects were investigated thoroughly. Women and men between the ages of 20 and 90 were studied, including both Caucasians and African Americans, who had varying levels of education, including 68 with some postgraduate training. They came from different socioeconomic groups. (Although people who volunteer for sex research studies may have more open and candid attitudes about sexuality than the general population, no data suggest that they are any more or less responsive.) To make physiological measurements of erection and

MEASURING SEXUAL AROUSAL IN THE LABORATORY   (CONTINUED)

vaginal arousal, Masters and Johnson instructed each subject to apply the penile strain gauge or insert the vaginal photoplethysmograph.

Thus far we have described some of the benefits of controlled laboratory procedures to measure human sexual arousal. But there are drawbacks. Laboratories aren't very friendly, informal places. Indeed, they are highly artificial compared with most other places people experience sexual arousal and response. Nonetheless, the data recorded in this controlled environment can usually be generalized to other places people experience intimacy. The data recorded and collected by Masters and Johnson do not seem in any way peculiar to the laboratory setting or more characteristic of their subjects than the general population. In fact, with only minor revisions in their four-stage sexual response cycle (e.g., by Kaplan, 1974), surprisingly little data have been inconsistent with their research.

Because subjects quickly get used to wearing a penile strain gauge or vaginal photoplethysmograph, these devices can be used also to measure the changes of sexual arousal during sleep. The changes described earlier in sleep were determined with laboratory data using these devices. For example, **nocturnal penile tumescence** (NPT) is a technical term used to describe the erections men have when asleep. Chapter 14 describes how erections observed to occur during sleep can be used to rule out physical causes of erectile difficulties in men and allow therapists to focus instead on psychological reasons for this problem. Similarly, vaginal photoplethysmography is useful for monitoring sexual arousal during sleep in women.

This way of thinking about sexuality has preserved its mysterious, private, and "special" attributes, but it hasn't helped us gain a useful, objective grasp of this basic aspect of personhood. Most people have difficulty separating the physiosexual aspects of their bodies from the erotic associations of arousal and response. For example, if you are accustomed to thinking of penile erection solely in terms of penetration during intercourse, then some common observations might seem confusing. Normal, healthy men have erections in their sleep every 80 to 90 minutes during the rapid eye movement (REM) sleep stage that accompanies dreaming. These dreams need not be sexual for these erections to occur, and it is, therefore, difficult to interpret these erections as erotic responses. Another example is that baby boys usually have an erection sometime during the first 48 hours of life, and some even emerge from the uterus with an erection. Again, it is hard to explain such erections as responses to erotic stimuli or thoughts. Similar findings occur with women. Normal, healthy women vaginally lubricate every 80 to 90 minutes during sleep, also during REM sleep. And similarly, baby girls vaginally lubricate sometime during the first few days of their lives.

Since the publication of *Human Sexual Response,* many people have gradually recognized that human sexual responses are just as "natural" as the functions of any other human organ system. Nonetheless, it isn't always as easy to *feel* that this aspect of human sexuality is natural as it is to think it. Although it is normal to be curious about sexuality, it is difficult to explore questions if one is uneasy about the subject matter.

It is difficult to suddenly change the way one thinks and feels about sexual matters. A person who feels self-conscious looking at a sexuality text in a bookstore might feel nervous in a close, intimate interpersonal interaction as well. It is difficult to have feelings about sex that are conservative and self-conscious in one domain of life but have feelings about sex that are uninhibited and liberating in another. This often colors how people approach sexual situations and how they give themselves "permission" to be sexual beings.

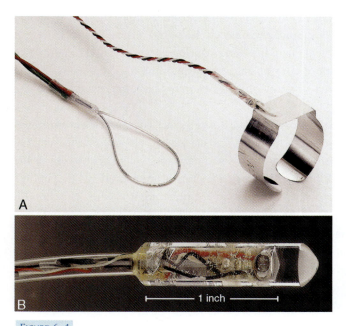

FIGURE 6-4   A. A penile strain gauge. B. A vaginal photoplethysmograph. These are two important tools in studying human sexual arousal and response in the laboratory setting.

BIOLOGICAL SUBSTRATES OF SEXUAL AROUSAL AND RESPONSE

A full understanding of what happens physically during sexual arousal and response requires examining the roles of the brain, spinal cord, and endocrine system in these processes. Although neural and endocrine function might seem "wired in," their activities depend heavily on how people acknowledge, evaluate, remember, and act on stimuli, and this is always highly personal.

The Central Nervous System

The central nervous system is composed of the **brain** and **spinal cord** (Fig. 6-5) Both are important in sexual arousal and response. Some neural pathways underlying sexual excitement are simple, while others are tremendously complex and involve one's personal sexual value system, as well as stimuli. The brain and spinal cord are both involved in perception, thinking, and motivation, which are all basic to most aspects of sexual functioning. Scientists are certain of two things about these structures: specific behavioral functions seem to be localized in fairly discrete areas of tissue, and different areas work together and coordinate their different contributions. In general, all *incoming* information from the sensory organs *ascends* from the body up the spinal cord and reaches specific areas of the brain. In contrast, body movements originate in *outgoing* nerve messages that descend from the brain down the spinal cord and to the muscles.

A basic neural function is the **reflex.** A reflex is the simplest stimulus-response connection in the nervous system. Sense organs gather information and send it to the spinal cord over specific nerve fibers. Nerve cells inside the spinal cord receive this information and process it. Nerve impulses originating in the spinal cord then travel back out to the body, such as to cause a muscle to contract if your finger has been pinched. Reflexes take place automatically and unconsciously; a person cannot "will" a reflex. Reflexes do not involve thinking. Although erotic stimuli can enter the central nervous system through all the sense organs, touch generally has the most important role in sexual reflexes. Sexual arousal in both women and men depends on several reflexes occurring inside the spinal cord. Let's examine how this works in an erection.

Touching, stroking, and rubbing a man's penis are examples of tactile stimulation often interpreted as erotic or sexual. This touch information is carried to an area in the lower spinal cord. A well-defined, discrete collection of nerve cells in the central nervous system is called a **nucleus.** A nucleus plays an important role in a sequence of events leading to an erection. Nerve cells in this nucleus send a message that eventually relaxes muscle fibers in arterial walls in the penis, allowing the arteries to swell as more blood fills them. This causes an enlargement of the corpora cavernosa (discussed in Chapter 3) and an increase in the length and circumference of the penis. Tiny

valves in the veins of the penis are compressed, allowing the blood that has engorged the penis to stay there. As long as this state is maintained, the erection continues.

Sexual arousal, however, is not the same kind of reflex as a knee-jerk elicited by tapping the knee. Sexual arousal is another category of reflexive response in the nervous system. Thought processes have much to do also with the development of an erection; fantasy alone may elicit the reflex. The brain, af-

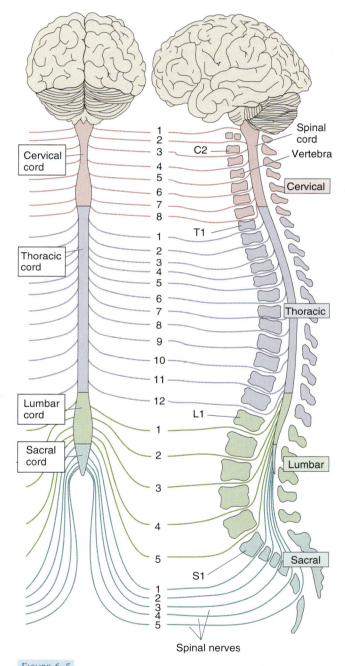

FIGURE 6-5 Cervical, thoracic, lumbar, and sacral regions of the spinal cord (left). The spinal cord is contained within the bony vertebral column (right). Spinal nerves are named for the level of the spinal cord at which they enter or exit.

ter all, *interprets* stimuli as erotic or non-erotic; the erection it-self is the reflex.

Just as erection depends on the normal functioning of spinal reflexes, ejaculation does too. Another spinal center controls the reflex involved in ejaculation; this one is located higher in the spinal cord, and the blood vessels of the penis are not involved. Continued tactile stimulation of the penis selectively stimulates this area of the spinal cord, which in turn sends signals to the internal sexual structures involved in the muscular contractions that eject semen from the body. As with the reflex of erection, cognitive factors are relevant. One's thoughts and personal interpretation of sexual stimuli may either assist or inhibit ejaculation. In other words, in both spinal reflexes, the brain is the key interpretive organ.

The neurological structures and processes underlying female sexual arousal and orgasm are presumably similar to those in men, although these events in women take longer, sometimes a lot longer. Women and men both should understand this important sexual difference. We use the word "presumably" because the neural pathways underlying the involvement of the spinal cord in female arousal and orgasm have not yet been fully investigated. However, a surprising discovery (Komisaruk, Gerdes, & Whipple, 1997; DeKoker, 1996) has shed some light on a nerve pathway that previously was not thought involved in sexual arousal and orgasm. An important nerve called the vagus courses through most of our internal organs. It is involved in such functions as vomiting, swallowing, and breathing. Because it does not come close to the spinal cord, scientists never considered it might have a role in sexuality. Reports of spinal-cord-injured women having orgasms, however, aroused attention in the scientific community. Despite the fact that these women had severed spinal cords, tactile stimulation in body areas above the level of spinal transsection seemed to reach the brain stem via the vagus nerve to give rise to orgasmic experiences. In these studies when women with lower spinal cord injuries engaged in genital self-stimulation for 12 minutes, increased thresholds to pain, increased heart rate, and increased blood pressure were measured; these commonly accompany orgasm. These women also reported menstrual discomfort during their periods. Apparently, sexual and other vaginal feelings can reach the brain through a pathway previously undiscovered. Similar research on spinal-cord injured men is currently underway.

As discussed in Chapter 3, despite the controversy surrounding female ejaculation, many women do in fact ejaculate, and fluid is released from the urethra at the time of orgasm. Such ejaculation is a predominantly local event involving stimulation of the Grafenberg area and the consequent pressure exerted on Skene's glands surrounding the urethra (Davidson, Darling, & Conway-Welch, 1989).

Up to this point, we have focused on the lower levels of the central nervous system. Yet some brain function is clearly involved in the perceptions of sexual stimuli and the arousal that sometimes follows (Fig. 6-6). But just exactly what does the brain *do* with erotic information? Note, first, that the brain

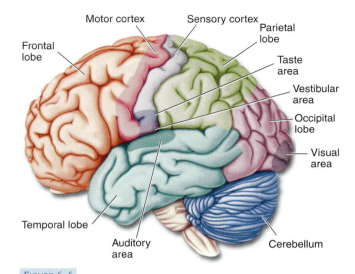

FIGURE 6-6 Lateral view of the human brain. Sensory areas indicate the locations in which incoming information is received and processed. Messages to muscles originate in the motor cortex. Our most uniquely human cognitive functions are mediated in the frontal lobes.

functions underlying sexual feeling and behavior involve *thinking,* or cognitive assessment. A person's evaluation of the environment, memories of the past, and emotional habits all clearly influence his or her sexuality and all involve brain functions.

One area of the brain with a large role in the emotional elements of sexual experience is the group of interconnected subcortical structures called the **limbic system.** The brain is divided down the middle by a central fissure into two cerebral hemispheres. These hemispheres have a wrinkled appearance and are covered by a layer of nerve cells just a few millimeters thick, called the *cerebral cortex* (the word "cortex" comes from an old Greek word meaning "bark"-the thin layer covering a tree). Our most "human" cognitive abilities are mediated by the cerebral cortex: learning, memory, judgment, perception, planning, and so on. The limbic system is a group of *sub*cortical structures, located underneath the cortex. Figure 6-7 illustrates the various structures of the limbic system. The limbic system plays a crucial role in the experience and expression of emotion. Scientists have discovered that electrically stimulating various areas of the limbic system promptly elicits erections in monkeys and the assumption of mating postures in rats. Electrical stimulation of other brain areas does not cause this effect. Apparently spinal cord reflexes, thinking, and subcortical functions all interact in the pleasurable aspects of sexual experiences.

The Autonomic Nervous System

As described above, sensory nerves carry information into the central nervous system, and motor nerves carry directions from the central nervous system to the muscles. Parts of the nervous system not included in the central nervous system are collectively referred to as the **peripheral nervous system.** An important part of the peripheral nervous system is the **autonomic nervous system;** "autonomic" means independent, au-

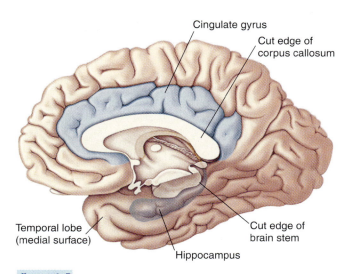

Cingulate gyrus

Cut edge of corpus callosum

Temporal lobe (medial surface)

Cut edge of brain stem

Hippocampus

FIGURE 6-7 The limbic system is a group of subcortical structures that are involved in the experience and expression of emotions—many relating to sexual stimuli.

tomatic, or involuntary. The autonomic nervous system controls many essential physiological functions without our being aware of its functioning, although it does have connections to the brain and spinal cord. Some of its activities are clearly related to sexual arousal and response.

The autonomic nervous system has two separate branches: the **sympathetic nervous system** and the **parasympathetic nervous system.** The former is composed of two chains of nerves and ganglia that run along both sides of the spinal cord. (A ganglion is an aggregation of nerve cells outside the central nervous system). The parasympathetic nervous system is made up of two localized neural centers at the top and the bottom of the spinal cord (Fig. 6-8). These two branches of the autonomic nervous system are anatomically separate and have different biological functions. In many ways, their functions are "antagonistic," that is, their activities are opposite one another. For example, the sympathetic nervous system is involved with "fight or flight" behaviors. It prepares us for emergencies, conflicts, or flight from conflict. Sympathetic arousal is associated with increased heart rate, increased blood pressure, increased breathing rate, and the stimulation of glucose production and release of glucose from the liver; these changes are adaptive at tense times. The hormones epinephrine and norepinephrine are released with sympathetic activation. In contrast, the parasympathetic nervous system helps the body return to normal after a fight or flight situation and keeps the body's physiological systems on an even keel throughout the day and night.

The autonomic nervous system is also closely related to sexual arousal and response. The parasympathetic nervous system's activities underlie sexual arousal and are involved in vaginal lubrication and erection. Once sexual arousal has occurred, the sympathetic nervous system mediates orgasm.

Overall, then, both the central nervous system and the autonomic nervous system are involved in sexual arousal and

response. While brain and spinal cord activity take place very promptly in response to sexual stimuli, the autonomic nervous system's responses take a little longer but are as important in the subjective experience of excitement and orgasm. Recent data also suggest that the sympathetic nervous system may be involved in perceptions of sexual arousal, as well as orgasmic experience. Historically, Kinsey, Pomeroy, Martin, and Gebhard (1953) suggested that sexual arousal in women was mediated primarily by the parasympathetic nervous system. Kaplan (1974) confirmed this finding but noted that orgasm results from sympathetic activation. However, Meston and Gorzalka (1996) demonstrated that the sympathetic nervous system may also play a part in arousal. Physical exercise plays a role in activating the sympathetic nervous system. These investigators found that subjects who had exercised vigorously on a bicycle had elevated levels of sexual arousal as measured by vaginal plethysmography when they later viewed erotic films compared with the control group. These effects were not apparent immediately after exercise but took about 15 minutes to take effect. These measured responses were purely physiological and were not accompanied by any *subjective* increase in sexual arousal.

Hormones and Sexual Arousal and Response

In the past, the nervous system and the **endocrine system** were considered separate and independent, but scientists today see these two important physiological entities as profoundly interrelated. Scientists today talk about "neuroendocrine" functions, because the nervous system affects glandular secretions and these hormones affect neural functioning. The effects of hormones can be highly variable. In some cases their action lasts only minutes, as in the case of a heart rate increase during moments of stress, threat, or excitement. In other instances, the effects of hormones occur over months or even years, such as with growth hormone secreted by the pituitary gland. Although the influence of hormones on behavior is clear and direct in animals, because humans have a well-developed cerebral cortex, most behavior is influenced much more by thinking and perception than simply by hormonal action.

As discussed in Chapter 3, tiny amounts of hormones can have a profound effect on sexual differentiation and the prenatal development of female and male body configurations. Specialists in the study of endocrine glands and hormones are called endocrinologists. This chapter will consider the effect of sex hormones on sex drive, arousal, and response. Hormonal actions can be both powerful and subtle at the same time. Human sexuality researchers make a distinction between the *organizing effects* and the *activating effects of hormones.* Organizing effects are ways in which hormones direct early physical development and, therefore, affect the anatomy and physiology of specific organs. Chapter 3 described how the prenatal secretion of androgens from a male embryo's testes causes the differentiation of external male genitalia and how the absence of this hormone fosters the differentiation of

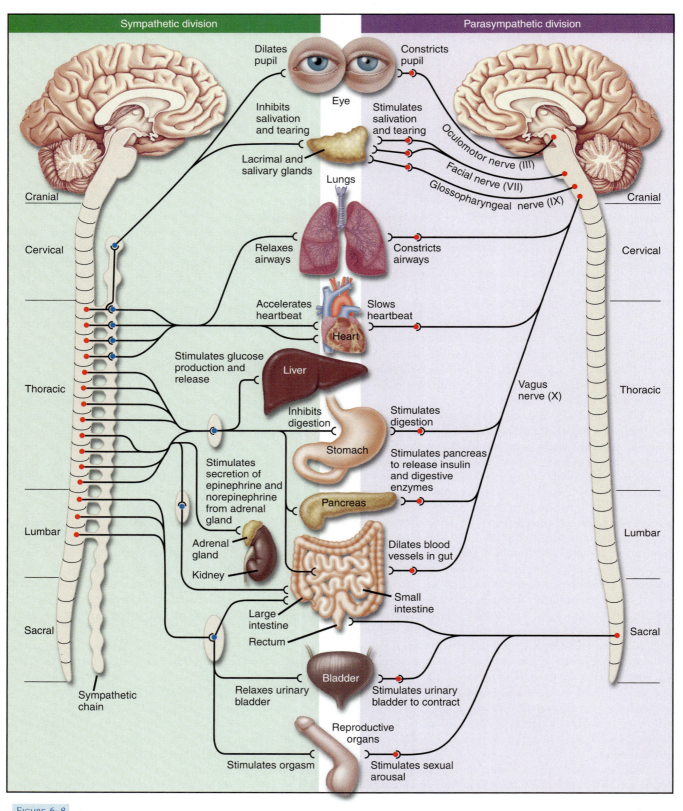

Sympathetic division

Parasympathetic division

Dilates pupil

Constricts pupil

Eye

Inhibits salivation and tearing

Stimulates salivation and tearing

Oculomotor nerve (III)

Lacrimal and salivary glands

Facial nerve (VII)

Glossopharyngeal nerve (IX)

Cranial

Cranial

Lungs

Cervical

Relaxes airways

Constricts airways

Cervical

Accelerates heartbeat

Slows heartbeat

Heart

Stimulates glucose production and release

Liver

Thoracic

Thoracic

Inhibits digestion

Stimulates digestion

Stomach

Stimulates secretion of epinephrine and norepinephrine from adrenal gland

Stimulates pancreas to release insulin and digestive enzymes

Pancreas

Adrenal gland

Vagus nerve (X)

Lumbar

Kidney

Dilates blood vessels in gut

Lumbar

Large intestine

Small intestine

Sacral

Rectum

Sacral

Bladder

Sympathetic chain

Relaxes urinary bladder

Stimulates urinary bladder to contract

Reproductive organs

Stimulates orgasm

Stimulates sexual arousal

FIGURE 6-8   The sympathetic and parasympathetic branches of the autonomic nervous system. The former manage the body's "fight or flight" responses to threats and stressful stimuli, while the latter help the body to return to normal after these types of experiences.

external female genitalia. In contrast, activating effects are the ways hormones affect the appearance or cessation of a specific behavior. Although organizing effects are easy to document experimentally, it is more difficult to prove the existence of clear and unambiguous hormone-behavior relationships in humans.

The hormone that has been most extensively studied in connection with sexual interest, arousal, and response is testosterone. Both women and men have this hormone. It is produced in a male's testes, in small amounts in a woman's ovaries, and in the adrenal glands of both sexes. Of course, men have far more than women. Investigators believe that testosterone has an activating effect on human sexual desire. Supporting evidence for this includes the fact that castration and antiandrogen drugs cause a pronounced lowering of a man's sex drive, although not always immediately. Because cognitive and psychosocial factors also play a powerful role in sexual desire, however, the lack of testosterone alone does not always immediately inhibit sexual desire in men. Another example of the impact of testosterone on male sexual desire is the sudden increase in sexual interest, and sometimes sexual behavior, that occurs with adolescence in males. Sex hormones not only have a powerful effect on changes in body configuration during this time but also are related to an increase in adolescent men's interest in the opposite sex. Again, testosterone does not act simply by itself; the wider psychosocial environment has tremendous influence on the form and direction of this sexual interest. Generally speaking, however, higher levels of testosterone are correlated with higher levels of sex drive and more frequent sexual activity.

One of the more interesting differences between women and men concerns the activating effects of the primary sex hormones. While the impact of testosterone on male sex drive is pretty clear, the same is not true of the effects of estrogen on a woman's sexual desires and inclinations. Although a woman's body produces relatively small quantities of testosterone, her body is far more sensitive to this small amount of testosterone than is a man's body (Bancroft, 1984). The small secretion of testosterone from a woman's ovaries and adrenal glands has an important impact on her sex drive, and generally, this "maintenance level" of testosterone secretion in women is meaningfully correlated with sexual arousal and responsiveness. During menopause, when there is at first a gradual decrease in the secretion of estrogen from a woman's ovaries and then later a profound decrease and ultimately a cessation of this hormone, testosterone secretion from her ovaries is diminished significantly as well. *Hormone replacement therapy* helps avoid some of the health problems that often accompany diminished estrogen secretion, such as osteoporosis and increased risk of coronary artery disease. Recently, some estrogen supplementation products include a small amount of testosterone, which has a generally enjoyable, facilitating effect on an older woman's sexual interest and responsiveness (Sarrel, Dobay, & Wiita, 1998). The decision to use hormone replacement therapy is made by the woman and her physician.

Heiman, Rowland, Hatch, and Gladue (1991) studied the effects of erotic stimuli (sexually explicit videotapes) on physiological and endocrine changes in women compared to women observing a neutral videotape. Physiological measures of sexual arousal were noted more in the women watching the videotapes with sexual content than in women watching other tapes. However, endocrine changes are more difficult to determine. The amounts of cortisol (an adrenal hormone), prolactin, luteinizing hormone, and testosterone in the bloodstream were measured before and during presentation of the erotic videotapes. Interestingly, these researchers found no differences between the two groups in any of the four hormones related to sexual stimulation from viewing the videotapes.

It is difficult to point to a direct, prompt cause-and-effect relationship between sex hormones and sexual arousal and responsiveness. It is risky to suggest that taking testosterone automatically helps someone with declining sexual interest and performance because this does not always occur. Even low doses of testosterone have some dangerous side-effects in older men, and it may promote the growth of prostate cancer. Also, the rate at which natural testosterone secretion diminishes in women and men is not always easy to predict. With other drugs available for the treatment of lack of sexual responsiveness, this issue may become less important in the future. Nonetheless, testosterone replacement therapy can, when properly used under medical supervision, have a facilitating effect on sex drive in both women and men.

In recent years, much has been written about the supposedly beneficial effects of low doses of *melatonin*. This hormone is secreted from the pituitary gland, and some investigators have suggested that melatonin may enhance sexual arousal and responsiveness. However, we know of no persuasive, systematic scientific investigations that demonstrate beneficial effects of this hormone on human sexual response.

Patterns of Human Sexual Response

The pioneering efforts of Masters and Johnson began with recording data without any existing scheme for categorizing and analyzing the physiological changes that accompany sexual arousal and response. These laboratory results led to the development of more comprehensive approaches to human sexual responses. The accuracy and reproducibility of these data along with the ingenuity of the research methods built the foundation on which most subsequent sexual research on erotic response is based. While later researchers criticized the lack of a psychological perspective in this work, the physiology of human sexual response serves as the basis for further cognitive and emotional analysis.

Masters and Johnson's Human Sexual Response Cycle

In all, 382 unmarried or married females and 312 unmarried or married males volunteered as subjects in this research, including 118 female and 27 male prostitutes. By Masters and

Johnson's own admission, their sample could not be called large or randomly selected, yet in many ways was representative of the wider population. Data from this sample for over 11 years revealed compelling consistencies in the four-stage sequence of arousal and response. Masters and Johnson emphasize that there is significant variation in responses among men and women, but what follows is true of most people most of the time (Fig. 6-9).

FEMALE SEXUAL AROUSAL AND RESPONSE
Excitement Phase

Erotic feelings build gradually over time, generally more gradually in women than in men. While a woman's thoughts certainly play a major role in sexual excitement, the discussion here will focus primarily on the body (Fig. 6-10). Heart rate and blood pressure gradually increase throughout the excite-

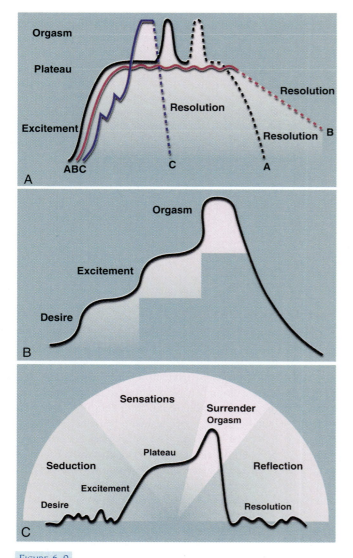

FIGURE 6-9   Three approaches to human sexual response. A. The Masters and Johnson sexual response cycle. B. The approach of Helen Singer Kaplan. C. The perspective of David Reed.

ment phase. **Vasocongestion** is the gradual accumulation of blood in blood vessels, in this case, in the vagina and lower pelvis. Because of this, the coloration of interior vaginal tissues changes. As blood accumulates, women often feel warmth and some swelling in the area, usually accompanied by a viscous vaginal secretion. This slippery liquid functions to facilitate comfortable penile penetration; physiological excitement in both women and men prepares for the comfortable entry of the penis into the vagina. This lubrication is somewhat alkaline, although changes during the sexual response cycle. As discussed in a later chapter, as women get older, there is progressively less vaginal lubrication. Accompanying these changes near the opening of the vagina are other changes deep inside. The innermost two-thirds of the vagina becomes longer and expands significantly. While lubrication, puffiness, and warmth are easy to notice, these deeper vaginal changes may not be apparent at all. During continuing excitement there is also a slight change in the orientation of the uterus with respect to the vagina; it seems to "sit up" a little and moves forward from its position before stimulation. While all this is happening, the labia minora and labia majora gradually become larger and softer and change to a darker, sometimes brownish or purple hue. The head of the clitoris becomes wider and the clitoris becomes longer. As sexual tension gradually builds, the head of the clitoris extends beyond the clitoral prepuce and is more exposed and, therefore, more sensitive to direct touch. Clitoral changes during excitement vary considerably among women. The length of the clitoral shaft may be more noticeable during self-stimulation of the wider genital area and somewhat less obvious during sexual intercourse.

During sexual excitement, a woman's breasts change (Fig. 6-11). Nipple erection occurs early during arousal, as does a gradual increase in the overall size of the breasts. Generally, the larger a woman's breasts are, the more apparent is this swelling in the excitement phase, caused by the increased flow of blood into the vessels of the breast. During excitement, the nipples may feel a bit harder while other breast tissue often feels softer to the touch.

In addition to vasocongestion in the genital area, a "sex flush" often appears over a woman's breasts, neck, and upper abdomen. As sexual arousal builds during the excitement phase, this change in skin coloration may become progressively more pronounced. For many, one of the pleasures of sex with the lights on is that these skin signs of arousal are more apparent, and people like seeing that their sexual sharing is producing a pleasurable response.

The Plateau Phase

With continued erotic stimulation, further physical changes occur along with the individual's perception of growing sexual pleasure. One of the most consistent aspects of the plateau phase in women involves the slight retraction of the clitoral shaft and glans beneath its hood. The exact extent and latency of clitoral retraction may depend on the nature and duration of sexual stimulation. For example, Masters and Johnson note

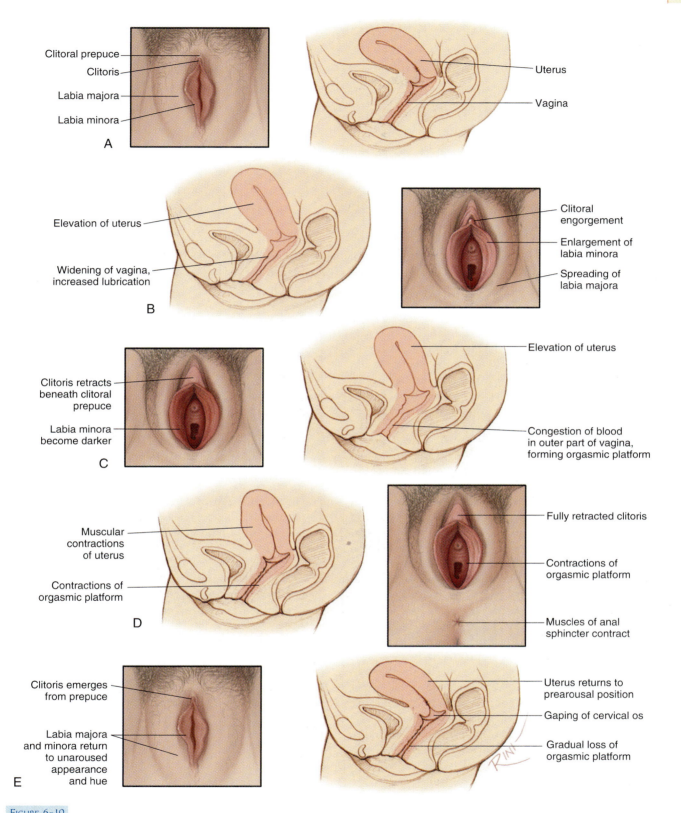

FIGURE 6-10 External genital changes during the female sexual response cycle according to Masters and Johnson: A. The unaroused female. B. Excitement. C. Plateau. D. Orgasm. E. Resolution.

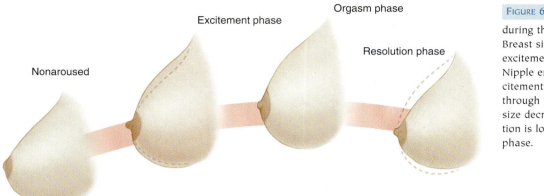

Nonaroused

Excitement phase

Orgasm phase

Resolution phase

FIGURE 6-11   Breast changes during the sexual response cycle. Breast size increases during the excitement and orgasm phases. Nipple erection begins in the excitement phase and continues through the orgasm phase. Breast size decreases and nipple erection is lost during the resolution phase.

that with sexual intercourse or fondling of the breasts, clitoral changes occur later in the plateau rather than earlier. In contrast, with pressing or manipulation of the mons veneris, clitoral retraction occurs earlier. In the plateau phase, the labia majora and labia minora become further engorged with blood and swell accordingly.

The most prominent physiological change during the plateau phase occurs in the outer third of the vagina. Masters and Johnson refer to this highly localized vasocongestion as an "orgasmic platform," which creates a significant narrowing to the opening of the vagina. This tightening effect creates a firm fit of the penis in the vagina, increasing tactile stimulation on the shaft of the penis and enhancing pleasure for both the man and the woman. If the woman does not have an orgasm, it may take as long as 20 to 30 minutes for the orgasmic platform to return to its usual dimensions. In the plateau phase, the uterus loses some of the elevation it gained during the excitement phase. In women who have a "tipped" or retroflexed uterus, these changes in the orientation of the uterus and cervix in response to erotic stimulation do not occur. Also in the plateau phase the inner two-thirds of the vagina becomes significantly wider and deeper. This "tenting effect" creates a small pool into which semen is deposited when the man ejaculates.

The areola of a woman's breasts swells so substantially during the plateau phase that it may look as though some of the nipple erection that occurred during the excitement phase has been lost, because much of the base of each nipple is concealed by the enlarged areola. Vasocongestion in the breasts causes further enlargement in the overall size of the breasts. This enlargement occurs much more in women who have breast-fed an infant than in those who have not; in women who have nursed, the breast may increase by as much as one-fourth its size (Masters & Johnson, 1966, page 29). The sex flush described earlier may grow in intensity or vividness, and muscular tension throughout the body may increase substantially. Heart rate, breathing rate, and blood pressure all continue to increase. The pulse rate may more than double from its normal resting rate during plateau.

Overall, the plateau phase represents a heightened state of sexual tension and desire and the experience of enhanced erotic arousal and enjoyment. Most individuals at this stage are fully aware that there is more to be experienced and savored. While it is appropriate and normal for the plateau phase to progress to the next stage (orgasm), it does not do so in all cases and may leave one or both individuals frustrated and feeling incompletely stimulated. This is discussed in the later chapter on sexual dysfunctions.

The Orgasm Phase

The sudden release of the tension that built during the plateau phase is an orgasm, in lay language also called "coming," "getting off," or a "climax." It is a powerful, pleasurable feeling that focuses the person's attention and thoughts entirely on sexual feelings and anatomy. In an evolutionary perspective, orgasms feel good because behavior that leads to perpetuation of the species is reinforced by intensely pleasurable sensations.

Because the clitoris retracts beneath its prepuce during the plateau phase, direct observation of this structure during orgasm is virtually impossible; Masters and Johnson never observed or recorded clitoral changes during orgasm. Nonetheless, powerful, pleasurable feelings often involve the clitoris during orgasm. As noted in Chapter 4, both clitoral and vaginal enjoyment may accompany orgasm. Rhythmic tensions frequently accompany orgasms, and these may spread throughout the pelvic area.

During orgasm specific changes take place in the vagina. There is a rapid loss of vasocongestion at the vaginal opening with the resulting loss of the orgasmic platform. Muscular contractions occur both at the orgasmic platform and in the musculature surrounding the anus and the urethra. Vaginal muscular contractions are rhythmic, strong, and in some cases prolonged, with almost a second between them in the beginning of orgasm. As these contractions continue, they are progressively farther apart and they grow less intense. A woman's report of the strength of her orgasm is generally correlated with the number and overall duration of vaginal muscular contractions accompanying orgasm. It is not unusual for more than a dozen vaginal contractions to accompany orgasm. Bohlen, Held, Sanderson, and Boyer (1982) measured the muscular contractions accompanying female orgasm and found that they lasted from 13 to 51 sec-

THE WORDS WE USE TO DESCRIBE ORGASMS

The language people use to describe arousal and orgasm is incredibly diverse and sometimes highly unique and personal. Throughout this book we have emphasized the importance of developing a good sexual vocabulary for communicating accurately and honestly about sexuality both with one's sexual partner and with health care professionals. Nonetheless, people naturally use a wide range of expression to describe something so intense and enjoyable. Some adults use cute expressions they learned as children because they have not learned a more precise way of describing these feelings. Other adults who do have a mature sexual vocabulary still enjoy using slang to describe their anatomy, behaviors, and feelings. While many are comfortable with the terms *penis, vagina,* and *testicles,* others talk about their *tallywacker, wazoo,* or *nuts.* Because the experiences of sexual arousal and response can vary so much among different people, it is natural that their way of talking about these things varies much as well.

People also use analogies to describe their sexual responses, describing their orgasms as "explosions," "flying," "throbbing," or "bursts of energy." A common analogy is feeling like a cork popping from a bottle of champagne (Proctor, Wagner, & Butler, 1974). Such expressions can be highly idiosyncratic. Because verbal descriptions of orgasms alone probably cannot fully communicate the power and intensity of this experience, *both verbal and nonverbal* aspects of orgasms say the most about what an individual is experiencing. The wonderful combination of words, heavy breathing, grunting, moaning, and vigorous pelvic thrusting might seem to "say it all" but still falls short of conveying the experience itself.

---

onds. The increased tension in the musculature of the orgasmic platform increases the tautness around the penis, helping keep semen inside the vagina to increase the likelihood of conception.

During orgasm, muscular contractions of the uterus have also been recorded, but these are irregular in intensity and duration and it is difficult to generalize about these. Generally, uterine muscular contractions begin high in the uterus and progress downwards toward the cervix. They begin at about the same time as the contractions of the orgasmic platform. Heart rate, breathing rate, and blood pressure generally reach their peaks during orgasm. Heart rate may reach 180 beats per minute, with a respiration over 40 breaths per minute. Blood pressures as high as 220/130 have been noted. Other involuntary motor behaviors may accompany orgasm, including uncoordinated movements of the arms, legs, neck, and torso. Some women arch their backs, and others may (sometimes embarrassingly) suddenly develop a cramp in their legs or feet. Uninhibited vocalizations or moaning are also common.

Whether orgasm derives from interpersonal manual stimulation, sexual intercourse, masturbation, or the use of vibratory aids, steady, continued stimulation is usually most effective in eliciting and prolonging orgasm. Many women never have orgasms during penis-in-the-vagina intercourse although they may do so readily during masturbation. It is often a good idea for a woman to communicate to her partner if they are doing anything that detracts from the gradual build-up of sexual tension and its release. Remember, again, that sexual arousal and response occur in a psychosocial/communication setting.

The Resolution Phase

In the resolution phase, the woman's body returns to its pre-excitement state. In later life resolution occurs more quickly than in women in their 20s and 30s, but the feelings of peace, satisfaction, and repose that accompany resolution are no less enjoyable. Many women report that in this phase they especially enjoy being held, cuddled, nuzzled, and caressed. The intimacy shared during intercourse now has a more emotional than physical texture.

The physical changes that occur during resolution are fairly straightforward. In a matter of seconds after orgasm, the clitoris returns to its usual unstimulated position beneath the clitoral hood. This occurs more quickly than the gradual dissipation of the orgasmic platform at the vaginal opening. The slight swelling in the size and diameter of the glans of the clitoris during arousal is lost very gradually. Masters and Johnson observed that this process may take as long as 5 to 10 minutes, or in rare instances up to 15 to 30 minutes. In a woman who entered the plateau phase but did not have an orgasm, clitoral enlargement may continue for hours after all erotic stimulation has stopped.

After sexual intercourse with ejaculation, if no barrier contraceptive method was used, there is an accumulation of semen at the back of the vagina, sometimes called the "seminal pool." During resolution, the cervix is "dipped" or immersed in the seminal pool, which facilitates the chances of sperm en-

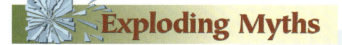

Exploding Myths

Good Sex Means Good Orgasms

Many women and men believe that orgasms are an indication that sex is enjoyable and fulfilling. While orgasms certainly feel good and leave most people with a wonderful feeling, they are not, in our opinion, the be-all and end-all of all sexual experience. Many women and men have wonderful sexual experiences without having orgasms or ejaculations. Nonetheless, there is a popular myth that orgasms are "proof" that men are good lovers and women receptive, sensuous, and responsive—that if a woman has sexual intercourse without having an orgasm, then something must be wrong with her, him, or them. The myth that orgasms validate a woman's affection or a man's effectiveness as a lover has unfortunately created an expectation among many woman that they have to "come" or their partners won't feel like "real men."

Because of this pressure to respond, many women and men at one time or another have faked an orgasm to show their partner that they are a good lover or because they knew no other way to end intercourse. One writer has suggested that men need some kind of indicator that their partners really liked having sex with them, and what better than a loud moaning or screaming orgasm (Zilbergeld, 1992). A popular writer has reported that of 40 women she interviewed, all said they had faked orgasms at least half the time they had intercourse (Brothers, 1982).

Ideally, women and men who make love together know each other well and understand the fact that sexual responsiveness "on demand" may have nothing to do with feelings of love, closeness, attachment, nurturance, and safety. Few might consider it "dishonest" to fake an orgasm, but authenticity and a nonjudgmental approach are important for genuine intimacy.

---

tering the uterus and subsequently the fallopian tubes to lead possibly to conception. The cervical opening may also widen slightly during resolution. The uterus descends a little to its position before sexual arousal. Heart rate, breathing rate, and blood pressure return to normal during the resolution phase. Any sex flush that developed will gradually dissipate. Many women experience noticeable perspiration during resolution as well, which can be quite profuse.

Finally, during resolution a woman's breasts decrease to their usual size, as engorgement of the veins diminishes throughout the tissue. The nipple retracts and the surrounding areola loses its swollen appearance, leading to the appearance that the nipples are again erect although they only look that way because more of the nipple is visible. This process takes 5 to 10 minutes after orgasm. Generally women who have not breast-fed an infant lose their breast enlargement more slowly than women who have.

In his book, *The New Male Sexuality* (1992), Bernie Zilbergeld comments that many women need to feel emotionally connected to their partners after sexual intercourse. Regardless of whether the intimacy was planned or not, many women say that these moments of close togetherness are very important and desirable. A man who abruptly separates himself physically from his partners after ejaculation sends an undesirable message: "I got what I want; I'm leaving." One woman in

Zilbergeld's study remarked, "For me, the buildup and the afterwards are at least as important as the actual sex. It's just a wonderful sense of connection that I have to have" (page 198).

MALE SEXUAL AROUSAL AND RESPONSE

Because a man's external genitalia are visible and erection is such a clear change, one might think that male sexual arousal and response are obvious. Yet sexual excitement, orgasm, and ejaculation involve a number of fascinating and complex physiological events (Fig. 6-12).

Excitement Phase

Erection occurs from vasocongestion in the pelvic area. Erection involves an elevation of the shaft of the penis and a slight retraction of the glans. The scrotum is drawn closer to the body, and its skin stiffens and "puckers" somewhat, and the testes are elevated. How quickly an erection takes place varies significantly, but it generally takes longer in an older man. (The effects of aging on human sexual arousal and response are discussed in Chapter 13). The nature and consistency of sexual stimulation affect the development of an erection, and some men need vigorous and prolonged stimulation while others become erect quickly with little or no physical stimulation. The type of erotic stimulation that fosters excitement also varies considerably. Visual, auditory, and tactile stimuli may all

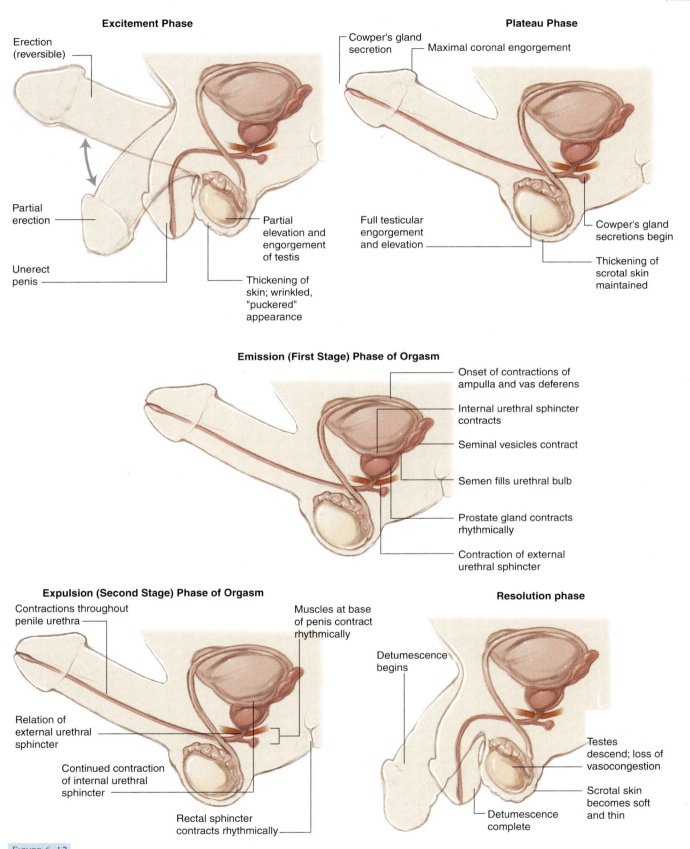

Excitement Phase

Erection (reversible)

Partial erection

Unerect penis

Partial elevation and engorgement of testis

Thickening of skin; wrinkled, "puckered" appearance

Plateau Phase

Cowper's gland secretion — Maximal coronal engorgement

Full testicular engorgement and elevation

Cowper's gland secretions begin

Thickening of scrotal skin maintained

Emission (First Stage) Phase of Orgasm

Onset of contractions of ampulla and vas deferens

Internal urethral sphincter contracts

Seminal vesicles contract

Semen fills urethral bulb

Prostate gland contracts rhythmically

Contraction of external urethral sphincter

Expulsion (Second Stage) Phase of Orgasm

Contractions throughout penile urethra

Muscles at base of penis contract rhythmically

Relation of external urethral sphincter

Continued contraction of internal urethral sphincter

Rectal sphincter contracts rhythmically

Resolution phase

Detumescence begins

Testes descend; loss of vasocongestion

Scrotal skin becomes soft and thin

Detumescence complete

FIGURE 6-12   Internal and external genital changes during the male sexual response cycle.

be involved, or fantasy alone may produce an erection. Distraction can lead to a sudden loss of tumescence. It is also normal for a man to experience brief periods in which the erection is lost but then regained.

Just as women's breasts change during excitement, similar changes sometimes occur in men's nipples. Masters and Johnson reported that 60% of their male subjects showed nipple erection, usually later in the excitement phase. Nipple erection may persist long after resolution, up to an hour or more. The sex flush also sometimes occurs in men, often developing late in the excitement phase or well into the plateau phase. Generalized muscular contractions often occur late in the excitement phase with both voluntary and involuntary muscular tension. As in women, heart rate, breathing rate, and blood pressure are also increasing.

The duration of excitement depends on the couple's interaction. When foreplay is leisurely and relaxed, arousal may build slowly. When it is more focused and urgent, excitement may develop suddenly. Different people have different preferences, but most couples like to get "in sync" with each other.

Plateau Phase

In the plateau phase, the penis further increases slightly in diameter. This is more obvious toward the glans. The penis may also have a slight color change at this time, becoming a bit darker, due to continued vasocongestion. This color change does not occur in all men and varies widely. As the plateau phase continues, a man's testes are drawn more closely to the body. Masters and Johnson explained that for men to experience full ejaculatory discharge of their semen, the testes must be fully drawn toward the body. If sexual interaction during the plateau phase is cut short and the testes have not been retracted fully before ejaculation, the semen leaves the body with less force. The testes also increase in size during the plateau phase, from 50% up to a 100% increase. This occurs due to vasocongestion in the testes; generally, the longer the plateau phase lasts, the larger the testes become, the higher they are retracted, and the more forceful this ejaculation is.

In the plateau phase the secretions of Cowper's glands often cause a visible accumulation of clear liquid at the tip of the penis; in some men this occurs in the excitement phase. Chapter 11 explains why this is one reason that coitus interruptus is ineffective for contraception. The nipples do not change much in appearance during the plateau phase. Generalized body tension continues to build, particularly apparent in the man-on-top position while he is supporting his weight and may feel shaky because of involuntary muscular spasms. Heavy breathing, a fast heart rate, and further increases in blood pressure all occur in the plateau phase. Loving and encouraging words can add much to this build-up of arousal, and one's partner generally feels an especially effective lover when hearing them! Sometimes, both women and men need to be reminded that "talk" isn't just another four-letter word (Zilbergeld, 1992, page 191).

The Orgasm Phase

Orgasm in men involves rhythmic contractions of tissues and muscles throughout the genitalia and pelvis. Muscles surrounding the urethra, the corpora cavernosa, and deep in the groin and hip area all contract to help force semen out of the body. Masters and Johnson showed that these contractions begin at intervals less than a second and become longer after the first few spurts of semen. These contractions continue at more irregular intervals for several more seconds, still releasing semen but with far less force. Learning about one's orgasms can be a very interesting exercise in self-awareness. Many men observe that the moments after the bulk of ejaculate has left the penis are the most intensely pleasurable. Orgasms can last from a few to many seconds. During this time there is little change in the size and position of the testes.

Orgasm in men is often accompanied by vigorous pelvic thrusting, involuntary muscular spasms, and shouting, grunting, or other verbalizations, although less dynamic responses are also common and normal. Just as women often feel a need to show that they have had an orgasm in order to reassure their partners of their ability as lovers, men often feel the same way.

In men, orgasm is often described as a two-stage process of "emission" and "expulsion." In the emission phase, seminal fluids are held momentarily at a point close to the tiny muscles surrounding the urethra where it exits from the bladder. At this point of "ejaculatory inevitability" a man knows he is about to ejaculate. In the expulsion stage, the rhythmic penile and pelvic muscular contractions begin, and semen is forced through the part of the urethra that runs through the penis. Some men feel the emission stage as "having an orgasm" and the expulsion stage as "coming."

If the man developed a sex flush, it may become more obvious during orgasm. Muscular tension during emission and expulsion become intense. Masters and Johnson recorded heart rates above 180 beats per minute in men during orgasm, and blood pressure and the breathing rate also peak at this time, although some men hold their breath while engaging in vigorous pelvic thrusting at orgasm. Many men perspire profusely after ejaculation, even if sexual interaction was not vigorous. The soles of the feet and palms of the hands are most likely to be wet with perspiration, often along with many other areas on the surface of the body. Masters and Johnson reported that about one-third of their male subjects reacted during orgasm with a significant perspiration.

The Resolution Phase

As a woman's body returns to its pre-arousal state during the resolution phase, so does a man's. The shortening and softening of the penis, called **detumescence**, occurs in two stages. The primary stage takes place soon after ejaculation, when the penis decreases in size but is still about 50% larger than it is when unstimulated. Later, the penis decreases in size to its unstimulated, usual size. After prolonged intercourse the primary stage of detumescence is extended and the secondary stage delayed. Generally, with intense, prolonged erotic stimulation, detumescence takes longer and the penis is slower to return to its unstimulated appearance. Masters and Johnson reported that if the penis is left in the vagina after ejaculation, detumescence of the penis may be delayed significantly, but if intimate closeness is interrupted and the man is distracted after intercourse, full detumescence may occur quickly.

After orgasm and ejaculation, men enter the **refractory period.** "Refractory" in this context means "unresponsive," and at this time continued erotic stimulation will not re-arouse the male, who cannot soon attain another erection. In younger men the refractory period may last an hour or so, whereas in older men it may last several hours or even a day.

During resolution, the testes return to their pre-excitement size and return to their usual lower position in the scrotum. Longer periods of erotic stimulation in the plateau and orgasm phases generally delay testicular and scrotal changes, and they may not return to their unstimulated stage for some time. Heart rate slows, breathing frequency decreases, and blood pressure returns to normal in the resolution phase. The sex flush dissipates very quickly.

Just as many women desire to be held and cuddled after intercourse, many men too report strong feelings of closeness and savor this personal time together, although much less has been written about this issue among men.

Helen Singer Kaplan's Three-Stage Model

Masters and Johnson's *Human Sexual Response* was published in 1966. Another way of analyzing the changes that occur during human sexual response was suggested by Dr. Helen Singer Kaplan in 1979. Kaplan was a sex therapist with a background, training, and experience different from that of Masters, a physician who specialized in obstetrics and gynecology and whose medical orientation contributed to laboratory-oriented ways of measuring the physiology of arousal and response.

Kaplan's conceptualization is different from that of Masters and Johnson in that she labels the first stage of arousal and response *"desire"* (Figure 6-9B). Kaplan felt psychological factors are critical early in a person's sexual excitement. The other stages in Kaplan's model are *"excitement"* and *"orgasm."* The physiological events occurring in Kaplan's three stages are the same as in Masters and Johnson's four stages, of course, but with a different conceptualization of the first stage, *"desire."*

THE DESIRE PHASE

Earlier we referred to the importance of a person's sexual value system and how it colors one's world and perceptions of erotic stimuli. Stimuli that for some are arousing, for example, may provoke anxiety and fear in others. Such differences depend on one's personal past as a developing child, adolescent, and mature adult. There are no certain, unvarying stimuli that carry the same sexual meaning for everyone. Therefore, desire is very idiosyncratic and personal and can be affected by many different considerations, including general health, psychological well-being, and medications.

Desire involves the mind. While Masters and Johnson observed and measured sexual arousal by focusing on its reflexive nature, Kaplan emphasized the importance of perception, memory, judgment, and other cognitive processes. Sexual desire also has a wilful quality, involving a purposeful decision to feel or suppress sexual desire. One who is tired or depressed, for example, might have to make a psychological effort to feel sexual yearning. Similarly, at times when sexual thoughts and arousal would be disruptive, one can focus on something else.

Kaplan's model clearly distinguishes between desire as a psychological issue and the solely physical first stages of response in the approach of Masters and Johnson. Both approaches are important and provide insight into human arousal and response.

THE EXCITEMENT PHASE

In Kaplan's second stage, vasocongestive responses of the pelvis and genitalia are prominent, corresponding to what Masters and Johnson discovered about penile erection and vaginal lubrication. A generalized, whole body increase in muscular tension (myotonia) is prominent during this phase along with a modest increase in heart rate, blood pressure, and respiration rate. For Kaplan, these physiological changes are continuous with the plateau stage, where sexual excitement continues to build. Kaplan's model also describes excitement and plateau as closely related and not separable in any meaningful way.

THE ORGASM PHASE

The third and final stage of Kaplan's model is orgasm, with the physiological changes described earlier. Resolution is not included in her scheme. While Kaplan appropriately emphasized the importance of cognitive and emotional factors preceding sexual excitement, it seems odd that she had little to say about similar psychological matters after two people have shared intimacy. Kaplan apparently felt that the return to preexcitement levels of physiological arousal did not comprise a coherent structure meriting a separate stage designation.

Thinking, Perceiving, and Sexual Arousal and Response

Masters and Johnson's and Kaplan's approaches to human sexual response are now classic and widely followed. In more recent years, new theories continue to be developed that emphasize perceptual and thought processes involved in how people perceive erotic elements in the environment and respond to them. This more recent focus on the psychological dimension is natural, since Masters and Johnson so thoroughly covered the medical and physical dimension.

Two of these newer approaches are those of David Reed (cited in Francoeur, 1991) and Eileen M. Palace (1995). Both of these models share something significant: a moment-by-moment attention to simultaneous events in mind and body. Reed developed what he called the *erotic stimulus pathway model* (Figure 6-9C). Reed built on the work of Masters and Johnson and suggested a sequence of changes he named *seduc-*

tion, sensations, surrender, and *reflection.* His model focuses on both physiological changes and the psychosocial environment . For Reed, desire and excitement are essential parts of seduction, which involves both attraction and charm. In seduction, people give themselves permission to think and feel sexually and attempt to present themselves in a way intended to be perceived as erotic by their someone else. While the word "seduction" is sometimes used to mean taking unfair advantage of someone, Reed used the term differently. The seduction process, therefore, involves arousal, which sometimes takes place over an appreciable length of time. The word "process" is important here: feelings of seduction often grow slowly, even imperceptibly,

during the development of desire, arousal, and focused sexual interest. Seduction is often prolonged and patient.

For Reed, *sensations* correspond to the latter part of excitement and the plateau phase as described by Masters and Johnson. During this phase people become acutely, sometimes hypnotically focused on erotic information from the senses. Many people report an enhanced acuity of touch, smell, and vision for erotic experience. One's interpretation of such perceptions is a cognitive experience accompanying other thinking about one's body and one's partner's body, but there is still often an element of primal feeling along with these more rational, interpretive experiences.

OUR PERCEPTIONS AND RESPONSES TO OUR PARTNER'S SEXUAL AROUSAL

So far we have looked at what happens in the bodies of women and men during sexual arousal and response. Most people are aware to some extent of what is happening inside themselves, but are men and women fully aware of the responses happening in their partners as well? Or are most people too caught up in their own feelings to pay much attention to exactly what is happening to their partners? At the outset we should note that men and women seem to differ, at least in our culture, in how easily they communicate sexual thoughts, feelings, and desires (Reinisch, 1990, page 101). In general, some women are not as comfortable initiating sex or verbally communicating their pleasures, annoyances, or outright discomforts during physical intimacy.

Misunderstanding what one's partner might like or desire is common. For example, during sexual excitement a man's erection may be obvious and the woman's vaginal secretions might be noticeable. Arousal in and of itself can be enjoyable, however, and either the woman or the man may not desire to promptly engage in penis-in-the-vagina intercourse. Just seeing that one's partner is excited does not necessarily mean one must proceed immediately to penetration. The same is true when a woman or man feels their partner approaching orgasm. Does this mean that they want to proceed as quickly as possible? Many individuals say their most enjoyable sexual feelings occur in a prolonged plateau phase. Couples commonly pause or delay the sexual build-up to enjoy it longer.

Because women often need a little more time to reach orgasm, it is a good idea for a couple to develop a clear pattern of communication by which a woman can signal her approaching readiness. This is important also as a couple gets older; Chapter 13 describes how with normal aging the plateau phase lasts longer in both women and men. One should not simply assume that one's partner is about to have an orgasm just because their pelvic thrusting is more vigorous. Talking to one's partner can be important for communicating one's feelings and responsiveness.

One of the most common incompatibilities in couples involves the final stage of response, resolution. Because this phase involves a return to pre-excitement levels of sexual feeling, some people believe that their partner is no longer interested in touching, cuddling, talking, or kissing. Actually, many people would like to continue to enjoy being close to their partners but have difficulty communicating this desire. With continued sexual stimulation some women can re-enter the plateau phase and have one or more additional orgasms. Most men, however cannot do this and enter the refractory period (Reinisch, 1990, page 83-84). It is a myth that men just want to nod off to sleep after intercourse and leave their female partners feeling alone. The more one understands the human sexual response cycle, however, the better one is able to communicate feelings, requests, and suggestions in a supportive, nonjudgmental way.

Reed's third stage is called *surrender.* Here one relinquishes restraint and gives in to the pleasures of the moment. One submits to high sexual arousal levels and yields to the desire for orgasm. During plateau, a person is more or less aware that orgasmic response is approaching but can delay or slow down that approach. In surrender, one stops such maneuvers and "lets go." "Surrender" in this context involves liberation and the free expression of sexual response. Not everyone can easily let go, however, and sometimes an excessive need for control and/or manipulation hinders full, uninhibited feelings of release. In Victorian times, for example, many men associated orgasm with loss of control over their own bodies and thereby felt guilt with orgasm. A young woman raised to think that "good girls" don't have orgasms may also feel guilt and ambivalence with building sexual arousal.

Reed's final stage is called *reflection,* which coincides with resolution. Reed's assumption here, with which we agree, is that it is common and normal for people to think about their behaviors. When intimacy has been fulfilling and liberating, one is likely to assess the experience as positive and may even feel more "sexually competent" the next time. If the experience involved feelings of shame, guilt, and failure, however, the person may become apprehensive about intimate relations in the future. Although reflection is a private experience, it is generally good to share one's feelings with one's partner and it often helps one feel better for doing so. In some ways Reed's scheme is a refinement of the work of Kaplan and Masters and Johnson.

The role of cognitive and perceptual processes in sexual arousal has been further explored experimentally by Palace (1995). This research emphasizes that becoming sexually excited is not primarily reflexive but that what one thinks and feels plays a major role. It has been found that generalized autonomic nervous system arousal may play an important role in sexual excitement. Palace demonstrated that viewing films that are likely to provoke anxiety or sexual excitement increases the likelihood that a person will respond physiologically to sexual stimuli, presumably because both anxiety and sexual arousal result from activation of the sympathetic branch of the autonomic nervous system. Interestingly, women subjects who were told that their physiological measures indicated sexual arousal when this was not true reported increased erotic arousal to sexual stimuli and also showed increased genital arousal. When this "false feedback" is combined with general autonomic nervous system arousal, these subjects reported high levels of erotic responsiveness and had elevated genital arousal measured by photophythsmography. In other words, believing one is sexually aroused may be sufficient to cause some physiological arousal even when the belief is based on false information. Palace's work supports the role of cognitive and perceptual events in arousal. This research was based on the responses of women to erotic stimuli and may not generalize to men. Palace points out, however, that men know when they are becoming erect and, therefore, have a clear indication of excitement. Women, in contrast, cannot directly see genital changes that indicate growing erotic arousal. Maybe Sigmund Freud was correct when he said our most sensitive erogenous zone is located between our ears!

The contributions of Reed and Palace are important because they demonstrate that people do not reflexively and unthinkingly respond to erotic stimuli. Our memories, preferences, thoughts, judgments, and perceptions play a central role in what "turns us on" and how we respond or do not respond. As we noted at the beginning of this section, humans take in information, evaluate it, and act on it, and this sequence of events can be both highly complex and personal.

FACTORS AFFECTING SEXUAL AROUSAL AND RESPONSE

A meaningful understanding of human sexual response ideally includes not only biological facts but also useful information about psychosocial issues and communication strategies. We call this a **climate of psychological safety,** by which we mean that two individuals approach a sexual experience willingly and without any suggestion of coercion or force. They feel comfortable in discussing sexual issues before, during, and after they make love and do not ignore any misunderstandings or incompatibilities that may emerge in any aspect of their relationship. Neither person feels that they are being "judged" by the other, both enjoy what the famous clinical psychologist Carl Rogers called "unconditional positive regard." In other words, they like, respect, and may love each other no matter what. People who enjoy a climate of psychological safety feel that they can be independent and part of a couple at the same time. A climate of psychological safety can be an important element of love, but people can also enjoy these mature relationship qualities without being in love (Table 6-1). Unless individuals feel safe, however, they will probably not be fully and comfortably receptive about intercourse or non-intercourse sexual pleasuring. (Hendrick & Hendrick, 1992; Byrne & Murnen, 1988).

Psychological Factors

Do our moods affect our sexual feelings and responsiveness, and if so, how? Can sexual excitement be willed by just think-

---

TABLE 6-1

Climate of Psychological Safety

Two individuals approach a sexual experience willingly, wilfully, and without any suggestion of coercion or force.

Two individuals feel comfortable discussing sexual issues before, during, and after they make love.

Two individuals do not ignore any misunderstandings or incompatibilities that may emerge in any aspect of their relationship.

Neither individual feels they are being judged by the other and both enjoy unconditional positive regard. They like, respect, and love each other without conditions.

Two individuals feel that they can be independent and still be part of a couple at the same time.

ing about sexual experiences? Can sexual arousal be involuntary and beyond our control? These questions involve the relationship between mind and body and the role of psychological factors in sexual excitement and orgasm. The mind stores recollections of thoughts, feelings, and actions, as well as their pleasurable or unpleasurable consequences. Because of the incredible human capacity for mental imagery and accurate recollection, people have a repository of their own sexual history, which affects their sexual behaviors.

Kaplan's model of sexual arousal begins with the idea of desire, which involves psychological aspects of sexuality more than just genital changes. But how is desire communicated? Earlier in this chapter flirting was described as one way. In addition, words spoken between people in intimate situations can play a big part in their excitement. How people verbally communicate their erotic feelings and desires has been systematically evaluated and reported. Wells (1990) assessed the kinds of language people find erotically arousing in intimate situations and found an interesting difference between heterosexual and homosexual individuals. Wells asked his subjects about their sexual references to male genitalia, female genitalia, intercourse, oral-genital stimulation, and manual stimulation of the genitalia. Many formal and slang terms were used by these subjects (heterosexual males, gay males, heterosexual females, and lesbians), and different kinds of people found different kinds of words erotic. Subjects were asked about their usage of formal terms (penis, vagina, clitoris, make love, fellatio, cunnilingus, masturbate) and common slang terms (dick, pussy, clit, fuck, blow job, eat, jack off). Although such terms are commonly used, Wells was unable to discover much about how these subjects used these terms with their spouses or lovers. However, he did discover that homosexuals in his study were more likely to use erotic expressions during sexual interactions with their partners and were also more likely to use slang terms for body parts and sexual acts than heterosexuals. Presumably, different communication styles are related to different types of climate of psychological safety. Some people are comfortable with slang and others are not, and neither is more or less "normal" than the other. People generally seem to find their own way to express desire and excitement.

Sexual imagery and fantasy are also associated with excitement and response. Sexual fantasies include recollections of previous sexual experiences and imagined sexual interactions with someone to whom one is attracted but has not been intimate with, sexual activities with strangers, or sexual activities thought unusual or "taboo." Most people fantasize during masturbation, and many also have sexual fantasies during intercourse; such fantasies may enhance an individual's arousal and responsiveness (Leitenberg & Henning, 1995). Many people need the stimulation of sexual imagery to have an orgasm during masturbation and look to erotica or pornography for this stimulation. Sexual fantasies may also focus on emotions that accompany sexual behavior.

Experts disagree whether sexual fantasies are a voluntary or involuntary aspect of sexual behavior. Fantasy can be provoked or stimulated but also frequently seems to happen on its own. All people do not have sexual fantasies, but those who do seem to experience them frequently. Smith and Over (1990) reported that men can be taught to enhance the vividness of their sexual fantasies, which heightens both physiological and subjective measures of arousal. However, other subjects who were given *general* instruction concerning imagery experienced no such enhancement when instructed to fantasize about sexual themes. Some writers suggest that sexual fantasies are a type of creativity and that they represent a basic human desire to explore our curiosity. Indeed, sexual fantasies have been viewed as a way of safely preparing for sexual experiences one has not had but has perhaps thought about exploring. Not everyone wants to act out his or her fantasies, however, and many may want to keep their fantasies highly private.

Fantasies may be involved in various aspects of the sexual response cycle. For example, a person might imagine a specific scenario that is erotically stimulating in order to heighten excitement or have an orgasm (Reinisch, 1990). Having and controlling powerful erotic mental images is very stimulating for many people, and this is not abnormal. If a person tries to actualize their fantasies in real life, however, this sometimes can be troubling, especially if the fantasy is not appropriate for their public image or self-concept. Although in some cases sexual fantasies develop into an obsession, this is rare. In these rare instances psychotherapy can help a person extinguish the forceful quality of such private erotic images.

Sexual fantasies have been explored in the laboratory, with physiological measures of arousal compared with the subjects' perceived strength of the images. In one study (Tokatlidis & Over, 1995), female subjects were presented with three different sexual themes and asked to fantasize about each. These were fantasies with images or activities involving genitalia, themes involving dominance during sexual acts, and themes involving sensual, non-intercourse experiences. The clarity of mental images and the subjects' focus on the content of the fantasy were related to the frequency with which these women had fantasies about these topics in the preceding year. Apparently, the more frequently a woman incorporated a theme into her sexual fantasies, the more evident it was in the subject's imagination and the more easily could the woman concentrate on specific attributes of the fantasy. Fantasies involving genital themes were generally most arousing, sexual power the next most exciting, and sensual scenes and feelings the least. Whether the results would be similar for men is a topic for further investigation (see Chapter 8, Table 8-2).

Another psychological aspect affecting sexual arousal is performance demand, or the "implicit or explicit desire for increased sexual performance" (Laan, Everaerd, Van Aanhold, & Rebel, 1993). This raises an interesting question: if we feel that someone else wants or expects us to behave sexually, does this facilitate or inhibit our arousal? Are we excited by being wanted or inhibited by concern for performing wonderfully? As discussed in Chapter 14 on sexual dysfunctions, performance demand can be potentially inhibiting, mainly for men. In a study of the impact of performance demand on arousal in women by Laan, Everaerd, Van Aanhold, and Rebel (1993), healthy women with normal sexual responsiveness were shown erotically explicit films or asked to engage in fantasy and were told to "try to become as sexually aroused as possible within 2 minutes and try to maintain it for as long as you can. Your level of sexual arousal will be recorded." Women in the control condition were told: "Focus on the sexual enjoyment or pleasure you might receive from the film (or your fantasy). Your level of sexual arousal is of no importance." Vaginal photoplethysmography was used to assess sexual arousal, and subjects were asked to rate their overall sexual arousal, their most powerful feelings of sexual arousal, their strongest genital feelings, and their strongest extra-genital sensations. By both subjective and physiological measures, those women given the performance demand experienced greater levels of sexual arousal. Physiological arousal was more pronounced in women observing the erotic film, and subjective arousal was greater in the women asked to fantasize. These data were similar to those recorded from men (Abrahamson, Barlow, & Abrahamson, 1989). This study showed that performance demand may play an important role in the sexual response cycle.

Sexual Experience and Sexual Responsiveness

Researchers have also asked whether individuals with many sexual experiences become sexually aroused more readily than those with fewer sexual experiences or who are virgins. A related question is whether those who become aroused more often get better at recognizing the signs of sexual excitement. Kilmann, Boland, West, Jonet, and Ramsey (1993) explored these questions using various self-report questionnaires. Subjects were undergraduate volunteers, who were placed in three groups based on their reported sexual experiences: virgins, those with between 1 and 5 casual sexual experiences, and those with 6 or more casual sexual experiences. The word "casual" was used in this study to describe an unplanned sexual encounter of individuals who had intercourse shortly after they met and who did not plan to even see each other again. The study polled 362 never-married undergraduate students, 85% of whom had reported at least one sexual encounter. The results were straightforward: subjects with more casual sexual experience did not rate themselves as more easily aroused sexually.

Whether subjective experiences can affect the magnitude or timing of sexual arousal has intrigued other investigators. Laan, Everaerd, Van Der Velde, and Geer (1995) sought to find out if a woman's awareness of her genital sensations while being shown erotic film images would contribute to her subjective reports of sexual arousal. The answer was yes: greater physiological measures of genital excitement correlated strongly with personal reports of sexual arousal. Women likely use two kinds of cues for evaluating their levels of arousal: their perceptions of external stimuli and their body's responses to those stimuli. These investigators reported that this relationship is clearest at low to moderate levels of sexual arousal and not so clear at higher degrees of arousal, perhaps because high levels of sexual arousal are more difficult to create and measure in the laboratory. The Laan et al. study did not explore this re-

lationship in men. Men, of course, can easily *see* and feel the physical manifestations of sexual arousal; their erections are generally obvious. Because there is no obvious reflection of excitement in women, women need to attend to more subtle indications of levels of arousal.

People can become aroused and have orgasms with or without a partner, of course, but shared sexuality is often more arousing if one's partner seems really involved in the love making. Both women and men think of partner involvement as extremely desirable, especially if it involves orgasm. Darling, Davidson, and Cox (1991) studied orgasmic response in women in relation to the timing of their partner's orgasm. These investigators surveyed over 700 women and discovered that when women experienced orgasm after their partners, they reported lower levels of physiological and psychological enjoyment. However, when women reported having orgasms before or simultaneously with their partners, their level of satisfaction was much higher. Women often do not have an orgasm at all during sexual intercourse; Reinisch (1990) reports that 50-75% of women who have orgasms through masturbation do not have them during sexual intercourse. This kind of information is helpful to couples who may not be aware of the timing of their responses and who might benefit by better verbal and nonverbal communication in their arousal and plateau stages.

Controlled experimental techniques have been used to examine whether a person can "will" or "suppress" sexual excitement through cognitive strategies alone. Mahoney and Strassberg (1991) reviewed the literature on this question and carried out experiments to clarify the issue of voluntary vs. involuntary control of sexual arousal in men. While penile erection is primarily under the control of the autonomic nervous system, there may also be a voluntary component to arousal (Herman & Prewett, 1974; Quinsey, Bergersen, & Steinman, 1976). A summary of the literature by Hatch (1981) leads to a few generalizations. First, many men can suppress the physiological signs of sexual arousal, even when presented with explicit sexual stimuli. Second, some men can "will" an erection, even when there are no obvious erotic cues present. This may be similar to how some people can use biofeedback to alter physiological functions, such as blood pressure or heart rate, that are generally thought beyond voluntary control. Although some people can do this, they have trouble describing just exactly how they do it. Facilitating or suppressing sexual arousal may involve similar processes.

Habituation

So far, we have seen that several psychological factors have a clear impact on the magnitude, latency, and duration of excitement. Another interesting psychological variable related to sexual arousal is **habituation,** a term that refers to diminished behavioral responses during repeated presentations of the stimuli that elicit them. We habituate, or get used to, erotic stimuli and have a lessened response to them the more we experience them, although perhaps only within restricted periods of time. Koukounas and Over (1993) asked male subjects either to watch the same 60-second erotic film segments or to engage in the same sexual fantasy for the same period of time. Participants repeated this procedure 18 times in consecutive trials, during which their penile circumference was continuously measured with a penile strain gauge and after which participants subjectively rated the eroticism of each film exposure and fantasy period. On the 19th and 20th trials, new film segments or fantasy themes were introduced. On the 21st and 22nd trials the subjects were again asked to focus on the earlier film segment or fantasy theme. Throughout the initial 18 exposures, subjects showed progressively less physiological arousal and lower subjective sexual arousal as they habituated to the stimuli. On the 19th and 20th trials with new stimuli and fantasy themes, both physiological and subjective measures of arousal increased significantly; this phenomenon is known as *dishabituation.* Finally, when subjects were re-exposed to the original film and fantasy, their physiological and subjective arousal levels returned to their lowered levels. Similar data regarding habituation have been reported by Meuwissen and Over (1990). In a different study, however, using color slides instead of film clips or fantasy, the amount of habituation recorded both physiologically and subjectively was significantly smaller than in these other studies (Laan & Everaerd, 1995).

Habituation may be a relatively common phenomenon. Many people in long-term monogamous relationships report that they find their partners less exciting and their sexual routines more routine and predictable, and even that they are somewhat bored with the physical aspects of their relationship. Women's magazines have frequent articles on how to "spice up your marriage." Even in long-term relationships, exploration, curiosity, and novelty are almost always appreciated and often invigorate patterns of sexual interaction that may have grown too predictable (Fig. 6-13).

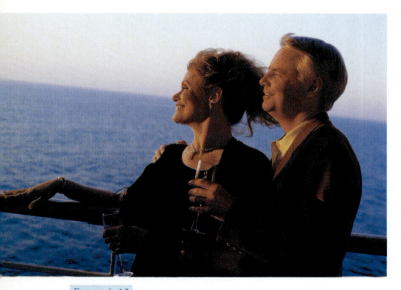

FIGURE 6-13   Sexual interest and inclination are usually lifelong patterns of behavior in women and men. Romance, affection, and intimacy at midlife offer enjoyment, as well as nurturance, for many couples.

Emotion and Sexual Arousal and Response

Just as our thoughts and fantasies affect sexual arousal, so too do our moods. Emotions such as anxiety, fear, or depression reflect clear changes in cognitive functioning and may also affect the activity of the autonomic nervous system. Many people find it difficult or impossible to feel sexual when they are anxious, fearful, hostile, or depressed, and these emotions also affect sexual arousal and response. These emotions are very common emotions and are often so troubling that many take prescribed medications to treat them. Studying the impact of these emotions involves methodological challenges. Should researchers rely on the findings of counselors and psychotherapists who study this issue in clinical settings but who, therefore, lack empirical evidence of the nature and extent of the disruptive effects of these emotions? Or can this question be explored reliably in the laboratory through short-term, artificial manipulations that may foster only temporary or insignificant levels of these emotions? Almost all sex therapists acknowledge the inhibiting impact of negative emotions on sexual arousal in both women and men.

A laboratory study by Hale and Strassberg (1990) demonstrated that when male subjects temporarily worried about avoiding electrical shock or critical feedback, their physiological arousal while watching erotic films was substantially lower than that of subjects not contending with these concerns. However, another study (Bozman & Beck, 1991) did not find significant differences in response between similar groups. Anxiety, of course, involves a pervasive but diffuse feeling of apprehension not specifically related to *particular* events—real, possible, or imagined. One of the problems of managing anxiety is that the person does not know exactly what (or who) causes it and, therefore, what or who to avoid. When people know exactly what they find problematic or threatening, this is called *fear.* Anxiety can be mild, moderate, or severe and is often difficult to describe precisely. Both Kaplan and Masters and Johnson have described the negative impact of anxiety, including anxiety that has nothing to do with sex, on sexual arousal. Chapter 14 on sexual dysfunctions discusses this topic further.

Depression also is a very common emotion. The effects of depression on arousability are not as clear as with anxiety. It is difficult to artificially induce depression in the laboratory. Still, Meisler and Carey (1991) found that men experiencing depression had diminished and delayed subjective sexual arousal, although penile tumescence as measured with a penile strain gauge was unaffected. It may not be possible to generalize results from such laboratory experiments to the population at large, however. Further, data regarding the relationship between depression and female sexual arousal are mixed. Some depressed women show delayed and diminished sexual arousal when presented with erotic stimuli, and others may have *increased* arousal. Further research is needed to elucidate the relationship of depression and arousal. It should also be noted that many depressed people take antidepressant medications,

Other Countries, Cultures, and Customs

SEXUAL AROUSAL AND PAINFUL STIMULATION IN ABORIGINAL CULTURES

In a true classic in the study of human sexuality, Clellan S. Ford and Frank A. Beach published *Patterns of Sexual Behavior* in 1951, which presented a cross-cultural analysis of sexual behavior in 191 different cultures, societies, and tribes on all continents. Their book is faultless by all scholarly standards. Although variations in foreplay and different types of sexual touch are discussed in Chapter 8, we will note here that approaches to sexual arousal differ significantly among different cultures. Behaviors that elicit sexual arousal in one part of the world may be utterly ineffective in another.

Ford and Beach point out that in our society women and men may "...pinch, scratch, bite, or otherwise bring pain to the partner" (page 55) during moments of keen arousal. When these behaviors are mild or moderate, the individuals do not feel threat or fear. While "rough sex" is practiced and even enjoyed by some people, when this behavioral pattern becomes habitual and abusive, it is plainly deviant. Ford and Beach speculate that although all humans may tend to be more assertive and physical during lovemaking, aggressiveness is not common in our own society. Their cross-cultural analysis of sexual behavior revealed that in some societies, however, this erotic/aggressive tendency is both magnified and accepted.

For example, the Siriono, a South American tribe, engage in extremely physical sexual interactions. The anthropologist A. R. Holmberg summarizes his research into the sexual practices of this group by noting:

> The sex act itself . . . is a violent and rapid affair. There are few if any preliminaries. Kissing is unknown, but oral stimulation is not absent; lovers have the habit of biting one another on the neck and chest during the sex act. Moreover, as the emotional intensity of coitus heightens to orgasm, lovers scratch each other on the neck, chest, and forehead, so that often they emerge wounded from the fray. Although people are proud of them, these love-scars sometimes cause trouble (in cases of extramarital intercourse), because they are visible evidence of the infidelity of a husband or wife.
>
> —HOLMBERG, 1946, 184, CITED IN FORD AND BEACH, 1951, 56

Ford and Beach offer more examples. Women of the Choroti, another South American tribe, routinely spit in their partner's face during intercourse, and women of the Apinaye (also of South America) frequently bite off parts of their partner's eyebrows and spit them off to the side with great fanfare. Other examples:

> Ponapean men [Oceania] usually tug at the woman's eyebrows, occasionally yanking out tufts of hair. Trukese women [Oceania] customarily poke a finger into the man's ear when they are highly aroused. Women of many societies bite the skin of the partner's neck, shoulder, or chest when sexual excitement is at its height. The red marks left on the skin may be a subject of jest; the Toda [Eurasia] greet any person who is so marked with the quip; "You have been bitten by a tiger."
>
> —FORD AND BEACH, 1951, 56

Of course, love bites, or "hickies" as they are sometimes called, are common in our own society too. These red or purple marks result from "suction kisses" and may persist a day or two (Reinisch, 1990, page 111).

which themselves can significantly diminish sexual arousal in some people who use them.

Anger is another emotion whose effects have been studied. Bozman and Beck (1991) studied the effect of anger on sexual arousal in men as subjectively and physiologically measured. In comparison to the control group and the subject group experiencing anxiety, participants who were angry had the greatest suppression of sexual arousal when presented with erotic audiotapes. These investigators believe that the anger experienced by many people impairs sexual arousal both psychologically and physiologically.

Biological Factors

Like psychosocial and interpersonal factors, many biological issues have a lot to do with sexual arousal and response. We have emphasized elsewhere that women experience cyclic changes in levels of female hormones before menopause, while men experience relatively steady levels of male hormones. Because different levels of female hormones are associated with mood changes and feelings of well-being, researchers have asked if women experience predictable changes in arousability in different phases of their menstrual cycles. Meuwissen and Over (1992, 1993) found that arousability does not differ across phases of the menstrual cycle. Both physiological and subjective measures of women's responses to sexual fantasies and erotic films did not reveal consistent, reliable differences in arousability through the menstrual cycle. Remember, however, that women vary much in their feelings of sexual receptivity during the menstrual cycle, and *expecting* to become aroused can often facilitate such arousal. There is nothing unusual about a woman who feels noticeable differences in arousability through the menstrual cycle. This research was done in a laboratory, and laboratory results are often different from those in other settings. Keeping a diary or personal journal would help one recognize whether such changes actually occur.

If the cyclic hormone changes in the menstrual cycle seem unrelated to sexual arousability, might hormone changes during pregnancy affect a woman's feelings of sexual inclination or erotic interest? Barclay, McDonald, and O'Loughlin (1994) reported on an extensive interview study that explored sexual interest and behavior during pregnancy. Twenty-five married couples participated during the first trimester of the pregnancy, and many of them also at the end of the second and third trimesters. The study revealed a significant decrease in sexual interest among these women through their pregnancies. Their husbands, however, reported no such decline in sexual interest. There was a notable decrease in the frequency of sexual intercourse through the pregnancy, although they commonly enjoyed non-intercourse sexual pleasuring. The diminished sexual interest in the women in this study may have been due to both hormonal changes during pregnancy and the potential physical discomfort of having intercourse with a notably distended abdomen.

Do oral contraceptives affect sexual arousability? Birth control pills artificially regulate levels of female hormones, which might have an effect on sexual arousability. This question is not as simple as it seems. Some oral contraceptives deliver a relatively constant level of female hormones, but others dispense different amounts of hormones during different phases of the menstrual cycle. Methodological questions are also involved, such as whether research dealing with the impact of oral contraceptive usage should be prospective or retrospective. Setting up questionnaire protocols before the period of study is generally better than relying on subjects' memories of their feelings of well-being and sexual interest in cycles once they are past. The data are far from clear.

Graham and Sherwin (1993) evaluated the effects of triphasic oral contraceptives on mood and feelings of sexual interest in a sample of women for whom the pill was prescribed to lessen premenstrual symptoms. Triphasic pills deliver different doses of synthetic female hormones during each of the first three weeks of a woman's cycle, with no hormone delivered during the fourth week. The women in this study who received oral contraceptives reported lessened sexual interest during and after the menstrual phases of their cycles. A subtle but important finding was that overall mood and sexual desire are independent of each other. The hormonal effects of birth control pills, therefore, had an adverse effect on both. In an earlier investigation, Bancroft, Sherwin, Alexander, Davidson, and Walker (1991) examined sexual experience and sexual attitudes among women who did or did not use oral contraceptives. Among the women in ongoing sexual relationships, those using oral contraceptives reported having intercourse more often and greater levels of sexual motivation and enjoyment, and evaluated their partners more positively than the women not using oral contraceptives. Finally, Warner and Bancroft (1988) noted that women using triphasic oral contraceptives were more likely to have rising and falling feelings of well-being and sexual interest compared with women using monophasic oral contraceptives delivering the same dosages of synthetic female hormones for 21 days of a 28-day cycle.

While these studies concern the relationship between oral contraceptives and feelings of well-being and sexual desire, that is not the same as a relationship between birth control pills and sexual arousability. Although Kaplan's model of human sexual response closely links desire and arousability, these studies did not actually measure arousability by either subjective or physiological measurements. Second, a relationship between oral contraceptives and sexual desire or arousability must also involve the woman's partner and the social and emotional characteristics of their relationship. Again, we emphasize that any meaningful study of sexual arousal should ideally consider an individual's whole psychosocial environment.

Legal and Illegal Drugs

Legal and illegal drugs are another interesting biological factor that affects sexual arousal and response. Drugs enter the central nervous system and affect our perceptions of erotic stimuli and our responses to them. **Aphrodisiacs** are substances that supposedly enhance erotic perceptions and sexual performance. In virtually all societies, people have sought such agents and have attributed magical or powerful properties to unusual substances, like ground rhinoceros horn. Although various drugs alter the intensity of physical sensations during sexual interactions, it is controversial whether any single substance has *singular and specific* effects in enhancing sexual arousal and orgasm. Because of simple expectancy, if one is told that a substance will enhance sexual feelings and response, a self-fulfilling prophesy may occur such that one perceives that effect even if any real effect is minimal or nonexistent. Finally, an agent that effectively stimulates sexual interest and response is not the same as an agent that nonspecifically lessens inhibitions, as discussed below.

Virtually all societies have discovered drugs that alter consciousness, including an enormous variety of substances. Even the most remote groups of people have discovered the mood and mind-altering properties of herbs, plants, fungi, and yeast fermentation. Societies everywhere perpetuated the use of such drugs through word of mouth, written records, and religious traditions. It seems the desire to alter consciousness is a cultural universal.

Alcohol is probably the most available mind-altering agent and is often reported to lessen inhibitions and enhance sexual feelings. But there are some serious risks associated with the use of alcohol. Adolescents and young adults often have a false sense of safety with alcohol because of its known potency and purity. Some young people assume that because they know the strength of what they are drinking and trust its purity in its manufacturing and packaging, then it *must be safe.* Alcohol is very different from drugs purchased on the street with little trustworthy information about their potency or purity. Even though people might not consciously think about it this way, most people just naturally assume alcohol is relatively safe since it seems such an accepted and pervasive part of our society. Yet alcohol does not affect everyone in the same way; people have different tolerances for it, and some people are at greater risk for developing a problem with alcohol.

The effects of alcohol on sexual feelings and behaviors are well known, even among those who don't drink, although those who do drink have a more accurate understanding of the effects (Bills & Duncan, 1991). Alcohol lessens a person's inhibitions and facilitates saying and doing things one might not otherwise say or do (Fig. 6-14). Although alcohol does not turn one into a completely different person, someone who becomes highly intoxicated is often surprised (and dismayed) to learn later about things they said and did "under the influence." Herein lies the dilemma for alcohol abuse related to sexual behavior: someone can put themselves into a state of mind in which they may be very open or even aggressive about expressing sexual thoughts and acting on sexual inclinations, and one can also facilitate another person becoming so incapacitated that she or he can not signal their lack of willingness to get into a sexual situation. The effects of alcohol depend on the individuals involved, of course, and their psychosocial setting (Table 6-2).

The effects of alcohol on human sexual experience and expression have been researched. In a study published in 1981, which analyzed the responses of 917 women over the age of 21 who represented the general United States population in demographic characteristics (Klassen & Wilsnack, 1986), most respondents stated that alcohol lessened their

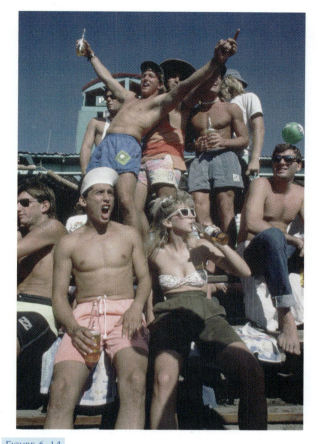

FIGURE 6-14 Alcohol often lessens inhibitions, including sexual ones. Alcohol use may contribute to contraceptive negligence, unsafe sexual behaviors, and aggressive behavior—not a very good combination.

sexual inhibitions and helped them feel closer to others socially and emotionally. Although many people believe that when drinking women become less discriminating about whether or when to have sex, only 8% of these women indicated this resulted from their drinking. However, 22% indicated that they became more sexually assertive and perhaps more active in "taking the lead" in suggesting sexual inter-

TABLE 6-2

Percentages of Acknowledged Male Offenders and Female Victims Who Reported Being Under the Influence of Alcohol During a Sexual Assault

	Reported Level of Inebriation		
	Intoxicated, %	"Mildly Buzzed," %	Total, %
Men	26	29	55
Women	21	32	53

From Abbey, A. (1991). Acquaintance rape and alcohol consumption on college campuses. J Am College Health, 39, 165.

Dear Dr. Ruth

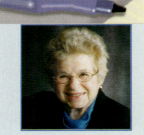

Question:

I know a glass of wine or two can be very relaxing before intercourse, but my girl-friend always drinks a lot before we make love. Why does she do this? Does this mean she's actually uncomfortable with me?

Answer:

More likely she's uncomfortable with herself. She may be having problems facing her own fears or feelings and is hiding them from herself by getting drunk. I don't know enough to guess about her mental state, but it is something that needs attention. Also, it wouldn't surprise me to learn she drinks at other times too in order to function in situations where she might feel a little nervous.

course. Disturbingly, fully 60% of these women reported they had been the object of another drinker's sexual aggression. Women in this study who drank daily and more heavily had the highest reported rates of sexual disinterest and the lowest rates of orgasm during intercourse. In other words, although alcohol may facilitate erotic interest and enhance sexual feelings, prolonged heavy drinking is associated with *diminished* sexual interest and responsiveness with a partner. Generally, lighter drinking is associated with more rewarding sexual experiences, according to these authors.

Crowe and George (1989) reviewed the literature on the impact of alcohol on both women and men and concluded that although alcohol may diminish inhibitions and enhance sexual arousal, it plainly suppresses physiological responses to sexual stimuli. This is understandable since in even moderate doses, alcohol is a depressant. These authors emphasize that the disinhibiting effects of alcohol are greatest with light drinking, and the physiological suppression is greatest with heavier drinking. Do individuals who drink with the *expectation* of enhanced sexual response experience more uninhibited, fulfilling sex? Generally, men who feel secure in their sexuality (who don't feel they need to get drunk to participate in sexual behavior) indicated that their expectation of enhanced sexual feelings predicted how much they drank (not too much), their maximum alcohol consumption (not too much), and the frequency of their drinking (not too often) (Mooney, 1995).

In a comprehensive analysis of the impact of alcohol on female sexual behavior, Beckman and Ackerman (1995) demonstrated that alcohol causes substantive changes in sexual behavior for only a minority of women, which contradicts the research of Klassen and Wilsnack (1986). In fact, alcohol may serve only to magnify one's "true" self when drinking. These authors emphasize that the *expectancy* for alcohol's effects is a very important factor in its actual effects. Although much has

been written about the effects of drugs on "risky" sexual behaviors, Beckman and Ackerman did not find alcohol consumption associated with these behaviors. Chapter 17 discusses this further in relation to sexually transmitted diseases and AIDS. These writers state, however, that heavy alcohol use is often associated with sexual victimization.

Recreational Drugs and Sexual Behavior

Cocaine, like alcohol, has generated both folk myth and scientific research regarding its effects on sexual functioning. Cocaine users often say it magnifies perceptions of sexual excitement and makes orgasms feel stronger and seem to last longer. Like alcohol, cocaine lessens a person's inhibitions, but as also occurs with alcohol, chronic cocaine use has unpleasant consequences. Kim, Galanter, Castaneda, Lifshutz, and Franco (1992) reported that the impact of cocaine on sexual arousal and response depends on several factors, including the form of the drug. Because of the extraordinarily high potential for abuse, dependency, and/or addiction with "crack" cocaine, much research has focused on it, although its actions are similar to the inhaled variety of this agent. Other variables affecting the impact of cocaine include the dose used, the frequency of use, the user's gender, the presence of a psychological or psychiatric disorder, and the individual's sexual value system. This research indicated unequivocally that prolonged and persistent use of crack cocaine fosters sexual *disinterest* and *dysfunction*, at least in a sample of psychiatric patients. As well, some subjects became more sexually promiscuous and acquired sexually transmitted diseases, perhaps because of diminished inhibitions. Another study of 100 women who were currently using cocaine or who had been in treatment for cocaine abuse assessed its supposed aphrodisiac properties (Henderson, Boyd, & Whitmarsh, 1995). The study clearly showed that crack cocaine is *not* an aphrodisiac and does *not* make women want to have sex. As in the study previously cited, these women reported higher levels of sexual dysfunction. Their rate of sexual dysfunction exceeded that of female alcohol abusers, perhaps in part because this sample was drawn from women receiving psychiatric treatment. Apparently, with both alcohol and crack cocaine, lessened inhibitions are not always accompanied by satisfactory sexual arousal and response and may even contribute to unrewarding intimate encounters.

Marijuana

After alcohol, marijuana is the most commonly used consciousness-altering drug and is the most common illegal drug. Marijuana has euphoric properties, meaning it fosters good feelings. As with other drugs used in sexual encounters, users often attribute aphrodisiac properties to marijuana. Although this agent may enhance mood and erotic sensations, it does not *create* them. Marijuana fosters a feeling of "time expansion" and may magnify sensory experiences; using marijuana may make a sexual experience seem to last a longer time and thereby contribute to sexual enjoyment. Additionally, this drug may seem to heighten perceptions related to sexual behavior. Although marijuana does not specifically increase sexual arousal physiologically, its effects likely depend on the person's interpersonal situation. In moderate amounts alcohol and marijuana "potentiate" one another's effects-one tends to magnify the effects of the other. Marijuana is not physically addictive, as are alcohol and cocaine. Nonetheless, frequently using marijuana or any drug in sexual activity may detract from the interpersonal qualities of the relationship.

MDMA

In recent years much has been written about methylenedioxymethamphetamine (MDMA), also called "ecstacy." People who use it often report that it stimulates sexual arousal. A large survey concerning MDMA seemed to confirm this (Cohen, 1995). Analyzing the responses of 500 subjects, Cohen found wide variability in the use of MDMA, with some subjects reporting a single experience and others in excess of 250 separate experiences. Respondents reported euphoria, feelings of increased energy, and sexual arousal as the most common drug effects, although many also reported unpleasant side effects such as nausea, headache, depression, and occasionally flashbacks. The effects of MDMA do not seem specific to the enhancement of sexual arousal but may be due to a generalized sense of well-being. Abuse is accompanied by a rapidly growing dependency, however, and extremely powerful cardiovascular and neurological activation. After several weeks, a person builds tolerance to this drug and no longer quickly or efficiently metabolizes it. Its by-products build-up in the bloodstream, sometimes causing hallucinations, delusions, and panic attacks.

MDMA is a type of amphetamine, called "speed" on the street. Amphetamines often stimulate a sense of euphoria. Most amphetamines are ingested in capsules or pills. Tolerance for amphetamines develops very quickly, and in only weeks doses that once created euphoria become ineffective and the user takes progressively larger doses to gain the same effect. At the higher levels of tolerance for amphetamines, people administer amphetamine intravenously. A study in Sweden assessed 27 men who had injected amphetamines intravenously and explored its effects on sexual functioning (Kall, 1992). All these men had participated in sexual activities while using amphetamines. Most reported enhanced sexual arousal, more intense orgasms, and prolonged intercourse. Whether these effects of amphetamines become less apparent with long-term usage remains to be seen.

Yohimbine

An interesting drug thought to have aphrodisiac properties is yohimbine. Although it has been available for many years for the treatment of high blood pressure, data about its effect on sexual arousability and responsiveness remain inconclusive. It comes from the bark of a tree that grows in West Africa, which some natives of this region eat in its natural, unrefined form to boost their sexual performance. The United States Food and Drug Administration approved a prescription synthetic form of yohimbine for the treatment of impotence. It was tested clinically with men, but it seems to enhance sexual feeling and responsiveness in women also. It is generally not prescribed for females, however, and never during pregnancy. Technically, it is in a family of drugs called MAO (monoamine oxidase) in-

AGENTS WITH SUPPOSED APHRODISIAC PROPERTIES—FOR WHICH THERE IS NO CLINICAL PROOF

Ginseng	Cantharides ("Spanish fly")
Mandrake	Amyl Nitrite
Vitamin E	Powdered Rhinoceros Horn
Jaipuri Plant	Oysters
Niacin	Vasopressin (a pituitary hormone)
Phenylalanine	Vitamin B6

hibitors and is related to reserpine, a powerful blood pressure-lowering drug that also has tranquilizing properties. Despite the fact that yohimbine is regulated by the FDA, it is advertised on Internet web sites.

Controlled laboratory data on the effects of yohimbine seem mixed, perhaps because men's arousal difficulties may result from physical causes, psychological causes, or a combination of both. Yohimbine has a beneficial effect on arousal in men with impotence due primarily to psychological difficulties but did not aid men who were impotent because of physical factors (Mann, Klingler, Noe, Roschke, Muller, & Benkert, 1996). Erections during sleep were not facilitated in this study. Carey and Johnson (1996) found through a statistical comparison of the literature on the effects of yohimbine that there was a general facilitating effect for the attainment and maintenance of erections. Rowland, Kallan, and Slob (1997) reported that this drug did not make any difference in the sexual functioning of men without sexual problems and had only mixed success in men with erectile difficulties; it had no effect on erections in sleep among men with erectile problems. Although physiologically this drug may stimulate blood flow into the penis and inhibit blood flow out of the penis, its effects in the laboratory are not always significant.

Overall, we are left with our original suggestion: sexual arousal is not simply a reflex that can be stimulated apart from cognitive assessment. Even drugs with an observed effect can have varying results. We should be suspicious, therefore, of claims for dramatic enhancement of sexual arousal through simple interventions.

ANAPHRODISIACS

While some drugs enhance sexual feeling and responsiveness, others inhibit or diminish arousal and may foster disinterestedness in sexual interaction. The term **anaphrodisiac** describes drugs that do this (Table 6-3). While some drugs are known to inhibit sexual arousal and are used specifically for that purpose (anti-androgens), others have similar actions as side effects of another intended drug action. A common example is some medications used to lower high blood pressure, called antihypertensives. Such drugs work through many different physiological mechanisms, and not all of them are associated with problems in sexual arousal and response. But some are, contributing perhaps to reasons some patients do not take their medications as prescribed. Some, but not all, antihypertensives cause erectile problems in men and delayed and/or diminished lubrication among women because of their effects on the autonomic nervous system.

Although some antihypertensives have an inhibiting effect on sexual arousal, other drugs do not interfere with arousal but make it difficult for a person to "lift off" the plateau stage and have an orgasm. This situation is a good example of the importance of an open relationship with one's physician for discussing such unwanted side effects and seeking a way around them . Taking mild tranquilizers with alcohol magnifies their effects and may render a person disinterested in sexual interactions.

Many commonly used antidepressants also inhibit sexual responsiveness to a varying degree. For example, most such drugs approved in the United States can cause loss of a previous pattern of orgasmic response. Although many people use antidepressants, few studies have been done of their effects on sexual arousal and response (Segraves, 1995). One investigation reported that over 40% of patients using various different types of antidepressants developed sexual problems as a result, with almost 20% of men using them reporting painful orgasms (Balon, Yeragani, Pohl, & Ramesh, 1993). Loss of sex drive, problems attaining and maintaining an erection, and delayed ejaculation were also reported (Hsu & Shen, 1995). One class of antidepressants, including Prozac, Paxil, and Zoloft, was clearly associated with many previously unreported sexual problems. Unwanted side effects can often be minimized, however, after enough time passes for the person to develop tolerance. Reducing the dose or changing the time of day the drug is taken may also help. In some instances the prescription is changed to a different antidepressant with fewer or no side effects.

Another example of an anaphrodisiac that may foster sexual disinterest is the large family of drugs called opiates, including codeine, methadone, morphine, and heroin. Synthetic opiates include agents such as Percodan, Demerol, and methadone. These drugs are usually prescribed to lessen pain, coughing, and diarrhea. Because opiates usually cause drowsiness and mental clouding, people seldom use them with the intention of heightening erotic sensations. At the same time opiates depress functioning in many areas of the central ner-

TABLE 6-3	
Some Common Prescription Drugs That May Have Anaphrodisiac Properties	
Antihypertensives:	Inderol (Propanolol Hydrochloride)
	Tenormin (Atenolol)
	Lopressor (Metaprolol)
	Corgard (Nadolol)
	Betapace (Sotalol Hydrochloride)
Antianxiety Agents:	Xanax (Alprazolam)
	Valium (Diazepam)
	Librium (Chlordiazepoxide)
	Klonopin (Clonazepam)
	Ativan (Lorazepam)
Antidepressants:	Prozac (Fluoxetine Hydrochloride)
	Paxil (Paroxetine Hydrochloride)
	Zoloft (Sertraline Hydrochloride)
Opiates:	Codeine
	Methadone
	Morphine
	Percodan (Oxycodone and Aspirin)
	Demerol (Meperidine Hydrochloride)

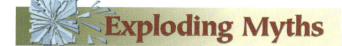

Exploding Myths

"Catching a Buzz Makes Me Feel Really Sexy."

Of all the legal and illegal drugs, the one mentioned most frequently as enhancing sexual experiences is marijuana. As we noted earlier, the common effects of marijuana include a sense of time expansion and heightened sensory experience. It may make pleasurable sexual feelings seem to last longer and be more intense. But the scientific research does not agree with anecdotal reports; some data may be surprising.

In 1979, Kolodny, Masters, and Johnson reported that in a sample of over 1000 women and men, over 80% of subjects who had used marijuana reported enhanced sexual experiences under its effects. However, sexual problems are also associated with marijuana usage, especially when it is used heavily and frequently. Kolodny (1981) found that among men who used marijuana daily, 20% reported some degree of difficulty in attaining and maintaining an erection. Comparable usage patterns in women did not seem associated with arousal stage difficulties, although occasional lack of vaginal lubrication did occur. Among female heavy marijuana users, menstrual irregularities were especially common. Data also indicate that chronic, heavy use of marijuana lowers testosterone levels in men (Kolodny, 1974) and lowered sperm production (Abel, 1981). These hormonal changes return to normal when marijuana usage is discontinued.

While many data indicate that marijuana usage is associated with increased rates of sexual activity, it is no longer thought that the drug itself "causes" this increase. Rather, marijuana use is seen as just one aspect of a "sensation-seeking" lifestyle in which more frequent sexual behavior occurs independently (Abel, 1981). In other words, more frequent sexual activity results from personality characteristics rather than the use of marijuana. And the research does show that overall patterns of sexual activity *decrease* with prolonged, heavy usage. Apparently, frequently "catching a buzz" can foster disinterestedness in a variety of human interactions.

vous system, they stimulate others, such as the vomiting center. Both natural and synthetic opiates thus have a profoundly disorganizing effect on sexual function (Spring, Willenbring, & Maddux, 1992).

Social Factors

Thus far, our discussion of factors affecting human sexual arousal and response has focused on psychological and biological factors. In addition, people function in wider social environments that involve expectations and norms about how and when erotic interests are to be channeled. As noted in a previous chapter, sex is a drive given *form and direction* by culture.

One of the most interesting and enigmatic issues affecting sexual interactions in the social domain is the notion of privacy. Privacy entails one's personal psychological assessment of freedom from intrusion, but norms that stipulate what is or is not appropriate in public are fundamentally social in nature. For most people, sexual behavior is intensely private and take place only where others cannot see or hear. Indeed, in addition to the general privacy protections of the Fourth Amendment

to the United States Constitution, state and local statutes often specify the fundamentally private nature of sexual interactions and what constitutes a "customarily private" place. (Incidentally, a car is generally not considered a "customarily private" place.) People often say they don't care much about what consenting adults do in the privacy of their own bedrooms, but what exactly does the term "privacy" imply?

Privacy is more complicated than just closing the bedroom door. Environmental psychologists and architects often view privacy as a capacity for boundary regulation and the control of information about oneself. The idea of "personal space" is less relevant when two people decide to allow each other into their most intimate space. Alan Westin (1967) suggested that privacy has four aspects. *Solitude* refers to being alone by oneself. *Intimacy* is another "level" of privacy, usually referring to more than one person (often just two) wanting to be alone and away from everyone else. Still more complex is the notion of *anonymity*, in which a person may seek to be and interact among others while at the same time desiring not to be known by name. Finally, *re-*

serve is a situation in which a person creates a psychological obstacle so that others cannot easily access them or their thoughts. Privacy thus is a mechanism for asking for space and time to be intimate with another person, as well as explore and collect one's own thoughts. Westin's scheme implies people have ways of signaling their lack of interest in interaction, or sexual interaction, with others. Most people find it difficult if not impossible to become sexually aroused unless they have privacy. The odd exceptions to this are covered in Chapter 18 on sexual variations and deviations.

Through history the nature of housing has evolved to accommodate increasing desires for privacy. In the Middle Ages, and well into the 15th and 16th centuries, extended families and strangers often lived in large, multi-purpose rooms. They ate, worked, played, slept, and made love all in the same place and within sight of one another (Rybczynski, 1986). As the middle class became more affluent, they could afford to occupy single-family homes in which different domestic activities took place in their own, separate places. Gradually, sexual activities became associated with explicitly segregated sleeping areas not shared by children or the extended family.

An even simpler way of thinking about what is private and what is public is our clothing. A connotation of the word *savage* involves being naked and making no effort to conceal one's genitalia and breasts. Indeed, the phrase "private parts" is used to refer to these areas. Just as "civilization" has fostered changes in domestic architecture and behaviors that are not by their very nature "public," civilization has also powerfully affected norms for nudity and styles of clothing.

ROLE OF THE SENSES IN SEXUAL AROUSAL AND RESPONSIVENESS

Science today is comfortable with the idea that the contents of our minds derive from our experiences. Aristotle claimed that it is through the five senses that all important information enters the mind for thinking and feeling. Yet philosophers have not always been so sure. In the mid-1600s, the famous French philosopher and mathematician Rene Descartes believed that the contents of the mind come from God and that interaction with the environment is only necessary to "activate" these thoughts, images, feelings, and moral certainties. While quite a lot of the brain is "pre-wired" before birth, behavioral scientists today accept that it is only through our senses that information enters the nervous system. This general position is called *empiricism,* and it represents a major historical trend in thinking about the development of the mind. Obviously sensory perceptions are a fundamental aspect of sexual experience. Vision, hearing, taste, touch, and smell are often all involved in the reception of erotic stimuli and the responses to these cues. Although people certainly can become aroused and perhaps even have orgasms by fantasizing, for the most part humans need sensory stimulation to fully experience eroticism and sexual excitement.

Sensory stimuli involve the immediate moment, but the brain also has stored literally millions of images and experiences in long-term memory. How a person receives and interprets sexual stimuli in any particular situation is affected by all the content of the mind at that time. Simply stated, old memories affect current perceptions. Some memories (both good and bad) are relatively permanent and persistent and even sometimes obtrusive. Memories can either enhance or inhibit what is happening sexually at the moment. Just as we can learn and remember new intimate or sexual recollections, however, we also have the ability to *unlearn* memories to prevent them from being distracting or troubling. Chapter 14 on sexual dysfunctions discusses this further.

Obviously, then, people are not "input-output" systems or machines whose behavior can simply be predicted on the basis of the current stimulus and emotional environment; in one way or another, sooner or later, the past plays a big part in one's present response to sexual stimulation.

Two of the sensory systems take up a great deal of the "brain space" in the cerebral hemispheres devoted to the senses: vision and touch. It is, therefore, not surprising that these modalities play so significant a part in behaviors essential to the perpetuation of our species.

Vision

Humans are often described as fundamentally "visual animals"; in other words, we seem basically dependent on visual stimuli and the functioning of our visual systems to move around in our environments and attend to the stimuli we need to notice to survive and procreate. A huge amount of the human brain is devoted to the visual system. The visual stimuli one finds sexually provocative, interesting, or exciting depend on culture and society's sexual customs. Some may speculate that humans evolved to attend visually to the sight of genitalia or breasts, but this cannot be proved. Still, the sexually evocative nature of genital display is acknowledged throughout the world, even in places where nudity is common for all. In other words, visual sexual cues play a big part in sexual arousal. "Intimate apparel," for example, suggests the power of visual and tactile stimuli to promise or imply sexual receptivity (Fig. 6-15). Even nonintimate apparel is often designed to display or accentuate parts of our bodies associated with sexual contact: the breasts, legs, and buttocks. Indeed, "augmentation" can be purchased to be inserted into the clothing to enhance the appearance of such parts of our bodies.

The earlier brief discussion of social influences on sexual arousal examined the notion of privacy. When it comes to sexual privacy and visually exciting stimuli, many people have learned a simple and interesting truism: to motivate someone to pay attention to a certain part of your body, cover it up or only reveal a bit of it. Psychologists use the term "incentive" to refer to the *promise or probability* of such reinforcement.

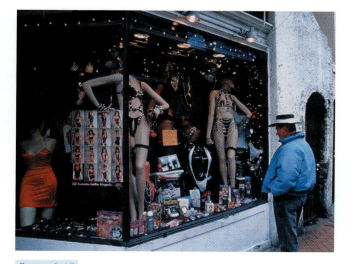

FIGURE 6-15   Many couples find exotic lingerie, sex "toys," and erotic books and videos an interesting way to add novelty and a little excitement to sexual interactions which have, perhaps, become a little routine.

Earlier we reviewed several laboratory investigations in which women and men watched videotapes with explicit erotic content, usually scenes of erotic touching or sexual intercourse; the subjects' physiological and subjective responses to these stimuli were then measured. In *virtually all* of these studies subjects of both sexes, various ages, differing socioeconomic status, and diverse educational backgrounds were aroused and attentive to these erotic stimuli. Still, in different cultures, people employ highly diverse strategies for ornamenting themselves in order to appear sexually "attractive." Humans are quite probably "programmed" to pay attention visually to sexual cues and respond accordingly physiologically and psychologically. As well, there don't seem to be any big differences between women and men in these responses, only that arousal often takes a little longer in women. Some data seem to indicate that women's subjective emotional responses to erotic videotapes and film clips is somewhat less than what men report to the same or similar stimuli (Mosher & MacIan, 1994), but it is unclear whether this finding can be generalized to the population as a whole. Remember also that Kinsey's studies found that women and men who had more formal education were more likely to have had more diversified sexual experiences, and that although there were significant differences between the sexes in his study, these seemed less apparent among better educated respondents; by Kinsey's own admission, better educated females were overrepresented in his sample. Perhaps women with more formal education are more likely to respond to visual erotic cues based more on their personalities and experiences and less on the basis of cultural stereotypes of women as less sexually inclined than men.

Touch

While vision tells us what is happening outside of our bodies, touch involves events right at the surface of our physical being.

In a sense, then, touch is a more intimate sense. The skin senses, as they are sometimes called, respond to both tactile stimulation (such as rubbing, pinching, and poking) and temperature changes. There are big differences in tactile and thermal sensitivity in various areas of the body. Some areas seem incredibly responsive to the slightest, briefest touch, while others are surprisingly insensitive. The most sensitive areas of skin have become associated with erotic stimulation and sexual pleasure, although less sensitive areas can take on erotic associations too if sexual stimulation has been paired with touching them. Chapter 2 explained the concept of erogenous zones, first introduced by Sigmund Freud. The primary erogenous zones (mouth, anus, genitals) have a very dense accumulation of free nerve endings close to the surface of the skin. This is why they are so sensitive. People also develop their own erotic "map" based on personal experiences of skin stimulation paired in time with sexual experiences. Although it is easy to focus on oral, anal, and genital stimulation as examples of sexual touching, remember that a gentle caress of the back, neck, cheek, or buttock is also often interpreted as highly enjoyable and erotic (Fig. 6-16). These are called secondary erogenous zones.

One aspect of the sense of touch is that it may all by itself fulfill powerful emotional and erotic needs. Humans might actually *need to be touched,* that is, there may be an innate longing for contact with others that is socially sanctioned in terms of what we learn is appropriate to "desire." Hollender (1970) studied this desire to be held, working with women who were suffering from anxiety disorders and depression. Dr. Hollender found that people differ in their desire to be touched, held, and cuddled. Yet many in the group he was working with thought of touch as necessary, not optional. In his sample of 39 subjects, 21 frankly stated that they had used sexual enticement with men in order to be held by them, which was what they most desired and enjoyed in their intimate encounters. Most in the entire group of subjects had made explicit verbal requests to be held. One woman described it in a most compelling and elegant way: "It's a kind of an ache . . . It's not like an emotional longing for some person who isn't there; it's a physical feeling" (Hollender, 1970, cited in Montagu, 1971). Hollender also reported that one of the subjects, a former prostitute, explicitly stated that she primarily used sex as a means to be held. If being touched alone seems such a potentially powerful human need, imagine the importance of tactile contact in relationships that are also sexually rewarding.

Related to the sense of touch is vibratory stimulation, which in the last few decades many women and men have incorporated in their intimate interactions; many also use vibrators alone during masturbation. Vibration (also called "vibrotactile stimulation") is perceived by many as highly erotic and arousing. Many people experiment with vibrators to learn more about their own sexual arousal and responsiveness and distinguish between the different stages of the sexual response cycle. Some people mistakenly think all vibrators are shaped like a penis or that women derive the most enjoyment from inserting them far into their vaginas. Actually, women consistently report that applying vibrotactile stimulation to their cli-

FIGURE 6-16 Patient, prolonged erotic massage is both a gesture of affection and caring, as well as an effective avenue of sexual stimulation.

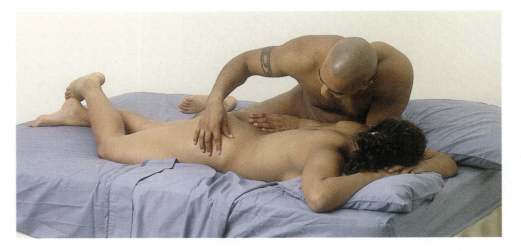

toris provides the most powerful pleasurable feelings. Vibrators are discussed in greater depth in Chapter 15 in reference to therapies for sexual dysfunctions.

In discussions of the importance of touch in a sexual context, the kind of touching must be defined. For example, there is a clear difference between genital and non-genital touching, which highlights the difference between the terms "sexual" and "sensual." Usually the term "sexual" is associated with genital feelings during intimate touching and intercourse, whereas the word "sensual" is far broader in its meanings. In some respects "sensual" refers to all enjoyments experienced through the senses, including exciting but also soothing experiences. A good example of a potentially very sensual experience is a backrub, especially when given by someone you love or like very much. The thermal and tactile stimuli of a body massage may be extremely calming on the one hand and sexually provocative on the other. Yet a backrub doesn't always arouse sexual excitement and may be experienced as a powerful pleasure on its own. In a sense, sensual touching can sometimes be interpreted as a "promise" of more intimate physical contact. While many people find it awkward to talk to each other during intercourse, verbal communication during sensual sharing is more common. Sensual enjoyments often serve to help create the climate of psychological safety many people feel important in order to fully and uninhibitedly enjoy one another.

An interesting study explored the perceptions of college women and men to a hypothetical situation: being the recipient of an uninvited genital touch from someone they knew on campus, a member of either the same or the other sex (Struckman-Johnson & Struckman-Johnson, 1993). Almost all of the female subjects indicated they would have an extremely negative emotional reaction to an unsolicited genital touch from someone of either sex, regardless of whether this touch was gentle or forceful. Men, however, reported virtually no negative reactions to either a forceful or gentle unsolicited genital touch from a woman but would have a highly unfavorable response to a touch from a man. Sexual touching, there-

fore, should be evaluated in a context of whether it is invited or uninvited, consensual or nonconsensual.

Hearing

Everyone likes to hear that they are appreciated and doing a good job. This occurs too with sexual interaction. Despite the primary and powerful roles of vision and touch in sexual arousal and response, most people find verbal erotic encouragement and praise highly arousing. Verbal expressions of affection are for many an essential first step in any interpersonal encounter with sensual and/or sexual meanings. Hearing that we are loved, exciting, and doing the right things to arouse our partner feels wonderful. We thus begin to see ourselves as *competent* lovers and grow more self-assured in our capacity to create pleasure in someone we care about. The old image of masculinity requiring that men be the "strong, silent type" is outdated. Both women and men appreciate verbal praise when they are enjoying sexual experiences. As well, both women and men have reported finding "talking dirty" highly arousing and an avenue for fantasizing during intercourse (Janus & Janus, 1993).

Good communication is generally an essential attribute of good sex and allows one to be able to tell or show someone else what one likes and when. Communicating such information is important, but perhaps not always during sex itself, when it might be interpreted more as a demand than a request. Listening to one's partner talk about sex when not having sex can provide much useful information in a nonjudgmental setting. Such information often clearly enhances excitement at a later time and helps to make shared intimacy more compatible with the needs and desires of two people. The same is true with communication after intercourse. Just as verbal praise and encouragement can stimulate a partner during sex, it can reassure and reinforce a partner after sex.

For many people verbal sexual encouragement is powerfully related to arousal and response. The number of 1-900 telephone numbers people can call to hear "sex talk" has exploded recently. Some men but virtually no women report using these "services." The caller pays a fee of $3 to $10 per minute (Fig. 6-17) to hear a prerecorded message or have a sexual conversation with an individual. The caller may disclose a sexual fantasy and typically masturbates while the other person speaks in a sexually explicit way to him (Glasock & LaRose, 1993). Chapter 18 on sexual variations and deviations discusses this further.

Generally speaking, verbally communicating one's good feelings about sex helps both partners enjoy each other more. Similarly, withholding positive and rewarding statements can cause both to wonder about the act of sharing. As discussed earlier, it is normal for people to use colorful language for communication about sex. Hearing such terms further enhances sexual arousal and responsiveness for many people (Janus & Janus, 1993).

Smell

People like nice smells, such as those associated with cleanliness, and most people find cleanliness a prerequisite to sexual intimacy, within a range of individual differences and preferences. In light of all the money and time people spend selecting perfume, cologne, and or after-shave lotion, it seems clear we think smelling good is an important aspect of good grooming and may enhance our "sex appeal." Relatively few personal grooming products are actually unscented. Recently, however, scientists are studying whether such products actually cover up

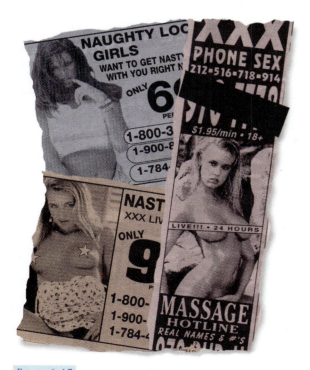

FIGURE 6-17 Hearing sexually suggestive conversation is highly arousing to many people. An enormous industry has grown by charging customers' credit cards in exchange for highly explicit sexual statements and directives.

normal human odors that convey information to others about our sexual motivations.

Pheromones are air-borne hormones whose effects are clearly seen in other animal species. Pheromones are usually detected through an animal's sense of smell, although they may also exert their effects through contact with the skin (Cohen, 1994). Some of these chemical agents act as sex attractants, whereas others may signal danger or simply mark a trail or territorial boundaries. Many insects, for example, secrete substances into the air that are received by nearby potential receptive mates, and when a female dog in the neighborhood goes into heat, male dogs nearby are aware of it and can be highly distracted. The possibility of human pheromones that may serve as sex attractants has long intrigued scientists and perfume makers. If humans actually did emit such substances into the air, much like the scent of our perspiration, would everybody be able to smell it? How close would they have to be? Would everyone be equally able to detect the scent? Would there be an immediate and automatic feeling of sexual "attention" or interest? If everyone were putting these chemicals into the air all day every day, how would we manage to think straight? The study of possible human pheromones has become an interesting and legitimate area of research. For example, as described in Chapter 4, scientists have wondered whether an important signal in the phenomenon of menstrual synchrony may be a very subtle menstrual scent, although no definitive proof or disclaimer of this possibility has emerged.

The question whether humans emit and/or sense substances that may signal sexual receptivity has stimulated some very interesting research. A study by Motluk (1996) involved presenting adult human males with the odors of a variety of fatty acids found in the vaginal secretions of women, one of which was found only during ovulation, while a control group was presented water vapor. The amount of testosterone in the saliva of these men was then measured. The men presented with the odors of ovulation secreted significantly more testosterone than the subjects presented with other vaginal scents or the water vapor. However, these results indicate only a physiological response to vaginal odors, not behavioral or cognitive responses, and do not mean that ovulation causes men to become more attracted to women. There is scant evidence that human pheromones exist that can initiate complex behaviors; the data seem to be highly suggestive but do not offer concrete, objective proof (Cowley & Brooksbank, 1991).

Our discussion of the role of sensory information in sexual arousal and response emphasizes a very important fact: during sexual interactions people receive much information perceptually, and it sometime requires focus to attend to any of this information. An appreciation of the emotional, cognitive, behavioral, and interpersonal aspects of sexual excitement requires paying attention to these various sources of information to grasp the subtle pleasurable texture of shared physical intimacy.

ISSUES INVOLVED IN SEXUAL AROUSAL AND RESPONSE

While the information presented thus far in this chapter is rather objective and noncontroversial, some aspects of normal human arousal and response involve much argument and disagreement.

The G Spot

One controversy regarding arousal and response has already been discussed: whether there is really such a thing as a "G-spot." Chapter 4 describes the functional anatomy of the female reproductive system and notes that many women report an area especially sensitive to touch located along the anterior wall of the vagina. Vigorous manual or penile stimulation of this area is thought to precipitate an orgasm different in quality from orgasms elicited through clitoral stimulation. Stimulation of the G-spot may trigger female ejaculation. We recall this issue here as a reminder of the controversial nature of these findings and the inconsistencies in the empirical data that both support and refute the G-spot hypothesis.

Multiple Orgasms

There is an interesting and important difference between the sexual response cycles of women and men during the resolution phase. As noted earlier, if erotic stimulation and inclination continue after orgasm in women, some will continue back to the plateau phase where they experience renewed building of sexual tension and have another orgasm. In some women, this can happen several times. Multiple orgasms may occur both during sexual intercourse and during masturbation as well. Even though such orgasms feel good, we believe multiple orgasms should not be the focused goal of all sexual intercourse. A sole criterion for sexual satisfaction would not account for the facts that rewarding, enjoyable intimacy can happen without an orgasm at all and that in many women, stimulation of the external genitalia after orgasm can be uncomfortable or even painful. If one orgasm is good, several are not necessarily better.

There is, of course, nothing wrong with a woman if she doesn't have multiple orgasms. She isn't sexually inadequate in any way. Women who do have multiple orgasms may have two or three during intercourse, and some have many more. In a study of over 800 female nurses, Darling, Davidson, and Jennings (1991) found that 42.7% of their sample had experienced multiple orgasms by masturbation, petting, or sexual intercourse. A few had multiple orgasms in all of these forms of sexual stimulation. Subjects were selected for this study because of their ability to verbalize their sexual experiences and their knowledge of basic sexual and reproductive anatomy. Interestingly, a number of important differences were found between subjects who had single orgasms and those who had multiple orgasms. Women who experienced multiple orgasms were more inclined to explore and experiment sexually and had orgasms by means of clitoral self-stimulation at an earlier age than did the women who had single orgasms. Further, multiorgasmic women were more likely to enjoy clitoral stimulation during intercourse, either by their partners or themselves, than women who reported single orgasms.

Since Masters and Johnson's description of the human sexual response cycle, investigators have believed that only women can have multiple orgasms. Men supposedly cannot because they experience a refractory period after orgasm during which no erotic stimulation, no matter how vigorous, can elicit arousal for at least a period of time. The duration of this refractory period depends in part on the man's age. Younger men have shorter refractory periods than older men. While a younger man may be ready for sexual arousal within an hour or two of an orgasm, older men may require several hours or even a day or two. The thinking about men not being able to have multiple orgasms has changed in recent years, however. Recall that orgasm is a two-stage process in men. It involves *emission*, during which the prostate gland, seminal vesicles, and part of the vas deferens contract and force semen into the urethral bulb where it is held temporarily. It also involves *expulsion*, during which semen is forced through the urethra and out of the penis. Some men have apparently learned the sensations associated with these two stages and have gained control over whether and when they will ejaculate. For example, if after emission has occurred, a man slows or stops his pelvic thrusting, he may enjoy intense erotic enjoyment without proceeding immediately to the stage of expulsion. Ejaculation is thus delayed. This is called a "nonejaculatory orgasm" and this individual will not experience a refractory period and may soon re-engage in sexual sharing and perhaps have another nonejaculatory orgasm or may finally ejaculate. Apparently the notion that emission must lead to expulsion followed by a refractory period is too simplistic.

More and more men are reporting their capacity for multiple nonejaculatory orgasms before ejaculation. Dunn and Trost (1989) studied over 20 men who were multiply orgasmic, having between 3 and 10 orgasms during prolonged periods of sexual intercourse. The men in this study could approach the point of ejaculatory inevitability and then "back off," pause, and continue having intercourse. Physically, these respondents had learned to separate the experience of nonejaculatory orgasm from that of ejaculation itself. Some of these men reported ejaculating more than once during prolonged sexual intimacy. While some subjects reported always having had this ability, others noted that they actively and purposely learned it through continued practice and experimentation. These men indicated that it was important to have a partner whom they knew very well and with whom they felt fully comfortable. Also, these men noted that their partner's responsiveness and the chance to enjoy intercourse at a leisurely pace were also important. The women with whom they had intercourse were just as interested in long-lasting intercourse and multiple orgasms as the men. Generally, as men get older and experience a prolonged plateau phase in their sexual response cycle, they are better able to discriminate between emission and expulsion and may be better able to control and delay their ejaculation. Studying multiply orgasmic men has shown that traditional beliefs and expectations about men's sexual responsiveness may be too narrow.

CONCLUSION

While the study of human sexual arousal and response has been clarified tremendously in the past 30 years through careful, empirical physiological measurements and observations, their very nature requires that they be approached with full awareness of psychological and social influences. The words "pleasure" and "sharing" are in the title of this chapter to emphasize these qualities, and any analysis of arousal and response that deemphasizes them is necessarily incomplete. This is one reason why Kaplan's thinking about the significance of desire as an essential aspect of sexual response in general is important. The language people use to describe excitement and orgasms says a lot about their general attitude toward our sexuality in general, although people often encounter difficulties trying to communicate comfortably and unambiguously about their responses to erotic stimulation.

This chapter covers the many and wonderful sensory experiences that accompany the human sexual response cycle to emphasize the many "inputs" people deal with in this intense interpersonal exchange called intimacy. These psychosocial and communication issues also help serve as an introduction to the discussion of love, affection, and intimacy explored in the next chapter.

Learning Activities

1. People experience sexual arousal as both inevitable and pleasurable under a wide variety of circumstances. Many people, however, have ambivalence and discomfort about their own sexual excitement. Speculate on personal, family, or other social factors that might foster a sense of uncertainty and anxiety about sexual arousal and orgasm.

2. Define the word "erotic" in your own words, and describe a scene in a movie you saw recently or a book you recently read that you feel is highly erotic.

3. When Barry McCarthy (1995) says that it is important to "take responsibility for one's own sexuality," what do you think he means by this phrase? Give an example of a behavior that illustrates this idea.

4. Flirting is a common way to express sexual interest and desire. Describe specific behaviors, gestures, postures, and facial expressions that you feel are flirting techniques.

5. Describe what type of person you think would be a volunteer in an experiment about sexual arousal and orgasm. Would *you* be comfortable applying a penile strain

gauge or vaginal photoplethysmograph to yourself? Why or why not?

6. You have learned that the sympathetic branch of the autonomic nervous system is associated with "fight or flight" behaviors and stimulates physiological changes that help us cope with emergencies, such as increased heart rate, increased breathing rate, and the channeling of blood sugar to our muscles. Speculate why this same branch of the autonomic nervous system is responsible for the neurological activities that underlie orgasm in women and men. Does there seem any relationship between orgasm and the "fight or flight" reaction?

7. When Masters and Johnson first published their research on the human sexual response cycle in 1966, their book was strongly praised by the scientific community. What criticism do you think this book might also have received from the scientific community?

8. Helen Singer Kaplan emphasized that human beings differ a lot in how they think about sexual desire. Since people learn about their own sexuality in the course of developing as adolescents and young adults, how do you think people begin to discriminate between "desire," "eroticism," and "sexuality?" What types of *experiences* might teach people about each of these?

9. Describe specifically your own concept of a "climate of psychological safety." Note the interpersonal, psychological, and social aspects of this concept and speculate about how it might change as one grows older.

10. Sexual fantasies are often portrayed in music videos. Describe a music video that does this and comment on the artistic and realistic (or bizarre) aspects of the scenes presented. Do you feel that this video was produced in "good taste," and what does this term mean to you?

11. The term "habituation" refers to diminished biological or subjective responses to continued, unchanging stimuli. Describe circumstances in which a couple might experience lessened sexual interest, excitement, and response over a period of time. What might they do to decrease the chances that the sexual aspect of a relationship could become boring and routine?

12. Describe what you have heard about the effects of prescription or recreational drugs on sexual arousal and response. Do you think these agents might really be aphrodisiacs, or could this be an example of self-fulfilling expectations?

13. Sometimes the *suggestion* of sexuality can be highly enticing and create keen sexual desire. One wag once said, "Statistics are like a bathing suit; what they reveal is interesting, but what they hide is vital!" What do you think about this?

14. Look at a number of women's and men's magazines, paying special attention to advertisements for perfume and cologne. Summarize the appeal of these ads. Is it beauty, cleanliness, sexiness, self-confidence, or playfulness that gets the reader's attention? What other personal qualities seem promised if you only buy the item?

Key Concepts

- The interpersonal context of sexual arousal and response involves the psychosocial context in which these behaviors occur and the communication patterns of the people involved.
- Spontaneous sexual expression is an important part of arousal and sexual anticipation.
- Flirting has elements of sexual assertiveness, is overt, implies invitation, and has an element of playfulness about it. Flirting is basically nonverbal and especially appealing if unconventional.
- Libido is a basic, primitive motivational force in the personality with sexual and/or aggressive aspects.
- The central nervous system is composed of the brain and spinal cord. The remainder of the nervous system is called the peripheral nervous system.
- Hormones are chemical substances produced in endocrine glands. They are secreted directly into the bloodstream, travel to some point distant from where they are produced, and change the rate of activity in some target organ.
- The organizing effects of hormones are the ways in which they direct early physical development and, therefore, affect the anatomy and physiology of specific organs. The activating effects of hormones are the ways in which they affect the appearance or cessation of a specific behavior.
- Masters and Johnson's sexual response cycle has four stages for the anatomical and physiological changes accompanying arousal and response in women and men.
  1. The excitement phase involves penile erection and vaginal lubrication in women. It prepares a couple for comfortable penetration.
  2. The plateau phase involves perceptions of building sexual tension and pleasure. Penile tumescence continues in men, and specific clitoral, vaginal, and breast changes occur in women.
  3. During orgasm there is a sudden release in sexual tension, usually followed by ejaculation in men and rhythmic contractions both at the entrance to the vagina and within the vagina itself in women.
  4. In the resolution phase, both internal and external male and female anatomical structures return to their pre-excitement states.
- Helen Singer Kaplan's three-stage model of human sexual arousal has three stages for *both* psychological and physiological changes in women and men.
  1. Desire refers to feelings of emotional attraction, attachment, safety, and an awareness of strong affiliative motives. Voluntary, willful feelings of closeness and excitement accompany the phase of "desire."
  2. Excitement corresponds to vasocongestive changes in the pelvis and genitalia and corresponds to penile erection and vaginal lubrication.

  3. The third and final stage of Kaplan's model involves orgasm and all the physiological changes that accompany this response.
- A more cognitive approach to sexual arousal is that of David Reed's, which he calls the erotic stimulus pathway model.
  1. In the seduction phase, feelings of desire, arousal, and focused sexual interest grow slowly.
  2. Sensations refer to an acute, hypnotic sexual focus on erotic stimuli and our perceptual responses to this information.
  3. In surrender, we relinquish our restraint and give ourselves up to the pleasures of the moment.
  4. The final stage, reflection, involves our subjective assessment of the fulfillment and enjoyments of the completed intimate acts in which we have just participated.
- When two individuals have approached a sexual situation willingly, willfully, and without any suggestion of coercion or force, they have created a climate of psychological safety.
- Sexual fantasies are a normal, creative avenue of experiencing sexual desire and in some ways help people mentally "rehearse" situations that may actually come about.
- Sexual arousal and response have both involuntary and voluntary aspects. While in some cases we seem to just "respond" unthinkingly, in others we give ourselves "permission" to pursue feelings of sexual enjoyment.
- Common emotions, such as anxiety, depression, and anger, all have the potential to diminish sexual arousal, response, and enjoyment.
- Privacy is an important social aspect of sexual arousal and response and involves the capacity to control spatial boundaries and the access others have to one's self.
- Empiricism is the philosophical approach that maintains that the contents of the mind derive from the inputs of the various sensory systems.

Glossary Terms

anaphrodisiac
aphrodisiac
autonomic nervous system
brain
climate of psychological safety
detumescence
endocrine system
habituation
limbic system

nocturnal penile tumescence
nucleus
parasympathetic nervous system
penile strain gauge
peripheral nervous system
pheromone
reflex

refractory period
sexual value system
spinal cord
sympathetic nervous system
vaginal photoplethysmograph
vasocongestion

$\mathcal{S}$uggested Readings

Beckman, L. J., & Ackerman, K. T. (1995). Women, alcohol, and sexuality. Recent Developments in Alcoholism, 12, 267-285.

Darling, C. A., Davidson, J. K., & Cox, R. P. (1991). Female sexual response and the timing of partner orgasm. Journal of Sex and Marital Therapy, 17, 3-21.

Darling, C. A., Davidson, J. K., & Jennings, D. A. (1991). The female sexual response revisited: Understanding the multiorgasmic experience in women. Archives of Sexual Behavior, 20, 527-540.

Ford, C. S., & Beach, F. A. (1951). Patterns of sexual behavior. New York: Harper and Brothers, Publishers and Paul B. Hoeber, Inc., Medical Books.

Henderson, D. J., Boyd, C. J., & Whitmarsh, J. (1995). Women and illicit drugs: Sexuality and crack cocaine. Health Care for Women International, 16, 113-124.

Hollender, M. H. (1970). The wish to be held. Archives of General Psychiatry, 22, 445-453.

McCarthy, B. W. (1995). Bridges to sexual desire. Journal of Sex Education and Therapy, 21, 132-141.

Montagu, A. (1971). Touching. The significance of the skin. New York: Harper & Row.

Rowland, D. L., Kallan, K., & Slob, A. K. (1997). Yohimbine, erectile capacity, and sexual response in men. Archives of Sexual Behavior, 26, 49-62.

7

Love, Affection, and Sexual Intimacy

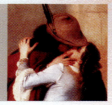

OBJECTIVES

When you finish reading and reviewing this chapter you should be able to:

1. Discriminate among the meanings of the terms, "affection," "attachment," "love," and "intimacy."

2. Discuss the psychological tasks involved in developing a relationship.

3. Explain the concept of "maturity" and discuss its seven distinguishing characteristics.

4. Discuss different styles of interpersonal attachment and give an example of each.

5. Summarize situations that may cause feelings of jealousy, and discuss how people cope with this powerful emotion.

6. Explore various meanings of *dependency, interdependency,* and *codependency.* Describe how two people relate to each other in these three ways.

7. Summarize Robert J. Sternberg's Triangular Theory of Love, giving examples of relationships in which passion, intimacy, and commitment are most prominent.

8. Describe how interpersonal relationships are enhanced or hindered by sex.

9. Define the "sexual double standard."

10. List and discuss potential benefits and drawbacks of having sex without being in love.

11. Discuss the special challenges of intermarriage and speculate how a couple might work together to minimize potential problems.

12. Discuss and give specific examples of principles of effective interpersonal communication.

13. Describe the requirements for productive negotiation between two people and give examples of each.

14. List productive ways of giving and receiving criticism during conflicts.

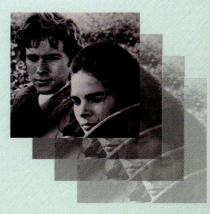

From Dr. Ruth

Many popular books categorize men and women as being from different planets or living on different planes. Comedians too often get easy laughs by poking fun at perceived differences between men and women. But while this topic may sell books and draw laughs, it also causes trouble because it gives people an easy excuse not to see others as they really are. Putting labels on your mate, rather than trying to really understand him or her, is a sure way to destroy a relationship, not build it up.

That's not to say that there are only physical differences between men and women. But if you are trying to make the most of your relationship with someone else, it is much more useful to concentrate on what you have in common than what separates you. Of course you've heard the phrase "opposites attract," and sometimes two people are attracted to each other because of differences. But it's one thing for two people to be attracted to one another and a whole different matter for them to stay together. So no matter what planet you think you're from, if you don't want to spend your life bouncing from one relationship to another, try to forge as many links to a potential lifetime partner as possible.

BASIC CONCEPTS OF LOVE, AFFECTION, AND INTIMACY

Just as sexual concerns seem to occupy us compellingly and frequently, so too do friendships and deeper intimacies. While many people are very curious about human sexuality, they are often less aware of or interested in the close association between a good relationship and good sex. We do not expect everyone to think this way too, but we hope this chapter helps you consider for yourself the importance of relationships.

This chapter examines theories about love and different kinds of love. Although much of the study of this subject has a focus on premarital counseling, we do not mean to suggest that only marriages make the best relationships. There are many different and successful kinds of relationships and forms of intimacy. In addition, since many relationships begin in the workplace, we will examine romantic attraction that occurs within organizations and the perceptions of managers and coworkers about such romantic attachments.

Finally we will note one assumption we made in putting together this subject matter. We believe that when people learn effective ways to relate to others, they will make efforts to improve the quality of their own relationships. People who apply this information to their own lives can, therefore, expect more rewarding relationships and better understand what "love," "affection," and "intimacy" mean to them personally.

"Affection," "Love," and "Intimacy"

Because people do not all have the same cultural, intellectual, and spiritual backgrounds, there are often big differences in how they conceptualize terms like "affection," "love," and "intimacy."

The word **affection** is often used to mean liking or fondness, usually without deep emotional or passionate connotations. Although this is a positive term, we generally use more serious and significant ways to refer to people who are very important to us. As "affection" involves good feelings about another person, "behaving affectionately" is the behavioral manifestation. Social workers, counselors, and psychologists teach us that people who give affection and receive it from others generally report their lives are going well and that they feel good about their relationships. We believe that affection is a sort of prerequisite for love and intimacy.

Love conveys a deeper meaning than affection. In 1962, the prominent psychoanalyst Erich Fromm wrote a little book that became one of the most popular books on college campuses for thirty years and remains popular and informative today. In *The Art of Loving*, Fromm examines the role of love in our lives and how it enriches our existence. He suggests that there are several different kinds of love, each with its own object and avenues of expression. Fromm discusses love between parents and their children, brotherly love, motherly love, erotic love, self-love, and love of God. He suggests that one's expression of love to another is an art that needs to be practiced to improve one's sharing of deepest affection and loyalty for another. Provocatively, he begins this book by noting many people's problem with love involves being loved rather than loving another. Because sexuality involves a mutual physical relationship between two people, we feel that the emotional sharing of a love relationship often enhances the mutuality of physical sex.

Fromm believed that we are all more or less fearful of separateness, the awareness of being utterly alone, and that sexual intimacy offers only a momentary relief from this universal human fear. The freely chosen object of human interpersonal attraction involves care, responsibility, respect, and knowledge (Fromm, 1962, page 26). *Care* is most commonly manifest in the love a mother gives her child. This kind of caring, according to Fromm, reflects a concern for the life and growth of the objects of our love. *Responsibility* concerns how we respond to the needs of those we love. These needs may be obvious or subtle, but if we love someone we generally are aware of them. *Respect* involves our desire to see others grow and mature without imposing upon them our expectations and goals for their development. *Knowledge* involves our knowing others as they really are, not as we think they are or would like them to be. Knowledge is based on respect for the separateness between any two human beings and the recognition that a deep, nonintrusive awareness of the other's authentic self is sometimes possible.

For Fromm, erotic love involves a desire for a temporary but complete and exclusive fusion with another person; it is the main route to real human intimacy. Although this psychoanalytic view may sound judgmental, it has value for helping one think about and clarify the role of sexuality in one's own love relationships.

The term **intimacy** also has unique and important connotations. Intimate relationships are typically characterized by a very close, warm relationship in which two people share very personal and private thoughts and feelings. There may or may not be a sexual dimension in an intimate relationship. Intimate relationships generally involve *sustained* affection or love, mutual trust, and a real sense of cohesiveness between partners (Prager, 1995). When we trust another person, we believe we will not be hurt, used, betrayed, or deceived. Intimate relationships are cohesive in that partners plan to spend time together and really like doing so, and have a sense of "we" in their affiliation. Affection, trust, and cohesiveness are all fundamental aspects of intimacy (Prager, 1995).

Working on Relationships

Relationships are held by married couples, cohabiting people, and single individuals. A relationship may have lasted many decades or a few short weeks, yet most relationships seem to have certain things in common. In a study of 94 married and committed (engaged or cohabiting) couples, Sprecher et al. (1995) isolated three primary areas clearly and consistently reported by people as fundamental to the quality of their relationship. Working to improve these areas had a highly beneficial effect on the satisfaction and commitment reported by

these subjects. These three areas are *companionship, supportive communication,* and *sexual expression* (Table 7-1). "Companionship" refers to doing many and different things with one's partner. The couple shares interests they find worth developing and enjoying together. "Supportive communication" involves both partners being willing to listen when the other needs to talk. The couple communicates nondefensively and without sarcasm, can discuss just about anything, and perceive that they have a lot in common. "Sexual expression" refers to being satisfied with one's sex life; the couple enjoys variety in their expression of physical intimacy, feels free to be sexually spontaneous, and feels that one's partner is very interested in them sexually. Although these investigators didn't start out studying how to work on a relationship, their findings revealed areas of importance for improving the quality of a relationship.

Regan and Sprecher (1995) asked a sample of 212 men and 348 women to judge the importance of a number of different factors in a marriage or long-term committed relationship. These researchers examined 22 different elements in a broad range of a couple's shared experiences: social status, personal attributes, sociability, expressiveness, and fulfillment of obligations. Both women and men in this sample generally agreed on what they valued as a contribution to a relationship. There were, however, a few interesting differences. Women valued emotional expressiveness in their male partners more than men did in women. It was also more important to women that their male partners got along well with the woman's family and friends and that men have the social status associated with well-paid employment. Physical attractiveness was the only characteristic valued more by men than women. Interestingly, men indicated that their partner's sexual fidelity was a more important contribution to the relationship than their own (Fig. 7-1).

TABLE 7-1

Reported Characteristics of High Quality Relationships

COMPANIONSHIP:	Enjoying many, diverse activities together.
	Developing and sharing mutual interests
SUPPORTIVE COMMUNICATION:	Mutual interests in one another's problems.
	Open, honest verbal and nonverbal communication.
	Difficult issues and concerns are not ignored
SEXUAL EXPRESSION:	Spontaneity and variety in physical intimacy.
	Being made to feel sexually attractive by one's partner.

From Sprecher et al., 1995.

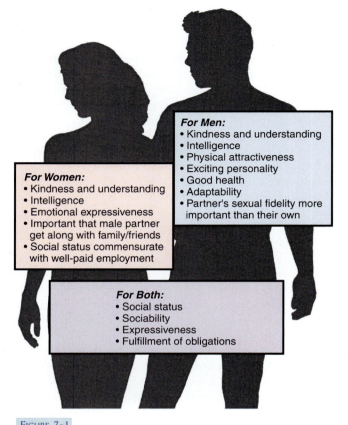

For Women:
• Kindness and understanding
• Intelligence
• Emotional expressiveness
• Important that male partner get along with family/friends
• Social status commensurate with well-paid employment

For Men:
• Kindness and understanding
• Intelligence
• Physical attractiveness
• Exciting personality
• Good health
• Adaptability
• Partner's sexual fidelity more important than their own

For Both:
• Social status
• Sociability
• Expressiveness
• Fulfillment of obligations

FIGURE 7-1   Women and men report that a number of characteristics are very important in a potential mate. Often these differ, but sometimes they are the same.

In general all important—and especially intimate—relationships have something in common: the challenge of being a fully participating member of a couple while still maintaining one's autonomy and developing one's independence. Because this challenge usually takes place within the context of a marriage or other committed relationship, it is worthwhile examining the "tasks" women and men face as they enter these bonds. Wallerstein (1994) isolated seven key challenges couples face during their early years together.

The first task a couple faces in developing a relationship bond is to change the nature of their connection with their families of origin and begin to create a sense of sovereignty as a couple. As people often maintain close contact with their parents, many women and men find it challenging to create a new family of their own independent of the expectations and traditions of their mothers and fathers. A second challenge is to develop a sense of "we-ness" in which the relationship is seen as much more than just the sum of the two. The strength and stability of a relationship are enhanced when a couple feels that together they possess resources that neither party has alone and that they can depend on these during tough times and daily frustrations and hassles. The third priority is to develop a sexual "style" that is mutually rewarding. Issues like

sexual spontaneity and playfulness, as well as the frequency of intercourse are exciting to explore together and present an important challenge for the development of candid sharing and good communication.

The fourth task in a new relationship involves the couple seeing the bond as a refuge of "safety and nurturance" (Wallerstein, 1994, page 649). Feeling protected from the threats and dangers of the outside world is basic to the feeling of safety that characterizes relationships people report to be rewarding and secure. The fifth challenge, which may not affect all people, involves creating a family while at the same time respecting the integrity and intimacy of the couple at the core of the group. Sometimes women and men selflessly give everything to the development of their children and neglect the maintenance that every relationship requires. Sooner or later this couple may find themselves feeling lonely and isolated from the children to whom they "gave" everything in the early years of their relationship. The sixth task requires that the couple build a relationship that is pleasurable and engrossing and that offers enjoyable distractions from the routines of daily living. Finally, the seventh task involves partners keeping and enjoying their early, idealized image of their significant other from when they were "young, crazy, and madly in love." Holding those moments and memories and enjoying them as sources of renewal and deep satisfaction is a manageable challenge in all relationships.

These tasks provide a clear general picture of what it takes to get a good start in a relationship, whether a marriage, a committed cohabitation arrangement, or another alternative. Wallerstein's approach was based on a longitudinal study in which 50 "happily married" couples were interviewed over the course of several years and reflects marriages that have lasted an average of 21 years.

THE DYNAMICS OF SOCIAL ATTRACTION

Before people feel affection, love, or a desire to be intimate with another person, they usually experience a less well defined emotion called **social attraction.** Social attraction is often the first stage in more meaningful relationships. Feelings of attraction between two people are actually comprised of several complex, interdependent elements. Social and behavioral scientists have isolated a number of important properties that affect whom we like and are attracted to. These include proximity, familiarity, physical attractiveness, similarity, and self-disclosure (Fig. 7-2). These elements can actually *predict* the types of people we are likely to be attracted to and want to spend time with.

Propinquity

"Proximity" (or the more technical term, "propinquity") simply means "nearness." People are more likely to become attracted to and like people they are near to. This is true in neighborhoods, dormitories, apartment buildings, and workplaces. After all, the more frequently you bump into someone, the more likely you are to learn about them, talk with them, and notice and appreciate their unique and interesting qualities. Studies have demonstrated that people living in student housing projects were far more likely to become attracted to their next-door neighbors than were people living in apartments further apart. In terms of friendships, dormitory roommates are more likely to like each other than are non-roommates. An opposite effect also can hold true, however: in apartment buildings, most residents say that of those neighbors they especially dislike, most live very close to their unit. These negative effects of proximity have been called "environmental spoiling" (Ebbesen, Kjos, & Konecni, 1976).

Familiarity

The more you see someone, the more familiar they become and the more likely it is that you may develop a genuine liking or attraction for that person. Generally, for example, you are more likely to know and become familiar with those who sit close to you in a class. Political candidates and advertisers similarly know that the more often you see their faces or products, the more likely it is that you'll vote for them or buy their product. The old saying that "familiarity breeds contempt" is wrong in this respect. Familiarity often leads to friendship and fondness.

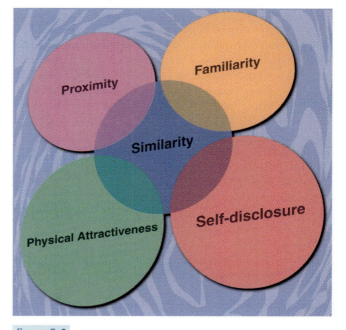

FIGURE 7-2 Social attraction is based upon a number of different, but interrelated qualities. These may grow or diminish in importance from time to time but all are consistent, important predictors of interpersonal appeal.

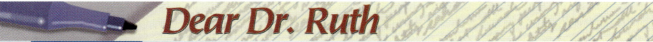

Dear Dr. Ruth

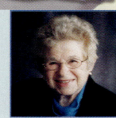

Question

When I was a little girl I thought I would grow up, fall in love, and share a wonderful life with a good and decent man. I am now 27 and have been through a number of very frustrating and unrewarding relationships with several guys. It seems that things always go really great at first, but then I begin to feel we never talk about anything really important, and eventually we don't talk very much at all. What can I do to have a better relationship? Is there something wrong with me, or do I just have bad luck?

Answer

Maybe your expectations are partly causing your relationships to end. You may be very interested in a certain thing, but that doesn't mean that the man you are with shares that feeling. You can't expect two people to turn into Siamese twins from dating a short while, or even from being married for a long time. Some people think that they have to find a partner who is a "soul mate." I don't know whether such a thing really exists, but maybe you'd be better off with a more realistic attitude. You have to work at a relationship. Think of love as a fire in a fireplace. It starts out with a big blaze, but unless you keep adding logs, it will burn out. If good conversation is important to you, make a point of stoking that particular fire. Buy tickets to a good play that you can talk about. Read a book and pass it on to him. Scout the newspapers for topics that you both find appealing. If you're willing to work at your next relationship, I feel certain that you can make it last longer.

Physical Attractiveness

Interestingly, in surveys in which women and men are asked to name and rank the qualities they find important in a potential mate, physical attractiveness is *never* at the top of the list. Factors such as "kindness and understanding" and "intelligence" seem much more important (Buss, 1985). This is true in a society that often seems obsessed with appearances, in which the media and advertisers encourage people's attempts to approximate societal conceptions of beauty. One should note, however, that there is often a discrepancy between how people rank personal attributes on such a list and how they behave in the real world everyday. In fact, good looks do matter and play an important role in the attraction between two people.

Some generalizations can be made about the role of physical attractiveness in social attraction, although attractiveness is difficult to define according to unambiguous, widely accepted attributes. Human tastes can be highly idiosyncratic, and those physical characteristics some people find highly attractive often leave others disinterested. Although we don't know how or why people develop their own ideas about attractiveness, large individual differences are undeniable. It is also very difficult to try to separate a person's physical attractiveness from their personality characteristics. Still, social and behavioral scientists have found that a woman's physical attractiveness is correlated fairly accurately with how frequently she dates. It has been shown that men put a greater premium on physical attractiveness in a potential date than women do. Further, when many different social and psychological attributes of two people are evaluated objectively (as a dating service might do), only physical attractiveness tends to predict how women and men will evaluate a date they had. Also of some interest is the apparent fact that women and men tend to date and marry others at a comparable level of attractiveness with themselves, just as they seem to select others with similar levels of intelligence (Feingold, 1988). Finally, research shows that attractive people are often seen as congenial, and congenial people are often evaluated as attractive.

Research has also shown that different considerations affect how people think about attractiveness in women and men. In recent years, for example, attractiveness in women has been associated with progressively thinner body shapes. Conformity to this standard has led to lower weights among college women, a large number of articles about obesity in the popular press, and an increase in eating disorders. Since the turn of the century our society has generally equated thinness with attractiveness (Silverstein, Peterson, & Perdue, 1986). Sociocultural standards of male attractiveness have also changed over the past generation. For example, since 1960 there has been a tremendous increase in health and fitness facilities and the number of men going to them. Messages in the popular press concerning body weight and attractiveness increased through the late 1970s and then gradually decreased over the following 15 years. Today's "ideal" male body is slender with good muscle tone and has not changed much over the past three decades (Petrie, Austin, Cowley, Helmcamp, et al., 1996).

More recent data suggest that African American women and men may associate body characteristics with attractiveness somewhat differently than Caucasian women and men. For example, Jackson and McGill (1996) found that African American men reported higher preference ratings for large body types and linked more favorable and fewer unfavorable characteristics with obese women than did Caucasian men. Both African American women and Caucasian women stated preferences for somewhat slender men, yet African American women associated fewer undesirable attributes with obese men than did Caucasian women. This study involved a relatively small sample of subjects, however, and a larger sample size would be desirable before generalizing from these data.

One more interesting aspect of attractiveness has been studied. Madey et al. (1996) studied whether the effects of alcohol include making members of the opposite sex seem more attractive. They found that when patrons in a bar were questioned at 10 p.m., 12 midnight, and 1:30 a.m., they reported significant increases in the attractiveness of opposite-sex patrons, but *only if they were not in a committed relationship at the time*. Apparently, relationship status also affects the perceived attractiveness of others. Attractiveness is often based on highly subjective personal feelings that can change from time to time.

Similarity

If two people are similar, are they more likely to be attracted to each other, or if they are attracted to each other, are they more likely to be similar? We know that when husbands and wives are similar to each other, they are more likely to report marital happiness and are less likely to divorce (Caspi & Herbener, 1990). Yet it is more difficult to determine whether similarity and attraction are *causally* related. Social psychologists have collected data that indicate that mutual attraction is an expected consequence of similarity (Byrne & Griffitt, 1973).

The term "assortative mating" describes how people pair off based on their real similarities (Buss, 1985). We say *real* similarities because often two people think that they are alike when in fact their commonalities are superficial and unrelated to important personality and other dimensions. A number of fairly straightforward demographic variables are important in assortative mating, including such factors as race, religion, ethnic background, age, and socioeconomic status. Nonetheless, people often think that differences instead of similarity lead to attraction. Do opposites attract? Is a person who is shy and reserved captivated by someone who is outgoing and self-assured? Captivated, quite possibly, but probably not genuinely attracted. The term *complementarity* is used to describe the inclination of some people to compensate for something absent in the other. Data collected over the last thirty years demonstrate conclusively that similarity is far more important than complementarity in interpersonal attraction and rewarding relationships. It's true: birds of a feather *do* flock together (Buss & Schmitt, 1993).

Self-Disclosure

Affectionate and loving relationships allow us to "open" and share what is on our minds and in our hearts without fear of criticism or rejection. The ability and inclination to engage in this safe sharing is called *self-disclosure,* and it is an important feature of mutually rewarding relationships. People generally feel comfortable self-disclosing when they are attracted to someone else, and one of the best signs that a relationship is maturing is an increasing amount of self-disclosure between two people. Of course, people more easily share those aspects of themselves about which they feel good, whereas it can be very difficult to share things they don't like about themselves or feel ashamed of. We generally open up to people who open up to us; in a sense, disclosure is a kind of trust. Sidney Jourard, who studied self-disclosure for decades, found that when we give up our defenses and let ourselves be known for who we really are, this tremendously facilitates the development of a loving relationship. This does not mean, however, that self-disclosure automatically awakens feelings of love in another person. Most people are put-off when someone they have just met tells them private things, for example. Nonetheless, feeling free and safe to share what's on one's mind can be extremely important in interpersonal attraction (Collins & Miller, 1994).

Attachment

Psychologist Gordon Allport (who is discussed later in this chapter) describes "emotional security" as one of the criteria of maturity. This term refers to emotional poise and a capacity to tolerate frustration. Emotional security also has much to do with how people affiliate with one another and establish relationships. Also important are one's personal past experiences with various kinds of attachments, as very often the past has a powerful effect on our present lives. An interesting approach to adult attachment styles derives from research exploring how infants bond with their parents (Bowlby, 1969; Ainsworth, 1989). Hazan and Shaver (1987) describe three *adult* attachment styles that mirror closely a number of infant-parent attachment styles. Mary Ainsworth has described three main infant-parent attachment styles: secure attachment, ambivalent attachment, and avoidant attachment. The same categories are useful in describing adult attachments, as shown in the work Hazan and Shaver:

- Secure attachment is seen in individuals who are not defensive with others and don't worry about depending on others. They don't have deep, enduring fears that others will desert them. Sexually, they enjoy long-term monogamous relationships and don't seem to need constant reminders and reassurances that they are loved and valued. People who make secure attachments are comfortable with their relationships but also feel they are whole, complete, and happy as individuals. They enjoy their own company and don't mind being alone.
- Individuals with anxious-ambivalent attachments are much less trusting and more likely to manifest jealousy and possessiveness in their relationships. They require constant proofs that they are someone's "one and only" and resent it deeply when the object of

their affection is with other people. People with anxious-ambivalent attachments have little idea how they would do on their own. They always see themselves as either with someone or between relationships, but never comfortably alone. These individuals do not appreciate meditative silence and solitude.
- Finally, people with avoidant attachments are not comfortable with intimacy and closeness. They do not find relationships enjoyable or understand how people can grow in relationships with others. They have little interest in establishing a climate of psychological safety with another person and have never learned to share their vulnerabilities without feeling defenseless and exposed. Sexually, they are likely to have brief, affectionless encounters.

Tidwell, Reis, and Shaver (1996) asked 135 undergraduate students with these three attachment styles to keep a social interaction diary for one week. They were to describe any personal or telephone interaction that lasted 10 minutes or more. Their results confirm the descriptions of these attachment styles above. Those with avoidant attachment styles described lower levels of intimacy in their interpersonal contacts, fewer good feelings, and more negative feelings as a result of their encounters with others, especially members of the opposite sex. They were also less likely to initiate such interactions. The authors suggest that avoidant types may go out of their way to minimize activities in which human closeness may occur. Those subjects with a secure attachment style described more intimacy, felt much better about initiating interactions with others, expressed more enjoyment and positive emotions as a result of their encounters with others, and also had fewer negative emotions in these interactions. Finally, subjects with anxious-ambivalent attachment styles reported experiences with highly variable outcomes, generally intermediate between the secure and avoidant types. Interestingly, these authors found that physical attractiveness had little to do with differing attachment styles. This study offers a glimpse into the daily experiences of individuals with different attachment styles, and generally supports the theoretical claims of Hazan and Shaver (1987).

Another study explored the relationship between a person's attachment style and important intimate relationships. Morrison, Goodlin-Jones, and Urquiza (1997) found in their sample of 368 community college students that subjects with avoidant or ambivalent attachment styles reported far more hostility in their interpersonal relationships than those with secure attachment styles. Additionally, those with avoidant attachment styles described themselves as less submissive in relationships. Respondents with a secure attachment style described themselves as more comfortable with interdependency in relationships and had few reservations about "leaning on" their significant other occasionally. Interestingly, the amount of time these subjects had spent in close relationships was not related to the effects of these different attachment styles. In another study of the effects of different attachment styles on the

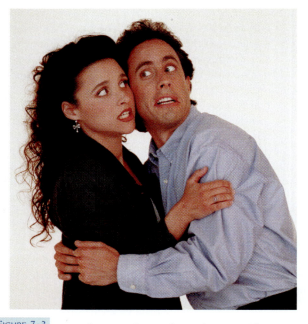

FIGURE 7-3 Even when people are obviously attracted to one another, they often remain a bit wary and vigilant despite their trust and affection.

interpersonal dynamics of a close relationship, Brennan and Morris (1997) found that securely attached college students were more comfortable in seeking positive feedback from those with whom they were involved, while those with other attachment styles didn't feel as comfortable in asking for this kind of validation.

We believe that these attachment styles have "face validity": one can read descriptions of how different individuals perceive social situations and act and can figure out which style corresponds most closely to one's own style. By learning about different attachment styles one may also better understand why one feels compatible or incompatible with others (Fig. 7-3). Can a person change her or his attachment style? We don't know of any research that has studied whether people can change their attachment styles.

Jealousy

As noted previously, people with anxious-ambivalent attachment styles are likely to experience jealousy and possessiveness in their interpersonal relationships. In fact, **jealousy** is a common, troubling emotion among most people regardless of attachment style. The daily news provides many stories of domestic violence in which jealousy has a major role.

Because attachment styles derive from infantile and childhood experiences with one's caretakers, some researchers have assumed that disrupted attachments early in life predispose an adult to feelings of jealousy. Clanton and Kosin (1991) studied this suspected connection and did *not* find any correlation or cause-and-effect relationship. Jealousy has received significant scientific attention only in the last two decades (Salovey, 1991).

Because jealousy so commonly affects relationships, and because sexual jealousy is so frequently implicated in violence and the dissolution of relationships, this topic deserves attention.

Jealousy involves fears and anxieties about betrayal and deception. To some extent, feelings of betrayal are similar in marriages, friendships, and social affiliations, although there are some differences among these different types of bonds (Shackelford & Buss, 1996). Generally, whenever one's significant other is involved with a third party, feelings of jealousy are likely to occur, even with brief, trivial social contacts outside of the relationship bond. The jealous person frets and worries, feels some uncertainty, and has problems understanding the "outside" attachment (Fitness & Fletcher, 1993). Stearns (1989) has suggested that according to contemporary social mores, confrontation is an unpopular way of dealing with jealousy and that people are far more likely to feel guilty about their feelings or to try to escape from the situation.

Another factor affecting jealousy is the duration of the relationship. Aune and Comstock (1997) found that the experience, expression, and perceived correctness of expressing jealousy increased with the length of the relationship. However, this study used a cross-sectional analysis of jealousy in groups of couples who had been together for varying periods, and the researchers point out that a longitudinal investigation is needed in which the development of jealousy is tracked more closely as it emerges in a relationship.

COPING WITH JEALOUSY

In Shakespeare's play *Othello,* jealousy is called a "green-eyed monster"—a fearful image for a human emotion (Fig. 7-4).

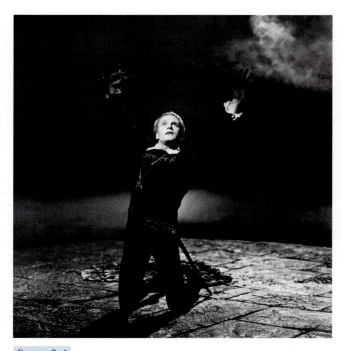

FIGURE 7-4 Sir Laurence Olivier plays Othello in Shakespeare's play of that name. This drama reveals some of the powerful and potentially destructive aspects of jealousy.

People affected by jealousy frequently behave in ways that show tremendous inner turmoil. Apparently, people in all societies experience jealousy (Clanton and Smith, 1977). In a large, comprehensive study, Guerrero, Andersen, Jorgensen, Spitzberg, and Eloy (1995) assessed how American undergraduate students report experiences of jealousy and how they communicate their feelings about jealousy.

Communicating feelings of jealousy can serve several functions. When people communicate their jealous feelings, they may gain information that helps reduce their feelings of uncertainty about their relationship and the "rival" relationship. Second, when a rival relationship and jealousy have hurt the primary relationship, many people want to repair the primary relationship, and clear communication about jealousy can help do this. Third, jealous feelings usually hurt a person's self-esteem if the person feels someone else is more important to his or her partner (Fig. 7-5). Clear communication is often an important first step in restoring one's self-esteem.

In rare cases, jealousy becomes part of a serious psychiatric disturbance referred to as the "Othello syndrome." In this condition the person's jealousy and/or belief in the sexual infidelity of their significant other reaches delusional proportions (Leong, Silva, Garza-Trevino, Oliva, Ferrari, Komanduri, and Caldwell, 1994). Patients suffering from the Othello syndrome have much hostility toward their partner, often including verbal threats and sometimes resulting in murder. The Othello syndrome is very rare but shows how compelling feelings of jealousy can become.

Depending on Others

The term **interdependence** describes how people feel an authentic concern for the happiness and welfare of their partner while at the same time remaining aware of their own needs and autonomy. Most social and behavioral scientists claim that true interdependence is not developed before young adulthood when one has a better understanding that to be in a good relationship with someone else, one must be at home with oneself as well. Interdependence is a basic attribute of mature intimate relationships. To depend on another person can be a genuine aspect of respect, esteem, and trust, or it can result from a deeper inadequacy and helplessness without the other. Just as real interdependence can occur in a robust and developed relationship, excessive reliance can present some problems.

There are interesting cross-cultural aspects in how people view the self in the social world and one's expectations and requirements of others. Because most Americans were raised within Western cultural traditions, our view of human action and achievement is generally individualistic. People are thought to succeed through their own efforts, and self-reliance is a celebrated societal norm. The "self-made person" has long been the image of worth and success in American society. But an interesting question arises. How does a woman or man enter the world of work everyday, knowing that their successes result from their own, and *only* their own efforts and skills, and then come home and effortlessly become part of a cooperative, sharing, collaborating wife/husband, or mother/father? Nonwestern

societies have more collectivistic values. In collectivistic cultures, such as Japan, cooperative contributions to the social or corporate environment are expected and rewarded. How the Japanese conceptualize the self is inherently different from how Westerners commonly do. Some researchers suggest the idea of

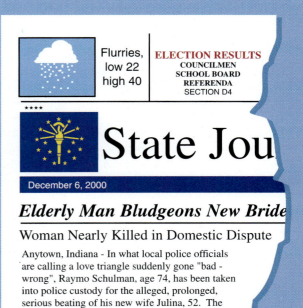

Flurries, low 22 high 40

ELECTION RESULTS
COUNCILMEN
SCHOOL BOARD
REFERENDA
SECTION D4

State Jou

December 6, 2000

Elderly Man Bludgeons New Bride

Woman Nearly Killed in Domestic Dispute

Anytown, Indiana - In what local police officials are calling a love triangle suddenly gone "bad - wrong", Raymo Schulman, age 74, has been taken into police custody for the alleged, prolonged, serious beating of his new wife Julina, 52. The Schulman's were married in June of this year and sources wishing to remain anonymous report that Ms. Schulman has been visiting her former husband regularly since that time. But three days ago when Julina returned home, her husband accosted her, tied her into a recliner in their family room, and beat her with his fists and an as yet unidentified blunt object for over 72 hours.

"I just can't believe she would cheat on me," Mr. Schulman was quoted as saying. "I've given her comfort and security and peace of mind and look what she goes and does! Nobody could take care of her as good as me, and the thought of her going back to that low-life, filthy man just made me lose my mind and my control and my pride."

Sources close to the story reveal that Ms. Schulman suffered broken facial bones, serious lacerations about the head and neck, and blunt force trauma to her chest, abdomen, and thighs. A number of her teeth had been knocked out. The medical examiner's office estimates that a significant period of hospiatalization will be needed to assess and treat Ms. Schulman's injuries. Love sometimes takes terrible twists in this small community in southeastern Indiana…

FIGURE 7-5 A "love triangle" can reveal violent emotions associated with jealousy. While this story might seem unusual in some respects, in fact it is based on a real incident. Daily newspapers have many unhappy stories similar to this one.

an *interdependent self,* in which people experience a greater sense of cohesion and membership with their wider environment (Markus & Kitayama, 1994). Interestingly, this concept is profoundly related to the idea of interdependency in close, loving relationships. We do not wish to make the idea of interdependency unnecessarily complex, but in order to talk about this issue between two adults, an understanding of larger social forces affecting our perceptions of one another is helpful.

In recent years, the term **codependency** has been used to describe relationships with an unhealthy dependency, often for a variety of different reasons. These relationships can be both unrewarding and frustrating and at the same time hard to get out of. Typically they do not involve mature intimacy, love, and sexuality. A codependent person is secure in their sense of being only when someone else defines their desires and wishes. They do not enjoy a sense of self unless their life is given up to the needs and desires of another person. In a codependent relationship a person feels bound psychologically to another person whose daily behaviors are motivated by a sense of urgency and compulsion (Giddens, 1992). Codependent relationships often involve substance abuse, alcoholism, gambling, compulsive sexuality, or another behavior pattern that is difficult to control. The term "codependency" has become a popular catchword and is often used loosely and inaccurately, often as a belittling label to characterize highly complex problems in an overly simplistic way.

The term *fixated* describes a situation in which two people have become addicted to their relationship with one another. The two people are unwilling or unable to create a full and rich life together and thirst only for the "security" of their bond. The tasks and routines of daily living take precedence over mutual growth and exploration in living. A fixated relationship is neither healthy nor enjoyable and seems remarkably resistant to therapeutic intervention.

THEORIES OF LOVE

Social and behavioral scientists develop theories about a wide variety of phenomena, and it's not surprising that a number of theories attempt to explain something as personal, emotional, and enigmatic as love. We will look at two such theories.

Sternberg's Triangular Theory of Love

We have already discussed many elements of attraction: proximity, familiarity, physical attractiveness, similarity, and self-disclosure. These are only the building blocks for intimate, enduring relationships, for clearly, there is more to loving than the sum of these components. Robert J. Sternberg (1988) has given us a useful way of thinking about different kinds of love. He suggests there are three key kinds of loving, which he represents schematically as three sides of a triangle: passion, intimacy, and commitment (Fig. 7-6). Passion involves powerful feelings that become obvious in romance, physical attraction, and a strong desire to become sexually involved. Intimacy is less "intense" and is reflected in the desire to feel close and connected and to form a meaningful bond. "Commitment" is as-

sociated with a time scale. On the one hand it involves a purposeful decision to love another in the present, but it also entails a strong desire to maintain that love over a long period of time.

Sternberg believes that the strength of our love depends on the independent potency of each of these three elements, while the particular kind of love we experience and the kind of relationship in which we engage result from the relative strengths of these three elements (Fig. 7-6). Table 7-2 illustrates how different types of relationships result.

PASSIONATE LOVE

Have you ever fallen "head over heels" in love? Passionate love is characterized by strong, preoccupying thoughts of the person to whom one feels powerfully attracted. Many people feel they are "floating on a cloud" and have a constant desire to see, be with, talk to, and make love with the other person. Passionate love can sometimes lead to reckless behavior, however, and it's still important to take precautions regarding contraception and STDs. People in a passionate relationship often feel "all wrapped up" in their feelings, and later, when the intensity of these feelings begins to ebb, as it inevitably does, some complain about being "suffocated" by the attentions of the other. The component of passion in love is very different from the other components of love Sternberg describes.

INTIMATE LOVE

Intimacy involves a genuine sense of liking one's partner and a desire to build together a more cohesive rapport. It involves sharing one's life with another in a candid, nondefensive way. Trust, patience, and tolerance are important aspects. A couple

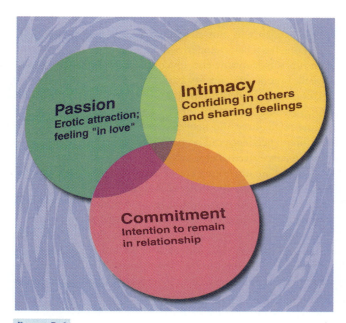

FIGURE 7-6 For psychologist Robert Sternberg, passion, intimacy, and commitment are three essential and interrelated aspects of love.

TABLE 7-2

The Triangular Theory of Love According to Robert J. Sternberg. Differing Combinations of Passion, Intimacy, and Commitment Result in Different Love Relationships

Type of Relationship	Component		
	Passion	Intimacy	Commitment
Liking	NO	YES	NO
Infatuation	YES	NO	NO
Fatuous Love	YES	NO	YES
Romantic Love	YES	YES	NO
Companionate Love	NO	YES	YES
Consummate Love	YES	YES	YES

After Sdoro, 1993, 689

genuinely enjoys developing their own communication style and becoming familiar with each other's imperfections and idiosyncratic characteristics—the things people rarely notice when first absorbed in intense passionate love. A sense of "we" develops, and the two look out for each other and try to avoid what irritates their partner. They try to anticipate each other's needs and desires and share a sense of humor. Respect is important in genuine intimate relationships.

COMMITMENT

People work hard together to build a commitment in a relationship. The two live in a climate of steady, enduring, confident affection for one another and strive to consolidate their union; they are partners. They deeply respect one another's privacy and enjoy sharing their partner with others in social settings. Trust and devotion are often at the heart of this kind of commitment. One would never take advantage of the other's vulnerabilities. They understand the inevitability of conflicts in daily living but do not feel these can harm their mutual esteem. They negotiate their differences fairly and with good faith. Of course, there are disagreements and differences in philosophy, yet they distinguish between significant and trivial concerns and work to resolve issues with focus and good will.

While Sternberg's components all seem positive, there may be some debate about how common or attainable they are and whether everyone shares the same vision that they comprise an attractive interpersonal relationship. To one degree or another, these three components may be present in all relationships, and in consummate love (which Sternberg believes is rare) all three are highly prominent.

A Typology of Love

The sociologist John Alan Lee has also explored the experience and expression of love (1977). Any typology may lead to the incorrect impression that people can be easily and unambiguously grouped into categories or that all of a person's behaviors conform to the defining attributes of a category. Keeping this caution in mind, let's examine Lee's six styles of loving.

Lee's first style of loving, *eros,* is based primarily on a person's physical appearance. There may be many different and sometimes enigmatic reasons why one feels a powerful love for another person, and these are often hard to describe clearly. Have you ever thought, "That person is *just my type.*" He or she may indeed be your type, but you may soon learn that your friends do not see this person in the same way you do. This is an "Eros lover," according to Lee.

The second style of loving is called *ludus,* which means "game playing." In playful love people do not commit to each other in a single, exclusive relationship but may enjoy many other relationships too that don't involve sharing deep feelings or highly personal aspects of themselves. These are friendships more than intimate bonds, although they may include sexual sharing.

A third style of loving, called *storge,* is a relationship that gradually evolves into a genuine feeling of attachment. This style of loving is slow, patient, tolerant, and enduring. In storge love, people explore a relationship they anticipate will eventually lead to a lasting devotion to one another.

Mania, Lee's fourth style of loving, involves a powerful romantic attachment involving passion and possessiveness. The person is obsessively preoccupied with the other person and constantly wants to be told and shown they are loved in return. They are highly anxious without this frequent reassurance and find it hard to focus on daily tasks and responsibilities because of their fascination with the person to whom they are attracted.

A fifth style of loving Lee calls *agape,* or "selfless love." This lover wants nothing in return for the expression of her or his affection. Just the experience of love itself is reward enough. The person feels truly alive and is unselfishly devoted to another person, with no urgency, jealousy, or clinging overprotectiveness in their feelings. They are both faithful and diligent in their expressions of love and take genuine delight in these behaviors and feelings.

Lee's last style of loving is called *pragma.* The word "pragmatic" means "practical," and the pragma lover seeks a partner who conforms to a number of sensible and often unromantic attributes. For example, a man may look for a woman who comes from an affluent family, is well-educated at a prestigious university, is pursuing graduate or professional training, and is comfortable in delaying a decision to start a family. Although this may not sound like love as it's usually thought of, some people do form relationships on this basis.

Lee's typology is interesting in part because it acknowledges that an emotion like love has different degrees and avenues of expression and involves a variety of experiences. Although most of us do not fit perfectly into one of these categories, it is an interesting exercise in self-examination to try to apply this typology to oneself. Both Lee's and Sternberg's theories are primarily descriptive, yet they may have some usefulness in helping people clarify their feelings for others or perhaps iron out problems in their relationships.

A Theory of Love and Sexual Desire

The theorist James Giles (1994) examined some of the complex connections between love and sexual desire, resulting in some thought-provoking speculations. Giles focuses entirely on romantic or passionate love and explores how sexuality gets mixed into these feelings. His perspective exclusively involves the *experiences* of loving and sexual desire and not their overt behavioral manifestations.

His analysis begins with a reference to the noted humanistic psychologist Rollo May (1969), who notes that "the paradox of love is that it is the highest degree of awareness of the individual self and the highest degree of absorption in the other" (page 62). Love is a dual self-awareness connected by the relation of desire. Giles then introduces one of the basic ideas of his theory:

> . . . at the very core of the experience of love lies a complex of intense desires involving the desire to be vulnerable before another person in order that one may be nurtured or cared for by that person, and, at the same time, the desire to have the other person vulnerable before oneself in order that one may nurture or care for that person. (p. 344)

Giles believes that intimacy, trust, and self-disclosure are all basic components of vulnerability. He suggests that in acting upon our sexual desires we bare our bodies to one another in *very much the same way* we bare our souls to one another when we share our vulnerabilities. In a sense, it is a physical kind of self-disclosure. And just as we share our nakedness, we caress one another and share our caring as well.

In his view, emotional vulnerability and physical self-disclosure and fondling are two sides of the same coin and complement one another in meaningful relationships. Either can exist without the other, but rewarding relationships usually involve both. Although Giles' speculations have not been explored by researchers for as long as Lee's and Sternberg's theories, they offer another significant way of thinking about the mysterious and awesome nature of love.

LOVE, SEX, AND RELATIONSHIPS

So far this chapter has dealt primarily with theories regarding the experience and expression of love in its different varieties and manifestations. Now we'll explore some empirical data and lifestyle issues about the role of love in different types of relationships. Because romantic love involves compelling feelings of closeness and attachment, much of this discussion focuses on this experience. The passionate component of love described by Sternberg has the characteristics of what most people mean by "romantic love." Hatfield and Rapson (1987) suggested that romantic love occurs in virtually all cultures and

FROM "ON LOVE" BY KAHLIL GIBRAN

Kahlil Gibran (1883-1931) (Fig. 7-7) was a Lebanese poet, philosopher, and artist. His book *The Prophet* (1923) contains many poems about virtually all aspects of our lives, and among the most poignant is a delightful work about love. Here are a few lines from that poem.

. . . When love beckons to you, follow him,
Though his ways are hard and steep.
And when his wings enfold you yield to him,
Though the sword hidden among his pinions
may wound you.
And when he speaks to you believe in him,
Though his voice may shatter your dreams as
the north wind lays waste the garden.
For even as love crowns you so shall he crucify
you. Even as he is for your growth so is he for
your pruning.
Even as he ascends to your height and caresses
your tenderest branches that quiver in the sun,
So shall he descend to your roots and shake
them in their clinging to the earth.
Like sheaves of corn he gathers you unto himself.

He threshes you to make you naked.
He sifts you to free you from your husks.
He grinds you to whiteness.
He kneads you until you are pliant;
And then he assigns you to his sacred fire, that you may
become sacred bread for God's sacred feast.
All these things shall love do unto you that you may know
the secrets of your heart, and in that knowledge become a
fragment of Life's heart.
But if in your fear you should seek only love's peace and
love's pleasure,
Then it is better for you that you cover your nakedness
and pass out of love's threshing-floor, Into the seasonless
world where you shall laugh, but not all your laughter,
and weep, but not all your tears. . .

—11-13

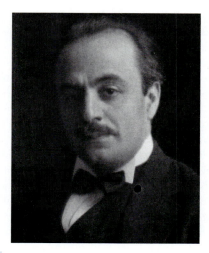

FIGURE 7-7 Kahlil Gibran, Lebanese poet, philosopher, and artist.

age groups. Jankowiak and Fischer (1998) found romantic love in 147 of the 166 cultures they studied. Apparently, cultural values, trends, and traditions cannot suppress this universal human experience. Still, the relationship between romantic love and long-term relationships has not always been obvious in human history.

As summarized by Brehm (1985), the ancient Greeks celebrated the power and pleasure of romantic love in both heterosexual and homosexual relationships but also acknowledged its irrational qualities. They believed that enduring, committed love relationships were incompatible with the excitement and passion of romantic attachments. Platonic love surmounted the urgency and lust of romantic love with an intellectual, austere rapport between two people; the appetite for the physical consummation of love just wasn't part of the picture. Similarly, the Romans viewed love as a complex recreational enterprise in which the chase was more fun than the capture. By the Middle Ages, a new tradition of love evolved: courtly love. Maidens were "loved pure and chaste from afar," and romance took on a highly idealistic quality. Knights pledged their loyalty to their ladies, went off to fight wars on their behalf, and returned to their idealized visions of purity and femininity, all of this supposedly involving a celibate, "higher" attraction than those carnal pleasures enjoyed by the peasantry. This was a common tradition in the Western history of love and romance until the seventeenth century, when the connection between love and marriage came to be seen as feasible and desirable.

This brief historical sketch shows that people's thinking about love has changed over time. Today, most people would react indignantly to the suggestion that love and marriage are unrelated. We certainly do not intend to tell you what to think about love, but we both believe that people's lives and relationships are tremendously enriched by love (Fig. 7-8).

Although we have reviewed the theoretical aspects of romantic love according to Sternberg, Lee, and Giles, we have not yet described the specific properties of ardent, passionate bonds. Pederson and Shoemaker (1993) sought to do this; they administered questionnaires to 177 college students and found five general aspects of romantic love: feelings of togetherness, expression of feelings, concern and communication, romancing and sensitivity, and spontaneity. Their subjects did not attribute equal importance to all of these, yet the responses clustered in these categories. Of course, these descriptions were in part a result of how the questionnaire was formulated and phrased, but these general feelings are clearly related to other concepts discussed throughout this chapter.

Another analysis of questionnaire data dealing with the dimensions of love (Aron & Westbay, 1996) confirmed Sternberg's earlier speculations about types of loving. This study isolated three central factors: passion, intimacy, and commitment. Aron and Westbay specifically analyzed interpersonal features associated with these three main factors. For example, phrases such as "gazing at each other," "euphoria," "butterflies in the stomach," and "wonderful feelings" were strongly associated with passion. Different descriptors were related to intimacy, including "openness," "feeling free to talk about anything," "being supportive," "being honest," and "showing understanding." Finally, commitment was associated with factors such as "devotion," "putting the other person first," "needing each other," "protectiveness," and "loyalty." Although often people claim it is too difficult to talk clearly and specifically

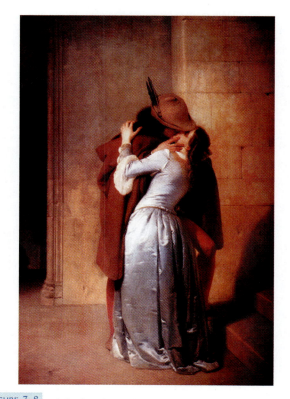

FIGURE 7-8 While the place of love in marriage has changed over the centuries, the central, enriching role of love in adult relationships is an age-old aspect of human nature.

about an emotion as "mushy" as love, careful use of questionnaires has shown it is possible to analyze and communicate these feelings. The research of Aron and Westbay demonstrates that there is a consistent, basic way that people understand love and that passion, intimacy, and compassion and their related attributes summarize some of the hard-to-explain qualities of love, as well as the feelings and behaviors associated with them.

Describing the overt actions of people in love is another matter, however. Lemieux (1996) found that in the responses of over 300 college students, romantic behaviors (excluding sexual interactions) seemed to cluster into five categories: enjoying mutual activities, sharing special occasions, offerings of gifts and tokens of affection, selfless behavior, and making sacrifices. The women in this study invested greater importance in these behaviors than the men, for reasons not entirely clear. Such lists of traits and behaviors should not, of course, be used as a "shopping list" of what to look for in a love relationship.

Idealization and Disillusionment in Romantic Love

How does the "average" person look at love today? Do people still believe it is a kind of madness or that it leads to frustration and dissatisfaction? Is love a diversion or entertainment? Does it inevitably involve some self-deception? Our culture clearly idealizes love, but do we have unrealistic expectations of it and its power to bond and enrich relationships?

Many people certainly do have unreasonably high expectations of a love relationship. Murray, Holmes, and Griffin (1996) suggest that enjoyable, predictable interpersonal relationships require a predisposition to see one's less-than-perfect partner in an enhanced, idealistic way. They call this a "positive illusion." They found that a relationship was most likely to continue over the course of their year-long study if both partners idealized one another. They also discovered that when two people idealized one another much at the beginning of the study, they reported *further* increased satisfaction with the relationship and a *decrease* in any conflicts or doubts they had at the outset. Interestingly, idealized partners gradually came to see themselves as their partners saw them. These researchers conclude that people may actually create the relationship they want over time, and that there may be a self-fulfilling prophesy in romantic attractions.

It seems as if love relationships involve an alternating awareness that one's partner is wonderful and perfect on one hand and human and fallible on the other. How do these apparently contradictory qualities coexist in the same person? Are we bound to find out sooner or later that the person we love isn't perfect? Judith A. Livingston (1996) explored the theoretical implications of these questions. A number of different things can occur when one finds out that the loved one isn't the perfect person once thought to be: the relationship may end, may continue with a more realistic, mature understanding, or may gradually fade away (p. 550). Livingston suggests romantic love is "enriched" by a balance between idealization and disillusionment, a balance that may change over the course of a relationship. However, sometimes a dramatic mismatch occurs between these two pictures of the other, leading to the rela-

Dear Dr. Ruth

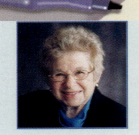

Question:

Can you help me with a question I've had for a long time? Is it "polite" for a woman to tell a man that she would like to have sex with him? Of course, I'm only talking about unmarried men.

People do seem to be more bold with each other these days, but I don't want to seem aggressive or cheap. Still, I am very sure about my feelings. I was raised to believe that "good girls" didn't express these feelings.

Answer:

Young ladies have always let men know how they feel, though not always in words. At one time, a dropped handkerchief was all it took, though these days dropping your handkerchief will only get it trampled on. But you don't have to rush off to the other extreme, either. Some men might find your boldness threatening, though others would enjoy it. My advice is to advance carefully. Remember, most women too do not like it if a man tries to go too far too fast.

Nonetheless, it is hard to make broad generalizations based on age alone. Because people are often grouped with similar-aged people when growing up, people naturally develop friendships and affectional bonds with others with whom they spend time. Elementary, middle, and high school classes usually include girls and boys of the same or highly similar ages, and the same is true in church groups and community centers. (As discussed in Chapter 12, however, things change somewhat in adolescence because girls begin pubertal development 1½ to 2 years ahead of boys and attract the attention of boys ahead of them in school.) In general, then, most people fall in love with and have relationships with others of a similar age despite what people say they prefer or seek.

The Role of Maturity in Adult Relationships

So far, we have explored characteristics of affection, love, and intimacy and how people work to enhance their interpersonal relationships. Behind this complex subject lies the assumption that we are talking about mature adults. If maturity is an essential attribute of rewarding intimate relationships, then we should explore its characteristics.

The psychologist Gordon W. Allport (Fig. 7-10) attempted to find the fewest important qualities of mature adults (Allport, 1961). He summarized what he believed were the six most important characteristics of mature individuals and emphasized that maturity is more a *process of personal growth and development* than a stable collection of traits. These characteristics are clearly important for creating and maintaining strong, loving relationships with others.

■ **Extension of the sense of self:** Mature individuals try to participate in important matters affecting the

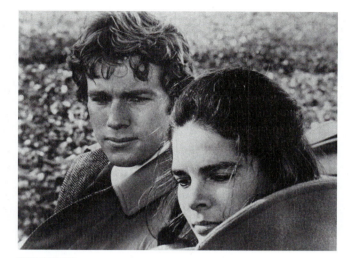

FIGURE 7-9 Ryan O'Neal and Ali McGraw in "Love Story" (1970), a powerful and emotional film about a young couple deeply in love. McGraw's character dies tragically in her mid-20s and she says, "Love means never having to say you're sorry."

tionship ending suddenly. For example, one person may have a desire for intimacy and commitment that is not reciprocated by the other, who may be disinterested in a devoted, long-term relationship. Such an incompatibility may be irreconcilable, and if these two people continue to see each other, the mismatch in their personalities may make the relationship unrewarding. Unlike Murray, Holmes, and Griffin (1996) cited earlier, Livingston believes that the greater one's idealization or sexual overvaluation of another, the greater will be the sense of loss, pain, and disillusionment later on. Does this mean that we are foolish to fall "head over heels" in love because the bloom of love will later be lost? Absolutely not. All intimate relationships involve some risk and potential loss. Remember the truism: "nothing ventured, nothing gained." Livingston also notes that one's idealization of another person is colored by early love and attachment experiences (Fig. 7-9).

The Role of Age in the Development of Relationships

People often wonder whether same- or similar-aged individuals are the "appropriate" objects of affection. In general, men tend to prefer women a little younger than themselves, while women often seek men their own age or a little older (Hayes, 1995). Many data support this conclusion (Buss, 1989; Kenrick & Keefe, 1992). Research supports this generalization among a variety of countries, ethnic groups, cultures, religions, and socioeconomic groups. This difference is apparent in self-reported preferences, marriage statistics, and personal advertisements in newspapers (Hayes, 1995), and it has been true throughout the 20th century. Researchers believe that youth enhances women's desirability as mates or marriage partners because men are more likely to evaluate younger women as more attractive. The greater social status and financial resources of older males make them similarly attractive to younger women.

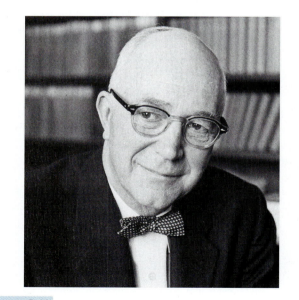

FIGURE 7-10 Gordon W. Allport, noted psychologist who developed a theory of the mature adult personality.

lives of other people. They try to incorporate diverse activities and endeavors into their lives. Their interests and actions may involve a passionate investment of time and energy. They are not self-centered or ego-centric.

- **Warm relating of self to others:** Mature individuals are capable of *intimacy* and *compassion*. While intimacy implies a capacity for important one-on-one relationships, compassion is a concern for and commitment to the wider community of humankind. Immature adults believe their personal experiences and emotions such as anxiety, depression, or guilt are distinctive and unique; no one else could possibly have the same emotions.

- **Emotional security (self-acceptance):** Allport believes that mature individuals have a capacity for "emotional poise." This includes frustration tolerance and avoidance of potentially hurtful impulsive acts. Mature individuals are at home with their emotions and accept their self-doubts calmly.

- **Realistic perception, skills, and assignments:** Seeing things as they are and not as one would like them to be is basic to maturity; those who consistently distort reality are not mature. Mature individuals also work to develop their abilities and seek arenas in which to apply their expertise. Mature people are "problem-focused." Scholars in many disciplines have noted the value of "losing oneself in one's work."

- **Self-objectification:** This technical term means "knowledge of self." Mature people know what they can do, what they can't do, and what they should do. They recognize their abilities, inabilities, and responsibilities. Allport also believed that mature adults have a sense of humor and can see the absurd in daily life, recognize it for what it is, and enjoy it.

- **The unifying philosophy of life:** Mature individuals have a workable, personal theory of life's meaning. It doesn't have to be complicated or sophisticated. When an individual's most important beliefs are obvious in her or his overt actions, they are living in accordance with their philosophy of life.

Few of us meet all these criteria all day every day. Allport believed, however, that just thinking about them from time to time indicates the desire to grow and mature. We believe they are also important in meaningful, intimate, loving relationships. Most of us want to be the best we can be in such relationships, but we don't always know exactly what that might entail. Allport's scheme still maintains its appeal and relevance since it was first published.

The Role of Friendship in Intimate Relationships

Most people believe it is important for people to become good friends before they become sexually intimate. As the terms "affection" and "intimacy" are difficult to define clearly and un-

ambiguously, so too is "friendship." Many see friendship as a necessary first step in a committed relationship, while others see friendship as what remains when an intimate relationship doesn't succeed. Can it be both? In one study of 270 college students, Parks and Floyd (1996) found that their subjects consistently attributed three main qualities to close friendships: self-disclosure, support, and shared interests and clear statements of the importance of the relationship. Generally, both females and males found these to be the most important features of closeness, as did individuals in various types and stages of relationships. About half of these subjects believed that "closeness" and "intimacy" have comparable meanings. These data indicate something important about close relationships: people like hearing from their significant other that the relationship is important. This is one of those simple, important things that we sometimes forget, but maybe we shouldn't.

Other characteristics of friendships serve to encourage and reinforce intimacy. For example, feeling one can confide in another and offer emotional support is associated with a close friendship more than a casual one (Derlega, Wilson, & Chaikin, 1976). Further, two people have to be *available* to each other in order to participate in self-disclosure, an important aspect of close friendships (Rawlins & Holl, 1987). The little hassles and disagreements among two friends are, as well, offset by the more important emotional intimacy of the relationship. People in intimate relationships also consistently report that sexuality is an essential aspect of their relationship as a whole (Blumstein & Schwartz, 1983); women and men are equally likely to report this.

"Our First Big Fight"

Conflicts are inevitable in close human relationships. People differ in their perceptions, expectations, and ways of approaching and solving disagreements. As difficult and troubling as arguments are, sometimes better understandings emerge from disputes. Siegert and Stamp (1994) analyzed the "first big fight" as a pivotal event in the early development of a relationship. They administered questionnaires to almost 250 undergraduate students, asking who had "survived" their first big fight, who had not yet had it, and who had ended a relationship because of it. These writers point out that relationships can grow and mature as a result of conflict or can end if both parties do not want to explore conflict resolution to improve their rapport, communication, and friendship. On the one hand, not everyone has the insight and motivation to learn from their mistakes and change their behavior; on the other, not all relationships should be preserved.

The first significant disagreement or argument can be a critical event or turning point early in a relationship. Siegert and Stamp discovered four common precipitating factors that commonly lead to the couple's first big fight.

- One key factor relates to the **point in time when one or both people begin to question their partner's level of commitment to their relationship.** Discovering that one's partner isn't equally invested in the future of the relationship can be a very unsettling discovery. When one person begins to pressure the other for this kind of commitment and their expectations are not met, a serious conflict arises almost immediately. This is especially true if the couple had been sharing sex on the assumption that a deep bond was developing.

- A second factor commonly leading to the first big fight is **jealousy.** Any third party, especially a former girlfriend or boyfriend, may provoke powerful feelings of jealousy and possessiveness that lead to an argument. Even if these concerns are not justified, the presence of the third person is often viewed as a real rather than potential threat. Because it is unusual for two people in an early relationship to discuss openly their jealousy, it often remains in the background but still affects expectations and perceptions.

- A third factor that often provokes a first big fight is a **violation of the general expectations of the relationship.** When certain routines and regular contacts develop early in a relationship, the couple often assumes they will continue and that both people will work to make it happen. But circumstances, living arrangements, and schedules change and present challenges. Will both partners continue to make time for each other? Will they continue to put the other first? Not always-and this realization can cause an argument in which one person accuses the other of "letting go" or "not taking this relationship seriously."

- Finally, simple **personality differences** can contribute to incompatibilities and differences that often cause a couples' first big fight. This may involve their religious, ethnic, racial, or socioeconomic backgrounds. For example, one person may have strong academic goals and work hard for high grades, while the other may be undecided about their goals and not too involved in their studies. Sooner or later this couple is going to have a major disagreement about the balance between academic and social pursuits in their lives.

These authors also identified a number of predictable consequences of the first big fight. This kind of an argument can provide the couple with new information that helps them clarify their feelings about each other and their relationship. People can learn much about themselves and others when they see what things they stand up for, what things they can compromise on, and what things for which they have flexibility and adaptability. Sometimes the urgency with which one's partner seeks a firm commitment can be surprising and unsettling, but this kind of information can come out of a big argument. Sometimes a conflict shows both that they are indeed dedicated to one another but have trouble expressing their mutual feelings.

A second interesting result of a couples' first big fight is a new awareness of their interdependence on one another. A couples' early arguments may highlight the delicate tension between two people striving to grow as individuals while trying to establish an alliance that may mature for many years. Independence and dependency often exist in a fragile balance, and a quarrel may highlight this tension and still reveal the seriousness of the partners' mutual affection. Another outcome of a couple's first big fight (presuming the couple stays together, and many do not) is that one partner may now know the other's vulnerabilities and areas of personal conflict, fear, or anxiety. Siegert and Stamp believe that fights focus a couple's attention on themes that may be problematic and will likely recur in the relationship. Knowing about these can be beneficial to the growth of the couple or may offer one person the weapon with which to hurt the other. Either way, a significant argument can quickly point out exposed and unprotected parts of the other person's personality.

Finally, what factors differentiate between couples who remain together after their first big fight and those who stop seeing each other? For those who stayed together, the first big fight significantly reduced their uncertainty about the strength and future of their relationship; for those who dissolved their partnership, the first big fight *increased* their uncertainty about the feasibility of the relationship continuing. Secondly, in couples who did remain together, the partners reported an improved ability to work together on issues concerning their relationship (Fig. 7-11). These couples recognized that there was always an opportunity for growth and improvement through the inevitable disagreements. Finally, Siegert and Stamp suggest that when two people stay together after their first big fight, they often believe the conflict derived from their *shared interactions,* while the couples who split up tended to see the conflict in terms of the fallabilities of two individuals acting independently. Although this study does not address all aspects of arguments in relationships, it reveals much about what it takes to work on a relationship and when it might be well to say good-bye.

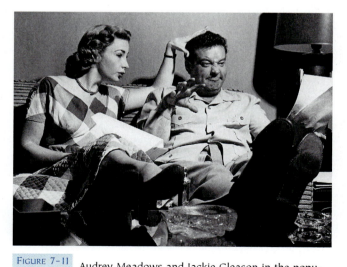

FIGURE 7-11   Audrey Meadows and Jackie Gleason in the popular television show "The Honeymooners" that aired in the late 1950s. As Alice and Ralph Kramden, these characters argue during every episode and each show ends with Gleason telling Meadows, "Baby, you're the greatest."

The "Double Standard"

People in rewarding relationships who enjoy shared feelings and an equitable division of labor often comment they "feel equal to each other." Neither a "leader" nor a "follower," a "boss" or an "underling"—just two partners exploring life and its challenges together as a team. As straightforward as this may seem, things have not always been this way. In the past many men had the subtle but unmistakable assumption that they were somehow entitled to things that their female partners were not, as if society had one set of standards for men and another for women. This came to be known as the **double standard** and has been the subject of much discussion and legislation. The double standard had a major effect on how people understood love relationships in the past. Because the double standard still affects how some people consider relationships and the opposite sex, it is worth examining this perplexing but persistent social issue.

The double standard has been institutionalized in some Western legal traditions. For example, in the English Divorce and Matrimonial Causes Act of 1857, there was a double standard in the provisions under which women and men were granted a divorce because of adultery. If a woman committed adultery, that act alone entitled her husband to divorce her. However, a woman could divorce her husband only if his adultery was combined with another marital misdeed. This inequality was later corrected in the Matrimonial Causes Act of 1923 (Holmes, 1995). This is but one example of how the double standard affected women's and men's rights differently (Table 7-3).

The sexual double standard remains an obstacle to equal rights and privileges within different kinds of relationships and even affects how young people formulate their ideas about what romantic love means for women and men. For example, Cimbalo and Novell (1993) found that for female undergraduates in their sample, traditional romantic behaviors, sharing daily activities, marriage and family issues, and religion were all a part of their attitudes about romantic love. In contrast, the males were more likely to emphasize shared sexual behavior, sexual experimentation, and the use of consciousness-altering agents as aspects of their romantic attitudes regarding women. In general, women are more likely to associate romance with security while men more readily associate romance with sex. While this study describes differences in *attitudes*, it remains to be seen if *behavioral* differences are similarly obvious. It would be interesting to see if this study could be replicated with a large sample of diverse young people.

Despite the legal gains women have made in educational and occupational arenas, there are still big differences between women and men in premarital sexual behavior. For example, Klassen, Williams, and Levitt (1989) noted that males are more likely than females to engage in premarital sexual behavior, to have more partners than their female counterparts, and to engage in sexual intercourse more frequently. Apparently our culture still has somewhat different expectations for females and males with respect to their "sowing their wild oats." We raise these issues because the double standard is often still a background issue contributing to assumptions and perceptions and perhaps still influencing relationships.

Growing Relationships Change

Commonly, people think that if they could just find that "special someone," they could simply build a good life together. Wouldn't it be nice if things were so simple? In fact, just as individuals grow over time and change, relationships do too; they grow, become stable or change, and sometimes end. Does love change over the course of a relationship, and do people have to work hard to maintain their attraction to and affection for one another? Researchers have learned some things about these issues but are still a long way from widely applicable generalizations.

Sprecher and Felmlee (1993) studied the role of conflict and expressions of love in relationships that were developing, stable, or dissolving in a large sample of college students (Table 7-4). They found that when relationships were failing, the partners involved demonstrated fewer expressions of love and affection and seemed less actively committed to maintaining the bond. There were more expressions of conflict and more ambivalence about being in the relationship. Something quite different occurred in relationships that were growing and developing. These subjects reported frequent expressions of love and affection and worked hard to sustain the new relationship; they understood the importance of making the other person feel valued and liked the same treatment in return. Interestingly, reports of conflict did *not* decrease in these growing relationships, but conflict seemed to encourage the couple to work hard at maintaining their relationship. Conflict was important in the learning process of the couple getting to know each other intimately. Just as people change over time, the relationships in which they are involved do too (Fig. 7-12).

Sprecher and Felmlee suggest it is a good idea for people in a developing relationship to understand the importance of be-

---

TABLE 7-3

"The Sexual Double Standard"—Different Expectations of Women and Men in American Society

WOMEN:
Romantic expectations of men emphasize security
Equitable sharing of domestic work
Focus on marriage and family values
Religious values are important in relationships
Passive deference to male authority
High degree of sexual selectivity
Infrequent desire for sexual intercourse
Hesitant in sexual experimentation

MEN:
Romantic expectations of women emphasize sex
Lack of involvement in domestic work
Focus on work and occupational values
Religious values peripheral to relationships
Active defiance of female authority
Low degree of sexual selectivity
Frequent desire for sexual intercourse
High interest in sexual experimentation

Based in part on Cimbalo & Novell, 1993.

TABLE 7-4

How to Keep a Good Relationship Growing

Express love and affection frequently and sincerely. Try not to feel constrained by traditional female and male roles and expectations.

Show an active commitment to mutual respect and open communication. Try not to discourage the expression of strong feelings.

Try to validate one's partner's uniqueness and importance. Enjoy the little idiosyncrasies that make a person special.

See conflict as an opportunity to clarify values and expectations, as well as mutual growth. Disagreements can lead to important understandings.

Mutual self-disclosure builds trust and a climate of psychological safety. It is important to feel comfortable about being vulnerable with those we love and trust.

Politeness and civility should never be taken for granted. We all like to be treated with respect no matter how well or how long we have known another person.

Try to maintain important friendships outside the relationship.

After Sprecher and Felmlee, 1993.

haviors that help maintain their association with each other. Self-disclosure, support, and shared interests are all maintenance behaviors that serve an essential function in building closeness, affection, and trust (Fig. 7-13). When two people are willing to occasionally discuss the quality of their relationship and examine problems together, the relationship will likely become even more rewarding and enjoyable and both partners will feel more commitment to one another. These writers emphasize that when two people are growing more serious about their relationship, they should *expect to experience more conflicts* as they more seriously explore one another's values. This is actually a good sign that they are growing more deeply into one another's lives and that their mutual growth requires frank exchanges of views.

LOVE AND AFFECTIONAL RELATIONSHIPS THROUGHOUT LIFE

When Robert J. Sternberg suggested that passion, intimacy, and commitment were the three basic components of loving, he no doubt knew that all relationships change over time and that each type of loving may play a different role in a couple's rela-

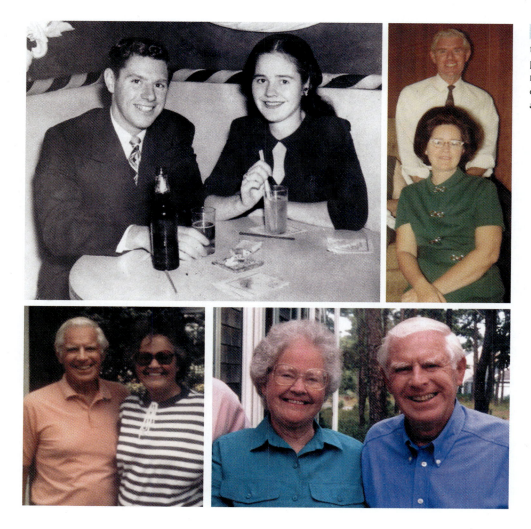

FIGURE 7-12 Relationships mature and change over time. The pleasures and priorities of newlyweds become new interests and enjoyments in middle and later adulthood.

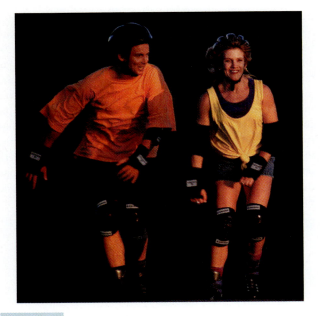

FIGURE 7-13 Exploring many shared interests together is an important way to build a relationship.

tionship as they grow together. The experience and expression of love is somewhat different for adolescents, young adults, mature adults, and the aging and elderly. It's simply not true that we all "lose the passion" as we get older. Because many marriages end in divorce, perhaps many people are unaware of normal changes in love and affection that occur over time and do not know how to handle them when they occur. That passionate interactions often become less frequent and intense with aging is no reason to believe the relationship is in trouble.

Special Issues Affecting Men Between the Ages of 20 and 40

Erik Erikson (1963) was an influential theorist about major developmental challenges throughout the life span. According to his theory, in young adulthood everyone, both female and male, grapples with the tension between intimacy and isolation. By "intimacy" Erikson meant the capacity to willingly enter close, mutual relationships in which one comfortably and non-defensively shares vulnerabilities with another person while still maintaining autonomy and a sense of individuality. "Isolation" is the failure to establish this psychological intimacy with a partner; the person is self-absorbed and feels they cannot enter any relationship in which they might be rejected. Traditionally, and to a significant extent today, women and men have somewhat different experiences in this stage. Many women work to establish a marriage, home, and family and are actively involved in the roles of wife and mother, while many husbands are investing most of their energy in their work.

Developing intimacy in young adulthood is a major developmental challenge, particularly for men (Colarusso, 1995). Many men in their late teens and twenties are more interested

in sexual activity than a deep intimate rapport with their partners; this is less true of women at this age or men later on in adulthood. Sexuality has a special urgency for most men at this time, and Dr. Colarusso believes that many men are not ready for truly intimate relationships until they reach their mid-twenties. This theorist believes that men transition into a more intimate rapport with women slowly, and that young men do not understand it is happening until they experience subtle feelings of loneliness during and after sex. After this change, most men have increased respect for their partners and come to associate sexual attraction with genuine love for the same person. These men come to see their partners as equals and become more comfortable with their growing interdependency. Because many women have been socially "scripted" to see sexual activity as a prelude to marriage and motherhood, they are often more cautious in sexual relationships that might be recreational, possibly accounting for the gradual increase in sexual intimacy occurring in females in this age group.

Many young men face another developmental challenge while these changes are taking place: fatherhood. Many young men in adolescence and young adulthood try to avoid the conception of a child. When they make a purposeful decision to become a parent, most young men say their feelings about sexuality change: "I've always enjoyed sex, but now that my wife and I are trying to have a baby it's totally different. I hope we can do it. It will be pretty awful if we can't" (Colarusso, 1995, p. 88). The implications of sexuality extend beyond him and his wife, and the connection between sexual intimacy and becoming a father is an explicit part of his life. Women too often gradually come to view the procreational role of sex as superseding its "recreational" role. These changes require time and growth and often are not easy.

Reappraisal During Early Marriage

The "7-year itch" is an expression traditionally referring to a period of marital uneasiness in one or both partners at about 7 years of marriage (Berman, Miller, Vines, & Lief, 1977). This is another of those familiar concepts about which there is relatively little serious research and systematic data. Common manifestations of this state include extramarital affairs (by both women and men), musing about marital separation, experimentation with one's lifestyle, and pervasive feelings of unhappiness with one's marriage (Berman et al., 1977). Some researchers (e.g., Levinson, 1986) describe an "age-30 transition," in which adults who have been married awhile reassess the "rightness" of their choice of a spouse and career. Because marriage and job comprise such large dimensions of many people's lives, this reappraisal can be very preoccupying. It is normal to wonder if we might "do better" in another relationship or job. In a sense, this is a process of exploring new alternatives when beginning to approach middle adulthood. Levinson (1980) describes various outcomes from the age-30 transition. A person may see that their marital and occupational choices are good and continue in their current lifestyle; a person may change direction in their job or marriage; or a person may make marriage and job choices they have not yet made.

Other Countries, Cultures, and Customs

ROMANTIC LOVE AMONG COLLEGE-AGE MEXICAN AMERICANS AND MARITAL LOVE IN LATER ADULTHOOD

Mexican Americans comprise a large percentage of the U.S. population, and researchers have wondered whether their beliefs and traditions regarding romantic love are similar to those of other Americans. One study explored this issue among college students in Northern California (Castaneda, 1993). A total of 83 students filled out surveys on their thoughts about love; 90% of these students were born in California, 5% were from other parts of the United States, and 5% were born in Mexico. They were asked, "What qualities and characteristics are important in a love relationship to you personally?" The subjects ranged in age between 18 and 46, with a median age of 21. Five different elements of romantic love emerged in the students' responses. This study had a small sample size, and, therefore, these data may not be generalizable to other Mexican Americans. Still, the results are interesting.

The aspect of love most frequently noted in this sample was *trust*. Trust was seen as essential to any loving relationship, and honesty was its central component. These students frequently equated trust with security in what Hazan and Shaver (1987) referred to as "secure attachment." The second most frequently mentioned aspect of a romantic relationship was *communication and sharing*, revealing characteristics of oneself and learning similarly about the other person. We have previously described this as "self-disclosure." These respondents noted that communication and sharing in a romantic relationship will not lead to judgements or rejection.

The third most frequent category of responses was *mutual respect*. This involves attributing high esteem to the other person and providing "special treatment." These subjects emphasized that when mutual respect is an aspect of a romantic relationship, partners can disagree without worrying about rejection; their differences are tolerated and lead to fruitful conflict resolution. The women in this study emphasized this importance more than the men. The fourth most frequent category of responses involved *shared values and attitudes*. The last category, *honesty*, was seen as evolving out of trust, communication, and sharing. Participants in this study remarked on the damaging effects on a relationship when honesty is lacking.

This study did not reveal any significant differences between Mexican Americans and other ethnic and cultural groups studied in relation to attitudes about romantic love. Nonetheless, it is always informative to learn about the similarities and differences in the many subcultural groups that live in the United States, especially since it is increasingly common for women and men from diverse races, religions, and ethnic and cultural groups to form relationships.

While these data reveal something about the romantic thinking of Mexican American college students, they do not necessarily indicate anything about people who eventually marry or how opinions about love and marital satisfaction may involve cultural differences. Contreras, Hendrick, and Hendrick (1996) studied this issue with survey responses from 54 Mexican American and 32 Anglo-American couples. They found a number of interesting differences between these groups with respect to marital love and satisfaction. Anglo-American respondents were more supportive of both responsible and idealistic approaches to sexuality than their Mexican American counterparts, perhaps because sexual matters are more obvious and pervasive in Anglo-American culture than in Mexican American culture. In terms of Lee's styles of loving, Mexican Americans described themselves as more game-playing and practical than Anglo-American respondents. Even though differences exist between subcultural groups, they may have little impact on the day-to-day functioning of the marriage or the contentment of both partners in the relationship (Fig. 7-14).

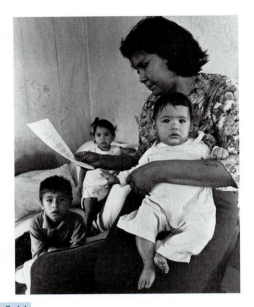

FIGURE 7-14 Despite important cross-cultural differences in parenting styles, it can not be argued that raising children is a common stressor within a marriage that can affect the relationship between a husband and wife.

Berman et al. (1977) conducted a questionnaire study at the Marriage Council of Philadelphia and found that couples in which one or both partners was between the ages of 27 and 32 and had been married for an average of 7 years sought marriage counseling almost twice as often as other age groups (Fig. 7-15). They pointed out that these couples were experiencing not boredom but communication and sexual problems that had persisted for quite some time. The partner experiencing the most inner turmoil usually initiated the decision to seek counseling. Often some specific precipitating event, like the death of someone close or a new friendship, stimulated a reassessment of the relationship and the desire to either repair it or move on. Events outside the marriage often led to examining the relationship, apparently because it could not support the person's attempts to cope with the new circumstances.

The Quality of Long-Term Relationships Through the Life Span

So far we have focused on the challenges facing young adults in the early years of marriage. Many marriages last decades, however, and researchers have examined how marital satisfaction or dissatisfaction grows or declines over the long haul. Does marriage keep getting better? Do people routinely become bored with one another? Is it common for women and men to lose their sense of passion or infatuation over time?

Psychologists and sociologists have discovered a "curvilinear" relationship between the amount of time a couple is married and their reported marital satisfaction. Generally marital quality is at a high level in the years immediately following the wedding, but slowly and gradually declines over the next 15 to 20 years, then begins to rise again. *Why* these changes occur is becoming clearer with research. Partners in a long-term relationship are less

likely to experience serious financial problems as they grow older together, men and women have often attained security in their jobs, and when children have left the home, women often enjoy more involvement in their careers, continued education, community and church involvement, and so on. Also, the often crushing responsibilities of raising children have diminished. Thus it is easy to see why in some cases the relationship improves (Berry & Williams, 1987; Pina & Bengston, 1993; Ward, 1993).

John Gottman, one of the best known researchers in "marital satisfaction," has described the factors that consistently detract from the quality of a marriage (Gottman, 1994). Analyzing videotaped interviews with married couples over 20 years, he found that while many people believe that anger is the most common cause of unsatisfying marriages, in fact it is not. Criticism, contempt, defensiveness, and stonewalling (refusing to discuss or negotiate problems) are far more harmful. Additionally, a lack of sharing power equally in the relationship has a highly negative impact. Generally speaking, when a couple cannot accept each other's differences, problems gain an enduring quality that makes them more difficult to solve.

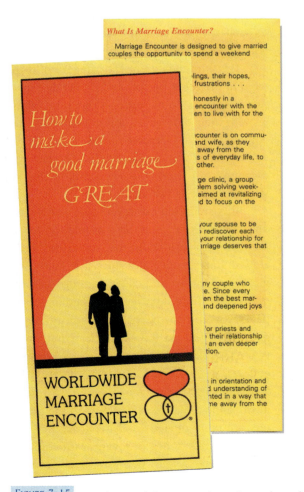

FIGURE 7-15 It is often said that "a good marriage takes a lot of work." Sometimes this "work" involves a couple participating in a marriage enrichment workshop of some kind.

Other Countries, Cultures, and Customs

INTERDEPENDENCE OVER THE LIFE COURSE IN JAPANESE AND AMERICAN MARRIAGES.

Americans often think marriage is similar in other cultures, which is not necessarily true. Ingersall-Dayton, Campbell, Kurokawa, and Saito (1996) described a number of intriguing similarities and differences between American and Japanese couples over the course of marriage, from extended narrative interviews with 11 Japanese and 13 American couples. The Japanese couples were married for an average of 43 years, the Americans an average of 47 years. The couples had an average of 2 children.

There are some cultural differences between the United States and Japan in terms of how interdependence changes over the course of marriage. In Japan, a marriage is more an agreement between two families than two individuals. Most of these Japanese couples lived their early years together in an extended family; all felt powerful pressures to conform to the customs of their elders rather than develop their marital relationship by themselves. Another important difference is the apparent lack of role equality in Japanese marriages. Males are more dominant and make virtually all significant decisions that affect the partners' lives together. While there are still gender inequalities in the U.S., they are far less apparent than in Japan.

Ingersoll-Dayton et al. explored three primary dimensions of these marriages: separateness and togetherness, negotiating roles in marriage, and negotiating intimacy in marriage. With respect to "separateness and togetherness," the marriages in these two countries began very differently; the Americans chose their spouses, and most of the Japanese couples had their marriages arranged, and for this reason, most of the Japanese women emphasized the difficulties in their early years of marriage. American wives devoted their early married years to their homes and families and later returned to work. Interestingly, throughout these interviews the Americans always used the word "we" to refer to their marriages, but this was virtually never the case among the Japanese.

Another difference between the American and Japanese couples concerned how they negotiated their roles in their marriages. The American couples were more interested in an *egalitarian* bond in which the woman and man shared equally in establishing and maintaining their relationship. In contrast, the Japanese marriages were based on *complementarity,* with each partner doing those things they were best at, without any effort for equality. Among the Japanese, roles were renegotiated over the course of the marriage.

There was an interesting difference between the Japanese and American couples in terms of their intimacy over the course of marriage. While the Japanese reported they enjoyed more time and emotional intimacy together the longer they were married, the Americans reported they sought more time to pursue their own interests in their later years.

Despite the methodological drawbacks to this study (i.e., only happily, once-married couples were studied), it described some interesting differences about couples in these two cultures. As U.S. society becomes more heterogeneous, such differences in racial, religious, and cultural perspectives on marriage will become more apparent. Clearly the nature of a "happy" marriage depends in part on a culture's customs and values.

While the afterglow of the honeymoon stays fresh for many couples for a long time, commonly the pressures of creating a home, starting a family, and beginning a career affect the quality of a marital relationship. Things do not inevitably get worse, but they do inevitably change. The tensions and stresses of parenting and the economic pressures confronting younger couples are challenges that also affect those who marry later.

Often as women and men age together through their 30s and 40s they have less time for each other and sometimes even drift apart. In a study of marital quality, Orbuch, House, Mero, and Webster (1996) found that as couples approach later life, their marriages seem to become more rewarding and relaxing because of lessened financial involvement in their children's lives and having attained security in their occupations. We should treat these data with some caution, however. First, the study was made only of first marriages. Because divorce and remarriage are increasingly common, more research is needed on how the quality of marriage changes in second or subsequent marriages. Second, this investigation was a cross-sectional analysis of couples who have been married for varying amounts of time. Couples were not "followed," or studied for long periods of time, which would be more informative. Also unanswered is the issue of how the quality of a marriage changes differentially for women and men. Such questions require more research but are important for a full understanding.

Intermarriage and Marital Contentment

The term **intermarriage** describes a marriage between two people of different cultural, religious, racial, or ethnic groups (Durodoye, 1994). This phenomenon is growing rapidly in prevalence and popularity in the United States, which does not have a longstanding tradition of comfortably tolerating inter-

marriage. For example, in the past, 40 of the 50 states at one time or another had laws prohibiting African-Americans and other groups from marrying individuals with European ancestry. Specifically, West Indians, Japanese, Chinese, Cherokees, Mongolians, Malayans, and Ethiopians were banned from marrying whites (Cretser & Leon, 1982). Now, over a million intermarriages occur in the U.S. each year, due in part perhaps to the dramatic increase in global business and education. Most research about intermarriage has been based primarily on relationships between blacks and whites and between Gentiles and Jews, but this situation is changing as intermarriage has become increasingly more common.

Are people who intermarry as happy as others, or do differences in racial, cultural, and religious customs create inevitable tensions that diminish the satisfaction of the relationship? Sociologists have found increased conflict among intermarried couples (Cottrell, 1990), although one would expect that people with any substantial differences would have a little more trouble getting along with one another (Fig. 7-16). McGoldrick and Preto (1984) suggest several factors that influence the marital satisfaction of intermarried couples:

1. The extent of difference in values between the cultural groups involved.

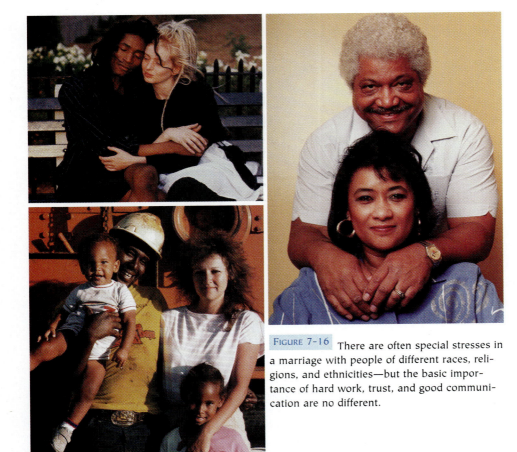

FIGURE 7-16 There are often special stresses in a marriage with people of different races, religions, and ethnicities—but the basic importance of hard work, trust, and good communication are no different.

2. Differences in the degree of acculturation of each spouse; couples are likely to have more difficulty if one spouse is an immigrant and the other a fourth-generation American.

3. Religious differences in addition to cultural differences.

4. Racial differences; interracial couples are most vulnerable to being alienated from both racial groups and may be forced into couple isolation.

5. The sex of the spouse; sex roles intensify certain cultural characteristics.

6. Socioeconomic differences; as Americans move upward in socioeconomic status, their cultural patterns tend toward the mainstream. Partners from different socioeconomic backgrounds or from cultures placing a differential value on socioeconomic status may have added difficulties.

7. Familiarity with each other's cultural context before marriage.

8. The degree of resolution of emotional issues about the intermarriage reached by both families before the wedding.

Other factors may affect the compatibility of intermarried couples, including different cultural values about taking care of and disciplining children, sexual expression in the relationship, and differences in food and beverage preferences (Romano, 1988).

IS FINDING THE "RIGHT" PERSON A MATTER OF GUESSWORK?

Affectionate, intimate, and sexual relationships can tremendously enrich our lives and promote our growth. Wouldn't it be wonderful if choosing a partner was a straightforward, simple process? In fact, finding the "right" person is often complex, risky, and frustrating, and a mistake can create problems for a long time. Again, we point out that marriage is not the only way a couple can bond, although studies of compatibility of two individuals are often based on premarital counseling. Should everyone undergo counseling before they marry to determine whether there may be some subtle but important differences between them? Absolutely not. But premarital counseling often reveals potential relationship problems. Discussions of differing perspectives on love, intimacy, and sexual concerns are often an important part of counseling. Some religious leaders offer counseling, as do other professionals. Colleges and universities often have a counseling center that can help. It's a good idea, if one has any doubts about entering into a lifetime commitment with another person, to examine these issues before finalizing the commitment.

What factors predict a rewarding long-term relationship? Current thinking focuses on something obvious but essential called "mindless moments" (Marano, 1997). Dr. John

Gottman believes it's the little things that really count. A good emotional rapport in any partnership seems to be built on hundreds of small kindnesses and considerations in the daily interaction between partners. These little courtesies build a solid foundation for weathering the inevitable common hassles of everyday life. Gottman believes that long-term relationships end not because some big, terrible thing happens but because the partners have not sustained their relationship by demonstrating their care and respect daily. Knowing this can perhaps help couples develop little ways of nurturing one another regularly. When problems do emerge, a couple with such a solid base in their marriage can better communicate nondefensively if one partner expresses a problem or dissatisfaction. Drs. Scott Stanley and Howard Markman have developed a 12-hour course that teaches couples to air their complaints without making accusations or becoming negative. A good marriage involves skills that can be taught and practiced. Other marriage communication courses also contribute to low divorce rates and greater relationship satisfaction. In one of the most remarkable innovations in premarital counseling, "community marriage policies" have evolved in many large American urban centers. Churches and synagogues of all denominations agree to perform weddings for only those couples who have had training in communication and conflict resolution (Marano, 1997). Since 74% of marriages in the United States are performed by clergy, this pact can affect a great many couples. As of 1997, 64 American cities had some type of marriage policy. Other marriage policies involve judges and magistrates as well.

Premarital Counseling Programs

Sullivan and Bradbury (1997) have shown that couples who participated in premarital counseling programs have better marital outcomes than those who do not. Why? Exploring this issue requires careful consideration of variables that put a couple at an above-average risk of marital strife (Karney & Bradbury, 1995). Important predictors of problems are (1) youth (below age 21), (2) income below average for age and educational attainment, (3) lower educational level (no postsecondary education), (4) parental divorce, (5) lower reported levels of marital satisfaction, (6) higher degrees of anxiety, (7) higher levels of stress, (8) physical aggression, and (9) persistent impulsive behavior. Couples in which a number of these are present are especially vulnerable to marriage problems, and when they do not have access to or receive premarital counseling, they are certainly at an increased risk for problems in their marriages.

An important issue concerns ways of recruiting into counseling those couples who are considering getting married and who have these factors. Generally speaking, once a couple considers getting premarital counseling, they eventually pursue it (Sullivan & Bradbury, 1977). Therefore, it is a good idea to provide information leaflets at locations where couples obtain marriage licenses and to make public service announcements on radio and television. Sullivan and Bradbury recommend that churches and other places of worship are logical choices to disseminate information about premarital counseling. Premarital counseling programs cannot prevent marriage problems if the people who need them don't participate in them.

Premarital Counseling and Marital Satisfaction

Larsen and Olson (1989) developed a lengthy questionnaire called PREPARE, which has been shown to predict which couples are likely to have marital problems and which are not. This simple paper-and-pencil test predicts with 80% accuracy those couples who eventually get divorced versus those who remain married. Various score categories on this questionnaire predict relatively well which couples will be happily married or unhappily married, those who will cancel or delay their marriage, and those who will become separated and/or divorced. Several aspects of the marital relationship are explored, including such issues as realistic expectations, personality issues, communication, conflict resolution, financial management, leisure activity, sexuality, children and parenting, family and friends, equalitarian roles, and religion. While these factors are not equally powerful in predicting marital compatibility, most offer a good indication of marital satisfaction or dissatisfaction. When engaged couples had similar views in these areas, they were more likely to be happy in their marriages 3 years later. This research demonstrates that the roots of serious marriage problems can be recognized long before they may become a serious obstacle to the growth of the relationship.

Interviews with people who have had premarital counseling provide additional information. Stucky, Eggeman, Eggeman, Moxley, and Schumm (1986) interviewed ten couples participating in a marriage enrichment program for newlyweds and 68 female graduates from a high school family life course, asking about their involvement in premarital counseling. They wanted to learn whether the respondents thought premarital counseling was an effective, realistic introduction to marriage. Despite the small sample size, important findings emerged. Two factors were found especially important in their assessment of premarital counseling: the number of hours they spent in counseling and whether participation was voluntary or not. Longer premarital counseling experiences were evaluated more positively and as offering a more accurate picture of day-to-day married life. Subjects who participated in premarital counseling as an independent, personal choice said they got a lot more out of it than others. The marriage policies described earlier that are implemented by local clergy may thus have an inherent flaw in that they remove much of the voluntary nature of premarital counseling. Interestingly, the Stucky et al. study found that the length of a couples' engagement was *not* a predictor of the effectiveness of premarital counseling.

Other approaches to premarital counseling take diverse approaches to exploring couple compatibility. Trainer (1979) developed a five-visit strategy for counseling and health-related issues. When time is limited and several important issues need to be covered, a method like this might be most effective. The first visit concerns the reciprocal, mutual, and contractual nature of marriage, along with important aspects of home life, including personality differences, money management, preg-

nancy, home management, and leisure time activities. This approach begins with the pragmatic aspects of living with someone else and sharing your lives, plans, and living space. Visits two and three focus on the partners' medical histories and a comprehensive physical examination for both. Various lifestyle issues are explored, particularly those affecting health, and plans are discussed for changing behaviors that impair health and longevity. Issues such as testicular self-exams, breast self-exams, and pap smears are raised. The fourth visit summarizes the first three visits in a wide-ranging discussion, followed by a discussion of relationship building. Verbalizing feelings, communication skills, and realistic expectations of marriage are explored. Later, 8 to 12 weeks after the wedding, a fifth session examines and solves any problems that may have emerged so far. Although this approach may seem rigid and regimented, when there is little time or enthusiasm for premarital counseling, this concentrated technique serves the needs of many couples.

Much premarital counseling is done by the clergy. Giblin (1994) introduces three approaches to premarital counseling from the perspective of the clergy. Each discusses the individual and joint expectations of the couple getting married, explores the history of the relationship and family influences on the engaged couple, and presents interpersonal skills that are important in marital relationships. The first approach is "the future glance," in which the counselor encourages a couple to share and clarify their vision of their future together. Realistic and unrealistic expectations are shared and discussed. The history of the relationship is reviewed, and paper-and-pencil surveys may be used. Two sessions may be needed to deal with all issues. The second approach, called the "the backward glance," focuses on each partner's family of origin. The influence of religious, ethnic, or geographic traditions is the starting point for fruitful analysis of how the past affects priorities and dreams in the present. Attention is given to how the partners' parents fought and resolved problems—an issue not usually discussed by people in love. Because one's parents' arguments and conflict resolution can have a powerful impact on a couple, they gain from understanding such differences in their backgrounds as early in their relationship as possible.

Giblin's third approach deals with "spirituality": the couple together investigates their notions about the meaning of their lives, their "mission" as spouses and parents, and the anticipated role of religious tradition in their home. While the couple may not have a religious orientation to life, they gain from discussing the importance of devotion in their interpersonal behaviors and world views. Of course, not all clergymen use this approach, but it is an example of a coherent way of doing premarital counseling that is compatible with religious perspectives on marriage.

PRINCIPLES OF EFFECTIVE COMMUNICATION

The term *relationship awareness* refers to the ability and inclination to talk about the attributes of a relationship. Women generally have a better relationship awareness than men and find it somewhat easier to talk about the quality of a relationship. In addition to talking about their feelings, couples need to talk about their opinions, thoughts, and world views as well. *Both* emotional and intellectual communication are important.

According to Gergen (1986), a second important characteristic of communication in close relationships is the *equitable division of labor.* Not everything always has to be equal, but fairness is needed in view of the time, skills, and abilities both partners bring to their relationship. When there is little communication about this issue, one or both partners may feel exploited, making further discussion more difficult.

Gergen suggests a third attribute of close relationships can be enhanced by good communication: *trust and the importance of "we."* Couples who believe that their partners behave with loyalty and fidelity report higher levels of love, happiness, and marital satisfaction; but they have to discuss their expectations clearly and sometimes frequently. Good communication is, therefore, needed. The importance of being a part of a couple depends on the recognition that they are a "we" as well as two "I"s.

A prerequisite for good communication, according to Gergen, involves *negotiating the rules of the relationship.* People more or less "invent" their understanding of their relationships, but over time a couple comes to understand their expectations of each other; acceptable and unacceptable behaviors need to be clear and comfortable for both partners. The trust they develop assures them that they will each abide by their agreements. For example, many couples never openly discuss extramarital sex. One who has firm feelings about this should be sure to discuss them with their partner and come to a mutual understanding of the implications of such behavior for the relationship.

A last necessity for good communication in a relationship is *equality in decision-making power.* Shared decision making is an important predictor of marital satisfaction. However, because many men have been socialized to think they must be in charge, they are often reluctant to share responsibility equally and their spouses often feel slighted. On the other hand, some women are brought up thinking that it is appropriate (if not necessary) to surrender authority to their male partners and passively accept the decisions he makes (Table 7-5).

In addition to these principles of good communication are a number of specific suggestions. Johnson (1987) summarized the distinctive features of effective communication:

- **Speak for yourself.** Take ownership for your remarks. They are not your parents' or friends' utterances, they are not representative of any doctrine—they are *yours.* Another potential problem is *speaking for no one,* in which you use such words as "it," "some people," "everyone," "they," or "one" instead of the pronoun "I." Don't refer to that big, anonymous crowd with statements that can be neither validated nor falsified.
- **Describe things objectively; don't judge subjectively.** Personal judgments can distort the accuracy of your statements. Focus on the other's behaviors rather

TABLE 7-5

Some Principles of Effective Communication

1. Each person in a relationship is responsible for his/her own growth as a person. Mature adults do not entrust their personal development to others.
2. It is essential to maintain one's independence while involved in a relationship with another.
3. Comfortably tolerating differences and imperfections reveals respect for one's partner.
4. Take some time every day to talk about a broad range of issues. Be supportive and clearly explain anything distressing. Be concise and do not repeat complaints.
5. Listen to your partner's complaints without interrupting.
6. Try to avoid being sarcastic. Avoid changing the subject when difficult issues emerge. Try not to be judgmental.
7. When a difficult problem has been solved, be sure to express appreciation.

than making inferences about their intentions (which cannot always be verified). While focusing on the behavior of others, *be brief, don't repeat yourself, and avoid sarcasm.*

- **Focus on the relationship.** Your statements about how you perceive the relationship are extremely important for your partner. Comment not about the other person but about your rapport with them. Saying, "I really enjoy how you let me relax with my own thoughts when I get home from work," is a statement about your partner's role in the relationship. Relationship statements can help your mate feel like an integral, contributing member of a strong bond.
- **Pay attention to different perspectives.** All too often, we see our world and others only through our own eyes and lose the capacity to see things from another's perspective. Fatigue, stress, frustration, or anxiety may color how we see things, and it is important to understand that different perceptions lead to different interpretations of things around us.

Nonverbal Communication

People can communicate thoughts and feelings in many ways without words. Nonverbal communication has been an exciting and active area of research for years. Although some obvious cues and signals are clearly conveyed during interactions, there are few clear, unambiguous gestures, expressions, or postures that reveal the thoughts of someone who doesn't want to communicate. One cannot "read someone's mind" by observing their nonverbal communication. People have similar facial expressions when experiencing certain emotions, but these do not precisely show what they might be thinking. For example, when someone won't look you in the eye, they may not be telling you everything on their mind. Body language and gestures are often highly personal mannerisms, however, and one should not infer too much from another person's posture or gestures. Learning to communicate well verbally leaves little to chance and causes the fewest ambiguities in interactions (Fig. 7-17).

How to Bargain Successfully

Differences in opinion or perspective often create situations in which two people have to resolve their differences through discussion or bargaining. Without successful skills in negotiation, two people may have poor communication, and their interpersonal disagreements could prove destructive to the relationship (Johnson, 1987). A few simple rules are useful for resolving these differences to the couple's mutual satisfaction:

- **Both people have to accept each other as equals at the outset.** To successfully bargain and resolve a conflict, partners must see one another as equals. In many marriages an odd and unproductive assumption hurts the couple's ability to successfully negotiate their differences: the person who earns the most is the boss. This creates a situation in which one person feels less important or influential than the other.

- **Both have an equal opportunity to state their views and concerns without interruption.** If something is troubling you and you want to get it off your chest, it is extremely frustrating if your partner tells you, "I don't want to hear what you have to say; I want you to listen to what *I* have to say." Denying another the chance to express their concerns is essentially denying their personhood and importance. It takes self-control and restraint to remain silent while your partner tells you something you might not want to hear, but unless you take turns with a frank exchange of views, nothing will be solved and both parties will feel angry and unfulfilled (Fig. 7-18).

- **Both parties get something and both give up something.** Disagreements in relationships require compromise, a basic value in human relations of all types. When you negotiate a ticklish situation with another person, be prepared to accept less than you might want, and understand that you may not be able to choose what you have to surrender. Although both partners may not be entirely pleased with a compromise, they do not feel exploited, used, or defeated. In a negotiation situation be clear in your mind at the outset about issues on which you will not compromise and go from there; but try to be reasonable and fair.

- **Everyone still has their dignity when it's over.** At the conclusion of a successful negotiation no one has been offended, insulted, or deceived. Both parties feel that they have treated the other fairly and honestly and feel good about the other's behavior, as well as their own. If there is a residue of rancor, further honest communication is extremely difficult. Much in any relationship has to be negotiated. As important as this negotiation is, people seldom learn how to do it well. We think the guidelines above are useful for relationships and even one's job.

Sexual Trust and Spontaneity

When two people have had a relationship over a significant amount of time, they often report that their physical intimacy has lost some of its early passionate excitement but that their

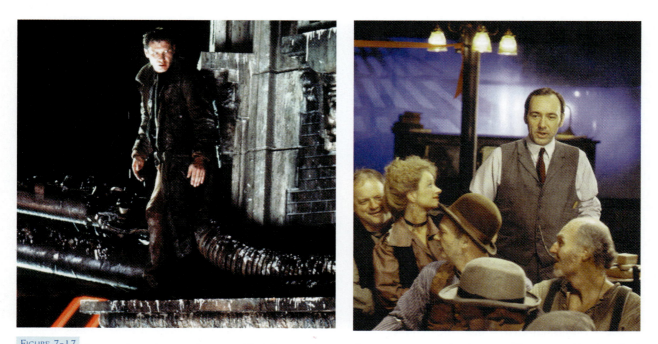

FIGURE 7-17 A person's posture, gestures, and facial expressions are important communication cues. Here actors Harrison Ford (left) and Kevin Spacey (right) depict strong, assertive, self-confident characters apart from their spoken words.

sexual communication continues to enliven and maintain their rapport. Often sexual sharing is a source of the bond of their relationship. It is often said that a couple's sex life is a microcosm of their broader life together. In other words, the conflicts, stresses, joys, and rewards that characterize their shared activities are also obvious in their sexual interactions. If a couple negotiates well, trusts one another, resolves conflicts when they arise, and shares what's in their hearts and heads, then most likely their sexual sharing also reveals this trust, love, flexibility, and spontaneity. In contrast, when two people have a relationship in which they do not perceive one another as equals, have trouble talking about important problems, can't seem to share their resources in working through obstacles, and behave in their roles in rigid and inflexible ways, these same issues are likely reflected in their sexual expression. Rarely does a couple enjoy terrific sex while the rest of their relationship is conflicted, frustrating, or punishing, at least not for very long.

Many people take better care of their cars than their relationships. Just as a car needs oil changes, tune-ups, and other regular upkeep to avoid a break-down, so too do meaningful interpersonal relationships and marriages require maintenance. It takes effort to preserve a quality bond between two people, and this effort is needed regularly, not just when the relationship seems at risk of a break-down. Any mechanic can tell you how much heartache you can save by doing a little *preventive* maintenance on your car. Marriages don't come with warranties or owner's manuals and maintenance schedules, and you can't buy any insurance to be helped at the roadside when your marriage fails. The very best kind of relationship maintenance is regular, honest, unselfconscious communication with which a couple prevents little problems from turning into big ones. The communication skills described in this chapter help to build a sense of solidarity between two people and reduce the ambiguity that can lead to misunderstandings and subtle worries.

Here is a simple exercise that can tell you a lot. Over the course of a few weeks, keep track of how much time you and your boyfriend/girlfriend/husband/wife spend talking with one another about important matters. Not the trivial things like which movie to go to or what to have for dinner, but really important things. Keep a little log in which you estimate how much time you take to talk about important matters and note the topics you explore. Most people will be surprised and dismayed to learn how little time they take to confront, discuss, and solve the truly important problems inevitably encountered almost daily.

Dealing With Anger

Anger is one of the most common, powerful, and perplexing of human emotions. The things that make people angry are as diverse as people themselves. Anger can have a significant impact on interpersonal communication. For a relationship to last and two people to take pride and delight in their togetherness, sooner or later they have to deal with anger and how to manage the experience and expression of anger.

People who are angry don't always *act angry*. A frank expression of anger is sometimes easier to deal with than more

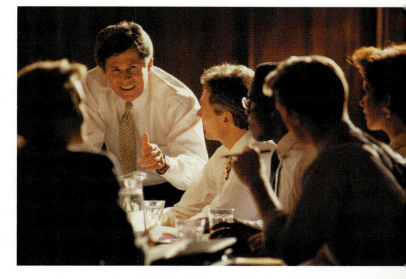

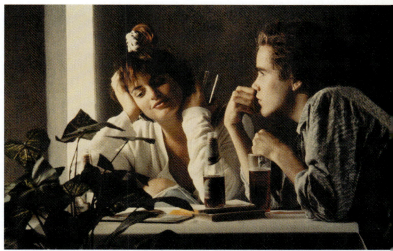

Figure 7-18 In genuine negotiation, all parties state their views without interruption, accept one another as equals, gain something and give up something, and keep their dignity and integrity throughout the whole process.

subtle or even devious expressions of hostility. A particularly difficult expression of anger is called **passive-aggressive** behavior. The person's remarks are nonviolent and indirect: instead of expressing their anger, passive-aggressive individuals may behave in a stubborn, obstructionistic, or deliberately ineffective way. The person may use caustic, sarcastic, or "catty" expressions instead of more honest angry expressions. Dealing with passive-aggressive people can be tremendously frustrating, and you must make an effort not to do what they want you to do: lose control.

Regardless of how hard you try, there will be situations in which you will get angry. You may feel that to be completely candid and forthright, you have to express your anger. Expressing anger in a productive, adult manner is hard for many people to do. Children are expected to get angry every time they are frustrated, but adults are not.

Frequent angry outbursts are often a sign of personal issues with which a person needs to deal, perhaps with professional assistance. On the positive side, when people get angry they often communicate that they will not let someone else take them for granted or be so uncaring about their feelings and interests. They are sticking up for themselves. When two people can express their anger, work through it, and solve problems together, their relationship is strengthened.

Offering and Accepting Criticism

Friction and misunderstandings are inevitable in close interpersonal relationships, and how one receives and offers criticism has much to do with whether anything good can emerge from differing viewpoints. Offering and receiving criticism are communication skills that require experience and practice for improvement. Doing this well allows a couple to enrich their problem-solving techniques and emerge the stronger for it. First you should ask yourself why you are criticizing someone close to you. If your intention is to hurt the other, then there's a different problem that needs to be solved. But if the intent is to work through a problem, you can learn to do this well. David W. Johnson (1987) formulated guidelines for accepting and giving criticism. These techniques can help improve virtually any kind of communication. We paraphrase his suggestions:

How to Accept Criticism

1. Listen carefully. Repeat the criticism in your own words so that you and your partner are sure about the nature of the conflict.
2. Try to see yourself as others see you. This change in perspective may show you something about yourself you didn't previously realize.
   You can learn something about yourself if you can do this.
3. Don't assume criticism is an assault on your behavior. Much criticism is intended to be constructive, but if we overreact negatively, good discussion doesn't result from it.
   Constructive criticism can be a way another person shows you how much you mean to them.

How to Give Criticism

1. Consider how the other person might accept your criticism. If you know a lot about the other person, tailor your message to fit their background and perspective.
2. Only speak for yourself. *Never* tell another person what others say about their personality or behavior; they can take care of themselves.
3. Only criticize actions or behaviors, never motivations or intentions. Never make inferences or guesses about what the other person is thinking.
4. Be clear and specific about why you think the other's actions are undesirable or ineffective. Describe your reactions to their behaviors and how they seem to be hurting your relationship.

5. Try to assess how the other person is receiving your comments, both while you are making them and later on. Following criticism with encouragement helps the other person feel better about themselves.
6. Try to focus on and mention positive attributes of the other person when making criticisms. This balance is only fair and shows your good intentions.

There's nothing really complicated about this. What is needed is some consideration and the intention to improve the relationship through shared feedback. Remember that criticism can avert big problems later on if issues are discussed when they first surface.

When People "Open Up" to Each Other

An earlier section mentioned self-disclosure, the way people reveal themselves to others. The ability to tell someone else your thoughts and feelings openly and honestly is very important in good relationships. Time and trust are necessary first ingredients of self-disclosure. The better you know someone, the more comfortable you are in sharing intimate aspects of yourself with them. Even among couples who have been together for years in good relationships, however, partners often keep some very private thoughts to themselves.

Social psychologists exploring the causes and effects of self-disclosure have discovered a few things relevant to good communication. For example, when people are anxious and worried, they usually find it easier to open up to others (Stiles, Shuster, & Harrigan, 1992). People often feel others will empathize with them and be supportive when having personal problems. When one person discloses to another, it is likely to be reciprocated, an effect called *disclosure reciprocity*. We don't like thinking our problems are unique, and when we share them with others they frequently try to reassure us with similar information about themselves. Strong bonds often form between people with similar problems. Some people are very good at getting others to self-disclose (Pegalis, Shaffer, Bazzini, & Greenier, 1994). They are good, attentive listeners who are verbally and nonverbally responsive to others. They enjoy sharing good, and sometimes intimate communication with others. They don't judge what they hear and seem able to validate others' feelings and thoughts in a sincere and genuine way.

Self-disclosure elicits trust in others, and this is essential in building a good relationship. When we don't have to consider every word we're saying, it is easier to relax and be more authentic with significant others. On the other hand, most people are skeptical and cautious when someone they don't know very well discloses information that seems highly personal and intimate (Collins & Miller, 1994). This kind of overfamiliarity may not help build a closer rapport between two people who are only casually acquainted. The person receiving the disclosure may think, "What am I supposed to do with this information?" While it may feel like a compliment for someone to open up to us, it may also involve a subtle pressure for reciprocal disclosure of private information we have no

Research Highlight

WHAT ARE PEOPLE LOOKING FOR?

Researchers have analyzed personal advertisements to learn about what women and men are looking for when they use this medium in hopes of starting a relationship (Cicerello & Sheehan, 1995) (Fig. 7-19). This study revealed something about *exchange theory,* concerning how people negotiate a "deal" in which one offers something in exchange for something from the other. In personal advertisements, men are far more likely to seek attractiveness and specific physical characteristics in a women while offering financial security. In contrast, women offer youth and physical attractiveness while looking for specific physical attributes and financial security. Women seek an older partner perhaps because age is typically associated with higher income, as well as personality attributes younger women might find reassuring and comforting in an older, and presumably more mature partner (e.g., knowledge, patience, skill, and wisdom) (Cicerello & Sheehan, 1995). Both women and men seek partners interested in health and shared professional and leisure interests. One surprising finding was that men frequently advertised emotionally expressive traits while women promoted their ambition and intelligence, representing something of a reversal of traditional feminine and masculine roles. The subjects in this study were self-identified heterosexuals; the women ranged in age between 23 and their "late fifties," and the men between 26 and 40. Whether these data can be generalized is an issue, however. The sample was entirely American, and racial differences were not assessed. Further, those who write personal ads may not be representative of the general population in significant ways. One also wonders whether the way people truly view ideal attributes in a potential mate correspond to the personal advertisements they actually write.

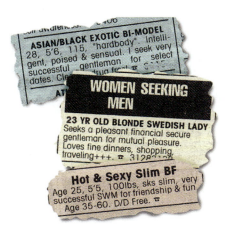

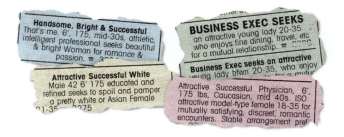

FIGURE 7-19 In personal ads, women often seek men with financial resources who are willing to impart them, while men typically look for attractiveness and particular physical characteristics. This is an example of "exchange theory."

desire to share. Self-disclosure is appropriate in a relationship that matures as two people come to trust and enjoy one another more and more over time.

Researchers have found that women are more inclined to self-disclose than men, for unclear reasons. Knowing this may help some women understand a male partner who seems too closed and private. Maybe traditional masculine socialization teaches males to keep their emotions *and their thoughts* to themselves. These traditional gender roles are softening, however, and men are becoming more similar to women in sharing their feelings and thoughts

Differences in What Women and Men Look For

Sociobiologists speculate that women and men have been driven by different evolutionary pressures with respect to procreating and caring for their progeny. Women have found it advantageous to mate with men with resources to provide for and protect their offspring, thus insuring the perpetuation of the woman's genes in subsequent generations. Men, of course, do not face the physiological costs of pregnancy or risks of childbirth. To get their genes into the next generation men would, therefore, seek someone young and fertile. Of course, these issues rarely affect how a person actually thinks when exploring a relationship with a member of the opposite sex. Yet this distinction may help explain the stereotypes that men want to have sex with many different women and women need to be more selective about their sexual partners because they carry the risks and costs of childbearing and childrearing.

If indeed this is part of our evolutionary heritage, such differences might be expected in personal advertisements. An analysis of over 1100 personal advertisements generally supports this evolutionary hypothesis (Wiederman, 1993). Men are far more likely to advertise their financial resources, as well as their honesty, sincerity, and integrity while at the same time seeking attractive (and presumably younger) women, a pleasing body shape, and a photograph. As noted earlier, women were more likely to offer men an appealing body, seek financial security, and look for honesty and sincerity in their potential mates. The men in Wiederman's study were more likely to look for women younger than themselves while women sought men older than themselves.

While body shape and attractiveness are commonly mentioned in personal advertisements, one "ideal" physique cannot be gleaned from these ads. Epel, Spanakos, Kasl-Godley, and Brownell (1996) analyzed 500 personal advertisements and found that women were less likely than men to publicize their body weight, and that lesbians were less likely to describe their bodies than heterosexual women. In contrast, gay and African American males were more likely to describe their body characteristics than other groups in this study. When women did advertise their body configuration, they typically conformed to current norms equating attractiveness with thinness.

What qualities do gay and lesbian individuals seek when they use print media to find partners? Hatala and Prehodka (1996) evaluated 396 randomly selected gay and lesbian personal advertisements and found males were more interested than the females in sexuality and physical attractiveness issues, while women seemed more concerned than men with personality characteristics of prospective partners. More systematic research is needed, however.

Personal advertisements have become very popular, for various reasons. Some people don't have the time to meet in other ways; they are at home, at work, or commuting to and from work. Other people say there aren't many "safe" places to meet others any more. The workplace is fraught with the threat of sexual harassment complaints (Slovenko, 1995). Finding someone can also be costly. "Interactions" is a dating club in Detroit that charges from $300 to $3,000 for finding a mate, depending on the length of the search process, the degree of selectivity, and the difficulties in finding that "perfect" desirable person. Dating clubs also often require applicants to sign waivers assuming no liability for an unsuccessful match or one with potentially harmful outcomes.

Romance on the Internet

In addition to personal advertisements, people are now exploring relationships on the Internet (Fig. 7-20). Something of a sexual revolution is taking place on the Internet, but not always with happy outcomes. Some people disclose many personal things about themselves to total strangers, maybe because they believe they will never see the person. It can be a big relief to get something off one's chest without worrying it may come back to haunt you in the future. However, much has been written about the inflated expectations of Internet

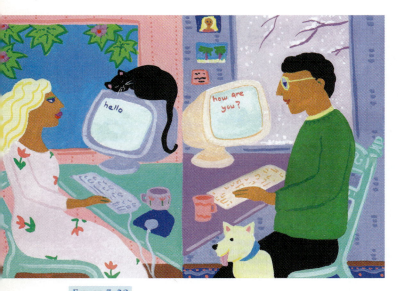

FIGURE 7-20 Meeting people and beginning a "relationship" on the Internet have become common. Yet certain risks are associated with such "friendships," and caution and patience are extremely important.

On the Lighter Side

PROS AND CONS IN THE PERSONALS

Many are still intrigued by the possibility that through personal advertisements, dating clubs, videos potential dates send to each other, and the Internet people can find that "special" person. Ellen Futterman (1996) summarized the pros and cons of these ways of meeting people:

> *Singles Groups Pro: A chance to get to know someone casually, in a comfortable setting.*
> *Con: You're stuck with a bunch of losers who couldn't get a date. Not as much exercise as a bowling league.*
> *Personals Pros: They've been around so long they're pretty tried-and-true. Safety in first face-to-face meeting.*
> *Cons: Have to weed through shorthand and the alphabet to find out the truth.*
> *SUMLWPSLS means Single Unemployed Male Living With Parents Seeks Leggy Supermodel.*
> *Video Pros: You can actually see what a potential mate looks like.*
> *Con: You can actually see what a potential mate looks like. And in person, fast-forwarding is not an option.*
> *Internet Pros: Hooking up to the computer-literate crowd while hitchhiking on the Information Superhighway was THE way to communicate in the early 90s.*
> *Cons: The early 90s are over. It's now been established that everyone in the chat room is 12 years old or under—except you.*

—FROM THE *ST. LOUIS POST-DISPATCH*, February 22, 1996.

"friendships," as well as bizarre and even dangerous outcomes to exploring relationships on-line.

The Internet gives many lonely people the opportunity for a form of human contact with others. Therapists and counselors are frequently hearing from lonely people who deal with their social isolation by making friends on the Internet. But this is not a relationship in the true sense of the word. Very little of what this chapter says about relationships is true of Internet "relationships." Very little effort is involved in making and keeping these contacts, and one is in total control of self-disclosures. A person can be as candid or deceitful as they please. People who use the Internet to "meet" other people often feel dissatisfied and unfulfilled by their reciprocal communications. Yet some become compulsively involved with Internet acquaintances and continue communication that is unfulfilling.

Computer dating has become big business. For example, at Match.Com based in San Francisco (http://www.match.com), for a fee you can publish a profile of yourself and read those others have posted. In 1997, Match.Com had 60,000 active users, 70% of whom are men and 30% women. Most are professionals over the age of 30 whose incomes are higher than average. Of course, many on-line relationships do find their way into the real world and result in compatible relationships and marriages. Nonetheless, it is important to be cautious. Following are safety tips for exploring relationships on the Internet, quoted from an article published in the *Guardian* by Jim McClellan (1997):

- Be patient. E-mail may seem like a very direct and immediate form of communication, but don't force the pace. Take time in establishing trust.
- Be sensible. When arranging real world first dates with online friends, no matter how well you know them, choose a public place and make sure someone knows where you're going.
- Be realistic. People can get carried away online and kid themselves they have found true love. Step back from things occasionally.
- Don't accept pressure and report any harassment to those maintaining the site.
- Look out for "passive language" or frequent use of "could", "should" and "would", apparently indicators of a potential lack of commitment or outright duplicity.
- Pay attention to choppy sentences or stories, where extraneous detail has obviously been edited out. Apparently online lies are often well rehearsed and the writer only includes the essentials.
- Guard your anonymity. Don't rush into revealing your real name and phone number. Avoid people who pressure you for those kinds of details.

■ Don't feel obliged to meet someone. It doesn't matter how long an online relationship has been going on - you don't necessarily have to take it into the real world if you don't want to.

—From the *Guardian,* February 6, 1997.

In addition, if you are thinking of meeting someone you have been communicating with on the Internet, it's a good idea to talk on the telephone first and to exchange photographs.

Internet "relationships" sometimes have bad endings. While the anonymity allows some people to be candid about their passions and tastes, successful outcomes are the exception rather than the rule (Lovey, 1996). Eventually solitude and loneliness become apparent to those hoping for something intimate and rewarding. At other times, behavior can get out of hand. For example, in 1996 James Wilson, age 15, from East Dundee, Illinois walked, bicycled, and rode a bus to get to Hingham, Massachusetts seeking another 15-year-old whom he first contacted on the Internet. Police found him just one block from the young lady's home and identified him as a missing person. He was returned to Illinois without ever meeting the girl he sought (Ferdinand, 1996).

In another case, an engineer from Philadelphia, Cary Bodenheimer, age 30, met a 13-year-old girl in Matteson, Illinois on the Internet and later had sex with her at a motel. He had initiated intimate contacts with other very young girls in the Midwest in a chat room for teens (O'Connor, 1996). Because cases like this are not unusual, Internet users should use every reasonable caution to avoid potentially terrible consequences. The Internet offers unsavory characters one more avenue to take advantage of youthful inexperience. Just as people who live in urban areas develop a "city sense" to stay aware of potential dangers around them, Internet users need to develop a "cyber sense" for the same reasons.

Nonetheless, there are extremely happy, compatible matches that begin on the Internet, and some people seem to find their "soul-mate" with surprising ease in this way. Sometimes, *not* having to face someone when talking to them can actually make it easier to be open and honest early in a relationship.

LOVE, ATTRACTION, AND ROMANCE IN THE WORKPLACE

Social scientists have learned from the study of assortative mating that apart from real or imagined similarities between two people, the amount of time they spend together is a powerful predictor of attraction. *Propinquity,* which means "nearness," is a useful concept for understanding why people who are apparently quite different strike up friendships that sometimes go much deeper. Because most adults spend more time interacting socially where they work than where they live, the work-

place is the most important arena in which adults form romantic attachments, and workplace romances are, therefore, worth studying. Researchers are interested in how and why romance flourishes in the workplace and what the outcomes are for the people involved, their superiors, and the organization as a whole. The results of such study are also applicable to higher educational settings, community organizations, the military, and religious groups.

Well over half of married women and most unmarried adult women work in this country. America's workforce is sexually integrated (Pierce, Byrne, & Aguinis, 1996). Pierce, Byrne, and Aguinis (1996) define a workplace romance as " . . . any heterosexual relationship between two members of the same organization that entails mutual sexual attraction" (p. 6). We are not discounting homosexual attractions and/or romances in organizations, but heterosexual relationships have been researched more fully. Working closely with someone who is attractive, articulate, and intelligent and has a good sense of humor quite normally leads to feelings of fascination. A detailed analysis of the literature on attraction in organizations (Pierce et al., 1996) found the following variables affecting office romances:

Attitude similarity
Propinquity
Repeated exposure
Job Autonomy
Organizational culture
Attitude toward romance at work
Job productivity
Worker morale
Worker motivation
Job involvement
Gossip
Promotion decisions
Relocation decisions
Termination decisions

These factors were isolated from a number of different studies using diverse research methods, including mail surveys, anecdotal reports, reports of expert panels, case studies, telephone surveys, and literature reviews. Clearly many workplace issues can bring people together in conversations in which they would discover similar attitudes, opinions, and world views. Such interactions would reveal to workers who their friends and supporters really are, and this familiarity and feeling of support could contribute to deeper feelings of affinity or infatuation. Physical appearance is also likely to be important, but we know less about how this variable operates in the workplace.

How do organizations react when employees are involved with one another? Although some take a restrictive approach and openly condemn such relationships, the United States Constitution entitles us all to freedom of association. An employment interview or organizational handbook are good sources of information about how a particular corporation, organization, educational setting, or military unit judges "office romances." The organizational culture

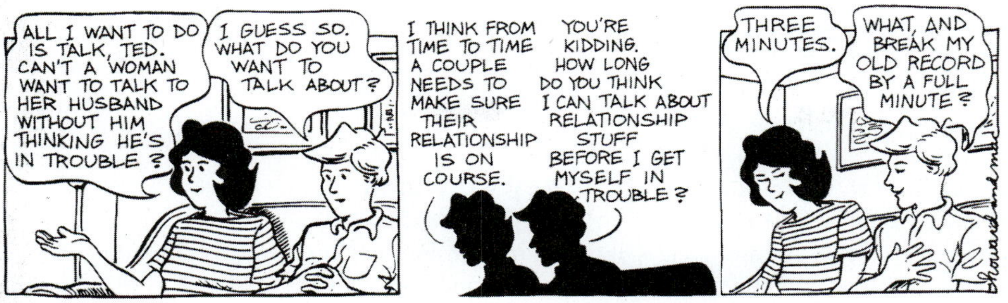

FIGURE 7-21 Preserving one's individuality while sharing a close, trusting, intimate relationship with another can be a challenge. As relationships mature, these challenges become less stressful and the way they are dealt with can reveal a deep and enduring bond between two people.

with respect to office relationships directly affects the likelihood of such liaisons developing. Where there are no prohibitions and workers feel free to flirt and banter, romances are likely to develop. But what happens when an organization explicitly forbids such relationships? Naturally they still occur but must be carried out with more propriety or even secrecy. Different organizations have different personalities, and the character of many interpersonal interactions is affected by such unwritten but powerful mandates. For example, Mainiero (1989) reported that office cultures that are "slow-paced, conventional, traditional, and conservative" generally dampen office romances, while those that are "fast-paced, action-oriented, dynamic, and liberal" are far less repressive of such relationships.

Do office romances affect how organizations function? A later chapter explores the issue of sexual harassment, but here we will comment on non-harassing relationships. Intimate relationships can have *both* enhancing and hindering effects. When a romance goes sour, it can certainly hurt the functioning of both small and large segments of the organization. Relationships other people don't know about are less likely to have any effect at all, but those that are public are likely to have direct effects on office functioning. Pierce et al. (1996) noted that the effects of a break-up of an office romance cannot be easily summarized. They report also that little is known about how long an average office romance lasts. The legal implications of terminations, promotions, and transfers related to office romances also involve many uncertainties. Brown and Allgeier (1995) surveyed a group of office managers to learn their perceptions of workplace romances. Most managers in their sample indicated that they were inclined to intervene in an office relationship when the two individuals were of clearly unequal status in the corporate hierarchy and when the relationship was hurting the quality and/or quantity of the group's efforts. Female and male managers were likely to respond similarly in these circumstances.

CONCLUSION

This chapter should help you think more concretely about the relationships you have had, are having now, and will have in the future (Fig. 7-21). Although it is not always easy to generalize about something as subjective as love, many aspects of relationships have been studied using rigorous methods of the social and behavioral sciences. The place of love in sexuality and the place of sexuality in love should now be clearer.

This chapter has had a rather social, interpersonal "flavor." The next chapter, however, will be quite different, as you will immediately see. As a matter of fact, the next chapter is the one students usually turn to read first.

Learning Activities

1. Many people have the idea that love is a mysterious, mystical, spiritual, and almost magical aspect of human nature. How did you feel to learn love is a serious and systematic area of scientific inquiry and that theories have been proposed to describe and define some of its attributes?
2. Sometimes, when people have known and loved one another for a long time, they seem able to finish each other's sentences. Have such people maintained their individuality in their intimate relationship?
3. Specifically, what do you mean when you think or say that a relationship "is going nowhere?" How long does it take to figure this out?
4. Perhaps you have read accounts in which women or men assaulted or even killed their partner after finding them with someone else. In your opinion, is extreme jealousy grounds for a plea of "temporary insanity?"
5. Describe your "first big fight" with someone with whom you were in love. How did it start? How did it end? Did it make your relationship stronger or lead to a break-up?
6. Feelings of frustration often cause one to criticize our partner's behavior. But frustration is a common, if not inevitable human experience. Is the way one deals with frustration in other areas of one's life similar to how one copes with sexual frustrations, or are there differences? If so, what are they?
7. People usually do not calmly proceed through a list of concerns when personal and deeply-felt difficulties disturb our communication, intimacy, or social interaction. What usually happens is more like this:

   She: "Come on, honey, just tell me what's wrong, so we can talk about it and work things out."

He: "I don't want to talk about it right now."

She: "I can tell that something is bothering you, and I'd like to help if I can."

He: "I said, I don't want to talk about it."

She: "I feel like you're freezing me out of something important that concerns both of us."

He: "Maybe some other time I can deal with this, but just now I have no desire to talk about it."

Is it a good idea to continue to "push the issue" in cases like this one? Does it seem that the person who refuses to discuss the matter is controlling the conversation?

Do you think this conversation would be different if it were the female who didn't want to discuss the problem?

8. Often a number of unspoken assumptions lie in the background of many important relationship issues, conflicts, and challenges. They may never be explicit to both parties but can be very powerful in controlling the communication between two people. Here are a few questions to help you to recognize some of these hidden suppositions in your own relationships.

    a. Do you believe that one person in a relationship is responsible for the other's happiness? If so, when the other person acts unhappy, what feelings do you have and how do you express them?

    b. Do you believe one person in a relationship is the "leader" and the other the "follower?"

    c. Do you ever find yourself "testing" the loyalty or affection of someone close to you? Does this person know they are being tested? How do you tell them that they have "passed" or "failed" your test?

    d. Do you believe that those who love you should "rescue" you from difficulties or protect you from them?

    e. Do you overtly or covertly compare your significant other to your mother or father? If you make this comparison to the other, do you do so to point out a deficiency in your partner's behavior?

    f. Do you frequently talk about the progress of your relationship, where it's going, or personal habits that might be hurting the relationship?

You can see how any of these issues might make it difficult to participate in a mature, communicative relationship where with unconditional positive regard and mutual acceptance. Do you recognize any of these communication habits in yourself or your partner?

9. Most of us know couples who have been married a long time, perhaps many decades. In your opinion, do these couples have fewer problems than younger couples? Do they handle their problems, disputes, and disagreements differently?

10. Write two personal advertisements. In one, describe yourself and highlight your best and most interesting attributes. Make the other an advertisement supposedly written by another person in whom you would be interested. Would you require a photograph? Rank the three most important characteristics you are looking for in another person.

Key Concepts

■ Intimate relationships involve sustained affection and love, mutual trust, and a sense of closeness and cohesiveness between partners. Intimate relationships involve the challenge of being a fully participating member of a couple while also maintaining one's autonomy and even developing one's independence.

■ Maturity is a process of personal growth and development, not an unchanging collection of traits.

■ Adult relationships can be described in terms of different attachment styles, including secure attachment, anxious-ambivalent attachment, and avoidant attachment.

■ Sternberg's triangular theory of love describes three primary components love: passion, intimacy, and commitment.

■ John Alan Lee has described a typology of six styles of loving: eros, ludus, storge, mania, agape, and pragma.

■ Relationship awareness refers to one's ability and inclination to talk about the characteristics of a relationship with a view to improving or maintaining its quality.

■ Equitable division of labor is an important characteristic of close relationships.

■ Trust and the importance of "we" are attributes of close relationships that can be enhanced by good communication.

■ Effective communication involves the following principles:
    Speak for yourself
    Describe objectively; don't judge subjectively
    Focus on the relationship
    Pay attention to different perspectives

■ Communication in relationships is enhanced by effective negotiating skills including but not limited to the following:
    Both people accept each other as equals at the outset
    Both partners have equal opportunity to state their views and concerns without interruption
    Both parties get something and both parties give up something
    Everyone has their dignity when it's over

■ Effective interpersonal communication includes learning how to accept and give criticism.

Glossary

affection	intimacy	passive-
codependency	intermarriage	aggressive
double standard	jealousy	social attraction
interdependence	love	

Suggested Readings

Blumstein, P., & Schwartz, P. (1983). American couples: Money, work, sex. New York: Morrow.

Fromm, E. (1962). The art of loving. New York: Harper & Row.

Harvey, J. (1995). Odyssey of the heart: The search for closeness, intimacy, and love. New York: Freeman.

Hendrick, C., & Hendrick, S. S. (1993). Romantic love. Newbury Park, CA: Sage Press.

Pennebaker, J. (1990). Opening up: The healing power of confiding in others. New York: William Morrow.

Prager, K. J. (1995). The psychology of intimacy. New York: The Guilford Press.

Salovey, P. (Ed.). (1991). The psychology of jealousy and envy. New York: The Guilford Press.

Sprecher, S., & Felmlee, D. (1993). Conflict, love and other relationship dimensions for individuals in dissolving, stable, and growing premarital relationships. Free Inquiry in Creative Sociology, 21, 115-125.

Wallerstein, J. S. (1994). The early psychological tasks of marriage: Part I. American Journal of Orthopsychiatry, 64, 640-650.

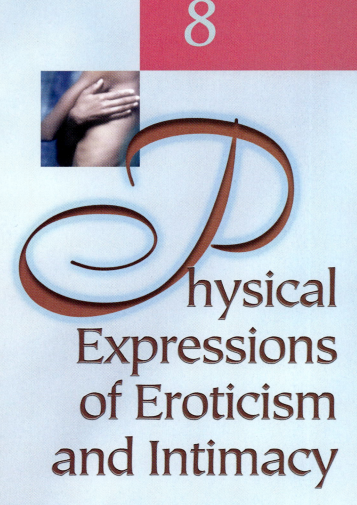

8

Physical Expressions of Eroticism and Intimacy

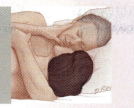

OBJECTIVES

When you finish reading and reviewing this chapter, you should be able to:

1. Explain various definitions of the term "normal" in reference to sexual expression.

2. Differentiate between "innate" and "learned" sexual behavior and explain the role of each in erotic feelings and behaviors.

3. Describe the diversity of human sexual expression, note the range of frequency of sexual intercourse, and summarize factors that influence how often people have intercourse.

4. Define "sexual scripts." Describe their characteristics and how they affect sexual behavior and what people find pleasurable.

5. Describe why individuals choose to masturbate. How can masturbating help someone learn about their sexual response cycle?

6. Explain why people who have an opportunity for sexual intercourse with a regular partner choose to masturbate?

7. Describe common motives behind sexual fantasy and explain why fantasy is so common. Explain differences in female and male sexual fantasies.

8. Describe why some people do not enjoy slow, sensual erotic touching. Explain why tactile stimulation can so powerfully create sensual pleasure and enhance shared intimacy.

9. Explain why kissing has such powerful sexual overtones and is both an expression of affection and erotic stimulant.

10. Describe why oral-genital stimulation is a controversial technique of sexual stimulation.

11. Explain why oral-anal stimulation and anal intercourse are high-risk sexual behaviors.

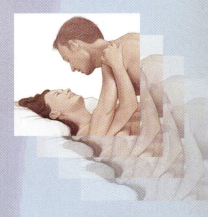

From Dr. Ruth

A young man once called me on my radio show and told me that his girlfriend liked to toss onion rings onto his erect penis as part of their lovemaking. I later told that story on David Letterman's TV show, and apparently many people passed it along at the office the next day. Suddenly, all across the country, whenever people mentioned onion rings, a little smile appeared on their faces.

While sex is certainly a serious subject and deserves serious study, it also brings a lot of pleasure to people and so deserves also to be thought of with a smile.

In the same spirit, we're including in this chapter some Top Ten lists related to sex. They are meant to inform, not to make you giggle, but it's okay if you find yourself smiling. It's only natural.

BASIC CONCEPTS OF EROTICISM

Welcome to your college course in human sexuality! We say this here because this is the first chapter in this book that many students look at. Commonly students beginning to study human sexuality think of the course as dealing primarily with intercourse and other sexual behaviors. Some students even are impatient to learn they won't study sexual intercourse until halfway through with the term. Nonetheless, the chapters that precede this one show that a richer understanding of sexual intercourse is based on those preceding topics. This chapter focuses on shared heterosexual intimacy and autoerotic sexual behaviors, but whenever appropriate we refer also to how these issues pertain to homosexuals.

What Sexual Expression is "Normal?"

The term "normal" has provoked and puzzled social and behavioral scientists for hundreds of years. Many offer definitions of "normal" sexual behavior, and others challenge those definitions. There is no one widely applicable definition of sexual normality that all professionals in the social and health sciences agree on. In reference to sexual behavior, many people wonder what "normal" sexual intercourse is or even whether oral-genital or anal sex is "normal" at all. In a *statistical sense,* normality usually refers to what most people are doing most of the time. In that sense, "normal" and "common" mean the same thing.

Regardless of how people behave sexually and their preferences for erotic stimulation, remember that the human brain has evolved to attend to pleasurable feelings, especially those involved in the perpetuation of the species, and that focus on pleasure suggests much sexual activity is "normal." As noted in Chapter 4, an enormous amount of subcortical brain tissue is devoted to the experience and expression of emotions. These structures are collectively known as the *limbic system.* The cere-

bral cortex is intimately involved in perception, memory, judgment, and language, to name a few cognitive processes that mediate daily behavior including social and sexual interactions with others. Recall also that the functions of the two branches of the autonomic nervous system, the sympathetic and parasympathetic, underlie sexual arousal and orgasmic response. We mention these functions of the nervous system just to remind you that the behaviors described in this chapter have their foundations in well-defined and clearly understood parts of the central and peripheral nervous systems.

Is Sexual Expression "Natural"?

Some people wonder why a chapter about the physical expressions of eroticism and intimacy even should be included in a text on human sexuality. After all, don't all of us do what "comes naturally?" Do we really have to be *taught* techniques of touching, kissing, oral-genital stimulation, or sexual intercourse positions? What's to teach? It is true that humans have evolved with innate, "genetically programmed" or "hardwired" perceptual, emotional, and behavioral mechanisms to ensure that human beings continue to have babies so that the species continues to exist. This chapter discusses many types of sexual activities that do indeed seem to come naturally.

Recall, however, the three themes underlying this entire text: education, motivation, and reassurance. This chapter, like others, is intended to teach you a few useful facts about individual and shared sexual intimacy, to motivate you to learn more on your own, and to reassure you about common "normal" variations in sexual expression. We can all always learn more, including about sexual thoughts, feelings, and behaviors. Few of us have received thorough instruction in how to touch our partner's genitals, stimulate them orally, engage in a variety of intercourse positions, masturbate, or touch a woman's breasts. While this chapter is informative about these issues, it assumes you already know something about these topics. Systematic instruction is indeed not necessary for most adults.

For the most part people really do know what to do "naturally." Still, sex books—especially those with clear, color pictures—sell well in part because people want reassurance that their sexual tastes and preferences are normal, and we think that such reassurance is very important. Finally, although people may all have the same innate motives for behaving sexually, that does not mean everyone enjoys all the behaviors and interactions described in this chapter.

Speculations About Evolution and Human Sexual Behavior

This book at different points includes the perspectives of different disciplines about human sexual behavior. Consider the interesting evolutionary commonality among human beings that distinguishes us from almost all other mammals, especially many primates: almost all people prefer having intercourse face-to-face while other creatures use the rear-entry position. How and why did humans evolve this way? This question has intrigued zoologists, evolutionary biologists, and sexologists for many years. No clear, correct answer to this question exists, but one popular writer has some very interesting speculations about this.

In 1967, the zoologist Desmond Morris published an important book called *The Naked Ape,* in which he explored possible behavioral relationships between our distant ancestors in evolution and ourselves. He explores possible and probable connections between prehistoric humans and modern people with respect to child rearing, aggressive behavior, feeding patterns, sexual behavior, and many other behaviors. He also examines in some detail why humans prefer having sex face-to-face. How did this happen? Why are we so different from our relatives on the evolutionary "ladder?" (Fig. 8-1). His speculations are interesting, although they are only theoretical suppo-

sitions not based on research, and they cannot be proved true or false.

In their enormous cross-cultural study of human sexual behavior, Ford and Beach (1952) reported that most (70%) humans throughout the world prefer the face-to-face position for sexual intercourse. More recent research supports this (Suggs & Miracle, 1993). Morris notes that most of our most important sexual signals and communication come from the front of the body: facial expressions and words, the appearance of erections in men, breast and nipple changes in women, and pubic hair and sexual flushing in both sexes. Virtually everything important and informative to one's partner can be seen in the front of the body. Such signals reveal arousal and readiness for penetration, effected then by the male moving to the female and entering her. Morris reminds us of something simple and significant: humans pair-bond, as only a few species do. That is, a person establishes a relationship with another person (generally only one at a time) for procreation. The identity of that person and his or her unique physical appearance are most obvious and apparent when viewed from the front. Pair-bonding, along with the development of spoken language, exert subtle but important evolutionary pressures to mate face-to-face. Although this is only speculation, the hypothesis is not unreasonable.

Other aspects of face-to-face intercourse also favor its becoming a human preference. Face-to-face intercourse allows more efficient stimulation of a woman's clitoris during penetration than the rear-entry position. As well, because the vagina is tilted forward in a woman's body, forming an angle with the opening to her uterus, frontal penetration more effectively stimulates the inside of a woman's vagina than rear-entry penetration. Morris also speculates that in rear-entry intercourse, males may have been attracted by the sexual signal of soft, fleshy buttocks. He suggests that these may once have served as a kind of "releasing stimulus" for sexual arousal in men—the signal that first caught a male's attention. In the gradual transition to face-to-face intercourse, this signal would have been replaced by a woman's breasts. Additionally, the frontal cue of the female's mouth and lips may have replaced the posterior appearance of a woman's engorged labia during sexual arousal. Morris even speculates that one of the reasons women in virtually all cultures color their lips is to attract attention to sexual interest or arousability. Similarly he thinks bras may have been developed in part to call attention to erect, symmetrical breasts for the same reason.

Common Sexual Behaviors

At various points, this book shares the results of sex surveys, although we always remind you of the pitfalls of survey research. Survey research provides much useful and interesting data about the variety of human sexual behavior, as well as some consistencies. As noted above, to Ford and Beach (1952), about 70% of people all over the planet prefer face-to-face intercourse. What other commonalities are there among most people? The most recent data from the Kinsey Institute (Reinisch, 1990) reveal that the intercourse position most

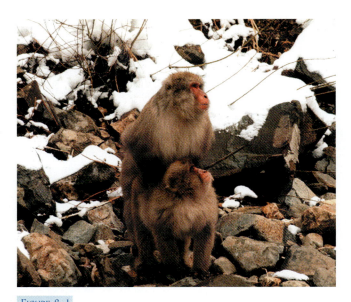

FIGURE 8-1   Non-human primates usually copulate using the rear-mounting position.

commonly reported by respondents is the man-on-top, face-to-face position, although the woman-on-top, face-to-face position is also quite common. Variety is common, however, and people usually explore different intercourse positions, such as sitting positions, the side-to-side position, and rear-entry positions. Later on this chapter illustrates and discusses these and notes how different positions differentially stimulate the inside of a woman's vagina and the clitoris.

Surveys also reveal something about how frequently people have sex (Tables 8-1 and 8-2). Of course, the average frequency depends on the person's age, marital status, and other characteristics. Beginning in 1988, the National Opinion Research Center started collecting data on the sexual behavior of Americans. Periodically, their figures are updated (Smith, 1991). Several interesting findings emerged from this large study. For example, by the age of 18, 97% of Americans have had sexual intercourse at least once. About 20% of Americans polled reported having no partners during the previous year, and on average, married adults had intercourse 57 times during the previous year. The frequency of intercourse tends to decrease the longer a couple is married. In a large, survey published by *Playboy* magazine (Hunt, 1974), married couples between the ages of 18 and 24 had intercourse an average of 3.25 times per week; those between 25 and 34, 2.55 times, those between 35 and 44, 2.00 times; and those 45 and over 1.00 time. We are presenting Hunt's data here because they do say something about the relationship between age and frequency of sexual intercourse among married couples. However, Hunt's study did not fully represent three segments of the American population: the poor, those living in rural locations, and those identifying themselves as political conservatives. Laumann et al. (1994) offer us more current data on this issue and our table includes their data regarding single individuals, those in cohabitation living arrangements, and married individuals as well.

The decision to have sexual intercourse may differ from the *desire* to have sexual intercourse, and different people have various personal "criteria" for sharing sex, especially when not married to one another. In 1997, Finkelstein and Brannick examined factors that may determine whether college students decided to have sexual intercourse. They studied 46 unmarried heterosexual women and 38 unmarried heterosexual men. Five factors were found to affect the decision to have sexual inter-

TABLE 8-1

Age and Frequency of Intercourse Among Married Couples

Age Group	Average Frequency of Intercourse Each Week
18–24	3.25
25–34	2.55
35–44	2.00
45 and over	1.00

After Hunt, 1974.

TABLE 8-2

Frequency of Sexual Activity and Marital Status

Never Married Singles

Males	Never	22%
	A few times each year	26%
	A few times each month	25%
	Two or three times each week	19%
	Four or more times each week	7%
Females	Never	30%
	A few times each year	23%
	A few times each month	26%
	Two or three times each week	13%
	Four or more times each week	7%

Cohabiting Couples

Males	Never	0%
	A few times each year	8%
	A few times each month	36%
	Two or three times each week	37%
	Four or more times each week	19%
Females	Never	1%
	A few times each year	7%
	A few times each month	32%
	Two or three times each week	43%
	Four or more times each week	17%

Married Couples

Males	Never	1%
	A few times each year	13%
	A few times each month	43%
	Two or three times each week	36%
	Four or more times each week	7%
Females	Never	3%
	A few times each year	12%
	A few times each month	47%
	Two or three times each week	32%
	Four or more times each week	7%

After Laumann et al., 1994.

course with a receptive partner: the length of the relationship or acquaintanceship, their awareness of the other person's prior sexual behavior, partners, and habits, whether the couple had been drinking alcohol, whether there was an expectation of intercourse, and the availability of condoms. Almost all respondents indicated that the availability of condoms was an extremely important factor in any decision to have intercourse. This list may not completely describe all factors involved in these sexual decisions, but they reveal something about "normal" American college students and what they are thinking about in such decisions.

Another study examined the attitudes of 51 unmarried women with high levels of sexual interest to determine the impact of these attitudes on their behavior (Sloggett & Herold, 1996). These women ranged from age 19 to 49 and were recruited into the study from college courses in human sexuality and conferences on sexual issues. Most indicated that sex was an important part of their lives, and two-thirds had sex with more than 10 men during their lives. The more important sexuality was in a woman's life, the higher was her reported sex drive and the more likely it was that she would have intercourse. Further, women with higher sexual interest engaged in sex more quickly with a new partner and reported higher levels of intercourse frequency. They also reported that they did not enjoy periods of celibacy in their lives. Interestingly, the higher the reported level of sexual interest, the lower was the level of sexual guilt experienced.

Data for men show higher rates of sexual activity than that reported by women. The 1991 U. S. National Survey of Men collected data on the sexual behaviors and habits of over 3,000 men between the ages of 20 and 39 (Billy, Tanfer, Grady, & Klepinger, 1993). Ninety-five percent of these men had had vaginal intercourse, with almost one-fourth reporting having been with more than 20 female partners. Older and better educated men had more partners than younger, less well-educated men. Among men who had never been married, 41% had not had intercourse in the month before the survey, and of divorced men, 32% had not had intercourse in the month before. About one out of five men in this sample had had anal intercourse at some time. Older Caucasian subjects were more likely to have given and received oral sex. Of all subjects, 1% had an exclusively homosexual orientation over the previous decade, with another 2% having participated in some homosexual behavior.

Reports of the frequency with which people have intercourse makes some individuals anxious. Often people wonder or worry whether they are having sex too often or too infrequently. Intercourse does not necessarily involve all the stages of the human sexual response cycle, however. For example, some men enjoy attaining an erection, penetrating their partner, and engaging in pelvic thrusting without an orgasm. These men still are considered to have intercourse. Similarly, women can become quite aroused and engage in a variety of sexual stimulative activities and be penetrated vaginally but not have an orgasm. Importantly, these men and women may report high levels of erotic satisfaction.

Women and men may differ in how frequently they enjoy having intercourse, regardless of their actual frequency. The sex drive also changes at times, depending on various inescapable pressures and stresses in life. More important than the number of times a couple has sex is their enjoyment of it. Having sex very often *isn't* very good if one partner feels forced to participate or if other important areas of life are neglected. Generally, couples with frequent sexual activity have had a high level of enjoyment for a long time, and the opposite is also true: couples who have intercourse infrequently have often shared this preference for some time. More isn't necessarily "better," and less isn't necessarily "worse."

Sometimes the frequency of intercourse is affected by other factors. When a couple is trying to conceive a child, the timing and frequency of their intercourse may be determined by the woman's fertility cycle or using fertility drugs. Similarly, if a man has a low sperm count and he and his partner are trying to conceive, he may be encouraged to avoid ejaculation for several days before his partner's period of peak fertility. Illness, convalescence, and the side-effects of various medications also affect a person's desire for intercourse. Birth control pills too can lower a woman's sex drive, and she may not desire intercourse as often as before (Crenshaw & Goldberg, 1996). All in all, key issues in intercourse and the variety of intercourse positions concern "quality" more than "quantity."

Motivation for Sexual Pleasuring and Intercourse

What is the human motivation for sexual pleasuring and intercourse? On the surface this seems a simple question with a simple answer, but there isn't just one good answer and it's not so simple after all. Some suggest that pleasure is the goal, or that orgasm is the goal of sexual interaction, or that pleasing someone else is the objective of intimate activities, and to some extent each of these is correct. In an earlier chapter we suggested that everyone is responsible for his or her own sexual enjoyment and responsiveness. Remember that sexuality is from time to time *both* a solitary aspect of one's personhood and a *shared* pleasure of a human bond.

There is clearly a difference between enjoying the sexual stimulation someone else gives one and being the person doing the stimulating, yet these aspects combine in rewarding sexual experiences. One is both thinking and feeling pleasure, safety, and validation and behaving in erotic ways so that our partner thinks and feels the same. This experience is an important objective of shared sexual experience. One writer (Kleinplatz, 1992) suggests that the most basic aspect of eroticism is the intention to please, stimulate, and arouse someone else. This writer views shared sexual experience as an *exploration* more than a direct path to known pleasurable goals. In other words, discovery may also be an important element of shared physical intimacy, or as Zen Buddhists say, *the journey is the reward.*

Perhaps this "journey" provides the keenest enjoyment of sexual pleasuring and intercourse. A later section discusses the role of sexual dreams and fantasies in a person's sexual responsiveness; for some, sharing these fantasies is a rewarding aspect of pleasing one's partner. By sharing physical pleasure, sexual fantasies, and erotic discovery one becomes part of a trusting, intimate relationship that includes mutual respect and sometimes genuine devotion.

Does all this mean that sex without love is a bad thing or that casual sex is an empty encounter? The previous chapter addressed this issue, although we encourage people to exercise caution in sexual encounters outside of committed relationships, we do not judge such behavior. We only want people to think clearly about their objectives in sexual expression, anticipate potential consequences for them and their partner, and make responsible, mature decisions.

Sexual Scripts and Sexual Behavior

In a play, actors recite their parts and behave as directed by the play's script. The "script" is a useful metaphor for a variety of human behaviors in diverse settings—an implicit set of suggestions and commands about how we're supposed to act in certain circumstances. Sexual scripts have become an active area of research. They are private guides for "appropriate" sexual thoughts, feelings, and actions in many settings. Much of how one thinks about masturbation, oral-genital sex, and sexual intercourse is affected by sexual scripts. Sexual scripts are powerfully affected by gender roles and how comfortable one is in them.

Simon and Gagnon (1986) suggested that sexual scripting takes place at three levels: cultural, interpersonal, and intrapsychic (Fig. 8-2). Cultural scripts affect our understanding of different roles and their enormous variety. Interpersonal scripts concern how we define or identify ourselves. Intrapsychic scripts reveal our understanding of different roles we do or might play in our lives. Gender role is a good example of a cultural sexual script: how people learn to behave "appropriately" as women or men in our society. Interpersonal sexual scripts affect interactions involving two people: what we think we "should" do in a specific situation and how the other person "should" act. Intrapsychic scripts more subtly involve our ability to imagine a different lifestyle and to think creatively about other identities. Sexual scripts are powerful and subtle as a framework for behaving within the norms of society.

Gagnon (1990) believes that virtually all interpersonal behaviors are scripted and that even sex researchers and those who write about sexual behavior are affected by the expectations inherent in sexual, gender-based scripts. Even when people try to keep an open mind and not judge people, Gagnon makes the important point that overt sexual behaviors, including masturbation, oral-genital stimulation, and sexual intercourse, reflect cultural, interpersonal, and intrapersonal scripts.

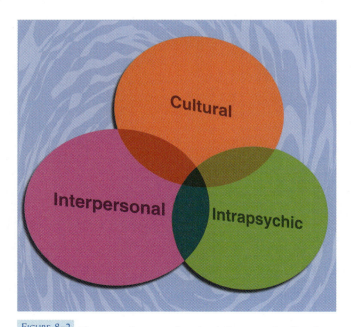

FIGURE 8-2   There are three overlapping influences of cultural, interpersonal, and intrapsychic scripts relevant to sexual experience and expression.

To make enduring changes in sexual behavior one first has to change the scripts, which can be very difficult. One can change behavior without changing scripts, but such changes are not likely to be permanent. Scripts can persist within a person for long periods of time.

Purnine, Carey, and Jorgensen (1994) used a questionnaire to learn about preferred sexual practices of heterosexual women and men, inferring that such practices would reflect the influences of sexual scripts. The men were found more sexually focused while the women were more romantically focused in their intimate interactions. The men were more likely to include alcohol and recreational drugs in their sexual interactions with women, and were more likely to want to share erotic literature with their partners. These were consistent differences in this large sample, but these results should not be considered aspects of the sexual scripts of all women and men.

Dating is a heavily scripted social behavior. There are things we feel we are supposed to do on a date and others that are inappropriate; we learn this while growing up in our culture. Alksnis, Desmarais, and Wood (1996) studied gender differences in the scripts of college women and men about dating, specifically about what "good," "bad," or "typical" dates are like. Males associated events with sexual connotations with good dates, especially if their partners behaved in sexually suggestive ways. Females associated sexually related events and remarks with less desirable dates. These results do not reflect scripts that all undergraduates have about dating, but they reveal something about unspoken expectations that may differ between women and men. Failing to understand these different expectations can lead to misunderstandings and bad feelings.

Many undergraduates go to Florida for spring break, and sexual encounters are often anticipated (Fig. 8-3). Mewhinney, Herold, and Maticka-Tyndale (1995) explored the sexual scripts and sexual behaviors of Canadian university students during spring break in Daytona Beach. In interviews students reported a common understanding that casual sex was common and that this behavior was more likely to occur and was more acceptable or "normal" during this time. Casual sex was not expected by all the students who reported having it, however. The sexual script for spring break was affected by the overall atmosphere of sexual permissiveness and anonymity, as well as the widespread consumption of alcohol. This is just one example of how sexual scripts affect sexual expectations and behaviors in a specific psychosocial environment.

Guilt and the Enjoyment of Sex

Guilt is a complicated issue. People conceptualize it, experience it, and perhaps act to eliminate it all in different and highly personal ways. Some things about guilt are common to most people, however. It is not considered a good feeling or emotion, and it can affect one's willingness to engage in sexual behaviors, to engage in sexual behaviors with certain people, and to fully enjoy intimate interactions. Guilt can be a powerful deterrent to sex and can completely eliminate any good feelings associated with eroticism and shared physical intimacy. Guilt is relevant to the discussion in this chapter because the ability to become responsive can be significantly impaired by the experience of guilt.

People feel guilty about a number of things related to sex: masturbation, petting, premarital intercourse, extramarital intercourse, homosexual inclinations, or even enjoying intercourse unrelated to planned conception, and other things. There may also be gender differences in what we feel guilty about sexually. For example, in the early 1970s, sociologists found that females felt significantly less guilt than previously about premarital intercourse (Bell & Chaskes, 1970). Guilt feelings can lead to conformity to social norms. Guilt involves the feeling that one has violated the morals, norms, and standards society (often represented by our parents) requires for cultural order. People also have guilt feelings about things that have little to do with society as a whole, often concerning sexual inclinations, feelings, and behaviors. Guilt is a major factor affecting sexual enjoyment.

Darling and Davidson (1987) found that guilt feelings diminish sexual satisfaction among adolescents and young adults. Lessened enjoyment can be psychological, physiological, or both. Guilt feelings can affect every phase of the sexual response cycle; they can impair arousal, lengthen plateau, prevent orgasm, and eliminate resolution when no orgasm takes place. Darling and Davidson found that over half of the females in their sample of American university students experienced guilt related to first intercourse. This guilt gradually lessened in later intercourse experiences, but many of these young women continued to feel guilty even if they did not have orgasms during intercourse. An important reason for these feelings was that in many cases they didn't particularly like the person with whom they had sex, and they perhaps found it more difficult to be sexually responsive. About 75% of both males and females reported feeling guilty about masturbation, and Darling and Davidson speculated that many were strongly influenced by older societal norms that discouraged genital self-pleasuring. Many of the females found that petting experiences adversely affected their psychological and physiological enjoyment of these behaviors. In another study of 45 married women ranging in age from their twenties to sixties, Keller, Eakes, Hinkle, and Hughston (1978) found that older respondents were more likely to report sexual guilt than younger subjects, perhaps reflecting older, more conservative sexual value systems. Studies like these imply that often situational factors more than religious or moral issues play a role in guilt feelings associated with sexual behaviors.

Pope John Paul II issued a 179-page encyclical called *Veritas Splendor* (The Splendor of Truth) (1993) (Fig. 8-4), in which he asserted that good is clearly and unambiguously good and that bad is similarly distinct and clear. He proclaimed that morals cannot be assessed situationally and that the Church's teaching offers salvation and freedom to the truly virtuous—an assertion at odds with the data from the social and behavioral sciences summarized in the previous chapter. Some evils are immediately apparent: genocide, slavery, and torture. However, the pope also labeled as distinct evils other behaviors that are of concern to more liberal Roman Catholics: the use of contraceptives, artificial insemina-

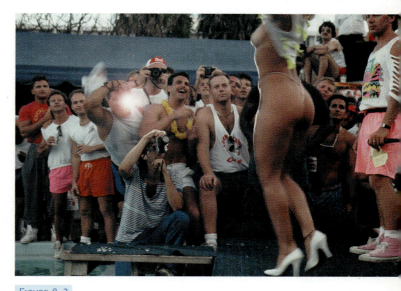

FIGURE 8-3 A beach scene in Florida during Spring Break. The combination of sun, skin, and alcohol often creates expectations of sexual activity.

tion, homosexual acts, masturbation, premarital sex, and abortion. For devout Catholics, these behaviors probably provoke powerful feelings of guilt. Of course, many of the world's religions make proclamations about sex that involve injunctions. John Paul II's encyclical, however, condemned many behaviors that professional and lay persons find acceptable

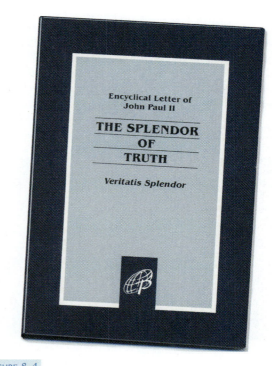

FIGURE 8-4 The papal encyclical Veritas Splendor (1993). This religious document reveals unambiguous judgments about many sexually related behaviors. Situational factors are not relevant to the interpretation of these actions.

and "normal." Of course conscience should be your guide, but one should understand how one's value system may create inevitable guilt feelings about sexual behaviors and how these feelings will have a negative effect on intimate behaviors and one's self-concept. In one sense guilt is actually an "instrument" used to encourage conformity with laws and doctrines basic to a social institution.

CELIBACY

Although this chapter focuses on physical expressions of eroticism and intimacy, not everyone enjoys having sex or experiencing sexual feelings. Many others choose not to masturbate or behave sexually with another person for personal or ideological reasons. These concepts too are important in a human sexuality course. Individuals who are asexual for any reason are not personally deficient; sex is always a choice and ideally never an obligation. The word *celibacy* comes from an old Latin word meaning a person is unmarried and, therefore, presumably not having sexual relations. As discussed in Chapter 2, historical and religious traditions emphasize marriage for sanctioning sexual activity. Modern definitions refer to the decision to abstain from sexual intercourse.

Partial Celibacy

Partial celibacy is a decision to abstain from sexual intercourse but not necessarily from masturbation. There are many reasons for partial celibacy. Some women and men wish to remain celibate until they marry because remaining virginal heightens their self-esteem. Others choose a period of partial celibacy because they need to "heal" after an unrewarding, abusive, or exploitative relationship. Some people lack sexual self-confidence, have anxiety about "performing well" sexually, and may fear intimacy because of the vulnerability it necessarily entails. Partial celibacy is also a good choice by those not using contraceptives because of the risk of an unanticipated preg-

nancy. Apprehensions about AIDS and other STDs are also good reason for many to be partially celibate for a time (Guinan, 1988). Just as many people very much enjoy the place of sex in their lives, others take equal delight and pride in their celibacy, and their choice is by no means a "second best" position. Some religious organizations encourage youth to pledge that they will remain virginal until they marry and to take pride in this personal commitment.

An organization called "Girls Incorporated" headquartered in Indianapolis has devised two programs intended to prevent adolescent pregnancy. The "Growing Together" program involves a series of parent-daughter workshops that teach and encourage family communication about several issues about teenagers' sexual behavior. The "Will Power/Won't Power" program teaches interpersonal skills to help young girls resist peer pressure for early sexual involvement. Postrado and Nicholson (1992) studied the responses of over 400 young girls between the ages of 12 and 14 on questionnaires regarding their sexual behaviors given on two occasions in the first year of their participation in these programs. The two programs were not equally effective in discouraging early sexual activity. While the young women in the "Growing Together" program were 2. 5 times less likely than others to participate in sexual activity during the study period, those in the "Will Power/Won't Power" program were just as likely as others to have participated in early sexual activity. Apparently, even when individuals are voluntarily receiving support and guidance in their sexual decision making, partial celibacy is not easy. In this study, the term "sexual activity" included other behaviors in addition to sexual intercourse, and thus some of these respondents may have been partially celibate while having some sexual activity. An issue addressed in neither study is whether participants delayed the decision to have intercourse or found the idea of having sex unappealing and had no plans for intercourse later on.

Complete Celibacy

A vow of complete celibacy is a requirement for church leadership in some faiths, including Roman Catholicism. **Complete celibacy** involves abstinence from both masturbation and interpersonal sexual behavior. To those who much enjoy sex this may seem a severe requirement, but many Roman Catholic clerics are comfortable with it and truly enjoy their celibacy or say they do (Fig. 8-5). Complete celibacy is part of a behavioral commitment to the complete devotion of a person's emotional and physical energies to doing good works for others. In ancient church doctrines, complete celibacy seems to derive from the implicit connection between sexuality and uncleanliness and sin and from an aspiration to personal moral perfection (Frazee, 1988). The justification for complete celibacy changed gradually throughout history (see Chapter 2). In the fourth century the Church felt that sexual behavior would have a detrimental effect on ministers performing the sacraments, and in the eleventh century new church policies were formulated because of the increased monastic influence in the church hierarchy. Church doctrines regarding complete celibacy for priests

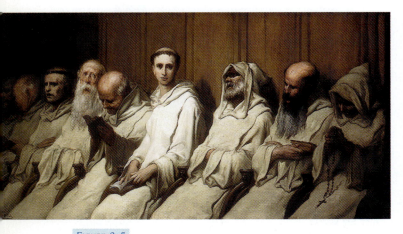

FIGURE 8-5 A vow of complete celibacy is one not undertaken lightly, especially by young people who are making a lifetime commitment to a religious faith.

and nuns remained unchanged from the twelfth to the twentieth centuries, even though there have been efforts to remove this prohibition on sex (Frazee, 1988). When nuns and priests leave their religious roles as spiritual leaders in the Roman Catholic Church, they often cite various factors contributing to this decision. While the constraints of complete celibacy are frequently mentioned as one reason, other matters concerning personal growth are just as frequently mentioned. Historically, Hinduism, Buddhism, Taoism, Shintoism, and Islam have also imposed celibacy on their religious leaders.

SEXUAL DREAMS

Our minds literally never rest. Our dreams contain real and symbolic imagery from our thoughts, feelings, and preoccupations. People have puzzled over the meaning of dreams since ancient times, and various explanations are offered. Some writers, such as Freud (1900), suggested our dreams are disguised attempts to fulfill desires that cannot be actualized during waking life. Others (Downing, 1996) believe dreams are attempts to solve problems and reach some understanding with "unfinished business" in waking life. Some dreams are highly arousing in an erotic way and filled with vivid images and occasionally lead to physiological arousal and orgasm. For some, the uncontrolled nature of this sexual imagery is upsetting, especially if the dream content is very different from how one sees oneself. Memories of erotic dreams can be persistent and puzzling. Sexual dreams are common, however, and do not necessarily reveal some aspect of personality. Although sexual dreams themselves are not erotic "behaviors," they can be part of one's sexual self-concept.

A Kinsey Institute (1990) report on sex notes that virtually all men and about 70% of women have sexual dreams, although only about half of these women have an orgasm during sleep. Erotic dreams may involve depictions of sexual practices or partners that are not part of a person's usual thoughts about sex. Remember that dream images do not always reveal one's "real" sexual desires, and disturbing dreams are not necessarily cause for concern or reveal some hidden problem. Still, dreams can help illuminate our understanding of waking experiences. One who is preoccupied with sex throughout the day should not be surprised by dreams that reflect this focus as well. **Nocturnal emissions,** or "wet dreams," are common in young men and men whose established pattern of sexual behavior is interrupted for some reason. They are called "wet" dreams because ejaculation occurs. Wet dreams involve erotic imagery that is often vivid and memorable upon waking. Because such dreams and orgasms are not under a man's conscious control, he should not feel guilty about the dreams. The stimulus for nocturnal emissions may not be entirely psychological, as tactile pressure of bedding against the penis may stimulate an erection and subsequent ejaculation. Kinsey's 1948 book, *Sexual Behavior in the Human Male,* reported that the highest incidence of nocturnal emissions occurs among men between the ages of 21 and 25 (71%). By age 50 only one-third of the men in his sample reported having wet dreams, and by the age of 60 only 14% reported them. The frequency of nocturnal emissions varies considerably. In Kinsey's youngest group of subjects (16 to 20 years old) some men had as many as 12 wet dreams in a single week, while others had only a few in a year. As with most sexual issues, there is variability both between and within individuals regarding these sexual experiences. Remember that men commonly have erections regularly throughout a night's sleep whether or not they are dreaming and irrespective of dream content. This is called **nocturnal penile tumescence** but is unrelated to nocturnal emission.

Women commonly begin having erotic dreams in adolescence. Vaginal discharges sometimes accompany these dreams, but many other factors also cause vaginal discharge, such as changes in hormone levels that are often dramatic at this age. There is no indication that women who have orgasms during erotic dreams are anxious or troubled by their responses, and women who are sexually active and comfortable with their intimacy generally feel good about nocturnal orgasms and tend to have more of them (Wells, 1986). Other data suggest that sexual arousal during sleep may be associated with anxiety (Henton, 1976), presumably because some subjects interpret their nocturnal orgasms as a result of their inability to suppress sexual urges. In a sample of 774 female undergraduates, Henton found that 22% experienced orgasms during sleep.

Sexual Daydreaming and Fantasy

Fantasy during masturbation and sexual intercourse can dramatically enhance arousal and responsiveness. Its role during intimacy with another is perplexing for some people: if you are having sex with someone, why would you have any need or desire to fantasize at the time? The role of fantasy in solo sex seems more obvious. Leitenberg and Henning (1995) published an exhaustive review of the literature on sexual fantasies that clarifies some issues about fantasies that are not immediately obvious. Because sexual fantasies (like dreams) are usually very personal, their content can illustrate the person's sexual value system in ways that their overt behaviors may not. The source of sexual fantasies is not always obvious. They may be stimulated by something one has seen or read or may be entirely imagined. Fantasies can arouse sexual excitement, and sexual excitement can arouse sexual fantasies. Leitenberg and Henning believe that sexual fantasies "appear to be deliberate patterns of thought designed to stimulate or enhance pleasurable sexual feelings regardless of whether the fantasies involve reminiscing about past sexual experiences, imagining anticipated future sexual activity, engaging in wishful thinking, or having daydreams that are exciting to imagine without any desire to put them into practice." (1995, p. 470).

Leitenberg and Henning note that women who fantasize during masturbation are more likely to experience orgasms more frequently during intercourse, and that men who fantasize frequently are also more likely to have orgasms during intercourse. Sexual fantasies help women and men become aroused and responsive during sexual sharing. People who report frequent sexual fantasies generally have fewer sexual problems and possibly more fully enjoy sexual activity.

Certain themes are more commonly reported in sexual fantasies: having sexual intercourse with someone you love, having intercourse with a stranger, having multiple sexual partners of the opposite sex simultaneously, exploring sexual behaviors you do not perform in real life, forcing someone to have sex with you or someone forcing you to have sex with them, reminiscing about a previous sexual encounter, visualizing scenes from an erotic movie, imagining oral-genital stimulation, being found sexually irresistible by someone else, having sex with someone famous, and many others. Apparently, our sexual fantasies are as diverse and creative as we are as individuals.

Gender Differences and Sexual Fantasies

Although women and men both have sexual fantasies, men fantasize more frequently than women (Jones & Barlow, 1990), especially with fantasies triggered by external events and those that occur spontaneously. With regard to sexual fantasies during intercourse or to become more sexually aroused, well over half of women and men in various studies report fantasizing very often or sometimes. Again, fantasy presumably heightens the ongoing pleasure of sexual intercourse for both women and men. There are, however, gender differences in the content of sexual fantasies. Men's sexual fantasies generally involve a more active role in a sexual interaction, and women's sexual fantasies involve more passive roles. Men see themselves as "actors" and women see themselves as "recipients" in erotic expression. Men focus more on highly visual, explicit sexual images, and women concentrate more on romantic, interpersonal, and emotional aspects of the shared experience. Men are more likely to fantasize about having sex with multiple female partners, although similar fantasies are not unusual among women. Women are somewhat more likely to have fantasies involving some element of sexual submission to a man, and men more frequently fantasize about "taking" or subduing their female partner (Sue, 1979).

Some fantasies are apparently stimulated by events in the individual's immediate environment. We often put ourselves in an environment in which we will be erotically stimulated and thus generate our own sexual fantasies. One way this is done is by reading erotic literature. Schmidt, Sigusch, and Schafer (1973) asked male and female university students to read an erotic story in which a young couple had sex and then measured the students' responses to this stimulus. Subjects rated the stories as somewhat arousing sexually and reported a generalized erotic excitement during the 24 hours immediately following. Both female and male subjects demonstrated physiological signs of sexual arousal while reading the story and reported some increase in sexual behavior, fantasy, and sex drive in the 24 hours afterwards. There were few differences between the women and men in this study, although the women reported a greater increase in sexual intercourse and sex drive than the men. Apparently, these subjects continued to think and fantasize about the story they had read, and these fantasies generally activated their sex drive and sexual behavior.

Just as people differ in other characteristics, our ability and inclination to create sexual fantasies varies. While some easily create and enjoy erotic images, others do not easily produce vivid depictions of sexual scenes in the "mind's eye." Tokatlidis and Over (1995) administered a paper-and-pencil test to assess differences in people's ability to create mental imagery to 119 women between the ages of 18 and 47 and assessed the relationship between these and genital and sensual arousal during sexual fantasy. Sexual arousal during fantasy was more clearly related to the subject's capacity to create vivid sensual images and their degree of absorption or involvement in those images than to their scores on this test. These investigators noted that the more frequently their subjects used certain erotic images in their fantasies, the more arousing were those images and the more clearly did they provoke physical enjoyment. Because men are thought to have more frequent sexual fantasies than women, one wonders whether women who more frequently fantasize erotically are more similar to men than to other women who do not fantasize as frequently.

Male sexual fantasies were studied systematically in a sample of 94 heterosexual men from 20 to 45 years old (Crepault & Couture, 1980). Roughly 60% of this sample were married, and all participants had lived with a woman during the previous year. All their subjects reported that they fantasized at times when they were not engaged in masturbation or sexual intercourse. Three-fourths reported that they engaged in sexual fantasies during intercourse with their wives or female partners. Two-thirds reported that they masturbated while fantasizing about erotic themes. Although the themes of their fantasies were not substantively different from those reported elsewhere, these data remind us of the role of such mental images in enhancing erotic pleasure during masturbation and/or sexual intercourse (Table 8-3).

The discussion so far has focused on common sexual fantasies. Little is known about the frequency or nature of sexual fantasies involving unusual or "deviant" sexual thoughts and acts. We will further discuss this in Chapter 19.

For many years telephone services have existed for stimulating sexual fantasies. Often someone on the other end of the line "talks you through" sexual fantasies, frequently involving the caller's masturbation while on the phone. Such services are sometimes called "dial-a-porn," and an immense amount of money is spent on this avenue of sexual fantasy and expression. Such services offer callers sexual control: the caller (who is paying the fee), usually a man, can ask for stimulating talk during masturbation, can say just how he wants to have intercourse, can ask for exciting vocal responses from the person called, usually a woman, or can imagine exotic forms of sexual experimentation. Telephone sex has become an addiction for many men. Although it might seem a "victimless" sexual pastime, the expenses some men incur can destroy their (and their family's) financial security.

Glascock & LaRose (1993) studied the female participants in these phone calls. In an analysis of 82 phone recordings, they found virtually no sexually violent topics, such as rape or involuntary bondage. Some men requested erotically

TABLE 8-3

Most Common Sexual Fantasy Themes

Female

Emphasis on nurturant touching, feeling, and caressing and partner arousal

Mental focus on physical arousal and feelings of emotional closeness

Mental images of a former or current sexual partner

Passive role in sexual behaviors—partner is doing something *to* them

Romantic thoughts and feelings involving love and devotion

Male

Impersonal sexual behaviors

High level of visual imagery—less focus on feelings and emotions

Sex involving little or no foreplay, proceeding quickly to intercourse

Visual focus on specific parts of partner's body

Sexual activity with great variety of partners

Group sexual interactions

Focus on specific sexual acts, i.e., fellatio

assertive behaviors from their female listeners, and these men apparently enjoyed a passive role in their fantasies. The most common types of phone calls involved male callers fantasizing a subservient role in a sexual situation or engaging in mutually enjoyable erotic stimulation ("I'll do this to you and you do this to me"). We include this subject here to show something more about the power of fantasies and suggest that auditory fantasies can be as powerful as visual ones.

As a final note, people who develop an addiction to phone sex find that it is astonishingly difficult to break the habit. If discovered by one's partner, like other addictions it can profoundly alter or damage a relationship. The partner may have difficulty understanding why the person would want to be "talked off" by a stranger on the telephone when they are offering love, nurturance, and their own sexuality. Like people with other addictions, people dependent on phone sex to meet their sexual needs are not easily helped with therapy. Often this problem is shockingly persistent and refractory to clinical assistance.

MASTURBATION AND AUTOEROTICISM

The terms "masturbation" and "autoeroticism" have related but different meanings. **Masturbation** refers to genital self-stimulation with some anticipation of an erotic satisfaction, although it is not always necessary for a person to stimulate his or her genitalia in order to experience orgasm; some women have orgasms as a result of breast stimulation alone (Masters & Johnson, 1966). Masturbation may also involve the use of vibratory aids, as well as erotic printed materials. The term "au-

toeroticism" has a broader meaning. Autoeroticism involves self-stimulation that may or may not involve external physical stimulation; it can refer to sexual feelings or thoughts with no outside stimulation at all. Autoeroticism may refer to the personal sensual "texture" of various sexual perceptions and feelings.

There has been much controversy about masturbation, and many people feel guilty about masturbating. An old-fashioned term for masturbation implies it is an entirely unwholesome behavior: self-abuse. Guilt about masturbation is often based on very old religious and cultural beliefs about the appropriateness of sexual response only for procreational purposes. It is sometimes viewed as a dismal alternative to sexual intercourse, and many people are shocked that others who have regular access to a sexual partner still choose to masturbate occasionally or even incorporate masturbation into their lovemaking. As noted in an earlier chapter, ancient Judeo-Christian religious traditions contributed negative meanings associated with masturbation. When the survival of a nomadic tribe depended upon the fertility of its women and men, anything that wasted a man's "seed" was seen as a threat to the survival and prosperity of the group. Throughout the history of Western civilization masturbation was viewed as a failure of self-control, a tawdry surrender to one's "baser" animalistic instincts. Recall the discussion of semen-conservation theory in Chapter 2: historical thinkers believed that masturbation wasted precious bodily fluids that had the potential to be channeled into virtuous thoughts and actions. The Victorians were decidedly uneasy about masturbation, and some people even made wire cages to cover a boy's genitals to thwart any attempt at self-stimulation.

"The best to you each morning!" Dr. J. H. Kellogg (1852-1943) (Fig. 8-6), who started the modern breakfast cereal industry, was developing a simple food intended to help people

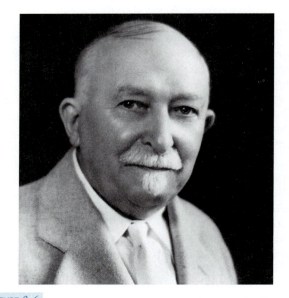

FIGURE 8-6 Dr. J. H. Kellogg hoped that marketing and selling simple cereals (like corn flakes) would help young adults better control their sexual urges and avoid the temptation to masturbate.

(usually young people) control their presumably hard-to-control sexual desires. Dr. Kellogg, the director of a large hospital, believed several factors clearly indicated a person masturbated regularly, including heart rhythm irregularities, stooped posture, and acne. For Dr. Kellogg these were certain signs the person was having trouble controlling her or his erotic urges and, therefore, masturbated. Most of the attention on this "scourge" of masturbation was directed to males; historically there was little acknowledgment that women masturbated or had strong sexual feelings at all. Kellogg believed that a bland diet would assuage these powerful inclinations and help to restore self-control and good mental health to those unable to handle their powerful sexual urges. Sylvester Graham invented graham crackers in the nineteenth century for the same reason: bland foods were thought to help control erotic feelings (Reinisch, 1990).

Between the 1890s and World War I, a more enlightened attitude toward masturbation gradually emerged, in part because of the lay public's interest in the developing science of psychiatry. Still, change came slowly and was relatively ineffective in neutralizing widely publicized historical misconceptions. Outrageous pseudoscientific claims about the adverse effects of masturbation can be traced back to the mid-1700s, when S. A. D. Tissot published *A Treatise on the Diseases Produced by Onanism.* (Technically, onanism can refer either to masturbation or coitus interruptus, withdrawing the penis from the vagina during intercourse and ejaculating outside of a woman's body.) Tissot believed there were catastrophic psychiatric consequences of "wasting" one's semen and suggested the loss of a single ounce of semen had the same effect as losing 40 ounces of blood. Such bizarre claims would be comical if it weren't for the fact that Tissot's book and teachings provoked untold guilt and misery. By the middle of the next century most people thought that masturbation caused insanity and many physical ailments, eventually encouraging Kellogg and Graham to explore dietary means of controlling this behavior.

In 1891, Dr. E. T. Brady was one of the first medical professionals to question Tissot's claims and noted that despite the supposedly compulsive quality of masturbation, it probably didn't do as much harm as had originally been thought. He stated, "But it is very probable that its importance as an influence has been greatly exaggerated, particularly in connection with the causation of insanity" (cited in Fishbein & Burgess, 1947). About this time a more cautious professional tone appeared in pronouncements about the effects of masturbation. As soon as scientists determined how common the practice was, it became apparent to all that there had been an enormous amount of exaggeration about all too human behavior. Today, most medical, social, and behavioral scientists believe that masturbation is neither psychologically nor physically harmful except when a compulsive feature of some psychological disorder.

Masturbation as a Learning Exercise

An important legacy of Greek and Roman civilizations is the belief in the importance of "know thyself" as a guiding principle for personal growth and development. We apply this dictum to both our intellectual *and* physical attributes. Just as many experts in human sexuality encourage you to examine your own genitalia with a mirror to gain a better understanding of what you look like, they also often encourage people to masturbate to learn more about how they respond to erotic genital stimulation. Let's look at an example of what masturbation can teach someone who has never masturbated or had orgasm in sexual intercourse with another person. You would probably have some difficulty understanding the human sexual response cycle in Chapter 6. It might not be clear what arousal and excitement feel like or how quickly or slowly these develop and their physical indications. The same is true with the plateau stage of the sexual response cycle, feelings of ejaculatory inevitability or imminent orgasm, penile or vaginal contractions, and the return to pre-arousal levels of excitement in the resolution stage. We are not urging everyone to start masturbating but are pointing out that masturbatory experiences can teach one much about how the body responds to erotic self-stimulation. Masturbation need not focus exclusively on the primary erogenous zones, as many find that their breasts, anus, or other body areas (particularly the mons veneris in women) are extremely sensitive and that stimulating them during masturbation may significantly heighten arousal and responses.

For those who feel they have something to learn about the sexual response cycle through masturbation, we recommend planning the experience to assure total privacy at a time when you are well-rested, free of stress, and free of interruptions. Masturbation can be a very informative exercise in sensual self-exploration, and interferences should be prevented. Whether to share your masturbatory experiences with another is entirely up to you. Mutual masturbation is considered by many a highly arousing and enjoyable alternative to sexual intercourse or an aspect of foreplay before intercourse. For two people who are unready to have intercourse but who want to share eroticism, mutual masturbation offers this opportunity without risk of unanticipated pregnancy or transmission of a sexually transmitted disease, provided the genitals do not come into contact and semen is not deposited in or near any body orifices.

Issues Surrounding Masturbation

For many years now, data collected about masturbation frequency reveal that among people who masturbate, males do so more frequently than females. Laumann, Gagnon, Michael, and Michaels (1994) polled women and men between the ages of 18 and 59 and discovered that the percentage of males who reported masturbating at least once a week (24.6) was far higher than for females (7.06) for all age groups studied. The frequency of reported masturbation declined significantly over the age of 50 for both women and men. This difference occurs among all age groups surveyed, regardless of marital status, educational attainment, religion, race, and ethnicity. The first Kinsey study in 1948 reported that virtually all males and about two-thirds of females masturbated at some time in their lives. These are grouped data, of course, and individual differences among people are not apparent. Certainly some women masturbate very frequently and some men never at all. The reasons for this large gender difference are obscure, which cannot be attributed to specific anatomical, hormonal, genetic, or psychosocial factors. It has been suggested (Hyde, 1979) that a protruding penis is more likely than a woman's clitoris to encounter incidental daily friction that may become associated with real or symbolic erotic cues in the environment. Supposedly this minor but persistent skin stimulation creates a perceptual readiness to acknowledge sexual stimuli that surround us. This hypothesis is worth testing empirically and systematically. In 1993, Leitenberg, Detzer, and Srebnik reported that in a sample of almost 300 introductory psychology students, the males reported masturbating three times more frequently than the females during their adolescent and early adulthood years. While these investigators noted that there is apparently no relationship between adolescent and young adult masturbatory experience and later satisfactoriness of heterosexual intercourse experiences, overall perceptions of sexual satisfaction, sexual arousal, or the incidence of sexual problems in later relationships, this may not always be true. For example, women who have trouble having orgasms may be helped significantly with guided instruction in various masturbatory techniques. Furthermore, individuals who report masturbating more frequently are probably more open-minded about their sexuality in general and thus more likely to report higher frequencies of sexual intercourse in marriage and greater satisfaction with the sexual component of their relationship. Masturbation has not been shown to "taint" one's later sexual experiences or the enjoyment one derives from those experiences.

Leitenberg, Detzer, and Srebnik speculate on the wide difference in frequency of masturbation between females and males and note that often women have orgasms more regularly and reliably during masturbation than during sexual intercourse. The lower frequency of masturbation by females, they suggest, may reflect traditional feminine sexual socialization that associates sexual satisfaction and responsiveness with shared intimacy and romance rather than masturbation.

Because genital self-stimulation begins in early childhood, the attitudes and responses of parents and caretakers to pre-adolescent masturbatory behaviors can set an emotional "tone" about genitally focused sexual pleasure. Stern reproaches, scolding, or even slapping a child's hand can cause the child to learn maladaptive emotional responses to intimate pleasures. Consider the confusion a youngster experiences if pain is consistently paired with pleasure. This situation is not likely to lead to unambiguous feelings of sexual enjoyment later in life, and the person may come to doubt the appropriateness of genital pleasure. Later in life this can cause real problems, as we'll discuss in a later chapter on sex-

ual dysfunctions. While growing up, these parental interventions may carry some troubling or perplexing double messages: "Your genitals are dirty; save them for someone you love."

For these and other reasons, youngsters frequently feel guilty about masturbation and sexual pleasure in general. Responsible, informed parents make a point of recognizing their children's sexual growth and development, and this can have positive effects on the youngster's emerging sense of self and favorable perception of their bodies and feelings from them. For some parents, this is a delicate process of reinforcing healthy feelings while minimizing a sense of shame or undue self-consciousness.

Guilt, Masturbation, and Sexual Fulfillment

Despite the fact that these are more enlightened times than the days of Graham and Kellogg, for many there is still a sense of guilt or shame surrounding masturbation. As noted above, because women have been socialized to believe that intimacy and romance are important for the unambiguous enjoyment of sex, masturbation conceivably provokes guilt in some women. Additionally, for someone raised to believe in sex-for-procreation, masturbation is viewed as a sexual behavior that does not result in conception or the birth of a child. Generally, females are somewhat more likely to feel guilty about masturbation than are males. Evidence suggests that women's guilt feelings are also more likely to detract from their experiences of sexual arousal and responsiveness. In a study involving almost 700 female undergraduates and recent graduates, Davidson and Darling (1993) found that subjects who reported guilt feelings about masturbation had more negative feelings about masturbation in general and were unlikely to report having good psychological and physiological reactions to their behavior. Perhaps more importantly, these women reported lower overall levels of sexual adjustment and satisfaction in their lives.

Davidson and Moore (1994) examined the socialization pressures many women feel to associate sexual pleasure with procreation or procreative behaviors. In a survey study of almost 800 never-married heterosexual women at a university, these researchers found of women who only masturbated, women who both masturbated and experienced sexual intercourse, and women who only had sexual intercourse but didn't masturbate, the women who only masturbated reported the highest levels of guilt about masturbating and engaging in petting behaviors. Among these three groups, the women who only masturbated were also most likely to report lower levels of comfort with their own sexuality and sexual satisfaction. These findings probably can be generalized to many other women in other settings too. In an age of potentially fatal risks associated with unprotected sexual intercourse, lessening the guilt associated with masturbation would seem a worthy objective for sex educators and other social and behavioral scientists.

Early Adolescent Masturbation Experiences

Thus far we have been discussing masturbation among sexually mature individuals that typically leads to orgasm. Fox (1993) points out an interesting similarity between early masturbatory experiences in prepubertal boys and clitoral manipulation and orgasm in early adolescent females. Fox interviewed 100 men who were willing to discuss their masturbatory experiences before reaching puberty and gaining the capacity for orgasm and ejaculation. Fully 82% of this sample reported that genital self-stimulation before puberty was accompanied by a prolonged "blissful" genital pleasure that could be maintained for 15 to 30 minutes. Because clitoral stimulation in women can lead to orgasm but generally not ejaculation, this writer analogized prolonged plateau-stage pleasure in females to this prolonged "blissful" pleasure in young boys. Because many men are unwilling or unable to discuss their early experiments in genital self-stimulation, collecting these data took Fox 15 years, and it may, therefore, be difficult to replicate this investigation readily. Although masturbation and intercourse are often ejaculation-focused activities for men, there is certainly a potential for prolonged pre-ejaculatory eroticism and orgasm; perhaps in the course of growing up, men have forgotten the highly pleasurable feelings that precede orgasm and ejaculation. The suggested similarity between this pleasurable state in men and plateau-stage enjoyment of sexual tension in women is intriguing.

Masturbation in Couples

People who think of masturbation as a "second best" form of sexual expression have difficulty understanding the place of masturbation in a relationship. According to Laumann, Gagnon, Michael, and Michaels (1994), 16. 5% of the married men in their sample and 4. 7% of the married women reported masturbating at least once a week. What is the motive to masturbate in a relationship? One partner's unreceptivity to intercourse may play a role, but other factors may occur as well. The effects of age, illness, and boredom may affect the frequency of intercourse, as well as a person's general level of satisfaction with the relationship. Sex researchers have identified the *pursuer/distancer relationship* in marriage as a source of conflict about sexual intercourse (Betchen, 1991). In this situation, one person chooses masturbation over sexual intercourse, leading to a vicious cycle in which one partner desires and pursues intercourse while the other distances him/herself and masturbates while alone. This situation often involves a purposeful manipulation of one's partner and can be seen as controlling and even emotionally abusive. This can be a maddening situation, particularly if the couple's communication skills are poor. The situation gets progressively worse as the pursuer persists and becomes more energetic and angry while the distancer removes him/herself further by masturbating even more frequently. The dynamics of this situation can be complex and may require the help of a counselor or therapist. Whenever one partner openly chooses masturbation over sex-

ual intercourse with their spouse, the pursuer/distancer scenario may be occurring. We discourage manipulating one's partner by either offering or withholding sex.

Masturbation isn't always problematic in a relationship, however. Generally, women and men see masturbation in relationships differently. Men often view masturbation as *supplementary* to regular sexual intercourse: an optional outlet for pent-up sexual energy. Incorporating masturbation into love-making is also a way to explore erotic pleasures with one's partner. In contrast, women report that masturbation has more of a *substitutive* role (Hessellund, 1976). When a woman's partner is unavailable, unwilling, or unable to have sexual intercourse, she may perceive masturbation as an enjoyable, substitute sexual outlet. Nonetheless, often one partner feels sexually inadequate if she or he finds out that their partner masturbates regularly and may view the behavior as a rejection of their sexuality.

Masturbating in the presence of one's partner allows you to show them exactly how and where you like to be touched, as well as how vigorously you prefer to be stimulated. Just as we can learn about ourselves through masturbation, we can also learn a lot about our partner.

Vibrators and Masturbation

Vibrators are manufactured in a variety of sizes and shapes, but vibrators are not necessarily the same as dildos. Technically, a dildo is any erect-penis-shaped object that may or may not vibrate. Stigma has long been attached to the use of vibratory aids in masturbation or during intercourse, with one partner feeling the other must "need something else" and "I must not be enough for him/her." Masters and Johnson (1970) advocated using vibrators to help people learn about their sexual response cycles, overcome inhibitions, and learn about themselves. Although there is really no substitute for the nurturance, love, and attachment of a good sexual relationship, vibratory aids can indeed enhance your knowledge of yourself and help explore interesting erotic dimensions with your partner. Masturbation with vibratory aids is *very common,* and there should be no guilt or misgivings associated with this means of sexual exploration.

Most scientific research on vibrators has involved women, but both women and men use vibrators during masturbation and intercourse. Women who use vibratory aids do not generally insert them deep into the vagina but selectively stimulate the external genitalia, the clitoris in particular. Davis, Blank, Lin, and Bonillas (1996) studied the use of vibrators in a large sample of women from age 18 to 75. Their questionnaire asked about why women use vibrators and the situations in which they do so. Women in their sample used vibrators mostly to increase their level of sexual pleasure and responsiveness, mostly during masturbation but frequently with a partner. Most reported that the orgasms precipitated by using a vibrator were stronger and lasted longer than those otherwise occurring during masturbation or intercourse. These women overwhelmingly reported that they very much enjoyed using

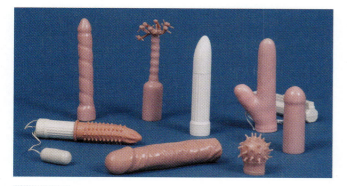

FIGURE 8-7 Vibrators are manufactured in a variety of sizes, shapes, and textures. When applied to the genitals or the anal area, vibratory stimulation is often perceived as keenly erotic.

Methods of Masturbation

Several methods of masturbation are consistently reported by women and men. The most common method of female masturbation involves stimulating the clitoris, often by touching or rubbing its glans or shaft, often while stimulating one's nipples manually. Vibratory stimulation of the clitoris and opening to the vagina is also quite common. The mons veneris is often rubbed or pressed during clitoral stimulation. Women do not usually insert objects into their vaginas during masturbation, although this is not "abnormal"; clitoral stimulation is generally preferred. Many women masturbate while lying on their back, and others lie on their abdomen while touching and/or rubbing their clitoris and mons veneris (Fig. 8-8).

Men usually masturbate by stroking the shaft of the penis up and down in a rhythmic manner. The glans is the most sensitive part of the penis, but most men do not usually grasp or stroke the glans, instead stimulating the shaft. Occasionally touching the glans increases sexual arousal. While most men masturbate this way, there are other means of penile self-stimulation. Some men lie on their abdomen and rub their genitals against the bedding. Some men also grasp or gently squeeze the scrotum during masturbation, but generally only the penis is used (Fig. 8-9).

Although masturbation is usually a solitary behavior, many couples enjoy mutual masturbation, either as a prelude to intercourse or as a shared erotic activity enjoyed for its own sake. Shared masturbatory behavior is highly arousing for many couples. Simultaneous manual and oral stimulation of the other's genitals is often highly erotic. Many couples enjoy the special intimacy associated with eye contact during mutual masturbation.

their vibrators. Additionally, most said that the clitoris was the preferred location for vibratory stimulation. For women who want to feel sexually self-sufficient, a vibrator offers control and reliability for erotic experiences and experimentation. Vibrators offer both supplementary and substitutive means of erotic self-stimulation.

Women who report using vibrators say a small amount of lubricant often enhances the pleasure. Vibrators are available from many pharmacies and mail-order businesses usually marketed as "massagers" (Fig. 8-7). One should not feel embarrassed to purchase a vibrator. If a couple uses a vibrator during shared intimacy, it should be washed thoroughly before the other uses it if it was inserted into a body orifice, but *should not be immersed in water.*

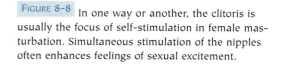

FIGURE 8-8 In one way or another, the clitoris is usually the focus of self-stimulation in female masturbation. Simultaneous stimulation of the nipples often enhances feelings of sexual excitement.

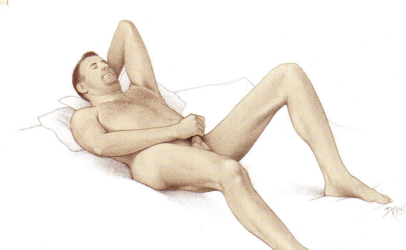

FIGURE 8-9 In male masturbation, the shaft and glans of the penis are stroked rhythmically. While men masturbate in many different ways, this is the most common.

DR. RUTH'S TOP TEN FACTS ABOUT MASTURBATION

1. Masturbation is free—free of cost, free of disease, and hopefully guilt-free. Everyone is entitled to their share of privacy to do with as they please, including having an orgasm.

2. Masturbation is an effective tool for women and men who want to learn how to have an orgasm. While partners can provide much pleasure, they may also be too distracting. A woman or a man who learns how to please herself or himself can share that knowledge with a lover.

3. Many married people masturbate because rarely do two people have the same level of sexual desire. There's no reason for one to be sexually frustrated or the other to feel forced to have sex, since masturbation is an effective alternative. Masturbation used to avoid sexual interplay with a partner can be a problem, but when used to supplement a satisfactory sexual relationship, there is nothing wrong with it.

4. A vibrator can help a woman reach an orgasm during masturbation. Occasionally she can use the vibrator to approach the orgasmic response and complete it with her hand or finger.

5. There's no limit to how often one can masturbate, though caution should be exercised to prevent it from becoming compulsive. Someone who reaches a point where the need to masturbate interferes with socializing, school, or work should reduce their masturbation to a level where they are in control of their urge to masturbate.

6. A couple watching each other masturbate is the only absolutely safe sex, as long as no bodily fluids touch the other person's body. There are many forms of "safer" sex, but condoms can break, people do cheat on each other, and any exposure to bodily fluids involves some risk.

7. While many people find sexual intercourse more satisfying than masturbation, others achieve a stronger orgasm through masturbation. They may be better able to cause the sensations that bring them to orgasm, or perhaps their senses are heightened when they focus entirely on their own feelings.

8. A man who masturbates under conditions that make him hurry might develop a tendency towards premature ejaculation. To gain control of when he ejaculates during intercourse, men should allow themselves more time. Masturbation not only brings pleasure but can also be a time for exercising control of orgasms.

9. Masturbation does not cause acne, hair to grow in the palms, or blindness. Masturbation may cause an irritation to the genitals, in which case using a lubricant is recommended.

10. The sexual fantasies people have while masturbating are just that, fantasies, and are usually unrelated to real life.

Other Countries, Cultures, and Customs

THE DHAT SYNDROME

Chapter 2 reviewed historical aspects of semen-conservation theory, the belief that depleting semen through intercourse or masturbation causes a depletion not only of energy but character and moral rectitude. Many Victorians believed that refraining from sexual expression except for planning conception was virtuous and that any "unnecessary" loss of semen weakened a person physically and morally. On the Indian subcontinent there is a similar "syndrome" called "dhat," in which men experience anxiety, lethargy, weight loss, and sexual dysfunction that they believe results from the loss of semen through masturbation or nocturnal emissions. In fact, these symptoms are associated with anxiety. This syndrome is common in India and Sri Lanka (Dewaraja & Sasaki, 1991; Joshi & Money, 1995).

Some men in India and Sri Lanka also develop significant anxieties about the contents of their wet dreams because they believe they cause a depletion of their energy. These apprehensions are similar to those of Victorians, perhaps related to the fact that the English occupied this part of the world extensively between the mid-1850s and mid-1940s. The possibility of similar anxieties in other world cultures would seem worthy of investigation.

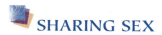

SHARING SEX

Interactive sexuality includes many activities: foreplay, oral-genital stimulation, heterosexual intercourse, anal stimulation, and intercourse. The following chapter deals with homosexuality and its expression; this chapter focuses on heterosexual interactive intimacy. Although we expect most readers to have some knowledge or experience in sexual matters, we believe you will learn some new things about the variety of heterosexual erotic motives and behaviors.

Throughout this book we've discussed the importance of a climate of psychological safety in sexual interactions. In most instances, sex cannot be enjoyed fully unless two people trust one another fully, have privacy, feel comfortable sharing their vulnerabilities, and don't fear the outcomes of their intimacy. Coercion is inappropriate in any sexual encounter, and any real or imagined force or pressure, physical or psychological, is inappropriate for rewarding sex.

The Importance of Touch

Although many people think of sex as involving one person penetrating another, shared touching, skin-to-skin, is an important and potentially very enjoyable aspect of intimate expression and should not be diminished because it doesn't seem as "serious" as intercourse. **Foreplay** is any of a number of activities in which two people engage before having intercourse, although these behaviors *need not always lead to intercourse* but may be enjoyed by themselves.

Because erotic touching is often a part of foreplay, many people wonder whether they are doing it well. Although there are no set guidelines on how to touch your partner, a few prin-

ciples characterize the kinds of touching women and men report they enjoy. Before considering the nature of sexual touching, however, the issue of **personal space** deserves mention. Everyone has a space surrounding their bodies they like to control, and people generally feel uneasy if others come too close or intrude into this personal space. Different factors affect how we regulate our personal space. For example, we usually don't mind if someone we like or love touches us, but often we are reserved or rejecting if a stranger or someone we dislike does the same thing. Personal space also varies over the surface of our body. Although we might not mind someone patting us on the back, we would be distressed and startled if a stranger put their hand on the inside of our thigh. The better we know someone, the more easily we negotiate reciprocal touching in progressively more private areas of our bodies (Fig. 8-10). This often takes time because we need to get to know one another better first.

Review: Erogenous Zones

An earlier chapter describes the erogenous zones, areas of the body that when stimulated yield keen sensual and sexual pleasures. We all share the same **primary erogenous zones:** the mouth, genitalia, and anus. Most sexual interactions involve some or all of the primary erogenous zones. The **secondary erogenous zones** reflect one's personal life experiences with tactile, sensual, and sexual pleasures, as one associates the stimulation of certain body areas with erotic meaning and feeling.

During foreplay people often like their partner to begin their caresses gently and in less sensitive areas. As foreplay becomes more active, most people gradually prefer firmer or more vigorous touching or rubbing in progressively more sensitive areas. When the skin is moist or a little slippery, skin

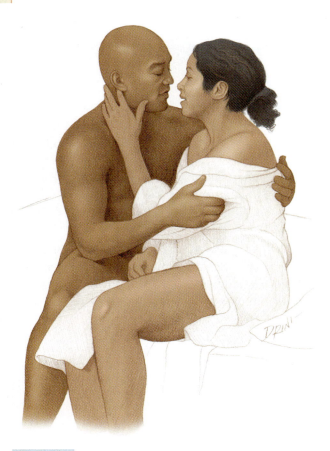

FIGURE 8-10 Reciprocal, non-intercourse intimate touching and caressing often create feelings of safety and trust in both partners and also serve to increase sexual arousal.

stimulation tends to be firmer and more deliberate and can also be more patient and leisurely. We will discuss erotic massage later in this section. Remember that everyone is unique, however, and what appeals to some might be boring or laborious to others. Generally it is better to err on the side of tact and care than be overly assertive and hurried. Prolonged foreplay is often desired by women and many men.

Foreplay facilitates comfortable vaginal penetration, although again, these behaviors need not lead to intercourse. It takes time for lubrication in women and erection in men to occur. When the woman is well lubricated and the man has a full, firm erection, vaginal penetration is easy. But with inadequate lubrication and an insufficiently firm erection, vaginal penetration can be uncomfortable and unrewarding. Therefore, a "take your time" approach seems best, even though patience is more difficult when a person is sexually excited. Open communication in foreplay lets two people share their affection and their bodies and have time to attend to their own arousal and responsiveness. Although scientific knowledge of human sexuality has increased greatly, some things *don't* change very much—such as this principle of sharing, which is as ageless as the human race.

Scientists have found big differences between men and women in sexual feelings and pleasures. Denney, Field, &

Quadagno (1984), studied a sample of 39 men and 49 women who were students in their early 20s. When asked about foreplay, sexual intercourse, or afterplay, the women reported that foreplay was the most important and enjoyable aspect of a sexual encounter. Men, in contrast, reported that intercourse was paramount. The women also said they would prefer to spend more time in foreplay and afterplay than did the men. These data confirm that while foreplay functions to facilitate comfortable intercourse, the diverse behaviors of foreplay may be enjoyed in their own right and do not always have to lead to intercourse. Why men and women report differences in this respect is unclear. Perhaps women are socialized more to associate sexual and sensual sharing and mutual pleasuring with traditional feminine personality characteristics. In contrast, men with a traditional masculine upbringing perhaps learn early that sex involves "doing something" to a woman rather than sharing something with her. Note that foreplay and afterplay typically involve more deliberate and attentive touching than sexual intercourse itself.

Most of the surface of our skin has the potential to contribute to erotic pleasure. Montagu (1971) raises the interesting hypothesis that our desire for sexual intercourse and intimacy is more basically a desire to hold and be held. From birth, some of our keenest pleasures come from feelings of warmth and gentle pressure on the surface of our bodies. Newborn babies who are not held and cuddled do not grow as quickly as those experiencing such stimulation. Earlier we noted that women often seek sexual intercourse in order to be held and cuddled afterwards. When asked about what they dislike about male lovers, women commonly complain that men are hurried and focused and do not understand the importance of unhurried touching and caressing. Studies of tactile sensitivity consistently demonstrate that females are more sensitive and have lower touch thresholds than men. This may explain in part why women seem more reliant on physical touch for sexual excitement while men depend more on visual stimuli.

Erotic Massage

While developing their sex therapy techniques, Masters and Johnson (Personal Communication, 1978) learned that when skin surfaces are moist or slippery, a couple is much more likely to engage in prolonged foreplay involving deliberate and thorough touching and caressing. As simple as this is, many couples still have difficulty with mutual tactile pleasuring. More recently there is a growing interest in erotic massage. Your local bookstore likely has simple, illustrated manuals with helpful suggestions for giving your partner an erotic massage.

There are many good reasons for exploring erotic massage with one's partner. One learns it is possible to be both relaxed and aroused, as careful, patient erotic massage can relax and excite you at the same time. Erotic massage also gives women and men the opportunity to enjoy prolonged touching along with visual enjoyment of your partner. Erotic massage also offers new foreplay techniques when a couple's usual activities have become predictable. Couples often fall into habits in their lovemaking, with little experimentation or exploration. Something new, like a sexy rubdown, can be even more stimulating because of its novelty. Patient touching and rubbing is an attractive alternative to foreplay routines that have lost their "zing." When coupled with low lighting, scented massage oils, soft music, and perhaps incense, couples are more open about what they like and communicate verbally perhaps more than in the past. And talking can be a very big turn on! Thinking we are pleasing our partner is one thing, but being told it clearly and with emotion is more fulfilling and stimulating. Leisurely massage often facilitates verbal communication, which further enhances excitement and pleasure.

Erotic massage also teaches us about areas of our bodies that are more sensitive than we might have thought, improving our understanding of our secondary erogenous zones and perhaps diversifying our personal sexual value system. We can enjoy our eroticism more fully when we share this kind of information with our partner. With massage two people take turns giving and receiving pleasure from one another, making it a more "equal" sexual sharing than some erotic interactions in which a man might typically "take the lead" because the man and woman have been socialized this way. Massage might begin with a shared bath or shower, or a few minutes in a whirlpool bath.

Massage can involve you showing your partner how you like to touch and be touched; taking turns can help both of you learn about your erotic "maps" and how vigorously or gently you prefer to be rubbed or fondled. Because many men have been raised to be assertive, they may have trouble getting used to being passive during shared touching but find it very enjoyable if they give it a chance. It may be difficult at first to refrain from acting on a desire to proceed more quickly, but the better one gets at this, the more delicious is the sensual pleasure associated with the massage. One can think of this in-

timate sharing as an erotic massage or prolonged foreplay, although those people who feel intimacy has to involve a "goal" may be more comfortable knowing where the process is going from the outset.

Erotic massage may involve genital or non-genital areas of the body, and deciding at the beginning can help both people focus on the sensations of tactile pleasuring rather than wondering what might be coming next. Non-genital massage may involve all areas of the body except the genitalia and anal area; genital massage focuses primarily on these parts of the body, although one might work up to it slowly with a full-body rub down. A helpful book on erotic massage (Inkeles, 1992) discusses creating an environment conducive to relaxed sensual sharing and explains the impact of massage on our circulatory, muscular, and nervous systems. It includes special techniques for massaging the back, the back of the legs, feet, front of the legs, chest, arms, hands, and head and face. The emphasis of this fine book is on massage as a relaxing, therapeutic form of sensual sharing. Figure 8-11 depicts one of the techniques it describes.

As discussed in Chapter 7, as we get older sexual arousal takes a bit longer. Erotic massage is an excellent way to prolong sexual sharing before intercourse and allows plenty of time to become fully aroused. Erotic massage is a special treat that some couples enjoy on special occasions. For others, it is a regular part of their sexual lifestyle. For a special someone in your life, you can make a "coupon" in an "I love you" card that they can redeem whenever they like. You will have given a gift, and they will have the pleasure of a special present awaiting them in the future, and both of you will have gained some control in the planning for a massage. Men who experiment with sexual massages too find they very much enjoy being touched—that tactile pleasures are not only for women (Zilbergeld, 1992).

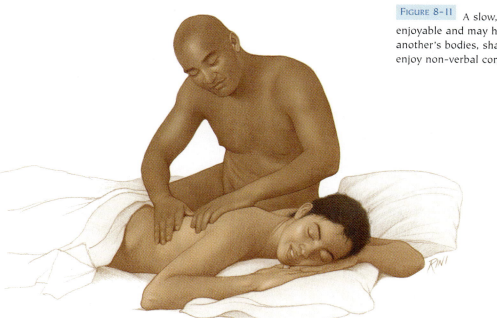

FIGURE 8-11 A slow, sensual massage can be very enjoyable and may help two people explore one another's bodies, share a sense of intimacy, and enjoy non-verbal communication.

Stimulating a Woman's or Man's Breasts

Of the secondary erogenous zones, the breasts, especially in women, are most often an erotic focus during sexual touching. Throughout this book we have mentioned the important connection between self-esteem and body image. A person who thinks that they are attractive to others is more likely to feel good about themselves. For some women, breast size, symmetry, and shape are an important aspect of feminine self-esteem and sexual self-confidence. Other women couldn't care less. For still others, breasts thought to be too large cause uncomfortable self-scrutiny. Our culture emphasizes this aspect of a woman's body. Yet there is no relationship between breast size and breast sensitivity or any other measure of sexual arousability and responsiveness. There are wide individual differences in breast sensitivity, but they are unrelated to breast size. As described in Chapter 4, despite sometimes large differences in breast size, most women have very similar amounts of milk duct tissue. Size differences primarily result from differing amounts of fat. Chapter 6 describes how nipple erection is common during sexual arousal, thus increasing the area of skin that can be stimulated, especially that very sensitive part of the breast.

Women often think that men are too rough when they caress their breasts. Good communication helps minimize this problem, but generally women appreciate it when their partner starts slowly and gently. During lovemaking many men stimulate their partners' breasts manually or orally, and many women stimulate their own breasts during masturbation. Reinisch (1990) summarized some of the data on breast stimulation and noted that even though most women receive some form of breast stimulation during foreplay or intercourse, only about half of them reported actually enjoying it. This is an interesting fact. Do most men stimulate their partners' breasts because they themselves like to or because they believe all women like to have their breasts stimulated? The answer is not known. However, some women who *do* report that they like this kind of touching have reported exactly how they like to be stimulated. For example, many women report that they enjoy a man starting slowly, putting his entire hand over their breast and pressing gently while moving their breast in slow circles, moving back and forth between the two breasts. As women become progressively more aroused, they prefer nipple stimulation with gentle touching, mouthing, or sucking. Remember that breast sensitivity often changes through the course of a woman's menstrual cycle, and a specific type of stimulation enjoyed at one time can be almost painful at another. Many women enjoy prolonged foreplay, and a woman's breasts offer a non-genital area of erotic focus for increasing the time a couple spends sharing erotic touching (Fig. 8-12).

Manual Stimulation of the Genitalia

Manually stimulating one's partner's genitalia is virtually universal in all cultures (Suggs & Miracle, 1993). Genital touching uses one of the most sensitive areas on the surface of the body, the fingertips, to stimulate another one of the most sensitive areas on the surface of the body, the genitalia (Fig. 8-13). People like their genitals to be touched gently or firmly, rarely roughly. One can touch one's partner's genitals for many reasons besides masturbation, such as with simple caressing and facilitating erection and lubrication. Genital touching during foreplay is a gradual penetration of an individual's personal space before more explicit genital penetration.

How do people like to be touched? Most women and men have similar preferences, with individual differences. Women, in one way or another, sooner or later, generally prefer the clitoris in manual stimulation, but again, most women like a man to gradually approach this very sensitive area. For

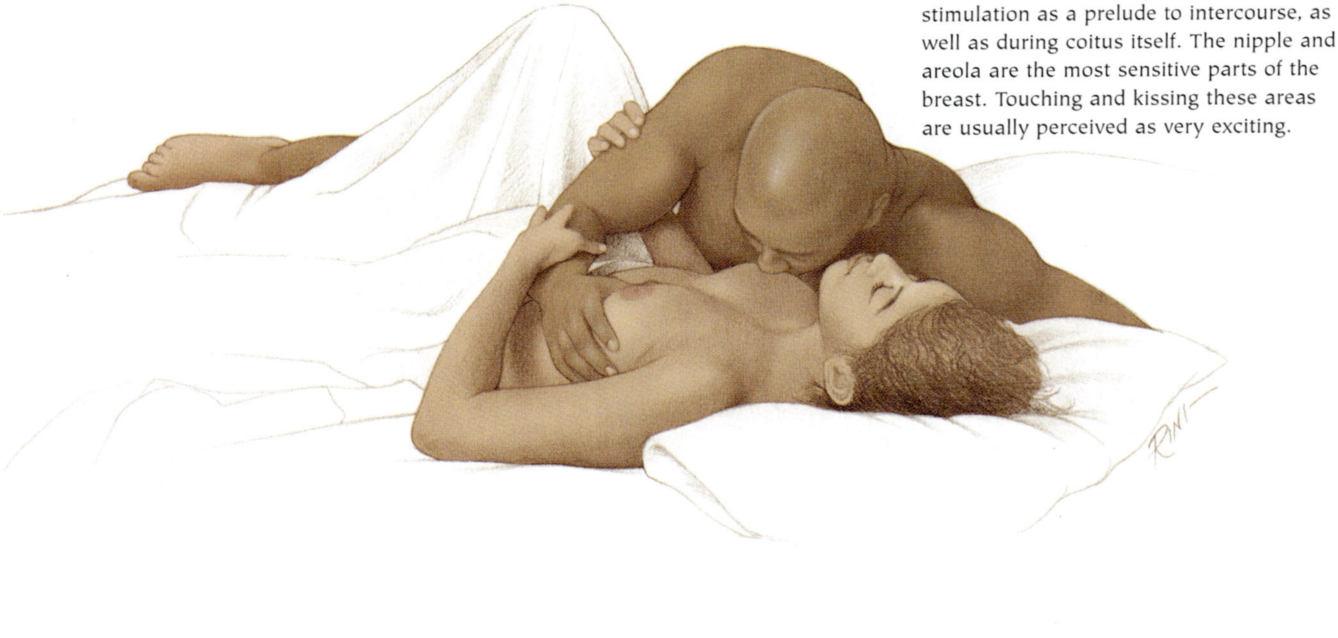

FIGURE 8-12   Most women enjoy breast stimulation as a prelude to intercourse, as well as during coitus itself. The nipple and areola are the most sensitive parts of the breast. Touching and kissing these areas are usually perceived as very exciting.

example, many women like to have the mons veneris rubbed or pressed, then the labia majora stroked. Of course, as women become progressively more aroused, vaginal lubrication increases, making the labia minora softer and more slippery. This usually makes it easier and more comfortable for a man to insert a finger into the vaginal opening, and many women report that they find this highly arousing and enjoyable. Going slowly and being gentle is very important. In their sex therapy techniques, Masters and Johnson (Personal Communication, 1978) described a "teasing technique" that includes manually stimulating a woman's external genitalia. The man caresses lightly the entire area surrounding the opening to a woman's vagina and then lightly moves his hand to her abdomen and continues this stroking, perhaps circling her navel. He continues to move his hand upward along her body and lightly touches her breasts, stimulating her nipples. Finally, he moves his hand back down toward her abdomen, and then further to her vaginal area, always being very delicate in his touching. Along with tender kissing and whispered expressions of affection, the teasing technique is often perceived by women to be keenly arousing.

Men too have differences and similarities in the way they prefer to be touched erotically. The glans of the penis and the frenum on its underside are the most sensitive areas of the genitalia. The area immediately surrounding the external urethral meatus is also especially sensitive. Men often take a few minutes to attain an erection, usually longer at mid-life or later. The time a man takes to become erect varies much, as does the gradual hardening of his penis. Some are very firm and others less so. All of these variations are common. Before erection occurs, men generally prefer gentler touching and stroking, especially along the shaft of the penis. The glans and frenum become more sensitive as arousal progresses, and stimulation of these areas is preferred after a few minutes of foreplay. As excitement builds, firmer stroking of the shaft of the penis is often enjoyed, beginning slowly and becoming progressively more rapid. The man should be aware of and communicate his changing level of sexual excitement; otherwise, he may ejaculate during vigorous penile stroking rather than penetrating his partner for sexual intercourse. Men would do well to communicate verbally or by some signal when ejaculation seems imminent. If the couple is planning to have intercourse, they often should proceed slowly so that the man does not feel the urge to ejaculate soon after entering his partner but can engage in mutual prolonged pelvic thrusting, offering both time to enjoy penetration.

While the shaft, glans, and frenum are the most commonly stimulated areas, some men say that gentle rubbing and squeezing of the scrotum are also keenly erotic. The testicles can be extremely sensitive to pressure, however, and care is needed not to press or squeeze them too much. Another area extremely sensitive to gentle touching and stroking is the skin between the back of the scrotum and the anus. There is a thin crease in the skin along this area, and touching it is usually perceived as highly enjoyable. This area is also highly sensitive in women. Because bacteria are commonly found around the

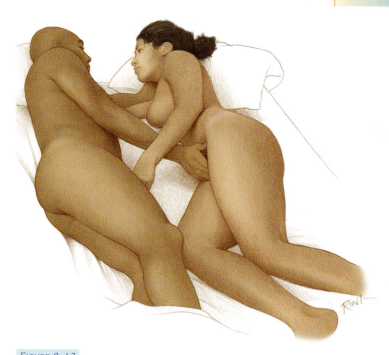

Figure 8-13 Mutual genital stimulation is a common foreplay behavior. Tactile stimulation can be very arousing and allows one's partner to feel an erection develop, as well as the occurrence of vaginal lubrication.

anus, it is important for this area to be clean, as discussed later. Women with long or sharp fingernails should be careful not to cause their partner any discomfort.

In addition to being touched by their partners, many people like to touch themselves during foreplay at the same time. Some people guide their partner's hand, and others supplement their partner's efforts. Don't feel bad if your partner stimulates themself while you are touching them. If they feel comfortable enough to manually stimulate themself while you are touching them, they must feel safe with you and fully exploring their own eroticism with you.

Kissing

Kissing involves questions of etiquette, expectation, and intention. Many people have implicit "rules" about kissing, although the "rule book" is not always clear. For example, many feel a first kiss is an important statement of affection that may reflect an intention to pursue the relationship further. Some also assume it is up to the male to make the first move, although this old custom is certainly changing. If a male attempts to kiss a female and she refuses, this may mean that she's not interested in him or just not interested right now. Acceptance of a first kiss implies that another will also be accepted. Kissing is a wonderful example of a complex human behavior that is both important and enigmatic.

In most cultures, people showing affection put their faces, lips, noses, or cheeks close together (Suggs & Miracle, 1993). This is true of women and men, women and women, and men and men. Cross-cultural differences in how people put their faces close together are intriguing variations on this compellingly consistent human behavior. There may be several reasons why variations on kissing evolved in different countries. First, kissing involves two people putting the most expressive areas of their bodies close together. Verbal communication, facial expressions, and the shared warmth of a hug and kiss communicate much. Second, remember that our mouths are a primary erogenous zone and have an enormous number of free nerve endings close to the surface of the skin: two people putting their mouths together are mutually stimulating an incredibly tender part of their bodies. The *reciprocal* nature of kissing is also important: we are stimulated at the same time that we stimulate another.

Kissing can convey both affection and intense eroticism. There is a delicate dance about how a kiss is offered and received. Kissing almost always occurs before sexual intercourse, except, interestingly, among prostitutes. A prostitute may engage in vaginal intercourse, oral-genital stimulation, or anal stimulation and intercourse but refuse to kiss a client. Kissing is very personal and perhaps involves a level of sharing and self-disclosure even more intimate than other erotic or genital behaviors. Some people think of kissing as a prelude to more serious sexual behaviors; others keep their lips locked in a kiss throughout sexual intercourse. Kissing is both an expression of affection and a technique of erotic stimulation. Kissing may be done with the lips only or may also involve inserting the tongue shallow or deep into the other's mouth. The terms "erotic kiss" or "French kiss" are often used to describe "deep kissing."

Because of traditional sex role learning, men are often encouraged to pursue their own sexual "style" and assume that women will follow their lead. Men were supposed to be sexually active and women reactive. Often women wait for a man to make the first move toward kissing. Implied in this unequal situation is an implicit understanding that women will gradually acquiesce to men who pursue kissing them. Margolin (1990) studied how undergraduate students respond to vignettes depicting females and males forcing a kiss on an opposite sex acquaintance who indicates that she or he does not want to be kissed. Subjects were far more supportive of females who persisted in trying to kiss refusing men than they were of men who persisted trying to kiss refusing women. These respondents were less sympathetic towards the men who said they did not want to be kissed, who apparently did not match commonly held stereotypes of sexual assertiveness. Yet there is no psychological, social, or anthropological reason in these scenarios to suppose that either the men or the women would naturally be more reticent to be kissed.

In closing this section, we note that in virtually all cultures, women color their lips in some fashion or otherwise make them more conspicuous. Irrespective of their skin color, women often color their lips in such a way as to make them stand out from the rest of their face, highlighting an expressive primary erogenous zone. The woman's motives may be various, including feminine self-confidence or pride in one's appearance. This practice may also draw attention to a woman's

speaking and gain more attention from those listening. The message from lip coloring or decoration is open to discussion, however. Magazine advertisements for lipstick convey much more than simply pride in one's appearance. Many such ads explicitly associate their product with sexual receptivity and attractiveness. Such ads give the reader the distinct impression that women thus depicted are more than just "kissable."

ORAL STIMULATION

Oral-genital stimulation is one of the most discussed and debated forms of shared eroticism. Some people have great difficulty even imagining orally stimulating their partner's genitalia or having their own genitals stimulated orally, while others find oral sex an exciting and richly rewarding form of sexual expression. Again, intimate behaviors among consenting adults in private places should be at the discretion of the participants, although "authorities" have argued about the legality of oral-genital stimulation for a long time. In some states oral-genital sex is a felony, meaning that those who perform these behaviors can be fined and imprisoned. Some laws against oral sex include a prison sentence of one year. While such penalties are rarely inflicted on consenting adults, the continuing existence of such laws says something about our heritage of sexual conservatism and the timidity of local legislators to change the laws to reflect current customs and behaviors.

Oral-genital stimulation and kissing actually have a lot in common. Both are expressions of affection and highly effective erotic stimulation techniques, and both involve the contact of highly sensitive primary erogenous zones. Just as depictions of sexual intercourse are sprinkled throughout the historical record of ancient Eastern and Western civilizations, so too are representations of oral-genital stimulation. These behaviors are as ageless as the variety of intercourse positions and other forms of erotic expression.

If the person's genitals are clean, oral-genital stimulation cannot be objected to on sanitary grounds. Like other forms of erotic expression, oral-genital stimulation is complex and diversified.

Social Scripts and Oral Sex

Earlier we discussed how sexual scripts affect sexual perceptions and the expression of eroticism. A script is much like an implicit "mind set" that plays a role in determining how we evaluate our psychosocial environment and how we behave and feel about behaving as we do. Oral-genital sex is certainly affected by one's sexual scripts. There seem to have been some changes in attitudes toward oral sex in the United States, however, over the last century. Gagnon and Simon (1987) examined changes in sexual scripts regarding oral sex in people born between 1928 and 1943 and those born between 1963 and 1967. The earlier data come from research carried out by the Kinsey Institute, published in Kinsey's *Sexual Behavior in the Human Male* (1948), and their more recent findings derive from interviews with over 1000 college students during the 1960s. Men in the older age group were far more likely to have

Research Highlight

USING A QUESTIONNAIRE TO STUDY ORAL SEX

Because of the sometimes controversial nature of oral sex and the fact that it is against the law in many states, it is difficult to learn how people view this intimate behavior. Andersen and Pollack (1994) developed a well-designed oral sex questionnaire that addressed how people think, feel, and behave with regard to cunnilingus and fellatio.

Andersen and Pollack administered their 52-item survey to male and female undergraduates at a large university on two occasions two weeks apart. Of the 336 participants, only 28 subjects had neither received nor performed oral sexual stimulation; these were then excluded from the study. The average age of these subjects was about 19 years. Subjects were asked to respond to each survey item on a scale of values ranging from positive to negative, evaluating each as "strongly agree," "agree," "neutral," "disagree," or "strongly disagree." Homosexuals were asked to respond to these items as if they were giving or receiving oral stimulation from a same sex partner. Following are some of the items that appeared on the questionnaire:

4. I enjoy performing oral sex because when I am performing oral sex I have complete control over my partner's responses.
5. I perform oral sex because of the pleasure it brings my partner.
11. I dislike performing oral sex because it is not a traditional form of sexual expression.
37. I don't enjoy receiving oral sex because I never achieve an orgasm.
42. When I want my partner to perform oral sex on me, I will physically guide his/her mouth to my genitals.
52. I enjoy receiving oral sex better than intercourse

—Andersen & Pollack, 1994, 132-133

These researchers found a very high test-retest consistency over the two-week interval between questionnaire administrations. Andersen and Pollack reported that there were seven general themes in their subjects' responses regarding feelings and behaviors associated with oral sex.

- **Performing oral sex.** These items dealt primarily with the enjoyment the person performing oral sex derived from the act.
- **Receiving oral sex.** These items concerned the personal sensual enjoyment the person receiving oral-genital stimulation derived from the act.
- **Orgasm.** These items concerned whether or how often the person receiving oral-genital stimulation had an orgasm during the act and how much they enjoyed and/or preferred this type of stimulation.
- **Partner's dislike.** These items dealt with the degree to which a person's partner liked or didn't like performing or receiving oral-genital stimulation and the impact of this preference on the person's overall sexual satisfaction in the relationship.
- **Persuasion.** These items concerned the degree to which a person felt they had to influence or persuade their partner to give or receive oral genital stimulation.
- **Control.** Feelings of being in control during sexual intimacy often play a big role in a person's overall sexual satisfaction, and this is one of the main themes that emerged from this research.
- **Traditional.** For some respondents, oral-genital sexual stimulation did not conform to a traditional view of sexual behavior and, therefore, was not considered fully appropriate or enjoyable.

As you can see, simply asking clear questions about oral-genital sexual stimulation can reveal a number of key themes that may motivate or inhibit an individual from this avenue of sexual sharing.

DR. RUTH'S TOP TEN FACTS ABOUT ORAL SEX

1. Many young people have the a misconception that oral sex is a good substitute for intercourse because it is safer. Although it certainly won't cause an unintended pregnancy, it does not prevent the transmission of disease. The likelihood of contracting a disease like AIDS seems lower than with intercourse, but it is not impossible, so it cannot be considered a safe form of sex. Fellatio performed on a man wearing a condom makes it as safe as intercourse with a condom, but holding a dental dam or piece of plastic wrap up to the vagina during cunnilingus to try to avoid contact with vaginal secretions doesn't add much protection.

2. While oral sex is much more common among young people today than in former generations, not every woman wishes to fulfill this common male fantasy. But as much as a man might desire fellatio, he should not try to pressure his partner into accommodating him.

3. Many women do not want to perform fellatio because they do not like the idea of having the man ejaculate into their mouth. Couples should discuss this, and if it bothers the woman, a man who promises not to ask for that particular ending to the act might be able to persuade his partner to perform oral sex.

4. Some men won't perform cunnilingus because they find female secretions distasteful (even with a dental dam). It is interesting to note that Buddhists believe female secretions to be energizing and harmonizing.

5. Whether myth or fact, some people believe that substances that enter a man's body affect the taste of his ejaculate. Eating red meat, smoking tobacco, and drinking coffee have been said to cause bad tastes, while eating celery or pineapple is said to improve the taste.

6. Whether it be a penis or vagina, cleanliness is often an issue for oral sex. Beginning foreplay in the shower or bath allows a concerned partner to personally attend to the cleanliness of the targeted organ and may lead to a greater willingness for oral sex.

7. The attitude that fellatio is somehow more "dirty" than intercourse permeates our society and is one reason some women are put off. Men should be careful about their attitude towards all types of sex and the language they use for all sexual acts. Women should similarly have this sensitivity with language and attitudes.

8. As men get older and lose their ability for psychogenic erections (without physical stimulation), they develop the same need for foreplay as women. Oral sex is a very good means to arouse a man, but if he has given only cursory attention to his wife's needs for foreplay in the past, she may not be as forthcoming with the attention that he now requires. As women age, diminished lubrication and delayed arousal are also common. Cunnilingus is a good way to apply a "natural" lubricant to the vulva.

9. While the sixty-nine position might seem an oral sex version of intercourse, since both partners are having their genitals stimulated at the same time, in fact many people find the attention they give to performing oral sex too distracting for them to fully enjoy receiving oral sex. For that reason, most couples who perform oral sex prefer for only one partner at a time to be on the receiving end.

10. While most states have removed the laws against sodomy and oral sex, in many states this activity is still against the law, though sometimes such laws do not apply to married couples. You can find out whether your state forbids this activity on the Internet (http://www. halcyon. com/elf/altsex/legal. html). Although I would never advise anyone to break laws, I certainly would advise you to maintain the utmost discretion if your state has banned oral sex.

had their early experiences with fellatio with prostitutes in brief superficial contacts than men in the younger group. Women and men in this older group had roughly equal rates of oral-genital contact with potential marriage partners. Among women and men born more recently, oral-genital contact was a much more frequent aspect of premarital sexual relations and was practiced about equally by both sexes. In both groups, oral sex was much more likely to be reported by women and men who already had sexual intercourse and was more frequently introduced by the man. Gagnon and Simon reviewed additional research published in the 1970s and 1980s and found another increase in the prevalence of oral sex in premarital sexual relationships during this time. It is interesting to note that the sexual freedom of the 1960s continued to expand, though more quietly, during the following two decades. Through the twentieth century oral sex became more established in the sexual scripts of American youth. While this research focused primarily on premarital sexual behavior, the authors noted that oral sex has also become a more common aspect of marital sex as well.

Cunnilingus

The term **cunnilingus** refers to oral stimulation, by either a man or another woman, of a woman's external genitalia and the opening to her vagina. Many women report they find cunnilingus a very effective form of erotic stimulation and often say it is more gentle than penile penetration of the vagina. During sexual intercourse the delicate and sensitive structures of the external genitalia are not usually stimulated directly, gently, or patiently, and the clitoris is not stimulated directly at all. Oral stimulation involves directly licking, sucking, or gently biting these responsive structures (Fig. 8-14). Additionally, and importantly, while a man is orally stimulating his female partner he generally is not approaching his own orgasm and, therefore, feels less urgency. Cunnilingus is a very "giving"

form of sexual intimacy for this reason. Many women need to fully trust their partner before they can feel comfortable with cunnilingus, yet once they do, they often find that they can have orgasms more easily through oral stimulation than during sexual intercourse. Many report frequent multiple orgasms. The clitoris is the preferred focal point of oral stimulation, especially with light or moderately firm licking. Many women also enjoy their partner inserting a finger into their vaginas during oral stimulation, especially touching the anterior wall where the Grafenberg area is located.

Fellatio

Fellatio is oral stimulation of the penis, and sometimes the scrotum, by either a woman or a man (Fig. 8-15). Most men report they find fellatio highly arousing and erotic either as a prelude to intercourse or instead of intercourse. Generally, men more frequently report enjoying cunnilingus than women report enjoying fellatio, although the reasons for this difference are unclear. Of course, there are many exceptions to these generalizations. Many individuals have never thought seriously about offering or receiving oral stimulation and are not attracted to these behaviors. However, some women who do not enjoy oral sex themselves *do* enjoy pleasing and stimulating their partner. Like cunnilingus, fellatio can be a very "giving" form of sexual intimacy. Many men report that they enjoy their partner nibbling or sucking the glans of the penis while stroking the shaft in a milking motion. Others prefer more vigorous sucking while fully penetrating their partner's mouth and/or throat. Saliva is a highly effective lubricant for oral stimulation in both women and men and may also facilitate comfortable penile penetration when intercourse follows oral-genital stimulation.

Whether to swallow or spit out the semen is controversial for some. This is purely a matter of personal preference, however, and not as important as the nature of the relationship between partners.

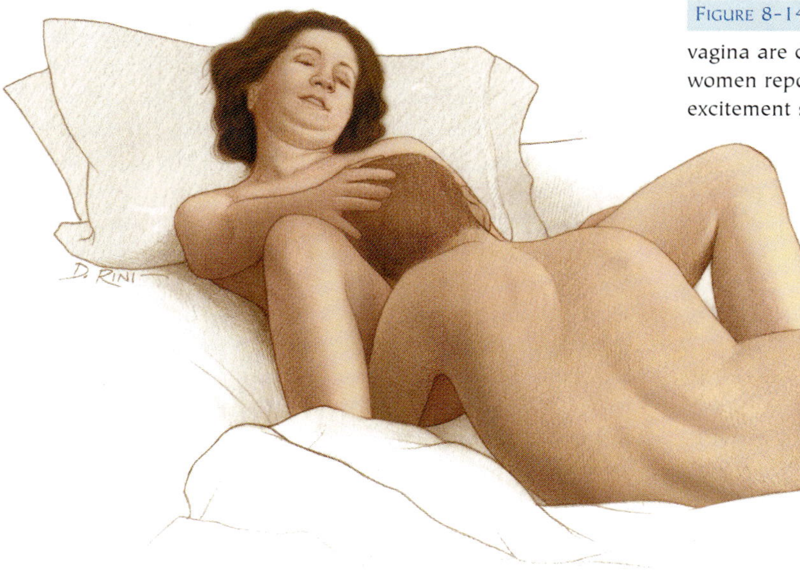

FIGURE 8-14 During cunnilingus, the clitoris and opening to the vagina are directly stimulated by a partner's mouth. Many women report that this is keenly arousing and enhances sexual excitement significantly.

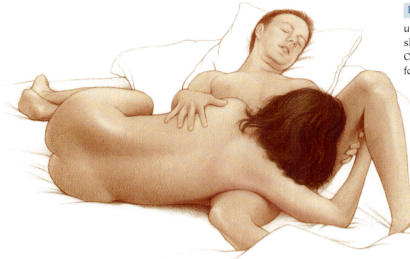

FIGURE 8-15 In fellatio, the glans of the penis is usually the focus of oral stimulation, although the shaft and frenulum are also extremely sensitive. Oral stimulation of the scrotum is very pleasurable for many men as well.

Mutual Oral-Genital Stimulation

Mutual oral-genital stimulation, colloquially known as "69" because of the configuration of two peoples' bodies engaged in this act, is for many a highly arousing and exciting form of sexual expression (Fig. 8-16). It offers two people simultaneous visual, tactile, olfactory, gustatory, and auditory elements of sexual stimulation. It may be a part of foreplay or engaged in for its own pleasures. When two people communicate their levels of sexual arousal, they can "synchronize" their arousal and climax simultaneously. Of course, not everyone enjoys this form of expression; we encourage couples to explore it or any form of sexual expressions only within a climate of psychological safety.

Oral-Anal Stimulation

Just as our mouths and genitalia are primary erogenous zones, so too is our anus. While oral-genital stimulation is very erotic for many people, oral-anal stimulation is similarly exciting for some also. Oral-anal stimulation is called **analingus,** but the colloquial term *rimming* is often used to describe putting one's tongue onto or inside of another person's anus. This is generally a form of unprotected sex because neither a condom nor a spermicide agent is used. It is especially important to be completely certain that your partner does not have an STD before engaging in this practice. We discuss this further in the chapter on sexually transmitted diseases and AIDS.

HETEROSEXUAL INTERCOURSE

Masturbation, mutual masturbation, touching and massaging, and oral-genital stimulation are all elements in a diversified and exciting sexual repertoire, although individual preferences vary widely. Such behaviors may be performed as foreplay or be enjoyed in their own right. Vaginal penetration is not the "be all and end all" of human sexuality. The technical term for sexual intercourse is **coitus,** derived from the Latin word for penis-in-the-vagina intercourse. For most people, vaginal penetration is the most common and preferred type of heterosexual sexual sharing. This section focuses on "heterosexual intercourse," and homosexual lovemaking is discussed more fully in the following chapter.

Sexual Scripts and Intercourse

Our sexual scripts often create in our minds various expectations about who should do what and to whom during intercourse. Because these scripts are part of our notions of "normal" sex, it is often difficult even to think of departing from these "rules" and anticipations. A major theme in this chapter, however, is that lovemaking is a highly personal and creative endeavor, and inflexible ways of thinking of sexual intimacy may stifle common human motives to explore new avenues of erotic sharing. For example, traditional male socialization often gives men the idea that they should "take the lead" during lovemaking, decide when and where the couple will have intercourse, choose foreplay activities, decide when it is time to move to vaginal penetration, choose which position to use, and with orgasm and ejaculation more or less determine when intercourse will be over. He may also see it as his prerogative to decide whether to share physical intimacy after intercourse is over. This, of course, is a very self-centered way of thinking about sexual intimacy. Implicit in this "traditional" way of thinking about sexual intercourse is the assumption that men are sexual teachers and women are sexual learners, and the teacher is always right. Because of the long-held double standard in our society, this way of thinking may have accurately described gender roles for most people in the past, but this outlook has rapidly become out of date and may interfere with candid sexual communication and a sense of shared enjoyment today.

Women and men can always teach things to one another and learn things from one another in all facets of their relationship, even though some men may feel threatened if their partner seems to know more about sex than he does. In the following sections are depictions of many different intercourse positions, some involving men playing a more active role and others with women playing a more active role. Our own philosophy is very simple: take turns! Being pushy in many areas of life is rarely received well by those around us, and sexuality is no different. The term *sexual assertiveness* describes this general attitude but can also refer to how otherwise polite and cautious behaviors are *perceived* by others. Sexual assertiveness is very much in the mind of the beholder. While it is important to be candid when communicating one's sexual feelings and intentions, this approach should include tact and tenderness.

Some perceive sexual intercourse in a serious way while others enjoy a more playful approach. For example, there are wide differences of opinion about talking during sex. Those who believe that intercourse is a somber or even spiritual experience might hesitate to talk easily about how they are feeling, their growing excitement, or to shout or make squeals of joy and pleasure. On the other hand, those who are comfortable and less somber likely find it easier to verbally share their feelings or cry, howl, roar, and cheer when having wonderful sensations. Everyone is unique, of course, and there is no one "best" approach to verbal communication during intercourse. Keep in mind that most people like to be told when they are doing a good job, however, and sex is no different. Talking during sex allows two people to tell one another exactly how they like to be touched and how vigorously. Talking lets them tell one another how good they are making each other feel, and of course this can be very reinforcing. While we respect a couple's desire to remain quiet during sex, verbal communication during intercourse can be a rich part of the intimate experience.

Another issue often arises about sexual intercourse: lights on or lights off? Again, people differ. Some feel that darkness affords a sense of safety and security or may protect one from looking shameful or embarrassed. In the dark, you don't worry about eye contact, and your partner can't tell if you are looking away in anxious self-consciousness. Others are aroused by mutual eye contact and are further stimulated by seeing their partner's sexual excitement revealed in facial expressions. This issue also involves how one feels about one's body. For someone with problems with body image, darkness offers security and safety. However, someone with a sense of pride in their physical appearance may be more willing to reveal private areas and take pleasure in one's partner's obvious enjoyment of their body. Many couples like something in between: a soft light, specifically candle light, during sexual sharing. Of course, it is untrue that most people have sexual intercourse only at night.

Different Ways to Have Sexual Intercourse

Sex is like music: there are many variations on different themes. Although a number of common positions are used for sexual intercourse, there are also many variations on those basic themes. The following sections describe common intercourse positions along with some common variations.

THE MAN-ON-TOP POSITION

The man-on-top position has also been called the "male superior" position, but that phrase has been interpreted by some to imply something "better" about this position for men because the man is above his female partner. Because of the hint of subjugation in that phrase, we find it somewhat unacceptable. In this position, a man is lying face-to-face on top of his female partner (Fig. 8-17). There are several common variations. The man might be lying flat on top of his partner with her legs spread apart but positioned flat on the surface. Or he might be kneeling over her with her legs elevated and wrapped around his hips, back, or shoulders (Fig. 8-18). This position offers men much freedom of movement, especially for vigorous pelvic thrusting. In some variations of the man-on-top position the man expends some effort supporting his body, however, especially if he is not lying flat on top of his partner. This

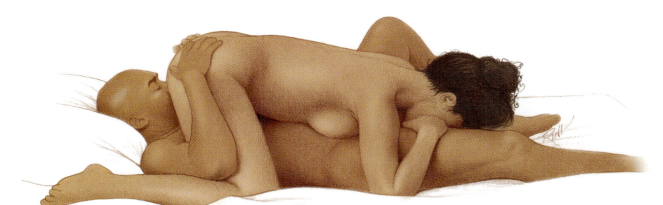

FIGURE 8-16 Simultaneous oral-genital stimulation, also called "69," offers both partners many highly arousing sensations and is frequently enjoyed before intercourse, or sometimes instead of intercourse.

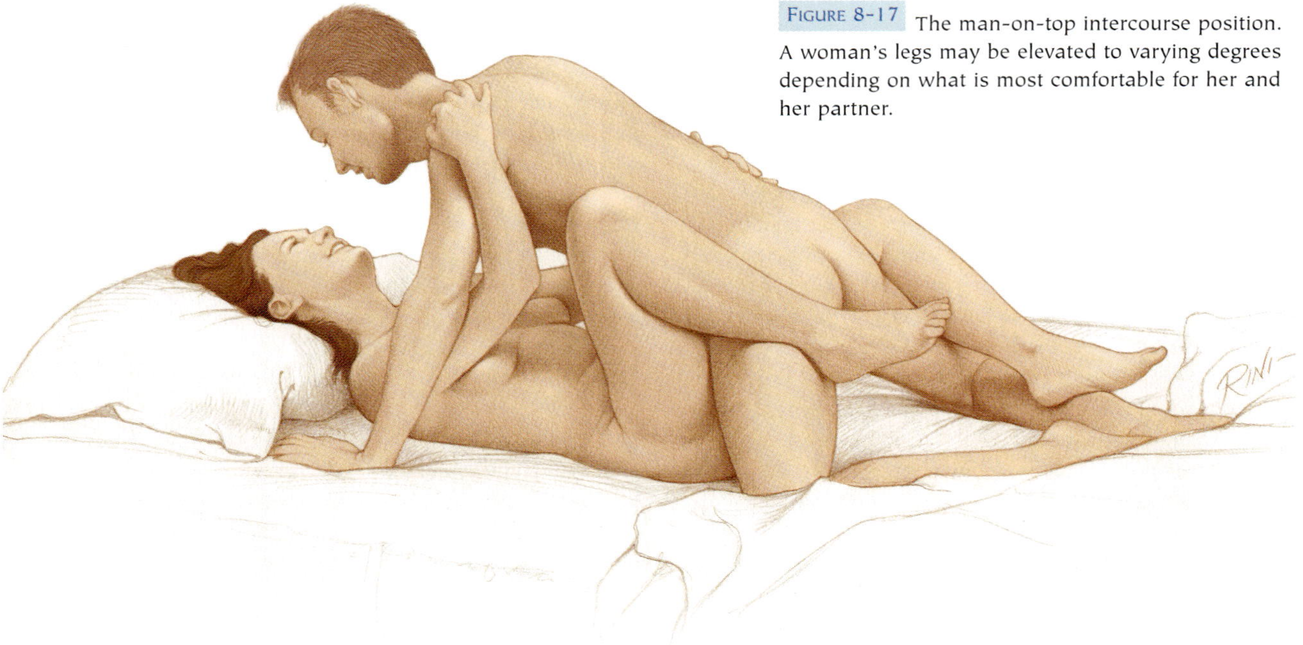

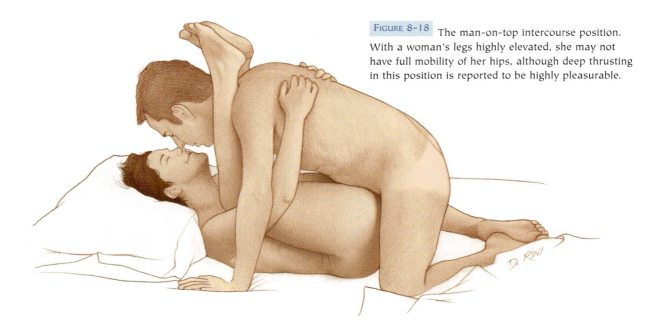

FIGURE 8-17 The man-on-top intercourse position. A woman's legs may be elevated to varying degrees depending on what is most comfortable for her and her partner.

muscular tension may make it difficult for some men to control or delay their ejaculation, as we will discuss in a later chapter on sexual dysfunctions.

For couples who like to kiss and look into one another's eyes during intercourse, this is a good position. The woman has the freedom to caress her partner's chest, buttocks, or other body areas during intercourse. If the man is using his arms and hands to hold himself up, however, he is not free to touch his partner while engaging in pelvic thrusting. This position also has the potential disadvantage of restricting female pelvic movements and restricts overall mobility for the woman. A woman lying on her back under her male partner is free, however, to use her hands to stimulate her clitoris during penile penetration of her vagina, or she may similarly stimulate her

FIGURE 8-18 The man-on-top intercourse position. With a woman's legs highly elevated, she may not have full mobility of her hips, although deep thrusting in this position is reported to be highly pleasurable.

Other Countries, Cultures, and Customs

AN HISTORICAL APPROACH TO THE "NATURALNESS" OF MAN-ON-TOP INTERCOURSE

As noted above, historical or religious traditions sometimes support the idea that the man-on-top position is the only appropriate or desirable way to have sexual intercourse. Any other position might give an "unnatural superiority" to the woman and thus alter her traditionally passive role. Clearly this is a male-dominated, paternalistic perspective likely to encounter strident dissent from any clear-thinking contemporary woman. Yet these supposedly "authoritative" pronouncements about how to have sexual intercourse are culturally interesting.

The man-on-top position is often called the *missionary position,* because this style of having intercourse seemed unusual to Pacific islanders who invented the expression to describe the behavior of religiously motivated Europeans having sex with island women. These islanders preferred the woman-on-top position and the rear-entry position and found the man-on-top alternative noteworthy and unusual (Reinisch, 1990). The term "missionary position" is still used frequently today. The authority attributed to men of the church was apparently manifest in this intercourse position, in which females were "subjugated" by their partners and positioned "beneath" them, as well as the islanders who were converted to this way of thinking.

Historically, a number of pronouncements have been made about the appropriateness of the man-on-top position. In his 1937 book, *The Sexual Life of Our Time,* Dr. Iwan Bloch is unequivocal about the "higher" or "human" aspects of this intercourse position:

> Passing to the consideration of the posture adopted during intercourse, we find in civilized man, who in this respect is far removed from animals, the normal position during coitus is front to front, the woman lying on her back with her lower extremities widely separated, and the knee and hip joints semiflexed; the man lies on her, with his thighs between hers, supporting himself on hands or elbows—or often the two unite their lips in a kiss. . . . The adoption of this position in coitus undoubtedly ensued in the human race upon the evolution of the upright posture. It is the natural, instinctive position of civilized man, who in this respect also manifests an advance on the lower animals. (p. 51)

Overall, masculine, paternalistic, and cultural influences all contributed to this being the "preferred" intercourse position in our culture. Attempting to justify this preference on the basis of the evolution of the human race is an additional interesting nuance.

---

partner's scrotum during penetration. Many researchers believe that the man-on-top position is best for enhancing the chances of conception. It may not be a comfortable position for either when the woman is pregnant. When youngsters and adolescents first learn about sexual intercourse, the man-on-top position is generally presented to them (by parents, peers, or in sex-education classes) as the prototypical form of having sex.

THE WOMAN-ON-TOP POSITION

In the woman-on-top position a woman sits or squats on her partner who is lying on his back. Her knees might be bent with the tops of her feet in contact with the bed, or in a variation of this position the soles of her feet are in contact with the bed as she squats over her partner's penis (Fig. 8-19). She may sit up or lean forward. Both partners can see each other's face and up-

per body as in the man-on-top position, but in the woman-on-top position both partners have their hands free to touch and caress one another. In some variations of this position, the woman lies flat on top of her partner with both of their legs straight and touching.

Many women enjoy the woman-on-top position because they have a greater range of motion and can more easily control the angle, rate, and depth of penile penetration. For example, she can move slowly and facilitate deep penetration or quickly with more shallow penetration. As in the man-on-top position, partners can easily kiss one another. In the woman-on-top position, she or her partner can also directly stimulate her clitoris manually during pelvic thrusting. He may also be able to easily caress or rub her buttocks and/or anus in this position, which many women find keenly erotic. Because the

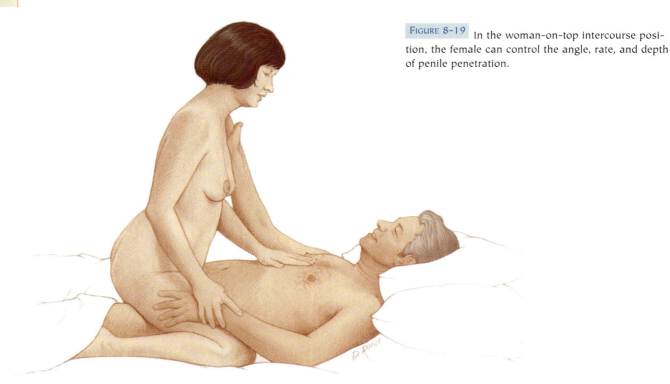

FIGURE 8-19 In the woman-on-top intercourse position, the female can control the angle, rate, and depth of penile penetration.

man does not experience as much muscular tension as in the man-on-top position, he can better control the timing of his orgasm and ejaculation. Just as there is nothing inherently "superior" about the man-on-top position for men, there is nothing inherently "superior" about the woman-on-top position for women. However, some men who are socialized to believe that it is the man's place and prerogative to be on top may feel uncomfortable being on the bottom and may feel unacceptably passive. Many people find it a good idea to take turns.

THE LATERAL-ENTRY POSITION

In the lateral-entry or side-to-side position, the couple lies on their sides facing one another (Fig. 8-20). Like other face-to-face positions, this gives a man and woman full visual access to one another and allows them to stimulate one another manually during vaginal penetration. Because both partners are lying on their sides, this position is a good one for couples during pregnancy. Because this position does not require as much energy or strength as other positions for sexual intercourse, it is also a good one during illness, disability, or convalescence. When two people desire a more relaxed, less vigorous style of lovemaking, the lateral-entry position is a good one. One of the reasons people report for having intercourse less frequently as they get older is simple fatigue. The lateral-entry position, because it is less taxing physically than other positions, is good in such situations.

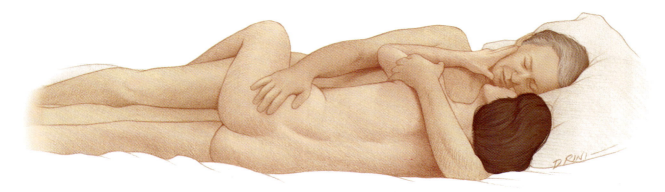

FIGURE 8-20 In the lateral-entry position, or side-to-side intercourse, neither partner supports their body weight. During pregnancy, illness, or convalescence this alignment is more comfortable and less strenuous than many other intercourse positions.

In addition to lateral-entry, face-to-face intercourse, a couple may also enjoy lateral-entry rear-entry intercourse while lying on their sides. In this variation of the lateral-entry position, a man lies behind his partner and penetrates her from behind while both are lying on their sides. This comfortable fit of two bodies is sometimes colloquially called "spooning" because of the image of two nested spoons. As discussed in a later chapter, the lateral-entry position is frequently recommended for couples experiencing sexual difficulties because it lessens muscular tension and allows more leisurely intercourse. Many couples find this position a little awkward, however, because it can restrict the full vigor of pelvic thrusting and full penile penetration is a bit difficult. Women who enjoy shallow penetration and rapid thrusting may find this position enjoyable.

REAR-ENTRY INTERCOURSE

Many couples report that rear-entry intercourse is extremely enjoyable and prefer this form of lovemaking to others; their reasons are not known, but many couples have this clear preference. In some respects, rear-entry intercourse is very different from the positions outlined previously. For example, a couple cannot see each others' faces during rear-entry penetration, and more stamina is required by both partners. The woman must support herself on her hands and knees while the man kneels behind her (Fig. 8-21). With neither partner lying on their back or side, this position can be a little more physically demanding than others. The man must reach around his partner's body to manually stimulate her clitoris or breasts, and this can be a little awkward. Because of what everyone has observed at one time or another, this position is sometimes called "doggy style" intercourse.

Rear-entry intercourse is unique in other ways too. For reasons that are poorly understood, men report more problems with ejaculatory control in this intercourse position than others, perhaps because of the muscular tension required to assume and maintain this posture and engage in pelvic thrusting simultaneously. Remember that during erection, the penis of many men is aligned at an upward angle, and because of this upward positioning the penis stimulates the anterior, or front, wall of a woman's vagina during penetration in the three positions discussed previously. However, when the woman kneels and the man penetrates her from behind, the upward angle of his erection selectively stimulates the *posterior,* or rear, wall of her vagina. Many women recognize the difference and find it highly arousing and pleasurable. In rear-entry intercourse, with coordinated movements during pelvic thrusting, both the woman and the man can engage in full, vigorous movements during each penile thrust, resulting in hard, deep thrusts (Fig. 8-22).

Rear-entry intercourse is also comfortable for obese people. Because significant abdominal mass may interfere with face-to-face intercourse positions, this alternative allows a more satisfactory and efficient means of penile penetration while still allowing a significant measure of pelvic mobility. This is not, however, the only or even the preferred position for sexual intercourse among obese people.

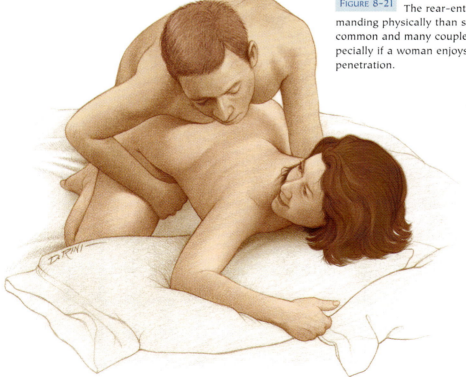

FIGURE 8-21 The rear-entry intercourse position is more demanding physically than some other positions, but it is very common and many couples especially enjoy this variation, especially if a woman enjoys having her clitoris massaged during penetration.

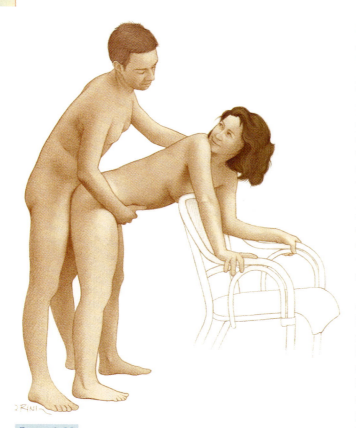

FIGURE 8-22 The rear-entry intercourse position is also often enjoyed with both partners standing.

One last comment on rear-entry intercourse; because male homosexual intercourse often involves anal penetration via a rear-entry position, it has been suggested that men who enjoy the rear-entry position for intercourse with women have latent, or hidden, homosexual tendencies. This is not true.

HETEROSEXUAL ANAL INTERCOURSE

Anal intercourse is a sexual variation, not a sexual deviation. It does not suggest a person or couple has any psychological problems or disorders. It is estimated that about one-third of women and men have tried anal penetration at least once, but the percentage of those who enjoy this sexual alternative regularly is not known. In one recent random telephone survey of heterosexuals in California (Erickson, Bastani, Maxwell, Marcus, Capell, & Yan, 1995), responses from over 2,000 women and over 1,500 men revealed that 8% of the men and 6% of the women reported having anal intercourse from one to five times each month in the year before the poll. If the woman has lost much of her vaginal muscular tone through repeated childbearing, anal intercourse can be a pleasurable alternative, especially for the male partner. Additionally, some couples who wish to avoid sexual intercourse during menstruation explore anal penetration at this time.

Remember that the anus is a primary erogenous zone; it contains a dense accumulation of free nerve endings and is highly sensitive. But unlike the vagina, the anus and internal membranes of the rectum do not produce secretions that lubricate this area and thereby make penetration more comfortable. Patient massage, manipulation, and fingering of the anus is often perceived to be highly pleasurable by many women, and slow penile penetration is more comfortable using a non-petroleum based sterile lubricant. Women who enjoy anal penetration often report that they prefer to slowly "back up" onto their partner's penis instead of passively receiving his thrusts (Fig. 8-23). Women often report that they have strong orgasms of long duration during anal intercourse.

Because bacteria normally inhabit the rectum, it is important for the man to not penetrate his partner vaginally after entering her anally, because this practice can cause a bad vaginal infection. If a couple wishes to have penis-in-the-vagina intercourse after anal penetration, it is very important for the man to wash his penis thoroughly with soap and water. Better yet, the man can use a condom during anal penetration

FIGURE 8-23 In heterosexual anal intercourse, slow penetration is very important. The use of a condom is generally recommended.

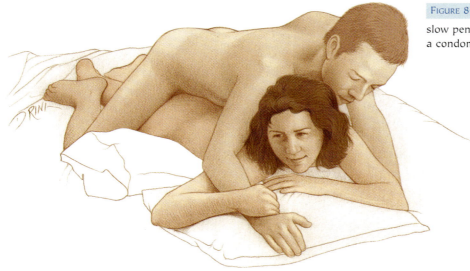

and simply remove it before vaginal penetration. Either way, it is important to keep rectal bacteria out of the vagina. The rectum can also contain the virus that causes hepatitis, another concern for couples exploring anal intimacy.

The AIDS virus also can be transmitted by anal intercourse. As discussed later in the chapter on sexually transmitted diseases, HIV is often found in a number of body secretions, most notably semen and vaginal secretions. During anal intercourse the delicate membranes of the rectum are sometimes slightly torn. Semen carrying the AIDS virus may, therefore, come into direct contact with the partner's blood stream, transmitting the virus from the man to the woman. Before exploring anal eroticism everyone should learn their partner's HIV status first. Just as using condoms is important in vaginal intercourse, this is also very important in anal intercourse.

SWITCHING POSITIONS DURING INTERCOURSE
Many people enjoy experimenting with more than one position during sexual intercourse, a simple way to introduce variety and reciprocity into physical intimacy. Switching positions during intercourse also helps avoid monotony that may come from too much consistency and predictability. Sexual etiquette is important in these maneuvers so that it does not seem that one partner is "instructing" or "directing" the other, thereby relegating that person to a more passive role than she or he might enjoy. In a good relationship both partners can feel safe and comfortable initiating novelty, and a tactful, tender approach is always appropriate. Changing positions during intercourse is easier if the two people are comfortable talking while having sex. Politeness and patience go a long way in reassuring one's partner that you aren't interested in a wrestling match. Changing positions can be spontaneous, not choreographed or planned, and comfortably informal. As with most aspects of shared sexuality, it never hurts to talk things over beforehand.

Psychosocial Aspects of Heterosexual Intercourse
Since this text takes a psychosocial approach to the study of human sexuality, we want also to look at this dimension of sexual intercourse. There are many cultural and societal aspects to this topic in addition to the technical and clinical elements. Although intercourse is an intense physical experience, women and men grow up in a culture, are educated in a society, and develop ideas about sex, women, and men throughout their lives. Culture thus has a significant impact on intercourse. Surveys of college students in the United States reveal that males are more open to premarital intercourse and oral sex than females, especially when they are not involved in a committed relationship (Wilson & Medora, 1990), but this generalization of course does not apply to all people all the time. How people feel about sexual behaviors has a lot to do with their overall perceptions about their genitalia and the relationship between their self-esteem and body image. One who is uncomfortable or feels shameful about genital sensations and pleasures is not likely to feel at ease in a variety of sexual situations. On the other hand, one who is "at home" with their body and fully enjoys the pleasures derived from genital stimulation is far more likely to enjoy expressions of interpersonal physical intimacy. This is exactly what Reinholtz and Muehlenhard (1995) found in a sample of 160 male and 160 female undergraduates. Students who reported more positive and fewer negative perceptions associated with genital stimulation were highly likely to engage in sexual activity, in particular oral-genital stimulation. These researchers reported that overall, men had somewhat more positive perceptions of their genitals and their partner's genitals than did the women in their sample. This is a simple but significant finding: People who like the feelings they get during genital stimulation are more likely to engage in a variety of sexual behaviors in which their genitals will be stimulated. This is perhaps all the more significant because human beings do not always behave in ways congruent with their feelings.

Anonymous questionnaire data have taught us much about how many young Americans explore various sexual behaviors and the interpersonal contexts in which those behaviors occur. Darling and Davidson (1986) explored some interesting and surprising things about male and female perspectives on sexual satisfaction in a large sample of university students. Among the respondents who were sexually active at the time of the survey, 67% of the males reported that they were "psychologically satisfied" after their first sexual encounter, while 28% of the female subjects reported similar feelings of fulfillment. When these individuals were asked about their *current* level of sexual enjoyment, almost 81% of the men reported a high degree of satisfaction while only about 28% of the women reported that they found sexual relations rewarding and enjoyable. Among the reasons men reported for discontent with the sexual aspect of their lives, the following stood out: too few opportunities to have sexual intercourse, a lack of an opportunity to have sexual relations with a variety of partners, and not enough opportunity to enjoy oral-genital stimulation. Discontents among the women were different: their partners did not attentively and effectively stimulate their breasts, intercourse was often uncomfortable, and some felt guilty, apprehensive, and fearful about having sex. These data suggest that the sexual experiences of young women and men may involve quite different feelings. This is important because these early feelings are the foundation on which later sexual experiences occur. If such a large discrepancy exists between women and men in their early adult years, what factors, if any, contribute to more similar feelings of sexual enjoyment as they get older? We will discuss this issue further in Chapter 13.

People usually report that they find orgasm to be one of the most pleasurable aspects of an intimate encounter. But people not only enjoy having their own orgasms—they want their partners to have orgasms too, and many feel that intercourse isn't entirely satisfactory unless their partner is aroused and responsive. Faking an orgasm gives one's partner the impression that they have been fully responsive when perhaps they have not. Because many people are performance oriented in sexual behavior, feeling that we have fully satisfied our partner can be very important. While both women and men can pretend to

DR. RUTH'S TOP TEN FACTS ABOUT SEXUAL INTERCOURSE

1. Some women naturally lubricate more than others. If intercourse is anticipated to last a while, then it is a good idea to have some lubricant handy because a woman's natural lubrication can dry up after a while and intercourse can become a painful, rather than pleasurable, experience.

2. It doesn't really matter who puts the penis inside of the vagina, as long as the woman is ready to receive it. If the man has trouble finding the right path, however, then the woman should certainly lend a helping hand.

3. If a man is not sure what type of thrusting a woman likes, then he should let her go on top. He can then note the types of motions she makes and be able to please her more when he's the one in control.

4. Not all intercourse noises come from the partner's vocal chords. Sometimes air and liquid inside the vagina can make various sounds, including a sound like the passing of gas. Rather than be quietly embarrassed by such sounds, admit them openly and share a laugh about them.

5. Placing a pillow underneath the woman's behind changes the angle of entry, which may make penetration easier, particularly if it is her first time. It also alters the sensations she feels and might make it easier for her to have an orgasm during intercourse. Remember that many women do not receive enough stimulation to their clitoris from intercourse alone to achieve orgasm.

6. Just because one partner isn't interested in sex doesn't mean that sex can't take place. There's nothing wrong with satisfying your partner without having an orgasm—as long as the person giving the orgasm doesn't feel pressured into it and they are content with the frequency of lovemaking in which they are sexually satisfied.

7. While many people desire simultaneous orgasms during intercourse, a couple shouldn't feel disappointed if this doesn't happen when they make love. It's more important that both partners derive satisfaction from the overall sexual experience than feel frustrated for not achieving this one feat.

8. While intercourse should not be rushed, so that both partners fully enjoy each other, there is nothing wrong with an occasional quickie. Sometimes making love within a short time frame, for example while changing clothes to go out to dinner, can be a very intense and satisfying experience.

9. One of the most important aspects of intercourse is what happens afterwards. Women take longer than men to become aroused, and they also take longer to come down from that plateau of arousal. If the process is a warm, loving one, their overall enjoyment is much greater. Consider the afterplay of one lovemaking session as the beginning of foreplay of the next.

10. Some people are bothered by the messiness of intercourse. Rather than cleaning up after lovemaking, try being proactive by placing a towel under you and another by the bed with which to wipe yourselves off. This way you can relax longer to enjoy the benefits of afterplay.

Other Countries, Cultures, and Customs

SEXUAL DIVERSITY IN FRANCE

The diversity of peoples' sexual repertoires has long received the attention of sex researchers. Since Kinsey's publications, investigators have been interested in the nature and variety of human intimate behaviors. The AIDS epidemic has given further impetus to the study of peoples' sexual behaviors as scientists sought to isolate potential high-risk activities. Messiah, Blin, and Fiche (1995) surveyed preferred sexual behaviors in a sample of almost 5000 respondents, age 18-69, in France. While their findings may not surprise you, the consistency of their data is compelling. Penis-in-the-vagina intercourse and erotic caressing were overwhelmingly represented in this sample while masturbation and anal penetration were rare. Somewhere between these two extremes were mutual masturbation and oral-genital stimulation. They found a reciprocity in these sexual behaviors; if one partner was inclined to provide one type of sexual stimulation, their partner was similarly disposed to return the favor. A limited number of sexual behaviors accounted for the vast majority of sexual interactions, and younger respondents were more likely to have more diversified sexual repertoires than their older counterparts.

have an orgasm, women do so more frequently, perhaps to validate the sexual skill and stamina of their partners (Janus & Janus, 1993). Whether most men's egos are really so fragile that they cannot deal with their partners not having an orgasm is a subject that might provoke lively speculation. Although there is little in the literature about faking orgasms, one report is interesting. Wiederman (1997) found that in a survey of 161 young women, over half had at one time or another pretended to have an orgasm while having sexual intercourse. These women generally perceived themselves as attractive and had more sexual experience (number of intercourse partners, oral-genital sexual experiences, intercourse at an early age) than those women who did not report feigning orgasms. The psychosocial context in which intercourse occurs includes the importance individuals attribute to their partner's responsiveness.

Because people in different life circumstances have multiple sexual partners, researchers have wondered whether a woman or man with multiple partners engages in the same or similar sexual behaviors with all their partners. This issue was addressed by Messiah and Pelletier (1996) in a sample of over 1500 heterosexuals, aged 18 to 69, who reported having sex with multiple partners. Most of their subjects' sexual repertoire was similar with all their partners. Vaginal penetration, body caressing, mutual masturbation, and oral-genital stimulation were all very common, regardless of which partner they were with. Masturbating oneself and anal penetration were rare among multiple partners. These researchers reported, however, that non-intercourse erotic touching and pleasuring and oral stimulation were reported more with non-regular partners. Women were less likely than men to report consistent condom usage while being intimate with multiple partners.

CONCLUSION

This chapter has presented much information about expressions of eroticism and physical intimacy to expand your knowledge base about the nature and diversity of sexual expression. We believe that a thorough and systematic examination of these "basics" is valuable. Understanding this material should enhance one's personal sexual etiquette, communication skills, and sharing of sexual pleasure.

Although this chapter has focused on heterosexual eroticism and intercourse, we are not implying that gays and lesbians are all that different. The next chapter deals specifically with homosexuality and the sexual behaviors of this very sizable group of people. You will soon see that the similarities between heterosexuals and homosexuals are more numerous and interesting than their differences.

Learning Activities

1. Speculate on why each of the following people might choose partial celibacy as a temporary lifestyle:
   - a seventeen-year-old high school student
   - a senior in college who had been involved in several monogamous sexual relationships over the last few years
   - a recently divorced woman who is head of a single-parent household
   - a man in his mid-50s whose wife has just passed away
2. Since Kinsey first published his surveys on sexual behavior in the late 1940s and early 1950s, couples have reported a

marked increase in the frequency and prevalence of oral-genital stimulation. Speculate on why this has occurred.

3. What nonmedical factors might discourage heterosexuals from exploring anal stimulation or penetration?

4. Some women believe that the man-on-top intercourse position is a symbolic manifestation of their historically submissive role in male-dominated societies. What do you think about this idea?

5. For some people, sex is not an important aspect of their relationship with another person and simply does not carry the urgency or priority as for others. Speculate on why a person might feel this way.

6. Clergy who participate in sexual intimacy with members of their congregation are apparently violating the spirit, if not the letter, of a confidential, helping relationship. This is also true of psychologists, teachers, social workers, and others. Many feel that they should be dismissed from their positions and prosecuted for sexual harassment. What do you think?

7. Many sexual interactions have certain things in common. In these interactions communication between the partners may involve **asking, teaching,** or **telling.** For example:

Asking: "What do you like?"
              "What would you like me to do for you?"
              "Do you find this uncomfortable?"
              "Would you rather I not do that?"

Teaching: "Watch how I do this, and then maybe you can try it."
              "If you do that a little more vigorously I think I would enjoy it more."
              "You might be going a bit too fast for me; try slowing down a little."

Telling: "Please don't do that; it makes me feel a little uncomfortable."
              "I enjoy that, but please be a little more gentle."
              "I'm not ready for that just yet."

What would you ask, teach, or tell in the following circumstances?

a. You have just had a sexual interaction you thought you would very much enjoy. But you feel disappointed and frustrated, and obviously were unresponsive.

b. You have begun a sexual encounter with someone you have been intimate with for a long time. You would like to be orally stimulated. You're not sure how to ask for this kind of stimulation. Does this seem to you a little like "begging?"

c. You find that having the lights on during sex is very exciting for you, but your partner consistently wants to have them off.

d. Your partner begins to relate to you a sexual fantasy he has found highly arousing, but you are shocked by its aggressive, egocentric quality.

e. As you perceive your partner's level of arousal building, her words shock you and seem coarse and obscene.

9. Speculate on the reasons a couple might decide to make a videotape of themselves having intercourse. Having made the tape, how might they incorporate it into their sexual lifestyle?

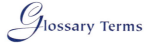

Key Concepts

- Sex, gender, and gender identity are all related to the object of our sexual feelings and our preferences in intimate behaviors.
- Acceptable and appropriate sexual behaviors maintain the privacy of those involved and do not generally involve coercion. Privacy implies consensual intimacy in customarily private places.
- Humans are generally considered not to have sexual instincts, and it is thought that our sexual preferences and behaviors result instead from learning and the influences of the psychosocial environment.
- Sexual pleasure is both a solitary aspect of our personhood and a shared pleasure in a human interpersonal bond.
- Sexual scripts are ideas that guide us about the appropriateness of certain types of physical intimacy and the people with whom we share those feelings and behaviors.
- Sexual guilt involves internalized feelings about what society deems "right" and "wrong" in our sexual desires and behaviors. Sexual guilt can significantly diminish any pleasure from shared sexual behaviors.
- Foreplay can involve any one of a number of behaviors in which two people engage before having intercourse. Tactile and oral stimulation are common foreplay behaviors.

Glossary Terms

analingus	foreplay	personal space
anal intercourse	masturbation	primary
coitus	nocturnal	erogenous
complete	emissions	zones
celibacy	nocturnal penile	secondary
cunnilingus	tumescence	erogenous
fellatio	partial celibacy	zones

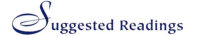uggested Readings

Comfort, A. (1972). The joy of sex. New York: Crown.

Friday, N. (1991). Women on top: How real life has changed women's sexual fantasies. New York: Simon & Schuster.

Hooper, A. (1992). The ultimate sex book. New York: Dorling Kindersley, Inc.

Morris, D. (1967). The naked ape; A zoologist's study of the human animal. New York: McGraw-Hill.

Peters, B. (1988). Terrific sex in fearful times. New York: St. Martin's Press.

Reinisch, J. M. (1990). The Kinsey institute new report on sex. New York: St. Martin's Press.

Westheimer, R. K. (1995). Sex for dummies. Boston: International Data Group.

Westheimer, R. K. (1988). Dr. Ruth's guide to good sex. New York: Crown Publications Group.

Zilbergeld, B. (1992). The new male sexuality. New York: Bantam Books.

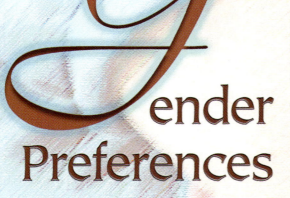

9

Gender Preferences

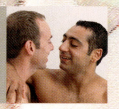

OBJECTIVES

When you finish reading and reviewing this chapter, you should be able to:

1. Explain the distinctions among "sex," "gender," and "gender orientation."

2. Define "homosexuality."

3. Summarize the historical, religious, and political foundations of contemporary thinking about homosexuality and the place of homosexuals in society.

4. Discuss Alfred Kinsey's notion of a "gender continuum" and describe his seven categories of gender orientation.

5. Define "ego-dystonic homosexuality" and discuss its distinguishing characteristics.

6. Describe current data concerning genetic, hormonal, and neuroanatomical aspects of the etiology of homosexuality.

7. Discuss psychoanalytic, psychosocial, and behavioral explanations for the development of homosexuality, and summarize the literature that supports and/or refutes these theoretical perspectives.

8. Summarize and discuss Bem's "Exotic Becomes Erotic" theory of sexual orientation and explain how it predicts the development of homosexuality.

9. Explain factors that motivate gays and lesbians to come out, and summarize the reasons homosexuals are often hesitant to disclose their gender orientation to others.

10. Describe the variety of gay and lesbian physical expressions of intimacy.

11. Define "homophobia" and describe the manifestations of gay-bashing in various segments of society.

12. Summarize the literature that examines the adequacy of gay parenting, and describe the unique problems lesbian mothers and gay fathers have raising their children.

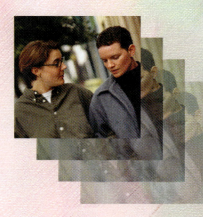

From Dr. Ruth

As you are about to learn, many studies have been done trying to figure out what attracts some people to members of their own sex. Many theories have arisen, but we still do not know for certain why this occurs.

I am as curious as anybody, I assure you, but the bottom line is that finding out is not all that important. If someone has a disease, you want to discover its cause in hopes of curing it, but being gay isn't a disease and doesn't require a "cure" or society's help in this respect. What gays do need from society is to be treated equally to everybody else. It is difficult enough being gay in our society without also feeling you're under a microscope to find out why you are "different."

On the other hand, the public does need to know more about what it means to be gay in order to eliminate the negative attitudes stemming from many complicated factors. As long as gays remain "they" rather than part of "we," they'll remain outsiders. This learning process is also important to gays because a homosexual or lesbian who is confused about his or her own sexual identity is likely to feel anxiety. So whatever your sexual identity, I urge you to read the material in this chapter carefully, with an open mind and an open heart.

Of all the issues explored in this book, homosexuality perhaps is most controversial and has evoked more arguments and strong feelings in the general public. In our society homosexuality is associated with anger, love, hostility, and compassion. This subject involves many things: gender orientation, self-concept, a way of behaving intimately, a stigma, and a badge or pride and self-assertion. This chapter will explore many diverse aspects of homosexuality. One objective is to clarify something you probably already know: sexual orientation concerns far more than just intimate behaviors. Sexual orientation is also a way we relate to our psychosocial environment: the friends we choose, whom we love, our professional relationships, our economic and political priorities, and our perspectives on the arts, media, and human relations.

A systematic discussion of homosexuality necessarily explores gay male and lesbian identities in a social environment that often stigmatizes minorities. The prejudice and homophobia with which gays have to contend ranges from the annoying and offensive to the dangerous and fatal. Homophobia is encouraged by various religions, a fact that seems contradictory to their spiritual aims. Homosexuality is more accepted in many other countries than in the United States. Because of the criticism and hostility many gays have to deal with, many are reluctant to "come out" and be recognized as homosexuals, and we will examine the stressors, adaptations, and challenges of this difficult decision. Coming out can affect occupational relationships or, as in the military, end one's career altogether. Because the rights of gays may be jeopardized, we will examine

a number of legal issues affecting homosexuality. Harassment of gays occurs in the work place, in colleges and universities, and in many neighborhoods.

Everyone lives and works in a wider psychosocial environment, and the nature of gay lifestyles in different social settings reveals much about this subculture. We will examine gay male and lesbian relationships, the current controversy over gay marriage, and the challenges of gay parenting. Some attention is given to sexual behaviors and techniques among gays in a discussion of physical intimacy. The gay community "takes care of its own," and we will describe gay neighborhoods and crime watch programs. The role of gays in the clergy and military round out our discussion of the social accommodation of homosexuality.

Because many people believe that being gay is a choice, social and behavioral scientists, physicians, and the clergy have debated the possibility and desirability of trying to change a person's gender orientation. Although our world is now more tolerant of homosexuality than only a generation ago, troubling and stereotypical depictions of gays still discourage an open-minded, objective assessment of homosexuals as individuals.

Chapter 3 explored issues involved in terms like "sex," "gender," and "gender identity." Our approach there did not deal with homosexuality or bisexuality *per se,* but in this chapter the relationship among these ideas is more fully discussed. Recall that the term *sex* refers to genetic maleness or femaleness; usually, but not always, one's biological/anatomical sex matches one's genetic sex. The term *gender* refers to something quite different: the psychosocial meanings and connotations attached to physical appearance. "Masculinity" and "femininity," referring to things that men and women supposedly think, feel, and do, are more related to "gender" than to "sex." This chapter also discusses the concept of *sexual orientation.* This term refers more to preference and behavior than to anatomy or self-concept. Sexual orientation explicitly involves who we desire to have sex with and whose eroticism we prefer and enjoy most. In a chapter on homosexuality, of course, sexual orientation here primarily concerns same-sex erotic attractions or, with bisexuality, erotic attraction to members of both sexes.

This overall approach to homosexuality involves the same three themes that have guided earlier chapters' exploration of human sexuality: the biological, psychological, and sociological aspects of attraction and behavior.

Let's begin the chapter with a definition of homosexuality. The one we offer here is by no means the only or even necessarily the most correct one, but it clarifies the basic issue behind a great variety of topics. *Homosexuality is the primary psychological and physical erotic attraction to members of one's sex.* We use the word "primary" because circumstances do not always allow one to act on all one's desires. Homosexuals desire and prefer sexual partners of their own sex in most instances. Further, "attraction" in this definition need not be a feeling that one acts on; one can be certain about it but not necessarily behave accordingly. This definition deals with feelings of sexual attraction, the context in which such feelings arise, and how people define themselves. In other words, many factors are involved in this definition.

Another introductory issue deserves comment. Since Sigmund Freud popularized the concept of the "unconscious mind," many people have a lingering suspicion that they could be feeling or desiring something (or someone) and not really "know" it. The term "latent" is often used to describe something not fully accessible to our conscious awareness, and many have speculated about whether a person can be a "latent homosexual" and not be aware of it. We doubt it. As we will see, rarely does anyone have entirely and exclusively heterosexual thoughts, feelings, and fantasies. Many things go through our minds from time to time, but it is highly unlikely that a person could have a *primary psychological and physical erotic attraction to members of one's sex* and not know it.

BASIC CONCEPTS

History, Religion, Politics, and Homosexuality

It is difficult to step outside of the perspective of one's historical era, especially when examining historical views on homosexuality. The word "homosexuality" did not even enter the vocabulary of Westerners until 1869, when the term appeared in a letter to the German minister of justice. The penal codes in Northern Germany were being revised, and some were considering making sexual contact between two persons of the same sex a crime. The person who wrote this letter, Karl Maria Kertbeny (1824-1882) (Fig. 9-1) was one of a few Germans at that time beginning to study the idea of "sexual orientation"

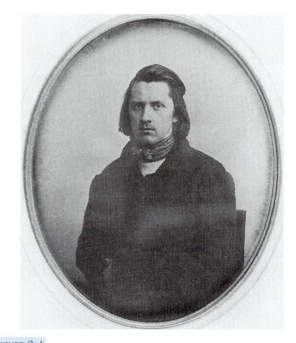

FIGURE 9-1   Karl Maria Kertbeny, who, in a letter to the German minister of justice in 1869, coined the word "homosexuality."

(Mondimore, 1996). Until this time, no historical documents referred to a category of gender orientation in a legal context similar to what today is called "homosexual." Neither was there any such category or term in the languages of ancient Greece and Rome. Of course, same-sex attraction existed, but society generally did not classify individuals with these preferences. This situation stands in contrast to the high visibility of gay issues in today's world.

The ancient Greeks thought and felt very differently about homosexuality than we do today (Fig. 9-2). They were at home with the idea that men would be sexually attracted to young men while being married to a woman and having children with her. Homosexual pleasure outside the marital bond was a norm. Marriage was the appropriate arena for having children, but homosexual eroticism outside of marriage was not only condoned socially but more or less expected. For the Greeks, an idealized homoerotic inclination occurred most commonly seen in relationships between older men and men in their late adolescent years or early adulthood (Mondimore, 1996). Once a young man passed this stage of life, he usually discontinued his homosexual relationships with older men, married, and had children. Today the term *pederasty* refers to such a relationship between older and younger men, or more technically, boys. In ancient Greece some men maintained an exclusively homosexual preference throughout their lives. Again, however, the Greeks had no special words to describe homosexual or heterosexual gender orientations, because they assumed that all men might have sexual feelings for members of their own sex. Interestingly, the Greeks had little to say about female homoerotic attractions, and we have very little

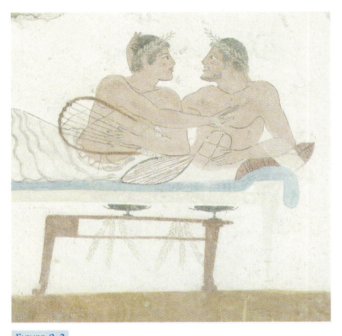

FIGURE 9-2 Homosexual love was an accepted and acceptable part of ancient Greek society.

historical evidence of the place of lesbian attractions in ancient times.

Much of this discussion of the historical aspects of homosexuality is drawn from the study by Mondimore (1996), who analyzes how successive historical eras viewed same-sex eroticism. This writer describes the "berdache," which in French means "male homosexual," in many Native American tribes. A berdache was a man who dressed and behaved as, and fulfilled the social roles and expectations of, a woman. Tribes throughout North America had berdaches, who had the high status of shaman in many instances. Female berdaches, as well, assumed and fulfilled the roles of males in their cultures. Whether male or female, berdaches were homosexual in the way we defined the term, and engaged primarily although not necessarily exclusively in same-sex physical intimacy. Berdaches were viewed by their societies not as either male or female but instead as a unique gender category. This phenomenon should be viewed within the general context of sexuality in Native American culture. Sexual expression among Native Americans was very comfortable and unself-conscious. Adolescent sexual experimentation and childhood sexual curiosity were totally acceptable aspects of growing up. Premarital, marital, and extramarital sexuality were expected and common. In this broader permissive context homosexuality was considered appropriate and, in the case of berdaches, even held religious significance. Native Americans, like the Greeks, had no discrete categories for heterosexual and homosexual inclination and behavior, except for the Aztecs in pre-Columbian South America. This civilization was extremely critical of homosexual behavior and grouped it with incest and adultery as major crimes against society. Those found participating in homosexual behaviors were put to death.

Mondimore's (1996) analysis of the history of homosexual expression encourages us to think carefully about our own categories of "heterosexual" and "homosexual." Our culture has created seemingly mutually exclusive groupings, but other cultures have had different visions of gender orientation. This writer believes that each different society "constructs" its own sexual mores and categories, and that comparisons between cultures may not fully account for unique social customs and pressures related to gender and sexual expression.

In several contexts this book has described the biblical origins of attitudes hostile to sexual behaviors not directed at procreation. We see this in historical prohibitions against masturbation and in connection with homosexuality. Because homosexual intimacy cannot result in progeny, the prohibitions against it are similar to those against masturbation. The Old Testament Book of Leviticus employs the word "abomination" to describe homosexual union, although other Christian tradition is less clear about homosexual behavior. Chapter 2 referred to the analysis by the historian John Boswell (1980) of same-sex marriage during the Middle Ages. Same-sex unions in many instances were encouraged and condoned by the church during this era, and same-sex bonds were often viewed as a "higher" form of affection and devotion than those between women and men. Homosexual priests were common in this period of church history. This tolerant attitude toward homosexuality in sacred and secular European society changed, however. By the early 1300s, a far more conservative (and punitive) approach to homosexuality was obvious in Europe, and this view has softened only moderately in many parts of the world in more recent times.

In 1997, for example, Amnesty International in a report titled "Breaking the Silence" documented murder, imprisonment, and torture of individuals because of sexual orientation. In Columbia, gay men and transvestites have been killed by death squads, and in Iran homosexuality is punishable by death and public stoning. Homosexual behaviors remain illegal in India, Nigeria, and Romania (*The Washington Post*, February 26, 1997).

Typically the most politically conservative segments of society are most hostile to homosexuality. Generally "conservatism" advocates maintenance of the political and social *status quo*, keeping things as they are—or as some people think they should be. There is usually little spirit of innovation in political conservatism, and little tolerance for diversity or divergence from conservatives' "accepted" notions of what is "normal." The political Right in the United States created a rhetoric that associates being gay with pathological behavior (Johnston, 1994). This assessment is viewed by some as an infringement on the civil rights of homosexuals. Such issues create one of the most contentious public debates of contemporary times. Recall the concept of "sexual fascism" discussed in an earlier chapter: a person's judging any sexual behavior that they themselves do not like as "bad" or "abnormal." Some have argued that the conservative political agenda is an example of sexual fascism.

Throughout most of the last several hundred years, homosexuality was not broadly perceived as a menace or threat to the social order. Bullough and Bullough (1997) noted a change in the scientific study of homosexuality from its early start in the 1860s to a different approach to these issues in the early 1970s. As objective and rational as scientists try to be, they cannot easily escape the "mindset" and existing paradigms of the era in which they live, and this is true also in the empirical exploration of different gender orientations.

The first person to develop a "scientific" theory of the etiology of homosexuality was Karl Heinrich Ulrichs (1825-1895), a German attorney and classical scholar (Fig. 9-3). Through much of the 19th century, homosexuality was studied primarily within medical science, in psychiatry in particular, as a pathological personality disorder, but physicians were not sure what caused it or whether it could be "cured." In the latter part of the 19th century, some important figures began to examine homosexuality with the primitive tools available at the time: case studies and clinical protocols of patients undergoing psychoanalysis. One of the first to speculate on the causes and nature of homosexuality was Havelock Ellis, introduced in Chapter 2. In 1897, Ellis published *Sexual Inversion;* "sexual inversion" was a term later adopted by Sigmund Freud to refer to gay males and lesbians. Ellis in this book reacted to the harsh laws against homosexuality in Great Britain in the Criminal Law Amendment Act of 1885 and the "Labouchere Amendment," which made male homosexual behaviors a misdemeanor punishable by two years of hard labor and anal intercourse a felony punishable by a life term in prison (Grosskurth, 1980). Ellis knew enough homosexuals to know this gender orientation presented no threat to society and believed it was time for a more dispassionate analysis. Ellis used thirty-three carefully documented case histories as the foundation for his book, which in later editions referred to the important early investigations of Magnus Hirschfeld (see Chapter 2) and Sigmund Freud.

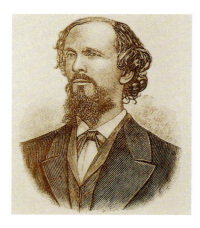

FIGURE 9-3 Karl Heinrich Ulrichs was the first person to develop a theory of the etiology of homosexuality based on his reading of history, literature, mythology, and human physiology.

No book like this had been published before. He dispelled the myth that homosexuality was a psychological disorder and hypothesized that genetic factors may play an important role in the etiology of homosexuality. He noted that many significant historical figures were homosexuals, such as Erasmus, Leonardo da Vinci, Michelangelo, and others (Grosskurth, 1980). While Ellis speculated that the prevalence of homosexuality in the general population was 2 to 5 percent, he cited no empirical data for this. His book, written primarily for physicians and attorneys, was one of the first serious efforts to explain the "normality" of homosexuals despite the repressive and hostile environment in which they typically live and work.

Between the publication of the first edition of this book (1897) and its last (1915), another serious study of homosexuality was published by Magnus Hirschfeld in 1914. Hirschfeld courageously explored the causes, nature, and lifestyles of homosexuals in Germany before World War I and between the two World Wars. He founded the Institute for Sexual Science and was instrumental in creating the World League for Sexual Reform (Vyras, 1996). In 1932 Hirschfeld traveled throughout the world in an attempt to legitimize the new science of "sexology," which in many ways resulted directly from the integrity and diversity of his research. His efforts were not always well received, and much of the criticism was obviously anti-Semitic. By the time Kinsey began his studies of sexuality in the 1940s, the systematic analysis of homosexuality was already well underway.

Several aspects of Alfred Kinsey's questionnaire dealt with the homosexual thoughts, feelings, and behaviors of his subjects. In interviews with these respondents he asked about pre-adolescent homosexual play, post-adolescent experiences, preferences and psychological reactions to same-sex interactions, sources of homosexual contacts, social conflicts experienced because of a homosexual identity, homosexual prostitution, and the subject's self-analysis of her or his own inclinations, appearance, conflicts, regrets, and future (Kinsey et al., 1948, pp. 68-70). Kinsey developed a rating scale (Fig. 9-4) to describe heterosexual-homosexual orientation, using these questionnaire items as a basis for individual gender-orientation ratings. Kinsey was careful to establish such ratings based on both "psychologic reactions and overt experience." In talking with women and men, Kinsey recognized that there were not two independent categories of heterosexual and homosexual orientations but that instead there is significant variation, experience, and experimentation. In creating his 7-point rating scale, Kinsey wrote:

It is a fundamental of taxonomy that nature rarely deals with discrete categories. Only the human mind invents categories and tries to force facts into separated pigeon-holes. The living world is a continuum in each and every one of these aspects. The sooner we learn this concerning human sexual behavior the sooner we shall reach a sound understanding of the realities of sex. (Kinsey et al., 1948, p. 639)

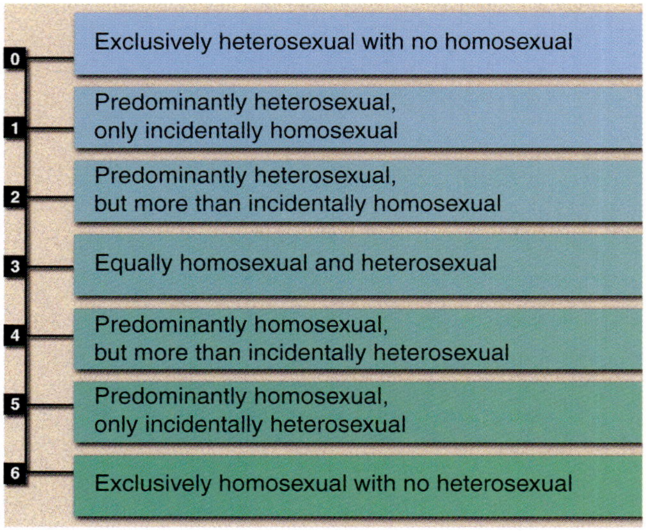

0	Exclusively heterosexual with no homosexual
1	Predominantly heterosexual, only incidentally homosexual
2	Predominantly heterosexual, but more than incidentally homosexual
3	Equally homosexual and heterosexual
4	Predominantly homosexual, but more than incidentally heterosexual
5	Predominantly homosexual, only incidentally heterosexual
6	Exclusively homosexual with no heterosexual

Figure 9-4 Alfred Kinsey was among the first to conceive of gender orientation as a continuum rather than a dichotomy. Here is Kinsey's rating scale of various gradations between exclusive heterosexuality and exclusive homosexuality.

Kinsey's scale assigned scores ranging from 0 to 6 for the following gender orientation descriptions; the descriptions are quoted from Kinsey's book.

> **0**   Exclusively heterosexual with no homosexual
> **1**   Predominantly heterosexual, only incidentally homosexual
> **2**   Predominantly heterosexual, but more than incidentally homosexual
> **3**   Equally heterosexual and homosexual
> **4**   Predominantly homosexual, but more than incidentally heterosexual
> **5**   Predominantly homosexual, only incidentally heterosexual
> **6**   Exclusively homosexual with no heterosexual

Kinsey and his coworkers speculated that 0 and 6 were opposites, as were 1 and 5, and 2 and 4. According to his interviews, Kinsey described 2% of his female sample and 4% of his male sample as exclusively homosexual. Kinsey had discovered something extremely important—that self-definition, overt behaviors, and psychological reactions were all basic to a gender orientation designation. Developmental and situational factors may also affect which of these categories describes a woman or man at any one particular time in their life. For example, some of Kinsey's respondents reported that they were exclusively heterosexual in one-on-one intimate encounters but had sexual contact with both women and men in group sex situations. The idea of a *sexual continuum* is one of Kinsey's more important contributions to the study of human sexuality.

Homosexuality and *The Diagnostic and Statistical Manual of Mental Disorders*

Since 1952 the American Psychiatric Association has published updated editions of *The Diagnostic and Statistical Manual of Mental Disorders.* For several reasons, this is an important and frequently consulted book. For each psychological problem, the defining characteristics are described and discussed. Its major diagnostic features are presented, followed by subtypes, associated descriptive features, relevant laboratory and physical examination findings, the impact of the client's cultural setting, age, and gender features. Also included are prevalence, incidence, lifetime risk, progression over time, pattern of family inheritance, and methods for differentiating the disorder from others with similar symptoms. Mental health care professionals must be fully versed with the *DSM.* As of this writing, the *DSM-IV* is the current edition. Professionals working with a wide variety of psychological and psychiatric disorders recognize that there are often subtle differences in the manifestations of these problems as society changes. This book is important in a discussion of homosexuality because until the American Psychiatric Association voted in 1973 to drop homosexuality from the third revision of the *DSM,* any sexual orientation other than heterosexuality was thought indicative of a mental disorder.

Descriptions and classifications of behavior, not to mention behaviors not socially sanctioned, are affected by current cultural norms and customs. Shortly after the American Psychiatric Association removed homosexuality from its compendium of mental disorders, the American Psychological Association did the same thing. Further, the American Psychological Association fostered the emergence of a new division within its organization, The Society for the Psychological Study of Lesbian and Gay Issues, which reflected its acceptance and sanctioning of serious psychological inquiry into gay and lesbian concerns. Since the early 1970s, the professionalization and legitimation of serious study into homosexuality have accelerated significantly.

That decision by the American Psychiatric Association required great deliberation and care. A study polled over 500 psychiatrists to assess their opinions regarding possible "causes" of male homosexuality (Vreeland, Gallagher, & McFalls, 1995). Among a wide variety of etiological factors, two were most frequently cited: genetic inheritance and exposure to inappropriate sex hormones prenatally—two factors that apparently minimize sociocultural influences on the development of this gender orientation. Additionally, when homosexuality *per se* was removed from the *DSM-III,* one category of homosexuality remained: "**ego-dystonic homosexuality.**" This diagnostic label describes a homosexual who is adamant and persistent in not wanting to be gay; the person has extreme, pervasive distress about their homosexuality. Some gays are unhappy and function poorly in their social environment because of prejudice. An important fact about the *DSM* is that insurance companies in most cases pay for counseling or therapy for clients suffering from disorders listed in this volume. Gays who live in a rejecting and hostile environment often need such clinical assistance.

There have been few systematic clinical investigations of the impact of a person's sexual orientation on the severity of their psychiatric symptoms. However, in one interesting study, 417 psychotherapists were presented with two different case histories of an imaginary patient who was said to be either a heterosexual or an ego-dystonic homosexual, both presenting with the same psychiatric symptoms (Rubenstein, 1995). There was a significant difference among these therapists in the seriousness they attributed to these two hypothetical patients; they believed that ego-dystonic homosexuals had more profound and troubling symptoms than heterosexuals with the same symptoms. Later, when discussing psychological aspects of homosexuality, we will further discuss ego-dystonic homosexuality. We raise the issue here only as an important professional and political issue in the history of the study of homosexuality. The *DSM-IV* directs therapists to diagnose clients with chronic, significant distress about their sexual orientation as "Sexual Disorder Not Otherwise Specified."

Discussions about ego-dystonic homosexuality stemmed primarily from the desire to remove homosexuality from the DSM, and many respected sex researchers and therapists do not believe the disorder actually exists. The DSM-III described the condition this way:

1. The individual complains that heterosexual arousal is persistently absent or weak and significantly interferes with initiating or maintaining wanted heterosexual relationships.
2. There is a sustained pattern of homosexual arousal that the individual explicitly states has been unwanted and a persistent source of distress.

—DSM-III, 1980, 282

Some professionals resisted including this "disorder" in the DSM-III simply because a person can be "ego-dystonic" about many things (some of which are highly trivial), such as acne or baldness. In other words, not wanting to have something is not, in and of itself, a problem. This argument has been put forward with compelling clarity by Suppe (1984).

The Nature and Timing of Homoerotic Self-Awareness

When does a person realize with some certainty that they are erotically attracted primarily to members of their own sex? Is this a subtle or sudden awareness? How does a person "process" this information or make sense of an inclination so different from what one's peers talk about? These and many other questions emerge in the thinking of gay males and lesbians, and they conceal or deal with them in highly variable ways. Often the awareness of being gay comes during adolescence, often in early adolescence. A young person recognizing this inclination often experiences an intense struggle with their social environment, especially in high school (Anderson, 1994). Often youngsters conceal this inner struggle indefinitely. Almost at the outset, the in-

dividual realizes that revealing one's homosexuality to others carries unpleasant risks. One's relationships with parents and siblings will be affected, often in tense and conflicted ways. One understands that their peer group will be critical and perhaps hostile, and that the development of homoerotic relationships involves many uncertainties. Some people try to downplay their revelation or feel they are just "going through a phase," minimizing the turmoil they may be experiencing (Anderson, 1994).

In one Canadian study, self-identified male homosexuals answered a questionnaire about the emergence of their gay identity (McDonald, 1982). Of the respondents 18% recognized their homosexuality before they had engaged in any same-sex behaviors. Additionally, 22% of the subjects accepted their homosexuality while involved in a long-term relationship with a man, while 23% accepted their homosexuality only after involvement in such a relationship. Interestingly, 15% of respondents indicated that they were still not comfortable with their gay identity. The subjects experienced a similar process of realizing their homosexuality and revealing it to others. While many gays go through these events in the same order, there is some variability as well. The "milestone events" in this process are one's awareness of homoerotic attractions, same-sex intimate behaviors, self-identification as a homosexual, having a long-term homosexual relationship, disclosing one's homosexuality to others, and gaining a positive self-concept as a gay person (McDonald, 1982) (Table 9-1).

The Nature of Theories and Research on the Etiology of Homosexuality

The next sections of this chapter explore psychological, biological, and social theories about the causes of homosexuality. No one category of theory is wholly satisfactory, but there is something of interest in these different approaches. Although individual researchers typically work with only one perspective, most scientists see this issue in an *interactionist perspective*. In other words, various theoretical perspectives together provide a sense of the origins of homosexuality, although no one view alone sufficiently explains exactly how someone becomes gay.

TABLE 9-1

Acknowledging Self-Awareness of Male Homosexuality

Self-labeling as homosexual without any gay intimate experience	18%
Self-labeling as homosexual while in an intimate relationship with another man	22%
Self-labeling as homosexual after long-term involvment in a gay relationship	23%
Subjects reporting unhappiness about recognizing their gay identity	15%

After McDonald, 1982.

Note: Not all subjects in this study could be readily classified in these four categories of response

From the beginning of the 20th century, social and behavioral scientists have speculated about the relative contributions of heredity and environment ("nature" and "nurture") in forming a mature human being. In some instances this has been a hotly debated issue. Estimates of the differential influence of these two factors vary, depending on the human attribute (i.e., intelligence, temperament, musical ability, etc.). The same is true about possible causes of a homosexual gender orientation. Some researchers believe that genetic, physiological, and hormonal factors are the primary factors determining homosexuality, while others believe that family, society, and processes of human growth and development provide a better explanation. As with other human characteristics, such heredity-environment debates fail to explain exactly why any one individual is a gay male or lesbian. Again, an interactionist perspective using the findings of both biological and psychosocial theories seems to offer a more useful and informative way of thinking about the etiology of homosexuality.

Because of the controversial and sometimes unpopular perceptions of homosexuality, one should recognize the difference between considering different causes and attributing *blame* to causes. Cause and blame are very different ways of thinking about why things happen. Another semantic matter should be clarified at this point: the nature of theories. Theories in science are *not* intended to be assertions about what is true or false, or right or wrong. Instead, useful theories summarize knowledge. They suggest the next logical step in investigating various phenomena and predict the results of that step. Of course, scientists don't always find what they expect, and therefore theories are constantly being revised. Overall, think of different theoretical approaches as making tentative, speculative claims, not "true" statements beyond challenge.

Ethical Issues in Studying the Causes of Homosexuality

Most scientists attempt to be thoroughly objective and keep their personal concerns completely separate from their research and the inferences they make from their data. However, in studies of the origins of homosexuality, often subtle biases creep into research conclusions. An example of this involves the role of biological factors in the development of homosexuality. Schuklenk and Ristow (1996) suggested that current biomedical research has so far failed to explain the origins of homosexuality and that there are important ethical questions in this area of research. For example, if a clear and consistent biological cause were found for this gender orientation, then, according to the gay activist Randy Shilts, being gay could be considered as natural as, say, being left-handed (Schuklenk & Ristow, 1996, p. 12). However, Schuklenk and Ristow point out that there is a difference between what is "natural" and what society views as "normal." If it could be shown that homosexuality was biologically natural, it is unlikely that society would then suddenly see it as normal. There is a still more subtle ethical issue involved. If it could be demonstrated that homosexuality was caused by a specific biological factor, would there be some temptation to find a "cure" for it? Would some then want to take action to

purposefully change an individual's gender orientation based on what they viewed as a biological "flaw"? Schuklenk and Ristow emphasize that scientific findings do not always lead to social enlightenment, especially in highly controversial issues.

Biological Explorations into the Etiology of Homosexuality

Research into possible biological causes of homosexuality involves three areas of inquiry: genetic factors, hormonal factors (including prenatal exposure to hormones or abnormal hormone levels), and subtle differences in brain anatomy between heterosexuals and homosexuals. These areas involve different questions and different research methods, although careful experimental design and control are essential in all. More than one type of factor might be involved, as well.

Any genetic analysis of behavioral differences among human beings must meet very specific criteria. McGuire (1995) has suggested that the following issues must be addressed:

1. Only valid, precise, quantitative measure of individual differences can be used.
2. Adequate methods must be employed in order to determine biological relationships.
3. Research subjects must be recruited randomly.
4. The sample size must be appropriately large so that valid inferences can be made.
5. Investigators must use appropriate genetic theories and models in interpreting their data.

McGuire notes that at the time of his writing, virtually all studies of a possible genetic basis for gender orientation failed to meet at least one of these important criteria; therefore, any inferences must be made cautiously. Keep these criteria in mind as we discuss the studies following.

There is some statistical suggestion of a genetic influence on the etiology of homosexuality. Studies of the gender orientation of twins reveal some consistencies in self-identified gays. Bailey and Pillard (1991) found that among male monozygotic twins, there is a 52% **concordance rate** for homosexuality, while for dizygotic twins the figure is 22%, a very significant difference. In a similar study examining female homosexuality, Bailey, Pillard, Neale, and Agyei (1993) reported concordance rates of 48% for monozygotic twins and 16% for dizygotic twins. Monozygotic twins (identical twins) are genetically identical, whereas dizygotic twins come from two ova fertilized by two sperm. Dizygotic twins ("fraternal" twins) are related like any siblings, but not identical genetically. Concordance rate refers to the percentage of twins who both manifest a characteristic. High concordance rates for monozygotic twins and lower but still significant concordance rates for dizygotic twins suggest a genetic role in the etiology of homosexuality. Yet, if homosexuality was based *entirely* on genetics, then concordance rates for monozygotic twins would be 100%. Different research varies somewhat in the reported concordance rates for monozygotic and dizygotic twins. Remember, however, that twins are usually reared in the same environment, which may also have an effect on gender orientation (as discussed later).

In 1993, Hamer, Hu, Magnuson, Hu, and Pattatucci reported that they had isolated five discrete markers on the X-sex chromosome that supported the possible role of maternal inheritance for male homosexuality. Two samples of subjects were studied in this investigation, 76 men recruited from an HIV clinic and 38 pairs of gay brothers who responded to a "gay publication" advertisement to participate in a research study. Questionnaires and interviews were used to determine which subjects were homosexual. Despite Kinsey's pronouncements on the non-dichotomous nature of gender orientation, subjects in this study were categorized as either heterosexual or homosexual. Among the subjects recruited from the HIV clinic, there was a higher incidence of homosexual maternal male relatives than homosexual paternal male relatives. Because a number of sex-chromosome linked traits, such as pattern baldness, are established to be inherited from one's mother, this finding seemed to make sense as an inherited trait. Additionally, 33 of the pairs of gay brothers all had the same five markers on the X-sex chromosome. This report of the possibility of a "gay gene" received much attention in the popular press, but this finding must be interpreted carefully. This study does point to the possibility of a region on the X-sex chromosome that may in some way be related to male homosexuality. Because of a number of methodological challenges, Bailey and Pillard (1995) believe genetic influences on gender orientation should be explored further. The data so far are somewhat stronger for male than female gender orientation. As simple as it may seem to recognize an X-chromosome correlate of homosexuality, attempts to replicate the work of Hamer and colleagues have not succeeded (Rice, Anderson, Risch, & Ebers, 1995). It seems that while genetic factors may play some role in the etiology of homosexuality, the psychosocial environment is also a determining factor.

IMPLICATIONS OF A GENETIC ROLE IN THE ETIOLOGY OF HOMOSEXUALITY

There has been much discussion about the possibility of changing traits that are genetically determined. For example, if gene therapies can "cure" someone with cystic fibrosis, some in the future may wish to alter the expression of genes implicated in homosexuality. This issue is especially controversial with respect to homosexuality because some in society view it as abnormal. Recently, some theologians have challenged theories of genetic foundations of homosexuality because they believe that a homosexual orientation is a wilful choice rather than an inherited trait or predisposition. Muir (1996), in the *Journal of Psychology and Christianity,* describes what he considers flaws in the methods and inferences in genetic and neurological research into the causes of homosexuality. He contends a genetic basis for homosexuality cannot be supported from an evolutionary perspective. Because people engaging in same-sex intimacy do not reproduce, he believes that Darwinian natural selection would not preserve behaviors that would not perpetuate the species. Religious condemnation of homosexuality has traditionally emphasized that this gender orientation derives from "faulty" environmental learning, failure in im-

pulse control, and other conscious choices. To such thinkers, a genetic role in the causes of homosexuality would minimize the role of these more "human" choices and make gays seem less accountable for their "deviant" gender orientation. Nonetheless, the role of genetic heritability in the etiology of homosexuality has been demonstrated in dozens of well-controlled, quantitative scientific investigations. As well, homosexuals are not *precluded* from reproducing and passing on their genes. Finally, one might ask whether it is society or biology that creates obstacles for homosexuals who wish to raise children.

HORMONAL FACTORS IN THE ETIOLOGY OF HOMOSEXUALITY

Chapter 3 described how during the period of prenatal embryonic development, even the tiniest amounts of some hormones can have profound and permanent effects on the form of the human body. Much current research has examined the possible role of prenatal hormones on a person's gender orientation. You will remember that in order for a genetic male to develop the appropriate internal and external genitourinary structures, testosterone must be present. For a genetic female to develop the similarly appropriate structures, *no sex hormones can be present.* Even trace amounts of sex hormones can have a tremendous impact on body form. As well, male and female hormones (specifically testosterone and the estrogens) contribute to many traditionally male and female personality attributes (aggressiveness, nurturance, etc.). Scientists have, therefore, wondered whether adult homosexuals have the typical amounts of "normal" sex hormones, or whether perhaps male homosexuals are deficient in testosterone and female homosexuals are lacking in female hormones. As of this writing, we know of no compelling empirical data showing that male and female homosexuals are abnormal in any hormonal sense. But much animal data has demonstrated that prenatal exposure to hormones can have a notable effect on an animal's later sexual behavior, in some cases fostering same-sex sexual activity. One must be very cautious when generalizing to humans from animal data, but in many ways the embryology and endocrinology of many sub-human species is similar to human embryological development. Some researchers think there may be a sensitive period during which exposure to hormones is especially important, and the sensitivity of the developing central nervous system to these hormones may fluctuate throughout embryological development. Thus the presence of prenatal hormones alone may not *fully* account for any effects on a person's later sexual preferences, orientation, or behavior.

While obvious enormous ethical difficulties prevent experimenting with prenatal hormones on human embryos, there have been informative "experiments of nature," as well as careful laboratory studies (Gladue, 1987) that provide persuasive data regarding the effects of prenatal hormone levels on subsequent gender orientation. Chapters 3 and 4 describe luteinizing hormone (LH), which is present in both sexes and related to the production of ova in women and sperm in men. When androgen is present prenatally at a critical period during embryonic development, male external genital differentiation occurs in genetic males, and subsequently the man's pituitary continues to produce consistent non-cyclic levels of this hormone. Genetic females, not normally exposed to androgen prenatally, have a cyclic fluctuation of LH throughout their reproductive years. Therefore, the lack of cyclic secretion of LH may indicate a "masculinized brain," while cyclic changes in LH levels may characterize the "feminized brain." Continuing along this line of reasoning, in women, rising blood levels of estrogen lead to an abrupt increase in LH secretion from the pituitary. However, men given an injection of estrogen do not show a corresponding increase in LH secretion from the pituitary. In other words, the masculinized and feminized brain responds very differently to estrogen. Do self-identified homosexuals have the same response to an injection of estrogen as the heterosexuals just described? The answer is interesting but not clear-cut. Gladue and colleagues (1985) reported that of the 14 men who identified themselves as distinctly homosexual, 9 (64%) showed an LH response to estrogen *intermediate* between that of heterosexual women and men, while *none* of the 17 heterosexual men in this study had this intermediate response pattern. Although this study used a small sample size, the results suggest an endocrine correlate of male homosexuality.

Still another interesting neuroendocrine difference was found between heterosexual and homosexual men by Gladue and coworkers. In the heterosexual men in this study an injection of estrogen decreased their normal production of male sex hormone, testosterone. However, in self-identified, distinctly homosexual men given an injection of estrogen, testosterone levels were notably depressed for significantly longer periods of time than in the heterosexuals. These data together point to a *possible* neuroendocrine role in the development of homosexuality in men, but most researchers emphasize that they can only suspect this connection and that a clear cause-and-effect relationship has not yet been identified (Banks & Gartrell, 1995).

Other research has examined the influences of prenatal *progestational drugs.* These are "pregnancy preserving" agents to help to prevent miscarriages in at-risk pregnancies. Collectively, these agents, referred to as *progestins,* interfere with the action of androgen prenatally. The use of one progestational drug, DES, or *diethylstilbestrol,* has known long-term effects on gender orientation. In a carefully done study Ehrhardt et al. (1985) reported that females exposed to DES prenatally engaged in more lesbian and/or bisexual activities during their lives than their siblings who were not exposed to this agent. Again, however, this does not suggest that prenatal exposure to DES *causes* the development of a homosexual gender orientation in women.

In summary, the experimental data on the effects of prenatal hormonal exposure on later homosexual gender orientation does not point to an unequivocal relationship; many factors apparently are involved. Remember that correlations do not reveal cause-and-effect relationships and that much of this research is *retrospective,* analyzing phenomena that have already happened and that, therefore, are not open to exploration of

suspected causative factors. Nonetheless, several studies have demonstrated an increase in homosexual and bisexual gender orientations associated with prenatal exposure to androgen or estrogen (Hines & Collaer, 1993).

BRAIN ANATOMY AND HOMOSEXUALITY

One of the more interesting and controversial findings in recent years in the study of homosexuality involves data suggesting neuroanatomical differences in the brain structure of heterosexual and homosexual men. However, for a number of reasons we must be very cautious about believing these differences are causally related to a man's gender orientation. The hypothalamus, a very small brain structure located close to the center of the brain, is involved in the regulation of many behaviors that help us survive (such as eating and drinking), as well as other behaviors related to the preservation of the species (such as fighting, fleeing, and sex). In 1991, LeVay reported that a particular nucleus in the hypothalamus was larger in men than in women and also larger in heterosexual men than in homosexual men. These data must be interpreted cautiously because they were derived from autopsy samples of subjects who had died of AIDS: 19 homosexual men and 16 heterosexual men. LeVay reported no differences in the size of this area of the hypothalamus in homosexual men and heterosexual women. LeVay's research involved one particular nucleus of the hypothalamus, the third interstitial nucleus of the anterior hypothalamus (Fig. 9-5). Other research (Swaab & Hofman, 1990; Swaab et al., 1992) reported that another part of the hypothalamus, the suprachiasmatic nucleus, was 150% larger in homosexual men who had died of AIDS than in heterosexual men who had died of the same cause. In addition to being substantially larger, the suprachiasmatic nucleus of homosexual men had twice as many nerve cells as the same area in the heterosexual men. As in the LeVay study, these data derive from autopsy tissue that potentially may have been affected in some unknown way by the AIDS virus. As well, because only adult brains were studied, there is no way to know whether the size differences were a cause or a consequence of gender orientation (LeVay, 1993).

Neuroanatomical data concerning the role of brain structures and gender orientation should be interpreted very carefully. For decades psychologists and neuroscientists have grappled with a controversy involving localization of function. This longstanding dispute centers on the question whether each localized area of the brain does one thing and one thing only, or whether many different areas of the brain all work together in mediating thinking, feeling, and behavior. Data have been collected that support both sides of the argument. In general, however, it is unusual for an area of the brain to be responsible for only a single aspect of human behavior, and the interconnections among various brain areas indicate a remarkable coordination of functions. Therefore, differences in the structure and size of only one or a few brain areas make the attribution of cognitive and behavioral functions to a single locus highly questionable. Further, scientists do not yet know how these various areas of the hypothalamus are linked, anatomi-

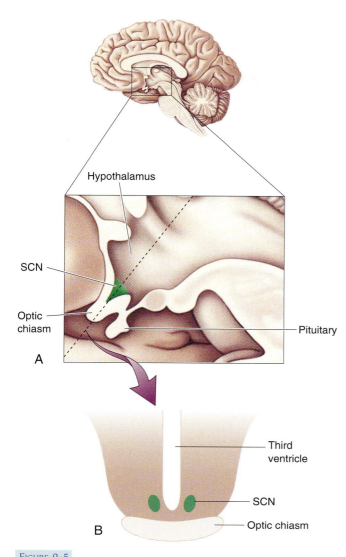

Hypothalamus

SCN

Optic chiasm

Pituitary

A

Third ventricle

SCN

Optic chiasm

B

FIGURE 9-5 The location of the hypothalamus within the brain, and the location of the suprachiasmatic nucleus (SCN) within the hypothalamus.

cally or behaviorally. One should be very careful about suggesting that specific anatomical differences in the brains of heterosexuals and homosexuals are significant, consistent, or well-understood. Other undiscovered variables may be involved.

Psychological Factors in the Etiology of Homosexuality

Through the last century, psychological approaches to possible causes of homosexuality have received far more attention than biological factors, in part because sophisticated physiological and endocrine techniques did not emerge until about 40 years ago. For example, only relatively recently have methods for measuring hormone levels in the blood stream become highly refined and accurate. Similarly, examining brain tissue in specific areas of the human central nervous system requires histological techniques that did not exist only a generation ago.

Prior to such developments, science relied heavily on psychological approaches to this issue. There have been many diverse and interesting approaches to possible psychological causes of homosexuality. Although some seem to make more sense than others, science progresses through the interplay and competition of many ideas, and all are important in the creation and revision of theories that drive research studies.

THE PSYCHOANALYTIC APPROACH

Recall that psychoanalysis began with the work of Sigmund Freud (1856-1939). The psychoanalytic approach involves three different dimensions: a theory of human growth and development, a theory of personality, and a method of doing psychotherapy. The focus here is on the theory of growth and development. Historically, psychoanalysts have not been renowned for keeping an open mind about psychological issues, perhaps stemming from Freud's own dogmatic personality. One prominent psychoanalyst noted that "homosexuals have numerous problems, and [that] no one reaches the final stage of exclusive homosexuality without serious inner conflicts, which remain, even if they are denied" (Fine, 1987, p. 90). Nonetheless, the psychoanalytic approach was among the first to explore the origins of homosexuality, and there is some value in reviewing this provocative theory.

In *Three Essays on Sexuality,* (1905), Freud writes about the development and nature of homosexuality. Freud believed, based on his clinical experience, that human beings are by nature *bisexual* and have both homosexual and heterosexual erotic inclinations. During psychological growth and development, heterosexual preferences and desires become prominent, but Freud believed that our homosexual urges never entirely disappear. This is similar in ways to Kinsey's seven-point scale emphasizing this gradation of erotic attraction. In Freud's psychosexual theory of development, children develop a deep emotional attraction to the parent of the opposite sex. This intense affiliation, according to Freud, is bound to be frustrated, and this web of attraction, affection, and conflict becomes the *Oedipal Complex* in boys and the *Electra Complex* in girls. These terms come from ancient Greek literature and describe son-mother and daughter-father enchantment, respectively. Ultimately, boys subconsciously redirect their desire to be loved to their father and thus identify with him. The term **identification** refers to a subconscious desire to become like someone we love, admire, or respect. This is not a wilful, purposeful "modeling" of behavior but occurs automatically and unthinkingly. Similarly, girls subconsciously alter their desire to be loved to their mother and similarly identify with her. The psychoanalytic perspective emphasizes the father in this triangle and suggests that a girl or boy who has a rewarding, trusting, open relationship with their father will not become a homosexual. However, no systematic, contemporary data support this broad generalization.

When, during the Oedipal or Electra conflict, a child does not fully identify with the same-sex parent, according to Freud, this situation ultimately becomes manifest in a homosexual gender orientation. The youngster identifies with the opposite-sex parent. Psychoanalysts believe that a homosexual is a person who has not developed beyond their Oedipal or Electra conflicts. One psychoanalyst (Fine, 1987) suggests that clinical evaluation of the sexual practices of homosexuals shows that a man who is passive during anal intercourse is symbolically offering his anus to another man instead of a woman's vagina and thus, in psychoanalytic thinking, is acting out his subconscious wish to be a woman. Similarly, a lesbian who uses a dildo to penetrate her female partner's vagina is said to be revealing her frustration in not having a penis of her own. (It is worth noting that in fact, most lesbians do *not* use dildos in their sexual interactions.) Although psychoanalytic approaches often reveal developmental problems, ultimately these are tied to peculiarities in family functioning, and research into this issue generally supports the pivotal role of parent-child interactive problems associated with homosexuality.

A well-known psychoanalytic analysis of the etiology of homosexuality was carried out by Irving Bieber (1962) and Cornelia B. Wilbur. To a large extent, both attribute a homosexual gender orientation to child-parent interactions. From an analysis of survey data from psychiatrists and male homosexuals, Bieber decided that gay males have a "close-binding" overattentive mother and a father who is remote and emotionally distant. The mothers were often described as "seductive" and "overintimate" and the fathers characterized as withdrawn or overtly hostile. Bieber also noted that the relationship between the parents of gay males seemed unrewarding and uncommunicative. Bieber suggested that a young man in this circumstance, when feeling attracted to a woman, would recall or relive a fear of his father's reprisal for taking away his mother's attentions. Speculations such as these are based on case studies and a retrospective approach and lack rigorous methodological controls; they should, therefore, be interpreted cautiously. For example, family patterns Bieber describes as potentially contributing to a male homosexual gender orientation also produce seemingly well-adjusted heterosexual men as well.

In 1962, Dr. Cornelia B. Wilbur, a psychiatrist at the Columbia University College of Physicians and Surgeons in New York, coauthored *Homosexuality: A Psychoanalytic Study of the Male Homosexual,* based on careful clinical study of 106 individuals. She described the early development of male homosexuality involving several consistent factors. For example, each parent has a unique relationship with a homosexual son that differs significantly from their relationships with their other children. She believes that the father is passive and indifferent and may contribute to his son's homosexuality through neglect of traditional male parenting roles and behaviors (Fig. 9-6). When the parents enjoy a stable love relationship with one another, however, homosexuality in one of their male children is unusual. In cases of female homosexuality, Wilbur notes that the mother is frequently a domineering figure in the family and extremely controlling in her relationship with her daughter. These mothers often engage in a chronic power struggle with their homosexual daughters, and the daughter almost always "loses." These daughters come to see their fathers as passive, detached, ineffective men. Dr. Wilbur

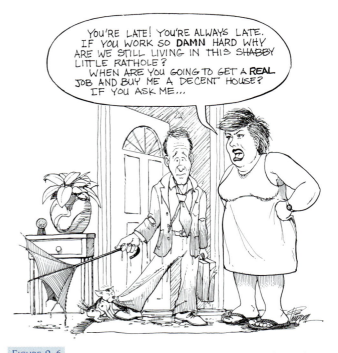

FIGURE 9-6 An early (and incorrect) theory of the etiology of homosexuality claimed that boys seeing their fathers acting passively with their dominant, assertive mothers would be more likely to become gay.

notes that even when many or all of these etiological factors are present, if a child has a good relationship with a sibling, the chances of an eventual homosexual gender orientation are substantially reduced. One last point: psychoanalysts generally believe that through the application of Freud's methods of psychoanalysis, a homosexual person can completely and satisfactorily change their gender orientation to heterosexual—a claim not supported by current data.

Behavioral Approaches to the Etiology of Homosexuality

In addition to biological and psychoanalytic approaches, a third perspective has received theoretical and empirical attention: the behavioristic approach. Often called "learning theories," these emphasize the profound and permanent importance of reinforced behaviors in the building of a person's thoughts, feelings, and actions. The consequences of our behaviors, these theorists believe, determine our thoughts, emotions, and actions. Proponents believe that biological factors, including genetic, hormonal, or anatomical factors, have little to do with a person adopting a homosexual or heterosexual gender orientation (Malott, 1996). Instead, a person's personal history and the behavioral contingencies of the environment are fundamentally responsible for the person's gender orientation. In essence, they say that we "are" what we have been rewarded for being. Behaviorists believe that one's biological characteristics and unique past are the backdrop against which the rewards of the current environment exert their effects. Therefore, according to behavioral theorists, while genes, hormones, and the brain have little to do with gender orientation, they cannot be left entirely out of the picture. Behavioral theorists believe that their approach can account for heterosexuality, homosexuality, transsexuality, and sexual variations and deviations.

Behaviorists believe that a person's environment provides the cues to stimuli that elicit behaviors, including homosexual behaviors (Greenspoon & Lamal, 1987). Behaviorists analyze the environment in which sexual behaviors occur, the behaviors themselves, and the sex of the participants, with the environment being the most important determinant. This approach is more quantitative and less qualitative than the psychoanalytic view. This approach explains the emergence of homosexual preferences over the course of growth and development. If typical childhood sexual curiosity leads a parent to reprimand, punish, or hurt a child, and that parent is of the opposite sex, behavioral theory emphasizes this opposite-sex hurtful experience and attends to the number and nature of such experiences through the childhood years. In other words, punishments and reinforcements accumulate over time to create in the child an expectation of reward or punishment associated with genital perceptions. What is important is the sex of the person causing the pleasure or pain and the consistency with which this is done. Behavioral theorists emphasize the importance and potential permanence of such experiences in the development of a young person's gender orientation.

Behavioral approaches to the etiology of homosexuality emphasize that an individual's first intimate heterosexual interactions are extremely important in the emergence of homosexual preferences. If those interactions involve feelings of shame, guilt, unreadiness, coercion, or repugnance, and if similar feelings accompany other heterosexual experiences, the individual is likely to gradually develop a receptivity to nurturant, loving interactions with someone of their own sex, even if at first these feelings are not associated with physical intimacy. In essence, if heterosexual contacts are not reinforcing, they are not likely to continue, for reinforcement is crucial in establishing and maintaining any behavior. The promptness of reinforcement is also significant. Delayed reinforcements are far less effective than immediate ones. If a person finds homosexual behaviors immediately enjoyable and reinforcing, any delayed feelings of shame, guilt, or self-recrimination are less important because they occur later on. As prompt reinforcements for homosexual interactions accumulate over time, intimate interactions with individuals of the opposite sex become less likely and less rewarding. In the behavioral approach, the acquisition of a homosexual gender orientation takes place very gradually over a long period of time.

There is one important and consistently reported aspect of gay self-identification that behavioral theories cannot explain: the fact that most gay men and lesbians are certainly and suddenly aware that they are erotically attracted to members of their own sex even before they have had any reinforcing physical contact.

Social learning theory (Bandura, 1965) suggests that people learn not only through their own behaviors and reinforcements but also through watching other people behave and experience reinforcements. This is sometimes called "observational learning" and is known to play an important role in many kinds of learning throughout the life span. Learning by watching instead of learning by doing lets us learn from other people's rewarding and punishing experiences without engaging in them ourselves. Social learning theory assumes that we imitate behaviors we observe and that some models are more influential in motivating our imitation of their actions. Although social learning theory has been an influential theory in the behavioral sciences for almost 40 years, we are unaware of any systematic application of this perspective to the origins of homosexuality, and it is unclear whether vicarious experiences may play any significant role. Because social learning theory has so powerfully explained a broad variety of other psychological phenomena involving interpersonal interactions, it may also be of some usefulness for exploring the etiology of homosexual preferences.

THE ROLE OF THE FAMILY IN THE ORIGINS OF HOMOSEXUALITY

Bell, Weinberg, and Hammersmith (1981) analyzed the etiology of homosexuality with emphasis on the interpersonal dynamics of the gay person's nuclear family of origin. This study used data collected from 979 homosexual women and men, compared with 477 self-identified heterosexuals. In this large, well-conducted study they demonstrated that when boys and girls do not accommodate to the common conception of maleness and femaleness, they are more likely eventually to assume a homosexual identity. However, these investigators emphasize that it would be premature and inappropriate to suggest that some families somehow "make" their children gay. For example, male respondents indicated that a close mother-son relationship was not very significant for the emergence of a homosexuality identity; nor was there a definable maternal personality among the mothers of gay men. Identification with the mother seemed entirely unrelated to the eventual emergence of homosexuality among males. Similarly, Bell and colleagues noted that the relationship between a boy and his father did not seem very significant in the origins of homosexuality. However, the homosexual males in this study *did* often perceive their fathers as cold and detached, as Bieber reported earlier.

In relation to family functioning, Bell and colleagues noted that homosexual males were no more likely than heterosexual males to come from homes in which their parents had a poor relationship. However, it was found that the mothers of male homosexuals had played a particularly dominant role in their relationship with their fathers. The nature of sibling relationships did not differ significantly between homosexual and heterosexual males. One important finding was the fact that boys who eventually adopted a homosexual identity were less likely to manifest stereotypically masculine traits and attributes while growing up. These researchers believe that sexual preference is generally determined in childhood and adolescence and that sexual behaviors in these stages reveal rather than cause a person's gender identity (p. 113).

This study explored similar issues in the backgrounds of female respondents. Women who reported poor mother-daughter relationships were less likely to identify with them, but this relationship in itself did not seem related to a later emergence of homosexuality, nor did the mother's personality seem causally related in any way to her daughter's homosexuality. The women in this study generally had relatively poor relationship with their mothers, however, describing them in highly unfavorable language, and were less likely to identify with them than were heterosexual women. The relationship of the homosexual women in this study with their fathers seemed unrelated to their eventual gender orientation. Even though these young women generally evaluated their fathers as weak and submissive, these characteristics were unrelated to their daughters' homosexuality. Bell, Weinberg, and Hammersmith did, however, point out that young women whose parents had a poor and apparently unrewarding relationship were later less likely to see heterosexual relationships in their own lives as potentially enjoyable, and this may have inclined them to explore homosexual intimacy. As among the men, the nature of sibling relationships for women was unrelated to the emergence of homosexuality.

Bell, Weinberg, and Hammersmith emphasized that gender preference is typically determined by the time a boy or girl reaches adolescence, even though they might not yet have acted on that preference. Most subjects in their study reported having homoerotic feelings of attraction about three years before beginning to explore same-sex physical intimacy. All had some heterosexual experiences and mostly found them unrewarding. This large, important investigation demonstrates it is extremely difficult to point to specific family influences with a clear impact on the emergence of a homosexual gender orientation. This strong body of evidence should discourage one from seeing too clear a cause-and-effect relationship between family dynamics and the etiology of homosexuality.

THE "SISSY BOY SYNDROME"

Often everyday observations are a source of ideas for scientific study. Such observations motivated Richard Green, a physician, to study young boys with an explicitly feminine demeanor. He noticed that their playmates called them "sissy," and he coined the phrase **"sissy boy syndrome"** to describe the 50 boys in the Los Angeles area whom he studied for 15 years. These boys often dressed as girls (94% by the age of 6 years), played with dolls, preferred female playmates, and often stated that they wished they had been born girls. However, unlike the transgendered individuals discussed in Chapter 3, most of Green's "sissy boys" later acknowledged their homosexuality. Technically, these children were described as "severely cross-gendered" (Bullough, 1994). These subjects were compared with a control group of boys who more obviously conformed to a traditional masculine identity (Fig. 9-7). Of the boys in the "feminine" group 75% ultimately adopted a homosexual gender orientation, while only one individual of 50 in the control group ultimately assumed a homosexual identity. While other investigators have studied feminine boys, Green's study was clearly the most comprehensive and took a longitudinal approach (Green, 1987). Green cautions against interpreting his findings too rigidly in terms of these young boys' relationships with their father, mother, siblings, peers, or early homosexual experimentation. Green also cautions parents from becoming distressed if their young sons sometimes dress-up like girls, play with dolls, or pretend that they are "mommy." Parents should not be distressed if their little boys avoid rough play and sports, because these preferences and personality characteristics are not necessarily ultimately associated with homosexual development. This careful scientist cautions his readers not to try to use these results as a guide to how to raise children to be heterosexuals. It is very risky to suggest that a few psychosocial variables will create a feminine little boy who will become homosexual. Data like Green's suggest that the interaction of genetic and psychosocial factors is sometimes obvious as early as age 6 in individuals who will later define themselves as homosexuals.

PARENTS' INFLUENCES ON THE GENDER ORIENTATION OF THEIR CHILDREN

Because homosexuals are often stigmatized in our society, many parents of gays and lesbians wonder whether they "did something" to "cause" their children to become homosexual. Golombok and Tasker (1996) investigated 25 children of les-

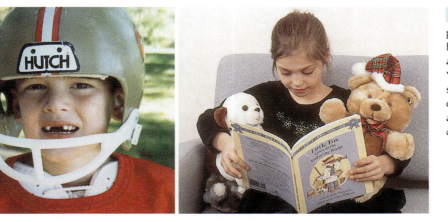

FIGURE 9-7 Early socialization pressures can powerfully affect how boys and girls think they are "supposed" to dress or act. Yet, despite these influences, some children are aware very early that their biological sex and identity are not always congruent.

bian mothers and 21 youngsters with single heterosexual mothers in a control group. In this longitudinal study the children were first studied when they were not quite 10 years old and again at about 24 years of age. These investigators used standardized interviews to try to learn if the parent's sexual orientation affected the eventual gender orientation of their child. During the first series of interviews, Golombok and Tasker analyzed general family dynamics and the children's gender role behaviors. Although the public often believes that homosexual parents raise children who become homosexual, this hypothesis was not supported by the results of this careful research. In the words of Golombok and Tasker:

> *Although no significant difference was found between the proportions of young adults from lesbian and heterosexual families who reported feelings of attraction toward someone of the same gender, those who had grown up in a lesbian family were more likely to consider the possibility of having lesbian or gay relationships and to actually do so. However, the commonly held assumption that children brought up by lesbian mothers will themselves grow up to be lesbian or gay is not supported by the findings of the study; the majority of children who grew up in lesbian families identified as heterosexual in adulthood, and there was no statistically significant difference between young adults from lesbian and heterosexual family backgrounds with respect to sexual orientation (p. 8).*

This study did, however, suggest that family environment may foster non-stereotypical thinking about gender orientation and an openness to sexual exploration. Indeed, a family's overall approach to sexuality and gender orientation issues may be important in the thinking of youngsters, especially in terms of tolerance and respect for sexual practices and preferences different from one's own. When the general family atmosphere regarding sexuality neither expressly promotes or rejects homosexuality, children may feel freer to experiment as their own sexuality emerges. Like other studies we have reviewed about the impact of society and the family on the development of a homosexual gender orientation, Golombok and Tasker cannot identify specific determining variables.

"EXOTIC BECOMES EROTIC": THE IMPORTANCE OF GENDER NONCONFORMITY

Since the important research of Bell, Weinberg, and Hammersmith was published in 1981, theories on the etiology of homosexuality emphasizing youthful experiences, especially family experiences, have become less persuasive. Yet some authors believe it is still too early to embrace exclusively biological theories. Daryl Bem (1996) developed a theory of sexual orientation that accounts for both biological and psychosocial factors, which he calls the "exotic becomes erotic" (EBE) theory. This is one of the more interesting and fruitful theories of sexual orientation to be introduced in many years, although it is too early to tell if the theory's basic claims will be supported by empirical evidence.

Following are the basic assertions of this theory (Table 9-2) (Bem, 1996). His original paper offers empirical support for each of these hypotheses.

A. Biological factors in themselves do not cause the adoption of a homosexual identity. Instead, they exert their influence through the child's overall disposition, such as tendencies to become aggressive or general activity level. Genetic influences on these aspects of human behavior are well known and thoroughly documented.

B. The child's temperament affects the kinds of activities the child enjoys and is likely to engage in consistently throughout her or his childhood. More active, dominant, assertive children will likely enjoy playing roughhouse and competitive sports. In contrast, more reserved youngsters will often prefer quieter, more social activities. In group settings such as preschools, children often play with others who like the same things. Thus boys often play with boys, who often have a more vigorous temperament, and

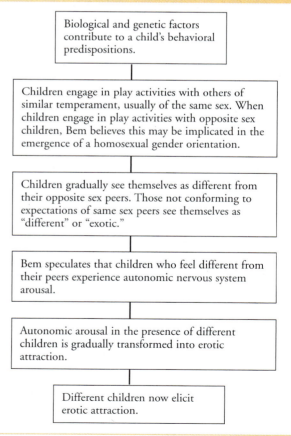

TABLE 9-2

Bem's "Exotic Becomes Erotic" Theory of Sexual Orientation

Biological and genetic factors contribute to a child's behavioral predispositions.

Children engage in play activities with others of similar temperament, usually of the same sex. When children engage in play activities with opposite sex children, Bem believes this may be implicated in the emergence of a homosexual gender orientation.

Children gradually see themselves as different from their opposite sex peers. Those not conforming to expectations of same sex peers see themselves as "different" or "exotic."

Bem speculates that children who feel different from their peers experience autonomic nervous system arousal.

Autonomic arousal in the presence of different children is gradually transformed into erotic attraction.

Different children now elicit erotic attraction.

After Bem, 1996.

girls play with other girls, who are more likely to enjoy more social interaction. When children engage in similar play with same-sex children, their activity is called "gender conforming." When, however, for one reason or another, children play with members of the opposite sex, this is called "gender nonconforming." Bem believes that the consequences of gender-nonconformity can be important in the emergence of a homosexual gender orientation.

C. As children grow up, they gradually see themselves as fundamentally different from opposite-sex peers. Eventually, they will perceive opposite-sex peers as "dissimilar, unfamiliar, and exotic" (Bem, 1996, p. 321). Similarly, children who do not conform to the expectations and customs of their same-sex peers feel these same-sex peers are different, or in Bem's words, "dissimilar, unfamiliar, and exotic."

D. Being with someone who is different can make a child feel uncomfortable, resulting in increased general nervous system arousal mediated by the activity of the autonomic nervous system (see Chapter 4 on the importance of the autonomic nervous system). The discomfort that many little boys feel around little girls is one example of this, but the same thing happens to effeminate little boys who are teased and antagonized by their gender-conforming male peers. Strong autonomic arousal may occur along with feelings of fear, suspicion, and avoidance. Bem suggests that children experience this increased autonomic arousal when with peers from whom they feel different. The child may be entirely unaware of this arousal.

E. The arousal associated with different children (exotic) is eventually transformed into feelings of erotic attraction. This is an example of an elementary psychological principle called "response generalization." Bem suggests that this occurs regardless of the source of the feelings of being different. This assertion is perhaps the most controversial of Bem's theory.

F. Erotic attraction is thus fundamentally based on experiences with those the child perceives as different and the autonomic nervous system arousal associated with this recognition.

To Bem, gender-conformity or gender-nonconformity is an extremely important factor in the development of a person's gender orientation in later life. Bell, Weinberg, and Hammersmith reported that the gay men and lesbians in their sample reported enjoying non-sex-conforming activities while children. In fact, among Bell, Weinberg, and Hammersmith's subjects, 71% of the gay men and 70% of the lesbians reported that as children, they felt very different from their same-sex peers (Bem, 1996, p. 323), thus seeing them as "exotic" and gradually developing an erotic attraction to them. As noted earlier, Bem's theory still needs to be tested thoroughly, but it does reinforce the claims and findings of the work done by

Bell, Weinberg, and Hammersmith and includes a biological emphasis (the activity of the autonomic nervous system) as well. Among current psychological approaches to the etiology of homosexuality, Bem's provocative approach will likely stimulate much additional research.

PSYCHOLOGICAL ASPECTS OF HOMOSEXUALITY

Heterosexuals often wonder what it's like to be gay. Gays are often stigmatized in our society and in some cases the victim of overt prejudice or physical abuse. No academic treatment of this subject can give us the full color and meaning of the feelings of alienation and isolation that may accompany being homosexual. This is true of the experience of anyone who has been the object of exclusion, derision, and discrimination. It is hard to understand the experiences of racial hatred, anti-Semitism, or gay bashing unless you have been on the receiving end of these ugly prejudices. No wonder many homosexuals are hesitant to openly admit their sexual orientation.

The process of revealing one's homosexuality to others is called "coming out" or "coming out of the closet." The word "closet" is important. Our closets generally contain our private possessions, out of the sight and awareness of others.

Coming Out in Adolescence and Young Adulthood

What does someone gain and lose by remaining in the closet or coming out? Both alternatives involve benefits and costs. By concealing one's homosexual gender orientation, one can "pass for straight" and thus avoid unpleasant and abusive experiences. At the same time, however, the person may feel that they are not being honest with themselves or others. Yet there are emotional costs in being honest with everyone instead of the discomfort of "faking" a heterosexual sexual orientation. By coming out, a person gives up the attribution of being "normal" in some people's eyes in exchange for feeling honest and being able to pursue gay relationships openly. Is it worth it? Only the individual in his or her own psychosocial environment can answer. Remember, according to Bandura's theory (1965) we often learn by watching what happens to other people instead of having to go through those circumstances ourselves. Gays who want to come out can observe the consequences for others who come out and perhaps make their decision accordingly. Observing others may help someone determine whether they are prepared, or prepared at this time, to disclose their homosexuality publicly. Coming out almost inevitably changes relationships with parents, siblings, and coworkers—and certainly with a spouse from whom a gay person has concealed his or her genuine feelings. It's a huge decision and is generally made gradually over a long period of time. On many college campuses gay, lesbian, and bisexual support groups offer support and guidance for young people agonizing over this decision.

Because in adolescence many young people are concerned with matters of identity, self-esteem, and their image in other people's eyes, coming out can be a troubling challenge. Most adolescents and young adults in their 20s want to be liked by others and sometimes go to extraordinary lengths to gain praise and recognition and avoid criticism and rejection. Homosexual adolescents and young adults are often very preoccupied with the challenge of revealing their authentic self to others while wanting to be liked and respected. Coming out does usually gain the praise and respect of the gay community, however. In addition to young people, many middle-aged women and men also have a tough time deciding to come out among their peers and coworkers.

Some writers have suggested that the developmental challenges faced by gay and lesbian adolescents are substantially different from and more complex than those for heterosexual young people (Rotherman-Borus & Fernandez, 1995) (Table 9-3). In addition to everyone's tasks of self-definition and identity formation, homosexuals confront four separate psychological tasks in the process of coming out. First, and perhaps most important, they must recognize and accept their homosexuality, often in an environment that denigrates and punishes homosexuals. Second, they need to explore their feelings within the local gay community, which is rarely a part of their school, church, or neighborhood network of friends. This exploration is often a secretive, solitary journey into feelings, behaviors, and relationships that do not conform to what most teenagers consider "normal." The individual may gravitate to gay neighborhoods and entertainment districts, hoping not to be seen by friends but hoping to learn more about their emerging homoeroticism. Brief, casual, exploratory sexual encounters often occur in this process, and Rotherman-Borus, Rosario, Meyer-Bahlburg, Koopman, Dopkins, and Davies (1994) estimate that 20% of males in these situations wind up trading sex for drugs. An increased risk of contracting HIV is another terrible aspect of this self-exploration. This search for clear self-definition has the beneficial effect of bringing adolescents and young adults to support groups and social service agencies that offer counseling and peer support, which can be critical at this time. Often, role models comfortable with their homosexuality offer guidance and acceptance without being exploitative.

The third step in this process of identity development involves telling other people of one's homosexuality. For reasons outlined above, concealing one's homosexuality is not surprising because of the aversive consequences that usually accompany its disclosure. Often homosexuals are abused physically by their parents when they come out (Hunter, 1990). While some families are eventually supportive and accepting, many are extremely hostile and rejecting. This form of family violence is rarely reported and is almost never prosecuted. After disclosure, the fourth step in the coming out process is becoming more comfortable with one's identity as a homosexual person. Rotherman-Borus and Fernandez (1995) believe that an adolescent or young adult who has come out will gradually develop a more favorable self-image and feel more at home with their homosexuality. The person's social scene changes dramatically. Gay men and lesbians become more careful to avoid places where they might be humiliated or hurt.

For some this process is a rocky road. As Rotherman-Borus and Fernandez emphasize, few concrete data are available that describe the ups and downs gays experience at this time. Radkowsky and Siegel (1997) suggested that the pressures and stressors of coming out and trying to establish an identity have an especially troubling effect on gay adolescents. These tensions make gay teens and young adults more vulnerable to loneliness, isolation, depression, and even suicide. To help these youngsters through this very difficult time, two things are essential, according to these authors. First is validation of what the young person is going through—an acknowledgment of their stresses and fears. Accepting the person's emotional and sexual feelings is tremendously important, not an issue to be taken lightly. People like to be told they are not peculiar, and this is especially true for these adolescents and young adults. Second, it is important for these youngsters to have an empathetic peer group of others who have experienced the same thing and can talk about their emotions and thoughts. With these two elements, the person developing a homosexual identity is less likely to feel isolated and alienated, and this is very important.

Coming out often involves an interesting and delicate interplay between an individual's desires for intimacy and for privacy (Ben-Ari, 1995). For many gays, it is difficult to have both at the same time, and intimate inclinations and behaviors rarely escape at least some degree of public awareness and scrutiny. It has been suggested that coming out would be easier if adolescents and their parents realized this delicate balance and shared their feelings with one another about both intimate and private needs. Ben-Ari explored the coming out process in a group of 32 adolescents (19 males and 13 females) and 27 of their parents (8 fathers and 19 mothers). Through in-depth interviews the gay males and lesbians were asked about their parents' and their own experiences in disclosing their homosexuality. The data revealed that coming out involves three phases, named "prediscovery," "discovery," and "postdiscovery." Two-thirds of this sample stated they were fearful about coming out to their mothers and fathers. What was most troubling was the fact that once they had disclosed their homosexuality, their revelation could not be retracted but would have permanent, long-term consequences. About half of these respondents indicated that they feared

---

TABLE 9-3

Psychosocial Tasks in the Process of Coming Out

Recognition and acceptance of one's own homosexuality

Exploration of personal feelings in the wider psychosocial context of the local gay community

Telling others of one's homosexuality

Becoming more comfortable with one's identity as a homosexual person

After Rotherman-Borus & Fernandez, 1995.

parental rejection. An interesting finding was that 63% of these adolescents indicated that they knew at least one of their parents knew they were gay before their disclosure. The most commonly stated motive for coming out was the desire to be honest with oneself and others. The delicate balance between intimacy and privacy was clearest in the postdiscovery phase of coming out. At this time the person felt fear of rejection on one hand and the desire for a more nurturant, honest relationship with their parents on the other. Ben-Ari emphasizes that parents can help their children by showing their understanding of this delicate balance between the desires for intimacy and privacy.

DOES FAMILY THERAPY HELP?

Families with serious problems often seek social and psychological assistance in clinical settings. A teenager or young adult's disclosure of homosexuality often creates tremendous tensions in the individual's family, regardless of the form of that family, sometimes leading to physical abuse. Can family counseling help in this very volatile situation? Saltzburg (1996) noted that when a child reveals her or his homosexual gender orientation, parents often suddenly withdraw their love, support, and nurturance. Family therapists believe that this is a crucial time in the parent-child relationship and that therapeutic intervention may help parents adjust to their child's sexual preferences. This is an important insight. Although the person coming out may need help, the parents often also need special support and counseling. Saltzburg believes that the first priority in the teenager's psychological well-being is that the adults responsible for the adolescent make every reasonable effort to try to understand their youngster's feelings and try to empathize with his or her emotional turmoil and uncertainty.

Many teenagers find it hard to reconcile their magnified sexual feelings with traditional, heterosexual family expectations and social norms. This situation makes it difficult for the person to conceal or suppress homoerotic feelings and more difficult still to engage in acceptable interpersonal relationships. These teens have few "appropriate" arenas for exploring this emerging aspect of their identity, and this impedes the development of a comfortable self-concept. Social pressures encourage these adolescents to "detach" their homosexual feelings from the rest of their personalities and get on with their lives. It is important for parents to respect the emerging sexuality and privacy both of the heterosexual children in the process of coming out. Saltzburg emphasizes that the parents of gay adolescents should make every effort to respect the sexual probing their children are likely to engage in, and this issue is often very important in family therapy.

Nonetheless, the hostility of the wider social environment to homosexuals discourages the adolescent sexual development that often occurs more easily among heterosexuals. Moreover, there are no widely accepted social vehicles for this development among gays; there are no "hay rides," dances, or skating parties for homosexual youth to socialize with one another. In short, social sanctioning is lacking for recreational and interpersonal activities for gay teens. This also makes it difficult for

parents to know what to do for "openers" to discuss and deal with their child's homosexuality. Saltzburg recommends that the family have a "special event" to recognize their child's gender orientation and show their support, such as a family trip to a gay/ lesbian bookstore to buy books about the homosexual subculture. Family therapy for adolescents who are coming out can help parents learn more about their child's feelings and thoughts and thus begin a dialogue about this important aspect of adolescent development. As of this writing, however, we know of no exhaustive research documenting the impact of family therapy on adolescents' adjustment to a homosexual orientation.

DIFFERENT PEOPLE COME OUT IN DIFFERENT WAYS

Acknowledging one's homosexuality can be a lengthy process, especially because of many subtle pressures to just "go with the flow" and do what most (heterosexual) young adults do and not question the obvious. But the "obvious" is different for some, and recognizing this occurs against a background of denial, lack of information, and myth. The following narrative by a gay man describes this process:

> I was eighteen when I first perceived myself to be homosexual. I was taking a shower in my college dormitory. I looked at a naked boy and was sexually excited. The sight of other boys had excited me sexually before, but this was the first time that I connected my response with the word "homosexual." A straight-A student, I was, in this respect, a slow learner.
>
> Being sexually excited by the sight of another boy made me aware that I was different, that "there was something wrong with me." I had never met a homosexual man, or at least been aware that I had met one. But I knew what every other Midwesterner knew in 1942: Homos were mysterious, evil people, to be avoided at all costs. And I was one. Often, when I thought of this, I would break out in a cold sweat. I couldn't be. I shoved the idea aside. When it cropped up, I thought: I must be the only homosexual in northern Ohio. It took me five years to discover that I wasn't. (Brown, 1976, p. 32)

This sensitively written excerpt reveals some of the confusion and certainty, doubt and clarity, that often characterize the process of acknowledging and accepting one's homosexuality. Note, however, that societal hostility to gays and gay issues is greater and far more politicized today than in 1942. Still, this example shows that one's personal revelation of a homosexual gender orientation generally proceeds slowly and tentatively. It is difficult both to feel a genuine affiliation with a segment of society openly reviled and to be certain of one's identity.

Although some writers have described the coming out process as a typical sequence of events (e.g., McDonald, 1982), there are significant individual differences among homosexuals striving for comfortable self-disclosure. The steps many gays take while coming out often blend together, including the following: realizing one's homoerotic attractions, exploring same-sex physical intimacy, self-labeling as a homosexual person, exploring affiliation in a long-term relationship, telling important others in one's life, and finally establishing an identity as a homosexual person. As straightforward as this seems, not everyone goes through these stages in this sequence. McDonald interviewed almost 200 gay males and found that 18% labeled themselves "homosexual" before ever engaging in same-sex erotic experiences. This figure is a relatively small percentage of self-identified homosexuals; far more individuals assumed they had a heterosexual orientation before having a same-sex erotic experience. Additionally 22% acknowledged their homosexual identity while involved in a long-term relationship with another man, and 23% assumed their homosexual identity only *after* becoming involved in such a homoerotic relationship. Further, 15% of these subjects reported that they had not developed a positive gay identity, although this researcher did not consider them ego-dystonic homosexuals. Although many gays go through similar stages when developing a homosexual identity, many do not, and McDonald's research highlights such differences. Although this researcher did not study the coming out process among lesbians, the findings of others indicate some subtle differences between gay males and lesbians.

Cass (1979) described a step-wise coming out process among lesbians, and Kahn (1991) tried to determine whether lesbians experienced stages similar to that of gay males. The questionnaire data from 81 subjects showed that women label themselves subjectively as lesbians at the same time they are exploring homoerotic intimate behaviors with other women. Kahn also found that subjects who held more open views about women's roles in society and homosexuality generally made better progress in identity development and could disclose their homosexual gender orientation comfortably. These findings indicate that women and men are similar in their gradual progression toward coming out, but that significant individual differences may exist.

Gay Male and Lesbian Lives in the Psychosocial Environment

People often think more about the physical dimension of relationships of gay males and lesbians than more basic interpersonal concerns, such as intimacy, social networks, and relationship dynamics. This is a prejudicial way to think about

Dear Dr. Ruth

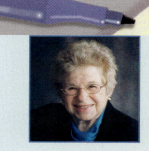

Question:

I am a 40-year-old accountant working in a large firm in New York. For years I kept my homosexuality a secret and was especially careful not to let anyone at the office know. But Dr. Ruth, I'm just tired of living a lie and want to be known and respected for who I really am. Still, I'm worried that my straight friends will want nothing more to do with me and that I could even be fired. Do you have any advice for me?

Answer:

This is a decision only you can make. Losing a good job is something I would fear, so my first reaction is to keep it a secret. On the other hand, if it really bothers you, considering how large the homosexual community is in New York, you could probably find another job, perhaps even with a company headed by a homosexual.

Of course, another approach is not to be overt about your sexual preference, but not to be paranoid about it either. As a single man not seen with a steady woman friend, you are probably already suspect. If you gradually let it be known that you had gone somewhere where homosexuals congregate, like Fire Island, for example, but still didn't allow yourself to be seen with a male lover, then your sexual identity could seep into everyone's consciousness without posing too much danger to your job or relationships. There would still be some risks, and you might lose some friendships, but if you take it step by step, I think that you can reveal your homosexuality without risking any serious damage.

Other Countries, Cultures, and Customs

ASIAN LESBIANS AND THE COMING OUT PROCESS

Just as female and male heterosexual roles differ in various cultures, so too does the acceptability of revealing one's homosexuality. Asian lesbians, for example, have a very challenging coming out process, especially among those who have been socialized and continue to live in an Oriental subculture. Chan (1987), based on her own clinical practice with Asian lesbians, described the powerful conflicts many of these women feel in their development of a homosexual identity. Individual counseling sessions and questionnaire data informed her report. In coming out, the Asian lesbian must deal with individual developmental issues, as well as cultural traditions and expectations.

For example, because Asian cultures are basically patriarchal and women have traditional subservient roles in their families and communities, it is difficult for them to assert their autonomy or find acceptance in roles other than those of wife, mother, daughter, or daughter-in-law. Exploring an individual identity outside the context of the family is difficult for many Asian women, and a homosexual identity introduces a conspicuously unusual challenge. Being anything but "traditional" is clearly conspicuous, and being a lesbian is anything but traditional. While it is appropriate for Asian men to establish an identity independent of their family roles (through their jobs, for example), this is not considered appropriate for women. Chan suggests that Asian lesbians are violating their culture's expectations of women in three ways. They willingly surrender the traditional roles of wife and mother. They decline to be defined through their relationships with men. And finally, they wish to be recognized through an affiliation with other women in a society that typically defines women's bonds through attachment to men. These three challenges comprise a coming out process quite different from that in the Western world.

Asian lesbians not only decline to be defined as subservient females, they instead claim autonomy as women who are partners of other women. Chan emphasizes that sexual matters are not commonly discussed openly in Asian cultures; therefore, coming out more or less forces recognition of an issue considered forbidden, as well as a "gender-inappropriate" preference. It is no wonder that Asian lesbians feel especially isolated in their societies, with such a high cost of coming out.

---

other people—to focus on their sexuality rather than their full personhood. It is even more biased when such analysis is done from a heterosexist perspective that may not be relevant. In the 1990s, *queer theory* (a term used by many gays) emerged as a way of viewing homosexuality from the perspectives of gays and lesbians. This approach de-emphasizes a person's gender orientation and recognizes that as long as homosexuals are seen as different or deviant there is a risk of cultural and political bias (Minton, 1997). Queer theory resists political domination rooted in homophobia. This approach emerged from the gay rights movement, based on the importance of homosexuals speaking for themselves, rather than gay and lesbian issues being presented to the public by "scientific experts."

Heterosexuals often wonder what gay and lesbian committed loving relationships are like. While society provides many idealized images of the traditional heterosexual nuclear family, we virtually never encounter depictions of loving long-term homosexual unions. Heterosexuals, therefore, have much

curiosity and odd speculations about the wider lives of gays and lesbians. Just as it is almost impossible to briefly describe most heterosexual lifestyles and relationships, it is very difficult to characterize "typical" homosexual lifestyles and relationships. Heterosexuals also find it hard to conceptualize the nature of devotion and commitment homosexuals enjoy without the standard societal ceremony of marriage. What is daily experience for homosexuals living alone or with partners in an environment of hostile treatment and homophobia?

The term "gay community" refers to both a typically urban spatial enclave and a sense of mutual support among homosexuals. A community is defined more or less by boundaries and markers. This is generally true of gay neighborhoods, but symbols of *social cohesiveness* also serve to define a community. There are many neighborhoods where many gays and lesbians reside in large North American cities (Murray, 1996). However, various institutions are more important in defining a community than simply the concentration of residents in an area. Gay bars, bookstores, restaurants, health clubs, health care facilities, travel agencies, crime-watch programs, and churches are institutions that give a community a sense of social cohesiveness. In many large cities a "gay yellow pages" helps members of the gay community support one another. Familiarity with such geographic areas and institutions is usually an essential aspect of gay and lesbian lifestyles in the U.S. A genuine sense of solidarity emerges in these places. In these areas gay males and lesbians establish relationship bonds that are the backbone of "gay pride, [gay] consciousness, and collective action." (Murray, 1996, p. 192).

The "primary group" for many homosexuals is composed of other gays and lesbians. The term "families we choose" has recently replaced the more objective, sociological term (Murray, 1996). As early as 1954, Leznoff described this self-segregated group of individuals: (a) unselfconscious and unrestrained practice of homosexuality; (b) a high degree of social isolation; (c) little or no concealment from any heterosexual primary group; (d) total involvement within homosexual society; (e) no conception of sexual variation as a threat to one's social position; (f) little concern with informal sanctions applied by heterosexual society.

Within these groups or "families of choice" gays and lesbians acquire an idea of appropriate normative behaviors, speech and gestural communication patterns, and the "rules" for meeting and dating others. These give the community a dynamic, changing quality continually reinforced by the willing conformity of its members. There is also an interesting commonality in the occupations many gay males and lesbians choose, commonly involving the allied health sciences, rehabilitation medicine, counseling, and teaching—areas commonly called the "helping professions."

Even the way language is used to describe homosexuals reveals the influence of the gay community in defining itself. For example, since 1988, the word *queer* has been used with increasing frequency to refer to gays born after the baby boom (Murray, 1996). Gays and lesbians use this term in a comfortable, unselfconscious way, but often heterosexuals use it in a derogatory fashion. Before the 1970s, the preferred term was *homosexual,* which was gradually replaced by *gay.* Terms such as *gay woman, dyke,* or *lesbian* drift in and out of vogue from time to time. What is important here is that self-description is an essential aspect of the gay community. Incidentally, Murray (1996) states that younger homosexuals sometimes use the term *queer* to provoke their elders, whom they see as insufficiently confrontational.

An interesting aspect of the psychosocial environment of gays is the importance of the "gay bar" as a place for social bonding. Both "unattached" gays and lesbians and gay and lesbian couples enjoy going to gay (as well as heterosexual) bars. Although many different institutions may exist in a gay community, in some cities or areas only gay bars signal to visitors that they are in such an area. Before the gay rights movement, gay bars were a place where gays could enjoy privacy, anonymity, and some protection from the scrutiny of law enforcement officials. Today, gay bars are a more open and accepted arena in which homosexuals can explore sexual relationships and sometimes find affection (Murray, 1996). Often a genuine solidarity and mutual recognition and acceptance are present in these establishments (Fig. 9-8).

After adolescence and young adulthood, most homosexuals have experience living in a relationship. According to Bell and Weinberg (1978), 51% of white male homosexuals and 72% of white lesbians and 58% of black male homosexuals and 70% of black lesbians report being in a relationship. Heterosexuals are often surprised to learn that gay relationships have the same frustrations, challenges, and joys as their own. Gay couples bicker about taking the garbage out or who messed up the checkbook. They argue about the inequitable division of domestic chores, saving too little or spending too much money, drinking, drugs, and differences in approaches to raising and disciplining children—all just like heterosexuals. Systematic assessments of homosexual couple lifestyles reveal no deep and fundamental differences from heterosexual couples. One wonders whether there is really such a thing as a unique gay "lifestyle" after all.

An important similarity between homosexual and heterosexual long-term relationships is frequency of sexual expression. Blumstein and Schwartz (1983) reported that for both heterosexual and homosexual American couples, the frequency of sex decreases with the length of the relationship, although the decline was more pronounced for homosexual couples. Overall, 45% of married heterosexuals had sex three or more times each week, while the comparable figures for gay males was 67% and 33% for lesbians. Among couples who had been together for at least ten years, the corresponding figures fell to 18% for married heterosexuals, 11% for gay males, and 1% for lesbians.

Another interesting issue is a notably different perspective on sex outside the relationship. Lesbians react far more negatively than gay males to the prospect of their partner having sex outside the relationship. Blumstein and Schwartz described particular aspects of a sexual relationship that seem especially

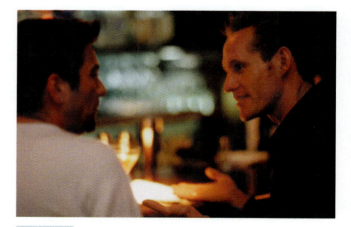

Figure 9-8 Gay bars offer privacy and a chance to relax in a place where one's gender orientation isn't criticized. In these safe, quiet settings many feel free to see old friends and explore new relationships.

important in homosexual relationships. For example, they found that lesbians who engage in oral sex report that they are more satisfied with their sexuality and their relationships (cited in Murray, 1996, p. 175). Additionally, these researchers report that males who perform anal sex on their partners are perceived as no more "masculine" than those who are passive during anal intercourse, and many couples "take turns" frequently.

Peplau and Cochran (1981) examined the values of gay men and the manifestations of these values in their relationships. With a questionnaire study of 128 men, they found that gay men differ conspicuously from both lesbians and heterosexuals in terms of sexual exclusivity. Fifty-four percent of the men in their sample had an intimate sexual encounter with someone other than their primary partner during the previous two months, compared to 13% of lesbians and 14% of women and men in college. More recently, however, the AIDS epidemic has fostered more sexual exclusivity among gay men. Peplau and Cochran also reported that gay men's relationships involved two prominent themes: personal autonomy and close attachment to another person. These are independent although related values, and neither necessarily rules out the other, and these values are similarly important in heterosexual relationships.

Queer theory encourages objective, non-judgmental comparisons between homosexuals and heterosexuals. One difference involves age preferences and partner choice among homosexuals and heterosexuals. Kenrick, Keefe, Bryan, Barr, and Brown (1995) analyzed almost 800 singles ads written by homosexual and heterosexual women and men, and their findings confirmed other research on this question. Heterosexual women in all age groups consistently seek men their own age or older, often several years older. Heterosexual men change their age preferences over time; younger men seek *both* older and younger women, but the older a man gets the more likely

it is that he seeks a younger woman. Homosexual men showed the same age preferences as heterosexual men, while lesbians revealed a preference pattern intermediate between the inclinations of heterosexual women and heterosexual men. These findings are important because they illustrate that homosexuals do not simply reverse heterosexual roles in their relationships, as is sometimes believed. These results were confirmed by another study by Over and Phillips in 1997.

One aspect of homosexual relationships that differs somewhat between gay men and lesbians concerns the duration and number of primary relationships. Generally, lesbians are likely to have had fewer sexual partners and to remain in committed relationships longer than gay males, at least until recently. Today, because of the threat of AIDS, fewer gay males are exploring casual sexual encounters, and more are becoming involved in a sexually exclusive relationship with another man (Kelaher, Ross, Rohrsheim, Drury, & Clarkson, 1994). The discussion in Chapter 7 of love, affection, attraction, attachment, and sexual intimacy is relevant also to homosexuals. The same issues are basic to the building of trust, commitment, and intimate sharing among gay men and lesbians.

Because gay relationships are rarely sanctioned by formal marriage ceremonies, may lack permanence, and rarely involve children to foster a sense of family and continuity, some people think gay men and lesbians grow "old, sad, and lonely." Dorfman and her colleagues (1995) explored whether aging and elderly homosexuals are more depressed and socially isolated than heterosexuals at the same age. In a sample of 23 female and 33 male homosexuals and 32 female and 20 male heterosexuals between the ages of 60 and 93, they found no significant differences between homosexuals and heterosexuals in these two areas. One important difference between these two groups, however, was the *source* of their social support. Among elderly gay men and lesbians, support came primarily from friends, while among the heterosexuals in the study support came mostly from families (Figs. 9-9 and 9-10).

Sexual Behavior and Techniques

The discussion of heterosexual intimate behaviors in Chapter 8 emphasized that fulfilling sex is usually an aspect of an enjoyable relationship. The same is generally true of homosexual lovemaking. Like heterosexuals, gay men and lesbians desire and enjoy non-genital sexual pleasuring. Being held and caressed is important to all of us, irrespective of our gender orientation. And just as sex among heterosexuals involves a variety of acts and positions, so too is there much diversity among homosexuals. The behaviors described here are not an exhaustive catalog of the range and variety of physical intimacy homosexuals enjoy.

Being touched and mutual touching are desired aspects of sex among homosexuals (Fig. 9-11). This involves both primary and secondary erogenous zones, as discussed in earlier chapters. Kissing, genital touching, and anal stimulation involve the primary erogenous zones, while caressing one's partner's chest, breasts, thighs, or buttocks stimulates secondary erogenous zones. Another important similarity between het-

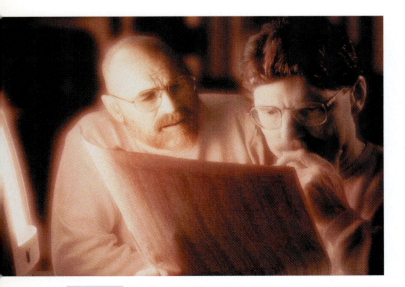

FIGURE 9-9 Lifelong gay and lesbian relationships are often no less supportive, nurturant, and loving than are heterosexual marriages.

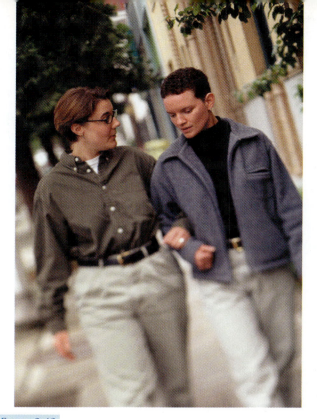

People in strong relationships enjoy doing many different things together with a wide network of friends. This is just as true for gays and lesbians as it is for heterosexuals.

erosexual and homosexual lovemaking is the desirability of foreplay to stimulate a gradual building of sexual tension, which is usually released at orgasm. Taking turns giving and receiving pleasure is basic to all varieties of sexual sharing. It has been suggested that because men know men's bodies better, and women know women's bodies better, homosexuals may better understand how their partner would like to be stimu-

lated, how vigorously, and for how long. Foreplay for homosexuals often involves mutual masturbatory behaviors, which may or may not result in orgasm; such stimulation often initiates erection in men and vaginal lubrication in women. Mutual masturbation is a common sexual behavior among homosexuals, which both partners often report they especially enjoy. Among lesbians, **tribadism** is a common form of sexual expression; two women stimulate one another's genital areas. This may include the vulva and/or mons veneris. It may involve the use of the hand or other body prominences, like hips or knees (Fig. 9-12). As mentioned in Chapter 4, compression of the mons is perceived by many women to be highly erotic.

Cunnilingus and fellatio are very common forms of homosexual intimacy, as among heterosexuals. The descriptions of these behaviors in Chapter 8 apply as well to same-sex lovemaking. Oral sexual stimulation and mutual oral sexual stimulation (the "69" position) are enjoyed and are frequently the preferred avenues of erotic expression among gay men and lesbians. As noted in the discussion of oral and mutual oral stimulation among heterosexuals, if both partners practice effective hygiene and have discussed their sexually transmitted disease (STD) history and HIV status, sharing these behaviors is generally safe. In the later chapter on STDs are discussed recommended precautions for oral and mutual oral stimulation.

Much has been written about anal stimulation and intercourse by gay men. Anal penetration is not always easy or comfortable, yet many gay men enjoy this sexual expression. Muscles surrounding the anus do not readily relax to allow comfortable insertion of the penis. Using a condom lubricated with nonoxynol-9 along with K-Y jelly often helps comfortable penetration. The passive partner (the one receiving penetration) should determine how things progress during anal sex. Men receiving anal penetration often report having orgasms (women, too, often have orgasms during anal penetration),

Mutual genital stimulation and masturbation are a common avenue of shared homosexual intimacy.

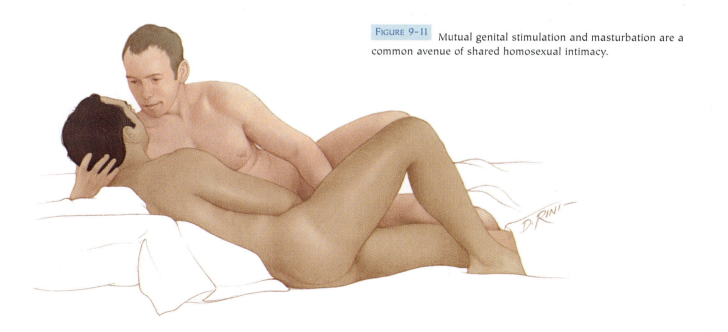

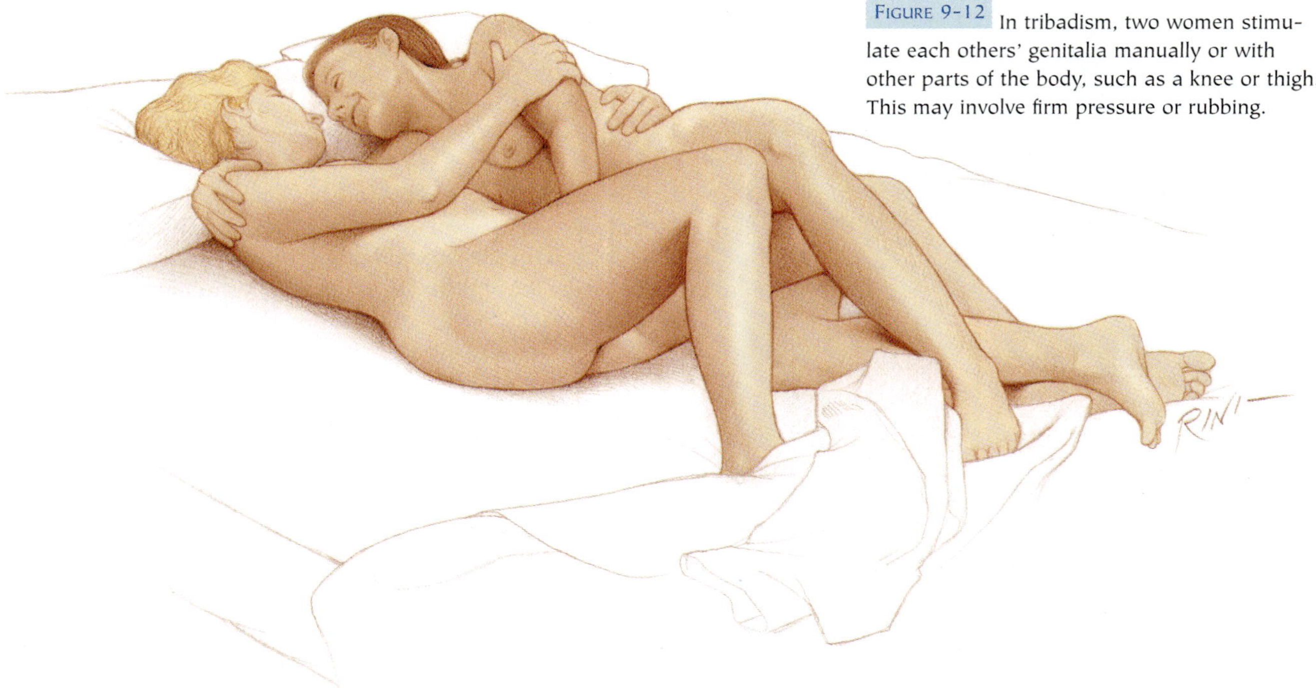

FIGURE 9-12 In tribadism, two women stimulate each others' genitalia manually or with other parts of the body, such as a knee or thigh. This may involve firm pressure or rubbing.

due primarily to the fact that the person's penis in the rectum exerts some pressure on the partner's prostate gland (or in women, the back of the vagina), which often lowers the threshold for orgasm. As we noted earlier, the rectum normally contains many bacteria, so the penis should be thoroughly washed after withdrawal before the couple re-engages in manual or oral sexual sharing.

Another kind of sexual sharing among gay men, called **interfemoral intercourse,** involves one man putting his penis between his partner's thighs, engaging in pelvic thrusting and often ejaculating there. Interfemoral intercourse can be enjoyed in either the face-to-face or rear-entry positions.

A highly controversial avenue of homoerotic sexual expression for both men and women is called **fisting.** Among women, one partner puts her closed fist into her partner's vulva, and sometimes the vagina. Non-petroleum-based lubricant is necessary to do this comfortably. Among men, one person places his closed fist into the rectum of his partner, often at the moment of orgasm. This behavior should not be undertaken with haste and impatience, nor should the insertion be too vigorous, for when penetration is abrupt and forceful, the rectum, vagina, colon, or anal sphincter may be damaged. Despite its somewhat violent nature, many homosexuals say fisting is an enjoyable intimate behavior, often interpreted as a tender and gentle gesture. Generally, however, most homosexual and heterosexual people do not find fisting an attractive sexual alternative. Serious health problems may result from this practice, including sudden cardiac irregularities (Reinisch, 1990).

Changing One's Gender Orientation

Earlier in this chapter we discussed different perspectives on the origin and nature of homosexuality. While some believe it is a wilfully wicked choice, others maintain it is determined by genetic, hormonal, and neuroanatomical factors. Still others think homosexuality has many potential contributory influences. As noted, one perspective contends that homosexuality is entirely a (misguided) choice and that homosexuals have the potential to change (with capable, insistent guidance) to the more common heterosexual gender orientation. Virtually all research, however, shows this assertion to be highly suspicious or plainly untenable.

Recall that homosexuality was removed from the DSM-III in the early 1970s, and subsequent revisions continue to omit it. It is not considered a personality disorder, sexual disorder, anxiety disorder, psychosis, or anything of the kind. It is today widely and generally recognized as an alternative sexual orientation. Nonetheless, there are still some who disagree with this position.

As noted earlier in this chapter, in the early 1970s many psychiatrists and psychologists believed that one form of homosexuality created a tremendous amount of subjective inner turmoil: "ego-dystonic homosexuality." This term refers to gays and lesbians who consistently and enduringly hate their homosexuality and have diminished self-esteem because of their gender orientation. They feel diminished by their sexual preference and aberrant in a heterosexual world. In such cases should clinicians try to "change" these people into heterosexuals, or help them adjust the best they can to their homosexual inclinations? When an individual's inner turmoil grows so great that it interferes with their occupational performance and interpersonal relationships, most counselors and therapists believe the person would benefit from clinical assistance. Indeed, many ego-dystonic homosexuals desperately want to change their gender orientation because they feel their lives would be easier and less complicated.

Other people believe that a homosexual gender orientation is a "moral lapse" rather than an authentic aspect of the self. Various clinical and religious voices have taken a very critical and often patronizing approach to homosexuality. In 1948 the prominent psychoanalyst, E. O. Krausz (cited in Chandler, 1993), said homosexuality should be viewed as a "compulsion neurosis," much like a person's inability to stop washing their hands dozens of times each day. With psychotherapy the homosexual could be "cured" of her or his homoerotic attractions and desires. Of course, today we know that this is simply not true. Moreover, it is unreasonable, if not frankly insulting, for homosexuals to be told that they need to "get a grip" on themselves, change their ways, and be like "everyone else."

Historically, the psychiatric "treatment" of homosexuals has been a popular enterprise. Irving Bieber and his colleagues worked with 106 homosexuals (1962). Many different psychoanalysts and psychotherapists engaged in prolonged attempts to change the gender orientation of their clients. About 70% of these therapists identified themselves as psychoanalytic in their approach; the remaining 30% saw themselves as more eclectic. In this sample, 72 patients self-identified as exclusively homosexual and 19% eventually claimed to have adopted a heterosexual lifestyle. Of the 30 patients who had originally self-identified as bisexuals, half claimed to have become heterosexuals. Generally speaking, the longer the patient was in therapy, the greater the chances of a change in gender orientation. Another report (Hatterer, 1971) followed 200 homosexuals over a period of 17 years. In this study 143 patients were evaluated between 1959 and 1969. The language used to describe the outcomes of this study is in itself quite telling. Of these 143 patients, 49 were described as "recovered," 19 were "recovered partially," while 76 still remained homosexual. The term "recover" implies that homosexuality is an illness from which one can recuperate. Despite such claims, which derive primarily from the psychoanalytic community, contemporary thinking in the social and behavioral sciences on this issue views with *extreme skepticism* the assertion that gender orientation can be changed by psychiatric treatment, regardless of the nature of that treatment.

Presently it is highly unusual to attempt through psychoanalysis or psychotherapy to change a person's gender orientation, sexual preferences, or preferred erotic behaviors. Still, the issue hasn't disappeared. For example, Whitehead (1996) wrote that lesbianism is "caused" by a young girl's problematic relationships with her mother, as well as her childhood and teenage friends. According to this writer, this fosters feelings of being different and lonely, which make the girl hungry for female affection and acceptance. These developmental events, along with homosexual experimentation and the "powerful" messages of the "political feminist left," more or less result in a woman "deciding" to become a lesbian. Further, this writer believes that the religious-therapeutic "healing community," once it becomes sensitive to these issues, can keep these lesbians from exploring even more radical homosexual alliances. The emphasis here is on "healing," i.e., returning the person to a more "normal" heterosexual identity. Similarly, Dallas (1996) argues for making every

clinical effort to change a homosexual's gender orientation to a heterosexual gender orientation because only the latter conforms to the Christian perspective on the "revealed truth."

The issue of trying to change a person's gender orientation is obviously not a simple or certain therapeutic enterprise, and the assumptions behind such attempts are often not based on psychological, medical, or sociological information. Few contemporary, reputable psychiatrists, psychologists, or licensed clinical social workers now make such attempts.

SOCIOLOGICAL PERSPECTIVE I: ATTITUDES OF VARIOUS GROUPS IN SOCIETY TOWARD GAYS AND LESBIANS

Now we will take a sociological perspective and examine gay male and lesbian identities in the social environment. We will explore the gay experience of being a stigmatized minority and the ways in which stereotypes depersonalize individuals with the belief that "they're all just the same." What is special, unique, and important about a person is taken away when someone lumps that person in some group and makes inaccurate assumptions about what the person is like. Stereotypes are even more rigid when they include generalizations about physical appearance, gestures, clothing, demeanor, and speech patterns and accents. Words like "queen," "fag," "dyke," or "lipstick lesbian" combine hostility with supposedly humorous connotation. When you're making fun of someone, you're not taking them seriously. Homophobia in our culture dehumanizes gay males and lesbians and detracts from their personhood, as well as their special skills, abilities, and aptitudes.

Homophobia and Gay-Bashing

Homophobia is a form of prejudice with clear public manifestations. Remember, of all the personal characteristics for which a person might be criticized, in many instances homosexuality is the most invisible (Mondimore, 1996). But consider all the bad things that can happen to a homosexual if or when she or he comes out: they could lose their job or be passed over for promotion (the "lavender ceiling" as Mondimore, 1996 refers to it), be rejected by their family of origin or current nuclear family, be assaulted, be expelled from the church in which they pray, or be left out of peer group activities in which they formerly participated. Some homosexuals, therefore, work vigilantly to keep their homosexuality a secret and remain in a state of constant anxiety about being "discovered." This has been called "stigma management." For most homosexuals, however, stigma management eventually takes more physical and psychic energy than the individual can manage. Often, coming out involves a decision to limit one's life as completely as possible to homosexual acquaintances, businesses, friends, socializing, and "safe" places to live. There are big differences, however, in how homosexuals confront and deal with societal homophobia and gay-bashing (Fig. 9-13).

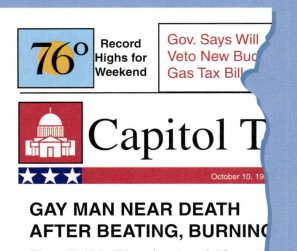

A

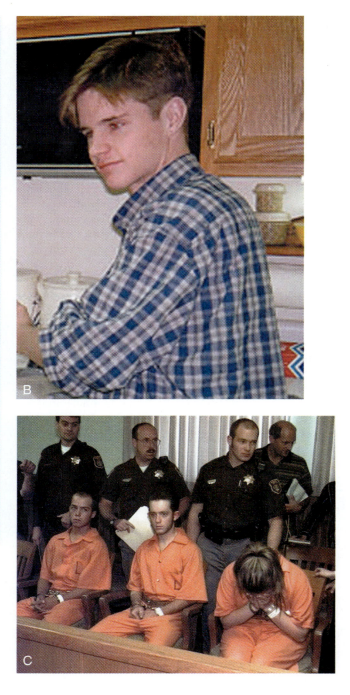

FIGURE 9-13   Matthew Shepard was beaten, tied to a fence post, and left to die in October of 1998 (A). This case received international attention as an example of a horrible hate crime motivated by homophobia. Matthew (B) was a student at the University of Wyoming in Laramie. Those accused of beating and killing him (C) were quickly apprehended. From left are Russell Henderson, Aaron McKinney (who was eventually sentenced to two consecutive life sentences for the murder), and Chastity Pasley.

Just as social scientists are not fully certain about how and why people come to hate any religious or racial group, the sources of homophobia are not clearly understood. Reinisch (1990) notes that people with homophobic views usually think that they don't personally know any homosexuals, have friends who are also homophobic, have less formal education, go to church more often than the "average" Christian American, hold inflexible opinions about female and male sex roles, and are highly dogmatic and authoritarian. In a sense, their overt hatred of homosexuals is their way of telling everyone they are "straight" and don't want to be confused with someone who

isn't. Homophobic individuals seem unable to understand that all male homosexuals are not effeminate, all female homosexuals do not look and act masculine, and that gay men and lesbians do not routinely solicit or molest youngsters, have a psychological disorder, or behave promiscuously. Homophobic individuals often do not understand that a person cannot "become" homosexual by interacting with homosexuals. Homophobia is difficult to confront and extinguish, even in well-educated segments of our society. In many ways, homophobia in society forces many homosexuals to live their lives in a clandestine way.

Many legal rights protect homosexuals, despite a hostile social climate. An important right is privacy, as described in the Fourth Amendment to the U.S. Constitution. Today, privacy is understood to include the information about oneself that others can obtain. We are all guaranteed the right to privacy, which includes gender orientation, as well as financial information regarding credit card transactions. The Constitution further guarantees rights to free speech, freedom of association, due process, and equal protection under the law. Despite these apparent protections, many gay men and lesbians contend with employment discrimination in getting hired or staying employed. Studies demonstrate that subtle anti-homosexual biases still remain *and have been upheld by the courts* (Portwood, 1995). While both the social and behavioral sciences and the legal profession have a tremendous storehouse of knowledge about human nature, empirical evidence from the former does not necessarily inform the latter.

The nature of the legal issue became especially obvious on May 20, 1996, when Supreme Court Justice Antonin Scalia dissented from the court's majority opinion that Colorado and its independent municipalities had the legal right to protect homosexuals from discrimination. The majority opinion was considered an important moment in the fight for gay rights throughout the country. In it the justices noted that homosexuals may indeed be a unique group of Americans whose fight for legal protections is one more modern manifestation of the civil rights movement.

Hostility Toward Homosexuals in Various Segments of Society

We would like to think that people in the social, behavioral, and helping professions are more accepting and non-judgmental about gender orientation issues, but this is not always the case. Many professionals who work closely with the public harbor homophobic feelings and exercise heterosexist biases when dealing with students, clients, or patients. When a person has been socialized to fear, dislike, or mistrust homosexuals, these feelings are slow to change if they ever change at all. Yet we should all be ever-vigilant to these feelings and biases in ourselves and do our best to prevent them from interfering with professional and occupational responsibilities. An example of such subtle prejudice was described in a sample of 187 social workers (Berkman & Zinberg, 1997). The mean age of their subjects was 46 years, meaning that many of these social workers were "baby boomers" educated in the supposedly liberal 1960s. These respondents completed a questionnaire designed to assess attitudes toward homosexuality and any heterosexist bias. The study revealed that 10% of the subjects had frank homophobic attitudes and most had clear signs of heterosexist biases. Because of the small sample size, these data may not represent society at large, however. Interestingly, the degree of homophobia or heterosexism in this sample was far less among social workers who had more contact with gay men and lesbians, indicating that "real life" experiences may help to dispel myths and prejudices about homosexuals. Berkman and Zinberg also found that social workers with deep religious convictions were more likely to manifest these tendencies. Perhaps most interestingly, social workers educated on homosexual issues were neither more or less likely to have homophobic beliefs and heterosexist biases. It is regrettable that professionals working with people with adjustment problems often have attitudes about homosexuals that are anything but objective and non-judgmental.

Like social workers, psychotherapists are expected to have an objective, non-judgmental attitude when working with homosexual clients or training other therapists. As Russell and Greenhouse (1997) noted, this is not always so. Homophobia and heterosexism can have powerful effects on a psychotherapist's training, the therapist's relationship with her or his clients, and perhaps the relationship between the therapist's own sexuality and rapport with their clients. During therapy training, both the training supervisor and the therapist-in-training ideally are aware of any hint of "homonegativity" in their thinking, feeling, or actions. This can be a challenge because psychotherapists no less than social workers are a product of their development and psychosocial environment, and this background frequently and subtly promotes the "normality" of homophobia and heterosexism. This can have a distorting effect on a psychotherapist's training and should be addressed and worked through during this complex educational process. Russell and Greenhouse believe that any psychological issue that supervisor and student conceal or resist dealing with is still an important aspect of training, whether or not it is openly discussed. Things about ourselves we consider "private" seldom remain private while undergoing psychotherapy, and clients are entitled to expect that their therapists have worked through any misgivings they may have about homosexuals or their own sexuality. This issue is important because gay men and lesbians with psychological problems often feel they have no place to go. Before beginning any therapy, the client is entitled to a candid informational interview with the therapist, and personal problems related to one's homosexuality should be expressed at this time to determine whether the therapist can deal with them professionally and effectively.

Homophobia is also present in educational settings. In some instances, homosexual adolescents risk public humiliation, harassment, and even serious physical abuse just by going to school. The New York City Board of Education opened the Harvey Milk School in April of 1985 in a church in Greenwich Village in order to protect gay males and lesbians from such abuses. (Harvey Milk was a gay activist elected to the San Francisco Board of Supervisors in 1978, and who worked for gay rights throughout California before being murdered by an apparent homophobe.) Most of this school's first students had dropped out of other schools because of harassment. In many instances, courts find for students who are victims of homosexual harassment. Jamie Nabozny was awarded $1 million by a Wisconsin jury because two high school administrators at his schools in Ashland, Wisconsin did nothing to protect him, even after he went to them repeatedly for help. They were found to have denied him his civil rights because they did not act to stop the violence. Due in part to the continual abuses in school, Nabozny attempted suicide three times (Reese, 1997). Across the country, an estimated 28% of gay and lesbian high school students drop out of school because of such threats and abuses. A recent Colorado survey indicates that 65% of the teachers polled had no college course that covered facts, concepts, and principles about homosexuality (Reese, 1997). Additionally, 82% had never had a seminar or professional training session about homosexuality. Because of these circumstances, a gay rights group, the Lambda Legal Defense and Education Fund, published a manual to deal with this problem in the schools. It is titled, *Stopping Anti-Gay Abuse of Students in Public Schools: A Legal Perspective,* and is available from this organization at 666 Broadway, Suite 12, New York, New York, 10012-2317. Students preparing for a career in education will find this an important addition to their professional library (Fig. 9-14).

Homophobia and heterosexism are present too in higher education. Indeed, gay rights issues are more visible and controversial than ever before on college campuses. Gay, lesbian, and bisexual organizations exist now at most colleges, although sometimes they are not formally recognized—sometimes as an indirect result of administrative homophobia. For any group to be granted office space on campus or a share of student activity monies, a list of the members of the organization usually must be submitted to the administration, which for gay, lesbian, and bisexual organizations could violate a student's right to privacy. Nonetheless, many young adults who are coming out don't mind being recognized as members of such a group. A report in the *New York Times* describes how two universities with religious affiliations dealt with gay members of the student body. The University of Notre Dame and its sister institution, St. Mary's College in South Bend, Indiana, denied

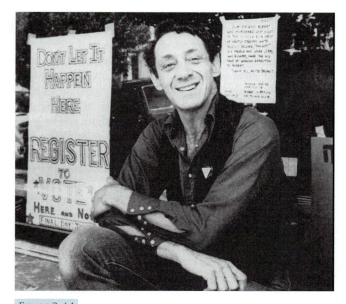

FIGURE 9-14   Harvey Milk, a prominent gay activist who was elected to the San Francisco Board of Supervisors in 1978. He was murdered on November 17 of that year, apparently the victim of a hate crime.

recognition to an organization for gay males and lesbians at the two institutions, claiming that "the group's purpose was inconsistent with the college's mission and the teachings of the Roman Catholic Church" (May 10, 1995). A different result occurred at Yeshiva University in New York City, a traditionally Jewish university, which recognized a gay and lesbian alliance, even though homosexuality is an infraction of traditional Jewish law. The president of Yeshiva noted that because its admissions policy was non-denominational, the institution was bound to meet the needs of "people who reflect a wide range of backgrounds and beliefs." In a case involving a campus organization for gays and lesbians at the University of South Alabama in Mobile, Judge Myron H. Thompson of the Federal District Court in Montgomery, Alabama, ruled that an Alabama statute that barred such organizations from receiving university funding was unconstitutional because it violated the students' rights to free speech and freedom of association (Dunlap, 1996). One would expect a growing recognition and acceptance of gay, lesbian, and bisexual organizations on college campuses throughout the country.

Exposure to self-identified homosexuals may enhance people's understanding of gays and lesbians. Geasler, Croteau, Heineman, and Edlund (1995) studied how a group of 260 college students altered their perceptions of homosexuals after attending a panel presentation by lesbian, gay, and bisexual speakers. The subjects in this study, between 18 and 48 years old, filled out a questionnaire. Many respondents reported that they had changed their attitudes toward homosexuals, at least to some degree, and many reported that their misconceptions and stereotypes about homosexuals were dispelled by their personal exposure to the panel's presentation. Many subjects noted areas of similarity between themselves and panel members and reported a better grasp of the problems and frustrations of homosexuals in our society. As often occurs, someone who interacts with people about whom they had a stereotype finds that their beliefs are incomplete or simply wrong.

For reasons discussed earlier in this chapter, some religious traditions are overtly hostile and unaccepting of homosexuality. The contemporary manifestations of this intolerance are not easily pinpointed, however. *Knowing about* this intolerance is different from *seeing its consequences.* Hunsberger (1996) found clear manifestations of religious fundamentalism, right-wing authoritarianism, and hostility in his analysis of Muslim, Hindu, and Jewish religions, as well as in individuals with Christian affiliations. Fundamentalism is similar with respect to homosexuality in many of the world's major religions. When a religious group feels antipathy toward homosexuality and gay and lesbian lifestyles, there can even be economic overtones. For example, in 1997 delegates to the Southern Baptist Convention voted by an enormous majority to boycott the Walt Disney Company because they felt the company had adopted policies supporting gay and lesbian rights. The leadership of this group discouraged its members from patronizing Disney theme parks, stores, and the ABC television network, owned by the Disney company (*Christian Century,* July 2-9, 1997). One Georgia pastor was quoted as saying, "If we approve this resolution, you have the moral obligation to go home, cancel your ESPN coverage, get rid of the A&E Channel, stop watching Lifetime television and never turn your TV to ABC, including *Good Morning, America . . . .*"

HOMOSEXUALS IN THE MILITARY

If under the United States Constitution homosexuals are entitled to full enfranchisement in American society, why has there been so much controversy in recent years about gays in the military? Of course, homosexuals have *always* been in the military, and everyone who has been in the military knows it. Homophobia often includes the mistaken belief that homosexuals cannot control their homoerotic desires and that this would prove catastrophic to morale, discipline, and combat effectiveness. The same could be said, but rarely is, about heterosexuals in the armed forces. There is no logical or empirical reason for this double standard, but resistance to gay males and lesbians in the military has been very strong. In a large, representative sample of Americans, 71% of women and 58% of men believe that homosexuals should be allowed to serve in the military (Gallup Organization, December 14, 1996). As with any prejudice, it is difficult to determine accurately what percentage of Americans hold homophobic beliefs. The reasons for this significant difference between women and men are not clear.

The scope of this issue is unclear. Senator Howard M. Metzenbaum was quoted in the *Congressional Record* as saying that:

> *According to the GAO [General Accounting Office], women constituted 23 percent of all discharges [from the U. S. military] for homosexuality, yet they represent just 10 percent of all military personnel. Officers constituted 14 percent of all those serving in the military, yet they represent just 1 percent of those discharged for homosexuality . . . . According to a Penn and Shoen 1991 opinion poll, 8 in 10 Americans believe that homosexuals should not be discharged from the military solely because of their sexual orientation . . . . According to the General Accounting Office, the military wasted $490 million that they spent recruiting and training the homosexuals that they subsequently kicked out over the past 10 years. (September 18, 1992)*

Certainly, this enormous issue impacts lives, careers, budgetary considerations, and public opinion. Whether homosexuality affects combat readiness and fighting effectiveness has not been determined through carefully controlled, long-term studies.

Changing the policies of the military would likely not lessen the homophobia in society as a whole. In 1997, in a sample of almost 1000 people polled by the Gallup Organization, Wyman and Snyder found that those who could express their personal values and beliefs, as well as what things about others caused them distress were generally in favor of lifting the ban on gays in the military. Still, polls frequently result in contradictory data, and it cannot be definitively stated what

the country as a whole wants, what the military as a whole wants, and what the gay and heterosexual communities want. President Clinton's "Don't ask, don't tell" policy generated much controversy without moving toward any resolution. Many gay and lesbian military personnel, often of senior rank and experience, have decided to come out while still in the service and tell their stories in newspapers and news magazines (Fig. 9-15). The lives and careers of these public servants are forever changed by their coming out. In October of 1997, the United States Supreme Court upheld President Clinton's "don't ask, don't tell" policy.

Speculations about what *might* happen if the ban on gays and lesbians in the military was lifted include concerns about "living in tight quarters" and "sharing a foxhole." Anxieties about sharing communal living areas and bathing facilities are also expressed. *Never* presented is a thorough description about what in fact *actually does* occur. The issue here involves the circumstances under which a minority group becomes influential, and there are good answers to that question. One of the best predictors of successful minority influence is *consistency;* persistent minorities often achieve their goals, if only because they open and stimulate wider discussion in society. Schacter (1951) discovered that a person in the middle of a contentious public discussion soon becomes the focus of media attention,

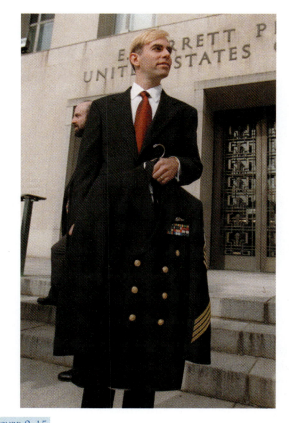

FIGURE 9-15　Senior Chief Petty Officer Timothy R. McVeigh leaving the U.S. District Courthouse in Washington, D.C. on January 21, 1998. McVeigh was discharged from the Navy for acknowledging his homosexuality.

Other Countries, Cultures, and Customs

GAYS IN THE MILITARY IN OTHER COUNTRIES

On January 5, 2000, Britain was forced by a decision of the European Court to lift its ban on gays in the military. A new code of conduct stipulates that "inappropriate sexual behavior between personnel on duty—and not a person's sexual orientation—would be a punishable offense" (Associated Press, *The Daily Press,* January 13, 2000 p. A8). In fact, the United States is unusual in not having legal policies for the rights and responsibilities of gays in the military. Other NATO countries have clear policies of non-discrimination or simply do not see an issue at all. The Associated Press reports on gays in the military in other countries:

Canada: Gays are full-fledged members of the Canadian armed forces. There are no special arrangements or considerations.

Israel: Has accepted gays into its ranks since a 1993 decision banning restrictions on recruiting. Occasional charges of discrimination are made, however, such as the dismissal last fall of a gay officer who had sex with a soldier on base.

Netherlands: Discrimination based on sexual orientation is prohibited by the constitution, and homosexuals serve in the armed forces. Harassment might sometimes occur but is not officially tolerated.

France: France has no official policy, but discrimination based on sexual orientation is prohibited by law. There is currently no debate on the issue.

Greece: Homosexuality is banned among officers in the Greek armed forces. An officer found to be homosexual is forced to resign his or her commission. Conscripts may be exempted if they are gay, although they may insist on serving.

Hungary: There are no restrictions on homosexuals serving.

Norway: There are no restrictions on homosexuals serving.

Denmark: Homosexuals were denied the right to serve until 1954. From 1955 until 1978, they could serve only in the Home Guard. In 1978, the Defense Ministry ruled that sexuality was not the government's business.

Italy: There is no official policy on gays in the Italian military, but gay men are often allowed exemption from Italy's compulsory 10-month military service if they admit they are homosexual and say they fear discrimination.

Finland: Has compulsory military service, but men may be excused on the grounds of homosexuality.

Sweden: There is no specific policy on gays in the military, and a Defense Ministry spokeswoman says it is not an issue in Sweden, which is generally liberal about homosexuality and gives legal recognition to gay partnership.

—Associated Press, *The Daily Press,* January 13, 2000, A8

which is what happened with the public discussion over gays in the military. Another important predictor of minority influence is *self-confidence.* Politely assertive members of a minority often give the public doubts about the position(s) of the majority (Nemeth & Wachtler, 1974) and encourage the majority to rethink its positions and strategies. Finally, when the minority is both self-confident and persistent, the majority begins to seem not to enjoy unanimous public support. It remains to be seen whether this process will occur with the pub-

lic debate over gays in the military, since the "don't ask, don't tell" policy is still relatively new.

Homosexuality in the Cinema and Television

The last two decades have seen a remarkable increase in the depiction of gays and lesbians in the entertainment and communication industries. Movies and television are now more comfortable with gay themes, characters, and actors and actresses.

These representations generally portray homosexuals as persons of worth and ability, and movies and television have done an excellent job of showing the agony and indecision accompanying the coming out process for individuals and their families. Dramatizations reveal the conflict of "passing for straight" when gays and lesbians feel that the revelation of their homosexuality would compromise their careers or social support system. The isolation and anger of being a stigmatized minority has been well portrayed. In the visual arts homosexuality is present in everyday thinking in America. Indeed, there is much optimism about the progress of homosexuals in assimilating more completely in our culture. The fact that serious homosexual subjects are portrayed with tact and candor indicates Americans may be growing more tolerant of homosexuality.

The film *Philadelphia* raised public consciousness about many stereotypes and misperceptions about homosexuals and the gay community. *Philadelphia* was presented to the public as the first "major studio production to deal with the subject of AIDS" (Brookey, 1996), although AIDS was merely the film's integrating theme and the movie showed much about homosexuality in general. Earlier, "queer theory" was described as a conceptualization of how influence operates in society along lines of gender and sexual orientation. *Philadelphia* presented this view with sobering and sensitive candor (Fig. 9-16). The film is about a capable young attorney in a large Philadelphia law practice; he is admired and his work respected. When he

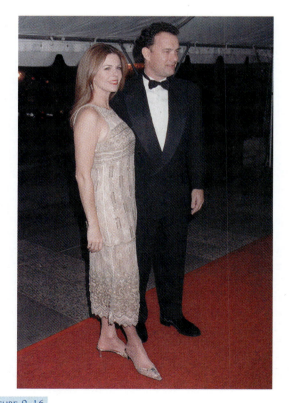

FIGURE 9-16 Actor Tom Hanks, star of the film *Philadelphia*, with his wife, Rita Wilson, arriving at the American Foundation for AIDS Research awards ceremony in New York in November 1998.

discloses that he has AIDS, he is terminated from the firm and sues to regain his position and livelihood. This movie touches on heterosexism in professional America, the cohesiveness of the gay community, the impact of AIDS on gay and heterosexual friendships, and the importance of death with dignity. This film "humanizes" gays and portrays a caring homosexual community that is anything but deviant. An important aspect of this film is also seen in other films and television programs: the family atmosphere of the gay community. When homosexuals are portrayed as part of some extended, mutually supportive "family," they are shown in a highly positive light (Brookey, 1996). This representation, however, may be another example of the claims of queer theory: power lies in heterosexual values and customs. Society might benefit by thinking more broadly about what a "family" really is.

Even when gays and lesbians are the primary focus of a television series such as *Ellen,* the same family values issue emerges. This is true of Ellen's relationships with gay and straight friends and the nurturant relationship she shares with her parents. This sitcom, like *Philadelphia,* shows homosexuals as non-deviant, productive members of society and as competent, serious people whose sexuality is only one aspect of their personhood. The modest but important popularity of *Ellen* mirrors the public's growing acceptance of gays and lesbians. An interesting aspect of this television series was that the actress who played Ellen, Ellen DeGeneres, came out as the show concluded the season. This *really* gave viewers something to think about: the actress and her character disclosing their homosexuality at about the same time. Before this disclosure, the audience could explain their interest in the show because of its clever scripts and poignant, off-hand humor. Then the show changed to something entirely different. What did it mean *now* if at school or work the next day you talked about what was on *Ellen* the night before? Did that suggest you were gay?

Homosexuality on the Internet

An enormous number of websites are devoted to homosexual issues and concerns, as well as heterosexual issues. As with most topics, such websites vary between the extremes of excellent sites and worthless misinformation. There are sites for chat rooms, gifts, matchmaking, message boards, book and movie reviews, entertainment, and gay and lesbian pornography. Groups such as the National Organization of Gay and Lesbian Scientists and Technical Professionals maintain websites. Support sites help gays in domestic partnerships. Recently, many businesses have focused on homosexuals as a powerful economic segment of the population with significant discretionary income, and gay literature increasingly includes advertisements designed specifically to appeal to gays and lesbians. Figure 9-17 depicts some interesting examples of this trend in marketing that are tastefully but plainly targeted to a gay and lesbian clientele. Of all the websites developed for the gay and lesbian community, some of the most popular deal with health issues and AIDS. Accurate and up-to-date medical data and drug developments frequently appear on the web before reaching weekly news magazines. The many websites on gay and les-

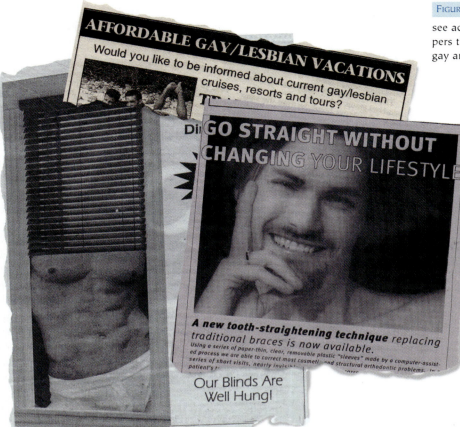

FIGURE 9-17   It is becoming more common to see advertisements in local and city newspapers that appeal primarily and obviously to a gay and lesbian clientele.

bian concerns reveal how the "information age" has helped a once-closeted segment of American society feel connected to an enormous support system and thus less isolated and stigmatized than in the past.

SOCIOLOGICAL PERSPECTIVE II: WITHIN THE GAY AND LESBIAN COMMUNITY

Up to this point, we have examined society's attitudes toward homosexuals. Now let's look more closely inside the gay and lesbian community itself.

Gay Marriage

When two people love each other, they often want their relationship recognized and sanctioned by society, and marriage has been the traditional way to do this. Historically and spiritually, marriage has been a bond between a man and woman that might lead to the birth of children and the improved security of the tribe or community. When two people of the same sex want to get married, many conservative elements of society resist, as has happened recently with more publicity and debate than in the past. Various state legislatures have

taken up the question of gay marriage or other civil bonds. This issue affects all states, however, because of the longstanding legal tradition that marriages performed in one state are recognized as legal in others.

There has been a tremendous resistance to gay marriage throughout the country, however, some taking the form of anti-gay marriage laws. For example, the Utah legislature passed a law specifically forbidding the sanctioning of gay and lesbian marriages that have taken place in other states. Similar legal wrangling is taking place in virtually every state. For a long time homosexuals sought legal recognition of their relationships, but only recently has there been a coordinated nationwide effort by the gay and lesbian community to influence lawmaking at the state level. Controversial debates surrounding gay marriage have occurred in California, Vermont, and South Dakota, where there was a concerted effort by the National Gay and Lesbian Task Force to influence the outcome of the legislature's deliberations. A group called the Human Rights Campaign Fund recently published the results of a poll that showed Americans are more vehemently opposed to gay and lesbian marriage than other gay rights issues, apparently because of the pronatalism implicit in marriage.

Since homosexuals have lived together in the past and have quietly enjoyed their private relationship, why is there a big push for gay marriage in recent times? It involves more

Research Highlight

LONG-TERM HOMOSEXUAL UNIONS

While many people think of long-term marriages as happy ones, less is known about long-term homosexual relationships. Little has been published about such relationships because large, representative samples are difficult to isolate and study. Other research methods can give us insights, however. In a careful analysis of this issue, Clark and McNeir (1997) wrote movingly of this subject in a long-term case study. They explored the special challenges facing gay men attempting to establish and maintain long-lasting, loving relationships. They comment that "urban gay ghettos" may even hinder such bonds among homosexual men.

Clark and McNeir discuss the challenges facing gay men who would like to develop responsibility and accountability in a sexually exclusive, mutually nurturing bond. These challenges are virtually identical to those heterosexuals face as they explore ways of living with and loving another in a trusting, supportive relationship. These writers emphasize that conflicts are an inevitable part of close human contact and that all of us, gay or straight, must accept that sometimes it is best to agree to disagree. Both homosexuals and heterosexuals often must work past uncertainties and anxieties from old, unresolved, and perhaps abusive relationships. Both must learn to trust each other despite these old memories. These writers note that a long-term relationship offers homosexuals some relief from sexual performance pressures in the gay bar pick-up scene. Like heterosexuals, those in long-term gay relationships must learn to deal with the non-sexual friendships of others without jealousy.

Since the psychosocial environment is often hostile to gays, Clark and McNeir emphasize the importance of the home, the entire domestic environment, as a safe refuge. Long-term gay relationships often involve feelings of safety and security from hostile, anonymous forces outside of the home. They claim that sexually exclusive, long-term homosexual relationships may not be the only ethical way to live as a gay couple, but it is one *good* way. Clark and McNeir include a number of "tips" that they feel facilitate long-term homosexual relationships. Note that these generally apply as well to heterosexuals.

- giving each other undivided attention, both communicating and listening well
- respecting each other and honoring each other's lives, both co-celebrating each other's successes and co-suffering and commiserating over each other's disappointments
- asking for and actually valuing the other's opinion and making appropriate changes in responses
- developing and nurturing shared values, . . . shared interests, . . . and shared life-giving commitments
- making choices and time commitments together or in consultation with each other; never deciding for the other one
- allowing each other individual space, but knowing when teamwork is crucial; cooperating
- being flexible, willing to give up certain less important things . . . in order to relax together; striving for harmony not by ignoring conflicts, but by sorting out what is important and what really is not
- talking through situations, disagreements, or misunderstandings to reach mutually agreeable solutions
- clarifying and apologizing whenever anger and frustration over something else . . . has been misdirected, thus assuring each other that anger isn't really meant for one of us and, conversely, learning when not to react or overreact to anger not really directed at us
- remembering to say "thank you" for the seemingly little things, such as a home-repair task accomplished or the house dusted and vacuumed
- remembering to say "I love you" in ways other than sex—with hugs, in friendly teasing, in words at the bottom of a reminder note or a to-do list or in a voice mail

—Clark & McNeir, 1997, 5

Other Countries, Cultures, and Customs

GAY MARRIAGE IN DENMARK

We don't know much about the success or permanence of gay and lesbian marriages because this is a new phenomenon in the United States. But gay marriage has been legal in Denmark since 1989, and a Danish study revealed that gay marriages have an extremely low divorce rate: only 17% in contrast to the 46% divorce rate of heterosexuals. This may in part be due to the fact that gays had been in their relationships longer than heterosexuals before they married and were generally older than the heterosexuals studied (Jones, 1997). The Danish psychologist studying gay and lesbian marriages, Dorte Gottlieb, believes that when two people have enough courage and conviction to marry, knowing their sexual orientation will be revealed on their official documents, they are probably highly committed to one another in the first place. This may help explain the permanence of some of these relationships.

than just wanting to have one's love recognized and sanctioned by law; it also involves economic benefits that typically accompany marriage. Such benefits include joint insurance policies, adopting children, filing joint tax returns, inheritance of jointly owned property, government benefits (Social Security) for surviving spouses and dependents, immigration issues, and spousal benefits in employment contracts (Shumate, 1995). Legal definitions of the term "spouse" are being debated, and recently many large companies have extended spousal benefits (such as health insurance) to the partners of gay and lesbian employees. Other issues arise too. In 1983 Sharon Kowalski was injured and became mentally and physically disabled. At the time she was involved in a four-year relationship with Karen Thompson. After the accident, Kowalski's mother and father denied Thompson visitation rights even though Thompson's visits likely would have benefitted her partner's recovery and long-term health. It took several years before the courts named Thompson Kowalski's legal guardian (Schneider & O'Neill, 1993) (Fig. 9-18).

Gay Parenting

Just as the issue of gay and lesbian marriages evokes strong feelings on all sides, gay parenting is a controversial subject receiving more attention in the press. Scientists have collected much data about the adequacy of gay parenting, and this evidence reveals virtually no substantive problems or deficits in comparison with heterosexual parenting. One methodological issue involves the fact that many homosexuals are single parents, and these parenting outcomes should not be compared with two-parent families because often there are significant differences. Divorce may also adversely affect a child's development, independent of the gender orientation of one or both parents. Data about gay parenting outcomes are important because issues, such as gay adoption, joint custody, and child custody by gay parents are pressing contemporary concerns.

Patterson (1997) explored the family and individual growth, development, and family adjustment of children 4 to 9 years old in the San Francisco Bay area, who had been adopted by or born to lesbian mothers. Overall, mothers in both situations adjusted well to parenthood and enjoyed good self-esteem. Their children also had adequate social development compared to their peers and had typical levels of self-

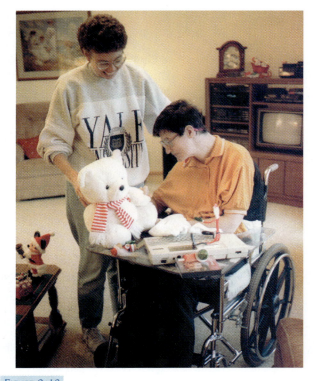

FIGURE 9-18 Sharon Kowalksi and Karen Thompson sharing Christmas in 1992. Cases such as theirs have prompted a reexamination of the rights of partners of gays and lesbians.

esteem. Patterson and Redding (1996) demonstrated that gay and lesbian parents are as likely as heterosexual parents to provide good home environments that foster appropriate development in their children. These writers believe that with the current state of knowledge on this issue, a parent's gender orientation alone is not very relevant for child custody disputes, visitation rights, foster care settings, and adoption, even though some courts rule against awarding child custody to a parent self-identified as a homosexual.

Because parents are role models for their children, social scientists are interested in the kinds of behaviors and values children of gay parents acquire. Hoeffer (1981) studied sex-role behaviors in 6- to 9-year-old children in lesbian-mother families, and the results reinforce Patterson's findings: lesbian parenting in itself has no unique, adverse developmental consequences. Indeed, Hoeffer discovered an interesting finding. Hoeffer presented children in lesbian-parent homes and children in heterosexual-parent homes with pictures of toys. Some were stereotypically masculine toys, others stereotypically feminine toys, and others gender-neutral toys. She asked the children to sort these pictures into three groups: those they most wanted to play with, or somewhat wanted to play with, or didn't want to play with. The mothers also were asked which toys they most, somewhat, or least wanted their child to play with. The children's preferences were predictable: boys wanted to play with boy's toys and girls wanted to play with girls' toys, regardless of their mother's gender orientation. The mothers' responses, however, were interesting. Lesbian mothers clearly preferred that their children play with both masculine and feminine toys, regardless of their child's sex. The lesbian mothers were more tolerant of their children's desire to play with any toy they chose to, while the heterosexual mothers clearly wanted their children to play with stereotypically gender-appropriate toys. Perhaps mothers who are more flexible about gender-orientation issues foster a similar open-mindedness in their children.

The Lesbian & Gay Parenting Handbook, an instructive book about gay parenting by April Martin (1993), includes much practical information about legal, financial, and ethical issues as well as artificial insemination, custody, surrogate pregnancy, and sperm donation. Numerous books too have been written for children to help them better understand gay parenting and its challenges.

Dear Dr. Ruth

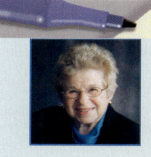

Question:

I'm writing to you because I don't know who else to turn to. I live on the north side of Chicago in an ethnic neighborhood near old friends and many beautiful churches. In the last several years a large number of homosexuals have moved into the area, opened shops and clubs, and parade around the streets shamelessly holding hands and kissing. We "old timers" are sick of it. Our neighborhood has been taken over. These homosexuals even elected their own candidate for alderman. What can we do to restore morality and good taste to our streets?

Answer:

No matter what your background happens to be, there was probably a time when your ancestors moved into this neighborhood of yours and displaced someone else who was already living there. In all probability, the "old timers" of that era were just as upset with your group as you are about the changes taking place. Though we speak of a melting pot, the fact is that our stew is full of lumps. Birds of a feather flock together because they share similar tastes. If our society was perfectly blended, there might be less friction, but there might also be less pleasure.

I think if you take a closer look at this "invasion" you'll find a lot of good things about it. I bet your neighborhood is undergoing a real revitalization. There are probably new shops, new restaurants and a new excitement. You might not feel totally comfortable with your new neighbors yet, but give yourself the chance to get to know them. In the end you might be very glad they picked your area to move into.

Gay fathering has been studied less than lesbian-mothering, but some things have been learned about the special challenges for gay men who want to raise children. Bozett (1981) noted that gay fathers have two different identities at two extremes of social "desirability": they are fathers and they are homosexuals. Bozett found that the nature and extent of the father's experience in the gay subculture affect how easily he assumes these two roles comfortably. Men who acknowledged their homosexuality before marrying women more easily adjusted to their gay and paternal identities than men who kept their gender orientation entirely clandestine before marriage. For these men to reconcile these different aspects of their lives, both the gay and heterosexual communities have to support their parenting efforts, and this is rare. Indeed, the gay-father identity clashes with three common attributes of the gay community: gays are typically single, form relationships that are generally brief, and are a youthful subculture (Bozett, 1991). Gay men with children in contrast, may have been in-

volved in a relationship with a woman long enough to have a child and may be old enough to be a parent of a child or adolescent. Gay fathers often find that new friends or partners are jealous of the time and attention they spend with their son or daughter; this is true as well among heterosexuals who have children, are unmarried, and begin to date.

When a gay male or lesbian has a child, issues of child custody and visitation may arise, and courts must establish standards for making decisions on such issues. Stein (1996), writing in the *Social Service Review*, notes that the "best-interest-of-the-child" standard is typically used by courts in rulings on custody and visitation and that this standard involves two issues. The court must consider any parental behaviors deemed potentially problematic for parenting. Although the parent's sexual orientation might be related to such behaviors, there may be problems in the home having nothing to do with the parent's homosexuality. The second issue is that many judges view homosexuality in itself a sufficient reason to

Other Countries, Cultures, and Customs

HOMOSEXUALITY IN CHINA TODAY

As political repression slowly subsides in China, tolerance for homosexuals seems to be slowly growing (Faison, 1997). Yet the psychosocial climate affecting gays and lesbians in China is quite different from that in North America. Recently, especially in China's larger cities, such as Beijing and Shanghai, gays and lesbians have begun to meet quietly in clubs in an environment free from historical prohibitions or government and police intrusion. The government seems to tolerate homosexuals because they do not organize and seek rights and freedoms. To the degree that they remain a "quiet minority," they are tolerated. Most gays and lesbians still conceal their gender orientation from most friends and family members. In 1992, an AIDS telephone hot line was set up in Beijing, and local authorities allowed books about homosexuality to be published. As long as homosexuals do not demand a public voice, they are let alone. Gay bars and clubs offer the chance to relax and just "be yourself," which is important for self-acceptance and establishing meaningful friendships with others. The problem of feeling isolated is more common in smaller, rural communities, however. The Chinese Psychiatric Association still believes that homosexuality is a type of mental illness, which in some cases is even treated by electric shock. Despite claims of a "cure" by some doctors, others criticize such methods on humanitarian and scientific grounds.

While journalists have described a picture of growing tolerance, scientific studies of homosexuals in China are rare, although recently, reforms have made it possible for social and behavioral scientists to begin exploring this subject. Pan, Wu, and Gil (1995) interviewed 165 self-identified homosexuals in four cities in China. Their characterization of homosexuality in China isn't that much different from that in our own society. Respondents report a wide range of sexual orientations and a large number of preferred sexual practices. Many are married with children and explore homosexual and/or bisexual relationships in secret. Although social scientists are just beginning to learn something about homosexuality in China, what has been learned so far tells us more about how human beings are similar than how they differ.

deny child custody and restrict visitation. A recent case in Virginia illustrates how complicated a custody dispute can be. On the one hand, the Supreme Court of Virginia believes that homosexual persons are not, per se, unfit parents, but on the other hand lesbian relationships often involve sexual conduct that is a felony in Virginia; on that account the court deprived a lesbian mother of the custody of her child. The justices apparently did not see the basic contradiction in their ruling (Stein, 1996). A similar legal tradition seems to be emerging in Colorado, where judges have decided against custody for lesbian mothers simply because they are lesbians (Duran-Aydintug & Causey, 1996).

Canadian courts have dealt with similar custody disputes, typically using the "best-interest-of-the-child" criterion. Casey (1994) has noted an irony in that Canadian courts frequently award child custody to lesbian mothers who have not "come out" but deny custody to women who are honest about their gender orientation. Canadian judges have given various reasons for denying custody to lesbian mothers: potential sexual molestation of the child, compromised psychosexual development due to exposure to homosexual adults, harassment of the child by peers, and fear of exposure to AIDS (Casey, 1994). The research of Charlotte Patterson, cited earlier, however, indicates that such problems are very unlikely to occur. Similar legal considerations have been addressed in the Netherlands, where official government reports address the adequacy of gay and lesbian parenting. van Nijnatten (1995) summarized these reports that no data indicate that gay and lesbian parents aren't at least as competent and committed as heterosexual parents and that it would be unwise to formulate or enforce any public policies excluding homosexuals from raising their children.

The Ordination of Gay and Lesbian Clergy

A slogan used by some gays and lesbians to raise consciousness about the presence of homosexuals in all spheres of American life is, "We are everywhere"—with the unspoken clause "whether or not you know it." The ordination of gay men and lesbians as spiritual leaders, for example, has been a contentious issue in many faiths (Fig. 9-19). Two assumptions are relevant here: (1) gay men and lesbians can enjoy a fulfilling life as spiritual leaders, and (2) gay men and lesbians have spiritual needs often best met through a relationship with a homosexual member of the clergy. Being a homosexual and being a spiritual person are certainly not mutually exclusive. Barret and Barzan (1996) noted, however, that because gay and lesbian lifestyles are often judged as sinful, homosexuals are not welcome in some religious communities. Barret and Barzan suggested that gay men and lesbians spiritually struggle to deal with both society's hostility to their homosexuality and their desire to explore their unique selfhood and connectedness with God. This is a special challenge for clerical counselors trying to help homosexuals reconcile these different awarenesses.

If traditional religious groups don't welcome homosexual congregants, imagine how they might feel about having a gay

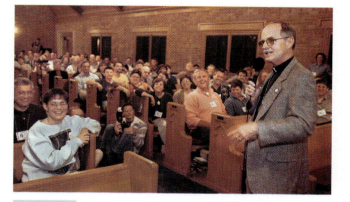

FIGURE 9-19 The Reverend Mel White, a gay pastor, works to eliminate violence against homosexuals. Here he addresses a group at the First Church in Lynchburg, Virginia. Gay and lesbian clergy work hard to meet the spiritual needs of those they serve—a big job when there are frequent signs of society's hostility against homosexuals.

or lesbian minister. Resistance to the ordination of gay and lesbian ministers seems common throughout the world. For example, churches in South Africa refuse to accept gay and lesbian clergy (Thiel, 1997). The 1997 constitution of South Africa makes discrimination illegal based on "race, gender, sex, pregnancy, marital status, ethnic or social origin, colour, sexual orientation, age, disability, religion, conscience, belief, culture, language and birth." Clerics maintain that the Bible and God's law prohibit churches from accepting homosexuals as congregants or ministers. In Great Britain, it was announced in 1977 that 19 bishops of the Church of England had knowingly ordained "actively gay priests, and 37 in all have knowingly employed or licensed such clergy" (Nowell, 1997). Yet in 1991 the Church of England adopted a statement on human sexuality that the church would "tolerate homosexual relationships among the laity, but not among the clergy."

In 1996 an Episcopal Church court convened a trial of a bishop for heresy. Walter Righter was charged with knowingly ordaining a "non-celibate homosexual" as a priest in 1990. Reverend Righter apparently violated a 1979 resolution passed by the Episcopal Church's General Convention that prohibited the ordination of sexually active gay and lesbian clergy. In 1996 the Archbishop of Canterbury and the Bishop of Guildford disagreed over the position of the Anglican Church regarding homosexuals. The Right Reverend John Gladwin of Guildford criticized church policy that stipulated that homosexuals are "wicked" individuals and argued that the church needed to reconsider its position that sexual relations are appropriate only in traditional marriages. George Carey, the Archbishop of Canterbury, maintained the church's more conservative stance (Wroe, 1996).

In churches throughout the world, gay ordination is at the center of an often passionate debate. Ironically, many members of a congregation are pleased with the caring, efficient professionalism of a pastor or minister until they discover that she or he is a lesbian or gay; then some feel they must leave the congregation.

CONCLUSION

Homosexuality is a broad and intricate topic in the study of human sexuality. We have explored the genetic, hormonal, neuroanatomical, psychological, and sociological aspects of this subject. Although the controversies involved are uncomfortable for some, controversy can motivate people to look at subjects in new ways. This chapter has raised many contentious points, findings, and perspectives, but we always encourage a fair and open-minded approach. Perhaps no other chapter in this book will generate stronger feelings and, we hope, the desire to learn more.

Learning Activities

1. Speculate how a homosexual person trying to conceal his or her gender orientation might feel when others use words like *faggot, fairy, homo, lezzie, or dyke.*

2. In 1990 CBS commentator Andy Rooney commented on a TV special that many of our behaviors hurt our health and can kill us, particularly, "too much alcohol, too much food, drugs, homosexual unions, cigarettes..." Comment on this public pronouncement, and speculate on the likely audience response to such a statement.

3. Here are a few well-known historical and contemporary figures known or thought to have their homosexual and/or bisexual preferences:

Pyotr Ilich Tchaikovsky	Leonardo da Vinci
Oscar Wilde	Michelangelo
Martina Navratilova	T. E. Lawrence (of Arabia)
Noel Coward	Gertrude Stein

   a. Do you think any of these people were so stigmatized by their homosexuality or bisexuality that the quality and/or quantity of their work was adversely affected?

   b. In which cases might an alternative lifestyle have had a positive influence on their careers?

4. Based on your *personal experiences and observations,* do you think that homosexuality is a mental disorder? Explain why or why not.

5. If homosexuals believe that counselors and psychotherapists would focus on their gender orientation instead of their specific emotional or psychological problem, how willing would they be to seek assistance? Similarly, if homosexuals believe that the clergy focuses more on their sexuality than their spirituality, to whom would they turn to meet their religious needs?

6. If, in your own experience, you have noticed that some gay males are effeminate in their mannerisms, which theory of the etiology of homosexuality might best explain this?

7. If a gay or lesbian person was extremely apprehensive about disclosing their homosexuality to others, what might be the *very best consequences* of their decision to come out? What would be the *very worst consequences?*

8. Should a public school system open a separate high school for gay and lesbian students because they are victims of gay bashing in traditional high schools? How might taxpayers react to this expenditure of public monies?

9. In America all citizens are entitled by law to freedom of speech, freedom of assembly, and the right to privacy. Over the years, many minorities have proclaimed the injustices with which they have been treated. Americans of various races, religions, and ethnic groups have spoken out about prejudice, discrimination, and biases. Do you think Americans are getting tired of hearing the concerns of all of these groups?

10. When long-term relationships and marriages don't "work out," a break-up can be a very difficult time for both people. Married heterosexuals often face legal issues and a need for counseling. Yet we never seem to hear very much about how people recover from the same situation in the gay community. Speculate on this situation among gays and lesbians. To whom do they go for support?

Key Concepts

- Homosexuality is the primary psychological and physical erotic attraction to members of one's sex.

- Alfred Kinsey described gender orientation on a sexual continuum ranging from exclusively heterosexual thoughts, feelings, and behaviors to exclusively homosexual thoughts, feelings, and behaviors.

- Regarding different etiological factors in the development of homosexuality, the interactionist perspective holds that different theoretical approaches work together to provide a workable idea of the origins of homosexuality.

- The localization of brain function perspective holds that each specific area of the brain does one thing and one thing only; this approach is controversial.

- Psychoanalysis refers to a theory of human growth and development, a theory of personality, and a method of doing psychotherapy. Sigmund Freud developed the psychoanalytic approach.

- In Freud's psychosexual theory of development, children develop a deep emotional attraction to the parent of the opposite sex. This web of attraction leads to the Oedipal complex in little boys and the Electra complex in little girls.

- Behavioral approaches to the etiology of homosexuality emphasize an individual's first heterosexual interaction in the emergence of homosexual preferences.

- Social learning theory suggests we learn not only through our own behaviors and reinforcement experiences, but also through watching other people behave and experience reinforcements.

- In the "Exotic Becomes Erotic" theory of sexual orientation, children growing up gradually see themselves as fundamentally different from opposite-sex peers. Eventually they perceive opposite sex peers as "dissimilar, unfamiliar, and exotic." Erotic attraction is fundamentally based on experiences with those whom the child perceives as different.
- Queer theory de-emphasizes a person's gender orientation but recognizes that to the extent that homosexuals are seen as different or deviant, society is likely to manifest a cultural and political bias.
- Homophobia is an irrational fear of homosexuals, the possibility of a homosexual encounter, or the recognition of homosexual inclinations in oneself.

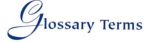

Glossary Terms

concordance rate
ego-dystonic
  homosexuality

fisting
identification
interfemoral
  intercourse

"sissy boy
  syndrome"
tribadism

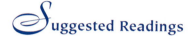

Suggested Readings

Burch, B. (1993). On intimate terms. The psychology of difference in lesbian relationships. Urbana, IL: University of Illinois Press.

Card, C. (1995). Lesbian choices. New York: Columbia University Press.

Hamer, D., & Copeland, P. (1994). The science of desire. The search for the gay gene and the biology of behavior. New York: Simon & Schuster.

Mondimore, F. M. (1996). A natural history of homosexuality. Baltimore: The Johns Hopkins University Press.

Murray, S. O. (1996). American gay. Chicago: The University of Chicago Press.

Plant, R. (1986). The pink triangle. New York: Henry Holt and Company.

10

Fertility, Infertility, Pregnancy, and Childbirth

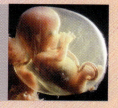

OBJECTIVES

When you finish reading and reviewing this chapter, you should be able to:

1. Distinguish between "fertility" and "fecundity."

2. Define "pronatalism" and explain its social manifestations.

3. Discuss the sequence of events in the fertilization of an ovum, its progression down the fallopian tube, and its implantation in the uterus.

4. Explain measures for increasing the chances of conception. Sketch a basal body temperature chart and explain where the chart indicates the period of peak fertility.

5. Describe the procedure of *in vitro* fertilization and explain why a woman might choose it.

6. Describe GIFT, ZIFT, and intracytoplasmic sperm injection, and note what fertility problems are most frequently treated with each.

7. Explain concerns people have about sexual intercourse during pregnancy, and describe medical opinion about this.

8. Outline the three stages of labor and describe the experience of mother and baby in each.

9. Summarize the *Roe v. Wade* Supreme Court decision, emphasizing elements that have been addressed by state legislatures.

10. Describe the different methods of abortion, the risks of each, and the time frame when health risks to the woman are lowest.

11. Summarize strategies for thinking critically about abortion, and characterize women most likely to choose an abortion.

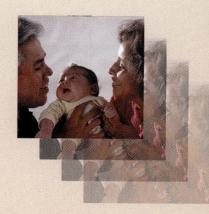

From Dr. Ruth

Pregnancy and childbirth are the most natural of processes, and you might think that by this point in history carrying a baby to term and delivering it would be a simple matter. As a mother of two, believe me when I tell you, it is not. Some aspects of pregnancy are incredibly wonderful, but there are days when you desperately wish someone would find a better way. Then again, when you talk to a couple who has been trying to have a child and can't, their pain quickly makes you realize how lucky parents really are.

I once interviewed several midwives for a book I was writing. One commented that for years she'd told expectant mothers that the period after childbirth would be difficult but manageable, and then she had her own child and couldn't believe how difficult taking care of a newborn baby actually was.

While pregnancy and childbirth are universal experiences, they are also very personal. Remember that as you read this chapter. At times you may feel you are reading a biology textbook, but this chapter contains information that can touch you very, very deeply.

Previous chapters have discussed many different aspects of human sexuality, including historical and philosophical issues, sex and gender, anatomy, physiology, and endocrinology. We have explored many issues related to sexual and reproductive health and well-being, arousal and response, love and relationships. The previous two chapters also dealt with physical expressions of eroticism and intimacy. All of these subjects are related to our thinking, feeling, and behaving as sexual beings. Now we turn to the related topics of fertility, pregnancy, and childbirth.

"Fertility" is a person's actual reproductive *performance,* that is, how many children they have brought into the world. "Fecundity," in contrast, refers to a person's biological *potential* to procreate. Fecundity involves ovulation in women and spermatogenesis in men, while fertility involves becoming pregnant, carrying a pregnancy to term, and giving birth. An earlier chapter's discussion of ovulation and spermatogenesis related to fecundity, while this chapter examines factors affecting fertility.

An important influence on how one thinks about fertility is society's attitude about becoming pregnant and giving birth. In virtually all cultures throughout the world childbirth is seen as a good thing. The uncritical promotion of the goodness and appropriateness of having children is called pronatalism. Although we believe that having children is wonderful if a man and woman want to do so, we also believe that becoming a parent is a choice and not a necessary requirement for a full life. Thus this chapter approaches parenthood as a choice, not an expectation or obligation. Of course, our culture applies many not-so-subtle pressures to have a baby. Many people in their twenties or thirties assume that it's "just time" to have a child—after all, isn't that what their mothers and fathers did? Often one's parents and in-laws make little comments such as, "I really love your new little kitten, but I'd rather have a grandchild. . . ." Our language includes phrases revealing an implicit expectation that one should have a baby: "I'm really excited by my new promotion at work, but I'm not sure I should take it. After all, my biological clock is ticking. . . ."

DECIDING TO BECOME A PARENT

When Is it Time to Have a Baby?

Parental, societal, and often ethnic and religious factors influence whether, when, and how often people have children. One of the world's foremost experts on psychological development in adulthood, Dr. Bernice Neugarten (Fig. 10-1), introduced the term "age clock" to refer to things we assume we should be doing at certain times in our lives. People often formulate (but do not often discuss) a "life plan" or "script" of the important events in our life's journey. Many people build children into their plans. But the issue of when to have children can involve several complicated factors. Should you have children when you're young and the chances of prenatal and birth complications are lowest? Should you wait until after college, or maybe after finishing law/medical/graduate/business school? Should you wait until you have paid off your student loans? Until you're settled in your career? Until you can move out of your apartment into your own home?

Note that even the preceding questions involve certain assumptions. Young people often assume they will experience

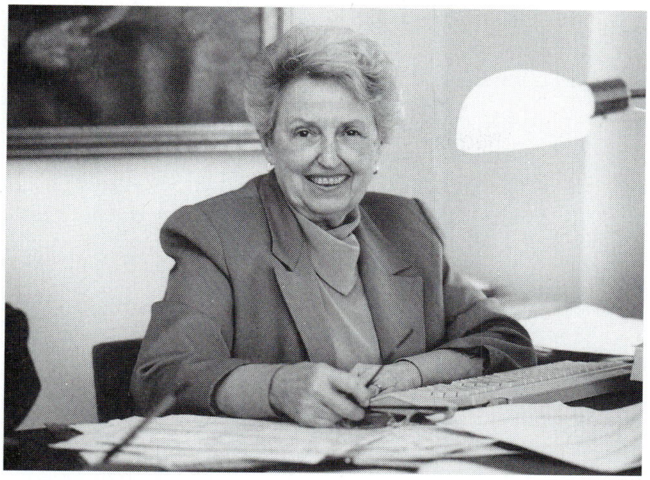

FIGURE 10-1 Dr. Bernice Neugarten, who developed the idea of "age clocks." These comprise a person's ideas about what they feel they should have accomplished or what they should be doing at certain "landmark" times in their lives.

only one period of educational training, one career, or one marriage. In fact, these assumptions often are not true anymore. Most people will have more than one job and more than one period of educational or professional preparation, and many people will have more than one spouse, and perhaps even more than one family. The point here is simple: having a child is a personal choice that is affected by many factors, some of which cannot be controlled.

Factors Affecting the Choice to Become a Parent

Every culture celebrates becoming a parent the first time with a tremendous ritual, a "solemn social act" (La Rossa, 1986). Although becoming a parent is a matter of free choice, society applies pressures to have children. The Judeo-Christian tradition encourages young people to be fruitful and multiply. On the other hand, economic factors may delay the decision to have a child. One's standard of living depends on how much money a couple earns, and often couples wait to have children after attaining a desired lifestyle.

As well, the arrival of a child is not always seen as a blessing. Glenn and McLanahan (1982) have noted that raising a child costs a *tremendous* amount of money. In November of 1999, the U. S. Department of Agriculture estimated that a low-income family will spend $115,020 raising a child born in 1998, an "average" family $156,690, and an upper-income family $228,690—not corrected for anticipated inflation. Additionally, parenting can be emotionally exhausting, frustrating, and thankless, and the presence of a child or children in a household can foster marital problems, conflicts, and power struggles.

Dear Dr. Ruth

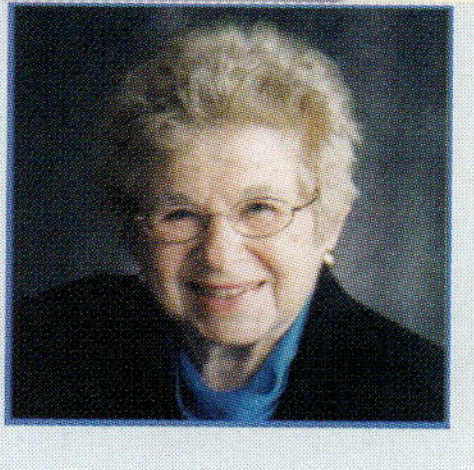

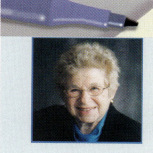

Question:

I am 28 years old, married, and the youngest of three sisters. Both my older sisters are married and have three or four kids. My husband and I want a family but don't think we're ready yet. But both our parents keep saying we're selfish and "wrapped up in ourselves" and it's starting to make me angry. I want to be polite, but firm too. What should I say?

Answer:

As a parent I too do not always agree with every decision my adult children make, but I try to follow an old German saying about grandparents: *Schweigen, Schlucken, Schenken.* This means grandparents should be quiet, swallow their advice, and give gifts. This applies also before becoming grandparents. As a couple, sit down with each set of parents and let them know, firmly but politely, that you plan to have children but that it is not their business to help you decide when. I know this may be difficult. But since they're not going to be there to change every diaper, wake up for every 2 AM feeding, or pay for every bill, it's not their decision to make. They won't be happy with this, but don't argue—just remain firm. Later on, if they still bring it up, just remind them of this discussion and close the subject. You are adults and nobody, not even your parents, can tell you when is the right time to have your children.

Nonetheless, motherhood has a respected status in our society, and wanting to be a "good mother" is for many young women an important part of their identity. More recently, being a "good father" has also gained more social status. In part a result of the feminist movement, women feel less obliged today to follow this imperative and to instead develop a sense of their self-worth apart from their reproductive "performance."

Couples often wonder what impact a child will have on their relationship (Fig. 10-2). Despite the many wonderful feelings of parenthood, there can be several unhappy consequences for a marriage. Bell, Johnson, McGillicuddy-Delisi, and Sigel (1980), cited in Abbott and Walters (1985), have enumerated many potential problems:

(a) lower morale of the parents, often due to fatigue
(b) less satisfying, less frequent marital communication
(c) less equal relations between husband and wife
(d) an increase in the number of rules mothers expect children to follow—although, interestingly, the number of rules diminishes in families of five or more
(e) a decrease in parental attention to other children
(f) an increase in family tensions
(g) less parental attention to the school progress of other children
(h) a decrease in parent-child closeness (except in later-born children)
(i) an increase in parental authoritarian behavior
(j) a decrease in maternal energy
—Adapted from Abbott and Walters 1985, 187-188

Still, most married adults have children, and these negative outcomes are most often balanced by the positive aspects of having a child:

(a) the joy of watching a child grow up
(b) reexperiencing one's own childhood
(c) a powerful sense of feeling loved and needed
(d) feeling one is playing a part in creating the next generation
(e) learning about child development
(f) perpetuating one's family's name and traditions

Many of us when young never question whether we will become parents; we simply assume that sooner or later we will. Having younger siblings in the household offers a glimpse of the pleasures and pitfalls of parenting. Adolescents when babysitting may begin to formulate a life script that includes behaviors they are "rehearsing" when caring for other people's children. Babysitting is like a "real-life role-play" of what many girls have done for years: playing with dolls. Similarly, taking care of a little brother or sister can teach one about infants and children and affect how one feels about becoming a parent. On the other hand, someone who experienced or observed abuse from a parent may have no desire to again be part of a nuclear family with children. The point here is that the decision to become a parent is personal and reflects one's life experiences.

Mature Parenting

It is ironic that it takes no personal maturity at all to become a parent but takes a lot of maturity to be a good, responsible parent. The discussion of love, affection, attachment, and rela-

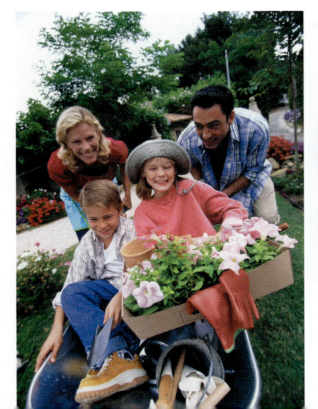

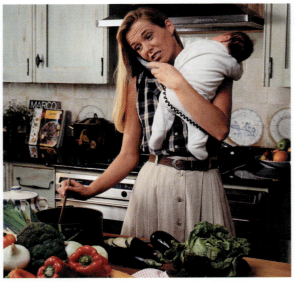

FIGURE 10-2 Children can affect a couples' relationship in different ways. While the experience of parenthood can be very enriching, children can require enormous resources in time, patience, energy, and money.

tionships in Chapter 7 included criteria of maturity in adulthood. Many of these are related to the decision to become a parent. Allport (1961) described *self-extension,* the concept many people have that there is more to life than just looking out for ourselves, taking care of ourselves, and enjoying as much personal pleasure as we can. From the day of childbirth, able parents are continually making personal sacrifices. Allport also wrote about *the ability and inclination to initiate and maintain warm, open relationships with others.* Intimacy and compassion are required to be a good parent, and a prospective parent gains from self-analysis about these qualities. Another important attribute of maturity is *frustration tolerance.* Parenting can be tremendously frustrating at times, and parents must be able to avoid acting aggressively when they become frustrated. Perhaps the most important characteristic of a mature adult outlined by Allport is a *clear set of personal values* that are important to you and obvious in the way you act. When deciding whether to become a parent, consider whether you have the necessary maturity for this difficult challenge. Parenthood requires a long period of selfless generosity, altruism, and constant care and concern, as well as effective long-term financial planning.

Pamela Daniels and Kathy Weingarten's book *Sooner or Later: The Timing of Parenthood in Adult Lives* (1982) is a good discussion about the decision to become a parent. These writers examine the question of "when" to choose to have a baby from different perspectives:

- **The Natural Ideal.** Many couples do not deliberately decide to have a baby. Instead, they share an unspoken intuition when they are prepared for this next step in their lives and marriage. Many couples can't remember discussing the subject; it was always an unquestioned assumption. Some couples decide to try to conceive immediately after marriage, based on religious tradition or expectation. These couples often feel the same way about having more babies. Usually the extended family happily expects the pregnancy and birth.
- **The Brief Wait.** Daniels and Weingarten found this strategy in every generation, race, and religious group in their American sample, especially among middle-class couples with a college education. This couple first wants to get to know one another better, leave the military, graduate from college or professional school, find their first job, travel, or purchase their first home. They feel it necessary to get settled before starting their family. Many young people enjoy their jobs and prefer to spend more time at work without feeling guilty about parenting responsibilities waiting at home. Some couples experience a brief wait because of a fertility problem.
- **Programmatic Postponement.** Some people feel that before they can choose to have a baby, they must grow up more themselves and develop their sense of self. Many feel that they do not yet fully understand the reciprocal expectations of a love relationship. This can be true of both spouses. "Psychological readiness" for parenthood is a common concern, as is the desire to experiment with different lifestyles first. Some couples want to build a strong, intimate marriage before they "invite" children into it. People who postpone having a child for these reasons often say they need more time to learn to manage their household, as is essential when a baby arrives.
- **The Mixed Script.** Often women and men want different things at different times, and couples commonly differ about whether or when to have a baby. This difference of opinion can affect the couple's interaction in many ways, not just in terms of contraception issues and pregnancy. Longstanding resentments and power struggles may occur.
- **No Scenario.** Many people simply don't have a plan at all regarding becoming parents. They may have only a vague idea of what they would like to be doing at different stages of their lives. They simply have a style of taking what comes.

Other studies of the timing of parenthood reveal interesting differences. For example, Hardy, Astone, Brooks-Gunn, Shapiro, and Miller (1998) followed over 1700 inner city children in Baltimore for 30 years and found that women who delayed the birth of their first child until they were at least 25 years old had babies with more fortuitous developmental characteristics and who were more self-sufficient as adults. The later birth of a first child is frequently associated with higher educational attainment of the mother (De Wit & Rajulton, 1992), which might enhance a woman's parenting skills.

Becoming a Parent in Later Adulthood

Not everyone's script is the same, of course, and many people will have more than one job, spouse, and family in their lives. More people are becoming parents with a second or subsequent spouse later in adulthood. Additionally, effective contraception is more inexpensive and convenient than ever before.

Women who say their "biological clock is ticking" mean several different things. Some desire to have a baby when the chances of prenatal and birth complications are lowest; others desire to have a child when one is young and energetic enough to handle the exhausting tasks involved. Still others would like to see their child grow up, marry, and have their own children. In contrast, men often want to delay the birth of their first child so that they can meet early career challenges and then have more time at home to enjoy their baby. In the last 100 years, more and more women have waited longer and longer to have their first baby. A century ago, married women in their late teens and early twenties commonly gave birth to their first babies. Today, more women wait until their mid- to late-twenties (Fig. 10-3). Many more women in their mid- and late-thirties are now having children, a trend true of both white and African American women (Turner, 1992). This is so

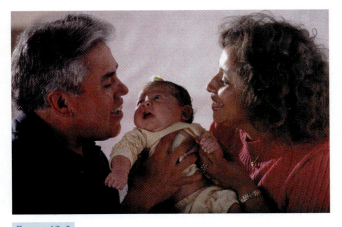

FIGURE 10-3   It is becoming more common for couples to delay a decision to start a family. Involvement in a career, second and subsequent marriages, and the availability of assisted reproductive technologies are some of the factors behind this change.

even though women in their 30s and 40s have greater risks of problems during pregnancy or childbirth.

Daniels and Weingarten studied women who had their first child in their 40s and found a fascinating and diverse group of parents. Many had purposefully delayed their decision to have a child for reasons such as those already described. The decision to become a parent at this age typically involves a sometimes bewildering array of medical technology and diagnostic procedures much different from what younger couples usually experience. These tests and techniques allow analysis of many common risks of later-life pregnancy. For example, "older" women have a higher risk of giving birth to a baby that is abnormal in some way, and amniocentesis can detect those cases in which problems may occur. While younger couples generally view the pregnancy's progression trimester by trimester, older couples often conceptualize their pregnancies in two periods: *before and after* the amniocentesis test (Daniels & Weingarten, 1982). Amniocentesis is discussed more fully in a later section of this chapter.

Daniels and Weingarten found that there were three general types of adjustment to the arrival of a new baby when the parents are at midlife.

- **A Supplementary Experience.** For new parents at midlife who saw the arrival of their newborn as a supplementary experience, the baby's requirements and the parents' resources seemed relatively well matched. Mom and Dad continued their prior roles and responsibilities and found time to love and care for the infant. Their established lifestyle was not overly disrupted, and they seemed able to carry out the additional, and sometimes unpredictable, tasks of first-time mothers and fathers. This is often true of younger couples too.
- **A Whole New Chapter.** For some parents, the demands of parenting were continuous and immense. These women and men entirely changed how they viewed themselves, their lives, and their marriage. Old

habits and behavior patterns no longer seemed flexible enough. The infant didn't join an existing family; it forced the creation of a new one (Daniels & Weingarten, 1982, p. 205). Again, this too is true of younger couples.
- **The Crunch.** In a third version of parenthood at midlife the new mother and father felt overwhelmed. They doubted whether their resources could meet the new demands of parenting. Previous expectations about babies, their marriage, their lifestyle, and being a parent were badly out of sync with the realities of having a child.

The arrival of a newborn at midlife can validate long-held hopes, lead to a whole new life, or create a frustrating awareness of inadequacy and unreadiness. The most common important difference between older and younger couples is that the financial status of the family is usually stronger among older couples. This may provide a greater sense of domestic comfort and security that can enhance parenting in ways younger couples do not often enjoy.

The Decision to Remain Childless

The decision to remain childless is not the same thing as infertility but is a deliberate decision. Because pronatalist biases are common in our society, people who decide that they do not want to have children are often viewed suspiciously by people who have children. They may be seen as self-absorbed adults who think of nothing but themselves—which, of course, is often false. In the years following World War II, for example, many couples, especially those with upward professional and economic dreams, purposefully chose voluntary childlessness (Boyd, 1989). Personal and occupational advancement after the war often led to the decision not to have babies. The same considerations are relevant today. In an extensive longitudinal study of young adults who decided to remain childless (Bram, 1985), two-thirds of the couples who chose this option still had no children 7 years later, while most of those who were delaying their decision to have a baby had children by this time. Generally speaking, people who decided not to have children reported a high degree of life satisfaction and were content with their decision.

A study in Australia (Callan, 1983) revealed that voluntarily childless couples perceived themselves as intelligent, practical, individualistic, self-fulfilled, and well-adjusted, while other individuals who had children described them as selfish, unusual, and to be pitied. Although some couples choose to remain childless as a temporary lifestyle consideration, others report that they experience conflicting demands of work, family, and traditional parenting roles and in general do not like children (Nave-Herz, 1989). Another study showed that American undergraduates felt couples who were voluntarily childless had a significant social stigma, as if these individuals were somehow deprived of a "normal" part of adulthood (Lampman & Dowling-Guyer, 1995). In contrast, couples who were involuntarily childless were frequently evaluated positively.

Jacobson and Heaton (1991) analyzed data from over 13,000 adults in the National Surveys of Families and Households (1987-1988) to reveal that 3.5 % of the men and 2.8 % of the women were childless by choice. This survey revealed variables associated with the decision not to have a child. More highly educated women were less likely to want to become parents, as were those not reporting a religious preference or affiliation, those who reported working more than 40 hours each week, and those who didn't want to work at all.

Recently a pattern of couples with dual income, no kids (DINKs) has become popular in the United States. Many DINKs know early in life that they do not want to have children, while others gradually develop this feeling. Some become DINKs because they delay the decision until it is too late or because they have become too comfortable in a lifestyle free of childrearing obligations. Some simply believe that they wouldn't make responsible mothers and fathers. Despite their well-intentioned motives, many DINKs are openly criticized by those who have children.

Preparing For a Healthy Pregnancy

A healthy young woman who is free of serious health problems, well-nourished, and receiving regular medical attention has an excellent chance of giving birth to a very healthy baby. Except for the mother's age, these factors involve time, care, and making informed decisions before and during the pregnancy. Yet good prenatal care is mostly common sense.

EFFECTS OF MATERNAL AGE

Biologically, a woman's best time to have a baby is during her 20s, although safe, uneventful pregnancies are common both before and after this "window of opportunity." Pregnancy during the teenage years carries a higher risk of complications during pregnancy and childbirth; some experts believe these risks are 4 to 5 times higher than for women in their 20s. After a woman reaches her 30s, the risk of having a child with Down syndrome begins to increase dramatically. With this chromosomal abnormality children have a flattened facial appearance, small folds of skin over the topmost portion of the eyes, a flattened bridge of the nose, small hands and fingers, and short stature. Down syndrome is associated with varying degrees of mental retardation, with an average IQ of about 50 (90 to 110 is normal). The chances of giving birth to a baby with Down syndrome at age 20 are about 1 in 1923, while the chances at age 40 are about 1 in 109 (Daniels and Weingarten, 1982). Scientists don't know exactly how age is related to Down syndrome, but it clearly is. Amniocentesis can tell a couple whether their fetus will be born with Down syndrome and allows them to consider terminating the pregnancy.

TERATOGENS

Anything that can harm the embryo or fetus in the uterus is called a *teratogen*. **Teratology** is the study of birth defects. Many prescription and recreational drugs can harm the developing embryo or fetus. Generally, a teratogen that affects the embryo (the period between the end of the second week of

pregnancy and the end of the eighth week) has the greatest impact because at this time the body's major organ systems are forming and beginning to function. Disruption of this developmental progression can have devastating and permanent effects on the baby's appearance, the functioning of its internal organs, such as the heart and brain, and even its survival. **Fetal alcohol syndrome,** for example, is a condition caused by women drinking alcohol during their pregnancy (usually 3 or more drinks a day) (Abel, 1981); babies are born with physical abnormalities and later often manifest psychological and behavioral problems as well (Fig. 10-4). Most obstetricians recommend that women drink no alcohol at all while they are pregnant.

According to the Council on Scientific Affairs of the American Medical Association (Report 15, June 1999):

> *Alcohol consumption during pregnancy is associated with smaller neonatal head size, neuropathological changes, and electroencephalographic disturbances. Children affected by fetal alcohol syndrome exhibit developmental delay, hyperactivity, delayed motor development, poor psychomotor performance, and visual-perceptual deficits.*

The effects of cocaine on an embryo or fetus can be catastrophic. Cocaine in adults can cause extreme fluctuations in blood pressure, and the same occurs in a fetus if its mother uses cocaine. However, because blood vessels are not yet fully formed in the fetus, rapid and extreme changes in blood pressure can cause vessels to rupture, and prenatal strokes in the fetus often result. Unfortunately, the baby may be born with partial or even complete paralysis, which will last throughout life. Children born to women who use cocaine during their pregnancy may also have learning disabilities and behavioral prob-

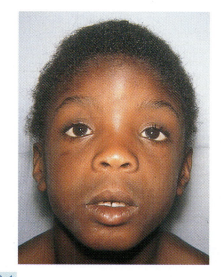

FIGURE 10-4   A child with fetal alcohol syndrome. Slow growth, heart abnormalities, widely spaced eyes, and mental retardation are often associated with this disorder. Problems with motor coordination and memory are also frequently noted.

lems that become apparent only years later. Heroin also can cause life-threatening problems for a newborn. Heroin used by a pregnant woman crosses the placenta and enters the fetus' circulatory system, and the baby is born addicted to heroin. Withdrawal from the addiction can cause serious problems, such as problems regulating body temperature, convulsions, and serious digestive disorders, and in some instances the infant may die as a result of heroin withdrawal.

Smoking tobacco is unhealthy for an individual in many ways, of course, and is especially harmful if a woman smokes during pregnancy. The risks of spontaneous abortion and prematurity are higher among smokers, and babies born to smokers typically have low birth weight. People who smoke also are more likely to drink, multiplying the potential hazards to the developing fetus.

EFFECTS OF DISEASE

Diseases affecting a pregnant women often adversely affect the embryo or fetus, as well. A common example is *rubella,* also called German measles. If a woman contracts this disease during the first trimester the baby is almost certain to be born deaf and have a malformed heart, abnormalities in eye structure, and bone abnormalities in the lower extremities. A woman thinking of becoming pregnant can have a blood test to determine whether she has ever been exposed to rubella and has antibodies. If she has not, she can be vaccinated against rubella before becoming pregnant, but a pregnant woman cannot receive this vaccination. Fortunately, most young children are immunized against rubella when they enter school.

EFFECTS OF STDs

A later chapter discusses sexually transmitted diseases in detail; here we only point out that several STDs can have devastating effects on the developing fetus. Women with syphilis pass the disease to their fetus through the placenta. If a woman has or acquires syphilis after the fourth month of pregnancy, its impact on the fetus is terrible. The infant will be born blind, deaf, and retarded, often with gross physical malformations—or born dead. All women are routinely tested for syphilis during their first prenatal visit, and many states require a blood test in order to get a marriage license.

In a woman with active gonorrhea at the time of childbirth, the infant will pass through an infected birth canal and the bacteria will infect the newborn's eyes. Therefore silver nitrate eyedrops are always applied (regardless of the possibility of an STD) or antibiotics used, or blindness can result. Babies born to mothers with active *chlamydia* run similar risks when they pass through an infected vagina and are more likely to develop an eye infection or pneumonia or die later of sudden infant death syndrome.

Women with active genital herpes during a vaginal delivery face a very serious potential birth-related outcome. Genital herpes is a viral STD, and about half of all newborns exposed to it during birth will develop encephalitis, a serious brain infection, and die. Half of those who survive are likely to be permanently blind. When a woman has an active outbreak of gen-

ital herpes, delivering her baby by Cesarean section avoids the risks of infecting the newborn.

The most serious sexually transmitted disease is AIDS. One fourth of the babies born to HIV-positive women have the virus at birth. It is not known why this happens to some infants and not to others. The virus is also present in the mother's milk. HIV-positive babies are born with head and face abnormalities and retarded growth.

EFFECTS OF EXERCISE

In recent decades health professionals have learned much about the benefits of maternal prenatal aerobic exercise. The American College of Obstetricians and Gynecologists recommends brisk walking, swimming, and stationary cycling as safe, health-enhancing forms of exercise during pregnancy (Table 10-1). Moderate tennis and jogging are also acceptable for women who engaged in these activities *before* their pregnancy and feel that they have the coordination and endurance to continue with modest exertion. Activities in which a pregnant woman might fall should be avoided. Brisk walking is a safe, convenient, effective form of exercise appropriate for virtually all women through most of their pregnancy. Exercise at high levels of exertion is unnecessary because even moderate activity can maintain cardiovascular fitness. Women should avoid exercise that would cause their heart rate to exceed 140

TABLE 10-1

Health Guidelines During Pregnancy

Dietary Issues

Fruits and vegetables: Eat four or more half-cup servings of fruits and vegetables each day, especially those rich in Vitamin A and natural fiber. Fruit and vegetable juices are also excellent.

Breads and cereals: Eat four servings of enriched breads and cereals each day. Select whole grain breads whenever possible.

Meat, eggs, and beans: Fish, poultry, eggs, red meats, nuts, and beans. These are all concentrated sources of protein. Eat three servings each day.

Dairy products: Milk, yogurt, and cheeses are all rich in calcium and protein. Drink four 8 ounce glasses of milk each day. Consult your physician if you can not eat dairy products.

Water: Drink 8 glass of water each day.

Weight Gain

Most doctors recommend a 25-30 pound weight gain throughout the course of pregnancy.

What You Should Avoid

Alcohol

Cigarettes

Medications unless prescribed by your doctor

Street drugs and narcotics

Caffeine

Exposure to sexually transmitted disease

What About Exercise?

Walking and swimming are excellent types of exercise for pregnant women. Stretching exercises developed especially for pregnant women are helpful too.

beats per minute and activities that would cause overheating (over 101° Fahrenheit). Saunas and hot tubs should be avoided throughout pregnancy because high body temperatures can cause some birth defects. The body temperature can exceed 102° Fahrenheit when in a sauna or hot tub. After the third month of pregnancy, a woman should avoid exercising on her back, which could cause a reduced heart rate, reduced blood pressure, dizziness, and a reduced flow of blood to the fetus (*The PDR Family Guide to Women's Health and Prescription Drugs,* 1994).

EFFECTS OF DIET

Nutrition is basic to women's overall health throughout life, and during pregnancy it also affects the development of the embryo or fetus. A woman's diet and the amount of weight she gains have a major impact on the baby's health. The ideal amount of weight to gain in pregnancy depends on what the woman weighs when she becomes pregnant. If she is underweight, the recommended weight gain is 28 to 40 pounds. Women of normal weight should gain 25 to 35 pounds, and overweight women should gain 15 to 25 pounds. Usually weight gain in the first trimester is 2 to 4 pounds (*The PDR Family Guide to Women's Health and Prescription Drugs,* 1994). Pregnant women should consume about 2,500 calories a day. Most people's diets have sufficient nutrients to support the developing baby, although usually pregnant women need an iron supplement. Folic acid, calcium, and zinc requirements also increase during pregnancy. Folic acid supplements are associated with normal development of the central nervous system and a low risk of spinal cord defects. Most obstetricians recommend vitamin supplements during the second and third trimesters.

THE DYNAMICS OF FERTILIZATION AND IMPLANTATION

Chapter 4 described factors that determine ovulation and spermatogenesis. **Fertilization,** or conception, refers to the union of a sperm and an egg. Until recently, scientists were not sure exactly how a sperm penetrates an ovum. Figure 10-5 depicts a normal sperm and a normal egg. Relative to their incredibly small size, sperm have an immense swim to accomplish before getting near the egg.

Fertilization usually occurs in the upper one-third of the fallopian tube after the egg is released from the ovary in the middle of a woman's menstrual cycle. After intercourse with a man with a normal sperm count, of the possible 500 million sperm left in the vagina, a total of about 400 sperm will reach the region of the fallopian tube containing the ovum. Sperm cells are among the smallest in the human body, measuring no more than about 2/1000ths of an inch. Eggs are much larger and are barely visible to the unaided eye, measuring less than 1 millimeter in diameter. Most reproductive endocrinologists believe that sperm remain motile and capable of fertilizing an

egg for 48 hours after intercourse, and sperm have been found swimming vigorously in the female reproductive tract several days after intercourse. Although it is a long swim from the vagina to the top of the fallopian tubes, sperm can reach the egg as soon as an hour after intercourse, although most take much longer. Sperm do not swim in random directions; there is evidence that ova secrete chemicals that attract sperm to the egg (Angier, 1992).

An egg contains half the chromosomes necessary for the creation of a new human being, as well as nutrients that meet the energy needs of the rapidly developing cell mass after fertilization. The ovum is surrounded with a thick, gelatin-like layer called the *zona pellucida.* To fertilize an egg, a sperm must first penetrate this sticky layer, but sperm are built to do this (Fig. 10-5). A sperm has three main parts: head, mid-section, and tail (see Fig. 4-27). The whip-like motion of the tail propels the sperm in a wiggle-like motion. The mid-section contains *mitochondria,* tiny little structures that break down carbohydrates to produce energy to fuel the long swim. Mitochondria are found in most body cells. The head of the sperm contains the chromosomal material for fertilization. A little capsule on the tip of the head, called an *acrosome* contains the enzyme *hyaluronidase,* which is essential for fertilization.

An ovum making its journey down the fallopian tube is covered with protective *cumulus cells.* Sperm surrounding the ovum must force their way through this layer of cumulus cells. Some investigators believe the ovum secretes a substance that attracts sperm during their final swim up the fallopian tube (Roberts, 1991). It is not known whether the ovum itself secretes an attractant substance or the fluids that surround it. Researchers are studying this issue in hopes of developing new treatments for some types of infertility or possibly advancing contraceptive technology. A sperm cell that has penetrated this layer of cells can bind to a sperm-receptor molecule in the zona pellucida. Investigators have discovered a specific protein molecule called P34H on the surface of human sperm that seems necessary for the early binding of the sperm to the zona pellu-

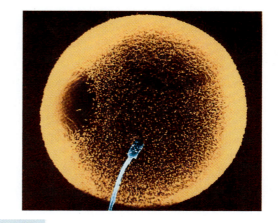

FIGURE 10-5 Scanning electron micrograph of a human sperm fertilizing an ovum.

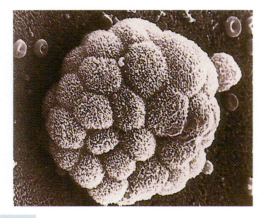

FIGURE 10-6   Scanning electron micrograph of a human blastocyst 4 or 5 days after the ovum has been fertilized.

cida (Itzhaki, 1996). This substance is added to sperm while passing through the epididymis. When sperm bind to the ovum, the acrosome releases its enzyme, which begins to break down the zona pellucida. A sperm cell that penetrates the zona pellucida then enters the ovum, and cell membranes of the egg and sperm fuse. This causes a chemical change in the tiny space between the egg and the zona pellucida that makes the sticky, gelatin-like covering impenetrable to other sperm so that the egg cannot be fertilized by more than one sperm. When the chromosomes from the egg and the chromosomes from the sperm become enclosed within two *pronuclei,* and these fuse, the fertilized egg becomes a *zygote,* and cellular division and development begin. All this takes place high in the fallopian tube (Fig. 10-6).

Scientists for decades have studied the timing of sexual intercourse in relation to ovulation and the most likely time to result in fertilization. The ovum remains fertilizable for about 48 hours after ovulation. Must sperm be present before ovulation for fertilization to occur, or can they be present any time during this 48 hour period? A systematic study of this question analyzed a sample of 221 healthy women who wanted to become pregnant after stopping taking birth control pills (Wilcox, Weinberg, & Baird, 1995). They kept daily records of when they had intercourse, and daily urine samples were analyzed to measure the metabolites of estrogen and progesterone to provide evidence about the time of ovulation. After 625 menstrual cycles in these 221 women (an average of 3 months for each subject), 192 became pregnant, with two-thirds of these pregnancies resulting in a live birth. Conception oc-

Other Countries, Cultures, and Customs

SEXUAL PRESELECTION OF MALES IN OTHER COUNTRIES

In many places in the world couples desire a boy baby. This is especially true in China, where couples are encouraged to have only one child and there are economic penalties for having two or more children. Coale and Banister (1994) studied cohorts (groups of people born in a similar time-span) in China of people born from the 1930s on. In every cohort studied there was a significant discrepancy between the numbers of males and females at the time of their first census. In China, as well as some other countries preferring males, there are thousands of "missing" female children. An implication is that girl babies have lower chances of surviving, probably as a result of selective infanticide of female newborns. Even today, proportionately fewer females are born, probably because of an increasing use of sex-selective abortion.

Liu and Rose (1995) studied the social characteristics of 809 couples attending a sex preselection clinic in Great Britain. The ethnic origins of many of these couples seemed to suggest cultural influences on the desirability of having a baby of a particular sex, usually male. Among these couples, 57.8% were of Indian origin, 32% were European, and 3.6% Chinese. Couples who wanted to have a boy already had an average of 0.09 boys in their family and an average of 2.70 girls. Couples wanting to have a girl already had an average of 2.46 boys in their family and an average of 0.14 girls. Obviously, the sexes of children already in the family strongly affect why people seek sex preselection, or "family balancing" as it is sometimes called. Interestingly, over 80% of these couples said that they wanted to have another child even if they could not preselect its sex. Generally, Asian and Middle-Eastern couples who visited the clinic preferred a boy.

Because there is less cultural pressure in the U.S. to have sons, many Americans do not readily understand the desire of people in other cultures to have a child of a particular sex.

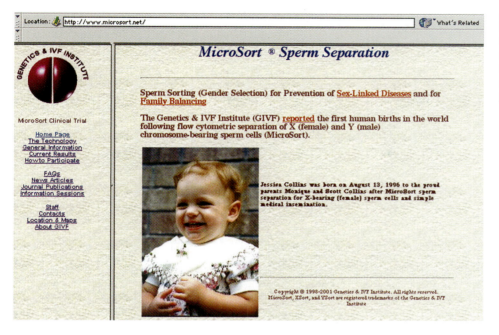

Location: http://www.microsort.net/　　What's Related

MicroSort ® Sperm Separation

GENETICS & IVF INSTITUTE

MicroSort Clinical Trial

Home Page
The Technology
General Information
Current Results
How to Participate

FAQs
News Articles
Journal Publications
Information Sessions

Staff
Contacts
Location & Maps
About GIVF

Sperm Sorting (Gender Selection) for Prevention of <u>Sex-Linked Diseases</u> and for <u>Family Balancing</u>

The Genetics & IVF Institute (GIVF) <u>reported</u> the first human births in the world following flow cytometric separation of X (female) and Y (male) chromosome-bearing sperm cells (MicroSort).

Jessica Collins was born on August 13, 1996 to the proud parents Monique and Scott Collins after MicroSort sperm separation for X-bearing (female) sperm cells and simple medical insemination.

Copyright © 1998-2001 Genetics & IVF Institute. All rights reserved. MicroSort, XSort, and YSort are registered trademarks of the Genetics & IVF Institute

FIGURE 10-7 Technologies are available that facilitate highly accurate sexual preselection. One common reason for using these involves balancing the number of girls and boys in a family.

curred *only* when intercourse took place during the six days *preceding* the day of ovulation, and pregnancy never occurred when intercourse took place after the day of ovulation, even though the ovum can survive for 2 days. In this study the timing of sexual intercourse was not related to the baby's sex. When intercourse took place 5 days before ovulation, there was a 10% chance of pregnancy occurring, rising to 33% when intercourse took place on the day of ovulation.

Choosing a Child's Sex

Many couples when asked if they want a boy or a girl say, "We don't care, just as long as it's healthy." Some couples definitely have a preference, however, for various reasons. In some societies a boy is desired to carry on the family name, work in the family business or farm, or assume a position of local political authority. Different societies attribute different levels of importance and privilege to males and females. For example, in the People's Republic of China, India, Bangladesh, and Egypt there are explicit preferences for male children. **Sex preselection,** as this is called, involves many ethical and medical issues.

Techniques exist that separate the two kinds of sperm so that one or the other can be used to selectively fertilize an egg using *in vitro* fertilization, a technique discussed further in a later section. Such techniques provide a means to predetermine the sex of the baby (Fig. 10-7).

Progression of the Fertilized Egg to the Uterus

Within 24 hours after the embryonic period begins, cells in the developing zygote begin to divide in a process called *cleavage*. The fertilized egg's journey down the fallopian tube takes about 6 days (Fig. 10-8). Then it implants in the lining of the uterus, the endometrium, which has been prepared by female sex hor-

mones to receive it. One day after fertilization there are two cells instead of one. On day 2 there are 4 cells, and on day 3 there are 8. When implantation occurs, the developing embryo is called a *blastocyst*. The blastocyst remains inside the zona pellucida until just before it implants itself in the endometrium; it actually "hatches" from this membrane. Soon after the blastocyst is implanted in the endometrium, profound changes occur in the tissue adjacent to it. The wall of the uterus becomes highly vascularized to ensure plenty of available oxygen for the fragile developing mass of cells. As described in Chapter 4, the corpus luteum produces large amounts of progesterone at this time to keep the endometrium soft, spongy, and healthy, thus further guaranteeing the continuation of pregnancy. The embryo once firmly implanted in the lining of the uterus begins to secrete a hormone called **human chorionic gonadotropin**, which stimulates the corpus luteum to continue its output of progesterone to support the early pregnancy. This continues until the 11th or 12th week of embryonic development, at which time the placenta itself secretes significant amounts of progesterone to maintain the pregnancy.

Sometimes the blastocyst is not implanted in the lining of the uterus but instead nestles into the peritoneal cavity surrounding the ovary or in the ovary itself, or it may get "stuck" in the fallopian tube. An increased density of blood vessels occurs also when implantation takes place where it shouldn't, for the continued growth and development of the embryo. Implantation occurring anywhere outside the uterus is called an **ectopic pregnancy,** which can be dangerous because the blood vessels surrounding the embryo in its inappropriate location can rupture and cause significant internal bleeding in the mother. Because these changes often cause abdominal pain and sometimes vaginal bleeding, medical intervention should be sought for these symptoms at any time during pregnancy.

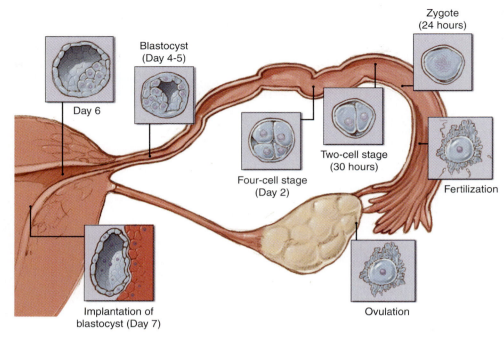

Zygote
(24 hours)

Blastocyst
(Day 4-5)

Day 6

Four-cell stage
(Day 2)

Two-cell stage
(30 hours)

Fertilization

Implantation of
blastocyst (Day 7)

Ovulation

Figure 10-8 After an ovum has been fertilized, it takes about 6 days to reach the lining of the uterus where it becomes implanted. Various stages of cellular division are taking place during this time.

Most of the time these early weeks of pregnancy proceed well. The pregnant woman seldom has any indications she is carrying an embryo. It is too early for the symptoms of early pregnancy, such as "morning sickness" or fatigue to become apparent. Still, some women say that they "just knew" that they had conceived at a particular time and are "aware" of life growing within them even at this early time. Although these mysterious thoughts and feelings should not be discounted, there are no physiological signs of pregnancy at this time. Data do support, however, that women who are trying to become pregnant are more sensitive to early signs of pregnancy when they do occur (Miller, 1978). Rita Seiden-Miller studied 49 women pregnant with their first child in three groups of subjects: those who had definitely planned conception, those who had "sort of" planned conception, and those who had not planned or anticipated conception. Women who "sort of" planned their pregnancy or didn't plan their pregnancy at all were far more likely to believe that they were pregnant only after receiving confirmation from their doctor. These data were collected before over-the-counter pregnancy tests became widely available, and confirmation today is as close as the local pharmacy.

INCREASING THE CHANCES OF PREGNANCY

Earlier chapters have already discussed some of the factors that facilitate or diminish the chances of pregnancy occurring. Little "specialized" knowledge is involved, and increasing the chances of becoming pregnant involves only a few simple, inexpensive measures. The key is determining as accurately as possible when during the menstrual cycle a woman is likely to ovulate. A couple who knows this can decide when to have unprotected intercourse. We believe pregnancies ideally begin only after a couple has spoken at length about having a child together and both agree they want a child. We also hope that a couple planning a child enjoys an open, communicative, monogamous relationship and shares each other's best interests. As well, they should be certain neither has a sexually transmitted disease. If there is a risk that the baby may inherit some genetic abnormality or problem, then the couple should first discuss the matter with their physician or a genetic counselor. Finally, a couple needs to have considered the financial obligations involved with having a baby.

Timing of Sexual Intercourse

We described earlier the research of Wilcox and colleagues (1995) that demonstrated that the chances of conception are highest after intercourse in the 5-6 day period preceding ovulation. These results have not been replicated, however, and there is still some controversy about a woman's fertility the day or two immediately after ovulation. Nonetheless, improving the chances for conception depend on determining exactly when ovulation occurs. A woman can learn in several ways when she is ovulating or about to ovulate, as we first described in Chapter 4.

First, recall that some women can actually *feel themselves ovulate.* A fertilizable ovum being released from the ovary is sometimes accompanied by lower abdominal discomfort called "mittleschmerz," which in German means "pain in the middle" (of her body, not her menstrual cycle). According to Wilcox and colleagues, having intercourse shortly before ovulation or on the day of ovulation provides the greatest opportunity for conception to occur. Ovulation is often accompanied by a clear, odorless vaginal discharge, which is usually obvious as a slight wetness in a woman's underpants, usually indicating that ovulation has just occurred. Since the chances of conception are best when sperm are already present when ovulation occurs, however, it is more helpful if the couple knows when ovulation is *about to happen.* Fortunately, this is relatively easy to do with a basal body temperature chart.

THE BASAL BODY TEMPERATURE CHART

The basal body temperature chart is described in Chapter 4 and only summarized again here. Figure 10-9 shows that the basal body temperature is relatively unchanging in the days before ovulation is about to occur. It is normally lower than the "normal" body temperature of 98.6° Fahrenheit. Just before ovulation occurs, the basal body temperature dips, sometimes as much a half to a full degree Fahrenheit. This clearly signals that ovulation is about to occur, probably in the next 24 hours. This is the best time to have intercourse to become pregnant. The next morning the basal body temperature has risen, sometimes by as much as a full degree Fahrenheit. This means that she *has* ovulated. The basal body temperature chart is a valuable tool to help a couple know when intercourse is most likely to lead to conception. The chart can also reveal that a woman is *not* ovulating, something she should discuss with her physician if she would like to become pregnant.

Note that Figure 10-9 illustrates a basal body temperature chart for a woman who ovulates regularly and lives a stress-free, healthy, orderly life. Many women will not have such an ideal chart, and many lifestyle issues can make a basal body temperature chart look relatively chaotic. Not all women ovulate regularly. Many women experience significant, intermittent stress throughout a monthly cycle. Catching a cold or flu or being chronically sleep-deprived also disrupts the temperature chart and can make it difficult or impossible to know if a woman has

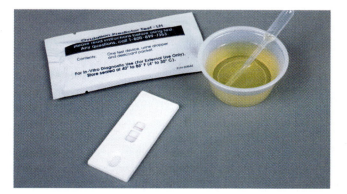

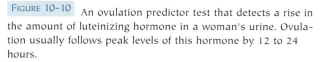

FIGURE 10-10   An ovulation predictor test that detects a rise in the amount of luteinizing hormone in a woman's urine. Ovulation usually follows peak levels of this hormone by 12 to 24 hours.

ovulated or when. Even women with highly regular menstrual cycles vary somewhat in the timing of ovulation because of stresses. Still, a woman who is not taking birth control pills and wants to know whether she ovulates regularly can use a basal thermometer to observe her cycle of fertility.

OVER-THE-COUNTER OVULATION PREDICTION TESTS

A more reliable way of predicting ovulation than using the basal body temperature method is to use an over-the-counter ovulation test kit (Fig. 10-10). Such kits can detect the increase in luteinizing hormone (LH) that signals that ovulation will soon occur; if the couple wants to conceive a child, the day of this increase is a particularly good time to have intercourse. Women vary in how much LH their pituitary gland secretes before ovulation and also in how long the elevated hormone level lasts. Kits sensitive to LH in a woman's urine are most likely to indicate when she is likely to ovulate. The kits available today include one type in which a test stick is exposed during urination and another in which a little cup is filled with urine and the test cassette added to it. Generally a number of urine tests are done over several days, and each kit comes with supplies for 5 or 6 tests. Different tests take from only a few minutes to as long as an hour to indicate the presence or absence of LH. Ovulation prediction tests cost more than over-the-counter pregnancy tests, but each kit includes several tests. The most sensitive ovulation prediction tests work very well in about 85% of the women who use them (*Consumer Reports,* October 1996). If a woman's release of LH is comparatively brief (less than 10 hours), she may need to test herself twice in one day to detect its presence.

CERVICAL MUCUS VISCOSITY

The word "viscosity" means "stickiness." Throughout a woman's menstrual cycle, regular changes occur in the viscosity of cervical mucus that indicate when ovulation is about to occur. Checking this is simple, takes very little time, and costs nothing, but it may be a less accurate indication of when ovulation is about to occur. The woman simply inserts a clean finger into her vagina and pulls out a small amount of mucus and rolls it between finger and thumb. Throughout most of the

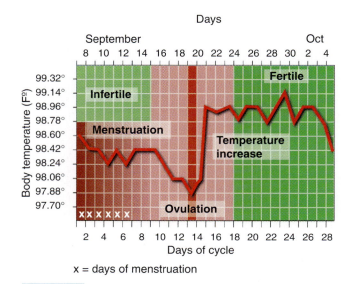

FIGURE 10-9   A basal body temperature chart, indicating cyclic changes in the early morning body temperature of a woman who is not using oral contraceptives.

menstrual cycle the cervical mucus is dense, white, and opaque. A day or so before ovulation, however, the cervical mucus is stringy, clear, and slippery. The woman may separate her finger and thumb and see a thin fiber of mucus between them.

For a number of days after a woman's menstrual period there is virtually no mucus at all. Then for several days the mucus is white or yellowish and thick, and then it becomes clear and stringy. When she is no longer fertile, the cervical mucus again becomes thick and cloudy. It takes time, patience, and practice to use this method to determine when one is ovulating, but it can be used in conjunction with ovulation test kits or basal body temperature charts to more accurately determine when the period of peak fertility is occurring.

Although taking one's temperature every morning or checking one's cervical mucus might seem inconvenient, anything that helps to predict ovulation can improve the chances of becoming pregnant, which can be important for a couple having difficulty having children.

A "Tipped" Uterus

In most women, the uterus tilts forward toward the bladder, but in one in five women it tilts backward toward the rectum. This is called a "tipped" or retroflexed uterus and for some women is associated with discomfort during intercourse. It was once thought that a retroflexed uterus might cause problems in conceiving, carrying or delivering a baby, but doctors now know this is incorrect (Reinisch, 1990). Because of the different orientation of the uterus and cervix with respect to the vagina, the chances of conception might be improved with rear-entry intercourse to provide a more direct path of sperm from the penis to the cervix. This way, there will be less leakage of semen from the vagina after intercourse and more sperm to swim through the cervix into the uterus.

Different Intercourse Positions

Except for women with a retroflexed uterus, the man-on-top intercourse position maximizes the chances of conception, especially with the woman drawing her knees up high toward her shoulders (Fig. 10-11A). It might even help to prop up her hips with a pillow during intercourse so that semen is deposited in direct proximity to the cervix at ejaculation. This position maximizes the opportunity for sperm to swim through the cervix. The man should ensure that his penis is as far inside his partner as possible when he ejaculates, should hold as still as he can during ejaculation, and should withdraw as slowly as possible. If the woman lies still on her back for up

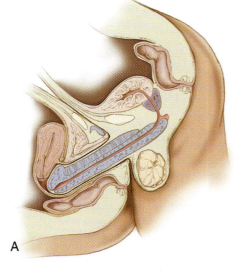

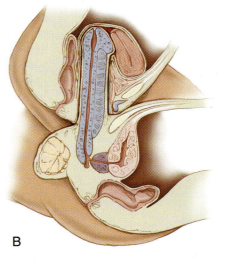

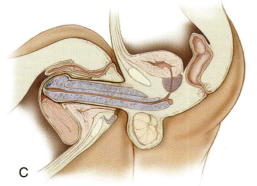

FIGURE 10-11 Cross-sectional drawings of three intercourse positions. (A) man-on-top, (B) woman-on-top, and (C) rear-entry. The man-on-top positions maximizes the chances of conception.

to an hour after intercourse, this minimizes the amount of semen that leaks out the vagina. Some physicians even recommend that the woman insert a tampon wrapped with plastic wrap into her vagina after intercourse to act as a plug to limit the semen that leaks out the vagina, but we know of no research studies showing this is effective. Generally, the woman-on-top position is less effective for conception (Fig. 10-11B), as is the rear-entry position (Fig. 10-11C). Note, however, that getting up right after intercourse does *not* necessarily lower the chances of conception, nor does having intercourse while standing up or in other positions, so no one should consider these "safe" positions when trying to avoid conceiving.

Stress and Fertility

Chapter 4 discussed some factors affecting spermatogenesis in men, such as high testicular temperatures that can reduce sperm production. The effect of environmental or psychosocial stress on fertility is less well understood in both women and men. Both animal and human studies have demonstrated that stress adversely affects fertility, although among humans this is most clear only at very high levels of stress, such as among inmates of concentration camps (Negro-Vilar, 1993). The effects of more common forms of stress are more difficult to ascertain. Generally speaking, people experience stress when they must make adjustments in their lives, and the greater the need for adjustment the greater the amounts of stress people report. Much of what is known about the effects of stress on fertility is anecdotal. One large, systematic study of the effects of stress on semen quality (Fenster, Katz, Wyrobek, Pieper, Rempel, Oman, and Swan, 1997) provided a better understanding of this relationship. These investigators studied the effects of job stress and life-event stress on semen quality. Sperm count, sperm motility, and semen volume seemed unaffected by job stress and most life-event stress. However, in men who experienced the death of a close family member, sperm motility was diminished and the number of abnormal sperm forms in their semen increased. Again, the impact of stress on fertility seems clearest at higher levels of psychosocial stress. Vartiainen, Saarikoski, Halonen, and Rimon (1994) studied the effects of lifestyle and personality factors in 191 healthy women who had not had a child. Women who had a low number of negative life events and few psychosomatic symptoms had higher than average fertility. It remains to be seen whether the reverse is true: whether a high number of negative life events and many psychosomatic symptoms are associated with fertility problems. Psychosocial stresses have been clearly related to changes in the progress of pregnancy, however. Vartiainen, Suonio, Halonen, and Rimon (1994) found that certain stressors were clearly related to complications of pregnancy, such as low birth weight. These included negative life events, anxiety, and physical and mental work stress. A woman's personality traits, strategies of coping with stress, and her social support system did not seem to offset the negative effects of these factors.

Some scientists speculate that the elevated levels of "stress hormones," which generally adversely affect our health, may also affect sperm production and ovulation. These hormones

are secreted by the adrenal glands and are often referred to as "catecholamines." More will be known about these effects in the future.

Eating Disorders and Fertility

A relationship exists between eating disorders and fertility. In virtually all mammals, food intake is closely related to reproductive capacity in females. If a woman eats too little, or far too little, her body automatically diverts resources from regular ovulation and menstruation to other functions related to survival. A woman's reproductive physiology depends on the hourly availability and breakdown of food. This is more important than her general body configuration or ratio of lean body mass to fat (Wade, Schneider, & Li, 1996). If nutrition is inadequate for any reason (famine, too much exercise, or eating disorders), temporary or long-term infertility results.

A study of 66 infertility clinic patients found 16.7% to suffer from an eating disorder (Stewart, Robinson, Goldbloom, & Wright, 1990). Because many women with eating disorders are of normal weight and appearance, and because eating disorders are stigmatized, these researchers caution gynecologists to explore more carefully patients' dietary habits and consider the possibility of eating disorders. Eating disorders can have many effects on a woman's reproductive functions (Stewart, 1992). These include a lack of ovulation, extremely light periods, lack of menstruation, lowered sex drive, temporary infertility, extreme morning sickness during pregnancy, small weight gain during pregnancy, small for gestational age newborns, low birth weight newborns, increased chances of illness in the newborn, and difficulties in breastfeeding. More so than ever before, obstetricians today are encouraged to inquire carefully about a woman's nutritional status and the possibility of eating disorders.

Discovering the Pregnancy

Women, men, and couples react in various ways to learning the woman is pregnant. Some women and men begin to assess the suitability of their home and car and consider their financial security; some are motivated to purchase unemployment or life insurance. Knowing one is about to become a parent is an adult reality and a significant transition in a person's psychological growth and development. A couple who shares society's pronatalism may feel they are more "normal" now and have entered a natural next stage in life. Of course, with an unplanned and unwanted pregnancy, people have very different feelings. Shock, fear, anger, anxiety, and depression may occur and may persist for some time. An individual who considers terminating the pregnancy with an abortion has much to think about and discuss and very important decisions to make. A single woman who plans to have and keep her baby may feel apprehensive and uncertain about the future and must consider the possibility of raising a child without a partner and what that means to her lifestyle and financial situation. It may be necessary to interrupt or terminate one's educational plans. In all situations, however, learning that one is pregnant is a milestone event in a person's life likely to be remembered, either warmly or with dismay, forever.

A COUPLE PREPARES FOR PARENTHOOD

Regular prenatal care is essential for a healthy pregnancy and the birth of a healthy child. Unfortunately in the United States, women of all ages, educational levels, marital statuses, and economic standing do not have access to capable obstetric care, and some women do not seek such services even when they are available, convenient, and affordable. Yet of all human life span stages, the prenatal period is the most important because events taking place now will affect the degree to which the child will have the capacity to reach its full inherited potential. Without good prenatal care, many kids just don't have a chance. Later sections will describe tests included in good prenatal care.

Knowing that one is about to become a parent raises many issues and priorities, and life will literally never be the same again. Most people re-think their roles and new ones they will soon adopt. Issues such as education and training take on new meaning, along with issues of job security, income, health care benefits, and financial planning. The couple begins to clearly define their responsibilities, obligations, and dreams in relation to a child. It's an exciting time, but at the same time a little frightening. The baby's arrival may reveal unrealistic expectations and dreams, and the couple may face some hard pragmatic decisions. If their relationship has not been strong up to this point, pregnancy and the arrival of a child seldom improve things, and a baby may reveal or exacerbate preexisting problems.

SEXUAL INTERCOURSE DURING PREGNANCY

Many couples wonder whether sex during pregnancy could in any way hurt the pregnancy or the embryo or fetus inside the uterus. Studies of the effects of intercourse during pregnancy have failed to reveal any adverse outcomes for the pregnancy, the birth process, or the newborn (Klebanoff, Nugent, & Rhoads, 1984). Most obstetricians tell their patients that so long as a woman doesn't experience discomfort, intercourse up to the beginning of labor is just fine. However, women who experience vaginal bleeding or uterine cramping are discouraged from having sex during pregnancy. Sexual interest generally declines among women as their pregnancy progresses, although not usually in their male partners (Barclay, McDonald, & O'Loughlin, 1994), and there is an overall decline in the frequency of sexual intercourse. Nonetheless, couples not having intercourse often engage in other avenues of erotic expression. Barclay, McDonald, and O'Loughlin (1994) explored the sexual expression of 25 couples during pregnancy and found that 19 of the couples continued to practice oral sex regularly and 3 had anal intercourse during pregnancy, illustrating that alternative, non-intercourse avenues of intimacy are not uncommon during pregnancy. In the past some people worried that intercourse during pregnancy might be related to premature birth, but a recent study (Kurki & Ylikorkala, 1993) found no

such statistical relationship in a sample of over 400 women. However, early delivery is statistically associated with frequent intercourse along with the presence of bacterial vaginosis (Read & Klebanoff, 1993).

Because a pregnant woman's protruding abdomen may make the man-on-top position uncomfortable, couples often explore other intercourse positions (Fig. 10-12). The side-to-side position (either face-to-face or rear-entry) allows the woman to comfortably recline on her side while being penetrated and also lets her partner caress her breasts and buttocks (Fig. 10-12a). Similarly, the woman-on-top and rear-entry positions allow comfortable intercourse without putting pressure on the woman's abdomen. Physical intimacy is often important in a couple's relationship, and there is little reason to significantly alter a couple's sexual expression during pregnancy.

DEVELOPMENT OF THE EMBRYO AND FETUS

Pregnancy Tests

A urine or blood test may confirm a pregnancy. Since both detecting a substance produced by the membranes surrounding an embryo, called human chorionic gonadotropin (HCG). Urine tests can detect traces of this hormone by the 21st day of pregnancy. Blood tests are more sensitive and can detect a pregnancy as early as 8 days after conception. Such tests are available from primary care physicians, gynecologists, and often local health departments, and home pregnancy tests available at drugstores are sensitive enough to detect traces of HCG in a woman's urine by the first day of a missed menstrual cycle. The amount of HCG increases rapidly during the first few days of pregnancy, doubling every two to three days (*Consumer Reports,* October 1996). These tests are quick and highly reliable although they may produce a false-positive result if a woman has recently given birth, taken certain fertility drugs, or had a miscarriage, when there may still be high levels of HCG in her blood even though she is not pregnant. In one type of home pregnancy test the woman puts the indicator in her urine stream, and in another she collects her urine in a cup and then tests it. Although the test directions indicate that they can be used at any time, the largest amounts of HCG usually occur in the first morning urine. The test registers the presence or absence of pregnancy in 2 to 5 minutes, and women are instructed to read the result right after the recommended waiting period because waiting too much longer allows a "positive" result to turn "negative." Most home pregnancy tests have good or excellent sensitivity and typically cost under $10 each. Women with a positive result should consider themselves pregnant and see their doctor to confirm the result. Women who are anxious to become pregnant may test themselves well before their period is due and obtain a false negative reading, although some available tests can detect traces of HCG in the urine well before this time (Fig. 10-13).

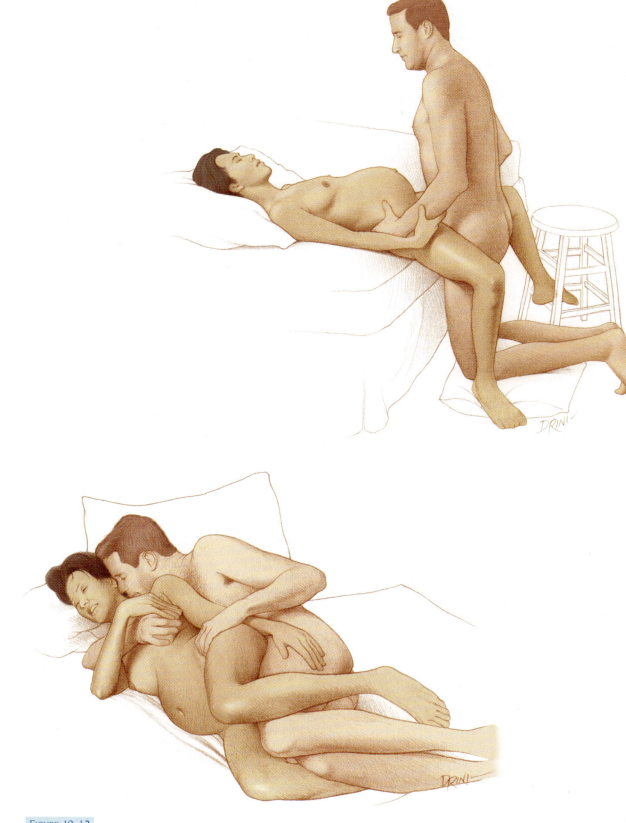

FIGURE 10-12   Intercourse positions that minimize pressure on a woman's abdomen are more comfortable for her as pregnancy advances into its later stages.

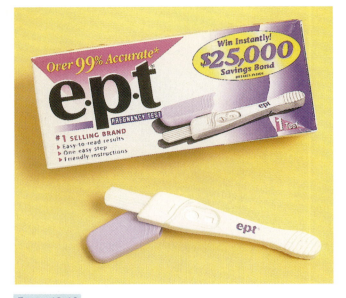

FIGURE 10-13   Over-the-counter pregnancy tests can be extremely accurate, but the user must follow the enclosed directions carefully. A number of factors can lead to false results.

Early Development

We have described so far the development of the fertilized egg up to implantation in the lining of the uterus. Now we turn to the development of the embryo and fetus and the most important changes occurring at different stages of pregnancy. The embryonic period begins at about the second week of pregnancy, when the woman generally doesn't yet know she has conceived. A missed period is typically the first sign of pregnancy, although women miss periods for various other reasons too, including emotional stress, extreme fatigue, significant weight loss, and illness. About 20% of women who are pregnant also have some periodic menstrual discharge during the early months of their pregnancies.

Sometimes fertilization occurs but implantation does not. This often happens because hormonal stimulation of the endometrium is inadequate to prepare it to receive this delicate, dividing mass of cells. When implantation does not happen, the zygote is expelled through the cervix without the woman even knowing that she conceived or that implantation failed to occur. Fertilization and implantation are different processes, and the former does not lead inevitably to the latter.

Research Highlight

NONSURGICAL TREATMENT FOR ECTOPIC PREGNANCIES

A fertilized egg does not always progress down the fallopian tube to the uterus but may instead begin to grow outside the uterus in the pelvic cavity or in the fallopian tube itself. As you know, this is called an ectopic pregnancy. Because of a recent dramatic rise in the number of young women in the United States having ectopic pregnancies, physicians have sought nonsurgical treatments for this problem, since surgical treatment has higher risks than most non-surgical treatments. One relatively new medical treatment holds promise for ectopic pregnancies.

A drug named methotrexate is commonly used in chemotherapy for cancer. It selectively seeks out and attacks cancer cells characterized by a high rate of growth and division. Administered in a much smaller dose to a woman early in an ectopic pregnancy, it similarly seeks out and selectively destroys the fast growing and dividing cells of an early embryo stuck in the fallopian tube or the pelvic cavity. This treatment has been used in recent years with good results in ending ectopic pregnancies without surgical intervention. Doctors can determine whether the methotrexate has worked by measuring the amount of HCG in the woman's blood, since elevated amounts of this hormone signal early pregnancy. If the level of this hormone falls suddenly, it may be inferred than the pregnancy has ended. When methotrexate is used and the HCG level does not fall, a second injection can be given.

In one study (Thoen & Creinin, 1997) of 47 women with ectopic pregnancies, 43 were treated successfully with methotrexate; 36 were treated successfully with a single dose, and 7 needed a second dose. Only 4 women required surgery after methotrexate therapy failed to end the pregnancy. In another review of methotrexate treatment of ectopic pregnancy, of 540 women treated with a single dose of this agent, 84% did not require further medical or surgical treatment (Yao & Tulandi, 1997). This is a promising treatment for ectopic pregnancy undergoing further testing and controlled clinical trials.

The period of the embryo extends to the end of the eighth week of pregnancy, at which time the fetal period begins, which continues until birth. As shown in Figure 10-14, the embryo doesn't look at all like a little human being. In fact, early in the embryonic period the developing conceptus looks similar to the embryos of most other animals with a backbone. As development continues, however, the human appearance becomes compellingly obvious (Fig. 10.14).

Miscarriage, or "Spontaneous Abortion"

Once a fertilized egg is implanted in the lining of the uterus, it doesn't always stay there. Separation of the fertilized egg from the endometrium is called a **miscarriage,** or **spontaneous abortion.** An estimated 20% of all medically documented pregnancies end in a miscarriage (Turkington, 1999). The term "abortion" technically refers to the separation of a developing embryo or fetus from the lining of the uterus. When this happens by itself, it is called a "spontaneous abortion," although the term "abortion" used by itself refers to a medical procedure making such a separation. About half of miscarriages happen before the woman even knows that she has conceived. The only indication that a miscarriage has occurred is usually an especially heavy period. Most women who have miscarriages are still able to become pregnant and have a baby in the future. The term "miscarriage" is usually used when a pregnancy is lost during the first 20 weeks; at a later time the term "fetal demise" is used. Any time a pregnant woman experiences vaginal bleeding, a miscarriage is a possibility, and the doctor should be consulted immediately.

Miscarriages result from a number of factors. Abnormalities in immune system functioning may play a role, as well as hormonal imbalances, illnesses (such as rubella, diabetes, or lupus), chromosomal abnormalities, and anomalies in the structure of the uterus and/or cervix (*The PDR Family Guide to Women's Health and Prescription Drugs,* 1994).

In those instances in which vaginal bleeding and abdominal pain accompany the rupture of the amniotic sac surrounding the embryo or fetus, the cervix then widens somewhat, followed by uterine contractions that expel the products of conception from the uterus. This is referred to as an *inevitable miscarriage.* Sometimes, however, if the uterus does not fully eject all the products of conception, an *incomplete miscarriage* results. In about 1% of pregnancies, none of the membranes, placenta, or embryo/fetus are expelled; this is a *missed miscarriage.* After incomplete and missed miscarriages, the cervix needs to be dilated surgically so that the contents of the uterus can be removed. This procedure, called a "D & C" for dilation and curettage, is usually performed between the 8th and 12th weeks of pregnancy. The same procedure is also used for different conditions, including some unrelated to pregnancy or miscarriage.

Obstetricians and gynecologists believe that women can reduce their risk of miscarriage with a few simple measures. The risk is lowered by not smoking, drinking alcohol, or consuming large amounts of caffeine. Exposure should be minimized to ionizing radiation and environmental toxins (arsenic, lead, formaldehyde, and benzene). Injury to the abdomen should be prevented, such as may occur in an automobile collision by compression against the steering wheel or by car seat belts. A pregnant woman should also talk to her doctor before using any medications.

Dealing with a miscarriage can be extremely difficult. Feelings of depression, loss, guilt, and remorse are common. Support groups and counseling can help a couple cope with this very real loss. Because the couple may begin making plans to conceive again, antidepressant or antianxiety medications should not be taken. While family and friends are usually aware of the woman's feelings, men also experience despondency after a miscarriage but seldom receive the same kind of support as their partners and often feel isolated. Keep this in mind the next time you hear of a friend who has miscarried.

Development of the Embryo

At the very beginning the embryo is not much more than a developing mass of cells, but this cellular proliferation and specialization occurs according to a carefully organized, genetically determined sequence of changes. Embryologists use the term *differentiation* to describe how these early developing and dividing cells group together according to their future functions. To simplify, these early cells can be considered in two groups: outside cells and inside cells (Fig. 10-15). The outside

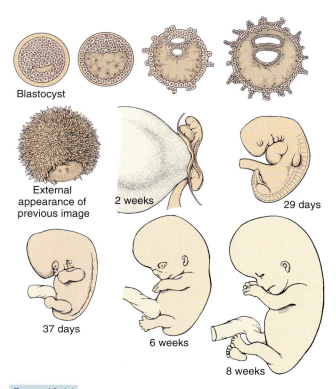

Blastocyst

External appearance of previous image

2 weeks

29 days

37 days

6 weeks

8 weeks

FIGURE 10-14   Stages of development of the human embryo.

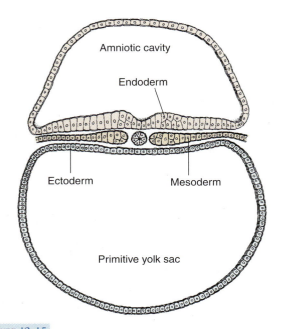

- Amniotic cavity
- Endoderm
- Ectoderm
- Mesoderm
- Primitive yolk sac

FIGURE 10-15   Differentiation of ectodermal, endodermal, and mesodermal cellular layers in the early stages of human embryonic development.

cells differentiate into protective and nourishing membranes: the amniotic sac surrounding the embryo and fetus, the chorion, the amnion, the umbilical cord, and the placenta. The placenta is a *semi-permeable membrane,* meaning that some substances can pass through it and others cannot. Many viruses and bacteria can cross this placental filter, but others do so less readily or not at all. Because the mother's circulatory system and the embryo's are linked, the carbohydrates, fats,

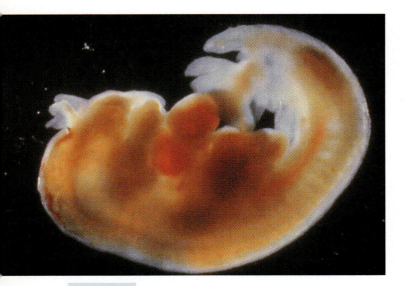

FIGURE 10-16   Photograph of a human embryo. Note the cephalo-caudal and proximo-distal directions of physical growth and development.

and proteins consumed by a pregnant woman reach the developing embryo and fetus through the umbilical cord. Nutrition for the developing embryo and fetus and metabolic wastes are exchanged through the placenta. The placenta also produces the hormones progesterone and estrogen, as well as HCG, which stimulates the corpus luteum to secrete progesterone and estrogen during early pregnancy until the placenta can take over this function. The developing baby is surrounded by amniotic fluid, which increases in volume throughout seven months of pregnancy and then diminishes a little in the final two months. Amniotic fluid is much like blood plasma. Amniotic fluid is always being produced, as well as being resorbed as the fetus involuntarily swallows it and absorbs it in its intestinal tract. The embryo's and fetus's metabolic wastes are absorbed through the umbilical cord and reach the mother to be excreted.

The "inside cells" eventually turn into the baby. Early in embryonic development three cellular layers form and begin to differentiate: the *ectoderm, mesoderm, and endoderm.* These become the body's major organ systems. The ectoderm eventually turns into the skin, the nervous system, sensory receptors, and some of the glands in the endocrine system. The mesoderm differentiates into the circulatory system, bones, muscles, excretory system, and reproductive system. The endoderm develops into the digestive system and respiratory system. Long before most women even know that they have conceived, many important embryological developments have already occurred. For example, the earliest structures of what will become the brain and spinal cord are already formed 21 days after fertilization. The cells that will become the baby's heart begin to differentiate at 24 days, with the early heart taking shape during the fourth week. The embryo's arms and legs differentiate between the fifth and eighth weeks, and the face begins to form then but does not yet have an obvious human configuration. At this early point in embryonic development, the cerebral hemispheres of the brain are two hollow sacs of very delicate tissue. At the end of the eighth week, the embryo weighs 1/30th of an ounce and is less than 1 inch long. Embryologists use the term *organogenesis* to refer to the formation and early functions of the internal organs in the first two months of pregnancy. During this time, the embryo is most vulnerable to birth defect-causing agents because any destruction or alteration of the embryo is multiplied many-fold with continued growth and development. If such destruction or alteration is profound, the developing embryo may not survive.

A human embryo's appearance (Fig. 10-16) looks obviously distorted compared to an infant's. Two principles of embryonic and fetal growth are most obvious in the early developing embryo. *Cephalo-caudal development* means growth takes place first and most quickly toward the head and later and slower toward the lower extremities; the embryo's head seems disproportionately large and its legs and feet are tiny. *Proximo-distal development* means growth takes place first and most quickly along the midline of the body and later and slower at the tips of the extremities (hands and feet). This is why the embryo's trunk seems so large while its fingers and toes are small. At the end of the period of the embryo, all the internal organs have been formed and to some degree have begun to function. Not until the 5th month of pregnancy, however, do they lie in their correct positions inside of the body.

Development of the Fetus

The Latin word "fetus" means "young one," and the fetus looks more like a baby (Fig. 10-17). The fetal growth rate increases dramatically, and all major organ systems are now formed and functioning. During the 3rd and 4th months of pregnancy, the rate of muscular development accelerates noticeably. The fetus grows more during the 4th month than in any month of pregnancy. At the end of this month, the fetus is 6 inches long, and all of the products of conception (external membranes and structures and the fetus itself) weigh 4 pounds. The heart of a 4-month-old fetus can circulate 25 quarts of blood every day. By the end of the 4th month of pregnancy, most women begin to feel fetal movement, although this varies. The earliest fetal movements don't feel like elbows or knees poking or shoving the inside of the woman's abdomen but rather like a faint, internal tickle.

By the 5th month of pregnancy, the fetus's skin is fully developed, but because as yet there is little fat beneath it, the fetus now has a frail, bony appearance. The earliest physiological manifestations of sleeping and waking now occur, and

hair, finger and toe nails, and sweat glands begin to appear. During the 6th month, the fetus can open and move its eyes, although the visual part of the brain responsible for seeing will not be fully developed for at least another 2 months. In the 7th month of pregnancy the brain undergoes its most dramatic rate of growth. There is a rapid increase in the number of nerve cells and maturation of pathways within the brain, as well as pathways connecting sense organs to the brain and the motor area of the brain to the body's muscles. Toward the end of the 7th month occurs a rather sudden appearance of neuronal connections (synapses) among nerve cells in the outermost cellular layers of the cerebral hemispheres, the cerebral cortex. Until this time there were few or no connections among nerve cells in the cortex, the part of the brain involved in the most "human" capacities: perception, memory, judgment, and problem solving. About 25 years ago a baby born at the end of the 7th month of pregnancy had a *fair* chance of surviving, but today a baby born at this time has a *good* chance of surviving, using sophisticated technology to assist in basic life functions. Many babies born even before this time can now survive through aggressive, high-tech medical intervention.

In the last two months of pregnancy, the fetus gains about 8 ounces each week as its body accumulates fat. During the last two weeks of pregnancy, the rate of growth slows as the pla-

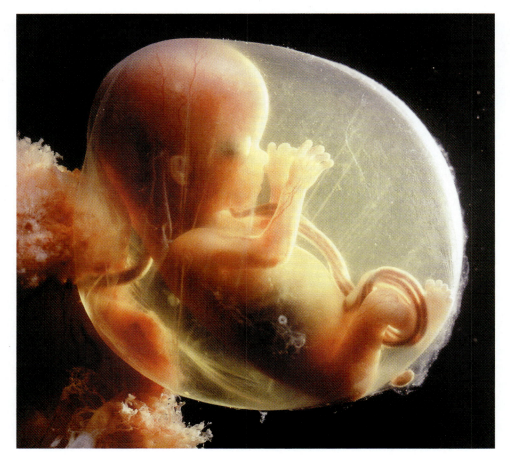

FIGURE 10-17 Human fetus. Cephalo-caudal and proximo-distal development are still obvious. Note the amniotic sac surrounding the fetus and the amniotic fluid within it. Portions of the placenta can be seen at left.

centa loses some of its efficiency and the uterus drops to a lower position in the woman's pelvis.

A Couple's Reactions to the Progression of Pregnancy

In late pregnancy feelings of excitement mingle with some normal apprehension and often impatience too. Many women feel they're just *never* going to have this baby. How women and men react to a pregnancy and each other during this time depends on many factors. Of course, not all pregnancies are anticipated, much less wanted. Such factors affect the feelings of women and men throughout the pregnancy. A couple who conceived through assisted reproductive technology is usually overjoyed at the prospect of becoming parents. Or a couple's alcohol and/or other substance abuse problems can dramatically affect how they acknowledge a pregnancy and its possible outcomes. The nature of the relationship between the mother and father obviously affects how they view pregnancy, birth, and parenting. Family, religious, racial, and ethnic traditions and customs also affect a couple's thoughts and feelings about becoming mothers and fathers. It is not unusual, for example, for members of an extended family to consider a young woman immature until she has had a child, with the birth of her baby an important rite of passage during early adulthood. If a woman has had a miscarriage or abortion, these past events may profoundly affect how she and her partner view the current pregnancy. Finally, what the couple knows about human sexuality generally and pregnancy and childbirth specifically influence their adjustment to the changes that are likely to occur in each of them through the next 9 months.

Feelings of anticipation and apprehension are common, especially during a first pregnancy. Generally, a woman's emotional reactions during the first trimester of pregnancy focus on physical symptoms (e.g., nausea, vomiting, fatigue), and feelings during the last trimester of pregnancy involve anxiety and emotional tension (Rofe, Blittner, & Lewin, 1993). The physical transition from not being pregnant to being aware of one's pregnancy can be dramatic. Later in pregnancy it is common to worry about the outcome of the pregnancy, the health of the newborn, and the adjustment to a larger family. Because of this we feel it is imperative for the father to be involved with the pregnancy from the very beginning. Although men differ much in their desire to be part of this whole process, most want to be involved. Women and men both enjoy the wonder of feeling new life move inside the uterus, and parent-baby bonding can be said to begin like this. Marriages often change when the focus of the relationship becomes the pregnancy, and sometimes this is difficult to handle, especially for men. Men may feel they are not the sole focus of their partner's attentions, and less frequent sexual intercourse may reinforce their feelings of becoming "peripheral" to the pregnancy. In some

Dear Dr. Ruth

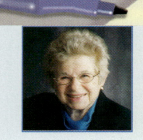

Question:

I am a 25-year-old woman. When I was in my teens and early 20s I was pretty wild. One time I had chlamydia, but I got treated and it's gone. I also drank a lot and even used LSD a few times. My husband really wants children, but I'm scared my past might catch up with me and the baby might be born abnormal. Can this happen?

Answer:

Because of your concerns, you should consider preconception counseling before trying to get pregnant. This will include talking about your medical history and having a physical exam. This is important for someone who has had a sexually transmitted disease or used drugs. If you don't already have a gynecologist, choose one for this exam. Since this doctor might be the one who delivers your child, you may want to interview several. Be completely honest and open with her or him about your past. If your husband will be going with you to the doctor and you don't want him to know some things about your past, call the doctor ahead of time and give those details then. Hopefully your past won't affect your present plans. Even if there is some problem, it is not likely to affect the health of a baby. Being completely open with your doctor greatly increases the odds both of becoming pregnant and having that healthy baby.

cases, a lot of time, money, and planning are invested in the pregnancy, with less time for one- on-one intimate sharing and romance. The pregnancy may also involve the extended family, with parents and in-laws sharing their (sometimes unwanted) advice, tips, and suggestions.

THE HEALTH OF THE FETUS

For centuries of recorded human history, events in the uterus were a mystery and a matter of much speculation, sometimes quite fanciful. Many old woodcuts and sketches accurately portray the physical appearance of the fetus, but many other illustrations show a miniature adult in the womb. Today's technology can tell us an enormous amount about the most minute aspects of the internal and external growth of the embryo and fetus. Diagnostic tests reveal much about the mother's and developing baby's health throughout the pregnancy. Obstetricians do everything possible to consider the woman's personal health history and any genetic considerations that may affect the development and birth of the baby.

Ultrasound Imaging

Ultrasound imaging allows doctors to visualize a developing baby without disturbing the pregnancy. High-frequency sound waves pass through the woman's abdomen and into the expanded uterus. Anything inside the uterus reflects these sound waves to produce an image revealing the embryo or fetus. Ultrasound allows a doctor to estimate the developing baby's age by comparing the size of various body parts with established growth norms and to keep track of its development in the womb (Fig. 10-18). *Intrauterine growth retardation,* which can be determined with ultrasound, is a complication in about 5% of all pregnancies; it is implicated in serious problems at or around the time of birth. The size, location, and efficiency of the placenta can also be determined. These are all good indices of normal or abnormal fetal development, and ultrasound helps determine when fetal monitoring equipment should be used (Hobbins, 1997). Ultrasound can also confirm an amniocentesis prenatal diagnosis of Down syndrome (Rotmensch, Liberati, Bronshtein, Schoenfeld-Dimaio, Shalev, Ben-Rafael, & Copel, 1997) and guide the doctor's insertion of the needle into the abdomen for this test.

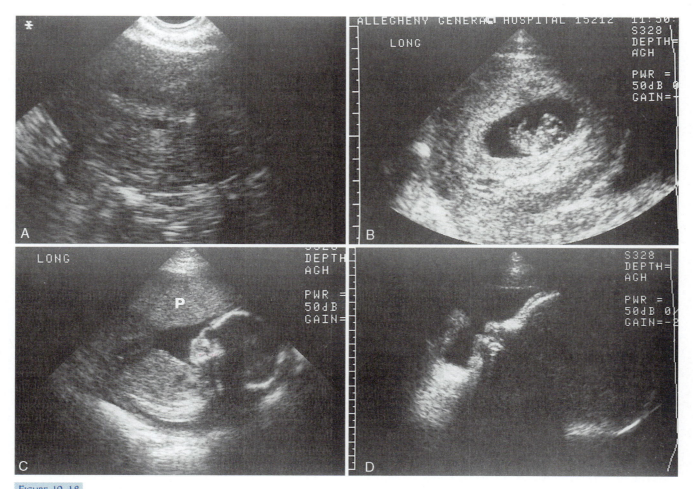

FIGURE 10-18 Four ultrasound images revealing the progressive growth and development of a normal embryo, and later the fetus. Significant specialized training is required to fully interpret images like these.

Ultrasound can confirm an early pregnancy, reveal the presence of more than one embryo or fetus, assess the efficiency of placental functioning, and determine the amount of amniotic fluid. Because many of the fetus's internal organs are visible with ultrasound, their form and function can be assessed long before birth, and sometimes problems are diagnosed and treated during pregnancy. The position of the fetus in the uterus can also be evaluated and may guide the obstetrician's decisions about how best to deliver the baby. Also, if the fetus's heartbeat cannot be heard or if fetal movement ceases, ultrasound can help determine if a problem exists.

Before an ultrasound test, the pregnant woman must drink a great deal of water and not urinate before the examination. For a pregnant woman this may cause some discomfort because of the pressure of the fetus on the bladder. Most couples are excited when they first see the image of their developing baby, and developmental psychologists note that bonding between parent and child can begin long before the baby is born. Eurenius, Axelsson, Gallstedt-Fransson, and Sjoden (1997) studied how women and their partners reacted to the results of ultrasound imaging during the second trimester of pregnancy in a sample of over 300 couples. The primary concern of most women and men in this sample was whether the fetus had any malformations. The couples in this study generally reported the test was a positive experience.

Ultrasound imaging can be problematic as well, however. For example, sometimes ultrasound suggests there is a problem, a physical deformity for example, when at birth the newborn is normal in every way (Angier, 1997). Similarly, ultrasound and other prenatal tests may indicate an entirely normal fetus when doctors and the parents later discover sometimes profound and catastrophic abnormalities. Some are concerned too about whether the ultrasound test itself might cause problems. Scientists have wondered about the impact of high-frequency sounds on the later visual and auditory performance of children. In a study of more than 3200 youngsters, however, no relationship was discovered between ultrasound testing and later visual and hearing problems (Kieler, Haglund, Waldenstrom, & Axelsson, 1997).

Amniocentesis

Another prenatal diagnostic tool, **amniocentesis,** can detect certain genetic abnormalities in the developing fetus. It is used for *genetic* abnormalities existing at the microscopic level of chromosome structure or the number of chromosomes in developing fetal cells. Unlike ultrasonography, this test is invasive. For some four decades, it has been used routinely to assess the fetus of pregnant women over the age of 35 because of their higher risk of conceiving a child with Down syndrome. In some cases younger women too are offered this test. The test is recommended also for some women who previously miscarried and for those who have a previous child with a chromosomal abnormality, or when either parent is a carrier of a potential inherited genetic defect.

As the fetus grows, many of its cells are sloughed off and remain suspended in the amniotic fluid surrounding it. Amniocentesis involves removing some of these cells in a fluid sample and examining their basic genetic characteristics. In most cases, amniocentesis is carried out in the 16th week of pregnancy, which can be well determined with ultrasound, but also as early as the 14th or as late as the 20th week. In the procedure, ultrasound is used to accurately locate the placenta and fetus. Then a needle is inserted into the uterus through the abdominal wall. A small amount of amniotic fluid is drawn out and sent to a laboratory where the cells are grown and examined for signs of genetic abnormalities. This usually takes about 10 days to 2 weeks. The procedure carries a small risk; a recent study of almost 2100 women revealed a risk of spontaneous abortion in a second trimester pregnancy of 1.3% (Marthin, Liedgren, & Hammar, 1997). Although amniocentesis can detect over 90 different genetic abnormalities, usually testing is done for only a few disorders, depending on the woman's age, sometimes the partner's age, and the family histories of both parents. Should the test reveal a serious genetic problem, the couple, with their obstetrician and perhaps a genetic counselor or clergyman, may consider the agonizing decision of having a therapeutic abortion.

Chorionic Villus Sampling (CVS)

When a fertilized egg is implanted in the lining of the uterus, its attachment is secured by microscopic fingers of tissue called **chorionic villi.** Because they grow from a protective membrane supporting the early embryo (the chorion), they contain the embryo's genetic material. Like amniocentesis, **chorionic villus sampling** (CVS) can detect many genetic abnormalities in the developing embryo. The significant advantage of CVS is that it can be done as early as the 8th week of pregnancy and the results take only a few days except when cells need to be cultured in the laboratory, requiring about 2 weeks. CVS is usually performed at 9 to 12 weeks. Ultrasound is used to locate the fetus and placenta, and a needle is inserted into the uterus either through the vagina and cervical opening or through a small incision in the woman's abdomen.

Doctors have generally considered the risk of spontaneous abortion to be about the same for amniocentesis and CVS, although a recent study indicates that the risk of spontaneous abortion may be higher with amniocentesis (Cederholm & Axelsson, 1997). In a group of 147 women undergoing amniocentesis and 174 having CVS, amniocentesis had a spontaneous abortion rate of 6.8%, while CVS had a rate of only 1.7%. This study also showed that in many cases, both amniocentesis and CVS do not reveal clearly the presence or absence of genetic abnormalities and a second test needs to be carried out. Women in this study receiving amniocentesis required retesting in 19% of cases, while those receiving CVS required retesting in only 5.2% of cases. All tests in this study were carried out between 10 and 13 weeks of pregnancy, a time often too early for clear results from amniocentesis. Even with these highly advanced technological tools, prenatal diagnostic testing can still be unclear. Both amniocentesis and chorionic villus sampling can detect several problems early in pregnancy, including the following:

1. Tay-Sachs disease—an inherited disorder of lipid metabolism
2. Cystic fibrosis—a deficiency of enzymes from the pancreas causing breathing difficulties, and excessive loss of salt through perspiration
3. Sickle cell disease—an abnormality in the shape of red blood cells
4. Neural tube defects (e.g., spinal bifida)—an abnormality of the spinal column with the protrusion of the spinal cord through the vertebrae
5. Chronic fetal hypoxia—respiratory difficulties due to a lack of oxygen
6. Potential for premature birth
7. Fetal lung immaturity
8. Various viral infections
9. Toxoplasmosis—a bacterial disease that affects the nervous system
10. Down syndrome—also sometimes called trisomy-21

Alpha-Fetoprotein

The fetus produces a specific protein molecule called alpha-fetoprotein (AFP). This substance can be measured in the mother's blood and tested usually in the 16th to 18th weeks of pregnancy. Elevated amounts of protein in the mother's blood stream could indicate a neural tube defect in the fetus that causes the spinal deformity *spina bifida*. In spina bifida the membranes surrounding the spinal cord, and sometimes the cord itself, protrude through the spinal column, forming a large protuberance along the person's back. This test cannot definitively indicate a spinal cord malformation but indicates the need for follow-up testing, possibly including amniocentesis, to rule out this and other problems. Very low levels of APF may indicate the possibility of Down syndrome. In a study of over 48,000 pregnant women with APF levels measured (Crandall & Chua, 1997), 2.2% had results indicating mildly, moderately, or highly elevated levels. In this sample 25% of those with mildly elevated levels gave birth to babies with spinal abnormalities, while 88% of those with moderately elevated levels and 98% of those with highly elevated levels had similar unfortunate outcomes.

With amniocentesis, CVS, and APF readily available to women seeking prenatal care and counseling, the chances of detecting genetic or nervous system abnormalities are good. Many pregnant women are anxious for a "guarantee" that their baby is developing normally and may request one or all of these tests, even when their age and personal and family health histories do not indicate the need.

Embryoscopy

The prenatal diagnostic tests discussed so far are only *indirect* measures of what is happening inside the uterus. In recent years, however, medical scientists have developed a method for direct, visual inspection of the embryo or fetus, and the results are dramatic and informative. Slender, imaging devices are now used inside the uterus in both pregnant and non-pregnant women. These instruments allow scientists to view a developing human embryo or fetus without compromising the pregnancy. **Embryoscopy** is carried out through the cervix or a small incision in a woman's abdomen. It is effective for diagnosing gross limb or facial abnormalities as early as the first trimester of pregnancy and is often performed along with amniocentesis (Reece, Homko, Koch, & Chan, 1997). The device does not enter the amniotic sac and involves only a low risk, with few if any adverse consequences for the mother or developing baby. Embryoscopy can also confirm problems that are only suggested through ultrasound. For example, embryoscopy has been used to verify conjoined twins ("Siamese twins"), a condition that may not be determined with certainty through ultrasound (Hubinont, Kollmann, Malvaux, Donnez, & Bernard, 1997). Embryoscopy has also been used to study the effect of prenatal trauma on the placenta, which usually results in small hemorrhages on the embryo's head (Quintero, Romero, Mahony, Abuhamad, Vecchio, Holden, & Hobbins, 1993). When CVS leads to a suspicion of damage to the placenta with potential harmful effects on the embryo, embryoscopy can demonstrate or disconfirm such a speculation.

Another application of embryoscopy may profoundly impact future studies of prenatal development and fetal health. The fiberoptic tube inserted into the uterus for imaging can include a thin needle to extract blood samples through the umbilical cord as early as in the first trimester (Reece, Whetham, Rotmensch, & Wiznitzer, 1993). Analysis of prenatal blood samples can help diagnose and possibly even treat congenital diseases in the first trimester.

Other Prenatal Tests and Health Monitoring

In addition to the sophisticated tests described above, routine blood and urine tests are also important for the health of the mother and developing baby. Blood tests for anemia are very important. Because women lose blood each month during menstruation, the doctor wants to establish that the pregnancy is beginning with enough iron in the woman's blood stream. Another test determines the presence or absence of Rh factor in the woman's blood. Urine tests help establish whether a woman has kidney problems or is diabetic. In routine prenatal examinations women are also screened for hepatitis B, syphilis, gonorrhea, and sometimes chlamydia. Because the virus that causes AIDS can cross the placenta and enter the fetus's blood stream, women who are at risk for AIDS are also given an HIV test during pregnancy. The doctor will also check on the woman's vaccinations, particularly for rubella. The pregnant woman also needs current vaccinations for tetanus and diphtheria.

Because a woman's weight is particularly important during pregnancy, many doctors recommend that a woman who weighs too little or too much attain a normal weight for her height and build and maintain it before becoming pregnant. Women who weigh too little are more likely to give birth to babies who arrive too early and are too small. Women who weigh too much are more likely to develop diabetes temporarily during pregnancy. Because there is a strong connection between low folic acid levels in a pregnant woman's blood stream and defects in the development of the neural tube, which will become the brain and spinal cord, doctors encourage all pregnant women to take a folic acid supplement daily. This is typically included in a prenatal "multivitamin."

Finally, the woman's blood pressure must be monitored frequently and carefully throughout pregnancy. High blood pressure is the most common cause of mid- and late-pregnancy fetal loss and is also implicated in inadequate prenatal growth and complications of childbirth. Fewer than 10% of pregnant women have high blood pressure, and in most the problem is not realized until it is noticed that they are retaining large amounts of fluid and have swollen fingers, feet, and ankles. In serious cases, an antihypertensive drug may be prescribed to bring down the blood pressure. Usually pregnant women are encouraged to eat a diet high in protein and low in salt and to stop smoking if they are still doing so. Untreated high blood pressure may lead to a condition called *preeclampsia,* in which kidney problems develop, leading to premature birth. Preeclampsia is also associated with kidney and liver damage and visual disturbances in the mother. Women who receive regular prenatal check-ups are unlikely to develop this problem or experience its serious consequences.

"High-Risk" Pregnancies

Pregnancy does not always go smoothly, and the term "high-risk pregnancy" is used to describe pregnancies in which bed rest and aggressive medical intervention may be needed at home or in a medical setting. Many obstetricians advertise their competence in managing high-risk pregnancies. Fortunately, few women have high-risk pregnancies. *Gestational diabetes* can cause the same problems for a newborn as long-standing diabetes, such as increased thirst, increased urination, and weight loss. Women at risk for gestational diabetes may be tested for this in the sixth or seventh month. Another problem requiring close attention is persistent vomiting. Although nausea and vomiting are normal in early pregnancy, if they continue throughout gestation a woman can become dehydrated and may experience kidney and liver damage. In very serious cases of chronic vomiting a woman may enter a hospital to receive intravenous fluids under medical supervision. *Vaginal bleeding* may be a concern in pregnancy, and bed rest is usually recommended. Vaginal bleeding occurring later in pregnancy is usually caused by some condition of the placenta or its attachment to the uterus.

Too little or too much amniotic fluid is another problem requiring close medical monitoring. If there is too much amniotic fluid, the doctor may perform amniocentesis to draw some from the amniotic sac. If there is too little, the fetus might press on the umbilical cord, and the doctor may wish to deliver the baby as early as is safe.

Another factor associated with high-risk pregnancy is Rh incompatibility. The Rh factor is a protein carried in the bloodstream. The Rh+ and Rh− versions of this protein are incompatible. If the mother is Rh- and the child's father is Rh+, the fetus too is Rh+; in this situation the mother's immune system reacts to the fetus as "foreign" tissue and manufactures antibodies that slip back into the fetus's bloodstream and destroy its red blood cells. In a first pregnancy, even if it doesn't come to term, there are too few antibodies to cause a problem, but in second and subsequent pregnancies the accumulated antibodies cause a serious medical condition. Women who are Rh- who conceive a child with a man who is Rh+ can receive an injection to neutralize these antibodies, keeping the baby safe.

Early rupturing of the membranes surrounding the fetus, intrauterine growth retardation, and *placenta previa,* a condition in which the placenta obstructs the baby's progress through the birth canal, also pose potential hazards. Multiple births, pregnancy in older women, and pregnancies that continue longer than they should also are high-risk pregnancies. Finally, in rare cases the placenta becomes partly or completely separated from the uterine wall. This condition, called *placental abruption,* is a genuine medical emergency requiring immediate, aggressive medical treatment. While a high-risk pregnancy requires close medical monitoring, these are a small percentage of pregnancies. If the pregnancy progresses through the first trimester without incident, the chances are 50 to 1 that the baby will be born with problems.

In most high-risk pregnancies, bed rest is recommended. Being confined to bed is seldom pleasant even when the woman knows it's the best thing for herself and her developing baby. Gupton, Heaman, and Ashcroft (1997) explored the perceptions of women staying in bed, through interviews and diaries of their experiences. Because of the complexities of high-risk pregnancies, doctors often want to ensure that the pregnancy does not continue longer than appropriate for the mother and her baby and induce labor, artificially stimulating labor with synthetic hormones or by rupturing the woman's amniotic sac. Rojansky, Reubinoff, Tanos, Shushan, and Weinstein (1997) studied 210 high-risk pregnancies and found that there were no increased risks caused by inducing labor in women with high-risk pregnancies nor an increased risk of needing a Cesarean section.

THE PROCESS OF GIVING BIRTH

Most babies are born after nine months of pregnancy, although many arrive early and some later. Although many pregnant women are excited and impatient about finally having their baby, they often feel anxious and concerned once labor begins.

In a vaginal delivery (Fig. 10-19), the cervix gradually thins to allow the passage of the baby's head through the birth canal. As discussed in Chapter 4, the uterus is a large, hollow muscle. During labor, the uterus contracts and relaxes rhythmically, and this gradually thins the cervix. Although the progression of events is predictable, every woman's labor is unique, and her second and subsequent labors differ from each other as well. Lower abdominal cramping that lasts about a half an hour even though the woman changes posture or position generally signals she has probably begun labor.

Most doctors ask the woman to come to the hospital when her contractions are about 5 minutes apart in a first pregnancy. During this time she should not eat anything or drink anything but clear liquids. First births take longer than subsequent ones because the cervix has not been fully stretched before, and this takes time. Before labor, the cervix has not opened very much, perhaps a centimeter or two. As labor progresses, the cervix opens significantly, until at full dilation it opens to a diameter of 10 centimeters (4 inches). As the cervix dilates, it becomes thinner; this thinning is called "effacement." This is usually enough for uncomplicated progress of the newborn out of the uterus, into the vagina, and out of the body.

Inducing Labor

Late in pregnancy, the infant is large and the placenta begins to lose its efficiency as a semipermeable membrane. If the baby continues to grow, passage of its head through the mother's pelvis may become difficult. For these reasons, the doctor may recommend inducing labor, which has become a common practice. If labor has begun and then stops, the doctor may rupture the amniotic sac or administer synthetic hormones to keep labor progressing. When labor is long and difficult, the risks of complications increase, especially for very young and older women.

When a pregnancy continues into the 40th or 41st week, obstetricians disagree about how to proceed. Some advocate inducing labor, whereas others use a fetal monitor to assess the baby's health and wait to see how things progress. The joke about doctors who induce labor so that they can deliver babies at their own convenience is rarely reflected by reality.

The Stages of Labor

Between a woman's first contractions and the emergence of the baby are three stages of labor. Most normal first births progress through these in 12 to 24 hours. Second and subsequent births usually take less time, sometimes much less time, because the cervix has already been fully stretched once. The first stage of labor, *active labor,* begins with the first contractions and lasts until the cervix is fully open, or effaced. The second stage of labor involves the emergence of the baby from the birth canal and is sometimes called expulsion. The final stage of labor involves the passage of the placenta and membranes, collectively called the afterbirth, through the vagina.

Active labor has three phases, with obvious changes as the woman progresses from one to the next. The following outline describes what happens to most women most of the time, but remember there are many individual variations.

- **Early Active Labor.** In this phase contractions are usually far apart, often 10 minutes or more. They are not always localized in the abdomen but often involve feelings of tightness in the back or groin. The timing and strength of these contractions vary much among different women. Women are typically told to stay

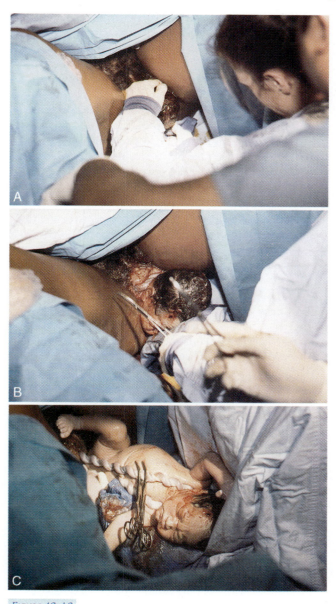

FIGURE 10-19   During a vaginal birth, the baby's head first "crowns" as it slowly emerges from the vagina (A), then the entire head and shoulders emerge (B), followed by the trunk, buttocks, and legs (C). The umbilical cord is being cut in (C).

home in early labor. The woman often feels excitement and anticipation along with some apprehension. During this stage the cervix dilates to about 4 centimeters (1.5 inches).

- **Active Labor.** Contractions now come about 3 minutes apart, and the woman focuses on her labor and is less buoyant and outgoing. She is more attentive to the strength and duration of each contraction. Each contraction lasts 45 to 60 seconds and is clearly focused in the abdomen. Women often report they "feel one coming," recognize when the contraction "peaks," and feel it "die down." The cervix dilates to about 8 centimeters (3 inches). The woman needs strong resolve to stay focused on each contraction, and many women use relaxation techniques and breathing exercises to cope. Many women find this aspect of active labor very uncomfortable and frequently request medication to ease their pain. Most prepared childbirth classes emphasize the difference between "pressure" and "pain," however. Pain medications are administered in doses that interfere as little as possible with the baby's vital functions while still providing some relief. Local anesthetics can be administered in the cervix, the pudendal nerve (which numbs the perineum and does not interfere with a woman's ability to "push"), the spinal canal, and the epidural space (the area between the spinal cord and the vertebral bones surrounding it). The couple often discusses these options with the obstetrician at some time late in pregnancy.

■ **Transition.** During this phase of active labor, the cervix dilates fully to a diameter of about 10 centimeters (4 inches) to allow passage of the baby's head. Most experts and mothers agree this is the most demanding stage of labor. Contractions are strongest and longest, with much less time between them. These contractions usually come every 2 to 3 minutes and last from 60 to 90 seconds. Women often feel very emotional and sometimes are irritable or even a little hostile during this stage, which often surprises their partner, who might be coaching her during labor.

After progressing through these stages of active labor, the woman is usually ready for a vaginal delivery. At the end of active labor the baby's head is firmly lodged in the birth canal. This is called "engagement," which begins the second stage of labor eventually leading to expulsion of the baby. The strength, duration, and frequency of contractions change, usually now occurring every 4 to 5 minutes. During this time women are encouraged to begin pushing with each one. Although most women are quite tired at this time, their excitement and anticipation usually offsets their fatigue and discomfort. Each contraction nudges the baby's head further along in the birth canal, with eventual stretching in the perineal area as the head descends from a position behind the woman's pubic bone.

The baby's head should emerge from the vagina slowly and gently, or the perineal area may tear a little. To prevent tearing, the obstetrician may make a small incision called an **episiotomy** between the vagina and rectum, which usually involves little or no discomfort. After the birth the episiotomy is repaired with a few stitches, and moderate discomfort may occur as this incision heals during the next week or so. Women who have strong feelings against having this procedure carried out should talk with their doctor about it so that efforts can be made to accommodate her wishes as long as medically advisable. At this time in the second stage of labor the woman is discouraged from forceful pushing and may be encouraged to breathe in a rapid, shallow way to avoid bearing down.

Because the bones of the cranium are flexible at this time and the head is soft, it is often squeezed a little during expulsion through the birth canal. The head should be delivered slowly, with care taken that the umbilical cord is not wound around the baby's neck. Then the remainder of the baby's body emerges. The delivery room is now very busy. Secretions are gently suctioned from the baby's nose and throat. Its breathing, heart rate, muscle tone, color, and reflexes are checked immediately and again 5 minutes later; this is called the Apgar score. Silver nitrate drops are placed in its eyes. The umbilical cord is clipped and cut. The newborn's footprints are taken, a first record of the baby's identity. During this period the placenta separates from the wall of the uterus, sometimes with the doctor's help, and emerges from the vagina. The placenta and the cervix are quickly examined to be sure that no tearing has occurred.

Cesarean Delivery

A **Cesarean section,** or C-section, involves a surgical incision through the abdominal wall and uterus to deliver a baby promptly rather than through the birth canal (Fig. 10-20). It is called "Cesarean" because Julius Caesar was supposedly delivered in this way, although many historians doubt this. The high number of such deliveries in the United States invokes much controversy, although this procedure can save the mother's life, the baby's life, and significantly decrease the likelihood of childbirth complications. Some of this controversy involves physicians' desire to minimize risks during delivery, even if it means surgically extracting the newborn "just to be on the safe side." Cesarean sections are usually performed when labor would be medically unsafe or physically too demanding for the mother, when the baby must be delivered as soon as possible and there isn't time to induce labor, when the baby is too large or positioned in a way that makes vaginal delivery hazardous, when there is a medical emergency, or when the placenta's position blocks the baby's progress through the cervix.

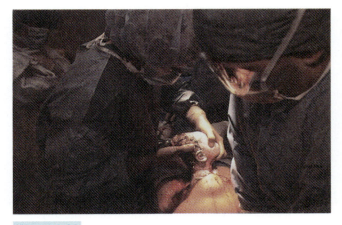

FIGURE 10-20   In this photograph of a Cesarean section birth, the newborn's head is gently removed from the uterus through an incision in the woman's abdomen. Some risks associated with a vaginal birth can be minimized with this procedure.

In most cases, an epidural block is used for anesthesia, and the surgical incision is made lengthwise or in a transverse manner. In an emergency the doctor may use general anesthesia to begin the delivery more quickly. Because a Cesarean delivery is an invasive surgical procedure, there is risk of surgical complications, such as postoperative infection, blood clots, and bleeding, and steps are taken to prevent these. Recuperation takes much longer than following vaginal birth. Doctors once thought that a woman who had a Cesarean delivery would also have to have C-sections for any subsequent deliveries, believing that the uterus with a healed incision would be too weak to progress through labor without rupturing. The thinking on this issue has changed, however. Most women today are encouraged to consider a vaginal birth after a Cesarean (VBAC), and about 60% of women who had a previous Cesarean delivery will have uncomplicated vaginal deliveries. This is a matter for a woman to discuss with her doctor. Many women feel vaginal birth is a fulfilling experience and prefer it when medically safe for her and her baby.

Birthing Alternatives

In recent decades doctors, new mothers, and other medical professionals have explored childbirth alternatives that recognize the desire of many parents to have their child enter the world in a setting less technological than a hospital. In the past only rarely were fathers invited into the delivery room to be present at the birth of their child and to offer emotional support and medical assistance to the mother. Now there are a number of birthing alternatives. We do not encourage women to have a baby in any particular way but do believe that a woman's decisions related to childbirth should be informed and based on knowing the different options.

Alternative birthing procedures do not necessarily offer mother or infant significant medical advantages over traditional strategies. However, couples who participate in Lamaze, Leboyer, or Bradley protocols report feeling better informed and more in control through the process of labor and delivery. Also, for a couple with concerns about possible effects of anesthetics on the baby, these methods offer strategies that minimize or eliminate the need for such agents.

GENERAL ANESTHESIA

Many women are very apprehensive about childbirth and desire general anesthesia. Since general anesthesia also affects the newborn, however, it may not be appropriate in high-risk pregnancies. If the woman has too much anxiety or if the pressure and discomfort are overwhelming, general or local anesthesia may be the best alternative. Women who choose these options are not bad mothers but are making a personal decision about a highly personal matter and should not be criticized for this.

THE LAMAZE METHOD

On a trip to the Soviet Union in 1951, the French obstetrician Fernand Lamaze discovered to his surprise that many Russian women going through labor did not require or request drugs to diminish pain. They managed their labor contractions by fo-

cused concentration on pleasant memories or objects in the labor room. They also used breathing exercises that kept high levels of oxygen in the bloodstream and allowed more control over the need to push, further minimizing pain. Of course, women delivered babies successfully for thousands of years without any anesthetics. The **Lamaze Technique** is a short course in prepared parenthood. Couples attend six weekly classes lasting about 2 hours each. All important pregnancy and childbirth topics are discussed. Women learn to focus their attention and use various breathing techniques. Their partners are coaches who offer help timing contractions, gently rubbing the woman's abdomen, encouraging them to concentrate, providing ice chips, dabbing their foreheads, and so on. The assumption is that couples who know a lot about labor and delivery know what's coming and what their options are at each step. Women who are relaxed and informed feel more in control and less apprehensive and thus experience less physical discomfort and less frequently request pain medications. Instruction concerning when and how hard to push eases the passage of the baby through the birth canal. Studies have demonstrated that women who take Lamaze classes report less discomfort during active labor (Leventhal, Leventhal, Shacham, & Easterling, 1989), and measurably higher pain thresholds during labor (Whipple, Josimovich, & Komisaruk, 1990). Lamaze instructors, usually women, are trained and professionally certified by the American Society for Psychoprophylaxis in Obstetrics.

THE BRADLEY METHOD

Robert Bradley, a Denver obstetrician, developed a childbirth method in the late 1940s that emphasizes relaxation exercises during labor but does not include breathing exercises as does the Lamaze method. Although fewer women use the Bradley method than the Lamaze method, both emphasize the importance of relaxation and education. Couples begin the Bradley method at about five and a half months of pregnancy and learn 12 different relaxation exercises, which help women better manage their discomfort during labor. As in Lamaze classes, couples meet weekly in sessions typically lasting 2 hours. The father also is the coach, encouraging and supporting his partner through the stages of labor and suggesting additional relaxation techniques if others become less effective. The Bradley method encourages women to change position frequently during labor and not lie on their backs. Taking a stroll or a warm shower are excellent diversions. Both the Lamaze method and the Bradley method are basic and simple.

LEBOYER DELIVERY

Other "natural" childbirth techniques that minimize or eliminate anesthesia have also become popular. The French obstetrician Frederick Leboyer developed an approach intended to minimize the stress of delivery for the newborn (Leboyer, 1975). Leboyer calls his method "birth without violence." He believes that spanking a newborn on its bottom to stimulate breathing and having silver nitrate drops immediately put into its eyes in a room of cold temperatures and bright lights is an unpleasant way to come into the world. Additionally, he be-

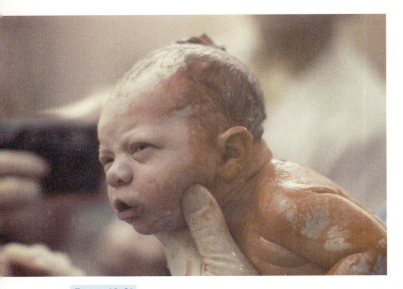

FIGURE 10-21   In the Leboyer method of childbirth, the newborn is gently taken from close skin contact with its mother to a warm bath. Lights are dimmed and soft music often played. Although medical assessment of the baby is very important, strong emphasis is placed on the newborn's comfort and its interactions with its mother.

lieves it is unnecessary and traumatic for the umbilical cord to be cut promptly after delivery. Instead, he believes that the cord should be left intact for several minutes to allow the newborn to get used to inhaling air before it has to do so on its own. Leboyer recommends that as soon as the baby emerges from the birth canal it should be gently laid on its mother's warm, bare abdomen and gently caressed. After a few minutes, the baby is placed in a warm bath to induce calm relaxation (Fig. 10-21). Harsh delivery room lights are turned off, and soft ones create a more soothing ambience.

Childbirth Settings

At one time in the past virtually all babies were born at home. Today, women have more choices for where they will deliver and the treatment and support they receive. Nonetheless, most women in America still prefer to have their babies in the hospital, often because this is the only place most obstetricians will deliver children and because of the technological resources available in case a problem occurs during labor or delivery. Because the traditional labor and delivery unit sometimes has a cold, impersonal quality, some hospitals have "birthing centers" with a more relaxed, home-like atmosphere. Labor and delivery typically take place in the same room, which is furnished more like a bedroom. Soft lights, curtains, carpeting, wallpaper, and home furniture replace the more austere fixtures of most hospitals (Fig. 10-22). But because the facility is located within the hospital, the doctor still has access to sophisticated equipment in case of an emergency, and the surgical suite is just down the hall.

Many women prefer home birth as a comfortable, natural option. If a complication or emergency occurs during labor or delivery, however, resources are few for handling it at home. Most obstetricians therefore do not deliver babies at home and generally recommend against the practice. This is not to say that home birth is a bad idea, but this birthing option must be considered very carefully by everyone involved.

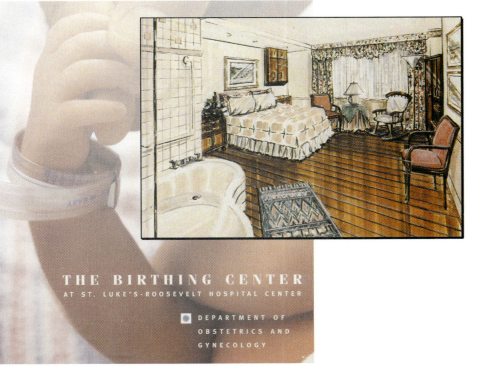

FIGURE 10-22   Many hospitals now offer birthing centers, which offer a more comfortable, "home-like" environment, so the birth of a baby can often be attended by friends and family members if the parents feel at ease with this.

In recent years many obstetricians have welcomed midwives into their practice. Midwives are thoroughly trained and certified to offer professional, nurturant care during labor and delivery. Controlled studies have demonstrated that midwives deliver babies that are just as healthy after birth as those delivered by obstetricians (Davis, Riedmann, Sapiro, Minogue, & Kazer, 1994). Many midwives work in hospitals and birthing centers, and others help with home deliveries. In many rural and isolated localities, midwives play a central role assisting women during childbirth when few other health care resources are available.

AFTER CHILDBIRTH

Many adjustments must usually be made after a baby is born, and often the whole household changes. Domestic space is allocated differently, sleep schedules change, and the whole concept of "free time" changes. Dealing with the demands of a totally dependent newborn can be daunting, and the relationship between the mother and father may be stressed at this time. People frequently say, "Your life will never be the same again"—and this is true. This adjustment process involves many changes, just a few of which we'll discuss here.

Postpartum Depression

Most women experience a normal period of sadness and irritability during the week or two after childbirth. Some cry more readily than otherwise. Women who stay in the hospital only briefly after giving birth are more likely to experience depression than those who stay in the medical setting longer (Hickey, Boyce, Ellwood, & Morris-Yates, 1997). This is an important finding, since health insurers generally discourage longer postpartum hospital stays. Feelings of despondency, discouragement, and gloom that are serious and persistent are called postpartum depression. Postpartum depression can last months. It has many of the same characteristics as any major type of depression: feelings of sadness, an inability to concentrate, psychomotor agitation, and a loss of enjoyment in things one formerly found enjoyable. Sleep irregularities and appetite increases or decreases may occur. Women who were anxious or depressed before or during their pregnancies are more likely to be depressed for a long period afterwards. Women with bipolar disorder (manic-depressive illness) or premenstrual syndrome are also more likely to experience prolonged depression after giving birth (Pariser, Nasrallah, & Gardiner, 1997). One can easily feel overwhelmed by the pressures of being a new mother coupled with the expectations of parents, in-laws, and one's spouse. *Everything* has changed. Although hormonal factors are thought to play a role in these feelings, this mechanism is not fully understood.

Viinamaki, Niskanen, Pesonen, and Saarikoski (1997) reported that women who had serious financial problems, a limited social support system, and relationship problems with their significant other were more likely to have chronic depression after childbirth. Interestingly, most of these women in their study chose not to become pregnant again. Many women recover from this depression fairly rapidly, however, and often have more children.

Before giving birth, many women and men are heavily involved in their jobs and families and enjoy a sense of accomplishment in both. Leathers, Kelley, and Richman (1997) demonstrated that the loss of this involvement has a large causative role in depression in both women and men after the birth of a baby. Social scientists have studied whether women in other societies experience postpartum depression similarly. Ghubash and Abou-Saleh (1997) reported that postpartum depression in the Arab world is comparable to that reported in both Europe and North America. Somewhat comparable data concerning postpartum depression have been collected in Japan (Tamaki, Murata, & Okano, 1997), Dubai (Abou-Saleh & Ghubash, 1997), and Brazil (Rohde, Busnello, Wolf, Zomer, Shansis, Martins, & Tramontina, 1997). Antidepressant medications are often used in the treatment of postpartum depression.

Breast and Bottle Feeding

A large percentage of time spent caring for a newborn is devoted to feeding, and the baby gets much more than nutrition while being fed. It gets the exclusive attention of the person dispensing the milk. Some psychologists believe that infant feeding instills a sense of trust in a child long before it can walk or talk. Virtually all nutritional needs are met by mother's milk, as well as by commercial formulas. Breastfeeding, which had become relatively rare after the advent of commercial products, is popular again. According to the U. S. Department of Health and Human Services (1996), 60% of American mothers breastfeed their newborns, many for some time into infancy. Breastfeeding has many advantages. Human milk is high in fat and low in protein, a good balance for a rapidly developing nervous system. Human milk has virtually all the nutrients a newborn needs until it is about 6 weeks old and also carries the mother's antibodies to diseases. Breast-fed babies have fewer colds, intestinal problems, and allergies than bottle-fed babies. Breast milk is more digestible than bottle formulas, and breast-fed babies make a smoother change to solid foods.

Most women who breastfeed their babies find their feeding interactions satisfying, although some women are uncomfortable or embarrassed about breastfeeding in public. Because breast milk is digested efficiently, the baby is hungry again in about 2 hours, compared to 3 or 4 hours in formula-fed babies. For working women who breastfeed, this can be a problem. Many women therefore combine breast- and bottle-feeding. A study by Horwood and Fergusson (1998) reported a link between how long an infant is breast-fed and later cognitive development and academic achievement in school (1998). About 1000 children in New Zealand were studied; the length of breast feeding was documented, and from 8 to 18 years of age their mental development and school performance were monitored. The longer these children had breast-fed, the higher were their IQ scores at ages 8 and 9. Reading ability and mathematical skill between ages 10 and 13 were similarly positively associated with length of breastfeeding. At the end of high school, academic achievement scores were also positively related to length of breastfeeding. The mothers of these children were a little older, better educated, and wealthier, but these factors alone did not account for these findings. Interestingly, in the recent past breastfeeding was more common among poorer American women. Today, however, women of all socioeconomic levels breastfeed their babies.

Resuming Sexual Relations After Childbirth

Obstetricians generally recommend that a couple not have sexual intercourse for six weeks after childbirth. The couple can explore a variety of nonintercourse expressions of physical intimacy, of course. Masturbation, mutual masturbation, and oral-genital stimulation are common alternatives. Since caring for a newborn can take up much of one's time and energy, a woman should not be surprised if she does not feel sexual for some time after childbirth. Sometimes an episiotomy needs a long while to heal, and until then vaginal penetration is probably uncomfortable. After a woman gives birth the low levels of estrogen in the bloodstream causes a thinning of the walls of the vagina, which can make penile penetration painful. Similarly, estrogen levels stay low while a woman breast-feeds. A non-petroleum-based lubricant, like K-Y jelly, can make intercourse more comfortable. The couple may also try intercourse positions that allow the woman to control the angle, rate, and depth of penetration, such as the woman-on-top position. Pelvic thrusting should be slow and gentle soon after childbirth. Women who delivered by Cesarean section need a prolonged period of abstinence from intercourse while the surgical wound heals. Men often worry about hurting their partners and women are apprehensive about penetration. If such worries persist a long time, a sex counselor or therapist can help.

For about two weeks after childbirth, women experience a thin red vaginal discharge called *lochia*. This is not menstrual discharge. In women who breastfeed, the return to cycles of ovulation and menstruation is delayed. Women who do not breastfeed start having their periods again in 2 to 3 months. Nonetheless, a woman who does not want to become pregnant again right away should not have unprotected sex at this time. The first periods may be spotty and irregular but over time become more routine and uniform. The couple should consider what kind of contraception they might want to use after the birth of a baby and make appropriate plans.

INFERTILITY: BROKEN DREAMS AND PROMISING REALITIES

Many people have a life script that includes having children, but what happens when we find out that we can't? Even before a person seeks assistance for infertility, they may wonder what they will do with their lives. Many of the landmarks of the adult years focus on children: buying a house, taking family vacations, purchasing life insurance, saving for higher educa-

tion, and looking forward to becoming a grandparent. Suddenly, a person needs a new script to provide direction and goals for their most energetic adult years. Being unable to have children can be a crushing awareness and often requires counseling, therapy, and values clarification. Chapter 1 included a vignette that highlighted such concerns and showed the stress and tension that young couple was experiencing.

Many people were raised in an environment that taught them that it is their "duty" to carry on the family name or family traditions. Discovering an obstacle to this end can be extremely disconcerting, and the person often feels they're letting someone down: their spouse, their parents, their extended family. Many people become depressed and angry and wonder, "Why me?" Women generally experience more guilt and anxiety than men (Benazon, Wright, & Sabourin, 1992). Infertility can negatively affect a couple's marital satisfaction and detract significantly from their shared sexuality. Infertility forces people to think more about the distinction between sex for procreation and sex for recreation. The pleasure of sexual intercourse is often diminished when a couple discovers a fertility problem, and the medical evaluation of infertility makes sex seem even more clinical and removed from erotic feelings.

Fertility is not a simple yes-or-no matter, however—not a simple situation in which women get pregnant easily or don't at all. Fertility and infertility are endpoints on a continuum of how easily a couple conceives a child and carries the developing baby to term. Some women become pregnant the first time they have unprotected intercourse, and some try for years to make the same thing happen, even with extensive medical assistance. Infertility is defined in different specific ways, but generally when a couple has had unprotected intercourse about twice a week for a year to eighteen months and have not conceived, they are often encouraged to have a fertility work-up with their physicians, usually a gynecologist for her and a urologist for him. About 1 in 6 couples in the United States meet this criterion and seek the counsel of their doctors. Fertility problems are very common, and fixing them can be time-consuming, expensive, and frustrating. Following are the CDC's percentages of women seeking infertility treatment in various diagnostic categories:

Problems in the Fallopian Tubes	31%
Endometriosis	14%
Problems in the Uterus	1%
Male Fertility Problems	18%
Other Factors (e.g., STDs)	21%
Unexplained Factors	15%

The number of medical specialists who advertise expertise and training in treating infertility is growing (Fig. 10-23). Gynecologists, urologists, and reproductive endocrinologists are all involved in some phase of infertility treatment. In many cities large clinics use the most modern advances in reproductive technology in the treatment of infertility. Many couple's desire to have a baby is very powerful, and many medical resources are devoted to this problem. In addition to frustration, a couple with a fertility problem frequently experiences impa-

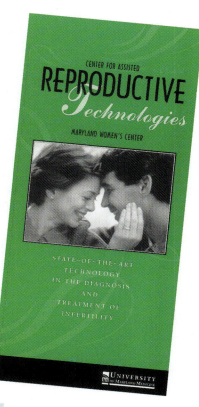

FIGURE 10-23 Many major medical centers throughout the United States offer couples a wide variety of assisted reproductive technologies.

tience. Doctors often move in a slow, careful, deliberate fashion, however, to determine the cause and best treatment for a couple's problem. We are surprised that in most instances of infertility, the woman undergoes extensive, and often expensive, medical testing before her partner is similarly tested. It may take many months of monitoring basal body temperature, noting the timing of ovulation, testing hormone levels in the blood, and determining that the fallopian tubes are open and that the uterus is normal before her partner has a semen analysis, which is a fairly simple and straightforward affair. It might be a good idea to evaluate both partners simultaneously to minimize feelings of impatience.

An Infertility Work-Up

The International Council on Infertility Information Dissemination has guidelines for couples who think they have an infertility problem. We include that information here but believe that one's own doctor is the best source of information for one's own case. This organization recommends consulting a reproductive endocrinologist unless one's obstetrician/gynecologist can fulfill all the following suggestions. A reproductive endocrinologist often can also manage both female and male aspects of infertility at the same time.

A woman's first visit should be scheduled during the first week of her menstrual cycle to determine her baseline levels of FSH and LH. Basal body temperature chart records can give the

doctor valuable information about her menstrual cycles over several months. The second appointment is scheduled on the day the LH levels surge, signaling that ovulation is about to take place. The woman is often asked to purchase and use a home ovulation kit and to contact the office the day the increased LH is obvious. In this visit she may undergo several procedures.

- **Cervical Mucus Tests.** The doctor assesses the viscosity of the cervical mucus, and a postcoital (after intercourse) test may be performed to determine how well the man's sperm are penetrating the cervical mucus. Additionally, cervical mucus is often tested for any bacteria that could pose a problem.
- **Ultrasound Examinations.** Ultrasound tests assess the thickness of the endometrium at the time of ovulation and follicle development in the ovaries. Fibroid tumors, ovarian cysts, or anything unusual in the shape of the uterus may be noted with this test.
- **Hormone Levels.** Blood tests can determine the levels of various hormones in the middle of the menstrual cycle and on the day of increased LH secretion. LH, FSH, estradiol, progesterone, prolactin, thyroid hormone, and testosterone are tested at this time.

Based on the results of this initial assessment, the reproductive endocrinologist may recommend the following tests. The fertility tests for men described below can be carried out at the same time these tests are performed on the woman.

- **Hysterosalpingogram.** A dye is injected through the cervix into the uterus and fallopian tubes. An x-ray is taken to determine if all structures and passageways are open without obstructions. For example, scar tissue blocking a fallopian tube will show up on this x-ray. This test can be mildly uncomfortable or painful.
- **Hysteroscopy.** If the doctor suspects some abnormality inside the uterus, she or he may insert a thin fiberoptic scope through the cervix into the uterus to visualize its interior. This outpatient procedure is usually done under general anesthesia.
- **Laparoscopy.** The fiberoptic scope is inserted into a woman's abdomen through the umbilicus (belly button), allowing the doctor to see the fallopian tubes and ovaries. When endometriosis is suspected, visualizing the lower pelvic region can determine whether this disorder is present.
- **Endometrial Biopsy.** A biopsy is the removal of tissue from some body area to examine it under a microscope for signs of disease. In an endometrial biopsy, a small amount of tissue is shaved from the lining of the uterus just before the period is expected. This test can reveal a problem during the luteal phase of the menstrual cycle that prevents a sustained pregnancy due to inadequate progesterone being secreted from the corpus luteum.

Overall, a fertility work-up involves precise procedures and alternatives that depend on the woman's unique circumstances

(Fig. 10-24). The couple should try to be informed consumers of medical services who understand good medical practices in the arena of reproductive endocrinology.

Just as various medical tests are used to evaluate female infertility, several tests are typically included in a fertility work-up for men. The urologist takes a thorough medical history, especially concerning situations, such as undescended testes, mumps after puberty, injury to the testes, or torsion (twisting of the spermatic cord). Prolonged exposures to high temperatures, radiation, or environmental toxins are assessed, as well as any history with prescription and recreational drugs and alcohol. The possibilities of diabetes and thyroid problems are also explored. A scrotal varicocele is a problem in the valves of the veins that carry blood from the testes, allowing blood to remain too long in the area. The increased temperature of the

testicle caused by the warm venous blood impairs the production of sperm. About half of all men with varicoceles have this semen problem, which may make fertilization more difficult; 40% of male fertility problems result from this disorder.

Semen analysis is the most important first step in the clinical assessment of male infertility. The doctor analyzes several semen samples (usually three over 6 to 8 weeks) to determine a baseline of sperm production and characteristics. Typically, the man is given a sterile, wide-mouth container and asked to masturbate into it. The sample is examined in the doctor's office within 2 hours. Avoiding masturbation and intercourse before collecting the sample can be important. With each day of abstinence up to one week, the volume of semen increases by 0.4 cc, and each day of abstinence adds 10 to 15 million sperm to each cc of ejaculate. A week's abstinence can affect total sperm count by 50 to 90 million sperm (Shaban, on line, 1997). The following specific characteristics of semen are analyzed:

- **Semen Volume.** If the total volume of ejaculate is below 1.5 cc, fertility is considered adversely affected. Conversely, a semen volume over 5 cc also lowers the chances of conception occurring, generally because higher volumes are often associated with fewer sperm per cc.
- **Sperm Count.** Approximately 20 million sperm per cc of ejaculate is considered the lower limit for fertility. Semen may contain as many as 90 to 100 million sperm per cc.
- **Sperm Motility.** This involves estimating the percentage of sperm in the ejaculate that are swimming, as well as the forward movement of swimming sperm in a straight path. Urologists believe that in normal fertility, about half of the sperm are vigorously swimming forward. Low semen volume and low sperm count can to some degree be compensated for by good sperm motility.
- **Sperm Form.** Ideally at least 30% of sperm have normal oval head sections, middle sections, and tails.
- **Other Factors.** White blood cells present in the ejaculate may signal an infection. Fructose from the seminal vesicles is necessary for normal sperm motility and action; the doctor may test for its presence.

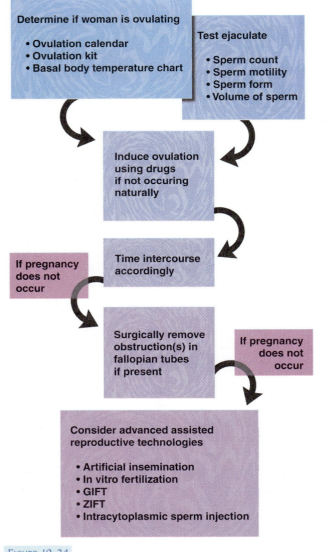

FIGURE 10-24   Some (but perhaps not all) of the steps that may be involved in assessing a woman's and man's fertility and some of the treatment alternatives for which they may be candidates.

If the semen analysis reveals deficiencies, blood tests will likely be used to measure levels of various hormones. The amounts of testosterone, LH, and FSH are determined, and sometimes also certain adrenal hormones, thyroid hormone, and growth hormone. In the postcoital test, the ability of sperm to penetrate cervical mucus is assessed. Cervical mucus is examined 2 to 8 hours after intercourse around the time the woman is expected to ovulate. The presence of sperm in cervical mucus shows they can penetrate the viscous fluid. A sperm penetration assay may also be performed, a test using a hamster egg to estimate how easily the sperm can penetrate a human ovum. This laboratory test gives doctors a good idea if assisted reproductive technologies will likely succeed. The doctor may also examine the acrosomes on the tips of the sperm's heads with an electron microscope to assess this structure. These sophisticated tests require skill and complex instruments and may not be appropriate or available for all men with fertility problems. Finally, the presence of bacteria in semen or prostatic fluid could signal the existence of a sexually transmitted disease that could cause reproductive problems.

A complete fertility work-up for a woman or man is time-consuming, complex, and expensive. Many health insurance companies do not pay benefits for infertility because they do not consider assessment and treatment of infertility "medically necessary," despite being a central psychological issue for those going through it. Psychological well-being is often poor for a couple experiencing infertility testing. They typically feel frustrated, impatient, and scared about their future if they cannot have a baby. These problems can be particularly devastating for less mature young adults. A later section discusses psychological counseling and support for couples being treated for infertility.

TREATMENTS FOR INFERTILITY

Of all but one of the assisted reproductive technologies described below, almost 80% of the women who use them have not had a previous live birth. Most women exploring these options are 30 to 40 years old. Half of all women using assisted reproductive technologies have a single-baby birth, 23.8% have twins, and 4.5% triplets or more babies. Younger women generally have higher success rates, and women over the age of 45 have very little success.

Ovulation-Stimulating Drugs

A common problem for couples who cannot readily conceive is that the woman does not ovulate regularly and predictably. In this situation the couple cannot know the best time to have sexual intercourse to maximize the chances of fertilization. The woman's basal body temperature charts may show she is not ovulating at all. In either situation, the reproductive endocrinologist may administer a drug to stimulate ovulation. The specific drug used depends on the patient's circumstances. Clomiphene (Clomid), the most commonly used drug, stimulates ovulation in 80 to 85% of women who use it, with 40 to 50% of them becoming pregnant. Ovulation-inducing drugs increase the chance of multiple births slightly because sometimes more than one egg is released during ovulation. Ovarian cysts are a side effect of this medication, and the doctor monitors for their development, typically with a pelvic examination. Women using Clomid often see indications of ovulation on their monthly basal body temperature charts and thus know when to have sexual intercourse. Because Clomid becomes less effective with continued use, many fertility specialists do not use this agent longer than three consecutive months. Clomid is also used to stimulate ovulation for *in vitro* fertilization techniques so that the doctor knows when eggs are available for removal.

Another ovulation-stimulating drug is "Pergonal," a synthetic version of FSH and LH. This agent is often followed by an injection of human chorionic gonadotropin (HCG). The FSH and LH in this drug replace or supplement a lack of these pituitary hormones that may be causing the failure to ovulate. It is used along with a basal body temperature chart and is also used to stimulate ovulation in women undergoing *in vitro* fertilization procedures. Clomid and/or Pergonal may not be appropriate for all women who are not ovulating regularly, if another medical condition rules this out.

Artificial Insemination

Artificial, or **intrauterine, insemination** is a treatment used when sperm cannot penetrate the woman's cervical mucus or swim fast enough through the reproductive tract. The cervix is completely bypassed in this procedure, and sperm are deposited directly into the uterus. If the man has a low sperm count or poor sperm motility, the couple may choose to use a donor's sperm to inseminate the woman. This procedure is also used by lesbians who want to conceive without having sexual intercourse with a man. This procedure is referred to as AIH (artificial insemination, husband) or AID (artificial insemination, donor). When donor sperm are used, the husband's consent is legally required. Semen is placed in a narrow cup and inserted through the cervix in a plug-like plastic device (Fig. 10-25) The device is removed several hours later by gently pulling a nylon thread attached to it. If the woman also is not regularly ovulating, Clomid may be used along with artificial insemination. The woman's basal body temperature chart

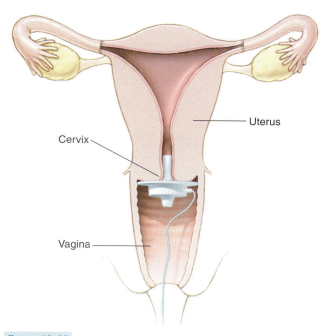

Cervix

Uterus

Vagina

FIGURE 10-25   Device used in artificial insemination. Sperm are deposited in the narrow cup that is inserted through the cervix and into the opening of the uterus. After 24 hours, the thin nylon thread is used to remove the device.

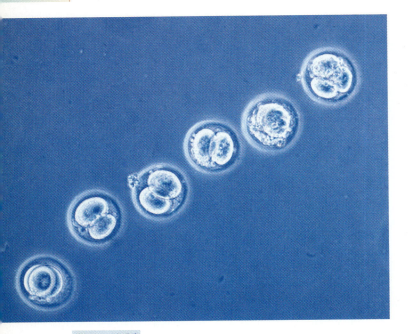

FIGURE 10-26 Normal cellular division of a fertilized human ovum. Note cellular division and increasing complexity of the developing cell mass. Each stage of cellular division is easy to recognize in the laboratory by trained technicians.

is used to inform the doctor when to use this procedure. Of all the assisted reproductive technologies, artificial insemination is the simplest and least expensive. This technique is about 74% effective when used for six menstrual cycles.

In Vitro Fertilization

In 1978 Lesley Brown of Oldham, England gave birth to her first child, Louise. Louise was a healthy normal baby although she was premature and weighed only 5 pounds and 12 ounces.

The only thing unusual about her was that Louise was conceived not in her mother's fallopian tube but in a sterile glass dish in the laboratory of Dr. Patrick Steptoe, a gynecologist, and his colleague Dr. Robert Edwards, an embryologist. Louise Brown was the first human conceived through *in vitro* **fertilization**. The phrase *in vitro* refers to an experiment outside the human body in a controlled scientific environment, in this case, a glass dish in the laboratory. Ms. Brown's fallopian tubes were blocked, preventing sperm and egg from meeting. A surgical attempt had been made to open her tubes but was unsuccessful. The couple desperately wanted a baby and were eager to participate in an experiment that then had not yet been successful in helping women like Lesley. Although the procedure seems simple, the hundreds of important details necessary for success had not yet been fully worked out.

Ms. Brown first received hormones to stimulate the development and maturation of eggs in her ovaries, eventually resulting in a fertilizable egg. Drs. Steptoe and Edwards performed a **laparoscopy** to look directly at her ovaries at the expected time of ovulation. They carefully removed a mature egg and placed it in a laboratory dish containing all the chemicals and nutrients normally found in the fallopian tubes at ovulation. Mr. Brown masturbated, and his sperm were promptly added to the dish. Could a human sperm fertilize a human egg outside the female reproductive tract? While the egg was being observed carefully for fertilization, Ms. Brown received injections of female sex hormones to prepare the lining of her uterus to receive the fertilized egg. Mr. Brown's sperm did fertilize his wife's egg, which then began to divide normally (Fig. 10-26). When cell division reached the blastocyst stage, the developing cell mass was gently inserted in Ms. Brown's uterus (Fig. 10-27). Hormone levels a week later signaled that the attachment was good, and the pregnancy was under way. Since this remarkable first *in vitro* fertilization and successful pregnancy, more than 20,000 babies throughout the world have been conceived through this

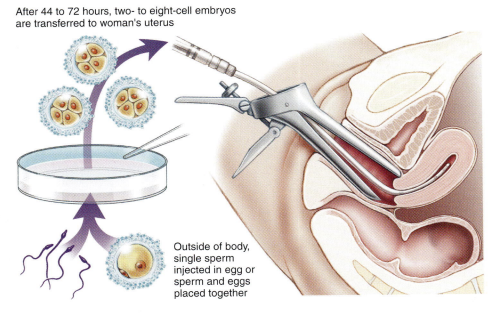

After 44 to 72 hours, two- to eight-cell embryos are transferred to woman's uterus

Outside of body, single sperm injected in egg or sperm and eggs placed together

FIGURE 10-27 In *in vitro* fertilization, ova are fertilized by sperm in a laboratory dish and are then transferred through a tube directly into a woman's uterus. Several such fertilized eggs are usually transferred during each attempt to conceive.

method. For more than two decades *in vitro* fertilization and other assisted reproductive technologies have given hope to many couples unable to conceive a child unassisted.

When Drs. Steptoe and Edwards began serious experimentation with *in vitro* fertilization, the chances of their success were extraordinarily small. Today in the United States, women who use this treatment for infertility can expect a 25% success rate of conceiving in any single reproductive cycle. In 1997 the Centers for Disease Control and Prevention summarized their research on assisted reproductive technologies; to date, these are the most accurate data available. In women under the age of 35, the success rate of conception for each menstrual cycle was 29.7%, for those between 35 and 39 the rate was 23.4%, and for those over age 39 the success rate was 13.2%. Clearly the woman's age is a very important factor in assisted reproductive technologies. These figures reflect *pregnancies per menstrual cycle.* The overall rate of live births is 19.9% (with multiple births counted as a single birth); this rate reflects the need to repeat the procedure four or five times on average. These data are for the use of the woman's own fresh (not frozen) embryos, not for donor eggs from other women. The CDC report includes the success rates for every licensed, certified fertility clinic in the United States and recommendations for choosing a fertility clinic in those areas where there is a choice. Of the different types of assisted reproductive technologies used, over 70% of cases employed *in vitro* fertilization. Success rates are significantly higher with fresh embryos than with frozen embryos.

Modern surgical innovations have simplified the removal of a woman's eggs for *in vitro* fertilization. Eggs are retrieved from the ovaries using ultrasound imaging and a needle in a procedure called *transvaginal oocyte retrieval,* which does not require a hospital stay or general anesthesia. The needle is inserted into the pelvic cavity through the wall of the vagina, causing only mild discomfort. After fertilization and early embryonic cell division occur in the laboratory, the developing cell mass is implanted into the uterus through the vagina and cervix. Women undergoing this treatment lie still for about an hour and can then go home.

The Atlanta Reproductive Health Center (1997) advises the following about *in vitro* fertilization:

- Undergoing *in vitro* fertilization does not usually damage a woman's ovaries.
- The doctor retrieve eggs only prior to ovulation, not afterwards.
- If the procedure does not result in a conception the first time it is tried, usually the woman must wait 2 or 3 menstrual cycles before trying again.
- The number of times *in vitro* fertilization is attempted is decided jointly by the couple and their physician.
- It is a good idea to have sexual intercourse in the weeks before an attempt at *in vitro* fertilization.
- Most fertility experts recommend that a couple abstain from sexual intercourse for two to three weeks after an *in vitro* fertilization procedure.

- Women are encouraged to remain sedentary for 24 hours after an *in vitro* fertilization procedure.
- From the time the woman's eggs are harvested, it takes approximately 13 days to find out if she is pregnant.
- There is an increased chance of multiple births with *in vitro* fertilization. About 1 in 4 procedures result in twins, and 2 to 3% in triplets. Because this procedure is complex and expensive, several fertilized eggs are implanted; typically not all of them develop into embryos, but sometimes some do.

Gamete Intrafallopian Transfer (GIFT)
In a different procedure called **gamete intrafallopian transfer** (GIFT), a woman's eggs are removed from her ovary and combined with sperm in the laboratory, as in the *in vitro* procedure, and then the unfertilized egg and sperm are implanted directly into her fallopian tubes through a small incision using laparoscopy (Fig. 10-28). This procedure is especially helpful for women who have one fallopian tube, endometriosis, damage to the cervix, or not enough cervical mucus. While estimates of success rates vary widely, GIFT is considered more effective than *in vitro* fertilization but is not recommended for all cases of female infertility. In the CDC's most recent report (1997), only 2% of assisted reproductive procedures employ GIFT.

Zygote Intrafallopian Transfer (ZIFT)
A drawback to GIFT is that the doctor cannot be sure that fertilization has taken place before inserting eggs and sperm into the woman's fallopian tubes. In **zygote intrafallopian transfer** (ZIFT) the harvested eggs and sperm are combined in the laboratory; after fertilization takes place, the zygote is placed inside the woman's fallopian tubes using laparoscopy (Fig. 10-28). ZIFT is also used rarely; only 2% of assisted reproductive procedures employ ZIFT.

The term *embryo transfer* is generally used to describe the placement of embryos into a woman's uterus through her cervix or directly into her fallopian tubes. This is not a very specific term and applies to several different assisted reproductive technologies. Ectopic pregnancies do not occur with either GIFT or ZIFT.

Injecting Sperm into Eggs
When a man has a very low sperm count, an egg can be harvested from the woman and an individual sperm injected directly into it, leading to fertilization, the beginning of cellular division, and early embryonic development (Fig. 10-29). This process is called *intracytoplasmic sperm injection,* (ICSI). After fertilization the zygote is transferred to the woman's uterus in the same manner as in *in vitro* fertilization. This is the least often used of the various assisted reproductive technologies described here. In about 1 in 3 attempts, this technique results in pregnancy and subsequent childbirth. This technique is commonly used for male fertility problems but involves some controversy. Because men are sometimes infertile because of a genetic disease, ICSI might inadvertently transmit such a disease

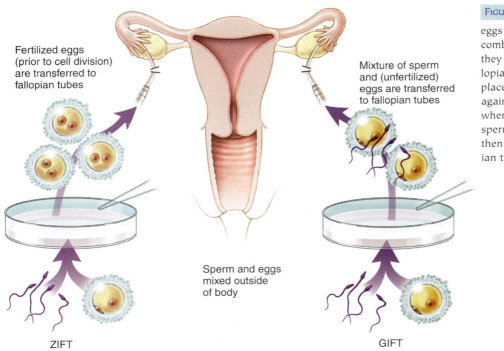

Fertilized eggs
(prior to cell division)
are transferred to
fallopian tubes

Mixture of sperm
and (unfertilized)
eggs are transferred
to fallopian tubes

Sperm and eggs
mixed outside
of body

ZIFT

GIFT

FIGURE 10-28   In GIFT a woman's eggs and her partner's sperm are combined in the laboratory and then they are inserted directly into the fallopian tubes, where fertilization takes place. In ZIFT ova and sperm are again combined in the laboratory and when the ovum is fertilized by the sperm and become a zygote, it is then inserted directly into the fallopian tube.

to the offspring; it may also be a factor in the development of reproductive abnormalities in the offspring. It has also been speculated that ICSI may damage DNA within the sperm used to fertilize the ovum. While these are only speculations, they are important concerns, and therefore ICSI is not always used when it might be appropriate.

Surrogate Motherhood

The word "surrogate" means "substitute," and a surrogate mother is a woman implanted with an embryo formed from another woman's ovum. When the woman can ovulate but cannot carry a pregnancy, surrogate motherhood is an option. It is also used when the woman cannot ovulate, with her partner's sperm used to inseminate a donor egg that is then carried to term by the surrogate mother. For example, in a woman who has had a partial hysterectomy, the uterus and fallopian tubes may have been surgically removed, but she still has egg-producing ovaries.

In surrogate motherhood arrangements, the woman who carries the embryo and fetus during pregnancy gives the newborn to its biological parents at birth. Her medical care and expenses are paid for by the biological parents, and she typically receives a substantial fee for undergoing the medical procedure and carrying the pregnancy. Complicated psychosocial and legal issues may be involved with surrogate motherhood, and the couple usually works with an attorney who is an expert in surrogate motherhood and assisted reproductive technologies. Laws governing surrogate motherhood vary among different states. One issue, for example, is that some women agree to a surrogacy contract expecting to hand over the baby at birth but later feel unable to part with the baby she has carried for so long. Many surrogate mothers want to maintain at least some contact with the child they gave birth to.

In a study in England, 19 surrogate mothers were asked why they offered their services to infertile couples (Blyth, 1994). These women were all in their 20s and 30s, and most had low socioeconomic status and little formal education. Of these 19 women, 6 planned to become surrogate mothers a second time, and 1 for still a third time. Only 1 did not give up the child after birth, and 1 carried the pregnancy of a close friend. The most common reasons for becoming a surrogate

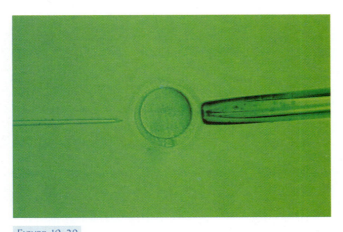

FIGURE 10-29   In ICSI, or *intracytoplasmic sperm injection*, a single sperm is aimed directly into a single ovum, which is then generally transferred to the woman's uterus.

mother were financial need and a deep curiosity about pregnancy. In all cases, the surrogate mother chose the parents for whom she worked. Five women reported significant problems giving up the baby, but only 2 said that they regretted the experience.

Counseling and Support for Infertile Couples

Because the prospect of not being able to have a baby is often devastating, many women and men dealing with infertility require significant emotional and psychological support. A diagnosis of infertility can lead to feelings of isolation and inadequacy, as well as financial hardship because of the costs of assisted reproductive technologies. Support groups of others sharing the same difficulties are often helpful. In 1974, Barbara Eck Manning, a nurse, founded the organization RESOLVE to serve this emotional and psychological need for women and men dealing with infertility and its treatment. Today, RESOLVE is a national organization maintaining a database of over 40,000 individuals and medical care providers, more than 50 chapters throughout the country, and a national staff. RESOLVE is a nonprofit organization with local chapters governed by volunteer boards of directors who are involved in infertility issues (attorneys, physicians, people who have adopted children, those who have had babies through assisted reproductive technologies, nurses, etc.). RESOLVE also advocates for comprehensive health insurance coverage for infertility treatment, since health insurance usually does not cover these costs (only 12 states mandate that health insurance companies pay for the costs of infertility treatment).

Couples who use assisted reproductive technologies and do not conceive are often emotionally exhausted, in debt, and demoralized and depressed (Stolberg, 1997). At some point they must decide when to stop and pursue other alternatives, such as egg donation or adoption. That is a difficult decision. Counseling often helps couples feel less isolated and may offer the friendship of those who have been successfully treated for infertility, as well as those who have learned a different perspective for their future.

Sperm Donation

Donated sperm are used to artificially inseminate a woman when her partner's sperm are lacking in some way and in some cases by women who do not desire intercourse. In the United States, reproductive technology is relatively unrestricted, and sperm banks vary in their quality control procedures. Some sperm banks may advertise that they have a large number of donors but may in fact have only a handful of donors. Sperm banks generally advertise that their semen has been repeatedly tested for HIV and other sexually transmitted diseases. They often keep detailed records of their donors, and a couple can stipulate specific attributes they want in a potential donor, such as educational attainment, ethnicity, blood type, hair and eye color, height, weight, and even occupation. One sperm bank makes available the first names of donors and their pho-

tographs. Some sperm banks even ask donors if they want to meet their offspring once they reach the age of 18. Frozen sperm or eggs can now be sent by overnight courier virtually anywhere on earth.

ENDING A PREGNANCY

Abortion is but one among many alternatives a woman or couple may choose when an unanticipated pregnancy occurs. Technically we are talking about "induced abortion," in contrast to "spontaneous abortion," or miscarriage, as discussed earlier. Abortion is one of the most controversial topics involved in the study of human sexuality. Our discussion will not concern abortion as a good or bad thing, however, or debate the legal issues. Regardless of people's different beliefs about abortion, everyone agrees this is a very big problem that affects many people, and no one sees abortion as a common, acceptable way to limit a woman's fertility.

The perceived need for an induced abortion arises in a number of different ways. The National Institutes of Health estimates that about half of abortions carried out in the United States each year result from some form of contraceptive "failure." This may mean that the contraceptive was not used consistently or conscientiously. Induced abortions are also sought as a consequence of sexual abuse, incest, rape, or simply a lack of good information about fertility and conception. When amniocentesis or chorionic villus sampling indicates serious abnormalities in the fetus, many couples also elect to terminate the pregnancy. Regardless of the reason, the decision to terminate a pregnancy should be approached with caution, care, and thorough consideration of alternatives, and many counseling opportunities are available to assist those who find themselves in this situation. Many rabbis and ministers are trained to help women and couples explore the various considerations in continuing or ending a pregnancy. Licensed clinical social workers, family doctors, family planning centers, and local health departments also provide help at this difficult time. Ideally, the woman's partner is attentive, available, and supportive as the two of them work through a complex decision-making process. The decision is up to the woman or couple, however, not someone else who tells them what to do for reasons that may not be their own. They should think about parenthood, about adoption, about abortion—carefully and cautiously, though time is somewhat limited. In most instances an abortion in the United States is legal only during the first three months of pregnancy. The risks to the mother rise dramatically after this. A woman who has an abortion during the first 12 weeks of pregnancy has a risk of death from the procedure of 1 in 400,000. However, after the end of the 16th week of pregnancy, the risk soars to 1 in 10,000. The longer a woman or couple delays in seeking counseling or other options, the fewer choices are available and the less time there is to decide.

The lack of comprehensive sex education in the United States has many unhappy consequences, one of which is unanticipated pregnancy. More than anywhere else in the developed world, American youngsters and adolescents are unlikely to learn about sexuality in primary and secondary schools, and one consequence of this inadequacy is the fact that 1 in 10 American women between the ages of 15 and 24 will become pregnant without wanting to. A large number of these pregnancies end in abortion; others end in miscarriage. While prominent voices in our society say abortion is a horrible, "murderous" action, those same voices frequently oppose sex education and even want to restrict the availability and usage of over-the-counter contraceptives. In other countries where excellent sex education is a basic part of a young person's education, the rates of adolescent pregnancy and abortion is far lower. For example, in the early 1990s, 97 of every 1000 American teens became pregnant, and 44 of these women chose to have abortions. In contrast, in Japan, only 10 of every 1000 teens became pregnant, and only 6 decided to have an abortion. Japan has an excellent sex education program for all elementary and secondary school children. Comparably low figures may be found in the Netherlands.

Just as the lack of good sex education has had a very negative impact on the health and well-being of young Americans, the lack of legal, medical abortions in the past had catastrophic consequences for women. "Back alley abortions" were common and frequently lethal before women obtained legally sanctioned reproductive freedoms in 1973 with the *Roe v. Wade* Supreme Court decision. Reproductive freedoms involve both public and private aspects of sexual behavior, and strong feelings about abortion have stimulated a strident public, secular, religious, and legislative debate. Almost everyone has an opinion about abortion, and that opinion is rarely negotiable. "Debates" about abortion seldom involve the kind of discourse that can change someone's mind.

Following is an excerpt from the landmark Supreme Court's ruling:

"(a) During the first trimester, the abortion decision and its effectuation must be left to the medical judgment of the pregnant woman's attending physician. (b) After the first trimester, the State, in promoting the interest in the health of the mother, may, if it chooses, regulate the abortion procedure in ways that are reasonably related to maternal health. (c) For the stage subsequent to viability, the State, in promoting its interest in the potentiality of human life may, if it chooses, regulate, and even proscribe abortion, except where it is necessary in appropriate medical judgment, for the preservation of the life or health of the mother."

This decision has provoked public debate for three decades, especially with respect to the question of when the embryo or fetus becomes a "person." A number of questions are involved in these difficult and perhaps unresolvable issues.

- What does the term **fetal viability** truly mean? Can any definition of this term take account of both the age of the fetus and the availability of sophisticated medical intervention?
- Does the term "woman" refer only to a female of majority age or to minors also?

- Does the term "maternal health" include both physical and mental health?
- The phrase "preborn baby" has been used referring to both the embryo and fetus. Is there any way to determine if this term is accurate and/or appropriate?

January of 1998 marked the twenty-fifth anniversary of the *Roe v. Wade* Supreme Court decision, and there was much media discussion of its impact on Americans. In a *New York Times/CBS News* poll, half of respondents said they felt abortion was murder, but one-third of these said it was often the best course of action in bad circumstances (*New York Times*, January 22, 1998). Many women polled seemed not to recognize the political dimensions of legal access to abortion, seeing it as a basic right of citizenship. Still, Americans today seem no more certain of the desirable legality of abortion than 25 years ago. A trend is emerging that argues that while abortions should still be legally available, stricter limits should be placed on those seeking them. The *New York Times/CBS News* poll revealed that 61% of respondents believed that abortion should be permitted during the first three months of pregnancy, but only 15% during the second trimester, and 7% during the third trimester. When subjects were asked whether abortion is an issue concerned primarily with the life of the fetus or with a woman's right to control her own body, 45% took the former position and 44% chose the latter. A quarter century of legalized abortion has not been able to resolve this dilemma.

The Decision to Have an Abortion

The abortion-or-birth decision can be agonizing. Women may make the decision with their partner but sometimes find themselves alone and isolated at this stressful time. Patterson, Hill, and Maloy (1995) studied a group of 55 women deciding whether to have an abortion; many of these women had made the decision on a previous occasion. Their data revealed that women who made their decision on their own coped with either outcome better than those who felt pushed, forced, or coerced one way or the other. Personal autonomy is clearly an important factor in this significant issue. In a study of 72 Israeli women, Slonim-Nevo (1991) found that most felt "sadness, ambivalence, confusion, and fear" while considering the birth-or-abortion decision. Most wanted to talk to a counselor. They wanted information about where they could obtain an abortion, how much it would cost, how they might pay for it, and how the procedure is performed. This sample of women clearly wanted emotional support, nurturance, and reassurance throughout the process.

Research has examined what types of women are most likely to seek an abortion (Henshaw & Kost, 1996). In an analysis of almost 10,000 abortions Henshaw and Kost found that women who are living with someone to whom they are not married or who claim no religious membership or affiliation are 3.5 to 4 times more likely to have an abortion as women of reproductive age in the general population. Non-Caucasians between the ages of 18 and 24, Hispanics, and women who are separated or have never been married have an elevated probability of an unplanned pregnancy, as do single women with low income, whose chances of becoming pregnant are about twice that of the population as a whole. This report revealed that Catholic women are as likely to have an abortion as women in the population as a whole, while Protestants are about 69% as likely and Evangelical or born-again Christians are about 39% as likely. Religion is not a predictor of likelihood of abortion, but there are correlations among different religious groups and their reported frequency of abortion.

Additionally, this study indicated that 58% of women who sought abortions were using some form of contraception in the month they learned they were pregnant. The number of women who became pregnant because of "condom failure" seems to be rising, perhaps because some couples do not know the correct way to use this generally highly effective method of contraception.

The great preponderance of evidence shows that women who have abortions do not experience many or serious emotional problems as a consequence (Rosenfeld, 1992). Women may experience ambivalence or even guilt, but the great majority feel profound relief. Still, some women have emotional problems or experience a major depressive episode after having an abortion. Generally, these women have abortions during the second trimester of pregnancy, have had previous abortions, already are experiencing psychological problems, such as anxiety, depression, or a personality disorder, and believe that they will not receive much support in their families or relationships. Women who have abortions because of medical problems or the discovery of a genetic abnormality in the embryo or fetus are more likely to develop a more serious depressive episode. Data show social support is a key factor in a woman's coping with feelings about an abortion. Women who perceive they have the support of their families or significant other feel more effective in managing their lives and report fewer psychological complaints after the procedure (Major, Cozzarelli, Sciacchitano, Cooper, Testa, & Mueller, 1990). Additionally, women who did not blame themselves or their partners for the need for an abortion adjusted much better than those who felt remorse for themselves or anger toward their partner (Mueller & Major, 1989).

Abortion Counseling

Abortions are performed in a number of different ways, usually depending on the length of the pregnancy. Abortions are legal in this country through the end of the 24th week of pregnancy. The earlier in pregnancy an abortion is performed, the lower are the chances of medical complications. Abortion is a serious surgical procedure that may involve discomfort and a brief period of recuperation. Few woman are negligent in using contraception because they believe that if they become pregnant "I could always have an abortion to get rid of it." Some women, feeling guilty about becoming pregnant or even denying that they are pregnant, wait far too long before seeking medical counsel or abortion services; this wait only increases potential risks inherent in the procedure. It is generally best to act as promptly as possible after receiving thorough, in-formed medical opinion and counseling. Some agencies offering "abortion counseling" have no intention of facilitating an abortion, however, but may in fact exert enormous pressure on women to "help" them decide to have their babies and perhaps give them up for adoption. Women who begin their search for information in the Yellow Pages may find a number of advertisements, including those for "abortion alternatives" that are very different from "abortion services."

Abortion Procedures

The overwhelming majority of abortions performed in the United States occur in the first 12 weeks of pregnancy. A blood test is first used to confirm the pregnancy. The most commonly used abortion method uses vacuum suction or aspiration to remove the contents of the uterus through a narrow tube (Fig. 10-30A). In general, the later the pregnancy, the larger is the tube used. Vacuum curettage, as it is called, can be performed in a clinic or a doctor's office; the process takes about thirty minutes and is performed under a local anesthetic. The cervix is first dilated, and then the endometrium and products of conception are evacuated from the uterus. When suction aspiration is performed within 2 weeks of a missed period, the procedure is sometimes called a menstrual extraction, which seems an especially low-risk form of abortion for teenage women. A soft, flexible tube is used in menstrual extraction. This procedure can be used until a pregnancy reaches the 9th week (Key & Kreutner, 1980; Meyer, 1983).

When abortion is performed at the end of the first trimester or the beginning of the second, a different procedure may be used. The cervix is dilated, but instead of suction a loop of wire called a *curette* is inserted into the uterus, and the endometrium and products of conception are scraped out (Fig. 10-30B). This abortion may be performed under local anesthesia in a hospital, outpatient clinic, or doctor's office. This procedure is similar to a dilation and curettage procedure (D&C) usually done in a hospital under general anesthesia. Another procedure is known as saline or prostaglandin procedure (Fig. 10-30C). In this instance, a needle is inserted directly into the amniotic sac. Saline or prostaglandins are then injected. Saline will cause the death of the fetus, while prostaglandins will initiate uterine contractions, which will eventually force the fetus out of the birth canal. After one of these agents is injected into the amniotic sac, the fetus is expelled within 19 to 22 hours. Women having this procedure are fully awake and have reported feelings of anxiety and anger when they observe a well-formed, dead fetus emerge from the vagina. These women also report more feelings of depression and anger. A D&C is also used for other gynecological problems, not exclusively for abortions.

A variation of the D&C, called a dilation and evacuation (D&E), is another type of abortion used during the second trimester (not shown). In this technique, the cervix is dilated and a combination of curettage, suction, and sometimes forceps is used to end the pregnancy. This is the technique most frequently used for second trimester abortions. At this point in pregnancy, the woman's uterus is softer and may more easily be torn or punctured, and therefore only experienced physicians should perform a D&E. Like the D&C, the D&E is usually performed in a hospital under general anesthesia.

In addition to surgical abortions are "medically induced" or "labor induced" abortions. In this procedure the physician injects saline solution (salt water) or prostaglandin, a chemical which naturally occurs in the body, into the amniotic fluid. This procedure is sometimes called a "saline abortion." Either substance in the amniotic fluid stimulates contractions like those occurring during labor, which force the fetus and placenta out through the cervix and vagina. This procedure is most commonly used when some gross abnormality is detected in the fetus after 16 weeks of pregnancy. It is performed in a hospital under local anesthesia, often after an ultrasound examination. In some cases, a D&C is performed afterwards to ensure the uterus is empty. The woman often stays in the hospital for a day or two afterwards. By 16 weeks gestation the fetus already looks somewhat like a baby, and seeing the fetus emerge from the vagina can be traumatic.

There has been much controversy about "late term abortions," which, under the provisions of the *Roe v. Wade* Supreme Court decision, may be prohibited by state laws, and in fact, many states have passed such laws. These abortions, performed after the 20th week of pregnancy, involve dilating the woman's cervix and extracting the fetus by its feet. Only about 1% of abortions in the United States occur after the 20th week. This procedure is typically used when the fetus is discovered to be profoundly abnormal in some way.

Drug-Induced Abortions

Drug-induced abortions are very different from surgical alternatives in the privacy they afford. Because women can be seen entering and exiting abortion clinics, they often feel conspicuous and worry about being recognized. Public exposure may also make them feel even worse about the situation. Taking a pill or receiving an injection in a doctor's office is a private experience, however, since no one need know why she is there.

Abortion-inducing drugs are called *abortifacients*. The best known and most controversial abortifacient is **mifepristone**, also commonly known as RU 486, the name under which it was first distributed in France. This drug works by inhibiting the effects of progesterone on the continuation of pregnancy. RU 486 can be used up to 9 weeks after a woman's last menstrual period and causes the early embryo to become unattached from the lining of the uterus and expelled through the cervix. As described in Chapter 4, without progesterone, the endometrium cannot become thick and fluffy and support the implantation of a developing embryo. French women seeking abortions far prefer RU 486 to surgical alternatives, although there are frequent side effects. Very heavy bleeding and cramping usually follow administration of this drug. RU 486 is delivered by an injection, and two days later a second injection of prostaglandin causes uterine contractions that force the embryo out. Mifepristone causes less discomfort than surgical abortions, and the risks to the woman are substantially lower. Mifepristone is effective in 96% of cases. This drug has been approved by the U.S. Food and Drug Administration. Anti-abortion activists have threatened to boycott other products of the company that manufactures mifespristone. The sale of this drug in the United States might be a moot point, however, since other drugs that do the same thing are already FDA approved and widely available, with highly predictable and safe abortifacient effects. They are already routinely used in this country. **Methotrexate**, a drug commonly used in cancer chemotherapy, and **misoprostol,** a drug used to lessen the chances of developing stomach ulcers related to anti-arthritic or pain medications, used together work the same as mifepristone. This combination has fewer side effects (occasional nausea and gastrointestinal symptoms) but is as effective as mifepristone in ending a pregnancy. Like mifepristone, it can be used up to the 9th week of pregnancy. As of this writing, the total cost of such drugs and

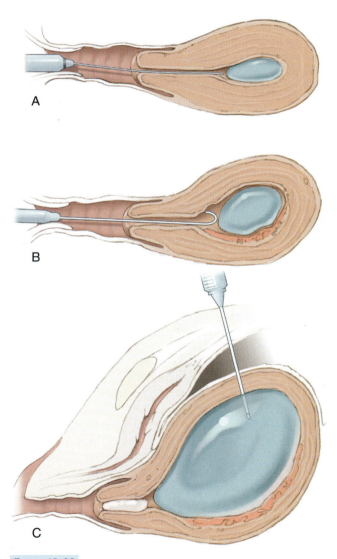

FIGURE 10-30 Schematic illustrations of three abortion procedures. (A) suction, or aspiration, (B) dilation and curettage, (C) saline or prostaglandin. The white plug in the cervix in (C) is laminaria, a sea weed derivative that helps dilate the cervix.

medical administration is approximately $350. In the rare event that a drug-induced abortion does not terminate the pregnancy, a conventional aspiration method is employed.

Anti-abortion proponents frequently claim that if having an abortion is as easy as taking a pill or having a shot, women will become more casual about having abortions and more negligent about using contraceptives conscientiously. No data support this assertion, however, and the suggestion that women would find it convenient to have an abortion reveals a lack of sensitivity to the distress, ambivalence, and guilt most women experience when considering or having an abortion. We feel it is important to be as nonjudgmental as possible about the trying circumstances in which many women find themselves at these times.

Fetal Viability

Most state and federal statutes on abortion allow abortions only before the point of fetal viability, that moment when the fetus can survive outside the mother. In the past this was considered to be at the end of the sixth month of pregnancy. Abortions after that time were performed only if the mother's life was endangered or her health seriously compromised. Now, however, fetal viability depends more on advances in medical technology than on the physiological maturity of the fetus. Neonatologists, doctors who specialize in the health of newborns, have extended fetal viability almost a full month earlier than two or three decades ago. As medical technology becomes even more sophisticated and interventions more effective, babies born even earlier will have a better chance of surviving. Therefore, the issue of fetal viability now has more to do with strategies of medical treatment than with the developmental status of the newborn. Infants born around the seventh month of pregnancy can now survive, and some born earlier have, with incredible patience and medical resources, survived as well.

Thinking Critically About Abortion

Critical thinking is a set of intellectual strategies used to sort through a complex issue to reach conclusions not clouded by emotions or attitudes. In contemporary culture you will be presented with facts, opinions, and sometimes the ranting of individuals who feel very strongly about abortion. Critical thinking skills help one analyze such information. Critical thinking skills involve addressing a number of questions about an issue:

1. What am I being asked to believe or accept?
2. What evidence supports the assertion?
3. Are there alternative ways of interpreting the evidence?
4. What additional evidence would be helpful to evaluate the alternatives?
5. What conclusions are most reasonable?

Following are a number of assertions people make regarding abortions and women who have them. Most of these are

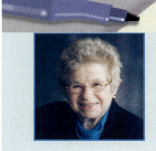

Dear Dr. Ruth

Question:

When a woman and man are having a child, the father often wants to be there when the baby is born. Do you think the man should be there when the woman has an abortion?

Answer:

Although the man may accompany his partner to the clinic and offer his emotional support, there is no reason to be in the room for the abortion procedure—unlike being there for childbirth. First of all, childbirth is a joyful occasion, while an abortion is anything but that. As well, labor can be a long process in which the man can be useful, helping the woman to breathe correctly, giving her rubdowns, giving her ice chips, etc., while an abortion takes only a short time and the man serves no purpose other than lending support. Doctors once resisted having husbands in the delivery room because the sight of blood often made them feel faint and because they could be a source of infection. Although doctors gradually accepted having men present for childbirth, I don't think most doctors would accept having a visitor hovering around during an abortion. But I think a man's wanting to be helpful and supportive is a fine reflection of his maturity and his desire to help his partner through a difficult situation.

Other Countries, Cultures, and Customs

ABORTION IN THE FORMER SOVIET UNION

The predicament and circumstances of women in some other countries and cultures is different from that in America in regard to abortion. The former Soviet Union, for example, differs profoundly from the United States in the frequency with which women seek and obtain abortions. Some abortion data are surprising or even troubling, but one must remember these two cultures have very different societal values and *huge* differences in access to reliable contraception. For many decades, abortion has been the primary method of limiting fertility among Russian women (Visser, Pavlenko, Remmenick, Bruyniks, & Lehert, 1993); little is known about how or whether this has changed since the break-up of the Soviet Union. In a survey of over 8000 Russian women in 1991, 41% used as their primary form of contraception withdrawal, the rhythm method, or douching—three not very effective birth control techniques. Among women under age 25, 35% reported using an IUD, but only 10% reported using birth control pills. Of all the women in this sample, 20% said that they primarily used a barrier method of contraception, in most cases condoms. For only 12% of these women was a doctor their main source of information about birth control, and only 55% of a sample of Russian gynecologists reported having been trained in family planning (Visser, Bruyniks, & Remmenick, 1993). Most surprising, 60% of that large sample of mainly urban, young, and well-educated women reported having had an abortion because of a contraceptive failure. Russian gynecologists, 83% of whom were women, suggested that so many Russian women have abortions because of a lack of contraceptive education, a lack of interest and involvement of men, and a lack of modern birth control methods, such as oral contraceptives. Only about half of these doctors fully understood how oral contraceptives work.

Popov, Visser, and Ketting (1993) summarized five questionnaire studies carried out in Moscow, Saratov, and Tartu. They found that between 1976 and 1984 very little serious psychological, sociological, or epidemiological research addressed contraceptive knowledge, attitudes, and behaviors in the former Soviet Union. Among the women in these large Soviet urban centers in this period, only 1 to 3% used oral contraceptives, and about 10% used IUDs. These factors probably explain the very high rate of abortion in Russia. There is a difference, of course, between having birth control and not using it and not having it available. Unfortunately, low-cost, effective, convenient contraception is still rare in Russia. Many Russians historically have been suspicious of and unreceptive to modern contraceptive technologies.

Another study summarized abortion statistics in Estonia, Latvia, Lithuania, Belarussia, and the Ukraine between 1970 and 1994. Very high abortion rates were found in all these countries, which were once part of the former Soviet Union and now are independent nations. Rates up to 142 induced abortions per 1000 women of childbearing age were found (Mogilevkina, Markote, Avakyan, Mrochek, Liljestrand, & Heilberg, 1996). These data indicate a gradually declining abortion rate since 1980, with 50 abortions per 1000 women reported in Latvia for 1994. Disturbingly, abortions and childbirths among adolescents are increasing in all these nations. Because of the high numbers of abortions, deaths due to complications during abortions are a troubling threat for these women. Because sex education has been proved successful in lowering the numbers of abortions elsewhere in the world, modern Russian health care providers advocate systematic sex education and abortion avoidance programs. The most recent data from Russia (Entwisle & Kozyreva, 1997), based on the Russian Longitudinal Monitoring Survey in 1994, revealed an abortion rate of 56 per 1000 women of childbearing age, plus or minus 12 abortions per 1000 women. This statistic is inexact because of the underreporting of abortions and differences in the design of various surveys in this project.

High abortion rates in a country that lacks availability of modern contraceptives makes one wonder why abortion is so prevalent in a country like the United States where birth control alternatives are easily accessible.

stereotypes. Critical thinking skills applied to these statements will lead to thinking more cautiously and realistically about abortion.

   a. Most women who have abortions are teenagers who do poorly in school.
   b. Women who have abortions don't care about the value of human life.
   c. Women who have abortions find it an easy decision to make.
   d. Women who have had an abortion quickly put it out of their minds and act as if it never happened.
   e. Women who have an abortion have no strong religious beliefs or convictions.

Planned Parenthood of America has compiled a profile of the "average" woman having an abortion. Following are some of the attributes of women having abortions, quoting directly from information provided at their website.

■ The majority of women obtaining abortions are young: 58 percent are under 25, including about 26 percent who are teenagers (aged 11-19); only 20 percent are aged 30 and older (Henshaw, 1992).
■ The proportion of pregnancies terminated by abortion is higher among unmarried women (56 percent).
■ Poor women are about three times more likely to have abortions than women who are financially better off.

In 1988, women of color had an abortion rate of 57 per 1,000, or 2.7 times the rate of white women (21 per 1,000). Abortion rates for minority women have increased considerably between 1984 and 1988—13% among minority women 15-19, 16% for those aged 20-24, and 6% for those aged 30-34.

■ Of the 1.6 million abortions obtained by U.S. women in 1988, 406,000 were obtained by teenagers. Women aged 18-19 have the highest abortion rate of any age group (64 per 1,000).
■ Teens are more likely than older women to have abortions during the second three months of pregnancy, when health risks associated with abortion increase significantly.
■ On average, women report more than three reasons that lead them to choose abortion: three-quarters say that having a baby would interfere with work, school, or other responsibilities; about two-thirds say they cannot afford to have a child; and one-half say they do not want to be a single parent or have problems in their relationship with their husband or partner. Seventy percent of women having an abortion say they intend to have children in the future.
■ Access to abortion services can be beneficial to young women's lives. A two-year study of 334 African-American teens showed that those who chose to terminate a pregnancy, in comparison with peers who opted to carry a pregnancy to term, were more likely to have stayed in school, economically better off, less likely to experience psychological problems, less likely to have subsequent [unanticipated] pregnancies, and more likely to practice contraception consistently (Zabin et al., 1989).

While the facts presented in this profile do not fully address all the stereotypes noted above, this accurate information about abortion is a good first step in thinking critically about the issues.

Privacy, Parental Notification, and Abortion

The issue of parental notification or consent before a minor can have an abortion is one of the most complex and controversial matters facing state legislatures today. Some abortion providers require that the parent or guardian of a young woman accompany her to the clinic and that both parties provide picture identification. This is true of surgical abortions, emergency contraception, and chemically-induced abortions. The *Roe v. Wade* Supreme Court decision gave individual states the right to pass laws to protect the health of the mother when abortions are sought. **Parental notification laws,** as they are commonly called, have been passed in at least 29 states, as of this writing, as lawmakers believe such statutes are necessary and in the best interest of the young woman.

In states requiring the involvement of at least one of the young woman's parents, teenagers who feel they cannot share their problem with their parents have a rather stark choice: go to another state for the abortion or try to win the approval of a judge to have the abortion in a process called judicial bypass. Either way, valuable time may be wasted, putting the woman at increased risk of complications associated with abortion, as well as higher costs (Planned Parenthood website, 1998).

It is important to consider family issues with respect to adolescent pregnancies. Almost one teenager in three between the ages of 15 and 17 does not live with both of their parents. About half of all teenage females being raised by their mothers have had no contact with their fathers during the past year. Over half of adolescents seeking an abortion report that at least one of their parents is already aware of their desire to abort their pregnancy; the younger the teen, the greater the chances that a parent knows the situation. About 75% of those age 15 or younger have told at least one of their parents, while 46% of those who are 17 have done so (Planned Parenthood website, 1998).

Taking personal responsibility for one's sexual and reproductive health may involve a number of legal, ethical, moral, and family concerns. We believe privacy and confidentiality in the medical setting are key issues for making mature and informed decisions.

CONCLUSION

There is a lot of information in this chapter that might someday educate, motivate, and reassure you. These are the three primary goals for this book. We are not encouraging you to become pregnant and have children, nor are we implying that parenting is a necessary part of being an adult in our society, for it is possible to enjoy a full and rewarding life without having children. However, since most of you will or already have had children, we believe that the information presented here is important for you and your baby-to-be.

In some people's thinking there is a big ideological gap between sexual arousal, intercourse, and response on the one hand and pregnancy, babies, and parenthood on the other. While the relationship of the two is necessary and obvious, it is normal not to associate the two at all times. Yet part of being a fully functioning adult involves understanding and foreseeing the consequences of our actions, and nowhere is this connection more important than in the connection between sexual expression and pregnancy. We quite literally reap what we sow. In the remaining chapters of this book, the connection between sexual arousal and response and the various contexts of sexuality in our lives may at first seem similarly remote, although such relationships will become clearer as these chapters present more information.

Learning Activities

1. People planning to become parents can have little certainty about the world into which their children will be born. Do decisions not to have children reflect an overly rigid obsession with control and an impractical desire to determine things well beyond our realm of influence?
2. Describe thoughts and feelings that might surface in a relationship when one partner learns that the other is infertile.
3. If you were a woman who waited until after the age of 35 to become pregnant, how would you feel if your obstetrician referred you to a specialist in "high-risk pregnancy?"
4. Do you think men are now more involved in the experiences of pregnancy and childbirth because they themselves want to be or because their partners want them to be?
5. Even though an infertility work-up for a woman is more extensive, expensive, and uncomfortable than a similar work-up for a man, why do you think that it is usually done on the woman first?
6. Very little is known about men's reactions to miscarriage. If the man has helped the woman through the progress of the pregnancy and its physiological changes, then he too may feel some emptiness, anger, or helplessness at this time. Men like women may view a miscarriage as a death. Unfortunately, men seldom have the opportunity to express their grief because the attention is devoted to the woman who is recovering from the medical procedures. Speculate on what support men might appreciate receiving at this time.
7. Crack cocaine is a powerful teratogen. Its effects on the fetus can be devastating, and permanent damage to the infant can occur:
   a. This agent causes immediate, pronounced vascular constriction in the mother and fetus, limiting the transfer of oxygen and nutrients through the placenta.
   b. The placenta is more likely to tear away from the wall of the uterus, in many cases initiating a premature delivery.
   c. Brain cells deprived of oxygen die in substantial numbers, which can result in behavioral problems and learning disabilities.
   d. Dramatic increases in maternal and fetal blood pressure often cause blood vessels in the brain of the fetus to rupture, with subsequent destruction of large areas of the brain. This prenatal "stroke" can leave the newborn permanently paralyzed, blind, or both.
   In your opinion, does the prenatal consumption of crack cocaine ethically constitute child abuse? If so, how should the legal system deal with the mother?
8. In early March of 1992, Dr. Cecil B. Jacobson was convicted of 52 counts of fraud and perjury for artificially inseminating patients at his northern Virginia fertility clinic with his own sperm, and lost his license to practice medicine. This case is an appalling breach of medical, legal, and ethical standards in the treatment of fertility disorders. In this case, 60 to 70 children may have been fathered by Dr. Jacobson.
   a. Should there be standards for prospective donors for artificial insemination procedures? If so, how should such standards be established?
   b. What procedures or tests should be used to assess the safety and suitability of each donor?
   c. If a child conceived by artificial insemination is born with a birth defect, who, if anyone, is liable?
   d. What measures should be taken to assure the anonymity of the donor?
   e. Should single women be able to choose to have a baby through artificial insemination with donor sperm?
9. Describe your personal feelings about home birth. Midwives point out that home birth is a safe, enjoyable, natural birthing alternative. However, if a problem occurs, immediate medical intervention involving sophisticated technological instrumentation may be required. Under what circumstances might you yourself consider home birth?

Key Concepts

- The uncritical acceptance of the goodness, normality, and appropriateness of having children is called pronatalism.
- Fertility involves a person's actual reproductive performance, while the term fecundity refers to their maximum reproductive potential.
- Parenthood ideally requires maturity, which involves self-extension, the ability and inclination to initiate and maintain warm, open, relationships with others, frustration tolerance, and a clear set of personal values.
- Embryologists use the term "differentiation" to describe how developing cells group together according to their future functions.

- The placenta is a semipermeable membrane through which some substances in molecular form can pass and others cannot.
- In cephalo-caudal development, the embryo's and fetus's growth takes place first and fastest toward the head, and later and slower toward the lower extremities.
- In proximo-distal development, the embryo's and fetus's growth takes place first and fastest along the mid-line of the body, and later and slower at the tips of the extremities (hands and feet).
- High-risk pregnancies include those pregnancies in which bed rest and aggressive medical intervention at home or in the medical setting may be needed to preserve the pregnancy.
- Labor involves three stages, during which the cervix becomes progressively thinner, the baby's head drops lower in the woman's pelvis, becoming "engaged" between her tail bone and pubic symphysis, and the newborn eventually passes through the birth canal. In the last stage of labor the placenta and other fetal membranes also pass through the birth canal.

Glossary Terms

amniocentesis
artificial insemination
    (intrauterine
    insemination)

Cesarean section
chorionic villi
chorionic villi sampling
ectopic pregnancy

embryoscopy (fetoscopy)
episiotomy
fertilization
fetal alcohol syndrome
fetal viability
gamete intrafallopian
    transfer (GIFT)
human chorionic
    gonadotropin
in vitro fertilization
Lamaze technique
laparoscopy

methotrexate
mifepristone
misoprostol
parental notification laws
sex preselection
spontaneous abortion
    (miscarriage)
teratology
ultrasound imaging
zygote intrafallopian
    transfer (ZIFT)

Suggested Readings

Brott, A. A., & Ash, J. (1995). The expectant father. Facts, tips, and advice for the dad to be. New York: Abbeville Press.

Eisenberg, A., Murisoff, H. E., & Hathaway, S. E. (1996). What to expect when you're expecting. New York: Workman Publishing.

Mahler, M. S., Pine, F., & Bergman, A. (1975). The psychological birth of the human infant. New York: Basic Books.

Nilsson, L. (1990). A child is born. New York: Dell Publishing Group, Inc.

Simkin, P. (1989). The birth partner. Everything you need to know to help a woman through childbirth. Boston, MA: Harvard Common Press.

Sussman, J. R., & Levitt, B. B. (1989). Before you conceive. The complete pregnancy guide. New York: Bantam Books.

11

Contraception: Making Choices or Taking Chances

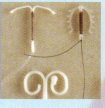

OBJECTIVES

When you finish reading and reviewing this chapter, you should be able to:

1. Describe historical examples of methods of contraception and note any contemporary parallels.

2. Summarize the issues a couple should consider when choosing a contraceptive that best meets their circumstances.

3. For each contraceptive method listed, summarize how it works, its effectiveness rate, and its advantages and disadvantages including side-effects and health risks:

   - Monophasic, biphasic, and triphasic oral contraceptives
   - Norplant
   - Depo-Provera
   - Spermicidal creams, foams, and jellies
   - Male condoms
   - Female condoms
   - Diaphragm
   - Cervical cap
   - Vaginal sponge
   - IUDs
   - Vasectomy
   - Bilateral tubal ligation

4. Explain which contraceptives are most effective in inhibiting the transmission of STDs.

5. Summarize why women and men might be negligent in using contraceptives correctly and consistently.

6. Explain what strategies emergency contraception involves and describe when a woman might need emergency contraception.

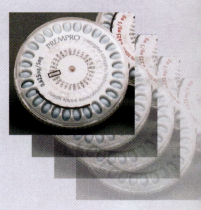

From Dr. Ruth

Since the time when I began crusading for the responsible use of contraception, unintended pregnancies among teens have gone down. Still, there are way too many such pregnancies, and it's still necessary to help people protect themselves from unintended pregnancy, as well as disease. I'm sorry there still is no absolutely perfect contraceptive—one that is cheap, easy to use, and without side effects, and doesn't detract from spontaneity or pleasure. Although medicine may some day reach the goal of perfection, effective methods do exist now, and the possible results of not using them are such that no one should ever engage in unprotected sex.

If you are sexually active now or hope one day to be, this is a chapter you should study thoroughly. No one loves babies more than I do, but I don't want to see you holding one you made until you are absolutely ready to do so.

The previous chapter discussed getting pregnant, being pregnant, and having babies. That chapter emphasized that sexual behavior has real consequences beyond the immediate sensual pleasures of intercourse. This chapter, in contrast, emphasizes that pregnancy is *not* a necessary, inevitable consequence of sexual intercourse. Only relatively recently in human history have people had the means and understanding needed to effectively control their procreation. However, having effective birth control methods and using them conscientiously are two entirely different things. Contraceptive choices take place within the context of a relationship. When communication in that relationship is poor, the couple may not make a successful decision about birth control if their ways of interacting are not open and honest.

Because so many areas of a person's life may be affected by their contraception decisions, a thoroughgoing discussion of different birth control methods is fundamental in a human sexuality textbook such as this. Therefore, this chapter is intended to help you consider, assess, and choose contraceptives based on your personal sexual value system and relationships. Contraceptive choices are highly personal, of course, and your reasons for using any birth control method are entirely your own or something for you and your partner to discuss.

This is a broad, diverse chapter covering many topics relevant to contraception. We believe that the more information you have about contraception, the less likely you will be to ever need to consider abortion counseling and services. It is very important for every child who comes into the world to be a wanted child.

HISTORICAL AND CONTEMPORARY CONTRACEPTIVE ISSUES

Fertility and Fecundity

As discussed in the previous chapter, conception and contraception involve issues of fertility and fecundity. **Fertility** refers to a person's actual reproductive performance: the number of live births a woman has had or the number of live births a man has fathered. **Fecundity** refers to a person's maximum biological potential to procreate. This chapter focuses on means by which women and men can limit their fertility and avoid pregnancy. As noted earlier, effective and convenient contraception has not been available for very long in human history. Indeed, one could argue that the use of contraception is a sign that a civilization is thinking about the quality of the lives of its members. Quality of life is less than optimum if the number of people far outstrip the local available resources. Presumably even ancient civilizations clearly understood the wear and tear on their women that accompanies frequent childbearing and made efforts to control fertility. On the other hand, the very survival of small, nomadic peoples depended on the fertility of their members. Throughout history there have been pressures both to procreate *and* to limit fertility.

Is There a "Population Explosion?"

For two generations social scientists have warned us of the frightening consequences of uncontrolled growth of the world's population. Explosive population growth fosters misery and substandard living conditions, and the consumption patterns of greater numbers of people contribute to global warming. In 1968, Paul Ehrlich in *The Population Bomb* claimed that unless humanity takes measures to control the rate of population growth, the world will suffer catastrophic consequences. Most Western, industrialized nations imagined impossibly dense urban areas. Famine in Third World countries received vivid press coverage. Today fertility rates in many areas of the world are beginning to fall.

Ben Wattenberg (1997) claims that the "population boom is going bust" and summarizes information from the United Nations publication, *World Population Prospects: The 1996 Revision.* For example, between 1950 and 1955, the global average number of children born to a woman was 5. This was truly frightening, since for the world to maintain an even population level only 2.1 children per woman are required. Between 1975 and 1980 the average number of children born to a woman had fallen to 4, and by 1995 the number had dropped to 3. Importantly, fertility rates are declining also in less developed countries. European nations, which enjoy a relatively comfortable standard of living, today have an average fertility rate of only 1.4 children per woman. Fertility rates are similar in Russia and Japan. Fertility rates are falling in sub-Saharan Africa as well. Worldwide, contraception now is often less motivated by trying to stem population growth and more by desires to improve the quality of life for oneself and one's children (Fig. 11-1).

A Brief History of Contraception

Throughout recorded history, people have sought ways to stop conception from occurring or to terminate a pregnancy (Fig.

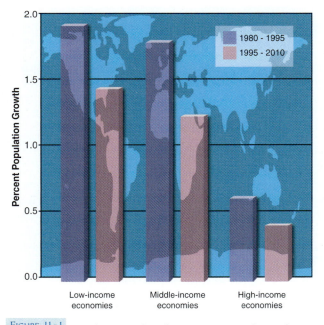

FIGURE 11-1   Fertility rates for all socioeconomic classes have begun to fall in many nations throughout the world. This trend has been apparent since 1985 and is expected to continue through 2010.

11-2). Methods that prevent conception are called **contraceptives,** and agents used to terminate pregnancy are called **abortifacients.** The ancient Greeks were fully aware of the distinction between these, according to Professor John M. Riddle (1997) of North Carolina State University. **Intrauterine devices (IUDs)** technically do not stop conception from happening but stop the implantation of a fertilized egg in the uterine lining. IUDs are, therefore, sometimes called **contragestational agents.** Ancient civilizations recognized peak periods of fertility during a woman's menstrual cycle and found ways to interrupt the cycle of sexual intercourse, conception, pregnancy, and childbirth. Because modern contraceptive solutions seem so sophisticated and ingenious, people often view past methods as "primitive" or "simplistic," but some ancient strategies were elegant and practical. Other historical methods of contraception were ineffective, harmful to a person's health, or even fatal. Modern contraceptives, in contrast, offer effectiveness, affordability, availability, convenience, and usually reversibility.

PESSARIES

A **pessary** is a vaginal suppository. Ancient pessaries were sometimes made of acacia tree gum. While this substance may have killed sperm, it probably worked by dissolving in the vagina and forming a seal over the cervix, thus blocking the progress of sperm. The oldest known written record describing contraception is the Kahun Papyrus, written about 1850 B.C. It notes a pessary composed of crocodile dung and fermented dough—not exactly a healthy mixture for delicate genital membranes! The great Greek physician Hippocrates apparently knew about pessaries, especially those that induced abortions. He discouraged other physicians from using them, perhaps because those used in his day were harmful to women. Centuries ago, some women in Constantinople inserted small natural sponges saturated with lemon juice into their vaginas. They acted as a barrier to sperm and created an acidic environment hostile to sperm.

PLANTS

For centuries, a wide variety of plants have been used as contraceptives and abortifacients. Before 370 B.C. a plant known as *silphium* was used as a contraceptive, although its method of use is unknown. Queen Anne's Lace was used for its contraceptive properties as long ago as the era of Hippocrates (about 430 B.C.). Modern scientists have shown that ingesting this drug blocks a woman's production of progesterone and can inhibit fetal development, although it is not used for this purpose by physicians. Other plants that have been used as contraceptives include onions, pomegranates, date palms, pine, cabbage, and juniper. Such plants are often dangerous because it is not always easy to correctly identify the plant, and its potency may vary. Some plants have unanticipated side-effects, and they are not nearly as effective as the methods described in this chapter.

INTRAUTERINE DEVICES

For thousands of years, people have known that a foreign object in the uterus can prevent conception or pregnancy. Arabs

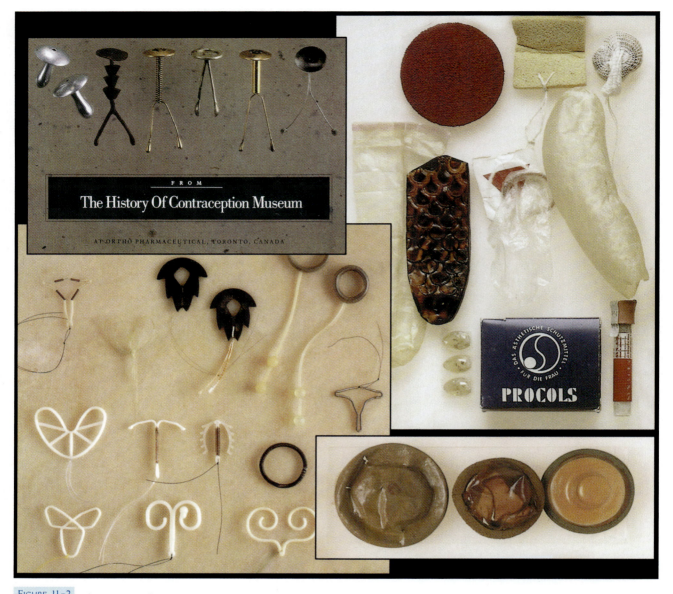

FIGURE 11-2 The History of Contraception Museum in Toronto, Canada, has displays of contraceptives that have been used throughout the world for hundreds of years.

were said to place date pits in a camel's uterus to prevent it from becoming inconveniently pregnant on long desert journeys. There are tales of Native American Indian women inserting dried pine needles through their cervix into their uterus to prevent pregnancy. Because the opening of the cervix is so narrow, inserting any object or IUD requires skill and may cause some discomfort.

CONDOMS

Throughout history men have used a variety of materials to cover their penises to prevent semen from entering the vagina. Historically, snakeskin, sheepskin, and linen have been used. For centuries animal intestines have been fashioned into con-

doms that made a reasonably good barrier and allowed excellent sensitivity, offering men the tactile experience of intercourse without apprehensions about pregnancy. In 1843 Charles Goodyear invented the process of "vulcanization," which allowed condoms to be manufactured from rubber. These had good sensitivity and were less susceptible to tearing than natural membrane (intestine) condoms.

DIAPHRAGMS

Before the development of oral contraceptives, **diaphragms** were the most popular female-controlled contraceptive method. In the past some women used a "block pessary," a wooden block with two concave indentations. They put this

THE HISTORY OF CONTRACEPTION MUSEUM

*I*n North York, Ontario, is the History of Contraception Museum, believed to be the only one of its type in the world. Here can be observed over 600 historical artifacts vividly portraying the ingenuity and creativity of ancient and more modern peoples attempting to prevent pregnancy. Exhibits include items from Asia, Europe, and South America. Visitors learn of the Ebers Papyrus, written about 1550 B.C., that methodically instructed women to grind up dates, the bark of the acacia tree, and honey to make a thick paste and apply it to the vulva before intercourse. This was an effective method of contraception, because acacia bark when it ferments turns into lactic acid, which is a highly effective spermicide, or sperm-killing agent.

The museum has an extensive collection of condoms, including fine linen ones worn in the days of the famous Casanova. Cloth versions were introduced by a Dr. Condom, personal physician to King Charles II, who apparently used lots of condoms. There are over 300 historical examples of IUDs in various shapes and sizes and made of a variety of materials, including jewels.

Oral agents for preventing conception did not begin with birth control pills. More than 4,000 years ago women in China drank mercury preparations to prevent pregnancy, and Indian women drank a tea made of carrot seeds. Some women in New Brunswick drank a kind of moonshine whisky prepared with dried beaver testicles. The relative effectiveness of these has not been documented thoroughly.

inside the vagina, making sure that one of these concave surfaces covered the cervix, creating a physical barrier. Later diaphragms made of metal and glass were awkward to insert and remove. Because of its shape, a diaphragm builds up suction over the cervix, making them even more difficult to remove unless they are made of pliable, flexible materials.

Margaret Sanger: A Pioneer in Contraceptive Rights for Women

Contraceptive devices and information became available not through a gradual social evolution but through an ideological revolution. **Margaret Sanger** (see Figure 2-15C) was born in 1883 of Irish-American heritage. Sanger's mother died from having had too many children, and Margaret had a pivotal role in raising her siblings. The central focus of her life was the dissemination of information and contraceptive devices that allowed women to decide if and when to bear children. Sanger coined the phrase **birth control.** Her passion for the cause was all-consuming. In 1914 she began publication of a newspaper, *The Woman Rebel,* in which she asserted her objectives in a bold, uncompromising manner. In the same year she published a pamphlet, *Family Limitation,* which has been called the "first modern marriage manual" (Wardell, 1980). She was not concerned about the moral sensibilities of those who were obstacles to her goal. In 1916 she opened in Brooklyn the first birth control clinic in the United States, which was promptly closed by the New York City Vice Squad, who threw Sanger in jail.

The public debate resulting from Sanger's evangelical approach to contraception availability occurred in the context of the highly conservative legal legacy of Anthony Com-

stock. Comstock had been the secretary of the New York Society for the Suppression of Vice. First locally, then regionally and finally nationally, Comstock advocated making it illegal to send contraceptive information and devices through the United States Postal Service, supposedly because these materials were obscene. Beginning in 1873 various versions of such "Comstock Laws" were passed throughout the country, and the last of these to be repealed was taken off the books in 1966.

Sanger was arrested in August of 1914 when the Post Office banned her newspaper after instigation by Anthony Comstock. Sanger faced serious, highly complex charges. She had only just turned 30 and was unprepared for the circumstances she faced, which included charges of rioting and incitement to murder. She left the United States for Canada and then London, where she met Havelock Ellis (see Chapter 2), who agreed with her agenda, if not her tactics. She returned to the United States in 1915 after Comstock's death and remained an advocate for available contraception for the rest of her life. In 1923 she founded the Birth Control Clinical Research Bureau in New York. This organization, staffed by a physician, gave care to all women, irrespective of their race or financial means. It merged with the American Birth Control League in 1939 and became the forerunner of today's Planned Parenthood (McCann, 1994). Hundreds of thousands of young women and men today enjoy the legacy of Margaret Sanger's courage, intelligence, and activism.

Margaret Sanger had to deal with an insidious issue. The most conservative sectors of society, including the law, medicine, politics, and the clergy, were almost exclusively male and openly opposed her goals and methods. In other words, the best educated and most advantaged professionals in America did not support the dissemination of contraception information or birth control services. Why? There is no easy answer to this question. Some have speculated that many men felt that if women were busy having and taking care of babies, they could do as they pleased at home and in society. American history is not unique in this respect. Contraceptive practices throughout the world virtually always focus on the fertility of *women,* not men.

The Development of Oral Contraceptives

Preceding sections summarize some of the historical milestones in the development of pessaries, IUDs, condoms, and diaphragms. These have been the methods used most commonly in the history of contraception. It wasn't until the middle of the 20th century that **oral contraceptives** became widely available. A pill a day—what could be simpler or more convenient? As oral contraceptives were refined, their incredible effectiveness and low cost became attractive reasons for using them. They are also attractive because they allow spontaneity: a couple could have intercourse without having to interrupt their intimacy to apply a condom, insert a diaphragm, or use some spermicidal foam, cream, or jelly.

Oral contraceptives were developed only after highly sophisticated techniques for synthesizing female hormones in the laboratory were developed. Synthesizing a hormone involves using chemicals to create a perfect replica of a hormone occurring naturally in the body. This involved complex biochemical techniques in the 1940s and 1950s.

The history of birth control pills involved three individuals involved in slow, painstaking research that ultimately led to the development of the pill. These were Gregory Pincus, M. C. Chang, and John Rock (Fig. 11-3), although many others were involved in research, development, and, importantly, public awareness. Once the complex biochemical problems were resolved (Birch, 1992), scientists needed courage and perseverance to explore the potential for oral contraceptives among humans. In 1951, Pincus and Chang, supported by a grant from Planned Parenthood, sought a synthetic version of progesterone called progestin. Such a hormone would "fool" a woman's physiology into thinking she was pregnant and, therefore, stop ovulation. After studying over 200 different substances, they isolated three steroids found in wild Mexican yams that proved highly effective in stopping ovulation in laboratory animals. John Rock then tried these compounds in contraception experiments at the Worcester Foundation for Experimental Biology in Shrewsbury, Massachusetts. It must have been very exciting for these researchers to carry out biochemical experiments while realizing that their results could completely change the nature of contraception throughout the world. In 1958, the Food and Drug Administration approved the first oral synthetic hormonal contraceptive.

At first, synthetic female hormones were used to treat a variety of menstrual disorders. The modern period of oral contraceptives began in 1960 when the FDA approved "Enovid" as an ovulation-inhibiting agent (Colton, 1992). The dosage of synthetic estrogen in these first pills was high by today's standards, about 150 micrograms per pill compared to 30 to 50 micrograms or less now. As the dosage decreased, the number and severity of side effects decreased substantially (Hedon, 1990).

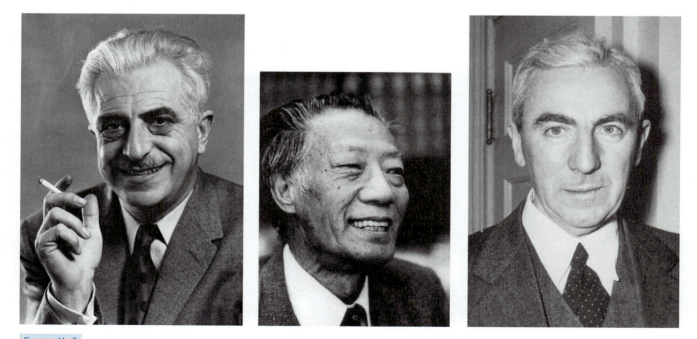

FIGURE 11-3   From left to right: Gregory Pincus, M. C. Chang, and John Rock, three pioneering researchers in the development of oral contraceptives.

Society's Perspective and the "Double Message" About Birth Control

Society seems to give many people, especially young people, a **double message** about birth control. On the one hand, those who use contraceptives to avoid giving or getting a **sexually transmitted disease** (STD) or being involved in an unanticipated pregnancy are commended for foresightful personal responsibility. On the other hand, many people believe they are planning to behave in a "wicked" way. Can these two attitudes about birth control be reconciled?

Many college students wish to be informed, safe, and accountable in regard to having sex. For women who haven't been to a gynecologist, and for men, the expedient solution is to use condoms. We have recommended condoms for many reasons for many years. Although some people are too quick to judge the foresightful behavior of being prepared with the advance purchase of condoms, most people will feel less embarrassed in making this purchase if they know they are acting in the best interests of both themselves and their partner.

Families, communities, and local health providers offer another confusing message, especially to adolescents and young adults. The message is sent that people often get carried away with the romance of the moment and neglect to use contraceptives. Family and health care resources are made available to "help out" these young people, who are often presumed to

TALKING ABOUT BIRTH CONTROL AT HOME

*A*lthough we both believe in the importance of accurate sex education in school, this of course does not always happen. Many parents prefer to teach their children themselves about all aspects of human sexuality, and their rights and wishes to do so should be respected. However, many parents don't actually do what they intend to do because they themselves are somewhat embarrassed about sexuality. Additionally, one in four American households is a single-parent, female-headed home, and for one parent to present accurate sexual information comfortably, openly, and honestly, often to children of both sexes, is a huge job. Even when parents are ready and willing to teach their children about sex, often they may not be well enough educated in this subject to do so well. One of the basic responsibilities of capable parenting involves learning much about sex to be able to teach one's child honestly and accurately.

As will be discussed in Chapter 12 on sexuality in childhood and adolescence, contraception is usually not an early topic to introduce to a child, but as she or he gets older it becomes more important. Children tend to be curious first about anatomical differences between females and males, and the mechanics of intercourse and procreation later on. Children who have a good grounding in these areas are then ready to learn about birth control. Talking openly and honestly with one's child about birth control teaches them that personal responsibility is an important value and that one should think about the consequences of behaviors and act accordingly.

It is necessary to speak with young children about basic anatomy and physiology, but birth control information won't make much sense. Similarly, a conversation about love, care, and commitment helps children understand the emotional context in which birth control is an intelligent, shared decision. When parents have done this, it is much less likely that a child will be embarrassed by this subject. Talking with children about contraception can bring together many aspects of human sexuality in a highly applied, practical way.

Talking with children in the home about birth control has another important advantage: they will be less likely to believe misinformation from their uninformed peers. Teenage peers are a notoriously inaccurate source of myth, superstition, and simply wrong information about preventing pregnancy. For example, a girl may be told that she cannot get pregnant the first time she has intercourse or if she and her partner have intercourse standing up. Many children receive little or no accurate sexual information at home and promulgate misinformation they hear from others; a child who doesn't have a good grasp of facts may be gullible and believe some of this nonsense. If the school doesn't offer correct, practical information about human sexuality and the peer group makes the situation even worse, then the home is the best place to begin. The next chapter includes some suggestions about how to do this.

be impulsive. But again there is the counter message: if you act beforehand to prevent an unanticipated pregnancy, you are suspect and some would even say immoral. Related to these confusing societal messages is another issue. Are contraceptives really all that available? Many people of all ages, married or single, are simply too embarrassed to make the public purchase of condoms or spermicidal creams, foams, and jellies. Some people would never buy birth control items in their own neigh-

borhood, and others fear they will be standing at the cash register when the salesperson calls out for a "PRICE CHECK ON CONDOMS AT REGISTER 3." The fact that condoms are available does not necessarily mean that they are accessible. Purchasing condoms from vending machines in washrooms offers privacy and is preferred by many. These machines should be installed in women's restrooms as well, since far more women buy condoms than men. In fact, the best-selling con-

---

MESSAGE FROM DR. RUTH: HOW TO TALK TO YOUR PARTNER ABOUT BIRTH CONTROL

Talking about contraceptive alternatives with someone with whom you are forming a close relationship can be difficult. Fear of an unanticipated pregnancy (or disease) usually won't scare you into having this conversation. But in the heat of passion you are less likely to think of the risks of unprotected sex. Even if one or both of you are already using contraception or have a condom, it is important to talk about it. For example, it is often a good idea to discuss the desirability of using a condom even if the woman is already using birth control pills.

Choose an appropriate moment to talk about contraception, but don't wait too long. The relationship should be at a point at which sex is at least a possibility before you broach the subject. But you must be prepared for the possibility of rejection. If the other person is not ready to have sex, he or she may be surprised when you bring the subject up and may reply awkwardly or brusquely. If so, shrug it off. Don't let this conversation, which is intended to help start a new chapter in your relationship, cause that relationship to end.

What's a good way to begin? I have a method for when people want to ask me a question but are reluctant to start out directly. I tell to them to say, "A friend has a problem." You can say something like, "My friend is going to talk to his girlfriend tonight about contraceptives, and boy is he nervous about bringing it up." How your partner responds will guide your conversation from that point. This approach opens the door for having *the* conversation, but it also won't hurt as much if your partner closes it.

Do your homework before having this conversation. Know about available contraceptive clinics and methods. If you plan to use condoms, a drugstore, Planned Parenthood office, or health department will do, but most other effective methods of birth control require seeing a medical practitioner, and it's a good idea to know what facilities are available in your area.

Convenience, effectiveness, and affordability are additional factors that may affect your contraceptive decision. Different couples face different things. Our only strong recommendation is that you discuss the subject in an open, informed way.

You may also need to discuss your partner's religious beliefs about the appropriateness of using birth control. For example, some religious doctrines discourage or prohibit using any method that interferes with conception as a consequence of sexual intercourse. "Natural family planning" methods are allowed but are generally less successful in preventing conception. Birth control methods that involve periods of abstinence are far less effective than those that do not.

One last point. if you are not in an exclusive, monogamous sexual relationship with your partner, a "barrier method" should be used every time you have sexual intercourse. These include condoms, female condoms, spermicides, the diaphragm, cervical caps, and vaginal sponges. Some couples like to take turns—the man using a condom sometimes and the woman using another barrier method at other times. Taking turns requires a couple to talk about when they want to make love, and any time a couple communicates about sex, their overall relationship is usually enhanced.

doms in America are packaged in a tasteful package with the silhouettes of a woman and man on the box. The intention to behave responsibly about birth control is not always easy to act on, and both intelligence and maturity are needed to act wisely to prevent unintended pregnancy.

Nonetheless, many people believe that if young people don't have contraceptives they won't have sex. This is entirely wrong, and there are *no* carefully collected, systematic data to support this nonsensical assertion. It is essential to acknowledge this fact rather than ignore it with the simplistic hope that young people will refrain from acting on one of the most powerful impulses we can experience.

Abstinence

For avoiding pregnancy, nothing works as well as **abstinence.** Abstinence means refraining from sexual intercourse and other sexual behaviors in which semen might come into proximity to a woman's genitalia. A person may decide not to have first intercourse until marriage or some point in the future or may take a "time-out" period from sexual intercourse. Although abstinence is a 100% effective means of avoiding conception, it is not always successful or reliable for a long period of time.

An earlier chapter distinguishes between partial and complete celibacy. Partial celibacy is abstaining from sexual intercourse but not from masturbation, and complete celibacy involves abstaining from both. The word celibacy is also used to refer to a decision not to marry. Abstinence is generally more similar to partial celibacy than complete celibacy. Abstinence is a *personal choice*. Often people choose abstinence for religious or spiritual reasons, for example, believing it inappropriate to have intercourse before marriage or except when planning conception. Many young people resolve, and some formally pledge, to refrain from having intercourse until they marry. Other individuals see abstinence as a period to think things through after an unre-

Other Countries, Cultures, and Customs

CONTRACEPTION IN JAPAN

There has long been a hesitancy in Japan to promote birth control pills because of the concern that immoral sexual behaviors might follow the wide distribution of oral contraceptives. Until recently, condoms and natural family planning strategies were the only approved contraceptive methods. A strong tradition of infant and maternal health care in Japan began in the Meiji period (1868-1912). Following World War II, these priorities became even more prominent in the government policies of this highly patriarchal country. Today, there is still little public discussion of sexual norms, reproductive policies, and oral contraceptives (Miyaji & Lock, 1994), although an interest in this birth control technology is more obvious.

Beginning in 1987, Japanese pharmaceutical companies encouraged researchers and medical practitioners to begin clinical investigations of low-estrogen oral contraceptives (Kuwabara, 1989), hoping to encourage the government to approve use of the pill. These pilot studies demonstrated no significant differences in the ways Japanese and Western women responded to these agents. Oral contraceptives were just as effective for Japanese women as for women in Western industrialized nations. But by 1991, only 1% of Japanese women of childbearing age had access to these agents, in effect because the government discouraged their use. Yet there seemed to be much public interest in low-estrogen pills at this time when the contraceptive failure rate in Japan was 25%. About 29% of Japanese women had had at least one abortion (Ogawa & Retherford, 1991). Although there was much interest in the pill, there was still some concern about potential side effects.

Despite this research, widespread oral contraceptive use is still banned. Japanese women have few options if they want to use birth control pills. One option involves using high-estrogen and progestin pills for contraceptive purposes, although these agents have been approved only for the treatment of menstrual disorders (Nagata, Matsushita, Inaba, Kawakami, & Shimizu, 1997). These pills were used by only slightly more than 1% of over 18,000 Japanese women in one study. Unfortunately, the risk of side effects from high-dose pills is greater than that of effective low-dose agents available in the United States. Most disturbing is the fact that among 35- to 49-year-old-women using high-dose pills, cigarette smoking is relatively common and likely magnifies the risk of cardiovascular disease. In Japan, as in most countries, governmental factors have a large role in contraceptive availability and decision making (Fig. 11-4).

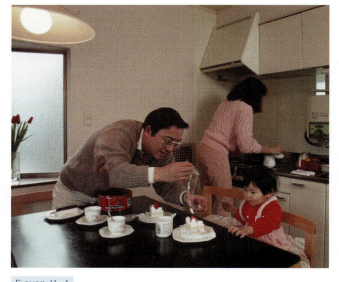

FIGURE 11-4   Oral contraceptives are not widely available in Japan. Condoms and "natural" family planning strategies are common. There is little public discussion about contraception in general. Still, Japan has one of the lowest birth rates among developed countries.

warding or exploitative relationship. A study that evaluated the success of sex education programs and contraceptive alternatives among adolescents (McKay, 1993) found that abstinence is highly successful for relatively short periods (perhaps a few weeks or months) but decidedly unsuccessful over longer periods (several months or a year). Another investigation revealed that girls perceive that they receive much more encouragement to be abstinent that do boys (Jensen, de Gaston, & Weed, 1994). Among girls, peer influence seems especially effective in encouraging abstinence. Other research has also reported a greater commitment to abstinence and less permissive sexual behaviors among girls than boys (DeGaston, Weed, & Jensen, 1996).

Several informational programs have been developed to offer teens and young adults exposure to a variety of sexual subjects. One such program, called Sex Respect, encourages abstinence more than informed, selective sexual behaviors. Goodson and Edmundson (1994) evaluated Sex Respect in accordance with criteria set forth by the Sex Information and Education Council of the United States and found the program incomplete in information, incorrect in some of its claims, and generally not meeting professional standards for a thorough sex education program. These professional sex educators consider focusing on abstinence instead of fully presenting the recommended content for a human sexuality course inadequate for people who might really need good sex information. Although programs, such as Sex Respect, might successfully encourage abstinence for brief periods of time, as of this writing, no available data from programs demonstrate long-term successful adherence to abstinence.

People give up abstinence for various reasons. Hopefully this is a genuine decision that has been considered carefully and thoughtfully, rather than a coerced decision made with a sense of sexual impatience or urgency. A period of abstinence

ideally ends when the person finds someone they can communicate with and trust completely.

Just as couples who rely on a form of birth control to prevent an unanticipated pregnancy should have a back-up barrier method available, people who are practicing abstinence might want to have a back-up barrier method available; condoms are probably best. Having condoms does not necessarily mean that one is planning to use them or to behave in any wrong way. Thinking ahead intelligently is always better than thinking back remorsefully.

Sources of Information About Contraception

People in many age groups and life circumstances need accurate contraceptive information and access to birth control alternatives. Teenagers, college students, and other adults can learn about contraception from many sources, and there seems to be a beginning trend toward including contraceptive information in school-based sex health programs. In a study of parents living in rural Ontario, Canada, over 90% supported family life education in the schools, and most respondents thought that children in grades 6 through 8 were old enough to learn about birth control methods (McKay, 1996). Even more of the parents believed that contraception information was basic to effective sex education in grades 9 through 12.

It has been shown that students enrolling in a sex education program for college freshmen at the University of Virginia were more likely to explore a sexually abstinent lifestyle. As well, both females and males who were sexually active were more likely to use a condom and were more careful using other contraceptive methods after participating in this series of lessons and discussions. Learning the importance of a variety of sexual subjects can have a demonstrable effect on behavior of young subjects (Turner, Garrison, Korpita, Waller, et al., 1994). In other settings too, young adults are talking about contraception and considering alternatives. Family practitioners have increased their role in contraceptive counseling (Heath, 1993). Because of changes in the structure of health care in America, many women consult their family doctor about sexual and reproductive issues rather than a gynecologist. Fortunately, most doctors listen to their patients carefully and offer their best counsel about selecting a birth control method. The point here is that couples who receive serious, complete information about human sexuality and birth control are in a much better position to talk together in an open, informed way to select and use a method acceptable to both of them.

CONTRACEPTIVE ALTERNATIVES

Any couple selecting the contraceptive method or methods best for them could benefit from a careful presentation and discussion of alternatives. Birth control methods fall into a number of broad categories, including barrier methods, intrauterine devices, hormonal alternatives, and chemical options. Some different methods may be used together, such as a spermicidal agent used with a barrier method. All four of these categories are reversible. Surgical contraceptive alternatives, such as tubal ligation and vasectomy, only sometimes can be reversed and, therefore, should be viewed as permanent options. For convenience, much of the material on contraceptive methods in the following sections is summarized in charts. Since cost is sometimes an important consideration, these charts include current costs, although prices are always changing and may not stay accurate.

In addition to allowing a couple to decide when or whether to have a child, contraception also affords them the ability to control the spacing of children. A couple may choose to condense or spread out over time their parenting activities. Some women and men want to have a first child out of diapers before a second arrives, while others want more than one child quickly in order to move beyond that early family stage more quickly. Some couples want to have only one child in college at a time because of the high costs of higher education. In other words, contraceptives offer some choices regarding child-rearing responsibilities and financial costs of raising adolescents (cars, car insurance, etc.) and young adults.

The following discussion of different contraceptive methods draws on two truly outstanding sources that you may consult if needed for additional information. The first of these is called *Contraceptive Technology,* by Robert A. Hatcher, James Trussell, and Felicia Stewart (1998). It is readable and provides everything you need to make a personal, responsible contraceptive choice. This is considered the "bible" of contraception among sex educators throughout the country. A second excellent source, available at most large bookstores, is *The PDR Family Guide to Women's Health and Prescription Drugs* (1994). Both of these include an enormous amount of useful information.

No contraceptive is perfect, and all have advantages and disadvantages. Yet there is an effective contraceptive for everyone, although using it consistently and conscientiously is a different matter. The two issues involved are finding the best contraceptive and being motivated to use it properly.

Hormonal Alternatives

Synthetic hormones used systemically or topically offer women a number of advantages and conveniences over many other types of birth control. Birth control pills, **Norplant, Depo-Provera** injections, and a new intravaginal implant called "the ring" are all extremely effective, have few troubling side effects for most women, and significantly reduce menstrual cramping and discomfort. Women must consult a physician to obtain these methods, however. Additionally, hormonal contraception offers women virtually no protection against STDs, which is important for a woman not in a committed, monogamous sexual relationship. This category of contraceptives involves both health risks and benefits.

Hormonal methods stop the ovary's production of mature, potentially fertilizable eggs. Because hormonal contraceptives deliver a daily dose of progestin and estrogen, or just progestin (Norplant and Depo-Provera), the woman's hypothalamus never receives a message to tell it to produce gonadotropin-releasing hormone (see Chapter 4). Therefore, the pituitary gland never receives a message to tell it to produce follicle-stimulating hormone (FSH) and luteinizing hormone (LH). Her ovaries thus never receive a hormonal message to initiate the events that eventually result in ovulation, and no ovum is released from the ovary. Hormonal methods block conception in another way also. These synthetic hormones cause a woman's cervical mucus to become so thick that sperm cannot swim through the cervix and enter the uterus. As well, distributed daily doses of progestin and estrogen or progestin alone block the thickening of the endometrium, so that even if by some rare chance ovulation and fertilization did occur, the fertilized egg could not implant itself in a soft, spongy uterine lining. Still, hormonal contraceptives are not quite 100% effective, and occasionally women using them conscientiously do become pregnant. Contraceptive research continues to seek improvements on existing methods.

Hormonal methods of birth control are also thought to offer some protections against cancer, although why this is so and what specific kinds of cancer are involved are a matter of debate.

Birth Control Pills

There are dozens of different kinds of birth control pills, which have various combinations of estrogen and progestins (Fig. 11-5). *Monophasic pills* have the same amounts of estrogen and progestin in every pill throughout the cycle, whereas *biphasic pills* have the same level of estrogen in every pill but increase the amount of progestin during the last 11 days of a cycle. *Triphasic pills* vary the amounts of both estrogen and progestin throughout a cycle. The distinctions among these types of pill might not seem significant, but physicians have good reasons for choosing one over another for a particular woman. Women might want to discuss the differences with their doctor. The

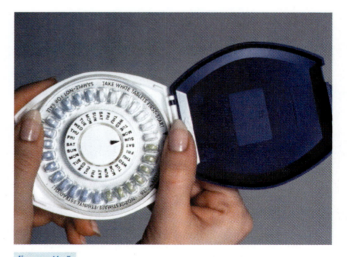

Figure 11-5 Oral contraceptives are packaged in a way that helps women remember to take their pills regularly.

pills should be taken at the same time of day every day. Additionally, if for any reason a woman vomits within 2 hours of taking her pill, she should presume that she has not absorbed her pill and should consider using a barrier method of birth control throughout the remainder of her cycle even though she is finishing that cycle's pill pack.

Birth control pills may also interact with other medications. For example, some antibiotics and phenobarbital may reduce the efficacy of oral contraceptives. Similarly, oral contraceptives can make other agents more toxic than when used alone, such as beta blockers (used to reduce high blood pressure), steroids, some antidepressants, and even caffeine. Therefore, it is very important for the woman to discuss with her physician any medications she takes or may take while using birth control pills. Finally, women using oral contraceptives should not smoke cigarettes. The combination increases the

SUMMARY OF ORAL CONTRACEPTIVES

Method: Oral Contraceptives

Expected Failure Rate if Used Consistently and Conscientiously: .1%

Expected Failure Rate if Not Used Consistently and Conscientiously: 3%

Advantages:

Extremely effective when used as prescribed	Diminishes menstrual discomfort
Does not detract from spontaneity during sex	Diminishes menstrual blood flow, offering protection against anemia
Can be used by most women	Easy to use
Offers some protection for ovarian and endometrial cancer	Easily reversible
	Thoroughly researched

Disadvantages:

Does not protect a woman against STDs	Side effects: headache, weight gain, breakthrough bleeding
Expensive for some users	Must be taken daily
Rare but potentially serious medical problems (see below)	Should not be used by nursing mothers for 6 weeks after childbirth
Can cause mood swings	

Side Effects: (Not everyone using the pills will have these)

Acne	Depression
Breast tenderness	Weight gain
Headaches	Nausea

Health Risks:

Heart disease and blood clotting disorders (rare)	Liver and gallbladder complications (rare)
Elevated blood pressure	Changes in cervical cells
Elevated blood sugar	Delayed return of fertility on discontinued use

Cost: $9.50–30. per month, depending on how they are obtained

For What Type of Person Is This a Good Contraceptive Choice?

Knowledge of partner's sexual behaviors and network	No family history of heart disease or blood-clotting disorder
Regular daily habits that foster conscientious usage	No current suspicion of reproductive system cancers
Under age 35 (health risks increase with age)	No kidney disease
	No high blood pressure
Have not had migraine headaches	No diabetes or pre-diabetic condition

Doctor's Visit Needed to Obtain This Method? Yes

risk of cardiovascular problems and may even increase the woman's chances of having a heart attack. Overall, birth control pills are extremely effective, convenient, and affordable, diminish menstrual discomfort, and offer some protection against ovarian and endometrial cancer.

Because women using oral contraceptives must remember certain factors, doctors have developed an acronym for when to consult them while using birth control pills. ACHES stands for these serious symptoms:

> A = abdominal discomfort
> C = chest pain, persistent cough, or shortness of breath
> H = headache
> E = eye problems, such as blurred vision
> S = severe leg pain (that might indicate the presence of a blood clot)

As safe and effective as oral contraceptives are, problems can occur, and women using them should be alert for any of these problems.

NORPLANT

Many women say that they have trouble remembering to take a birth control pill once a day. Among sexually active women, forgetting the pill can lead to pregnancy. Norplant is a kind of hormonal contraceptive that is implanted so that the woman need not take a pill every day. Six thin capsules are inserted beneath the skin on the underside of the woman's upper arm (Fig. 11-6). These capsules are made of a combination of plastic and silicone called Silastic and contain only progestin, specifically levonorgestrel. A local anesthetic is used to numb the skin when the capsules are implanted. One of the benefits of Norplant is that the woman is fully protected within only 24 hours after insertion of the capsules. Gradually levonorgestrel diffuses out of the capsules into the woman's circulatory system. Physicians prefer

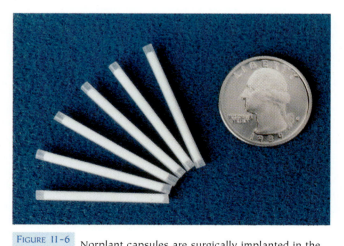

FIGURE 11-6   Norplant capsules are surgically implanted in the skin on the underside of a woman's arm. This method of contraception is effective for 5 years.

to implant Norplant in the 7 days since the woman's menstrual cycle begins to be sure that she is not pregnant at the time. Norplant is effective for five years, and then the capsules have to be surgically removed. This is sometimes not easy, since scar tissue often surrounds them. Within a day after removal, the woman no longer has contraceptive protection. The Food and Drug Administration first approved Norplant in late 1990.

A study compared the effectiveness of birth control pills and Norplant in a sample of 112 adolescents who were 18 years old or younger; half used pills and half used Norplant (Berenson, Wiemann, Rickerr, & McCombs, 1997). After one year, 34% of the subjects who were prescribed oral contraceptives were still using them, compared to 91% of Norplant users, probably because removing Norplant is far more involved than simply discontinuing pills. Women who stopped taking their pills typically cited a variety of side effects, including nausea, headaches, loss of sex drive, and aggravation of existing depression. Because they stopped, 25% of the women in the oral contraception group became pregnant during the 12 months of the study. Among subjects choosing Norplant, none became pregnant during this time. More than 80% of subjects in both groups reported side effects, irregular menstrual bleeding (annoying but not serious) being the most common. This side effect was more common in Norplant users. Additionally, Norplant users gained more weight than birth control pill users during the study and also had more abnormal pap smear results. Although side effects seemed to diminish during the second six months of the study in oral contraceptive users, there was little decrease in side effects among Norplant users. These data emphasize the importance of counseling for women considering Norplant, including a full discussion of the side effects. In women of different ages, irregular menstrual bleeding and spotting was the reason most commonly given for discontinuing Norplant usage (Kaunitz, 1996). Still, the effectiveness of Norplant far surpassed that of birth control pills in these young women.

When Norplant was first introduced in 1990, doctors thought it was less effective for women weighing more than 154 pounds. The capsules have since been modified, however, and effectiveness is no longer related to body weight.

DEPO-PROVERA

Although some women are a little suspicious about systemic contraceptives, Depo-Provera, a contraceptive injection taken in the buttocks once every three months, has proven very popular and effective (Earl & David, 1994). Some women can't take birth control pills because of health-threatening or annoying side effects, and many women experience abnormal mid-cycle bleeding that makes Norplant similarly unacceptable. Depo-Provera offers these women another choice, and having more choices is a good predictor of successfully avoiding unintended pregnancies. More than 30 years ago, Depo-Provera was used to treat endometrial and kidney cancer, and in the following two decades its reliable

SUMMARY OF NORPLANT

Method: Norplant

Expected Failure Rate if Used Consistently and Conscientiously: .09%

Expected Failure Rate if Not Used Consistently and Conscientiously: .09%

Advantages:

Extremely effective	No need to interrupt physical intimacy
Most women can use it	Absence of side effects related to estrogen
Lasts for 5 years	Minimizes menstrual discomfort and cramping
Women do not need to remember to take a pill every day	May reduce risk of pelvic inflammatory disease
	May reduce risk of endometrial cancer

Disadvantages:

Does not protect a woman against STDs	Capsules may be visible in very thin women
Expensive for some users	Outpatient surgery required for removal
Greater likelihood of abnormal pap smears than with birth control pills	May increase chances of irregular mid-cycle bleeding

Side Effects:

Headaches (most common side effect)	Breast tenderness (rare)
Enlargement of ovaries	Nervousness (rare)
Dizziness	Nausea (rare)
Weight gain	Acne (rare)

Health Risks:

Irregular menstrual bleeding	Blood clots or blockages in blood vessels (rare)
Abnormalities in ovarian follicles	Local infection during insertion or removal of capsules
Ectopic pregnancy (rare)	

Cost:

May be as high as $750 at insertion but averages less than five years' use of oral contraceptives. Average monthly cost is only $12.50.

For What Type of Person Is This a Good Contraceptive Choice?

Women who frequently forget to take birth control pills	Women for whom pregnancy might be catastrophic for the newborn:
Those who can pay the initial cost	Alcohol dependency
	Opiate addiction
	Women with HIV or AIDS
	Women who are habitual child abusers

Doctor's Visit Needed to Obtain This Method? Yes

---

and convenient contraceptive effects were recognized. Depo-Provera is a synthetic hormone called depot-medroxyprogesterone acetate, which is very much like the progesterone produced in the ovaries. It is used by more than 9 million women in some 100 countries. Four injections a year, each taking just seconds, is an attractive contraceptive alternative for many women. About 2 weeks after the injection a woman has the full contraceptive effects. The amount of this synthetic hormone in the bloodstream remains high for about a month and then stays constant for the next two months. A woman who cannot visit her doctor exactly at the end of three months can have the injection early without adverse effects or loss of effectiveness. Following each three-month dose is a period of about 4 weeks during which contraceptive effectiveness is still high, but it may not be safe to use this "grace period" often.

Research Highlight

LEGAL AND PUBLIC HEALTH SCHOLARS DEBATE NORPLANT COERCION

Since it was introduced in 1990, many Americans have been concerned that the courts might coerce or mandate Norplant use for women who have a large number of children out of wedlock, who use addictive substances during pregnancy, who are HIV positive or have AIDS, or who have a history of abusing their children (Table 11-1). Alarms of "social control" were voiced almost immediately. A *Philadelphia Inquirer* editorial advocated the use of Norplant as an agent in the "fight against black poverty" (December 12, 1990). To our knowledge as of this writing, four women convicted of child abuse have had Norplant implanted as a probation requirement. Because most of the women who involuntarily receive this contraceptive are single parents, black, and poor, there may be reason to assess charges that Norplant can be used as a vehicle of population control among some women.

As of this writing, however, the situation does not seem so insidious (Davidson & Kalmuss, 1997). As of 1997, no state had laws making welfare benefits contingent on using Norplant. There is less discussion in legal circles about judicially coercing Norplant usage. For example, forced Norplant insertion is now illegal in Illinois, and a judge in California has been disciplined for forcing a young woman to receive Norplant as a condition of her probation. Although it is possible that some health care professionals are subtly promoting Norplant for some of their patients, no available data support this assertion. In a study involving more than 2000 low-income women in Dallas, Pittsburgh, and New York City who were thinking about changing to a different contraceptive, these subjects did not report feeling forced, coerced, or encouraged to select Norplant over other options, such as birth control pills, Depo-Provera, or sterilization. Indeed, fully 45% of this sample selected Norplant of their own free will. Of these 2000 women, only 3 reported that they felt somewhat forced to select Norplant. Convenience, effectiveness, and duration of effect were the primary factors for selecting Norplant (Davidson & Kalmuss, 1997).

Research also demonstrates that suspicion about Norplant may be related to wider public attitudes about contraception in general. For many years data have indicated that people are more wary about contraceptives that affect a woman's entire hormonal and metabolic chemistry than about barrier methods of contraception, the use of spermicides, or IUDs (Piepert & Guttmann, 1993; Silverman, Torres, & Forrest, 1987). This may be because of some of the side effects of hormonal contraceptives noted earlier. Additionally, after Norplant was introduced to the public in 1990, the media tended to over-report adverse side effects while saying much less about women who experience no problems. In short, fears of Norplant coercion are largely exaggerated, and the women thought most likely to be forced to use it frequently choose it of their own accord.

TABLE 11-1

Controversial Legal Issues Surrounding Contraception and States' Rights

Some state legislatures have legal requirements to mandate the use of contraception among women who have abused drugs during pregnancy, those who have been found guilty of child abuse, and those who were on welfare. Here are a few examples:

Kansas

In 1991 the state legislature considered granting women on welfare a one-time grant of $500 for Norplant and $50 per year as long as Norplant was used. This bill was defeated.

Another bill mandated Norplant insertion among any fertile woman convicted of narcotics possession. This bill died in committee.

Louisiana

In 1991 the state legislature considered a bill which would grant women on welfare $100 per year if they used Norplant. The bill was amended to award this sum to any woman on welfare who used any method of contraception. The original bill ultimately mandated that Norplant would be provided at no cost to any woman on welfare. The amended bill died in committee.

South Carolina

A Senate bill introduced in 1991 gave courts the power to mandate Norplant usage among women who gave birth to infants who tested positive for drugs. This bill was referred to the judiciary committee and no action was planned.

From Ravi Srinivas, K., & Kanakamala, K. (1992). Introducing Norplant: Politics of coercion. Economic and Political Weekly, 27, 1531–1533.

SUMMARY OF DEPO-PROVERA

Method: Depo-Provera

Expected Failure Rate if Used Consistently and Conscientiously: 0.03%

Expected Failure Rate if Not Used Consistently and Conscientiously: 0.03%

Advantages:

Extremely effective

Most women can use it

Lasts for 3 months

Women do not need to remember to take a pill every day

No need to interrupt physical intimacy

Absence of side effects related to estrogen

Minimizes menstrual discomfort and cramping

May reduce risk of pelvic inflammatory disease and endometriosis

May reduce risk of endometrial cancer

May cause cessation of menstruation

Disadvantages:

Does not protect a woman against STDs

May delay return of fertility for up to 2 years upon discontinuation of usage

Cannot be discontinued during the 3 months of its effectiveness

Side Effects:

Headaches (most common side effect)

Depression

Dizziness

Weight gain (more pronounced the longer you use it)

Breast tenderness (rare)

Nervousness (rare)

Nausea (rare)

Health Risks:

Irregular menstrual bleeding

Possible loss of bone density (still under clinical investigation)

Ectopic pregnancy (rare)

Some drug interactions (rare)

Cost: Less than $50 per injection (average monthly cost less than $15.)

For What Type of Person Is This a Good Contraceptive Choice?

Women who frequently forget to take birth control pills

Women who are careful about using condoms in nonmonogamous lifestyle

Active women who can offset possible weight gain and bone loss

Women who make and keep regular appointments for injections

Doctor's Visit Needed to Obtain This Method?   Yes

Contraceptive choice should be an informed decision. Yet a study of over 800 women in large family planning clinics in the United States indicated that when it comes to choosing among oral contraceptives, Norplant, and Depo-Provera, women do not always have accurate information (Cushman, Kalmuss, Davidson, Heartwell, & Rulin, 1996). The data from this study reveal that women who choose oral contraceptives and Norplant consistently report that they feel Depo-Provera is less convenient and effective than the other two methods. Since Depo-Provera is indeed highly effective, some contraceptive counselors are concerned that women may not have all the information they need to make a good personal birth control choice. Additionally, some women in this sample using oral contraceptives and Norplant had inaccurate information about the cost of Depo-Provera and its side effects.

Spermicides

A number of chemical agents called spermicides, when used in low concentrations, are highly effective at killing sperm (Fig. 11-7). Sperm are fairly fragile and are easily killed or disabled by a change in temperature, moisture, acidity, or alkalinity, or even by light. Spermicides must be reliably effective, not irritating to delicate genital membranes, and non-carcinogenic.

Other Countries, Cultures, and Customs

ONCE-A-MONTH INJECTABLE CONTRACEPTIVES

Beginning in 1994, once-a-month injectable contraceptives underwent testing in many countries including Thailand, Egypt, Mexico, China, and El Salvador. These are estrogen-progesterone combinations that have been marketed under a number of names: Deladroxate, Cyclofem, Mesigyna, and Chinese Injectable No. 1 (Koetsawang, 1994). The first of these, Deladroxate, was used extensively in Latin America but promptly taken off the market because in a number of animal studies it caused breast cancers in dogs and unusual pituitary growths in rats. Cyclofem and Mesigyna were found to be highly effective and relatively free of side effects. Chinese Injectable No. 1 had poor contraceptive effectiveness when used once a month, but when its initial dose was doubled, its effectiveness was comparable to other injectable contraceptives. With a revised dosage schedule, Chinese Injectable No. 1 had low pregnancy rates, but many more recipients stopped taking the injections than with either Cyclofem or Mesigyna (Sang, Shao, Ge, Ge, Chen, Song, Fang, He, Luo, Chen, et al., 1995). The advantage of a once-a-month injection over Depo-Provera's once-every-three-months schedule is better regulation of monthly menstrual cycles. But even with once-a-month drugs, irregular bleeding is still the most common problem and the main reason women stop taking the injections.

Testing of these once-a-month injectable contraceptives was undertaken in Egypt between 1989 and 1992 (Hassan, el-Nahal, & el-Hussein, 1994). Almost 1100 women used Cyclofem and Mesigyna, and ratings of the acceptability of these drugs were very high. Many subjects reported that they would be willing to pay for the injections at the end of the trial period. Subjects who discontinued use reported a number of reasons, such as a perceived lack of social support for being conscientious with birth control and their husband's unsupportive attitude about contraception. Some cultures exert powerful social pressures to have many children. Women who stopped taking the injections were more likely to have experienced side effects.

Once-a-month injectable contraceptives have also been tested in Mexico, with rates of effectiveness and user satisfaction comparable to those in other countries. They were also compared with the Depo-Provera once-every-three-month regimen (Bassol, Hernandez, Nava, Trujillo, & Luz de la Cruz, 1995). In women using both types of injectable contraceptives, regular ovulation returned within three months after the last injection. The side effects of injectable contraceptives are generally similar to those of oral contraceptives, although the effectiveness is somewhat better and there is no risk of a woman forgetting to take the pill daily. As of this writing, research continues to improve the acceptability of once-a-month injectable contraceptives.

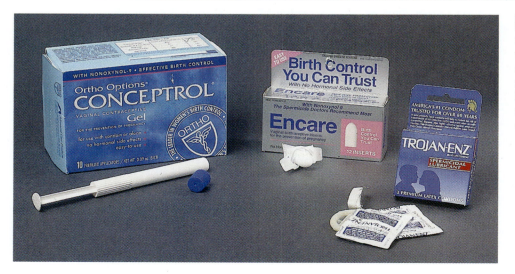

FIGURE 11-7 A variety of affordable contraceptive suppositories and gels are available over-the-counter. They are most effective when used with a barrier method of contraception, such as the male or female condom.

Spermicides are manufactured in a variety of forms: **suppositories, gels, cream,** or **foam.** To be most effective they should be used along with a barrier method of contraception, such as a cervical cap, diaphragm, or condom. These barriers keep the spermicidal substance in a place where it can work most effectively to kill sperm.

The most common spermicidal agent in use is nonoxynol-9, which is available in the forms noted above. Many prelubricated condoms are sealed in a small envelope containing nonoxynol-9. Using spermicides alone should be distinguished from using them with barrier methods of contraception. When used alone they have an unacceptably high failure rate (pregnancy occurs frequently). Spermicides used

with barrier methods have a combined effectiveness that is quite high. This information in the Summary of Spermacides box refers to the use of these substances alone, not in conjunction with any barrier contraceptive method.

One popular form of spermicide is small squares of film saturated with nonoxynol-9. These are placed inside the vagina, near the cervix. This 2 × 2 inch (5 × 5 cm) film dissolves in just a few seconds. Contraceptive film should be inserted into the vagina at least 15 minutes before intercourse. Its effectiveness depends on the care the couple takes to insert the film in adequate time to dissolve before intercourse. A recent study showed that when women applied contraceptive film inside their vaginas near their cervixes and their vaginas were

---

SUMMARY OF SPERMICIDES

Method: Spermicides

Expected Failure Rate if Used Consistently and Conscientiously: 6%

Expected Failure Rate if Not Used Consistently and Conscientiously: 21%

Advantages:

Somewhat effective (better than nothing)

Easy to purchase; readily available; sold in many places

No prescription or doctor's visit needed to obtain

Minimal, rare side effects

Protects against some STDs

Convenient to carry around in purse, backpack, or glove box

Can be used with partners who might resist using a contraceptive

Effective intercourse lubricant

Disadvantages:

May not protect against HIV

Must plan ahead of time to obtain and use

Could interrupt sexual spontaneity

Unpleasant taste or oral numbing during and after oral-genital stimulation

Side Effects:

Occasional allergic skin rash (rarely serious)

Health Risks:

May cause sloughing off of cervical cells

Minor irritation of cervix

Cost:

$5 to $10 depending on the type of spermicide selected. Each package may contain 6 to 12 doses.

For What Type of Person Is This a Good Contraceptive Choice?

People who can not afford or do not have access to family planning services

Those who cannot depend on their partner to use contraception

Women and men allergic to latex and not using hormonal contraception

Those who want to act independently in using birth control

Those who don't mind interrupting foreplay to use contraception

Women willing to take time to read instructions carefully

Women sufficiently comfortable with their bodies to insert these products

Doctor's Visit Needed to Obtain This Method? No

then washed with saline solution at varying times later, the amount of nonoxynol-9 remaining in the vagina could be measured (Mauck, Allen, Baker, Barr, Abercrombie, & Archer, 1997a). These investigators found amounts of spermicide well above that required to immobilize sperm up to 4 hours after the film was inserted, suggesting that nonoxynol-9 is apparently effective for quite some time. This study was carried out in the middle of each woman's menstrual cycle, when sperm normally have an easier time penetrating cervical mucus and entering the uterus. In addition to nonoxynol-9, benzalkonium chloride has been proved an effective spermicidal agent (Mauck, Baker, Barr, Abercrombie, & Archer, 1997b).

While nonoxynol-9 effectively kills the bacteria and viruses that cause STDs, whether it also kills HIV is still debated. Intense research continues and should soon answer whether this agent is effective in combating the virus that causes AIDS.

Barrier Methods of Contraception

This section explores a number of different contraceptive methods that involve a physical barrier or obstacle that prevents sperm from reaching an egg. These are the oldest historical forms of contraception and generally have fewer side effects than other alternatives available today. Although they are less effective and less convenient than hormonal contraceptives, they still are popular and when used with spermicides are extremely reliable. In the past, a wide variety of barrier methods were used. For example, African women once used the pods of the okra plant as a sort of vaginal pocket into which the man ejaculated; this ancient method has some striking similarities to the female condoms used today. Roman women used the bladder of a goat in somewhat the same way.

Barrier methods of contraception are popular today because they are also highly effective in preventing STDs. Women using birth control pills, Norplant, Depo-Provera, or IUDs sometimes want their partner to use a condom as well, to lessen the risk of contracting an STD. Many barrier methods are simple to use, making them appropriate for individuals with mild mental retardation or diminished psychological capacity. Some mentally retarded women do not always remember to take birth control pills or to return to their doctors regularly for Depo-Provera injections, and they may not tolerate the side effects of Norplant. Mental health professionals have had good success teaching them to obtain and use condoms properly.

With barrier methods of contraception, it is essential for women and men to plan to obtain them, have them handy, and use them every single time they have sexual intercourse. Some types of barrier methods need to be applied not too long or not too soon before intercourse. We like some types of barrier methods because they require a couple to talk about their shared contraceptive responsibilities, and the couple may take turns apply-

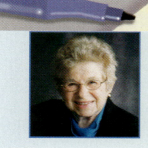

Dear Dr. Ruth

Question:

Whenever my girlfriend and I have intercourse, she insists on using both a condom and a spermicidal foam. Isn't that unnecessary? Won't either one or the other be plenty of protection?

Answer:

Neither is 100% effective in preventing an unintended pregnancy, and using both methods together does increase their effectiveness, although this is not always necessary. Studies have shown that careful condom use can be very effective. Other types of contraceptives are even more effective than either condoms or foams, and she could try one of these, but these more effective contraceptives offer no protection against STDs. The most important thing, however, is that you both are protected and that you both have confidence in the method you use. If you use only a condom and she feels some doubt, that could interfere with her enjoyment of having sex with you. So my advice is not to make a big deal about it. If she wants to use two methods, go along with it. If your relationship deepens or perhaps even leads to marriage, then you can discuss together what contraceptive is best for you as a couple. For now, continue using whatever makes her feel comfortable. Just make sure that the foam you use will not deteriorate a latex condom. I believe most contraceptive foams are safe, but check the packaging.

ing condoms or inserting diaphragms for one another. When both people are involved in contraceptive decisions the chances of a slip-up are smaller. Remember that inconsistent use of birth control pills may require use of a barrier method of contraception for the remainder of a particular cycle.

CONDOMS

A condom is a thin, flexible sheath that fits snugly over a man's erection and is rolled down to the base of his penis. Condoms are sometimes called the old veterans of contraception. In one form or another, condoms have been used for centuries. As technology has advanced, so too have the materials from which condoms are made. They were once made of rubber, then latex, and now various polymers as well. These changes provided greater tactile sensitivity, and thus men were more willing to use them. Along with the protection condoms offer against STDs, this has led to the great popularity of condoms and wide willingness to use them.

Condoms can be bought in many places today, unlike in the past when one had to ask a pharmacist. Condoms are available in grocery stores, discount stores, convenience stores, and vending machines in restrooms in college and university student centers. Local community health departments may provide condoms without charge.

Condoms are typically sold rolled up in sealed plastic, paper, or aluminum wrappers. Many, but not all, are sold with added lubricant, usually nonoxynol-9 (Fig. 11-8).

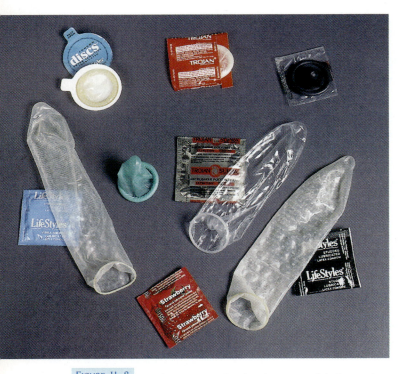

FIGURE 11-8 Condoms are made of various materials (natural membrane, latex, polyurethane) and are sold in a wide variety of colors, shapes, and textures.

Condoms should *never* be used with a petroleum-based lubricant, such as Vaseline, which can make them tear. For extra lubricant with a condom, a non-petroleum lubricant should be used, such as surgical lubricant sold under the name K-Y jelly. Generic and store brands of surgical lubricant are generally just as good. Although barrier methods of contraception must be kept handy, men should not keep condoms in their wallets. Sitting on a condom for days, weeks, or months can make it more likely to break. Most condoms are made of latex, although some natural membrane brands (made from sheep intestines) are also available but cost significantly more. Although some men report that natural membrane condoms offer better sensitivity, the difference is generally considered insignificant. Also, latex condoms do a better job of protecting against viral and bacterial STDs. When examined under very high magnification, both latex and natural membrane condoms can be seen to be porous, but the pores in latex condoms are significantly smaller than those found in natural membrane condoms and, therefore, offer better protection against bacterial and viral STDs, such as HIV (Vinson & Epperly, 1991). These pores are much too small for sperm to swim through. Although condoms offer excellent protection against unintended pregnancies, they are not 100% effective in preventing STDs. (STDs are discussed in depth in Chapter 17.) Since one can never be certain that a potential sexual partner is free of HIV, it is always a good idea to be protected against this fatal disease.

Although condoms are easy to use quickly and correctly, some men do not use them correctly in every respect. Following are guidelines for using condoms most effectively:

1. Always use a new condom for each act of intercourse, even if only a little time has passed since the first intercourse.
2. Before applying a condom, with thumb and forefinger pinch closed about an inch of it before unrolling the rest. This creates a reservoir tip to hold the ejaculate. Some condoms are designed with a reservoir tip, but it's still a good idea to do this.
3. Unroll the condom completely down the penis, all the way to its base.
4. Never penetrate your partner with your penis until the condom is applied.
5. After intercourse, hold the condom at the base of the penis before withdrawing from your partner. This prevents any leakage into the vagina that might otherwise occur.
6. Store condoms in a cool, dry place. The used condom can be wrapped in tissue with its wrapper and disposed of in the wastebasket.

Despite jokes to the contrary, condoms are available basically in only one size, which comfortably accommodates virtually all men. Some brands may be up to 20% longer than other brands, however.

SUMMARY OF MALE CONDOMS

Method: Male Condoms

Expected Failure Rate if Used Consistently and Conscientiously: <3% (if used with spermicides)

Expected Failure Rate if Not Used Consistently and Conscientiously: 12%

Advantages:

Readily available

Inexpensive

Offers excellent protection against STDs

Often lubricated with spermicide

Different colors, textures, and flavors offer variety

Encourages a couple to talk about and plan to use contraceptives

Disadvantages:

May not protect against HIV

Must plan ahead of time to obtain and use

Could interrupt sexual spontaneity

Generally discourages oral sex (fellatio) due to taste of latex

Requires partner cooperation

Some men claim a loss of sensitivity

Must apply condom before penetration

Side Effects:

Occasional allergic reaction to nonoxynol-9 (rarely serious)

Rare latex allergy can be extremely serious

Health Risks:

Generally none

Cost:

Free or very low cost at local health departments

$1.50 for three to $10 for a dozen

For What Type of Person Is This a Good Contraceptive Choice?

People who cannot afford or do not have access to family planning services

Men who cannot depend on their partners to use contraception

Those who want to act independently in using birth control

Those whose lifestyle might involve multiple sexual partners

Women who have trouble tolerating hormonal contraceptives or IUDs

Women who forget to take birth control pills

Women starting oral contraceptives and needing a barrier method for one month

Doctor's Visit Needed to Use This Method?   No

In May 1995, *Consumer Reports* evaluated about 40 different brands of condoms, describing the type of lubrication each used (if any), the concentration of nonoxynol-9 used (if used), the length and width in millimeters of each brand, the thickness of the latex used, and cost. The condoms were tested to see how easily they could break or tear. Condoms are not all equally resistant to breakage, and some are clearly superior to others while a few are frankly inferior. Often the thinnest condoms broke most easily. Consumers should, therefore, be careful about purchasing condoms advertised as "supersensitive," "superthin" or "ultrathin." On the average only 2% to 5% of

condoms break, and this usually results from using them incorrectly rather than some problem in the condom itself.

What to do if a condom breaks? Couples using condoms should know what to do in case this happens. First, both partners should wash their genitals with soap and warm water and should urinate as soon as possible to further reduce the risk of acquiring an STD. If the condom breaks after ejaculation, spermicide if immediately available should be applied promptly. A doctor can prescribe special birth control pills that can be used as a "morning after" contraceptive (see later section). Using condoms correctly as outlined above, however, is the best way to avoid breakage. A study of 41 licensed female sex workers in Nevada, where visitors to legal brothels are required by law to use condoms, found that during the nine days being investigated, not one condom broke. Additionally, only 0.6% of condoms fell off during sexual intercourse, and 3-4% slipped either during intercourse or during withdrawal. Although the effectiveness of condoms in blocking the transmission of HIV is still being debated, over 20,000 HIV tests had been conduced on licensed prostitutes in Nevada through 1993 and *none* tested positive (Remez, 1996). In a study of 932 sexually active American unmarried women between the ages of 17 and 44, 67% reported that disease prevention was their primary reason for using condoms (Anderson, Brackbill, & Mosher, 1996).

FEMALE CONDOMS

After years of research, in 1993 the United States Food and Drug Administration approved the first version of a **female condom**, sometimes called a "vaginal pouch," for use (Fig. 11-9). It is a long, flexible sleeve of polyurethane that is inserted into the vagina, up against the cervix at one end and at the introitus at the other. The penis is introduced through a flexible ring at the opening. The ring at the opening to the vagina affords a barrier for the labia majora and the interior of the vagina. Female condoms are not as convenient to use as male condoms, are not as readily available, and are more expensive. But for a woman who wants autonomy in contraception, the female condom offers an alternative. A woman has to be very comfortable with her body to use the female condom correctly and reliably, however. Women who don't like to touch their genitals, who have misgivings about masturbation, and who dislike tampon insertion and removal may not be comfortable inserting the female condom. People often choose different contraceptives because of such personal differences.

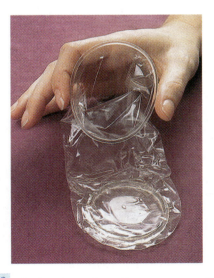

FIGURE 11-9   The female condom offers women excellent protection against sexually transmitted diseases (STDs) and unanticipated pregnancy, as well as autonomy in sexual and reproductive choices.

The female condom is not as effective as the male condom. American and Latin American women in monogamous sexual relationships tested the female condom as their only form of contraception for 6 months (Farr, Gabelnick, Sturgen, & Dorflinger, 1994). Among these 328 subjects, 22 Americans and 17 Latin Americans became pregnant, yielding an "accidental pregnancy" rate of 12.4% and 22.2%. Among women using the female condom consistently and correctly every time, the accidental pregnancy rates were 2.6% for the Americans and 9.5% for the Latin Americans. The failure rates may be due to inadequate spermicide; not all female condoms come lubricated with spermicide. In addition, some women may not leave the female condom in long enough after intercourse. None of these women reported any troubling side effects from using the female condom. The investigators concluded that this contraceptive was comparable to other barrier methods and also offered some protection against STDs. Other research concludes that many women do not enjoy using the female condom (Sapire, 1995) and have difficulties using it correctly. Women frequently report that they find its appearance unappealing, and some women do not feel comfortable enlisting the cooperation of their partners when inserting or removing it.

The female condom is made of polyurethane, which is less likely to break or tear than latex condoms. Polyurethane also seems to offer better sensitivity than latex, and this can be an advantage over male condoms. Body warmth seems better perceived through polyurethane as well. On the other hand, couples may notice squeaking and other unusual sounds during intercourse and might feel somewhat distracted.

A study in Kenya of women using the female condom concluded that many African women very much like using this contraceptive (Ruminjo, Steiner, Joanis, Mwathe, & Thagana, 1996). The women in this sample visited private gynecologists. Fully 84% of them indicated that they had very positive experiences with the female condom, and two-thirds said that they liked this form of birth control better than male latex condoms. More than half reported that they would use this contraceptive in the future if it became widely available and easily obtained. Some women had complaints, however. Some thought it was too large for easy insertion, and others thought it messy; some thought it reduced sensitivity substantially. Some of the male partners of these women disliked the female condom and discouraged its use, although this might also occur with other female barrier methods of contraception, such as the diaphragm or the cervical cap. Because the female condom is a relatively new form of birth control, it is still not clear what type of woman is most likely to use it. One study (Sly, Quadagno, Harrison, Eberstein, Riehman, & Bailey, 1997) pointed to some of the factors that contribute to its use, however. The female condom was evaluated more favorably by women who were currently living with someone, those who had had an STD in the past, those who had been tested for HIV, those who saw no difference in their degree of contraceptive control compared with the male condom, and those who didn't know

Summary of the Female Condom

Method: The Female Condom

Expected Failure Rate if Used Consistently and Conscientiously: 5% if used with spermicides

Expected Failure Rate if Not Used Consistently and Conscientiously: 22 to 26%

Advantages:

- Readily available
- Inexpensive
- Offers excellent protection against STDs
- Often lubricated with spermicide
- Encourages a couple to talk about and plan to use contraceptives
- Offers women some autonomy in taking responsibility for contraception

Disadvantages:

- May not protect against HIV
- Must plan ahead of time to obtain and use
- Could interrupt sexual spontaneity
- May discourage oral sex (cunnilingus)
- Requires partner cooperation
- Must insert condom before any penetration
- Use sometimes accompanied by squeaking sounds

Side Effects:

- Occasional allergic reaction to nonoxynol-9 (rarely serious)

Health Risks:

- Generally none

Cost: $3 to $4 each

For What Type of Person Is This a Good Contraceptive Choice?

- Women who cannot afford or do not have access to family planning services
- Those who cannot depend on their partner to use contraception
- Those who want to act independently in using birth control
- Those whose lifestyle might involve multiple sexual partners
- Those who have trouble tolerating hormonal contraceptives or IUDs
- Those who forget to take birth control pills
- Those starting oral contraceptives and needing a barrier method for one month

Doctor's Visit Needed to Use This Method?   No

---

very much about it and wanted to try something new. Although its advantages are quite compelling for some women, it is still too early to know how popular this form of birth control will become.

THE DIAPHRAGM

Diaphragms have been used by women for over 150 years and were the first reliably effective barrier method of contraception for women. Although less popular (and some think less convenient) than other methods of contraception today, many women are comfortable with diaphragms and see little reason to try something else. Diaphragms are shallow, flexible latex cup-shaped devices with an outer flexible ring (Fig. 11-10). In some diaphragms the rim is flat, while in others it is a coiled spring. The ring bends easily for comfortable insertion and removal. While not highly effective, with a failure rate es-

timated at about 18%, careful use can reduce this rate to about 6%. To be most effective, the woman uses the diaphragm with spermicidal jelly, inserts it properly, and leaves it in place for a prolonged period of time after intercourse. The flexible latex cup fits over the cervix, prohibiting sperm from entering the uterus (Fig. 11-11). It is held in place by vaginal muscles. Because the size of the cervix varies among women, a diaphragm has to be sized by a physician or other health care professional.

Learning to use a diaphragm properly involves some care. First, about a teaspoon of spermicidal jelly is evenly distributed around the inside of the cup and its rim. Using too much spermicide causes the diaphragm to slip out of its proper location. While lying on her back or perhaps standing with one leg elevated, the woman bends the rim between her thumb and forefinger and inserts it into her vagina at an angle toward the

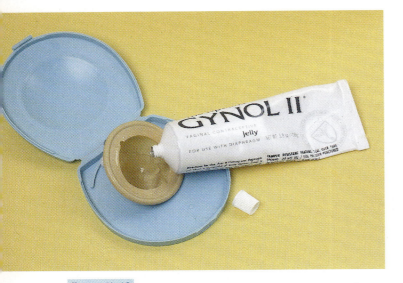

FIGURE 11-10   A diaphragm (in its plastic case) with a small amount of contraceptive jelly inside of it. Diaphragms are manufactured in various diameters to fit snugly over cervixes of different sizes.

lower back. She advances the diaphragm as far as possible and then checks to see that the front of the rim is behind the pubic bone. After inserting the diaphragm, she inserts a finger into the vagina to be sure that the cervix is completely covered. If not, she takes the diaphragm out, applies a little more spermicidal jelly, and tries again. Because this takes some practice, most doctors take the time to work with the woman learning how to insert the diaphragm. Some doctors give the diaphragm during this office visit, while others write a prescription for a local pharmacy. As with any skill, the more one does it, the better one gets and the fewer re-insertions are necessary. As with the condom, both partners can participate. Some women find that their partner can prepare and insert a diaphragm more efficiently and quickly than they can themselves. The diaphragm may not be the best contraceptive device, however, for women who are not thoroughly comfortable with their bodies.

Women who use a diaphragm need to be foresightful about having intercourse. The diaphragm should not be inserted more than 6 hours before intercourse. After this amount of time, if intercourse will occur, more spermicide should be introduced to the vagina. Many spermicides come with small plastic syringes that make this easy. The woman must also leave the diaphragm in for at least 6 hours after intercourse, but not longer than 24 hours. This ensures that the spermicide has killed all the sperm deposited in the vagina. Leaving the diaphragm in too long, however, may increase the risk of a vaginal infection. Removing the diaphragm is easy. The woman simply inserts a finger into the vagina and places it under the rim and pulls gently. A little suction may have built up beneath it, but this does not indicate a problem.

Women who plan to use a diaphragm should consider some additional issues. Changing positions frequently during intercourse is not a good idea because this may dislodge the diaphragm. The woman-on-top position is more likely also to dislodge it. Finally, a woman who gains or loses more than 15 pounds might need a different size diaphragm.

THE CERVICAL CAP

In one form or another, the **cervical cap** has been used since 1838 when it was developed by a German gynecologist. Like the diaphragm, it fits tightly over the cervix, but it is a thicker, thimble-shaped little cup, usually made of rubber or plastic (Fig. 11-12). In the late 1970s and early 1980s, The National Institute of Child Health and Human Development conducted a 3-year study of 2400 women to assess the effectiveness of cervical caps and determine whether any unanticipated

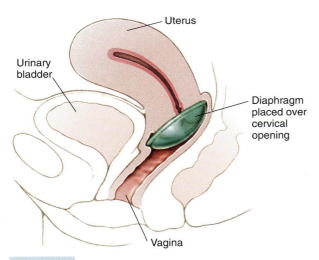

FIGURE 11-11   The position of a diaphragm that has been inserted correctly. Note that it snugly covers the cervix, blocking the progress of sperm into the uterus and fallopian tubes. Proper sizing and insertion of the diaphragm are essential.

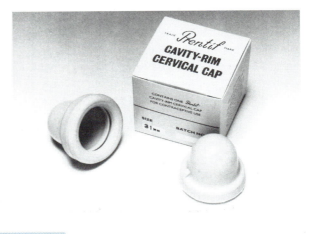

FIGURE 11-12   Like the diaphragm, the cervical cap fits snugly over a woman's cervix.

SUMMARY OF THE DIAPHRAGM

Method: The Diaphragm
Expected Failure Rate if Used Consistently and Conscientiously: 6%
Expected Failure Rate if Not Used Consistently and Conscientiously: 18%
Advantages:

Readily available

Inexpensive

Low cost of continued use

Encourages a couple to talk about and plan to use contraceptives

Offers women autonomy in taking responsibility for contraception

Disadvantages:

May not protect against HIV and other STDs—insufficient data at this time

Must plan ahead of time to obtain and use

Could interrupt sexual spontaneity

May become dislodged while changing intercourse positions

Requires partner cooperation

Must be inserted before any penetration

May become dislodged while using the woman-on-top position

Should be resized if a woman gains or loses over 15 pounds

May be difficult for obese women to insert correctly

Side Effects:

Occasional allergic reaction to nonoxynol-9 (rarely serious)

Health Risks:

Generally none

Cost:

Approximately $35, not including doctor's visit, which may cost $90. Yearly re-checks of the diaphragm cost approximately $75. Depending on how frequently a diaphragm needs to be replaced, this method averages less than $12. per month.

For What Type of Person Is This a Good Contraceptive Choice?

Highly conscientious, foresightful women

Those who cannot depend on their partner to use contraception

Those who want to act independently in using birth control

Those who are very comfortable with their bodies

Those who have trouble tolerating hormonal contraceptives or IUDs

Those who forget to take birth control pills

Those starting oral contraceptives and needing a barrier method for one month

Women with reduced financial means

Doctor's Visit Needed to Use This Method? Yes

side effects might occur. Before this, little information was available on the safety and effectiveness of the cervical cap, which usually had to be ordered from the United Kingdom.

Because cervical caps fit tightly over the cervix, there were initial concerns that prolonged use might lead to abrasions and possibly to cellular changes, but this fear proved unfounded. These contraceptives were approved for use in this country in 1988. Like diaphragms, cervical caps require the use of spermicides. Some women find the cervical cap a bit more difficult to insert and remove than a diaphragm, especially those with

an elongated vagina. Cervical caps also seem to become dislodged more easily during intercourse than diaphragms. Because different women have cervixes of different size, a physician must fit the device and instruct the woman how to insert and remove it. Although cervical caps have some disadvantages, they can be left in place for up to 48 hours, and additional applications of spermicide are not necessary when a couple wants to have sex (Weiss, Bassford, & Davis, 1991).

Some women have trouble obtaining cervical caps, mostly because they are not as commonly used in this country.

SUMMARY OF THE CERVICAL CAP

Method: The Cervical Cap

Expected Failure Rate if Used Consistently and Conscientiously: 6%

Expected Failure Rate if Not Used Consistently and Conscientiously: 18%

Advantages:

Readily available

Inexpensive

Low cost of continued use

Encourages a couple to talk about and plan to use contraceptives

Offers women autonomy in taking responsibility for contraception

Good birth control alternative for a woman who has urinary tract infections with a diaphragm

Can be applied up to 48 hours before intercourse

Less messy than a diaphragm

Only a small amount of spermicide needs to be used

Offers protection against some STDs

Disadvantages:

May not protect against HIV—current data inconclusive

Must plan ahead of time to obtain and use

Could interrupt sexual spontaneity

May be difficult to insert

Some women have trouble obtaining the right size

May become dislodged while changing intercourse positions

May require partner cooperation

Must be inserted before any penetration

Not readily available everywhere

Some health care providers have not been trained to insert it

Side Effects:

Occasional allergic reaction to nonoxynol-9 (rarely serious)

Health Risks:

Possible tissue abrasion/erosion of the cervix

Cost:

Approximately $45 plus office visit, which may cost approximately $90. Depending on how frequently a cervical cap needs to be replaced, the average monthly cost of this method is less than $15, including the cost of spermicidal agents.

For What Type of Person Is This a Good Contraceptive Choice?

Highly conscientious, foresightful women

Those who cannot depend on their partner to use contraception

Those who want to act independently in using birth control

Women who are very comfortable with their bodies

Those who have trouble tolerating hormonal contraceptives or IUDs

Those who forget to take birth control pills

Those starting oral contraceptives and needing a barrier method for one month

Women with reduced financial means

Doctor's Visit Needed to Use This Method?   Yes

Sometimes the woman's partner reports a little discomfort during intercourse, presumably because the penis bumps into the cap during pelvic thrusting (Secor, 1992). Early hopes for high effectiveness of the cervical cap have not, unfortunately, been realized. When one brand called "Fem Cap" was being developed in 1992, it's anticipated failure rate was estimated at 4.8% (Hatcher & Warner, 1992), but later data showed a rate of at least 6%, with far higher failure rates for inconsistent usage. More recent data reveal a failure rate of 10–13% for perfect, careful use (Trussell, Strickler, & Vaughan, 1993). Continued testing of the cervical cap also revealed that it is much less effective in women who have given birth, with some data indicating a failure rate as high as 26–27% (Trussell, Strickler, & Vaughan, 1993). Presumably, once the cervix has been stretched in childbirth, the cervical cap is less likely to remain snugly in place during and after intercourse. Women who have used both the cervical cap and diaphragm generally report it is a bit more difficult to use the cap.

The dome of the cap should be filled about one-third with spermicidal jelly. Spermicide should *not* be applied to the rim of the cap because this might prevent the suction needed to keep the cap in place. The cap is then inserted as far as possible into the vagina with the dome pointing downward toward the opening. The woman inserts her forefinger into the vagina and pushes the cap snugly onto the cervix, and checks that she can feel the opening to the cervix through the wall of the cap. Because some women have a little trouble doing this, health care professionals can provide a small application probe to help insert the cap into the proper location. The cervical cap can be applied up to 48 hours before intercourse and should remain in place at least 8 hours afterwards. When having a period, the woman should use another contraceptive method because the menstrual discharge can break the suction between the cap and the cervix. The cap is removed by inserting the finger into the vagina and giving the cap a nudge to break the suction. The rim of the cap is lightly tugged and the cap gently guided out. It should be washed with soap and water and dried thoroughly. A cotton swab is used to dry behind the rim. As with latex condoms and diaphragms, petroleum-based lubricants would cause the cervical cap to disintegrate and, therefore, should not be used.

Before being fitted with a cervical cap, it's a good idea for a woman to have a Pap smear so that the doctor has a baseline with which to compare later Pap smears. A woman who has had a miscarriage or a baby probably then needs a different size cervical cap. A cervical cap can generally be used for up to 2 years before it needs to be replaced.

THE VAGINAL SPONGE

Until fairly recently, the **vaginal sponge** offered women another over-the-counter birth control alternative. The sponge is a circular piece of synthetic soft foam impregnated with **nonoxynol-9.** It is about 2 inches (5 cm) in diameter and has slight indentations in the center of both sides. It has a little string loop that makes insertion and removal easy (Fig. 11-13). The sponge acts as a physical barrier to the cervix (but not as tightly sealed as a diaphragm or cervical cap) and slowly disperses spermicide inside the vagina. It isn't the best over-the-counter contraceptive. In women who have had vaginal births, its failure rate is as high as 28%, far less effective than all of the barrier methods discussed so far, but of course it is better than not using any method. When the sponge is used correctly and consistently, its failure rate is comparable to that of the diaphragm or cervical cap, around 17% (Trussell, Strickler, & Vaughan, 1993).

As of this writing, however, the vaginal contraceptive sponge is no longer being sold—for reasons of economics more than safety or effectiveness. The company that manufactured the sponge was directed by the federal government to make some modifications in its manufacturing plant that were

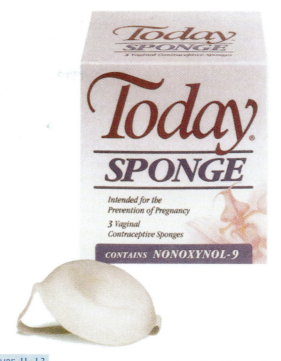

FIGURE 11-13   Sponges were once popular, affordable, and convenient, although not as effective as other contraceptive alternatives. They were taken off the market, but there is much interest in distributing them again.

extensive and expensive. Instead, it simply stopped making the sponge. It is anticipated that by the time you read this, some other company will purchase the right to manufacture the sponge and production will resume, using the original spermicide, nonoxynol-9, or some other agent.

The earlier chapter on sexual and reproductive health issues discussed toxic shock syndrome in relation to the use of different types of tampons. When the sponge was first introduced, some were concerned that it too might promote the growth of the bacteria that cause toxic shock syndrome, *Staphylococcus aureus.* However, carefully controlled studies demonstrated that this does not happen if the sponge is used as directed (Stumpf, Byers, & Lloyd, 1986). One study did demonstrate that consistent use of the sponge was more likely to lead to recurrent bouts of bacterial vaginosis (Mengel & Davis, 1992). Investigators also explored what women are most likely to use this contraceptive technique. Women who reported the highest satisfaction with the sponge generally had never been married and had fewer children. Sponge users reported that they were favorably impressed by advertisements for the sponge, perhaps more so than by their doctors. Finally, women who used the sponge did so more consistently correctly than women who used diaphragms (Harvey, Beckman, & Murray, 1989).

Because spermicides are known to offer some protection against STDs, studies have examined whether a concentrated source of nonoxynol-9 might offer special protection. In one

SUMMARY OF THE VAGINAL SPONGE

Method: The Vaginal Sponge

Expected Failure Rate if Used Consistently and Conscientiously: 17%

Expected Failure Rate if Not Used Consistently and Conscientiously: 26%

Advantages:

Offers women autonomy in taking responsibility for contraception

Can be used without a man's awareness

May offer protection against some STDs

Can be inserted up to 24 hours before intercourse

Disadvantages:

May not protect against HIV

The woman must plan ahead of time to obtain and use

Must be inserted before any penetration

Not readily available everywhere

Side Effects:

Occasional allergic reaction to nonoxynol-9 (rarely serious)

Occasional vaginal dryness

Health Risks:

None generally

Cost: When available, approximately $3 each

For What Type of Person Is This a Good Contraceptive Choice?

Women who cannot depend on their partner to use contraception

Those who want to act independently in using birth control

Those who are very comfortable with their bodies

Those who have trouble tolerating hormonal contraceptives or IUDs

Those who forget to take birth control pills

Those starting oral contraceptives and needing a temporary method for one cycle

Doctor's Visit Needed to Use This Method?   No

---

study of 74 Nairobi prostitutes who were at high risk for acquiring HIV, use of the nonoxynol-9 vaginal sponge did not reduce the risk of infection (Ngugi, Holmes, Ndinya-Achola, Waiyaki, Roberts, Ruminjo, Sajabi, Kimata, Fleming, et al., 1992). A new vaginal sponge has been introduced in France containing three different spermicidal agents: nonoxynol-9, benzalkonium chloride, and cholic acid. In a pilot study of 20 women using this form of birth control, none became pregnant during the year they used it. This particular combination of spermicidal agents has been shown to have inhibitory effects on HIV and its spread through sexual contact (Psychoyos, Creatsas, Hassan, Georgoulias, & Gravanis, 1993). As of this writing, this vaginal sponge is not distributed in the United States. Because the sponge was once readily available in the United States, however, researchers speculated that it would be a popular alternative for women who could not afford to visit a doctor for contraceptive counseling or birth control pills. In fact, this was not the case. In a large study of black and Hispanic inner city female adoles-

cents in New York City, the sponge was the form of birth control least likely to be used (Diaz, Jaffe, Leadbeater, & Levin, 1990). In fact, the sponge was used less often than no method of birth control at all and even the rhythm method and withdrawal. Availability does not translate into usage.

Contragestational Agents

As noted earlier, a foreign body inside the uterus may prevent a fertilized egg from being implanted and thus stop a pregnancy. Even today, researchers are not fully certain how IUDs work. When researchers examine the fallopian tubes of women using an IUD for signs of fertilized eggs, they almost never find any. Some scientists think that IUDs create a minor, chronic inflammatory reaction inside the uterus that is somehow lethal to sperm. Because of the uncertainty about whether conception actually occurs, IUDs are sometimes called "contragestational agents." There is renewed interest in this form of contraception today, which is safe, effective, and thoroughly tested.

On the Lighter Side

CONTRACEPTIVE MYTHS

We believe that accurate information about birth control is serious business, especially for those who might not be so careful about using it. As available as contraception is in our country today, and as simple as it is to use correctly, a number of rather odd or outrageous myths still exist about how to avoid an unintended pregnancy. Here are some of the more unusual things we have heard over the years. Remember: these *don't* work!

Myth 1. **A Woman Should Put Ice Cubes in Her Vagina After Intercourse.** In addition to this being decidedly uncomfortable, only seconds after ejaculation sperm have already made their way through the cervix and into the uterus. As noted earlier, putting anything into the vagina after intercourse seldom diminishes the chances of conception occurring, and douching may actually increase it.

Myth 2. **After My Girlfriend and I Have Sex, She Can Use Her Muscles to Push out All of My Sperm.** While some women have excellent vaginal muscle tone, there is no way a woman can expel all of her partner's ejaculate after intercourse.

Myth 3. **You Can't Get Pregnant if you Have Sex in a Hot Tub.** Oh, yes you can. The inside of the vagina is separated from the outside by many membranes and folds of skin that keep semen reserved within, even when a couple has intercourse in a hot tub. Don't count on the hot water or the chemicals in it to act as spermicidal agents.

Myth 4. **You Can't Get Pregnant if you Have Intercourse Standing Up.** Some people believe that all of a man's sperm will flow out of the vagina if the couple has sex standing up. This is certainly not true. Sperm enter the cervix very quickly after ejaculation takes place. *Any* sperm that enter the vagina can fertilize an ovum.

Myth 5. **Yellow Dye Number 5 Lowers a Man's Sperm Count.** We have no idea where this myth came from. But apparently enough people believed it that the Pepsi Company, which makes "Mountain Dew" (colored with yellow dye number 5), released a statement denying that men who drink Mountain Dew have a lowered sperm count or otherwise are less able to impregnate their partners.

Myth 6. **The Rhythm Method Refers to how a Couple Moves During Intercourse.** No. The rhythm method involves using a basal body temperature chart to determine a woman's most fertile time during her menstrual cycle. Some adolescents mistakenly believe that if a couple does not move "in rhythm" during intercourse, the woman can't get pregnant.

We would be interested in hearing from you if you have heard of other odd myths about preventing pregnancy.

Several different IUDs are used in the United States today (Fig. 11-14A). One of the most common, the Copper T-380A, sometimes called ParaGard, is a plastic T-shaped object with each arm of the T about 5/8 an inch (1.75 cm) long. Fine copper wire is wrapped around the base of the T, and copper tubing surrounds both top arms. The IUD contains barium sulfate to be visible on an x-ray of the woman's uterus if necessary. This IUD is effective for up to 8 years. The copper gradually dissolves over the years, working in a number of ways to inhibit fertiliza-

tion. Traces of dissolved copper magnify the inflammatory response of the uterus and create an environment throughout the woman's reproductive tract that is hostile to both eggs and sperm, much less a fertilized zygote. The amount of copper released daily is extremely small, about one-thirtieth of an adult's recommended daily allowance. Allergic reactions to copper are very rare. Another common IUD, called the Progestasert, is also shaped like a T. Its base contains progesterone, which is released gradually every day. This progesterone significantly increases the

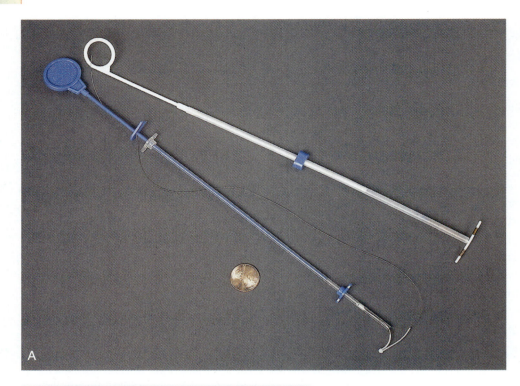

FIGURE 11-14 (A) Two different IUDs, the "Copper-7" (with blue tubular applicator) and the Copper T-380A (with white tubular applicator). Below (B) is a plastic model of the uterus illustrating the location and orientation of the Copper T-380A IUD. Note the two string filaments protruding through the cervix of this model. These are trimmed after the device is inserted by a doctor.

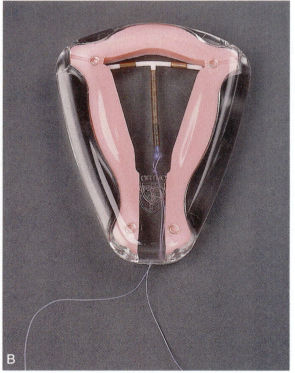

Many women like IUDs because they don't have to do anything with this highly effective contraceptive. For women who tolerate the IUD well and experience no complications, this is an extremely effective form of birth control. Among women using IUDs that gradually release copper, only 2 out of every 1000 become pregnant in the first year of use. Among women using ParaGard for a full 8 years, the failure rate is only 1.5 per 100 women. Convenience and effectiveness are strong selling points for many women who use the IUD.

Nonetheless, IUDs are not generally recommended for women who have not had children because of potential complications that could cause infertility. Woman who have an STD or who have multiple sexual partners and, therefore, have an increased risk of getting one are also not good candidates for IUDs. Further, if there is any chance that the woman might already be pregnant, an IUD definitely should not be used. Finally, women with a history of frequent pelvic inflammatory disease should not consider an IUD.

Other conditions too should discourage a woman from considering an IUD. Women who have chronically severe menstrual cramps and who lose large amounts of blood during their periods are not good candidates for the IUD, nor those with known or suspected cervical or uterine cancer. Women with clotting problems, anemia, or a history of IUD expulsion (they do sometimes come out) are generally discouraged from trying an IUD. Finally, women who got pregnant in the past while using an IUD should consider other contraceptive options.

All IUDs have two long threads that extend through the cervix into the vagina. If the woman or her partner cannot feel these threads before intercourse, the IUD may have been expelled without her knowing it, as can occasionally happen. The couple should then use a barrier method of contraception. Get-

thickness of cervical mucus, so that the cervix becomes highly impermeable to sperm in addition to the inflammatory response. Doctors recommend that the Progestasert be replaced every year, because the progesterone inside it is gradually used up. Although both of these IUDs are shaped like a T, there is an enormous variety of sizes and shapes of IUDs.

SUMMARY OF THE INTRAUTERINE DEVICE (IUD)

Method: The Intrauterine Device (IUD)

Expected Failure Rate if Used Consistently and Conscientiously: 0.1-1.5%

Expected Failure Rate if Not Used Consistently and Conscientiously: 0.1-2%

Failure rates vary for different types of IUDs

Advantages:

Effective and convenient

Does not change usual menstrual cycle pattern

Easy to determine if properly positioned in the uterus

Disadvantages:

No protection against STDs

Cramping and heavy menstrual discharge, especially when first inserted

Cannot always know if your doctor is experienced in inserting IUDs

Insertion can introduce bacteria into the uterus

IUD may be ejected or become incorrectly positioned in the uterus

Insertion or removal can be uncomfortable

Side Effects:

Cramping and heavy menstrual discharge

Health Risks:

Despite suspicions, no demonstrated relationship with pelvic inflammatory disease

Possible perforation of the wall of the uterus

Rare allergic reactions to copper

Vaginitis and cervicitis more common in women with IUDs

Occasional temporary low blood pressure and low heart rate after insertion

Cost:

$150-$200 for the IUD plus $200-$400 for insertion

With yearly gynecological check-ups costing approximately $100, this method of contraception costs approximately $15 per month over the 5-year life of an IUD

For What Type of Person is This a Good Contraceptive Choice?

Women who cannot depend on their partner to use contraception

Those who want to be independent in using birth control

Those with trouble tolerating hormonal contraceptives

Those who forget to take birth control pills

Women who are allergic to latex or nonoxynol-9

Women who have had children

Women and their partners who are comfortable checking to see that the strings are correctly positioned before having intercourse

Doctor's Visit Needed to Use This Method?   Yes

---

ting an IUD is a relatively straightforward process. Some tests are commonly performed first to ensure the woman does not have an infection and is not pregnant. A Pap smear is commonly done at this time. A woman who is not pregnant can have an IUD put in any time during the menstrual cycle. Women are encouraged to take a nonsteroidal anti-inflammatory agent (aspirin, ibuprofen, or naproxen sodium) to minimize any discomfort or cramping that commonly follows IUD insertion for 12 to 24 hours. While most women experience some discomfort during the insertion of an IUD, many do not. The doctor might use a local anesthetic in or around the cervix to minimize soreness. A very narrow tube containing the IUD is inserted through the cervix, and the device is deposited in the uterus. The IUD unfolds into its T-shape, and the doctor checks that the strings attached to it are in place (Fig. 11-14B). The procedure takes about 5 minutes. The entire

IUD should be completely inside the uterus, and the woman should not be able to feel it when she checks that the strings are in the proper place. A little bleeding or spotting is common after insertion and should not be cause of concern. The woman sees the doctor again in about six weeks to ensure everything is alright. The IUD is effective immediately. The first period after the insertion of the IUD is generally heavier than usual.

There are various times when a woman may decide to have an IUD inserted. A woman who has had a miscarriage during the first three months of pregnancy but no unusual complications can have an IUD inserted three weeks later. A woman can have an IUD put in immediately after either vaginal and Cesarean births if she chooses. A woman who is breast-feeding her newborn can have an IUD inserted six weeks after birth. Finally, an IUD can be inserted six weeks after childbirth if the woman is not breast-feeding, is not pregnant, or her period has not yet resumed. So there are a variety of circumstances that may contribute to the use of an IUD in connection with a miscarriage or live birth. IUDs are made of highly flexible plastic that can be comfortably removed if a woman decides that another method of contraception is more appropriate for her lifestyle. For women who want to become pregnant soon after the removal of an IUD, recent data indicate that women who have used copper IUDs usually promptly become fertile again (Singh & Ratnam, 1997).

Today, IUDs are safer and have fewer side effects than ever before, and they should not be so quickly ruled out as a possible birth control alternative. However, a woman and her doctor should consider a few things first. As described earlier, IUDs are not the best form of contraceptive for women with certain conditions or lifestyles (Odlind, 1996). Women using copper IUDs should expect a particularly heavy menstrual flow, although this is less likely in women using hormonal IUDs. In fact, hormonal IUDs are also used today to help manage the sometimes very heavy menstrual discharge associated with menopause (Coleman, McCowan, & Farquhar, 1997). In women in New Zealand and Australia hormone-releasing IUDs have been shown to be highly effective in treating heavy menstruation and fibroid tumors, which are among the most common causes of hysterectomy around the time of menopause.

Because IUDs usually stay in the body for an extended period, researchers have studied whether chronic irritation of the endometrium might play a role in the development of endometrial cancers. Two recent studies have demonstrated that prolonged use of intrauterine devices presents no increased risk of these cancers (Sturgeon, Brinton, Berman, Mortel, Twiggs, Barrett, Wilbanks, & Lurain, 1997; Hill, Weiss, Voigt, & Beresford, 1997).

Sterilization

All the contraceptive alternatives discussed so far are reversible. People can start and stop using them as their life circumstances or health change. Voluntary surgical sterilization, the most common method of birth control in the world, is *irreversible*, however, and people who consider it should think of it that way even though contemporary surgical techniques offer some success in reversing these procedures. In countries that penalize couples for having more than one child, such as China, sterilization is common and culturally encouraged. In women, **bilateral tubal ligation** involves clipping, tying off, or disconnecting the fallopian tubes through electrocautery (using an electrical current to melt both ends of the fallopian tube tissue closed). In men, **vasectomy** uses the same surgical methods to interrupt the vas deferens to make it impossible for sperm to enter the ejaculate. These forms of voluntary surgical sterilization are discussed separately below.

WEIGHING THE DECISION

One of our most essential freedoms is to decide whether and when to have children. Previous chapters have discussed the decision many people make not to have children and the subtle pronatalist pressures in this and other societies. The decision to render one's self incapable of becoming pregnant or of impregnating someone else should be approached carefully, gradually, and with full information. Some people simply don't want children and want a certain way to ensure this will never happen; for them, surgical sterilization is often an attractive contraceptive alternative. Nonetheless, modern lifestyles often change. People no longer have one period of educational training, one job, one career, one marriage, or one family. Many people develop new professional skills, change jobs several times, have more than one career, marry more than once, and have children with more than one spouse or partner. Therefore, one should consider possible future changes, such as being married a second or later time to someone who very much wants to have children, after one had chosen sterilization in an earlier marriage. As noted earlier, tubal ligation and vasectomy can be reversed, but the procedure is expensive, rarely covered by health insurance, and not always successful. Many things could lead to a change of mind about being sterilized. People get divorced when they were sure they would stay together forever. Young women and men die unexpectedly. Children sometimes die, leaving their parents childless. Because of all these situations the decision to become infertile should be made rationally and carefully.

Voluntary sterilization should be discussed with one's partner when appropriate. Not long ago many states had laws forbidding voluntary sterilization without the signed consent of one's spouse. These laws were recognized as potentially discriminatory and a violation of the Fourth Amendment right to personal privacy. Often young people who grow up as victims of abuse, poverty, deprivation, and chronic misery promise themselves that they will never bring another life into such a world. Health care professionals often strongly discourage voluntary sterilization among young people who have not had children, and may even refuse to perform the procedure. Doctors like others in private business have the right to refuse their services.

BILATERAL TUBAL LIGATION

Bilateral tubal ligation in women is sometimes called "tying the tubes." It is a low-risk surgical procedure with an extremely low fatality rate, about 4 in every 100,000 women. This risk is lower than that of other long-term forms of birth control and even the

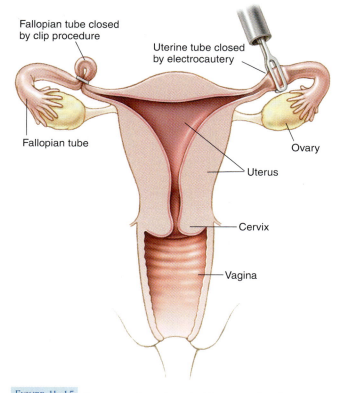

Fallopian tube closed by clip procedure

Uterine tube closed by electrocautery

Fallopian tube

Ovary

Uterus

Cervix

Vagina

FIGURE 11-15 Two procedures for tubal ligation. The clip procedure is illustrated on the left side and electrocautery is shown on the right side.

health risks of being pregnant and giving birth. The surgical procedure is relatively straightforward. In one variation, the gynecologist makes a small incision near the pubic symphysis to expose both fallopian tubes. The tubes are drawn through this small opening, tied or clipped or cauterized, and then placed back into the lower abdomen and the incision stitched back up again (Fig. 11-15). In another variation, called "band-aid" surgery, the small incision is made close to the navel, and carbon dioxide or nitrous oxide is then gently pumped into the lower abdomen to expand it slightly. A laparoscope is inserted into the abdomen to visualize the woman's fallopian tubes. A surgical instrument is advanced into the body cavity through the laparoscope and cauterizes the fallopian tubes, disconnecting them.

Many women decide to have their tubes tied immediately after delivering a baby, since they are already in a surgical setting and they may be sure that the baby they just had will be their last. Because tying or cauterizing the fallopian tubes prevents the meeting of a sperm and egg, this procedure is effective immediately. The operation has no effect on ovulation, and the woman continues to produce a mature, fertilizable egg each month, which simply dissolves and is absorbed into the woman's body. Because the ovaries continue to function normally, they continue to produce female hormones, at least until menopause. For reasons that are not completely clear, women who have had a tubal ligation have a somewhat smaller risk of developing ovarian cancer.

Although voluntary surgical sterilization is generally irreversible, in very rare instances the two disconnected ends of a fallopian tube grow back together, reestablishing the woman's fertility without her knowing it. No one is sure why or how this happens, but it occurs so rarely that it should not be a concern for someone thinking about having her tubes tied.

VASECTOMY

Men also often reach a point in their lives when they are sure that they do not want to have any more children. After the surgical procedure known as a vasectomy, there is no way for sperm to leave the man's body, although the other elements of semen are still in the ejaculate. Men who have had a vasectomy report no change in their erotic sensations during ejaculation.

In a vasectomy, a local anesthetic is used to numb the man's scrotum, and a small incision is made on each side of the scrotal sac (Fig. 11-16). The vas deferens is gently drawn out through the incision, cut, and the two disconnected ends tied off. Sometimes the doctor cauterizes the tubules to seal the ends. The procedure takes only about a half an hour and is typically done in a urologist's office rather than in a hospital or outpatient surgical center. Vasectomy is the most common form of birth control in the United States. It is much less expensive than bilateral tubal ligation and much less complex surgically. In couples who have all the children they want, the men are, therefore, more likely to have a vasectomy than the women to have bilateral tubal ligation. As noted above, vasectomy does not affect a man's sexual pleasure or interfere with the ability to attain and maintain an erection. The incidence of complications after a vasectomy is low. In rare cases, a man may develop epididymitis, a painful localized infection of the epididymis that is effectively treated with antibiotics.

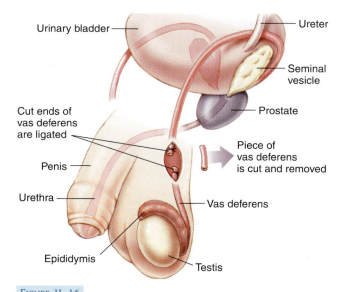

Urinary bladder

Ureter

Seminal vesicle

Cut ends of vas deferens are ligated

Prostate

Piece of vas deferens is cut and removed

Penis

Urethra

Vas deferens

Epididymis

Testis

FIGURE 11-16 Procedure for vasectomy. In addition to cutting the vas deferens and tying off its two ends, electrocautery also may be used.

NO-SCALPEL VASECTOMY

In the early 1990s, a new vasectomy procedure called the "no-scalpel vasectomy" gained attention. It had been used in China since 1974 (Li, Goldstein, Zhu, & Huber, 1991) and is sometimes referred to as a "Li vasectomy" because Dr. Shunqiang Li developed the method. In this procedure a small clamp is attached to the skin of the scrotum surrounding the vas deferens, holding it steady. A sharp, curved hemostat is used to make a tiny puncture in the skin of the scrotum. The vas deferens is gently drawn through this little hole and cut and tied or cauterized; the vas deferens on the other side is then pulled through the same opening and the procedure repeated. No sutures are required to close the tiny hole, and the surgical wound is only about 2 mm wide. Bleeding and infection after the procedure are extremely rare. Even more surprising, this minor surgery takes only 5 to 11 minutes. The only drawback to this procedure is that it takes a long time to learn how to do it skillfully. By 1997, more than 60 million no-scalpel vasectomies had been performed in 26 countries. Data show that this procedure has significantly fewer complications than a conventional vasectomy. An analysis of 1000 no-scalpel vasectomies carried out in Mexico showed that fewer than 2.1% had any postoperative bleeding or blood clotting beneath the surface of the skin, and in *none* was there any infection at the site (Arellano Lara, Gonzalez Barrera, Hernandez Ono, Moreno Alcazar, & Espinosa Perez, 1997). Although different surgical approaches are still advocated, this particular vasectomy procedure is quite effective and has advantages over the conventional procedure.

SUMMARY OF VOLUNTARY SURGICAL STERILIZATION

Method: Voluntary Surgical Sterilization

Lowest Expected Failure Rate:

Vasectomy: 0.1%   Tubal Ligation: 0.5%

Typical Failure Rate:

Vasectomy: 0.15%   Tubal Ligation: 0.5%

Advantages:

Highly effective   Permanent

Disadvantages:

No protection against STDs   Some people have trouble accepting their infertility

Occasional complications during surgical procedure

Side Effects:

Soreness following surgical procedure

Health Risks:

No consistent health risks

Cost:

As of this writing: Bilateral Tubal Ligation: $1300 doctor's fee +

Vasectomy: $850 doctor's fee + $85 initial consultation $125 initial consultation

For What Type of Person Is This a Good Contraceptive Choice?

Those who cannot depend on their partner to use contraception   Women for whom childbearing would be life-threatening

Those who want to act independently in using birth control   People at risk of passing along serious genetic disorders

People who are certain they do not want children or more children

Do You Need to Go to a Doctor to Use This Method? Yes

Continuing Developments in Contraceptive Technology

A new version of Norplant has been tested in Taiwan. Norplant-2 uses only *two* capsules instead of the six first used in the U.S. These new capsules are slightly longer than the originals, but inserting and removing two capsules seems easier. These rods are effective for 3 years and seem to have the same side effects as the original Norplant. A one-rod version called Implanon is being tested, and another version called ST-1435 is being tested in Brazil. These have a failure rate of about 1% and act by stopping ovulation and thickening cervical mucus. Other new implantable technologies being investigated are biodegradable pellets and microscopic spheres that are injected and release hormones directly into the bloodstream; these are effective for 1 to 2 years, but possible side effects are not yet fully known. These would be irreversible forms of birth control until the hormones are depleted.

Because Depo-Provera has been such a popular contraceptive, research has focused on developing other injectable methods of birth control that would minimize side effects of Depo-Provera: irregular bleeding, inconsistent monthly periods, and slow return to fertility upon discontinuation. It is thought that women would comply with monthly injections to gain these improvements.

A new device called the vaginal ring has been undergoing extensive clinical testing. It is made of Silastic and is 50-55 mm in diameter. Some types include only progestin while others contain a combination of progestin and estrogen. This device is positioned high in the vagina. The type with combination hormones can be comfortably left in place for 21 days, then removed for 7 days, with a typical period following. The ring can be removed for a couple of hours, but once the ring is removed, blood levels of progestin soon begin to drop.

Creams containing progestin that can be absorbed through the skin are also being developed and tested. Nesterone is a form of progestin that cannot be taken orally because it is rapidly broken down by the liver. A small amount of cream containing this hormone spread over a woman's abdomen on a daily basis is absorbed slowly into her bloodstream, causing a consistent level in the blood. This may become a good contraceptive option for women who are breast-feeding because the hormone will not reach the mother's breast milk (Blaney, 1995).

New progestin synthetics developed in the laboratory are being tested clinically for contraceptive effectiveness. Two such agents, desogestrel and gestodene, have undergone testing. The former is available in the United States, but the latter is not and as of this writing is still being tested in Europe. These agents compare favorably in effectiveness with products already on the market and have low rates of mid-cycle bleeding. However, both are associated with a higher risk of blood clotting problems than pills currently in use and, therefore, should be considered only with caution, especially if the woman has any personal experience or family history with clotting abnormalities.

While oral contraceptives generally act on the woman's pituitary gland, altering its secretion or FSH or LH, a different group of drugs is being tested that act on the hypothalamus. Because the hypothalamus gives instructions to the pituitary to produce FSH and LH, altering this chemical message could result in the pituitary not receiving the message or becoming less sensitive to it. Various strategies are currently being explored to affect the output of gonadotropin-releasing hormone (GnRH), but clinical tests may not begin for many years.

IUDs under development offer women a highly effective contraceptive with less menstrual bleeding than occurs with many current varieties. One of these, the Levonova/Mirena is a T-shaped, hormone-containing IUD device that releases a very small amount of progestin daily and is effective for 5 years or more. As of this writing it is not yet available in the United States, but clinical data from Europe are highly promising. An innovative development in IUD technology, called the Flexi-Gard, is a long thread surrounded by 6 short lengths of copper tube. One end of the thread is sutured into the lining of the uterus, holding the copper wire inside, and the other end of the thread protrudes through the cervix, allowing the woman to determine that her IUD is correctly in place. Its effectiveness, expulsion rate, removal rate, and continuation rate are comparable to or better than IUDs now available. Five-year data on FlexiGard are not yet available, so its period of effectiveness is unknown. Other more conventional IUDs are also being developed and tested. The Copper T 380 is estimated to be effective for 10 years.

For years researchers have tried to develop a contraceptive vaccine that could be injected and offer a prolonged period of effective birth control. Such a vaccine would contain antigens to prevent fertilization and/or implantation. It is unlikely, however, that such an agent will be available for many years. Two fundamental issues are that it will be difficult to determine how long such an agent would work and when and how easily it could be reversed. Nonetheless, research has focused on three different types of contraceptive vaccines. The first would offer immunity against human chorionic gonadotropin, the second against the substances secreted by the zona pelucida surrounding the mature, fertilizable ovum, and the last against proteins that cover the surface of sperm. Anti-human chorionic gonadotropin vaccines would destroy a blastocyst long before a woman had any idea that she had conceived. Vaccines affecting the zona pelucida would work by making it impossible for a sperm to bond with and enter an ovum. Vaccines acting on proteins covering sperm would make them clump together so that they could not swim toward and penetrate an ovum. This has been an active area of research interest since the early 1990s, with testing ongoing in laboratory animals.

There have also been improvements in condoms that offer an alternative to people with allergies to latex. In 1995 a polyurethane plastic condom was introduced with a cost similar to that of latex condoms. It is still too new for there to be sufficient data about its effectiveness and ability to prevent pregnancy and the transmission of STDs.

A new diaphragm called Lea's Shield is also undergoing clinical testing and may have reached the market by the time this book is published. It has a little valve that allows air to escape during insertion, creating a tighter, sealed fit over the cervix. It will be some time before it is known whether this modified diaphragm is effective and popular.

The innovations described above mostly involve women only. Innovative contraceptive methods for men are apparently many years away. Injections of testosterone enanthate suppress the secretion of the hormones necessary for spermtogenesis, but injections must be given weekly to be effective. Implants, patches, creams, pills, and vaccines are all under investigation as birth control alternatives for men, but virtually all of this research is in a very early stage. Additionally, little is known about possible side effects of these alternatives. For example, a substance called gossypol, which is derived from cottonseed oil, has been studied for years. At first scientists were excited about it, but then it was discovered that it caused irregular heart rhythms in many men, and others experienced fertility problems later on. Developing effective, contraceptive alternatives free of side effects remains a challenge to medical researchers.

PROTECTION AGAINST STDs

The previous discussions of various birth control methods have mentioned their different effectiveness in protecting women and men from giving or getting STDs. No contraceptive method offers complete assurance that a person will not receive or transmit an STD or infestation. Chapter 17 describes sexually transmitted infections and infestations in detail. If a person's sexual lifestyle involves having intercourse with a number of people, especially individuals not known very well, a consistent effort is needed to be protected against both unintended pregnancy and STDs during *every sexual encounter, even if it doesn't involve penis-in-the-vagina intercourse.*

Male latex condoms lubricated with nonoxynol-9 or some other spermicidal substance offer excellent protection against both bacterial and viral STDs. The female condom's effectiveness against STDs when used with a spermicide is also thought to be extremely good. The diaphragm and cervical cap are also barrier methods and are usually used with a spermicide, but both leave a woman's external genitalia unprotected if her partner is not using a condom. Although the cervix is blocked and semen cannot enter, many bacteria and viruses, such as syphilis or genital herpes, may still cause infection. Spermicides alone can also offer some protection against STDs but to be most effective must be used along with a latex condom. Different spermicidal products may contain different amounts and different concentrations of nonoxynol-9 or some other spermicidal agent, such as benzalkonium chloride or sodium cholate. Read the product's label carefully to find out which products contain more concentrated quantities of these agents. The labels of condoms lubricated with nonoxynol-9 do not usually contain information about the amount or strength of the spermicide

Of course, birth control pills, Norplant, voluntary surgical sterilization, and the IUD offer no protection against STDs. Uninformed women sometimes do not understand why they need to use *both* a condom and one of these methods of

birth control, especially if they are more concerned about not becoming pregnant than about not contracting an STD. In a large obstetrics and gynecology department at the University of Athens, over 10% of adolescents using oral contraceptives were diagnosed with chlamydia; the figure for young women whose partners consistently used condoms was exactly 0% (Creatsas, 1997). Recent data from the Center for Disease Control indicate that when women are encouraged to use latex condoms for HIV/STD prevention, consistent condom use increases significantly, and women who were using birth control pills continued to use them as well (*Morbidity and Mortality Weekly Report,* May 2, 1997). Aggressive educational programs help diminish the incidence of HIV and other STDs when women are counseled regarding the importance of correct, consistent condom usage. Other data paint a less rosy picture, however. Over 500 young women using Depo-Provera in 17 clinics in southeastern Texas were studied for nine months. period. Of those who used condoms before they began Depo-Provera, almost half said that after they began their injections they rarely or never used condoms again. It is not clear, however, how many of these women were in exclusive sexual relationships. Only 18% reported that they used condoms consistently while taking Depo-Provera injections (Sangi-Haghpeykar, Poindexter, & Bateman, 1997), perhaps because these were having intercourse with multiple partners.

Recent data indicate that some women may be especially sensitive or allergic to spermicides, such as nonoxynol-9. In these women the spermicide may irritate the delicate membranes of the vagina and actually *increase* the chances of acquiring an STD. The more spermicide used, and the more concentrated the dose, the greater the chances of this unusual eventuality (d' Oro, Parazzini, Naldi, & Vecchia, 1994), and this is an issue that has recently received much attention in Africa in connection with susceptibility to HIV.

Couples in a long-term, exclusive, monogamous relationship have no need to use a condom if the woman is using oral contraceptives unless she forgets to take one or more pills. But life holds surprises, temptations, and frustrations. A later chapter discusses extramarital affairs, for example. In any case, if a sexual relationship is not exclusive and monogamous, the possibility of contracting an STD always exists, especially if condoms are *not* used. This involves complex issues. It involves relationships, trust, and communication. It is important to use latex condoms lubricated with nonoxynol-9 whenever there is any possibility or risk of contact with a partner one does not know well or who might be suspected of promiscuous sexual behavior. With HIV one also has to be concerned whether a partner was promiscuous 5 or 10 years ago.

METHODS THAT DO NOT WORK VERY WELL

Although a wide variety of effective contraceptives are available to people with different lifestyles and needs, many use ineffective or meaningless approaches to birth control. Typically people use such methods because they are uninformed or misinformed. Inadequate sex education is the most important factor in poor decision making about birth control. Parents often cannot accept that their children are becoming sexual beings and resist and delay talking with them about many sexual issues, especially contraception.

Someone who believes that sexual activity is meant only for procreation and is not planning on having children is also likely unprepared for the eventuality of sexual intercourse. Human beings are not perfect decision makers, however, and despite their convictions and value system, people may find themselves in a sexual situation and behave in a way they had not anticipated. We are all fallible and make mistakes. Abstinence as a form of birth control does not always work very well.

Some believe douching after intercourse can be a form of contraception, but this is highly ineffective and unreliable. Although some douches may have a weak spermicidal effect, fluid introduced into the vagina under pressure will likely propel any sperm deposited there through the cervix and into the uterus, thus actually *increasing* the chances of conception. An earlier chapter discussed the health implications of frequent douching and noted that it may not only increase the chances of conception but also increase the chances of acquiring an STD. Stories are told too about the use of sometimes highly caustic agents being used as douches, such as carbonated beverages and detergent solutions, which can have very negative effects. Such practices are to be strongly discouraged.

Coitus interruptus, or withdrawal, is another highly ineffective attempt at contraception. When a man inserts his erect penis into a woman's vagina and engages in pelvic thrusting, he may be depositing large numbers of sperm there without even knowing it long before ejaculation occurs. Even men who are highly disciplined and frequently practice withdrawal cannot know when fluids are moving through the penis and into their partner. In addition to being ineffective as a contraceptive, coitus interruptus offers no protection against STDs.

Another method that works very well but only when practiced exactly as required is called the lactational amenorrhea method, or LAM for short. If a woman breastfeeds her new baby exclusively, she will not become pregnant for up to 6 months if her menstrual period has not returned. To use LAM as a method of contraception, several conditions must occur. The woman must breastfeed her baby on demand, which often means 6 to 10 times a day and at least once during the night. She must use both breasts. She must be certain that no more than 6 hours has passed since her baby's last feeding. She should be ready to use another contraceptive method if her period returns unexpectedly during this regimen, although according to Hatcher et al. (1998) about 80% of women ovulate before having their first menstrual period after childbirth. For this reason, LAM is generally not considered a highly reliable contraceptive method. When the baby begins to eat other foods or breastfeeds less frequently, LAM is definitely an ineffective form of birth control. Obviously, this technique offers no protection against acquiring an STD. Women sometimes develop sore nipples from frequent breastfeeding and stop rather abruptly, suddenly increasing their chances of becoming pregnant.

CONTRACEPTIVE NEGLIGENCE

Having contraception and using it consistently and properly are sometimes two very different things. The terms "adherence" and "compliance" are used to refer to behaviors that follow medical advice. Most doctors and health care professionals are concerned with how adherent their patients are in taking their medicine and taking care of themselves in other ways. They are also concerned about consistent, correct use of contraceptives. Not everyone using birth control does so *exactly* as they should, and many people are negligent about it. Why? This question has frustrated social and medical scientists for decades. We have already described a double message in society's attitude toward contraceptive use, especially among teens: if you are behaving responsibly about contraception and disease prevention, you are planning to be bad. But **contraceptive negligence** is a more complicated issue and affects many people with troubling consequences. Several investigators have explored this subject (Kanter & Zelnik, 1973; Miller, 1976; Tanfer & Horn, 1985), and their findings are summarized here. Although this topic obviously involves both women and men, most studies have focused on women.

Ambivalence About Becoming Pregnant

Many adolescent females and young women are ambivalent about becoming pregnant. They are not sure that having a baby wouldn't improve their lives. Being a mother seems to bring with it a clear identity, a more organized and routine lifestyle, adult status in some people's eyes, and possibly a spouse too. Many young women believe that having someone to love and take care of will help them grow and develop as well. They may have seen siblings or friends become pregnant and saw that parents, friends, and social services seemed only too ready to help. Although we have been discussing contraception primarily in biological terms, several important psychological and sociological issues affect a person's willingness to learn about birth control and use it correctly.

Social scientists have found four basic characteristics of young women who are ambivalent about using birth control. First, they tend to be passive individuals. They are often easily influenced and do not always have solid personal values on which they act. They can be talked into things. Second, they often have religious conflicts about birth control. Several religions, both Western and Eastern, emphasize sex for procreation and de-emphasize or are critical of sexual expression when conception is not planned. Many of these women feel they don't even need to think about birth control since they are "certain" that it doesn't affect them. Third, some women are very curious about pregnancy and anxious to experience what it's like to carry a human life within them. Finally, women who fear they might be sterile are often ambivalent about using birth control. Vaginal and reproductive system infections leave some women with doubts about whether they will be able to conceive. The popular press frequently publicizes declining fertility rates, the impact of STDs on fertility, and the fact that common STDs have no symptoms. Therefore, many young women who have been sexually active worry about whether they will eventually be able to have babies. In a sense, they are tempting fate to see if they are healthy.

Other Factors Behind Inconsistent Contraceptive Usage

Parents commonly say things like this to their children: "If you ever get pregnant, don't bother coming home again!" Built into statements like this is an escape hatch for youth in an environment of oppressive parental domination or physical or sexual abuse. Adolescents and young adults, therefore, know exactly what to do to get out of an intolerable domestic situation. In a sense, some use sex to remove themselves from what they perceive as a dangerous or unrewarding home. One problem with this approach is that for this person, the relationship with her partner and their willingness or preparedness to be parents is not as important as getting kicked out of the house. In such a case it is difficult to be optimistic about the baby's future or the permanence of the bond between its mother and father.

Another factor that sometimes contributes to a less than careful approach to birth control involves the beginning or ending of relationships. People often feel they don't need birth control "yet" when they are just starting to see someone or "anymore" when they are terminating their relationship. Young people thinking about contraception when they first meet someone and feel attracted to them feel that planning contraception would be like admitting a reckless willingness to do something "bad." They incorrectly believe that not doing

anything about birth control will diminish the chances to have intercourse. We're all human, however, and frequently have problems with delaying immediate gratifications. On the other hand, a person who breaks up with someone often feels bitter and unwilling to even consider getting into another relationship for a long time. So why keep taking birth control pills anymore if life for the foreseeable future won't involve sex? Yet often they form a new relationship much more quickly than expected, often spontaneously, just at this time of not being very careful about birth control.

Another factor is that many doctors and health care professionals have personal biases about the appropriateness of counseling unmarried adolescents and young adults about birth control pills and other means of avoiding conception. Unwittingly, such professionals are saying to their patients, "You're not at a point in your life when that sort of thing is necessary, are you?" The patient, therefore, is unlikely to take time to learn about different forms of contraception or to plan that they really might need birth control now or in the near future. Women who feel they are not receiving the services they want from their doctor should seek a different health professional.

Finally, women and men, married or unmarried, who are less likely to use birth control often share certain characteristics. They often have had less formal education. They are more likely to have a rural residence and/or rural origins. The reasons for this are not quite clear, although many rural areas lack easy access and close proximity to family planning services. They are more likely to lack stable, well-paid employment. Such individuals are also likely to feel rejected by more affluent and powerful segments of society (Table 11-2).

Dear Dr. Ruth

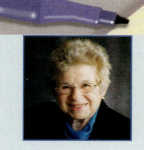

Question:

Sometimes I just don't understand myself. I am 24 years old and a woman. I don't use birth control because I truly don't plan on having sex. But after I've had a little to drink, I get myself into a sexual situation with some guy without any contraception and wind up having intercourse anyway. This has happened to me several times. Why do I keep doing this??

Answer:

There are two issues here. The contraceptive issue is simple to fix. All you have to do is to carry a condom in your purse any time you may be in a situation where this might happen to you. But having casual sex repeatedly is more serious. If you can't break yourself of this habit by yourself, I would definitely advise seeing a therapist. The consequences of your actions could be very serious.

TABLE 11-2

A Summary of Factors Contributing to Contraceptive Negligence Among Young Women and Men

Little Formal Education
A Pattern of Rural Residence and/or Rural Origins
Lack of Consistent, Well-Paid Employment
Feeling Rejected by More Affluent, Powerful Segments of Society

EMERGENCY CONTRACEPTION

The discussion of birth control so far has involved measures taken *before* unprotected intercourse occurs. In recent years, medical, legal, and social discussions about contraception have expanded to include interventions that take place *after* unprotected intercourse. For many reasons, planning ahead is the better alternative, but women should understand their options if they ever want to take contraceptive measures after intercourse. **Emergency contraception** involves ways to reduce the chance of pregnancy after sex. Emergency contraception can be accomplished in different ways, such as by using what the media often calls a "morning after" pill. Many professional organizations, including the American College of Obstetricians and Gynecologists, the Association of Reproductive Health Professionals, the American Medical Association, and the American Medical Women's Association, support the distribution of information about emergency contraception. Their materials provide the information in this section.

There are several circumstances in which emergency contraception may be appropriate. Unintended pregnancies are a huge social problem, affecting at least 3 million women, mostly adolescents or young women, each year in the United States. Emergency contraception is an effective way of reducing the number of unanticipated pregnancies and the abortions performed as a consequence.

There are three primary emergency contraception strategies: emergency contraceptive pills, progestin-only pills, and the insertion of a copper IUD. Emergency contraceptive pills are large doses of regular combination birth control pills. This treatment must be started within 72 hours of unprotected sex. Two elevated doses of these pills are taken 12 hours apart. This therapy has been thoroughly researched, and one's personal physician, gynecologist, or student health center can provide more information. Oral contraceptives containing only progestin are also effective emergency contraceptives, but treatment must be initiated within 48 hours of unprotected intercourse. This alternative may have fewer side effects than combination pills. Finally, a copper IUD inserted within 5 days of unprotected intercourse is also an effective emergency contraceptive. Emergency contraceptive pills are thought to work by inhibiting ovulation or making the endometrium unreceptive to the implantation of a fertilized egg if ovulation and fertilization occur. Another emergency contraceptive pill, RU-486, initially used with high success throughout Europe, has just been approved for distribution in the United States by the Food and Drug Administration.

Available data show that emergency contraceptive pills prevent pregnancy in about 75% of cases of unprotected intercourse. The effectiveness rate may depend on exactly when in a woman's menstrual cycle the unprotected intercourse occurred. No serious side effects or long-term complications have been proven associated with these pills, and there are no health risks associated with using emergency contraceptive pills repeatedly. It is unusual for women to use emergency contraceptive pills repeatedly, however, or as a regular back-up to contraceptive failure or contraceptive negligence. About half of women using emergency contraceptive pills experience nausea and approximately 20% vomit—the only common side effects. Because these pills may interact with other medications (i.e., anti-seizure agents, antibiotics, anticoagulants, and antidepressants), the woman should speak with her physician about these or any other prescription medications she is taking.

In a few situations follow-up counseling might be desirable after using emergency contraceptive pills. Any indications of complications should be discussed with the doctor, such as the menstrual period not starting within three weeks of the beginning of this therapy. Remember that these pills are only a contraceptive and cannot prevent an STD.

PRIVACY ISSUES, CONTRACEPTION, AND GYNECOLOGICAL CARE AND COUNSELING

Birth control issues and choices are private matters for women of any age but particularly raise privacy issues for adolescents. Although here we are primarily discussing teenage and young adult women, many of these issues are relevant to both women and men and a variety of medical problems and circumstances.

Women who are minors frequently feel that they cannot talk with their parents about contraception or make an appointment with a physician to obtain birth control pills. This is one reason it is important to talk about sexual issues in the home, since whether or not young people get contraceptives, eventually most will need them. Oral contraceptives require a doctor's visit, and often young women wonder whether this will be held in confidence, especially if she believes her parents are against her adolescent sexual experimentation. A study by the Alan Guttmacher Institute in the early 1990s revealed that only 12% of the young women in their sample had a medical visit before or in the same month when they had intercourse for the first time. Only 11% made a visit 1 to 3 months after first intercourse, and 5% 4 to 6 months after first intercourse. These data are powerful proof that most young women do not seek contraceptive counseling or contraceptives when they become sexually active. One reason is that they feel they cannot ask a parent to accompany them for such a reason or go by themselves. It is a ticklish matter for a young woman to privately make an appointment to see a physician and pay for the service without her parents' awareness. Clearly this is a significant part of the problem of unintended pregnancies among teens.

Many young people are not aware that their local health departments, community health centers, and Planned Parenthood Offices typically offer excellent medical care and counsel for very reasonable costs. We are not urging young women to go behind their parents' back, but they should know how to take care of themselves when confronted with complex, expensive, and emotional issues involved in becoming sexually active.

Many young women do not know their medical records are confidential. Even when a minor's parents pay for her visit to the doctor, the parents do not have a legal right to find out why she went and what happened in the doctor's office. If a prescription is written for birth control pills, neither the doctor nor the pharmacist can legally tell anyone about the prescription. One's medical records can be obtained by a third party only if the person signs a release making them available to someone else or they are subpoenaed by a court in a legal matter concerning the person's health. In the vast majority of cases, therefore, whatever transpires between a young woman and her doctor remains confidential. According to the Medical Records Privacy Protection Act, revised in 1996, strict practices and procedures afford all patients primary control of their medical information and records.

Confidentiality issues involved in the medical treatment of minors touches on a wide variety of issues, such as suicide prevention, treatment of STDs, and substance abuse (Thompson, 1989). In a survey of 131 family practitioners in Illinois addressing common ethical issues for doctors, the top concern was contraceptive counseling and prescriptions (Dayringer, Paiva, & Davidson, 1983).

Among lawyers, the Mature Minor Doctrine is a common-law rule that permits mature teenagers to give their own consent for medical care even if they have not yet reached the age of majority (Sigman & O'Connor, 1991). The Mature Minor Doctrine says that parental consent is not needed for emergency medical treatment, treatment of STDs, drug treatment, mental health treatment, pregnancy, and contraception. In the early 1980s adolescent civil rights were broadly incorporated into the Mature Minor Doctrine in such a way that the autonomy and well-being of the teenager held primary importance (Silber, 1982). In a large, urban California school district, Schuster, Bell, Petersen, and Kanouse (1996) asked over 2000 high school students whether they had spoken with their doctors about sexual behaviors and various risk prevention issues. The purpose of the study was to determine whether and to what degree teens trusted their doctors with such confidential issues. The results are interesting: 39% reported talking with their doctors about avoiding contracting HIV, 37% said they had discussed using condoms for heterosexual intercourse, 13% asked about the proper way to use a condom, and 8% reported having been given condoms by their doctor. Fully 68% said that they were confident that any discussions they had with their doctor about birth control would be kept confidential, and 44% felt discussions about a pregnancy would be kept confidential.

We believe that it is very important for everyone to assume personal responsibility for their own reproductive health and contraception, although in some cases this may prove difficult, expensive, or possibly embarrassing. Yet local, highly professional alternatives are usually available. The local health department or Planned Parenthood office is usually an excellent resource.

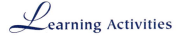

CONCLUSION

Safe, reliable, effective, affordable, and convenient contraception is relatively new in human history, existing for less than 100 years. Ideally, contraception decisions are personal and considered carefully with the participation of one's partner. There is a contraceptive method appropriate for every personality and lifestyle. Yet there is also much misinformation and myth about contraceptives. Many people who know they should be using birth control do not do so reliably. Emergency contraception is a more recent development and is effective in many situations. Everyone is entitled to privacy for contraceptive counseling and birth control.

*L*earning Activities

1. This chapter discusses the effectiveness of latex condoms both as contraceptives and as protection against STDs. Condoms are inexpensive and available and do not require a doctor's visit. Why is there controversy about the appropriateness of television advertising for condoms? In your opinion how could condoms be tastefully marketed on this medium?

2. In many communities, local school boards have decided that the family life curriculum should not include contraception. Speculate how they might have reached this decision despite high rates of teen pregnancy in this country.

3. By far, women in America buy more condoms than men. Suggest some reasons why this is true. Do you think that a man might feel uneasy at his partner's taking charge by purchasing condoms? Some men tell women, "If I wear a condom, I can't feel very much." An appropriate female reply could be, "If you don't, you won't feel *anything at all*." Comment.

4. In the past, involuntary sterilization was performed on mentally retarded adolescents and young adults in the hope that this would eliminate genetically transmitted retardation. Because this deprived people of their constitutional freedoms, it is no longer practiced. Try to describe the social justification for a systematic practice of involuntary sterilization. Could you foresee a situation in which such measures would be appropriate?

5. This chapter uses the phrase "contraceptive counseling," especially in reference to the doctor-patient relationship. Cassata (1982) summarized what is known about doctor-patient communication generally. Following are some things to consider when a person talks to a health care professional about choosing and using a method of birth control.

   a. Patients forget much of what the doctor tells them.
   b. Instructions and advice are more likely to be forgotten than other information.
   c. The more the patient is told in a short period of time, the greater the proportion he or she will forget.
   d. Patients will remember: (a) what they are told first and (b) what they consider most important.
   e. Intelligent patients do not remember more than less intelligent patients.
   f. Older patients remember just as much as younger ones.
   g. Moderately anxious patients recall more of what they are told than highly anxious patients or patients who are not anxious (Cassata, 1982).

   Considering this information, describe an effective message for a teenager or young adult seeking contraception counseling and birth control from their family doctor or gynecologist.

6. In 1991 Darlene Johnson, at the time 27 years old, was convicted of beating two of her five children. She was married and pregnant at the time. Judge Howard Broadman of Tulare County in California offered her probation instead of prison if she agreed to have Norplant implanted. She refused. In your opinion, was the judge's offer legally and ethically appropriate? Why or why not?

7. In some areas, high school and college clinics make condoms available to students at low or no cost. What is your opinion of this practice? Describe the advantages and disadvantages of this practice.

8. Virtually every society in the world has more, and more diversified, contraceptive methods for women than for men. Do you think this emphasis is justified? Why or why not?

- Many young adults perceive a double message from society about contraception. On the one hand, they are taught to be foresightful and take responsibility for their own behavior, but on the other, buying contraceptives apparently means that they are planning to be "bad."
- Contraceptive negligence is more likely among individuals who, for one of a variety of reasons, are ambivalent about becoming pregnant or may actually want to become pregnant to remove themselves from troubling life circumstances, such as a hostile, abusive home environment.
- Abstinence is refraining from sexual intercourse and any and all sexual behavior in which semen might come into the proximity of a woman's external or internal genitals.
- The Mature Minor Doctrine permits a mature teenager to give his or her own consent for medical care even if they have not yet reached the age of majority.

Glossary Terms

abortifacients	fertility
abstinence	intrauterine device (IUD)
bilateral tubal ligation	Margaret Sanger
birth control	Mature Minor Doctrine
cervical cap	nonoxynol-9
coitus interruptus	Norplant
condoms	oral contraceptives (birth control pills)
contraceptive negligence	
contraceptive	pessary
contragestational agents	prostaglandins
Depo-Provera	sexually transmitted diseases
diaphragm	
double message	spermicidal foams, creams, gels, suppositories
emergency contraception	
fecundity	vaginal sponge
female condom	vasectomy

Key Concepts

- Fertility is a person's reproductive performance, involving the number of live births they have had or contributed to.
- A person's maximum biological potential to procreate is their fecundity.
- Any device or behavioral strategy that minimizes or eliminates the chances of conception following sexual intercourse is a contraceptive, often referred to as birth control.
- There is an appropriate method of birth control for every lifestyle and personality.

Suggested Readings

Day, N. (1995). Abortion: Debating the issue. Springfield, NJ: Enslow.

DePuy, C., & Dovitch, D. (1997). The healing choice: Your guide to emotional recovery after an abortion. New York: Simon & Schuster.

Drife, J. O. (1997). The benefits and risks of oral contraceptives today. New York: Parthenon Publishing Group.

Hartmann, B. (1995). Reproductive rights and wrongs: The global politics of population control. Boston, MA: South End Press.

Juhn, G. (1994). Understanding the pill: A consumer's guide to oral contraceptives. Binghamton, NY: Haworth Press.

Riddle, J. M. (1997). Eve's herbs: A history of contraception and abortion in the west. Cambridge, MA: Harvard University Press.

World Health Organization. (1987). Barrier contraceptives and spermicides: Their role in family planning care. Geneva, Switzerland.

12

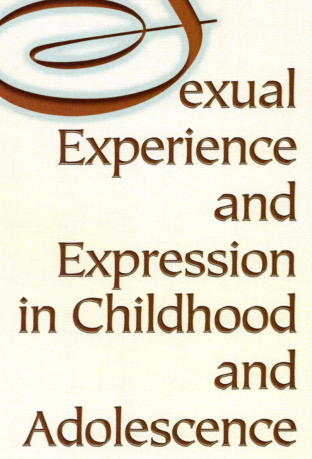

Sexual Experience and Expression in Childhood and Adolescence

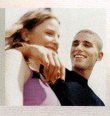

OBJECTIVES

When you finish reading and reviewing this chapter, you should be able to:

1. Describe the underlying assumptions of the psychoanalytic, psychosocial, and social-learning theories of human growth and development.

2. Explain the five basic concepts of Freud's psychosexual theory of development.

3. Describe the five stages of Freud's psychosexual theory of development, noting the relevant erogenous zone in each.

4. Describe the eight stages of development of Erikson's psychosocial theory of development, noting the positive and negative outcomes of each.

5. Summarize the basic principles of social learning theory and explain the importance of vicarious learning and feelings of self-efficacy in growth and development.

6. Discuss the difference between identification and complementation in the sexual development of girls and boys.

7. Analyze and discuss the long-term effects of childhood sexual experiences on later development during adolescence and adulthood.

8. Explain the relationship between exposure to effective sex education in childhood and later sexual behavior.

9. Explain four important socialization tasks and note their relationship to sexual development and expression during adolescence.

10. Explain the endocrine and physiological factors that precipitate puberty in females and males, and describe secondary sexual characteristics that appear.

11. Review reasons adolescents use or do not use contraceptives consistently.

12. Describe the decline in the double standard among teenagers in the United States.

13. Summarize the stresses of acknowledging one's homosexuality during adolescence.

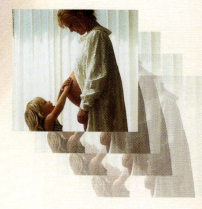

From Dr. Ruth

When I tell people that we now know that a male fetus in the mother's womb can have an erection and that a female newborn can lubricate vaginally and show signs of clitoral erection, the usual reaction is surprise. We don't think of a fetus, infant, or child as having a sexual side because they're not fully developed sexually. But in fact they are sexual beings, and if babies didn't wear diapers most of the time the signs would be more apparent.

I don't bring up this subject to shock people, but I want people to see that sexuality is a natural and important part of every individual—starting with infancy and maturing through childhood and adolescence. No one should feel guilty about having sexual feelings, since our sexuality is innate and a baby experiencing sexual sensations couldn't be more innocent. Although that fact does not give us permission to have sex whenever and with whoever we want, the feelings our innate sexuality engenders should not be a source of shame or embarrassment. Instead, we should seek to understand our sexuality throughout the life span, beginning with early childhood and adolescence, so that we can be fulfilled in all our human dimensions and avoid the problems that can become associated with sexuality at various ages.

We are all sexual beings from birth to death. This is not to say that we all have sexual intercourse throughout our adult lives, or that we all masturbate in childhood and later, or that we are preoccupied with eroticism and sensuality during every waking moment. However, from earliest infancy we are very aware of physical pleasures and that our bodies are highly sensitive to various tactile stimuli that we enjoy and want to experience repeatedly. This chapter will explore the experience and expression of sexuality as we mature through infancy, childhood, and adolescence. Maturation refers primarily to biological ways we change as we get older, and experience refers more to social influences.

People are sometimes baffled by discussing the sexuality of infants and children. Certain areas of our bodies are keenly responsive to touch, however, and these primitive pleasures are the foundation of what later takes on sexual and erotic meaning. Our personal sexuality develops over time, and this chapter will discuss various factors that influence that development. We begin with several psychological and sociological theories that describe the role of sexuality in human growth and development. These theories offer us valid and useful perspectives for interpreting sexual development. These theories also provide the broader context in which research is conducted on child and adolescent sexuality. We will examine the role of pleasure and pleasurable stimuli as powerful, ever-present motivators in sexual experience and expression.

The emergence of sexuality in childhood is generally easily observed and understood, although many parents are uneasy about acknowledging this aspect of their child's growth and development. Childhood is that period extending from about age 2 to about age 12, although many individual differences in development occur. Childhood ends when puberty begins, which occurs at different times for different people. In early childhood, youngsters begin to show interest in or may be overtly curious about anatomical differences between females and males, and they start asking questions. Once children enter school they often become less interested in sexual and gender issues, although their psychological and social development certainly continues. How children learn about sex in their families is important, as are the benefits of good sex education. Although this chapter is not intended as a practical guide for parents talking with children about sex, that topic is explored briefly.

Because the emergence of sexuality in adolescence is a large, rich topic, most of the chapter is devoted to the issues involved. During these years the relationship between self-esteem and body-image becomes especially important. This takes place along with developing socialization skills and the onset of puberty and the appearance of secondary sexual characteristics. While all of this is going on, adolescents are exploring masturbatory behaviors and various shared sexual experiences. While this is happening, teens are also often learning about sex in other places, such as their peer group, the home, family life education courses, and sometimes church-based sex education courses.

A major challenge for adolescents involves learning to behave responsibly in sexual expression, and learning about contraception is an important dimension. We will look at the consequences of teen pregnancy for these young women, their partners, their families, their communities, and society in general. We will also examine another aspect of responsible sexual behavior, avoiding sexually transmitted diseases, and the consequences of delayed diagnosis and treatment of these disorders.

Finally, we will discuss adolescents who face additional challenges as they come to acknowledge bisexuality or homosexuality. Most teenagers want to be liked and be similar to their friends. Because most teens are heterosexual, those with an alternative sexual orientation have difficulty being honest with themselves and their acquaintances and, therefore, often feel alienated. We will examine the pressures and stresses on these teens and the adjustment they ultimately make either coming out or staying in the closet.

Several important theories usefully describe human growth and development. Fairly predictable changes occur in sexual development during childhood and adolescence that can be understood within the context of developmental theory. These theories help explain normal and sometimes unusual aspects of sexual development. Three differing views are presented here: the psychoanalytic approach, the psychosocial approach, and social-learning theory. These three have guided research for decades.

THEORETICAL APPROACHES TO DEVELOPMENT

Underlying Assumptions

Psychoanalytic theory, or psychodynamic theory, is a Freudian approach to human growth and development. Freud believed that our adult thoughts, feelings, and actions are powerfully determined by subconscious forces of which we are unaware or have only a dim awareness. The term "psychoanalytic" refers to three different things: a theory of personality, a theory of development, and a method of psychotherapy. Freud was honest when he told his patients that psychoanalysis would probably not help them feel any better but that they would better understand why they were miserable! Freud believed that the basis for our personalities and sexuality is firmly established by age six, and after that it is extremely difficult to change ourselves in any meaningful way. This is not a very optimistic approach to human growth and development. Freud's theory emphasizes innate, biological drives and the pleasures we derive when they are satisfied or the frustrations we experience when they are not.

In contrast, the **psychosocial theory** emphasizes the impact of the social environment on human growth and development. The best known proponent of this approach was Erik Erikson, who felt lifespan development occurred as we confront challenges as we get older. How we resolve or fail to resolve these challenges at one point may or may not affect how we handle later ones. But unlike Freud, Erikson deemphasized the role of sexuality in development and believed that people can change, for the better or worse, whenever motivated to do so.

The third theoretical approach is **social-learning theory,** which is in a way an extension of the psychosocial perspective. Albert Bandura is the best known proponent of this theory. He believes that the rewarding or punishing consequences of behaviors shape one's development. However, he also believes that people can grow, change, and improve by observing the consequences of other people's behavior. Although we are obviously affected by the outcomes of our own actions, we can learn and change by watching what happens to others.

These are the basic assumptions of these three theories. Now we will examine each theory in detail.

The Psychoanalytic Approach

Sigmund Freud (1856–1939) is frequently misinterpreted, and people often have an opinion about him without every having read any of his original works. Yet Freud was a lucid and entertaining writer. He was among the first explorers of the mind to demonstrate and document that infant and childhood experiences can profoundly affect adult thoughts, feelings, and actions. His psychoanalytic theories deal with the development of emotional states and the impact of those states on adult functioning. Let's look first at basic issues that run through most of Freud's work (Table 12-1).

TABLE 12-1

Five Key Freudian Concepts

Determinism	The belief that *ALL* adult thoughts, feelings, and behaviors have their roots in childhood experiences before the age of 6 years. They cannot be substantively changed after that time. In essence, this is a denial of free will.
Libido	A basic, primitive motivational force in the personality. Its manifestations typically center around the expression of sexuality and aggression.
Erogenous Zones	During infantile and childhood development there are areas on the surface of the body that, when stimulated, yield keen sensual pleasure. These include the mouth, anus, and genitalia. Children desire complete and consistent stimulation of their erogenous zones.
Fixation	If, in the course of normal growth and development, a child's erogenous zones are *not* completely and consistently stimulated, later in life that individual will try to compensate for this lack or inconsistency of erogenous zone stimulation.
Sex	While we commonly associate the term "sexuality" with "genitality," Freud was not so ready to do so. Instead, Freud used the word "sexuality" in pretty much the same way we today use the word "sensuality." He used this word to refer to good and powerful feelings which come from various areas (erogenous zones) on the surface of the body.

Determinism. Through his psychotherapeutic experiences, Freud concluded that adult thoughts, feelings, and behaviors are completely determined by infant and childhood frustrations and overindulgences. The personality is fully formed by age 6, after which no real changes can take place. If all that we think, feel, and do is determined, we have no real free will as adults. What went before determines the here and now, as well as the future.

Sexuality. Freud used the word "sexuality" somewhat differently from its contemporary meaning. We consider the feelings we derive through stimulation of our genitals as sexual. Freud did as well, but he also included what we would call "sensuality." In other words, good feelings that come from our genitals and other areas of our bodies have sexual meaning. Freud's critics often fail to appreciate his use of the term sexuality.

Libido. Freud coined this term to refer to a basic, primitive motivational force in our personalities leading to sexual and aggressive inclinations and behaviors. The term is often used today to refer to a generalized "sex drive," but for Freud its meaning is more diverse. Libido is focused in different body areas as we grow through infancy and childhood and into adolescence.

Erogenous Zones. These are the areas in which libido is invested as we grow up. We earlier distinguished between primary and secondary erogenous zones. We all have the same primary erogenous zones: mouth, anus, and genitalia. Our secondary erogenous zones develop through our personal sexual and sensual experiences and may differ from person to person. As infants, children, and adolescents develop, they have one main primary erogenous zone at a time.

Fixation. Freud believed that infants and children are powerfully motivated to seek complete and consistent stimulation of their primary erogenous zones. This, of course, is impossible. No baby, no matter how pampered or indulged, can enjoy this constant stimulation. All infants and children must necessarily deal with incomplete and inconsistent stimulation of their erogenous zones. Freud thought that later in life people try to make up for past inadequate erogenous zone stimulation or to re-create excessive stimulation. For example, a baby who received inadequate and inconsistent nursing or bottle feeding might when grown up try to make up for this and develop eating habits leading to obesity. According to Freud we may become fixated at one stage of psychosexual development.

Freud's Psychosexual Theory of Development

This theory is highly deterministic, focusing on innate drives and tendencies, and based on the biological pleasures derived from physical stimulation of the erogenous zones. Freud formulated this theory from therapy sessions with adults suffering various psychological problems, most of which today would be classified as anxiety disorders. His work was controversial in part because he emphasized sensual and sexual pleasure in the highly proper and repressed Victorian era. This was a time when attributing erotic or sensual inclinations to infants and children was considered almost criminal. Freud said that much

of an infant's or child's behavior is motivated by the pleasure principle, an unrestricted desire to pursue keenly enjoyable feelings. Infants and young children do not understand which pleasures society considers appropriate; they just want pleasure. Reaching that understanding is a common developmental task in all cultures. According to Freud, the pleasures one seeks change as one develops through different stages (Table 12-2).

The Oral Stage. This stage lasts from birth until about 1 year of age. The mouth is the primary erogenous zone; in Freudian terms it is heavily invested with libido at this time. Oral pleasures and stimulation are highly sensual for the baby. Infants explore their world by trying to put many things into their mouths. This theory sees nursing as a keenly sensual or erotic experience.

The Anal Stage. Between the ages of 1 and 3, a child's anus is the primary erogenous zone. Retaining or expelling feces is highly pleasurable, even sensual. Children are toilet trained during this stage and often manipulate their parents and caretakers by appropriately or inappropriately learning when and where to urinate and have bowel movements. Some parents are tough, coercive, and inflexible about this process, while others take a more relaxed, flexible approach. Freud believed that different personality types emerge because of different parental styles of toilet training.

The Phallic Stage. From about ages 3 to 6 libido is focused for the first time in the child's genitalia. Freud described different developmental paths for boys and girls. Boys begin to

TABLE 12-2

Freud's Psychosexual Theory of Development

Stage	Ages	Characteristics
Oral	Birth–1 year	Libido is invested in the mouth, making oral stimulation (sucking) a sexual experience. Enhances maternal attachment.
Anal	1–3 years	Libido is invested in the anus. Expelling and retaining feces yields sexual pleasure. Conflict between physical urges and demands for social conformity.
Phallic	3–6 years	Libido is now invested in the genitals. Subconscious desire to consummate a sexual relationship with the opposite sex parent. Fear of reprisal causes identification with same sex parent and learning of sex roles.
Latency	6–12 years	No erogenous zones. Libido directed into socially appropriate activities.
Genital	12 years and older	Libido is again invested in the genitals. Desire to consummate a sexual relationship with a member of the opposite sex.

discover erotic pleasures through genital self-stimulation, or masturbatory behaviors. Freud suggested that a boy at this age has unconscious fantasies of a sexual relationship with his mother and sees his father as a rival for his mother's affections. He comes to fear his father, believing that his penis will be removed, which Freud called castration anxiety. The boy resolves this anxiety by identifying with his father. Identification is a subconscious desire to become like someone whom one loves or admires. By trying to become more like his father, he also seeks to be the central focus of his mother's affections. Freud believed that this identification process is extremely important for how children learn their sex roles. Freud called this process the **Oedipal complex,** named after the Greek play in which Oedipus unknowingly kills his father and marries his mother. As males learn socially accepted sex roles and develop heterosexual interests, they effectively resolve their Oedipal complex.

Instead of the Oedipal complex, girls go through the **Electra complex,** named after another Greek figure who helped murder her mother. In Freud's theory, when girls realize that they are different from little boys because they lack a penis, they desire one; this is called penis envy. Because of this perceived inadequacy, the girl is subconsciously motivated to seek a sexual relationship with her father and to become the sole focus of his intimate attentions. Freud believed females had less opportunity to successfully resolve this conflict and felt that women are, therefore, less psychologically mature than men.

Stories about men who never marry but remain totally devoted to their mothers throughout their adult lives and men who want to find a woman just like their mother, or women who want to marry men just like their fathers, are often interpreted in terms of a Freudian unresolved Oedipal or Electra complex. Heterosexual preferences are one outcome of the successful resolution of these complexes.

The Latency Period. Freud believed that after the age of 6, one's psychosexual development is mostly complete and the foundations of later erotic inclinations or fixations have been laid. Between the age of 6 and the onset of puberty there is little sexual development; he called this the latency period.

Freud may have been mistaken that there is little happening in children in this stage. Although sex and eroticism might not be on their minds, they show sensitivity to a number of sexual issues. For example, this is a time of active sexual curiosity when many children begin to play a game of "You show me yours, and I'll show you mine." During this stage many children actively or distractedly engage in genital self-stimulation. A common feature of the latency stage, however, is a psychological repression of erotic interest in members of the opposite sex, a time of what is called homosocial friendships. Girls and boys at this age generally create and maintain same-sex friendships and cliques and typically decline the chance to play with kids of the opposite sex.

The Genital Stage. Freud believed that at the onset of puberty, libido is again invested in the genitalia, and erotic stimulation begins to take on a more adult dimension. The genitalia are again the primary erogenous zone. He thought that to become psychologically an adult, a person must be in-

clined to initiate and maintain a heterosexual relationship culminating in sexual intercourse.

■ ■ ■

Although few now believe everything Freud wrote about sexual development, he was undeniably an important, and for a very long time lonely, pioneer in examining the relationship between early sensual experiences and later sexual adjustment and behavior.

Erikson's Psychosocial Theory of Development

Erik Erikson (1902–1994) studied with Freud but gradually came to disagree with him about the importance of sensual pleasure in psychological development. He believed that Freud's theory was too biological and deterministic and that it de-emphasized the importance of the social context in which psychological development occurs. His own view (**Erikson's Psychosocial Theory of Development**) was that human growth and development depended largely on the relationship between unfolding innate behaviors and how the wider social environment responded to the individual because of those behaviors. Erikson suggested that people develop through eight different stages between birth and death; the first five are described here, and the remaining three stages in the next chapter. Erikson was among the first to suggest that psychological development is a lifelong process. As long as we live we can grow, change, and improve. He also emphasized anticipatory development: someone who knows something about the major developmental challenges ahead can prepare for them and not be as challenged by such changes in one's life. Following are the first five stages, in which sensual, sexual, and intimate awareness and development also take place (Table 12-3).

Basic Trust Versus Mistrust. This stage begins at birth and lasts until the age of 1. An infant whose discomforts are anticipated and/or promptly removed, who is cuddled and played with, and who is cared for well begins to learn that the world is a safe place and others can be trusted. If, in contrast, the baby's discomforts are not anticipated or allowed to persist, if the infant is ignored or treated in an aloof way, if parental involvement is inadequate or inconsistent, then the baby gets an entirely different message: the world is not a safe or supportive place.

Autonomy Versus Shame and Doubt. From 1 to 3 years of age, infants and toddlers learn more about the consequences of their behaviors. When children are told or shown that they can be competent and self-sufficient in their play activities, feeding behaviors, toilet training, and interactions with others, they get the important message: "You can handle this on your own." However, if caretakers are overprotective of the child, do for it what it can do for itself, or belittle its early attempts at independence, the child then gets an entirely different message: "You can't do anything on your own but need other people's help to get things done."

Poor outcomes at one stage do not necessarily predict poor developmental outcomes in the next stage, nor do suc-

TABLE 12-3

Erik Erikson's Eight Stages of Psychosocial Development

Psychosocial Stage	Approximate Ages	Developmental Tasks
Basic Trust vs. Mistrust	Birth–1 year	Coming to understand that the world is a safe, rewarding, attentive, nurturant place with predictable rewards and pleasures.
Autonomy vs. Doubt	1–3 years	The child can now make choices and decisions; she or he is an independent person. Overly restrictive parents can hinder this.
Initiative vs. Guilt	3–6 years	The child first manifests ambition and social responsibility. Learning about future roles and larger social institutions.
Industry vs. Inferiority	6–12 years	Develops a capacity for productive work, pride in one's efforts, cooperation, and finishing the tasks one begins at home and in school.
Identity vs. Identity Confusion	Adolescence	Develops a cohesive sense of self. Understands need for conformity and desire for independence all at the same time.
Intimacy vs. Isolation	Young adulthood	Develops the ability to love and work without losing one's self in either domain. Will not change the self just to please others.
Generativity vs. Stagnation	Adulthood	Desires to leave the world a better place than she or he found it. Make important family and social contributions a symbol of one's life.
Integrity vs. Despair	Old age	To look back over one's life and be able to say that one has always done the best they could with resources available when they had to.

cessful developmental outcomes at one stage necessarily predict successful developmental outcomes in the next stage. Babies who are mistrustful at age 1 may become highly autonomous and independent by age 3.

Initiative Versus Guilt. Between the ages of 3 and 6 years, children play in ways that show they are learning about the roles and occupations of their society. This is a time when children talk about what they're going to do when they grow up. How parents and caretakers respond to them is very important, because they give the child one of two different messages: either "You can do it!" or "Don't bother trying because that's for someone who's better than you." The first message instills in children a sense of initiative or ambition, but the second leads to feeling blameworthy and inadequate.

Industry Versus Inferiority. At about the same time Freud said children were going through the latency stage, Erikson saw them confronting a different developmental challenge. He believed that between the ages of 6 and 11, children are learning to develop skills and competencies, to take pride in their efforts, and perhaps most importantly, to finish what they start. Feelings of having abilities and skills become more important at this time, and a sense of self-sufficiency begins to emerge. Children who do not feel especially good at anything or who are frequently criticized, however, come to feel inadequate and inferior to others. The distinction between industry and inferiority includes both manual and intellectual abilities. Again, the delicate interplay between the child's talents and a supportive or punitive social environment is important in Erikson's theory.

Identity Versus Role Confusion. When children reach adolescence, they become preoccupied with a new psychological challenge, the question "Who am I?" This is the first time the issue of identity emerges, and it is frequently accompanied by other hard questions, such as "Why am I here?", "What is my purpose in life?", and "What is the meaning of life?" Desperate as a young person might be to find unambiguous answers to these difficult, existential questions, none are likely to emerge at this tender age.

In this stage, teenagers also often deal with a conflict between being asked to be dependent and wanting to be independent. This conflict can make things very difficult at home. This is also often the first time a person is asked to change some aspect of themselves so that they will be loved, liked, or cared for, and this can be a difficult challenge. In addition to all these issues, sexual identity also becomes a preoccupation at this time. Issues of sexual orientation, sexual self-confidence, and early feelings of love and intimacy are a big part of adolescents' growth and development during this stage.

■ ■ ■

Erikson's theory overall is highly optimistic. When unhappy or traumatic events occur at one time during development, individuals always have the opportunity to put the past behind them. This nondeterministic approach emphasizes self-determination throughout the lifespan, a clear departure from the Freudian perspective. Additionally, gender identity and sexual awareness are important in the stage dealing with identity versus role confusion, an issue that continues into young adulthood and middle adulthood. Anthropologists who examine lifespan development in other cultures typically find that Erikson's theory highly predicts life changes over time in a variety of world cultures. As well, an analysis of the biographies of well-known public figures generally supports this general view of the lifespan. As we grow and refine our sense of ourselves as sexual beings, the challenges Erikson outlined are important in guiding our social and intimate interactions with others.

Social Learning Theory

The last theory we will examine in relation to sexual development in childhood and adolescence is *social learning theory*. Just as the psychosocial approach is an extension of the psychoanalytic model, this theoretical perspective is a refinement of the psychosocial model. While all specialists in growth and development attest to the importance of rewarding and punishing consequences of behaviors, social learning theorists believe that we also learn by watching others and noting the consequences they experience because of their actions. We learn vicariously through observations of others. Presumably, we are wondering and thinking about what they must be thinking and feeling as we watch them. An important figure in social learning theory is Albert Bandura, who advanced the concept called modeling, in which one purposefully tries to behave like someone else. We do this because we have seen others behaving and enjoying positive or pleasurable consequences of their actions and we would like to experience the same. Whereas modeling is a deliberate process, we also sometimes unconsciously try to be like someone else. This is called **identification,** defined earlier.

But of course, we don't model every behavior that seems rewarding to others. People are more likely to model another person's actions if they feel inexperienced or unsure of themselves and observe positive behavior by someone practiced, confident, and competent or like themselves. Bandura (1977) emphasized that much cognitive processing is involved in modeling one's actions after someone else's. For example, one must be interested in observing another person in the first place, must remember their behavior and review it periodically, and at some time in the future recall their actions to use them as a guide for one's own behaviors.

Bandura described the importance of self-efficacy, our feelings of competence and control in our lives. Social and behavioral scientists have suggested that social learning theory is very important for how we learn sex roles in our society, modeling our actions after competent same-sex parents and other role models. This process is usually well underway by late childhood. Although this theoretical approach de-emphasizes biological, deterministic, and nativistic factors, this is not a major shortcoming. Social learning theory emphasizes the family and peer group, as well as other well-known figures with whom youth identify. This approach helps explain how we learn to behave as women and men in our society. A later chapter examines in more detail how explicit sexual modeling, such as watching an X-rated video, can influence sexual behaviors and one's idea of acceptable and enjoyable intimate interactions.

Theories of Development in Perspective

These three categories of developmental theories are the most useful for explaining how behaviors change over time as a result of maturation and experience. None of them is necessarily better than another, and each is well-suited for explaining different developmental events throughout infancy, childhood, and adolescence. They describe the biological, interpersonal, and social backdrop against which sexual development takes place and a context for understanding the physical and social rewards associated with erotic feelings early in life.

These three models also complement one another. While Freud's theory deals with the pleasure principle and apparently primitive drives to enjoy good feelings and avoid anxiety, Erikson has a broader perspective concerning the ways in which these elementary, biological, and nativistic concepts fit into a child's or adolescent's relationships with others. Still more broad is social learning theory, emphasizing the impact of other's behaviors, including the behaviors of those whom we do not know.

Another common thread runs through these three seemingly very different views of human growth and development: the strong desire of humans to experience good feelings and pleasures and to minimize experiences of bad feelings and punishments. This desire for pleasure has powerful and persistent motivational qualities, and these theories remind us that many of our behaviors, significant or trivial, are organized around the pursuit of positive emotional experiences and the avoidance of punishing or painful ones. The power of sensual pleasure is very straightforward in Freud's theory: stimulation of our erogenous zones feels good and we do everything we can to make it happen. Incomplete or inconsistent stimulation of erogenous zones is perceived as unpleasant. In Erikson's theory, good feelings or pleasures derive more from positive psychological and social interactions with others, especially parents and caretakers. Feeling good about ourselves and our abilities and being validated for good achievement are extremely important in early and middle childhood. Good sexual self-esteem later in life is clearly related to feeling good about ourselves, being able to trust others, and feeling confirmed by those to whom we feel attracted. Additional ways of thinking about pleasure derive from social learning theory. We come to feel in control of our lives because we pay attention to the consequences of our own actions, as well as the outcomes of other people's behaviors. Modeling our behavior after those whom we love or admire plays a powerful role in building self-esteem, and we find pleasure in ourselves for doing this. The concept of pleasure, broadly or narrowly defined, is one of the common denominators of these three influential perspectives on human and sexual growth and development.

SEXUAL FEELING AND EXPERIENCE IN INFANCY

Infancy lasts until about age 2, roughly until the baby can walk and begin to use language meaningfully. Until language abilities are well developed, we have only indirect ways of learning about a child's thoughts or feelings regarding genital stimulation and the erotic feelings that may or may not result. We must make inferences about their thoughts and feelings based on observable, measurable physical changes that accompany any stimulation that adults might call "sexual."

Infancy as a Time of Innocence

Freud's view departed from the longstanding social views originating with the French philosopher Jean Jacques Rousseau (1712–1778), who believed that infants are not infinitely manipulable and trainable by their parents but instead are inherently good, "noble savages," endowed by God with an instinctive sense of right and wrong and an inborn tendency to grow in an orderly, predetermined way. Rousseau believed that this instinctive moral demeanor could be, and frequently was, undermined by harsh, repressive interactions with parents. Left alone, he argued, children will develop an ethical, moral, pure outlook on life. Freud's "modern" outlook clashed dramatically with this older tradition and was hard for scholars and clinicians to accept. Even more important, while Rousseau saw children as the active creators of their own futures, Freud instead saw children as profoundly affected by every experience. While Rousseau's view of maturation was optimistic and benign, Freud saw psychosexual development as fraught with inevitable problems. Freud's theory seemed an assault on the "babe in arms" view of infancy and childhood, and the critics of his day were unwilling to recognize the importance of the pleasure principle even in infants and children.

Sexuality as a "Natural Function"

As discussed elsewhere, people often do not consider human sexuality a natural physiological function but instead associate sexuality entirely with erotic or titillating stimuli and contexts. The broad view of sexuality considers not only the obvious biological aspects of sexual development but its psychosocial dimension as well. As noted earlier, boy babies often have erections at birth or in the first day or two, and girl babies are often born lubricating vaginally or do so in the first few days of life. Further, when their diapers are removed, both male and female babies often reach for their genitalia and touch, rub, or caress them. This self-stimulation has a casual, unfocused quality. Genital touching is obviously pleasurable, and babies promptly learn to touch themselves when their diapers are removed and while being bathed. These early experiences do not involve coordinated, rhythmic pressing or rubbing, but only uncoordinated grasping or rubbing. Because adults have had different experiences with genital self-stimulation, they often attribute feelings and motives to infants that they are unlikely to have, and these misattributions should be avoided whenever possible.

In addition to genital self-stimulation, infants frequently engage in pelvic thrusting movements simultaneously and have been observed to have "spasms" that look like adult orgasms. These behaviors have long been of interest to pediatricians and child psychologists. Fleisher and Morrison (1990) studied five girls between the ages of 7 and 27 months of age who engaged in "masturbatory posturing" while rubbing their pubic area on a parent's knee or a firm object while lying on their sides. This experience involved an irregular breathing pattern, flushing of the skin on their faces, and obvious perspiration. While some episodes lasted only a minute or so, others went on for a few hours. The parents of these infants were alarmed and perplexed by these behaviors, which medical tests showed did not result from abdominal discomfort or seizures but were plainly autoerotic. In another study, Bye and Nunan (1992) used recordings of brain wave activity and videotapes to demonstrate that such behaviors are not seizures but may in fact result from self-stimulation activities. Other researchers (Wulff, Ostergaard, & Storm, 1992) reported moaning, grunting, and facial flushing in two babies, 5 and 6 months old. Again epileptic seizures were first suspected as the cause, but these responses also were again associated with infant masturbatory behaviors. In none of these reported cases were penile or vaginal emissions noted.

Obviously new parents might be somewhat alarmed seeing their baby behave in these ways, but the parent or caretaker's responses to this behavior could be very important. It would be unwise to roughly jerk the baby's hands away from its genitals or slap them. Care should be taken to avoid creating an association between pleasurable genital sensations and discomfort; such associations can be extremely persistent and might affect a child's or adolescent's interpretations of sensual or sexual pleasure many years later. From the perspective of social learning theory, infants are not too young to establish an association between genital stimulation and pain; this is simply an example of classical conditioning.

With infants Freud was probably right: the pleasure principle determines many of the baby's early experiments with self-stimulation and may entirely govern the experience of sensuality in this stage. Parents have difficulty accepting such behaviors in children and often need to remember that infants are nonverbal, emotional, egocentric beings who have not yet learned society's notions of right and wrong. In this sense babies truly are "innocent."

SEXUAL EXPERIENCE AND EXPRESSION IN CHILDHOOD

New mothers and fathers often enthusiastically describe and compare their children's motor development, interested in whose baby stands first or walks first. This is true of personality, social, and motor development. Parents are proud of their child when he or she learns to ride a bicycle without training wheels. Parents eagerly describe how their kids learn language and use words in interesting ways. The same is true of children's cognitive development and how they begin to think and engage in problem-solving behaviors. But rarely is there spoken a word, question, or observation about sexual development in childhood. Many parents simply deny the development of their children as sexual beings. Nonetheless, parents impart some of their own sexual value system in subtle but significant ways. As discussed in an earlier chapter, one's sexual value system is the sum of everything with an erotic meaning for a person. Parents play a large formative role in the development of their children's early sexual value system. Chapter 3 described how a child's earliest conceptions of sex, gender, and gender roles derive from close interactions with a parent or caretaker. The issue here involves the child's early sexual behaviors and experimentation. An earlier chapter also describes scripts, which in this context are patterns of thinking about how males and females are supposed to behave or think appropriately about sex. While people derive many scripts from their parents, society powerfully reinforces some scripts while overtly ignoring others. Our sexual scripts involve our emotional responses to sexual stimuli, and these are subtly incorporated into our sexual value systems. Think of scripts as quiet, internal instructions to help us interpret and act on certain facets of our environment.

Fisher (1988) described a personality dimension related to sexual scripts. Children who gradually develop a sense of pleasure and interest in sexual feelings and behavior demonstrate erotophilia. This is a spontaneous, uncensored delight in erotic stimuli and perceptions. It is innate and early in life is uninfluenced by social notions of what is supposed to be proper or appropriate. Erotophilia is similar to Freud's pleasure principle. When parents and caretakers are punitive, rough, and coercive in response to the child's sexual experimentation, erotophobia may then emerge as a prominent personality feature. Overt fears and subtle anxieties become associated with matters having a sexual connotation. Erotophobic children grow up to have a restricted and nervous approach to almost anything with a sexual meaning. For example, they are less inclined to try to avoid unanticipated pregnancy and do not feel comfortable buying condoms. They might even be hesitant to take a college course in human sexuality. Erotophobic individuals generally have difficulty dealing with their own child when it comes to teaching basic information about sex.

All too often, childhood sexual experiences are written about in ways that suggest their traumatic, involuntary nature and long-term terrible consequences. Less is known about children's normal sexual curiosity and experimentation. Here we will examine what is common and normal among children between the ages of 2 and about 12, or the beginning of puberty. At this time, the earliest manifestations of erotophilia or erotophobia are already apparent. As soon as children become aware of the general physical differences between girls and boys, they are very curious about genital differences as well. This interest in the opposite sex and curiosity about members of the same sex is normal. Often this is more than simple curiosity. Kinsey (1948) noted that virtually all boys and about 20% of girls engaged in some form of sex play as children, especially with other children their own age. These data were collected from adults recounting their childhood experiences with others their own age. Since Kinsey's original research, more recent data reveal the same or even higher prevalence of sex play among same-aged, prepubescent girls and boys. Kinsey defined the term "sex play" as involving manually touching the genitalia of another child, although rough-and-tumble play too can have sexual overtones, as can the game of "playing doctor." Another common finding among prepubescent boys is group masturbation (sometimes called a "circle jerk"); remember that participation in such activities in no way predicts a

person's later sexual orientation. Many parents have happened upon their child with other kids in the neighborhood in a game of "let's pull our pants down!" Children are very interested in their anatomical differences long before they have any interest in the procreative or intimate aspects of sexual behavior. Children's sensitivity to stereotyped gender differences also follows later in their development.

Common Sociological and Psychological Aspects of Childhood

Sexual interest and experimentation do not take place in a vacuum but occur against a backdrop of common developmental changes. To fully appreciate sexual development in children, one must first understand typical children's behavior, especially between the ages of 6 and 11. Although not all children at this age manifest the behaviors described below, many do; these should be interpreted in a general sense and not viewed as developmental requirements early in life. These characteristics occur in the latency stage of Freud's psychosexual theory of development.

Repression of Erotic Interest in Members of the Opposite Sex. In childhood, children are likely to avoid close intimate or nurturant contact with members of the opposite sex. Little girls and boys pretty much stay in separate groups. While sexual curiosity may earlier have been an obvious focus of social interactions with same-aged acquaintances, this is less common in middle childhood.

Strong Homosocial Friendships. Freud noted the importance of strong, same-sex friendships during the middle childhood years. This is a time when both boys and girls have a best friend. They spend much time together, may have frequent "sleepovers" together, or maybe even get into trouble frequently in one another's company. In these same-sex friendships children often begin to whisper about the other sex and wonder what in the world they are up to. The development of sexuality in childhood does not necessarily have a heterosexual focus.

Early Perceptions of the Desirability of the Traditional Marriage Script. In middle childhood (ages 6 to 11) children are watching their parents or caretakers carefully and beginning to formulate feelings about whether they'd like to be married and have a family themselves one day. Of course, many children also see things in their home that might dissuade them from marrying or having children. Children witness and vividly recall all types of domestic occurrences. Some may involve genuine affection and deep mutual respect and reciprocity. Others might involve anger and hostility, as well as guilt, jealousy, and physical abuse (Fig. 12-1). A child's earliest thoughts about the meanings of sexuality take place within many different kinds of families with more or less rewarding environments.

Preoccupation With Rules, Order, and Organization. For the first time in a child's life, she or he is impressed with the idea that facts and physical objects can be meaningfully organized into categories based on similar characteristics (like a coin collection). Children gradually come to see the world as a somewhat orderly, predictable place.

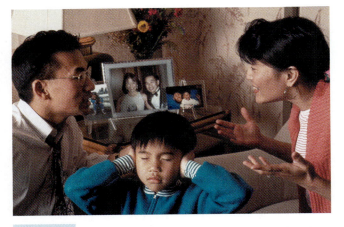

FIGURE 12-1 Before adolescence, children begin to develop their thoughts about the future and the desirability of being married and the nature of relationships between women and men.

Aggressiveness and Inconsiderate Behavior. A predictable aspect of development in middle childhood is that children are frequently cruel to one another and not always respectful of others' possessions. Children can be unaccountably mean to animals and each other. While common, these behaviors are by no means acceptable, nor should they be tolerated lightly. These behaviors are not directly associated with sexual development but are part of the psychosocial backdrop against which such development occurs.

Learning, Practicing, and Feedback

Social learning theory predicts that as children learn sex role behaviors, they will model people whom they perceive to be competent, nurturant, and authoritative. This "practicing" is an important part of a child's sex role development. How others respond to the child's actions may reinforce these behaviors, or in some cases these actions may be ignored or punished. In a very real sense, before adolescence children are testing out their notions of sex-appropriate behaviors before they ever begin to participate in a relationship with someone of the opposite sex. Sex role learning has been a very active area of research in the social and behavioral sciences, and many temperamental and family variables have been shown to powerfully affect this long and subtle process. Such factors as the presence or absence of a father in the home, whether dual parenting is loving and consistent, birth order, and relationships with siblings and peers all affect the ways in which children begin to act on their notions of what it means to be male or female. We earlier defined *identification* as the subconscious desire to become like someone we love, admire, and respect. This is a fundamental aspect of sex role learning that takes place subtly over many years. For Freud, it was one of the most important factors in sexual development. Identification occurs without the child being aware of it; it is subconscious. Modeling, on the other hand, is a more purposeful attempt to mimic another person's behavior, appearance, or demeanor.

Although most approaches to sexual development emphasize the importance of identification, another psychological and sociological process happening at the same time, called *complementation,* receives less attention. It is at least as important as identification in middle and later childhood. Complementation involves ways in which children make purposeful attempts to understand not only their own sex roles but also those of the opposite sex. Although during middle childhood there is often a repression of erotic interest in members of the opposite sex, children are often still trying to understand members of the opposite sex. Complementation is behind much of the sexual curiosity commonly seen in children in this stage, especially their curiosity about the genitalia of the other sex. As children become aware of the more obvious sex differences between girls and boys, their understanding of temperamental and emotional differences is developing as well, and complementation is involved here as well. Just as children are becoming aware of society's stereotypes about women and men and begin to subtly explore and practice behaviors congruent with these, they are also keenly aware of the stereotypes that describe attributes of members of the opposite sex.

Acting affectionately towards members of the opposite sex is also a basic aspect of complementation, for it reveals a child's sensitivity to ways in which women and men like to be treated. These behaviors are also important early examples of the building of mutual trust and reveal an understanding of respect and empathy. Modeling is very important as children see their parents hugging, holding hands, kissing, and simply helping each other get through the day in many little ways. Children who see mommy kiss daddy good-bye on her way to work are witnessing much more than a casual ritual; they are seeing attentive caring on a consistent basis, and who would argue that this isn't appreciated or important?

Learning About Sexuality in the Family

The family, regardless of how it is defined, is usually the first arena for sexual socialization, the first place where sexuality is discussed, taught, or ignored. The peer group is important, of course, but much implicit sexual instruction and learning occur long before a child has a peer group in elementary school. Walters and Walters (1983) analyzed the importance of the family for how children learn about sex and what information they eventually acquire. They believe that most mothers and/or fathers overestimate the content and specificity of what their children hear, remember, and learn about sex. They make the important point that young children have trouble understanding what they cannot see; this is not always obvious to parents and caretakers. For example, simply being told about sperm, eggs, and fertilization generally makes little sense to a child before adolescence unless clear, colorful visual aids are used. Similarly, the processes of embryonic and fetal development are hard for children to conceptualize without a concrete visual reference. Therefore, parents may not understand the state of their child's knowledge, and children may have an only nebulous, incomplete understanding of what their parents are trying to convey. This is true even with the most progressive, well-intentioned parents and the most curious, observant child. This fact is a starting point for the role of the family in sex education. If children find it hard to understand what they cannot see, think of the challenges of trying to explain a subject like contraception to children between the ages of 6 and 11.

Although fathers have become more involved in a variety of parenting activities, mothers are still the main source of information about sex for most children (Walters & Walters, 1983). In fact, as discussed later, high school students report that they would prefer to learn about sexual matters from their parents. Because as a general rule new learning builds on older learning, it is especially important that the earliest information be clear, correct, and understandable. As children develop thoughts, feelings, and behaviors related to sexuality in general, and their own sexuality in particular, certain key principles are involved:

- This whole process usually takes place without the child being fully aware of what is happening. Much early sexual learning is unconscious, and sometimes children actually know more than they think they do.
- Sexual learning begins at birth, as soon as babies begin to associate sensual pleasures with nurturance, physical enjoyment, and, as Erikson would note, a basic trust in others. It would be a mistake to think that children do not learn about sexuality until they produce or comprehend language.
- Parents, as the primary caretakers, are basic to the whole process. During early childhood, children may have many meaningful and potentially informative interactions with peers, other caretakers, and preschool staff, but the primary emotional-communicative relationship is with the parent or parents. One of the most fundamental aspects of responsible parenting is teaching a child about human sexuality.
- Even though people don't intend to, they sometimes convey information and emotions about sexuality that might not be entirely helpful or positive. Everyone has some anxieties about sex, and it is often hard to refrain from expressing or implying these. The more accurate information we have, however, the less likely it is that our verbal or nonverbal communication will include unintended, counterproductive messages.

Lewis (1973) demonstrated that effective sex education in the home can have very positive and long-lasting effects on children and adolescents. Indeed, this kind of information can protect children against misinformation and even premature sexual experimentation later in adolescence. Children who receive serious sex education in the home are more likely to begin sexual experimentation later and more cautiously. Those who do not receive such information are more likely to begin their sexual experimentation early and less cautiously, if not promiscuously. Lewis (1973) notes four important beneficial outcomes of a wide variety of sexual subjects being discussed in the home during childhood.

- Children will have more information about sexuality, and their information will be less subject to the distortions frequently introduced by the peer group. This will eventually make them less susceptible to myths that can misguide behavior.
- Children will find it easier to ask their parents questions about sex, as well as share their thoughts and feelings about sexual issues that might perplex or disturb them. If these subjects are not taboo, there is better sharing of facts and feelings.
- Children will be less likely to misinterpret their parents' statements on sexual subjects and will be better informed about their parents' sexual value systems. Children will have a clear and accurate perception of the ethical and/or moral dimensions of their parents' feelings about sexual subjects.
- Children will begin having sexual intercourse later in adolescence or young adulthood.

Even though it is difficult for many parents to talk to their children about sex, the benefits of doing so and the potential hazards of not doing so are too great to ignore. Therefore, we include here guidelines for parents of children and adolescents to help them anticipate questions and respond effectively. These are intended only as recommendations that can be useful and help alleviate the nervousness out of those little "talks" that many parents dread.

Guidelines for Talking to Children and Adolescents About Sex

Many mothers and fathers expect their child will come to them and ask questions. This does not always happen, and when it does, the questions are often brief and lack any clear context. Following are guidelines for talking with children and teenagers about sexuality.

Be Proactive. Don't wait for your child to raise questions about sex, because often they won't. Sex educators advise taking advantage of teachable moments when they arise, even with children who are not yet in elementary school. These are obvious little events that give parents the appropriate opportunity to raise an issue, ask a question of their child, or probe the child's level of awareness or understanding about a sexual topic. Such discussions early on prevent the peer group from first conveying its misinformation and myths. For example, the family cat having kittens is an obvious teachable moment, but many other opportunities are less obvious. A child may show some curiosity when seeing an undressed manikin in a store, offering the opportunity to comment on anatomical differences and the importance of privacy. Stories on the evening news often involves subjects, such as *in vitro* fertilization, unconventional family lifestyles, adoption, AIDS and other STDs, teen pregnancy, rape and child abuse, and sexual mischief by public figures. Being aware of and using such teachable moments helps you know your child's level of understanding about important sexual subjects (Fig. 12-2).

Don't Worry About Being Nervous. In fact, being a little nervous can be a good thing when talking with children about sex. It is much better to fumble and stutter a little, and perhaps even blush, than to say nothing at all or to give an overly smooth, polished presentation. If your child usually sees you behaving in a competent, authoritative way, seeing you a little nervous sends a very important message: *this must really be important.* Being nervous can offer an important nonverbal meaning to supplement the facts you are offering.

Children Do Not Do Everything They Are Told. Any parent can tell you this, but for some reason people mistakenly believe that if you tell children and teenagers about human sexuality, this will make them more likely to begin sexual experimentation and exploration. In fact, the exact opposite is usually the case, and you are fostering a more thoughtful, informed, analytic approach to sexual topics.

The Issue of Non-Obscene Art. Most parents are justifiably worried about their children being exposed to illustrations of nudity or sex acts and often take steps to be sure that their children and teenagers are not exposed to such illustrations in

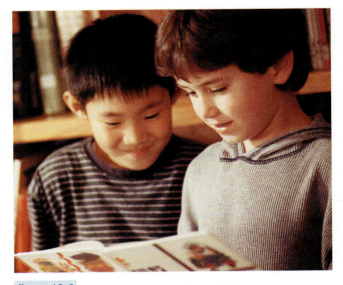

FIGURE 12-3 On those occasions when children encounter non-obscene art, they reveal a simple and genuine curiosity that is unrelated to the eroticism adolescents or adults might perceive.

print and electronic media. There's an important distinction between pornography and non-obscene art, although it's not always easy to express the difference. (See Chapter 19 for more detail.) Generally, non-obscene art may include pictorial representations of nude adult women and men. It does not, however, include pictorial representations of nudity in children, oral-genital stimulation, anal penetration, sexual intercourse, forced sex, or obviously deviant behaviors—these images generally conform to what is considered obscene art or pornography. Again, the distinction is not always clear and unambiguous; courts have tried to be specific and unequivocal about the differences between non-obscene and obscene art but have been unable to devise clear and unambiguous definitions agreeable to everyone.

When children (specifically, children before adolescence) encounter non-obscene art, they usually respond with a spontaneous, child-like curiosity: "Wow, look at that!" (Fig. 12-3). We are unaware of any evidence of long-term adverse effects of occasional, situational, or accidental exposure to such materials by preadolescent children. However, with persistent exposure or when children encounter pornography, the long-term results may be more uncertain or problematic, although cause-and-effect results from such experiences are not clear. Interestingly, when children get to adolescence without ever having encountered non-obscene art, their emotional reactions are frequently exaggerated. This does not mean, of course, that parents should leave non-obscene art where their children will find it. But parents should not be too concerned if their children happen upon such images on occasion. In fact, such exposure may actually prevent a more magnified emotional response later on to tasteful depictions of nudity in women and men.

Children visiting art museums often show a keen attentiveness to representations of nudity in paintings or statues.

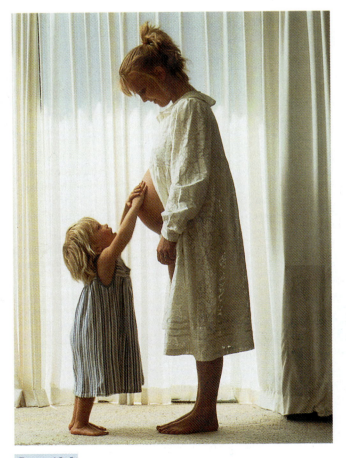

FIGURE 12-2 Early in childhood, children are curious about anatomical differences between women and men, as well as the very obvious physical changes that accompany pregnancy.

Often these are quite graphic and portray passionate expressions of affection. Do not steer your child away from these, but note the simple curiosity of children when they notice the nude human form. Art museums can provide teachable moments, as can art books in your personal library.

Answer Questions When They Are Asked. It is always best to answer questions when they are asked and in the appropriate terminology. A child's questions often have no obvious context, so it is best to answer only the question that is asked and not add more details until they are asked for. If your daughter asks you what a sperm is, for example, tell her. But note that she is not yet asking about eggs or how sperm and eggs get together, so provide only the information requested because the child won't know what to do with the rest. A child's questions about sexual matters are often very specific and represent all the child is asking about. Details about a broader context might be confusing.

The terms and language you use to describe body parts and sexual interactions are very important. Habits of language create habits of thought. Many families have cute expressions for the genitalia of little girls and boys, but a child who is old enough to point to any body part and name it is old enough to learn to say vagina or clitoris. A good working sexual vocabulary is associated with genuine self-esteem.

Sexuality Is a Natural, Intimate Aspect of Being Human. Younger children (usually between 3 and 5 years of age) often focus on anatomy and differences between women and men. Later (between 8 and 11) their curiosity will shift to reproduction, and only later to avenues of sexual expression. It is important to emphasize the normality and naturalness of sexual feeling and expression and to affirm its role in genuine human intimacy, closeness, and trust. Although it is important to talk about penile erection, vaginal lubrication, ejaculation, and so forth, it is also very important to put these clinical, physiological responses within the context of a good relationship and meaningful communication. Sexuality is a fundamental aspect of our humanness, and older children and teenagers can appreciate this. You can also have this discussion in a religious or spiritual context, if you feel more comfortable doing it that way.

Pleasure Is a Basic and Important Aspect of Sexual Expression. Sexual experiences feel good for an evolutionary reason: to promote reproduction. We respect that some people feel sex is solely for procreative purposes. Nonetheless, the keen pleasures associated with sexual experience and expression are often fundamental to bonding, tension reduction, relaxation, and a full sense of oneself (Fig. 12-4). People have sex for recreation, as well as for procreation, and discussions with children and adolescents would be incomplete without acknowledging this fact. Ignoring or evading this issue might perpetuate connotations of sex as "naughty" or "dirty" that children learn all too readily. The enjoyment of sexual pleasure includes also the rewarding feelings associated with *giving* sexual pleasure.

Privacy and Lack of Coercion Are Basic to Sexual Expression. This issue is discussed in other chapters, but this is also a central point to make when talking with children and adolescents about sex. Sexual interactions are, by law, fundamentally private behaviors of consenting individuals in places where they cannot be seen or heard by others. With children we often use the phrase "private parts" to refer to those parts of our bodies involved in sexual stimulation and enjoyment. Children need to understand that only family members or "special" people should see their nudity and that anyone who in any way forces them to reveal themselves or participate in sexual activity is most definitely behaving inappropriately and they should tell someone in authority about it.

This list of issues is by no means complete, and one's personal circumstances affect how sexual concerns are introduced and taught in the home. Again, we are not suggesting everyone should handle these issues in one certain way, though there are common issues one should be prepared to deal with in the home. Family and religious values and traditions often enter into these discussions, and only you can decide how to couch sexual concerns within the context of these beliefs.

■ ■ ■

In a revealing study, King and Lorusso (1997) distributed questionnaires to almost 700 college students and their parents. Over 500 of the parents returned the same questionnaire deal-

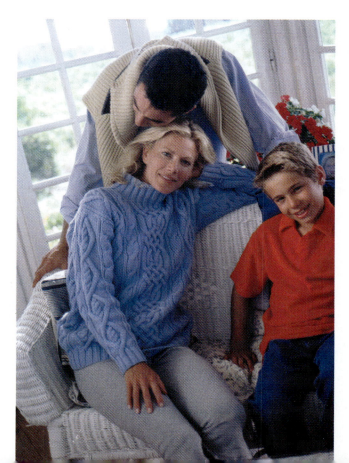

FIGURE 12-4 Sexuality is often an important aspect of a mature, diversified relationship between two adults who share their lives with each other.

sues. About 60% of these students reported that they had never had a meaningful, informative discussion about sex with either of their parents. Most felt that the reason was a poor climate of communication and personal feelings of embarrassment. However, their parents had somewhat different memories, and 60% of them reported that they had had such discussions. Among those parents who reported that they had not spoken to their child about sex, most said that it was because they felt that it was the responsibility of their spouse to do so, essentially letting the child's sexual education in the home to be skipped over altogether. Among students who reported that they had had good, instructive talks with their parents about sex, virtually all of their parents said the same thing. For both female and male students, it was the mother in the overwhelming majority of cases who took the initiative in such talks. Most of these students said that sexual discussions had been ongoing over several years, rather than having one big talk about sex. About half of the students noted that they had begun to talk with their parents about sex before their thirteenth birthday, while 40% of them didn't start talking with their parents about sex until they were between the ages of 13 and 15, which in our opinion is much too late. We find these data distressing because many parents are adamant in not wanting their children to receive family life education courses in their schools because they say they will teach their children themselves. But as these data show, parents frequently do not take the initiative to do this.

Long-Term Effects of Childhood Sexual Experiences

Earlier in this chapter the concept of determinism was described as a basic building block of Freud's psychosexual theory of development. In this approach infantile and childhood sensual experiences are said to have permanent effects on later personality development. Researchers have studied the extent to which this may in fact be the case. Bauserman and Davis (1996) analyzed self-assessments of college undergraduates with respect to their childhood and adolescent sexual experiences. Some of their experiences were rated as positive, others negative, and still others with attributes of both. As predicted, students whose child and adolescent sexual experiences were rated positively showed greater erotophilia in their sexual value systems and were more tolerant of sexual behaviors in others, as well as in their own sexual repertoire. Further, they seemed to enjoy greater sexual satisfaction in their lives. These students seemed to be more accepting of sexual experimentation at earlier ages than their counterparts whose experiences were either negative or mixed. Although these data support the fact that positive childhood and adolescent experiences have effects later on, one notes that our recollections of events early in our lives are often incomplete or simply wrong. Importantly, social learning theory is also supported by these data. This is a complex issue, with much in the popular press in recent years questioning the accuracy of childhood sexual memories, especially in connection with suspected sexual abuse. A critical and cautious attitude is necessary when making any broad generalizations based on findings such as these.

Other issues are involved regarding sexuality when there are children in the home. Our students and audiences often ask about the long-term effects of parental nudity on children. Many adults wonder or worry whether being seen naked by their children might in some way harm them psychologically or predispose them to sexual problems or unusual behaviors later in life. Similarly, parents are sometimes concerned about potential long-term effects on children of sleeping in their parents' bed or inadvertently witnessing their parents having sexual intercourse. Okami (1995) analyzed clinical opinion and scientific data on these subjects and emphasized that very few careful studies have been done on these subjects. Much of what is thought about these issues is based on the professional perspectives of clinicians, which in itself is sometimes enough to lead people to view these issues as a "problem" when in fact they may be just variations on normal behavior. Okami notes that opinions about children being exposed to nudity fall into two very different categories. On the one hand, some feel that this type of stimulation might be too vivid for children and perhaps become a source of later problems. Importantly, however, some counselors and therapists believe that the social setting in which exposure occurs is more important than the exposure *per se*. At the other extreme on the spectrum of opinion on this issue are experts who believe that children being exposed to parental nudity, especially same-sex parental nudity, may in fact enhance bonding and identification with the same-sex parent. It is interesting that although childhood exposure to parental nudity is undoubtedly a world-wide phenomenon, there are very little systematic empirical data about the nature of children's experiences in this common family context. Okami, Olmstead, Abramson, and Pendleton (1998) believe that claims of negative developmental outcomes associated with early childhood exposure to parental nudity and accidental observation of parental sexuality are greatly exaggerated, even when exposure occurs before age 6, as shown in a sample of teenagers questioned between the ages of 17 and 18 (Fig. 12-5).

Another common family issue involves reasons children often want to crawl into bed with their parents during the night and the impact of this behavior on both the child and parents. This is sometimes referred to as co-sleeping and is the source of much consternation among parents. There is some debate between specialists in the social and behavioral sciences and parents about the nature of these experiences and the long-term effects on children (Bennett, 1992). Anthropologists and sociologists refer to co-sleeping in a family as the "family bed." One view of this common phenomenon emphasizes that co-sleeping enhances a child's feelings of family intimacy, while others simply suggest that children will have fewer sleeping problems if they can sleep with their parents. These psychoanalytic views emphasize that children who co-sleep with their parents enjoy some very keen comforts and gain a powerful feeling of security that cannot otherwise be readily felt when the house is empty, dark, and quiet. Nonetheless, few scientists have devised and tested ideas about the impact of co-sleeping in large, random, representative samples of girls and boys. Yet co-sleeping is prevalent in other cultures with apparently few or no adverse developmental outcomes.

Earlier we noted that parents often have trouble accepting their children's sexuality. Similarly, children have trouble accepting their parents as sexual beings. Two important studies have probed this delicate issue (Hoyt, 1978, 1979). The term "primal scene" is frequently used to describe witnessing one's parents having sexual intercourse. In a sample of 345 college students, 18% reported either having seen or heard their parents having intercourse. On average, these respondents reported that they were about 12 when this happened for the first time. Generally, the older the child was when happening upon parental intercourse, the better was his or her long-term emotional reaction. Another study (Hoyt, 1979) found that in a sample of 25 female and 25 male undergraduates, 28% reported that they had seen or heard their parents having intercourse. In both of these studies, witnessing their parents' sexual intimacy did not affect their later sexual adjustment or overall outlook on life.

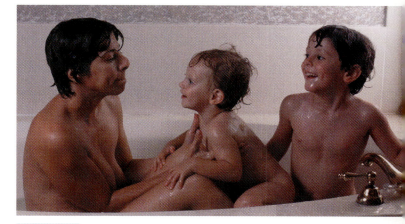

FIGURE 12-5 Many homes reveal a positive, healthy, unselfconscious approach to nudity, while at the same time teaching the importance of privacy in everyday life.

Research Highlight

HOW DO CHILDREN INTERACT SEXUALLY?

Much of what is known about children's sexuality is based on observations of children's sexual explorations and anecdotal evidence with very consistent themes. However, an important investigation described in detail various professionals' opinions about sexual behavior among children and the recollections of a large number of undergraduate students (Haugaard, 1996). This study by Dr. Jeffrey J. Haugaard involved anonymous questionnaires sent to 160 pediatricians, 141 masters or doctoral level psychotherapists, and 163 4-H club leaders. Questionnaires were also sent to authors of published articles about child sexual abuse, as well as elementary school teachers. In all, 337 questionnaires were returned. Anonymous questionnaire data were also recorded from 664 undergraduates.

In the first part of the study, professionals were asked to rate whether specific behaviors were acceptable for males and females in three different age groups: 4 years old, 8 years old, and 12 years old. The data in Table 12-4 show that a number of behaviors considered normal and acceptable for 4-year-old children were considered far less appropriate for children in the two older age groups, perhaps because of the common perception that children are innocent and have not yet developed an eroticized sexual value system. Some of the data reported here indicate child sexual abuse.

Undergraduates were asked to report whether they had engaged in a number of sexual experiences, such as exposing their genitals, fondling nongenital areas, fondling genitals, or having intercourse during three different age stages: ages 1–6 years, 7–10 years, and 11–12 years. These data are shown in Table 12-5.

In general, various sexual behaviors are less appropriate as children grow older, probably due to the perception that such activities in younger children are experimental and are not associated with the erotic implications of similar behaviors later in development. This research is important because it is based on the reports of a large, diverse, representative selection of professionals, as well as the recollections of a large sample of undergraduates. Similar data concerning common sexual behaviors among children have also been published by Friedrich, Fisher, Broughton, Houston, and Shafran (1998).

TABLE 12-4

Percent of Professionals Responding That a Behavior Is Acceptable for Male Respondents, Female Respondents, and Total Respondents[a]

	4-year-olds			8-year-olds			12-year-olds		
	Male	Female	Total	Male	Female	Total	Male	Female	Total
Undressing together (%)	91	86	88	34	54	42	10	22	15
Showing genitals (%)	77	80	88	24	39	31	7	21	13
Fondling nongenital areas (%)	69	70	69	39	52	45	33	39	35
Fondling girls' breast areas (%)	27	34	30	6	16	10	10	20	14
Fondling genital or anal areas (%)	16	20	18	2	9	5	5	10	7
Oral-genital contact (%)	3	4	3	1	2	1	1	2	1
Digital penetration of vagina or anus (%)	3	6	4	0	3	1	2	3	2
Attempted or simulated intercourse (%)	3	8	5	1	3	2	2	5	3
Intercourse (%)	1	2	1	0	1	0	1	2	1

Male respondents n = 137; female respondents n = 189; total respondents n = 337 (11 respondents did not specify their gender).

[a] From Haugaard, 1996.

These three issues regarding sexuality, children, and the home environment have generated controversy and sometimes dire predictions about the possible long-term adverse effects of these experiences for children and adolescents. However, when systematic empirical data are discriminated from clinical opinion, there is in fact no substantive proof of negative outcomes of these almost inevitable aspects of growing up in a functional nuclear family. Until more scientific evidence is collected on these issues, any claims should be made only with caution.

Sex Education and Sexual Behavior

Because there is often a big gap between what is taught in school and what is remembered or becomes a part of a person's behavior, it is important to determine the measurable long-term effects of sex education on the sexual behavior of young people. Because of the AIDS epidemic in this and many other countries, the World Health Organization has undertaken a "Global Programme on AIDS" and has published a report on this subject (Grunseit, Kippax, Aggleton, Baldo, & Slutkin, 1997). This work analyzed the results of 52 different studies on the relationship between HIV/AIDS and sex education and sexual behavior in young people. This research was conducted throughout the world. Of these, 47 investigations evaluated the effects of educational programs. Twenty-five found that such educational programs neither increased nor decreased the amount of sexual behavior, pregnancy rates, or the prevalence of sexually transmitted diseases in this population of respondents. On the other hand, 17 studies demonstrated a relationship of sex education with a later age of first intercourse, fewer sexual partners, fewer unanticipated pregnancies and a lower prevalence of STDs. Only 3 studies reported increases of sexual behavior related to these educational programs. These investigators emphasized that not all of these studies provided informative data and that it was difficult to compare investigations because of the diverse research methods employed.

TABLE 12-5

Percent of Undergraduates Reporting Each Experience, by Gender

	1–6 Years Old		7–10 Years Old		11–12 Years Old	
Type of Experience	Male	Female	Male	Female	Male	Female
Exposing genitals (%)	38	39	41	30	29	16
Fondling nongenital areas (e.g., back, stomach) (%)	19	19	30	26	37	31
Fondling genital areas (%)	11	9	11	10	17	10
Intercourse (%)	1	1	4	1	3	1

Male respondents n = 199; female respondents n = 465

However, the overwhelming opinion on the behavioral effects of sex education is that such programs do not encourage promiscuity. However, there are compelling and important data suggesting a cause-and-effect relationship for beneficial effects of sex education programs on the behavior of young adults.

Sex Education in the Schools for Adolescents

There is much political controversy about sex education in the schools, even though most Americans favor sex education for teenagers in school (Greydanus, Pratt, & Dannison, 1995). Earlier we emphasized the importance of sex education in the home as a basic, essential first step in a child's learning about the body, affection, and sexual expression. We also discussed a troubling inconsistency in those who resist sex education in the schools: they say they will do it in their own homes but frequently do not, or do an inadequate job. While parents and schools are arguing these issues, teenagers clearly think that sex education meets a very important need in their lives. In a Canadian study, Cairns, Collins, and Hiebert (1994) explored the self-perceived needs of 81 teenagers from age 14 to 20 regarding a comprehensive school health education program. Their opinions were sought about the importance of 15 different general needs. Of these 15 different needs, the respondents ranked sex education as the third most important, just after their desire to learn more about coping with personal problems and dealing with family relationships. These data probably reflect the thinking of many teenagers in many communities in the industrialized world.

Although it is beyond the scope of this text to describe a complete curriculum in sex education for teenagers, certain topics should ideally be important parts of such a curriculum. The essential topics are anatomical and physiological differences between females and males, sperm production in males, ovulation and menstruation in females, the process of conception, methods of contraception, sexually transmitted diseases and their prevention, masturbation, where to get contraception, where to receive abortion counseling, and HIV/AIDS education. We believe these are only the most essential components of sex education for teenagers—other topics also can be important. Comprehensive, well-organized sex education programs can have a big role in changing adolescent sexual behavior and encouraging teens to clarify their moral perspectives and sexual value systems (Greydanus, Pratt, & Dannison, 1995). In a study of 220 rural Canadian parents of public school children, more than 90% agreed or strongly agreed with the importance of offering sex education in schools as early as 6th grade (McKay, 1996). These parents felt that a number of important topics ought to be presented beginning in the 6th grade, including such issues as sexual orientation, methods of birth control, moral beliefs about sexuality, abstinence, STDs and AIDS prevention, puberty, reproduction, sexual abuse, rape, and the attributes of good interpersonal relationships. While parents thought that children at different ages are better suited for different topics, by the time their children reached 9th grade, they recommended virtually all ten topics in the questionnaire for inclusion in the curriculum. Although a number of specific subjects can be included in a sex education curriculum, content centers on four general themes: biological information, information about human sexuality in general, guidance for personal decisions about engaging in intimate behaviors, and the independent, autonomous young person's thinking and behaving (Schraag, 1989).

Asking youth in their early adolescent years what topics they are interested in learning about reveals several focal areas. Ryan, Millstein, and Irwin, (1996) asked 159 adolescents between 11.4 and 13.4 years of age what they wanted to learn about in their health education program. This group produced 200 different questions. Most of their questions (88%) dealt with biological aspects of human sexuality, reproductive and genital physiology in particular (52%). Only 6% of the questions had anything to do with the psychosocial setting in which sexual behaviors take place. The message here is simple: with limited time for sex education in the schools, a focus on biological, physiological, and reproductive issues will go a long way toward answering questions that many youth are too shy to ask. Of course, other important areas also need exploration, but this study reveals the areas students are most likely to be curious about.

Proponents of comprehensive sex education for adolescents cite both scientific reasons on the one hand and emotional and moral ones on the other (Ehrhardt, 1996). They say that useful information must somehow be conveyed to young people, who need it despite a variety of objections. One noted sex researcher, Anke Ehrhardt, believes a sex education program should be designed, discussed, and evaluated according to a variety of risk behaviors. The risk of being involved in an unanticipated pregnancy, the risk of contracting a sexually transmitted disease, and the risk of contracting HIV generally get a youngster's attention and perhaps motivate more cautious approaches to sexual behavior or even abstinence. Even the risk of feeling rejected is often a salient aspect of a teenager's thinking. Although risks often are associated with fears and anxieties, they indeed may be a point around which a constructive sex education curriculum can be organized (Table 12-6).

TABLE 12-6

Risky Sexual Behaviors That May Contribute to Unanticipated Pregnancy, Receiving or Transmitting an STD, or Acquiring HIV

Sexual intercourse without a condom

Vaginal penetration prior to the application of a condom

Sexual intercourse with a latex condom lubricated with a petroleum-based lubricant

Coitus interruptus

Oral ejaculation

Anal intercourse without a condom (both insertive and receptive)

Sexual behavior with someone one does not know very well

Another challenge for sex educators involves striking an appropriate balance between moral, ethical, and value-oriented issues on one end of the instructional continuum and practical, applied matters on the other (Dailey, 1997). An overemphasis on the former may help young people clarify their feelings and thoughts about sexual behaviors but may not help them act intelligently and take self-protective measures against very real and ever-present dangers (Fig. 12-6). In the end, sexual behaviors hold central importance in our interactions with others. Additionally, Dailey (1997) says sex educators face a tricky but important challenge of being honest and open about the pleasures of sexual behavior while also recognizing the importance of mature, foresightful decision making. Teenagers are often suspicious of sex education that ignores or minimizes the place of pleasure in sexual behaviors. An in-depth interview study of 19 British sex educators revealed that virtually all of them held negative opinions about teenagers engaging in sexual behaviors (Pitts, Burtney, & Dobraszczyc, 1996). Data like these are an important reminder that not just any health education teacher, or any teacher at all, is temperamentally qualified to teach this subject, regardless of their background, training, and credentials.

SEXUAL EXPERIENCE AND EXPRESSION IN ADOLESCENCE

Sexual experience and expression in adolescence is a huge subject, and we can only discuss it generally in a text with this broad a focus. Simply stated, sexuality is the central focus of adolescent development, and puberty is its main event. Words are limited in accurately describing the first stirrings of sexual feeling, especially when it is all mixed up with one's preoccupation with appearance, friendships, and the influence of the family.

One of the more subtle but significant preoccupations of most adolescents is body image, which is often closely related to self-esteem. This is usually the first time in a person's life when they form an image of themselves and their attractiveness, based on how attractive or "normal" they think they look

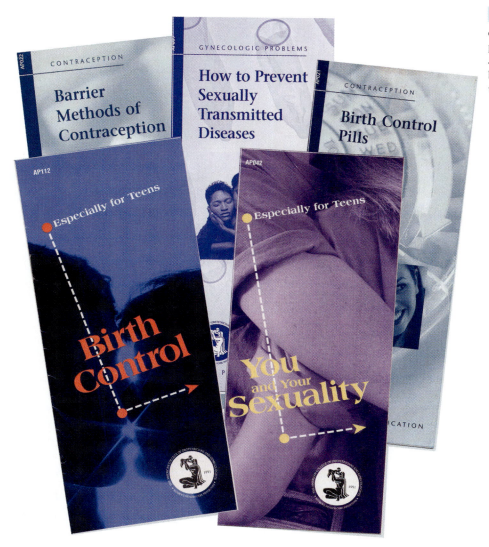

FIGURE 12-6   The American College of Obstetricians and Gynecologists publishes many readable, practical, authoritative brochures that can be both helpful and informative for teenagers.

to others, usually others their own age. Most adolescents are brutally critical of their own appearance and magnify their perceptions of even the slightest blemish or unusual feature. Teenagers look at their faces, their complexions, their bodies, and their rate of pubertal development and often compare themselves to the unattainable images presented by the advertising industry. No wonder kids can be so hard on themselves and each other! This constant self-scrutiny lasts many years and affects a young person's feelings about their desirability and acceptability among their peers.

Many adolescents often wonder about "who they are." This is a time of identity development, which Erikson believes is the basic psychological challenge of adolescence. Figuring out one's identity can be a large, long-term task, and teens face inevitable challenges while they are trying to do this. For example, there is frequently a mismatch between who a youth thinks she or he is and how others see and relate to her or him. This illustrates the influence of the psychosocial environment on adolescent sexual development. Such misattributions can make things difficult for a teen. An adult who looks at a 17-year-old female with large breasts, a small waist, and maturing hips may assume that this young woman (a) likes her body, (b) has lots of boy friends, and (c) is beginning to enjoy sexual experiences, when in fact, none of these may be true.

Psychosocial Sexual Development

Perhaps because the physical changes of puberty can be rather dramatic and occur very rapidly, it is tempting for social and behavioral scientists to focus on these alterations in body shape, size, and configuration at the expense of the broader psychosocial environment in which these are taking place. Yet the environment plays a profound role in motivating, regulating, or even extinguishing many of our behaviors. By adolescence most people are making good progress on the "socialization tasks" that are so important at this time. Although such tasks challenge us throughout our lives, from when we usually begin grappling with them after entering elementary school, during adolescence people first gain some mastery of them. Following are some of the key challenges.

Impulse Control. By the teen years, ideally children have learned to regulate and control their expression of aggressive feelings and, according to Freud's psychosexual theory, sexual feelings. By this time people are expected to refrain from acting on every aggressive and sexual feeling or inclination and learn to moderate or suppress the behavioral expression of these often strong feelings. We better anticipate the consequences of our actions and behave accordingly. Some teenagers openly admit that they feel stronger and better about themselves because they perceive there is strength in restraint.

Frustration Tolerance. The term "frustration" describes the unpleasant feelings we have when we find ourselves blocked in progress toward some goal. These goals can be significant and important or even relatively trivial, but generally people don't like feeling stopped. Psychologists, sociologists, anthropologists, and criminal justice experts know that a com-

mon response to frustration is aggression. One of the hard things about growing up is learning to suppress aggressive feelings when frustrated. This is especially important as teenagers begin to explore the sexual dimension of relationships and messages to "stop" in necking and petting situations. It is imperative that adolescents learn to suppress any aggressive inclinations they might feel at these moments.

Delay of Gratification. Another central challenge in human growth and development involves learning to put off small, immediate rewards in exchange for bigger, better ones at a later time. Delay of gratification is a basic part of morality, ethics, and conceptions of good conduct in society. This idea is behind some prohibitions against premarital intercourse. Children are not very good at delaying gratification, but as we grow into and through our teenage years, we are expected to learn the importance of this challenge (Fig. 12-7).

Learning to Live With Uncertainty in Our Future. Children are impatient about wanting to know what they will be doing later, tomorrow, or this weekend. If a child asks,"Mommy, can we go to the movies on Saturday?" and the mother responds as many parents do, "We'll see..." this is usually an unsatisfactory answer for a child. It's as if the child were saying, "No, Mom, I've got things to do, places to go, and people to see, and I need to know NOW." By adolescence children can better deal with this kind of uncertainty, especially in how meaningful relationships unfold and develop.

■ ■ ■

Learning to deal with physical changes, the attributions others make about teenagers, and early exploration of sexual feelings and interaction all take place against this backdrop of psychological and social development.

The child's family is very important for the child's sexual development. As we noted above, parents (a single parent or two parents) often have great difficulty accepting their adoles-

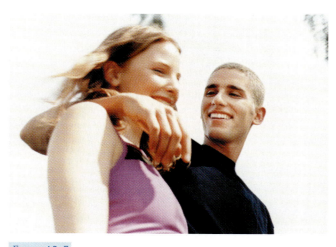

FIGURE 12-7 The challenges of impulse control, frustration tolerance, and the delay of gratification can be particularly difficult for adolescents as they begin dating and learn more about their own sexuality.

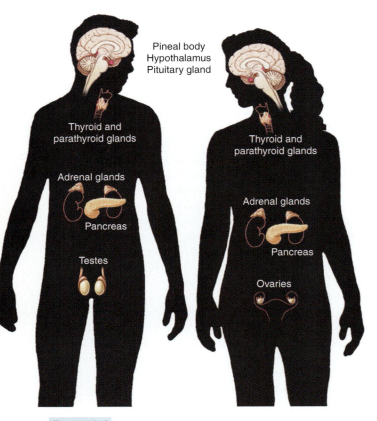

Pineal body
Hypothalamus
Pituitary gland

Thyroid and
parathyroid glands

Thyroid and
parathyroid glands

Adrenal glands

Adrenal glands

Pancreas

Pancreas

Testes

Ovaries

Figure 12-8   The brain and endocrine system work together to produce and regulate the hormones responsible for the appearance of secondary sexual characteristics in female and males.

cents as sexual beings, adolescents have similar problems accepting their parents as sexual beings. While this is common, it is rarely ever discussed openly and candidly. For many men, the idea of "some kid putting his hands on my daughter" is utterly unthinkable, even though his daughter might really want that to happen. For many mothers of teenage boys, the idea of some young woman "luring" their son into intercourse is similarly appalling. Parents rarely see their adolescent as the *active agent* in teenage sexual activities but usually see the other youngster as the one who is tempting their daughter or son into something they would never think of doing. Although teenagers sometimes take advantage of others sexually, it is naive to think that all adolescent sexual experimentation comes at the instigation of someone else.

Puberty in Females and Males

Puberty is the time when secondary sexual characteristics appear. The term "secondary" describes physical changes that result from increasing levels of sex hormones in the bloodstream, which come from the ovaries and testes as a result of stimulation from the pituitary gland. The following sections discuss the nature and timing of the appearance of these secondary sexual characteristics for females and males. There are significant individual differences involved in puberty, and there are many vari-

ations among youngsters of the same age in these changes. As described in Chapter 4, various brain and endocrine structures are intimately involved in a variety of developmental changes involving the female and male reproductive systems. Increases in sex hormones can really be quite dramatic. In boys in early adolescence the level of testosterone is 18 times higher than in childhood, and in girls at this time the level of estrogen is 8 times higher than in childhood (Malina & Bouchard, 1991).

These hormonal levels play a central role in the physical changes accompanying puberty (Fig. 12-8). There is also a subtle but compelling relationship between these changes and the moodiness that often accompanies adolescence. This is often obvious as young women begin menstruation, and it is no less obvious in the surliness or aloofness we see in young boys.

Generally speaking, puberty begins 1 1/2 to 2 years earlier in females than in males. Puberty can begin at 9 1/2 or 10 in girls and 11 or 12 in boys. Because of this, females are more likely to appear more adult-like at an earlier age than are males. This affects their socialization experiences and is likely one of the reasons that adolescent girls generally spend time with boys who are older than themselves.

While it is easy to see how pubertal changes begin during the early teens, data are beginning to accumulate that some very subtle hormonal signs of puberty begin long before this time. In both sexes a relatively weak hormone from the adrenal glands, dihydroepiandrosterone (DHEA) seems instrumental in setting the stage for the onset of puberty at about age 10. Beginning at about the age of 6, levels of this hormone rise steadily and reach a peak at around age 18. The term *adrenarche* refers to the start of the rise of DHEA levels at age 6. This hormone increases the activity of oil-producing glands in the skin, as well as a growth spurt at this time. Investigators also believe that increases in this hormone are responsible for the earliest psychological experiences that begin with attraction, then merge into desire, and only later lead to the inclination to act on sexual feelings (Marano, 1997), all taking place before and during early puberty. Although more attention has been devoted to studying the action of estrogen and testosterone, apparently the adrenal glands play a larger role in the early development of puberty than previously thought.

Pubertal Changes in Females

As levels of adrenal and ovarian hormones begin to rise in the bloodstream, a number of predictable physical changes begins to occur (Fig. 12-9A). Although the following list may seem to imply an order, in fact these events overlap in time significantly.

1. **Enlargement of the Breasts.** Breast development begins in late childhood, at about age 10, with what is known as the "bud" stage. At first it involves a slight enlargement and thickening of the areola, and then the tissues beneath it.

2. **Appearance of Straight, Pigmented Pubic Hair.** Puberty involves the appearance of two different kinds of pubic hair. At first, around age 11, fine, downy pubic hair appears high in the genital region.

It is often straight and wispy with only a slight accumulation. Often it covers the pubic symphysis.

3. ***Maximum Rate of Body Growth.*** Between ages 13 and 13 1/2, girls grow faster than at any other time during all of postpubescent life. Often, just prior to this dramatic growth spurt, a girl may gain some weight and appear a little chubby, but this is entirely normal.

4. ***Appearance of Kinky Pubic Hair.*** The second type of pubic hair to appear is a moderate to dense accumulation of kinky or curly pubic hair, which covers all of the genital area, usually by age 13 or 14. This pubic hair may be dark or light. There is great variation among girls in the appearance of this type of pubic hair.

5. ***Menarche.*** Menarche is a girl's first menstrual period. The average age of menarche in the United States is just under 13 years, but there is much variation among girls in this. Girls who are overweight often begin having their periods earlier because body weight is thought to be an important trigger for menstruation; this is sometimes called the "Frisch-Revelle hypothesis." During the first year a girl is having periods, many of her periods will be anovulatory, that is, they may involve a menstrual discharge but they do not indicate that ovulation has actually occurred.

6. ***Other Body Hair.*** Late in adolescence other body hair becomes more apparent. For example, axillary hair (arm pit hair) or hair on a girl's arms and legs becomes more obvious.

Remember the important relationship between self-esteem and body image. As these changes are occurring, a young girl is often beset by common anxieties about her attractiveness to others or the degree to which she conforms to social conceptions of beauty. Young women are usually much less aware of one another's pubertal development than are young men, because society often affords young girls more privacy than young men. For example, in high schools, girls in physical education classes often have private ceramic or canvas shower stalls and can cover up when showering after class. Boys more often have group showers. Boys might feel just as self-conscious about their development as girls, but in general, they are not given the privacy girls enjoy.

PUBERTAL CHANGES IN MALES

As in girls, the pubertal changes in boys are also happening at the same time (Fig. 12-9B). Because puberty begins in boys around ages 11 or 12, in early adolescence among boys and girls of the same age, girls will appear far more mature than boys. By the 7th grade the pubertal differences between the sexes are already quite obvious.

1. ***Increased Growth of the Penis and Testicles.*** At about the age of 11 or 12, the penis and testicles begin to get larger. This is a gradual process and takes several months to become obvious. But the

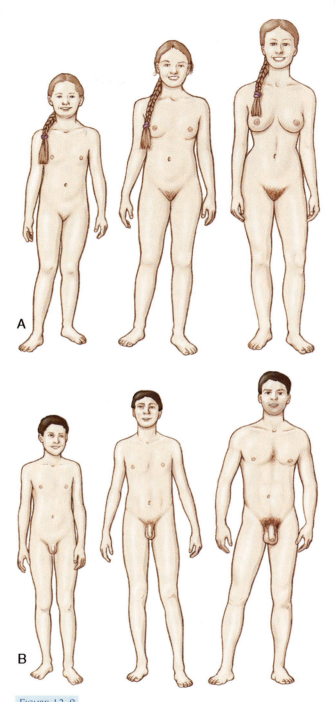

FIGURE 12-9 During puberty, girls develop into young women (**A**), and boys develop into young men (**B**). These changes create a change in body image and self-esteem. Young people are sensitive to the ways others respond to their physical develop-

difference between juvenile and adolescent genitalia is quite obvious, and many boys are a bit secretive and uncertain about these changes.

2. ***Appearance of Long, Downy Pubic Hair.*** Soon after the penis and testes have begun to increase in size, long, soft pubic hair begins to appear, typi-

Dear Dr. Ruth

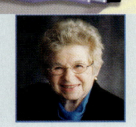

Question:

I am a college freshman and share a dorm room with two other girls. I have a question about being undressed in front of them. I have lots of brothers and sisters, and we were all comfortable about dressing and undressing in front of one another. So in the dorm when I come back to our room from the shower I usually just take my robe off, dry off, and get dressed. No big deal; it's just us girls and the shades are down. But wow! Both my roommates really freaked out when I did this the first time, and I guess I offended them. On the other hand, I really don't see a reason to hide from same-sex friends every time I get dressed or change clothes. What do you think?

Answer:

Relationships, whether between lovers, siblings, friends, or roommates, always involve compromise. If everybody did exactly as they pleased without regard for others, we'd live in a very chaotic world. So the question you have to decide is how important it is to you to live with your own style versus living with your roommates who happen to have a different style. There's no right and wrong here. There's nothing wrong with walking around naked in front of them, but there's also nothing wrong with them wanting to be more modest. Would it really bother you greatly to take underwear with you to the shower? Or is it worth the effort to "teach" your roommates to be less modest? My advice is to talk it out a bit, if both sides can keep an open mind, and try to arrive at the best compromise.

---

cally around age 12. While some of this covers the scrotum, much of it appears high in the genital area, above the penis but below the pubic symphysis. In many cases, this hair is so fine it is barely visible.

3. ***Appearance of Light, Soft Hair Above the Upper Lip.*** This is the first sign of facial hair and is not thick and tough as hair that will later grow there. These hairs are soft, but very obvious, especially if a young man has dark hair.

4. ***The First Appearance of Sideburns.*** After the first signs of facial hair have appeared, sideburns get darker and thicker. By about the age of 13, most young men need to shave about once a week, some more often. For some young men shaving is a ritual that affirms their developing sense of masculinity, and they shave more frequently than needed.

5. ***A More Definitive Appearance of Pubic Hair.*** Just as young women have two kinds of pubic hair, young men do too. The moderately dense accumulation of kinky pubic hair becomes obvious for the first time around age 15, although there is much

variability among adolescent males in the density and distribution of this growth.

6. ***Deepening of the Voice.*** Because of changing thickness of the vocal cords, a young boy's voice begins to change obviously although somewhat unpredictably during adolescence, a change that is usually not completed until about age 16. These changes often increase self-consciousness in an already nervous young man.

7. ***Lateral Spread of Pubic Hair.*** As development continues, pubic hair spreads slightly toward the crests of the pelvic bones. This is often accompanied by a general increase in the density of hair along the inside of the thighs and between the lower border of the navel and the pubic region.

These events are the main changes in a boy's puberty, but as he ages through his teens he manifests some signs indicating the end of puberty and the beginnings of young adulthood. These include such changes as:

8. ***The Genitalia Reach Their Adult Size.*** Toward the end of the teens, the penis, testes, and scrotum

attain their adult dimensions. By about age 18, this part of the body is decidedly adult. Genital development often lags behind the production of mature sperm, however. By the time most boys have reached the age of 14, there are fully formed, motile sperm in their ejaculate. In some, this occurs much earlier. In most cases, *nocturnal emissions,* or wet dreams, begin to occur about a year after a boy has ejaculated for the first time. Nocturnal emissions are not always accompanied by erotic dreams.

9. ***The Mature Hair Pattern.*** By the end of an adolescent's teens, his eventual adult hair pattern may already be obvious. Some young men begin to show signs of baldness during their early 20s. If a boy has inherited a gene for pattern baldness, its influence may already be obvious during later adolescence or early adulthood.

10. ***Other Body Hair.*** The last of the secondary sexual characteristics to become obvious is an assortment of terminal body hair. Hair on the arms, legs, chest, back, and lower back are the final physical changes of puberty. Here again, there are wide individual and racial differences in the density of this hair.

Now we turn our attention to the various solitary and shared sexual behaviors of teenagers and the implications and consequences of those behaviors. Our psychosocial approach emphasizes the important interaction between these biological changes and the environment in which they occur.

Exploratory Sexual Behavior Among Adolescents

We begin with a very simple but far-reaching fact: vulnerable adolescents are at the highest risk of behaving in reckless sexual behaviors (Gordon & Gilgun, 1987). Youth who lack authoritative information about sex, who lack firm parental boundaries, who have problems with self-esteem, or who feel excluded from interesting educational and occupational opportunities are far more likely to try to prove their autonomy and worth through sexual activity. Often these young people have been abused psychologically, physically, or sexually. Members of minority groups are especially vulnerable to the temptations of irresponsible sexual behavior. These disenfranchised youth are far less likely to use contraception conscientiously or to engage in safe sex on a consistent basis. They run greater risks of acquiring sexually transmitted diseases, and in delaying being treated when they suspect they might have one. They are more likely to be involved in an unanticipated pregnancy.

Petting. The term "petting" usually refers to touching and manual stimulation of another's body, but most especially the breasts and genitals. Usually petting is preceded and accompanied by kissing, and it is a virtually universal prelude to more serious sexual interaction. It is a type of sexual exploration and is by no means exclusive to teenagers. Male adolescents are more likely to engage in petting behaviors than are females. De Gaston, Weed, and Jensen (1996) reported that girls

are more likely than boys to report that sexual urges are controllable. As adolescents begin to participate in petting, issues of boundaries, wills, and limits become a part of sexual thinking, discussion, and the ways teens conceptualize what is permissible in their own minds.

Masturbation. Almost all adolescent boys and one-fourth to one-third of adolescent girls masturbate and in several surveys report having done so at some time during the past few weeks. Virtually every study of adolescent sexuality reports higher rates of masturbation among boys than girls. Nonetheless, it is difficult to make true, useful generalizations about any aspect of teenage sexuality. Sample sizes vary in size and composition, and data collected just a few years apart can be quite different for a number of unknown reasons. Therefore, it is impossible to offer data that describe definitively what adolescents do, how often, and why.

Masturbation is entirely different for teenagers than for children. While children touch themselves in an almost random, distracted way, teens touch their genitals in a far more goal-oriented, coordinated, planned fashion. Most teenagers who masturbate fully intend to precipitate an orgasm for the pleasure it entails. Childhood masturbation is rarely orgasm-focused. Early during the teenage years, boys masturbate often, and then somewhat less as they get older. Among girls there is an opposite trend: far less genital self-stimulation early and more later on (Oliver & Hyde, 1993). Adolescent masturbation is entirely normal and in no way affects psychosocial functioning or is physically injurious. Because teenagers are often somewhat secretive about their sexual development, they do not often talk with one another about masturbation and may feel somewhat unusual because they have seemingly discovered this autoerotic behavior on their own. Good sex education can help diminish the guilt that sometimes accompanies masturbation. While masturbation is primarily a solitary behavior, mutual masturbation among adolescents (both heterosexual and homosexual) is common. Mutual masturbation involves two individuals masturbating one another to orgasm, although this term can also be used for two or more people who masturbate in the visual presence of one another. While these behaviors may make some people uncomfortable, we believe they are far preferable to intercourse among people who feel unready or who wish to avoid unanticipated pregnancy or a sexually transmitted disease. Mutual masturbation allows people to feel sexually excited and responsive without having to worry about these other very real sources of anxiety.

Finally, masturbation is also a good, risk-free way of learning about one's sexual arousal and response. Teenagers can learn about the sexual response cycle (arousal, plateau, orgasm, and resolution) through genital self-stimulation. This is an important understanding, and its value to teens should not be minimized.

Sexual Intercourse. Social and behavioral scientists know that first intercourse is a special and important event for many adolescents. For many, it is the first time they have shared physical intimacy within the context of an affectionate interpersonal relationship, although for others it can be a brief, me-

Dear Dr. Ruth

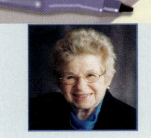

Question:

I have a question about masturbation. I am a boy and 14 years old. I masturbate, and it feels good. I am very private about it. But at church they said that masturbation is a sin, so I went to the library and read about it in one of your books, and you said you don't believe that it's a sin. You said it's normal and healthy. So I'm trying to decide who's right and who's wrong.

Answer

There are many different religions in this world, and they have very different ideas about things, so if I gave advice based on a religious concept I'd always be offending somebody. Let's not think about religion for a moment. In terms of normal health, there is absolutely nothing wrong with masturbation. It doesn't hurt anyone, and in many cases, if a boy doesn't masturbate, he's more likely to have wet dreams, which shows the power of strong sexual urges.

Now let's look at the religious part of your question. Many religions are based on the Bible, which does say men should not masturbate. In my own view, the Bible gives a lot of advice about how to live, and some of that advice we may choose to follow whereas other advice we can simply disagree with. After all, we've learned a lot about health and human psychology over the last few centuries, so we can't expect every idea from the past still to be relevant. I believe you should be permitted to relieve your sexual tensions through masturbation, but if your personal religious feelings are that masturbation is wrong, you should know that refraining from masturbation also does no harm.

chanical, unrewarding "coupling" of little real significance. For some it may involve feelings of failure, humiliation, or exploitation. It may be a gesture of rebellion against parental authority and control or a personal exploration of one's sensuality and eroticism. People often remember their first intercourse experience vividly because it is frequently invested with these types of thoughts and feelings. This section will discuss some of the factors surrounding non-coerced first intercourse and the circumstances that foster regular sexual intercourse among teenagers. In the last few decades, teenagers have been having their first intercourse experiences earlier and earlier. By the time teenagers have reached the age of 18, about half report having had intercourse, and the number increases to a minimum of 80% by the time they have reached the age of 20 (Seidman & Reider, 1994). Many motives are involved in the decision to engage in sexual intercourse during adolescence. The desire to explore and experiment sexually is certainly important, and often youngsters gain a sense of enhanced self-esteem by feeling desired. Others use their bodies to get a sense of validation and proof of their attractiveness. Additionally, some adolescents engage in sexual intercourse as a gesture of

rebellion against their parents or other authority figures. Other kids are lonely and will do whatever they have to in order to receive even brief attention or affection from others.

There are some interesting racial, ethnic, and gender differences in the age at which adolescents have intercourse for the first time (Leigh, Morrison, Trocki, & Temple, 1994), although such statistics may be somewhat inaccurate due to biases in data that depend on self-reports. One example of this may be found among African American males, fully half of whom say they have had intercourse by age 15. Among Caucasian males in the United States, half report having had intercourse by the age of 17, significantly later. Among females the situation is a little different. Half of African American females say they have had intercourse by the age of 17, whereas half of Caucasian and Hispanic American girls report having had intercourse by an only slightly older age, 18 (Michael, 1994).

Many parents worry about whether and how often their teenage sons and daughters are having sexual intercourse. This can be a concern when an adolescent has a "steady" girlfriend or boyfriend. In reality, teenagers having sexual intercourse within a single, exclusive relationship actually experience some benefits over those having intercourse with multiple partners. These individuals are far more likely to use contraception regularly than teenagers who explore their sexuality with a number of different partners (DeLameter & MacCorquodale, 1979). Additionally, young women in these relationships are much more likely to have orgasms during their sexual interactions with their steady boyfriend than are girls who have intercourse with a number of different boys. In fact, teenagers in long-term relationships who are having intercourse may in fact be far more conscientious about birth control, and the experience may be more mutually rewarding than that of their peers who are engaged in sexual activity with multiple partners or more casually or with less forethought (Fig. 12-10).

Oral-Genital Stimulation. Another common expression of sexual intimacy among teenagers is oral-genital stimulation. Fellatio and cunnilingus are common preludes to intercourse or are practiced by themselves often in this age group. In recent years much has been learned about this avenue of sexual expression among adolescents. When young people view their bodies positively and enjoy affirmative perceptions of their genitalia, they generally are more likely to engage in oral-genital stimulation and to report that they find these activities enjoyable (Reinholtz & Muehlenhard, 1995). In a study of over 2,000 urban high school students, about 10% of those who identified themselves as virgins had reported they had had oral-genital sex; this suggests that many teenagers who are not having sexual intercourse are not inactive sexually (Schuster, Bell, & Kanouse, 1996). Just as fellatio and cunnilingus are enjoyable varieties of sexual expression for adults, they are reportedly similarly practiced and enjoyed by teenagers, even those who have never had intercourse.

Outercourse. Earlier in this book we commented on sexual **outercourse,** which refers to the mutual enjoyment of a variety of sexual behaviors except for vaginal penetration. Many teens who are frightened of an unanticipated pregnancy or a sexually transmitted disease explore other ways of enjoying their eroticism with someone else. This is especially true because many adolescents are very nervous about obtaining and properly using condoms. For these reasons, many sex educators feel it is important to introduce the acceptability and advisability of non-intercourse avenues of sexual sharing (Genius & Genius, 1996). Outercourse is another form of "heavy petting," except that heavy petting frequently precedes sexual intercourse. While the parents of teenagers are typically apprehensive about their children's emerging sexuality and the various behavioral expressions it may take, they would do well to consider the possible consequences of openly criticizing *all* forms of sexual expression and experimentation (Fig. 12-11).

Issues Surrounding First Intercourse Among Adolescents

When social and behavioral scientists explore the reasons and motives for first intercourse by teenagers, several responses are consistently offered. Adolescents make a personal decision to engage in sexual intercourse when they believe they are in love,

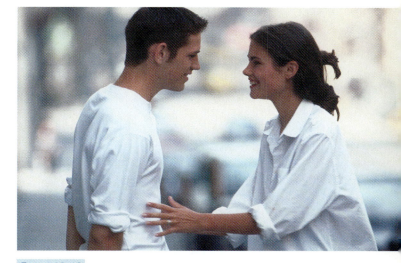

FIGURE 12-10   Teenagers in trusting, long-term, sexually exclusive relationships are far more likely to be conscientious about the use of contraceptives if they choose to share physical intimacy.

are curious and seek excitement, and enjoy feelings of sexual arousal (Traeen & Kvalem, 1996). Data suggest that emotional issues are more important to females, while physical pleasure is more important to males. In a large sample of Norwegian adolescents between the ages of 16 and 20, when asked their rea-

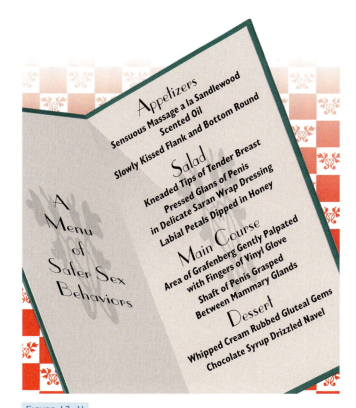

A Menu of Safer Sex Behaviors

Appetizers
Sensuous Massage a la Sandlewood Scented Oil
Slowly Kissed Flank and Bottom Round

Salad
Kneaded Tips of Tender Breast
Pressed Glans of Penis
in Delicate Saran Wrap Dressing
Labial Petals Dipped in Honey

Main Course
Area of Grafenberg Gently Palpated
with Fingers of Vinyl Glove
Shaft of Penis Grasped
Between Mammary Glands

Dessert
Whipped Cream Rubbed Gluteal Gems
Chocolate Syrup Drizzled Navel

FIGURE 12-11   There are many types of non-intercourse intimate pleasuring that do not involve the risk of sexually transmitted diseases or unanticipated pregnancies.

Other Countries, Cultures, and Customs

SEX AND ADOLESCENTS AROUND THE WORLD

Researchers have wondered whether the expressions of emerging sexuality among teenagers are unique to the customs and norms of the particular culture in which they occur, or if there are some important commonalities in sexual development among teens throughout the world. In fact, there are both similarities and differences.

In the 1950s, the cultural anthropologist David Marshall studied the people who inhabited a very remote island called Mangaia in the vast collection of Pacific islands broadly known as Polynesia. By modern Western standards, sexual development during adolescence on this island is very unusual (Marshall, 1971). For example, with puberty comes clear, direct instruction about many sexual behaviors. Both girls and boys are taught in great detail virtually everything they would need to know to begin exploring their sexuality with a healthy knowledge base of information. As a young boy's external genitalia begin to grow, a ceremony called *superincision* is held in which the skin on the dorsal side of his foreskin is cut open and retracted so that the glans of his penis is exposed. Both girls and boys are given explicit instructions about a number of different sexual techniques and positions. Boys are taught how to mouth and suck a woman's breasts, as well as perform cunnilingus. Boys learn stimulative techniques likely to precipitate orgasm in their partner, as well as to delay their ejaculation. Girls are encouraged to be active, enthusiastic sexual partners and given pointers on how to do this.

After this period of formal instruction, a period of active experimentation begins. Adolescent males engage in a practice called "night crawling," in which they leave their homes late at night and slip into the communal sleeping area of a young girl's family, seeking out the teenage daughter and having sexual intercourse with her. Other family members (perhaps more than a dozen) feign sleep but are attentive to sounds that might indicate that their daughter is enjoying the attentions of this particular young man. Both boys and girls are openly encouraged to have sexual intercourse with many partners in order to find someone with whom they feel compatible. He noted that half of all young couples marry because of an unanticipated conception and that there is an extremely high rate of births out of wedlock (over 19%). Marshall's anthropological research was carried out during the 1950s and published in 1971, but we are unaware of any more recent reports about these adolescent sexual practices since that time.

Adolescent sexual behavior has been a focus of other research as well. One study of Korean youth (Youn, 1996) indicated that the prevalence of kissing, petting, and intercourse is notably higher for boys than girls. These males also had a far larger number of partners in these three behaviors. Of those teens who were having sexual intercourse, most began at about the age of 18. In this culture the prohibitions against premarital sex are strong, and this behavior is seen as *highly* undesirable. Therefore, the subjects in this study (about 850 of them) in all likelihood significantly underreported the frequency of sexual intercourse. Despite these negative sanctions, about 23% of the boys and about 10% of the girls (average age almost 19 years) reported having had intercourse at least once, and among those who did, 37% of the males and 55% of the females noted that their most recent intercourse experience was during the last month.

Another study explored the sexual behaviors of adolescents in Malaysia in 1986 (Zulkifli, Low, & Yusof, 1995). These data were collected from 1200 adolescents between the ages of 15 and 21 in a large urban area, Kuala Lampur. Of these subjects, all but 19 people were unmarried. Among these unmarried teenagers, only 9% reported having had sexual intercourse. Older individuals were more likely to have had more, and more diverse, sexual experiences than their younger counterparts. Among the 521 youngsters who were dating, 20% had had sexual intercourse, 44% had participated in necking and kissing, and 35% reported having engaged in petting. Importantly, among those who had had intercourse, inconsistent contraceptive use was common.

sons for having sexual intercourse, the most common response was "because my partner wanted me to." In this society, if young girls do not want to have intercourse, boys won't press them. In this there may indeed be some interesting cross-cultural differences worthy of more careful study. As noted above, the desire to feel attractive, to be loved, and perhaps to exert personal control are other possible motives affecting the decision to have intercourse the first time.

Adolescents and Contraceptives

Regardless of whether teenagers get contraceptives, most will need them at one time or another. Remember that those receiving systematic, comprehensive sex education are more likely to begin their sexual experimentation later and more cautiously (Jacobs & Wolf, 1995). Chapter 11 discusses contraception in detail, but here we will look only at developmental issues involved. An interesting source of information about teenagers and contraceptive use is *Sex and American Teenagers,* published by the Alan Guttmacher Institute in 1994. This organization is a clearinghouse for information dealing with women's reproductive health issues. We here summarize information from that document. Since 1982, more teenagers use contraceptives for first intercourse. In 1982 only 23% used a condom in first intercourse, 13% used coitus interruptus, and 52% used no contraceptive method at all. However, by 1988, fully 48% used condoms during first intercourse, 8% used coitus interruptus, and 35% used nothing. This is an enormous change in only 4 years, probably prompted by concerns over HIV/AIDS. These data primarily involved teenagers between the ages of 15 and 19. We hope teenagers are getting better all the time at using contraceptives and that sex education curricula prompt even more widespread practice of these extremely important self-protective behaviors.

The bad news in the Guttmacher Institute's 1994 report was that sexually active women are waiting much too long before they consult a physician or family planning clinic for information about contraception or birth control itself. The following data describe young women between 15 and 19, based on a sample of over 3,500,000 individuals. Of this number, only about 12% saw a health care provider before or during the same month they had intercourse for the first time, while 11% did so between 1 and 3 months after their first intercourse experience. Additionally, 5% did so between 4 and 6 months, 12% between 7 and 12 months, 29% waited at least a year, and fully 31% had not sought contraceptive counseling or services at the time the survey was taken. The parents of female adolescents seem less encouraging and foresightful as they might be when it comes to thinking ahead about the possibility of their daughters becoming sexually active, and this might reflect the parents' personal uneasiness with the subject matter. While improvements in thinking proactively before first intercourse are cause for optimism, health professionals are still dismayed and perplexed about why so many young women wait so long to explore contraceptive counseling and/or alternatives.

Several factors may account for inconsistency in contraceptive usage in this unique population of young people (Fig. 12-12). Teens often assert their autonomy somewhat inconsistently over time, fail to use contraceptives they feel are inconvenient or cumbersome, and may seek peer acceptance through contraceptive negligence. Short-term relationships with several different partners keep the social scene fluid and, therefore, less predictable. These factors contribute to less than perfect contraceptive compliance and to a large number of unanticipated pregnancies.

Finally, an important aspect of the psychosocial environment involves the influence of parents and caretakers. This chapter begins with an overview of social learning theory and the importance of observing the behavior of others and learning from their actions, or vicarious learning. We learn by paying attention to what happens to other people when they behave in certain ways. Social learning theory does not seem able to help explain why adolescents do or do not use caution in their use of contraception. Birth control, after all, is not something you actually *see other people do.* You pay attention instead to what they say or imply. We really know very little about the way teenagers talk to one another about sex, much less important an issue than birth control. The same issue is involved in the impact of a parent's pronouncements about sex and contraception: adolescents do not generally see their mothers, fathers, or significant others us-

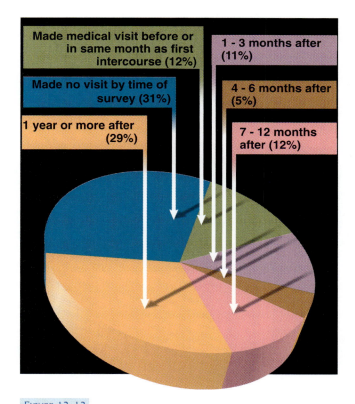

FIGURE 12-12 Despite access to contraception among adolescent and young adult females in the United States, there are still substantial delays in seeking birth control and counseling.

ing or discussing birth control. In fact, most social and behavioral science theories have not proved very useful for predicting who will or won't be careful about birth control alternatives or explore contraceptive counseling. A more fruitful theory is needed to guide investigations in this area.

Teenage Pregnancy

The United States has the highest rate of teen pregnancy among developed countries in the world. In a nation with the health care resources we enjoy, how could this happen? What is happening here that causes 1,000,000 unintended teen pregnancies each year? Scholars of human sexuality emphasize that this estimate of one million unintended teen pregnancies per year is actually low. There is no simple answer to this question, and no simple way to address the problem. Regardless of how one feels about teenagers having sex, or feeling or thinking sexually, about this there is no disagreement: this is a very big problem. It is an expensive problem, as well as one that affects lives, families, and futures. We have already examined some of the reasons why teenagers have sexual intercourse, and a large number of diverse reasons are involved. Yet why does the United States have the highest rate of teenage pregnancy among the developed nations of the world? Following are just some of the factors discussed over the last few chapters.

Very Often, Inadequate Information About Sex is Presented in the Home. Temperamental, religious, and intellectual factors affect what parents talk to their children about, when, and how specifically.

Family Life Education Programs in the Schools are Often Inadequate. Without authoritative information about sex at home, school is a reasonable place to expect solid facts and guidance to be given about sexual feelings, behaviors, and risks. As has already been noted, this does not always happen. For the most part, family life education courses are incomplete in content and make no pretense of discussing feelings and apprehensions that may be involved in adolescent sex.

The Peer Group Is an Untrustworthy Source of Information About Sex. The only thing worse than a teenager being sexually uninformed is a group of uninformed teenagers who are together frequently. Myth and misinformation are common in adolescent conversations about sex. For example, it is not uncommon for teens to tell one another that they can't get pregnant if they have intercourse in the middle of their menstrual cycle—the very time of highest fertility.

Planning to Behave Responsibly Is "Planning to Be Evil." Teenagers who are foresightful about contraception are often made to feel guilty, bad, or "dirty" if they plan to take precautions to avoid pregnancy or STDs.

Teenagers May Not Feel That Contraceptives Are Available. The fact that condoms, vaginal suppositories, films, and foams are available over-the-counter does not mean that people who need them find them easy to purchase. Often a feeling of guilt or stigma is attached to being seen buying these items. And who can ever tell who's watching. . . .

Peer Pressure Is Powerful. No one wants to feel odd or different from their friends. Teens dress, talk, and "hang out" in the same ways. Their alcohol and drug use patterns are plainly influenced by peer pressure and so is resistance to authority, academic motivation, and the perceived need to "prove oneself" sexually. Feeling alone and isolated is particularly painful for teens, and if having sex and talking about it makes one popular and important, then that indeed will often happen.

What are the consequences of teenage pregnancy? The Guttmacher Institute (1994) provides a sobering look at this subject. Teenage women (ages 15–19) who are sexually active and do not use contraception have a 90% chance of becoming pregnant over the course of one year. The phrase "sexually active" is hard to define precisely because intercourse is often impulsive and/or unplanned among adolescents, and there is no set number of acts of intercourse per week or month that define one as being "sexually active." The pregnancy rate rises to 95% for young women between the ages of 20 and 24, and returns again to 90% for women between 25 and 29. The younger the adolescent, however, the more likely it is that she will become pregnant and have her baby without being married. In fact, 81% of first births among teenagers between 15 and 19 take place among unmarried girls, while the comparable figure is 59% for females between 18 and 19, and 27% for women between 20 and 24.

Most people who have babies say that they want the "best possible life" for their child. Yet the median family income is quite low for teenagers who had their babies when they were under 19 and started a family. There is a clear relationship between age at the birth of a first child and the subsequent economic well-being of the family with the child. The Guttmacher Institute has reported median family income levels according to the age of a woman at the time of the birth of her first child. If a woman has her first baby when she is 19 or younger, her median family income will be approximately $17,600. However, if she is between 20 and 24, the comparable figure rises to $24,000, and if she is 25 or older the median income is $36,400 (Fig. 12-13). Although these data were compiled with 1987 data and the raw numbers may have increased since, the trend is clear and there is little reason to think the income differences according to age have changed substantially since. Although the term "family" is somewhat imprecise and may involve a single mother, a young married mother, being part-time or full-time employed, and so on, regardless of how the term "family income" is defined, the data related to the consequences of teen pregnancy are not hopeful.

We already noted that the United States has the highest teen pregnancy rate in the developed world. The Guttmacher Institute report reveals 97 out of every 1000 15–19-year-old women in the United States become pregnant each year—roughly 1 in every 10 girls in this age group. The comparable figure in England and Wales is only 46, and the figure is only 10 in the Netherlands and Japan. Sweden, Denmark, and Finland have rates between 25 and 35. The problem in the U.S. clearly has not been solved by any amount of threat, humiliation, or restrictiveness. Clearly, those nations who give serious, systematic family life education early in elementary school and present age-appropriate sexual subjects throughout adoles-

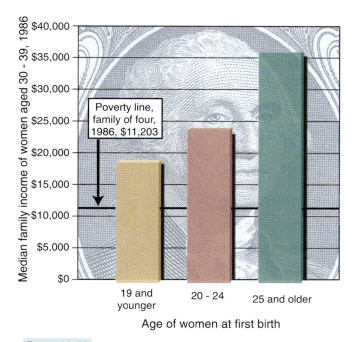

FIGURE 12-13   The age of a woman at the birth of her first child may have an enormous effect on her subsequent median family income.

cence have teen pregnancy rates *far lower* than the United States, in some cases, only 10% of our rate. However, it would be simplistic to suggest that sex education alone *causes* a lower rate of teen pregnancy without examining the impact of other variables, such as the availability of contraception and broader cultural attitudes about adolescent sexuality.

What happens to the 1,000,000 teenage girls who become pregnant each year? Of this number there are approximately 428,000 abortions, 288,000 out-of-marriage births, 142,000 marriages (most of which will not last 5 years), and 142,000 miscarriages. The miscarriage rate is so high because teenage girls are *4 to 5 times more likely to have pregnancy complications* than women in their 20s. Some sex experts describe teen pregnancy as "babies having babies" because adolescent women are still growing and developing and are not yet physiologically mature adults. What happens to the babies? Guttmacher Institute data (1994) indicate that 87% of teenagers who have their baby will keep it. Only 8% give it up for formal, legally binding adoption, and 5% place their child informally with someone in their extended family: a parent, a grandparent, or even an older sibling. Teenage motherhood profoundly affects young women. Approximately 80% of these women will drop out of school, 90% are unemployed during the year after giving birth, and 72% receive some form of public assistance.

In the past decade there have been signs that teenagers are becoming more foresightful in anticipating their first intercourse experiences and preparing for them. In the late 1970s, about 47% of teens used some form of birth control during first intercourse, and this figure rose to 65% by the late 1980s (Mosher & McNally, 1991). In most cases, this involved the use of condoms, but many more youngsters began using the pill as well. Coitus interruptus was still a common method of birth control during first intercourse, despite the fact that it doesn't work very well. This is certainly an issue that should be addressed in all family life education programs.

Sexually Transmitted Diseases in Adolescence

A later chapter examines sexually transmitted diseases in depth, but here we would like to comment about the special pertinence of STDs to teenagers. A key issue involves why teenagers are so vulnerable to getting and transmitting STDs. One reason is that age-appropriate information about STDs is not often conveyed clearly, completely, and nonjudgmentally. The mere thought of contracting an STD is so terrible that most teens simply suppress the thought, "tune out," or ignore the risk altogether. After all, most adolescents genuinely believe that only "bad" people get "bad" diseases, and accepting that they might get such a disease would be just too painful. Threats of terrible diseases resulting from sexual behaviors does *not change adolescents' behaviors for very long, if at all.* Fear rarely motivates enduring behavioral changes. Social-learning theory predicts that observing the consequences of STDs among their peers would be far more important and influential in modifying their behavior than adults trying to scare them. Just as many teenagers are pregnant for a long time before they tell anyone, many teenagers have STDs (knowingly or unknowingly) for a long period of time before they seek treatment. Even then, they often don't know where to turn.

What makes adolescents especially vulnerable to getting or transmitting STDs? There are a number of different reasons.

Delusions of Invincibility. A delusion is a false belief but one that is often held tenaciously. **Delusions of invincibility** are the false belief that bad things only happen to other people, never to oneself. Bad things happen to poor people, people of another race, people with less (or more) education, people who live in another part of the city, or people who are careless or just plain unlucky. " But not to me. I'm special." For example, people who neglect to put on their seat belt while driving often truly believe that because they are a good, careful driver, nothing bad could possibly happen to them. These false beliefs contribute to teenagers' negligence about both contraception and genuine risks of contracting STDs.

Poor Understanding of Irrevocable Acts. Growing up includes learning that all problems can't be solved, all mistakes can't be fixed, and all painful, embarrassing situations can't be remedied. Sometimes we're just stuck with a bad situation, can't make it better, and have to live with its consequences. Sometimes this is true for a little while, sometimes for the rest of our lives. Teenagers often believe that an STD can be easily and painlessly remedied, but at some point they learn that this is not always possible.

Teenagers who have a good understanding of the symptoms of different STDs are in a better position to seek effective medical treatment promptly. For example, 7 out of 10 women with the most common STDs, chlamydia and gonorrhea, will have no obvious symptoms at all in the early stages of these in-

Other Countries, Cultures, and Customs

SEXUAL BEHAVIOR AMONG AMERICAN INDIAN FEMALE ADOLESCENTS

One of the important themes of this book is that sexual behavior is most meaningfully viewed within its broader psychosocial context. Personal factors, family expectations, and community standards all powerfully affect sexual exploration among teenagers in all societies. The sexual behaviors of female adolescent Native Americans, one of the most important subcultures in American society, have been studied only recently (Murry & Ponzetti, 1997). Slemenda (1978), in studying young Navajo women, found that many held a traditional attitude toward sexuality in which pregnancy is seen as a healthy, normal part of adult life and should be accepted as such. Those who used contraception had assimilated more fully contemporary American social mores and expectations. Additionally, young traditional Native American women perceive sexual behavior as equivalent to entering a committed, sexually exclusive relationship (Attneave, 1982). However, many young assimilated Native American males do not have similar beliefs about the permanence and importance of this commitment. Some Native Americans live in a culture with explicit collectivistic goals, thereby minimizing individual tastes and preferences. Among the Omahas, for example, high fertility rates and large families are thought to help perpetuate tribal values and customs.

One recent study (Murry & Ponzetti, 1997) based on information from 130 young women has shown that on average, Native American adolescent females are about 12 years old at menarche and, on average, have sexual intercourse for the first time when they are 15. Most begin dating shortly after their 16th birthday, and the average age at which a significant portion of the sample (42%) first become pregnant is 16.4 years. Although this age may seem unusual to some, these researchers emphasize that often our opinions about what "should" happen during adolescent sexual development are affected by white, middle-class values, such as the idea that intercourse is "supposed" to happen within the context of a committed, loving relationship. Among the women in this sample, however, a steady dating relationship was not seen as a prerequisite for sexual intercourse (Murry & Ponzetti, 1997, p. 82).

For most of these young women, the family was an important socializing agent for learning about sexual issues. For example, 70% reported that their parents shared sexual information with them regarding how pregnancy occurs, 65% received information about menstruation, 34% were taught about a variety of contraceptive alternatives, and 39% received information about STDs. Most of these subjects also received information about sex in family life education courses in school. In all, these findings illuminate the sexual development and behavior of a significant subculture in our country.

---

fections: no pain, discharge, or lesions. A woman harboring one of these STDs without knowing it can also transmit it unknowingly. Further, if the woman delays treatment for a long time, scarring of the fallopian tubes may occur, which can render her sterile. Knowledge about STDs is, therefore, important if teens are to recognize and act on the earliest symptoms. Teens and adults both should realize that if they are sexually active and have had unprotected intercourse with a number of partners, they should see a health professional for a checkup for STDs—as well as begin using protection.

Promiscuity and the Double Standard

The word "promiscuous" has negative connotations. Very conservative people often view anyone who has premarital intercourse as promiscuous, although the word means different things to others. As we use the term here, promiscuous behavior has three fundamental elements. It typically involves nonselective sexual intercourse with several or many other people. Second, these encounters do not often involve foresightful planning about contraception or the avoidance of STDs. Indeed, promiscuity often involves high-risk sexual behaviors. Third, the person rarely feels any emotional attachment, affection, or love associated with sexual intercourse with these multiple partners.

Social and behavioral scientists cannot state with certainty why some adolescents become sexually promiscuous; probably there are many reasons. It is difficult to examine this issue apart from high-risk sexual behaviors, other problem behaviors (such as alcohol and substance abuse), and the psychosocial context of the adolescent's life (Biglan, Meltzer, Wirt, Ary, Noell, Ochs, French, & Hood, 1990). Because adolescence is a time of emerging sexuality, adults often believe that teenagers are more promiscuous than they actually are. Still, few teens today believe that two people have to be married to each other for sexual intercourse to be "right." Most teenagers believe in the notion of "permissiveness with affection" (Reiss, 1960). In other words, when two people feel and express genuine affection and mutual respect for each other, adding a sexual dimension to their relationship feels normal and appropriate. Different people have different personal criteria for just how much "affection and mutual respect" is involved, but only rarely do adolescents favor sex without affection.

Teenage sexual intercourse takes place within the wider context of the youngster's whole life, however. For example, promiscuous sexual behavior is frequently associated with antisocial behaviors, cigarette smoking, and the use of illegal drugs and alcohol. These factors also predict nonuse of condoms among teenagers (Biglan, Meltzer, Wirt, Ary, Noell, Ochs, French, & Hood, 1990).

In this context, as in other contexts we have discussed, there is a sexual double standard, an unwritten assumption that different expectations apply to females and males for what is "right" or "appropriate" sexual behavior. Historically, society has been far more accepting (if not openly encouraging) of sexual behavior by adolescent boys than by adolescent girls. Boys are supposed to "sow their wild oats," while girls are supposed to "save themselves for marriage." That's clearly a double standard. The fact that promiscuity has traditionally been attributed to females more than to males tends to hold females more accountable for sexual activity and may diminish the role males

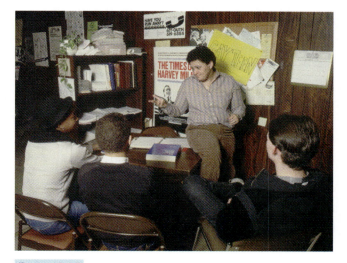

FIGURE 12-15 For gay and lesbian teenagers, peer support and acceptance can make coming out and developing one's identity a more comfortable process.

play in sexual activity, as well as its consequences (Dankoski, Payer, & Steinberg, 1996) (Fig. 12-14). This double standard began to decline in the late 1970s, and today most girls and boys do not believe in different "appropriateness" of sexual behavior for the sexes before (and after) marriage (Ferrell, Tolone, & Walsh, 1977). In fact, an important study supports the idea that teenagers are *not promiscuous*. Zelnick, Kantner, and Ford (1981) carried out a national study and found that most adolescents who had sexual intercourse had only a single partner, and only 10% reported having three or more partners.

Emerging Homosexual Identities in Adolescence

The earlier chapter on homosexuality discussed some of the unique challenges facing homosexual teenagers and young adults as they try to come to terms with their sexual orientation and "come out" to their friends and families. Two very stressful developmental challenges face gay and lesbian teenagers: the importance of acknowledging their sexual orientation on one hand, and the significance of developing an individual sense of identity at the same time, which is a central challenge of being an adolescent. For gay teens, these two tasks are virtually impossible to separate from one another (Fig. 12-15). Earlier we cited the work of Radowsky and Siegel (1997) that found that socially stigmatizing gay teenagers is highly likely to disrupt their development of a sense of identity and a solid feeling of self-esteem. They concluded that personal relationships with peers and family members are likely to be adversely affected because of this. As a consequence, gay teens are especially prone to depression, loneliness, and feelings of isolation. They may

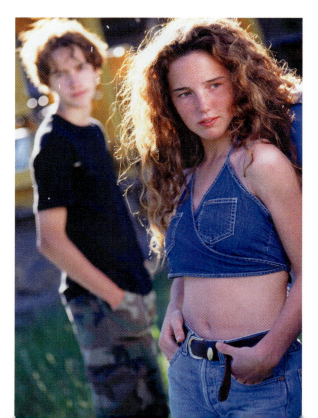

FIGURE 12-14 Since the late 1970s, the sexual double standard among adolescents has declined. Teenagers today are likely to make sexual decisions without regard to historical social conventions for females and males.

also be more likely to contract AIDS and commit suicide, according to these writers. Working to develop a sense of oneself and come to terms with one's homosexuality is certainly an enormous task, especially among youngsters who may not be very mature to begin with. Other writers have also reported that lesbian, gay, and bisexual young people are at an increased risk for the development of physical, emotional, and social problems (Kreiss & Patterson, 1997). In addition to the problems outlined by Radowsky and Siegel, substance abuse, sexually transmitted diseases, problems in school performance, being rejected by their families, and homelessness occur far more often than among heterosexual adolescents. Faulkner and Cranston (1998) also report that high school students who have engaged in homosexual acts are more likely to fight, to be victimized by physical violence, to use alcohol often, to explore illicit recreational drugs, and to attempt suicide.

One of the most important factors for gay and lesbian teens dealing with these developmental and sexual orientation challenges is family support. When mothers and fathers first find out that their daughter or son is gay, they often abruptly withdraw their support, and when that happens very little productive communication can occur. In such cases, professional assistance can often be very helpful in getting everyone's thoughts and feelings out in the open where they can be shared, discussed, and perhaps even resolved agreeably (Saltzburg, 1996). Coming out takes place in a wider psychosocial setting, and the family is a key mediator of society's expectations and judgments. Psychological intervention may be an excellent starting point for the disclosure and resolution of these difficult developmental challenges. In addition, one writer has suggested that school nurses may play an important role in preventing verbal harassment and physical violence directed at gay and lesbian students (Adams, 1997). Preventing these problems in the setting in which they are most likely to occur makes good sense.

Even an institution as conservative about homosexuality as the Roman Catholic Church has acknowledged the difficulties of being an adolescent beset with same-sex feelings and inclinations. A pastoral letter from the U. S. bishops titled "Always Our Children" asks mothers and fathers of gay children to avoid all moral condemnation and instead be supportive, loving, and tolerant (Allen, 1997). The bishops' belief is that the Catholic community could be more "welcoming and sensitive" than it has been. While the clergy clearly do not support homosexual lifestyles or rule out the possible effectiveness of therapy in changing a person's sexual orientation, their plea is for more tolerance and love and improved parent-child relationships. This accepting spiritual perspective could be extremely helpful for many teenagers with religious values.

CONCLUSION

This chapter has covered a broad range of topics. Although adolescents are usually thought of as emerging sexual beings, sensual pleasure has a role also in infant and child development. The goal here has been to describe and explain sexual development and the factors that enhance or inhibit its normal progression. Biological change over time is intricately interrelated with the wider psychosocial environment in which biological development occurs. This chapter has explored what it means to be a "sexual being" from the time we are born, and the relationships among self-esteem, body-image, and sexual behavior throughout adolescence.

The next chapter continues the discussion of sexual development throughout the life span, focusing on the young adult and adult years and then on sexuality in later life. This discussion of sexuality will explore the context of an intimate relationship that is psychologically mature.

Learning Activities

1. Now that you have read a summary of Freud's psychoanalytic approach and his psychosexual theory in particular, speculate on why people frequently criticize Freud's approach to development.

2. Social-learning theory maintains that we often try to imitate the behavior of other people, especially those whom we perceive to be competent, attractive, and effective. Do you think people commonly learn about sexual behavior by watching sexual scenes in movies or videos?

3. You and your partner are having a quiet, informal dinner with friends when your five-year-old daughter comes in to kiss you good-night and asks, "Mommy, what's a penis?" What do you do?

4. People are raised in different environments with different attitudes about the appropriateness of nudity in the home. Some parents and siblings are quite open and comfortable about being undressed, while others grow up in homes with great secretiveness about nudity. What were your own experiences about nudity in the home while you were a child? Would you create a home environment any different than the one you came from in this regard? Why or why not?

5. Many people grow up in homes in which parental conflict, or even abuse, is a consistent aspect of the domestic setting. Describe how this might affect a child's perceptions of the opposite sex and later inclinations to become involved in a "serious" relationship. Is there any aspect of your current relationship that reminds you of something unpleasant in your family of origin? If so, what is it?

6. This chapter offers a few guidelines for talking with children and teenagers about sex in a "best case" scenario. What role did your parent or parents play in your learning about sex? Did they make you feel comfortable or uncomfortable? Did they tell you too much or too little?

7. Children frequently engage in "sex play" or otherwise express their sexual curiosity. Did you as a child participate in any of these activities with same-age youngsters? If so, do you feel that the experience had any long-term harmful effects (or benefits) for you?

8. Try to remember your thoughts and feelings when you first realized you had reached puberty. Did you feel especially self-conscious? Did you attempt to conceal your physical changes?

9. As teenagers begin sexual exploration, they generally experience an unwritten, mutually understood sequence of progressively more physical, intimate behaviors, culminating in sexual intercourse. The first gestures have in the past been referred to as "getting to first base." Continuing with this baseball metaphor, try to articulate your understanding of "first base," "second base," "third base," etc.

10. If you were to design a sex education curriculum for high school students, what topics would you present and at which grade levels? In your opinion, are there any sexual issues high school freshmen are just not ready for?

11. Effective contraception is a shared responsibility between a man and a woman. Describe ways in which adolescents can together obtain and use different contraceptives. Why do many adolescent boys commonly say that birth control is the girl's responsibility?

13. Describe what it means to have a "good reputation" in terms of one's sexual behavior, and similarly, what it means to have a "bad reputation." Do you think that one's reputation is an accurate reflection of one's behaviors, or only the actions others *think* one is engaging in?

ℋey Concepts

- Freud's notion of determinism implies that all adult thinking, emotions, and behaviors are set as a result of infantile and childhood experiences.
- Freud used the term sexuality in the same way we use the term sensuality today.
- According to psychoanalytic theory, libido is a basic, primitive motivational force in the personality.
- Erogenous zones are areas of our bodies in which libido is invested as we grow up. Stimulation of erogenous zones yields keenly sensual pleasures.
- If, in the course of growing up, an infant's or a child's erogenous zones are not completely and consistently stimulated, the individual may become fixated at that stage and try to symbolically re-create the pleasures experienced at an earlier time.
- Freud's psychosexual theory of development claims that infants and children go through five successive stages as they grow up: the oral, anal, phallic, latency, and genital stages. Each of the stages except for the latency stage has a primary erogenous zone associated with it.
- For social learning theorists, feelings of competence and control in our lives, known as self-efficacy, are extremely important in human growth and development.
- Children who gradually develop a sense of pleasure, interest, and enjoyment in sexual feelings and behavior acquire

erotophilia. In contrast, children who learn to associate sexual feelings with pain, coercion, or humiliation develop erotophobia.

- The subconscious desire to become like someone whom we love, admire, and respect is known as identification. In contrast, complementation refers to the ways in which children make purposeful attempts to understand not only their own sex roles, but also those of members of the opposite sex.
- In adolescence, for the first time in the lifespan there is an important connection between self-esteem and body image.
- Exploratory sexual behaviors among adolescents occur for a number of reasons that reflect family values, peer-group expectations, self-esteem, and social norms.
- Whether or not adolescents receive contraceptives and/or contraceptive counseling, they will need them.
- Fear of illness and embarrassment are typically not sufficient to change an adolescent's behavior with respect to being involved in an unanticipated pregnancy or contracting a sexually transmitted disease.
- Gay teenagers have special challenges of trying to be honest with themselves about their identity and at the same time appear to be "just like everyone else."
- Promiscuity involves nonselective sexual intercourse with several or many other people. These encounters do not often involve foresightful planning about contraception or the avoidance of STDs. There is rarely any feeling of emotional attachment, affection, or love associated with sexual intercourse with these multiple partners.

𝒢lossary Terms

delusions of invincibility	identification	psychosocial theory
Erikson's psychosocial theory of development	outercourse	puberty
	psychoanalytic theory	social-learning theory

𝒮uggested Readings

Gravelle, K., & Gravelle, J. (1996). *The period book. Everything you don't want to ask (but need to know).* New York: Walker and Company.

Harris, R. H. (1994). *It's perfectly normal.* Cambridge, MA: Candlewick Press.

McCoy, K., & Wibbelsman, C. (1992). *The new teenage body book.* New York: The Body Press / Perigee Books.

Meredith, S. (1985). *Understanding the facts of life.* London: Usborne Publishing Ltd.

Roberts, E. (Ed.) (1997). *Am I the last virgin? Ten African American reflections on sex and love.* New York: Aladdin Paperbacks.

Westheimer, R. (1998). *Dr. Ruth talks to kids.* New York: Aladdin Paperbacks.

13

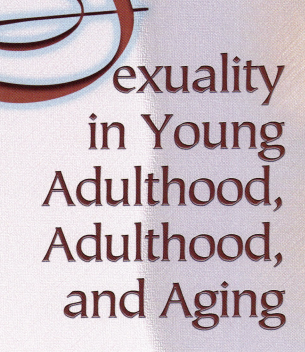

Sexuality in Young Adulthood, Adulthood, and Aging

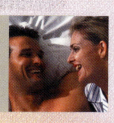

OBJECTIVES

When you finish reading and reviewing this chapter, you should be able to:

1. Discuss the major developmental psychosocial challenges of youth and adulthood according to Erik Erikson, and note the role of intimacy in each.

2. Describe the basic assumptions of sexual strategies theory, and speculate on the evolution of social strategies that create permanence and protection for females and tacit approval of wide sexual experience among men.

3. List the stages in the Sarrels' theory of sexual and intimacy changes through the adult years.

4. Describe the nature of sexual interaction during the early years of a committed relationship, and discuss the attributes of relationships that last a long time.

5. Summarize the reasons people have extramarital affairs, and explain patterns of infidelity among men and women.

6. Discuss myths surrounding sexual expression in later life, critically evaluating each.

7. Discuss the role of continued sexual behavior within the context of Erikson's stage of *integrity versus despair*.

8. Define "climacteric" and discuss its most obvious manifestations in women and men.

9. Summarize the hormonal and physiological changes that accompany menopause in women and describe how women might cope with these.

10. State the benefits and risks associated with hormone replacement therapy for the symptoms of menopause.

11. Review the physiosexual changes in later life for women and men and how they affect each stage of the sexual response cycle.

12. Summarize some the of special challenges facing gay and lesbian older individuals.

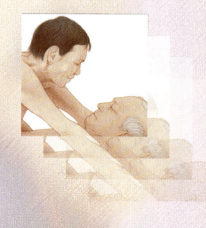

From Dr. Ruth

Some people imagine marriage as a blissful state starting with the romantic haze of the wedding day and continuing as a series of slow-motion embraces against a backdrop of gorgeous sunsets. But if these people examined the marriages around them, they'd have a better grasp of what marriage is really like and realize that the average couple spends a lot more time in slippers and curlers than in tuxes and gowns.

But isn't it better to be an incurable romantic? I like being an optimist, but I also know that if two people enter a relationship with unreasonable expectations, the odds are they're more likely to become disappointed by the truth than to keep their romantic vision. A little realism is required in a successful long-term relationship because none of us is perfect, and there is no such thing as the perfect marriage. But a perfect world would probably be very boring, and it's the differences among us, even the little defects that we all have, that make life, and marriage, interesting.

The same thing is true about sex. Some who have never engaged in sex with another person expect it will be like what they see in the movies. The lighting will be perfect, the sheets silky, and when that orgasm comes, the earth will move. To those of you who hold this fantasy, I'm sorry to be the bearer of disappointing news, but it's not going to be that way. In fact, the first few times you make love with someone, the level of enjoyment may be rather low. This is more often true for women, since there is a good chance at first that they will not experience an orgasm. But don't be disappointed if fireworks don't go off the first time you make love. Take hope from the fact that as your relationship develops, as you both learn what pleases the other, sex can improve significantly and become something you can continue to enjoy together until you are in your 90s.

As you read this chapter, think about how these issues of adult sexuality relate to your own life. If you're still wearing rose-colored glasses, take them off and have a fresh look around you. If you have idealized expectations about your perfect mate, consider how they may be affecting your relationship. If you are single and someone proposes cohabitation or marriage to you, imagine what your response might be and why you'd give that answer. Love and sex are such emotional issues that we all may have problems dealing with the reality of our situations. So as you study the information in this chapter, take some time to reflect on how these ideas relate to you and how you might make some positive changes in your present or future relationship.

Until a few decades ago, many social and behavioral scientists considered adulthood as a relatively stable, uneventful time of life with few predictable choices, changes, and challenges. But we now know that this is by no means the case. As Erik Erikson (1968) (Fig. 13-1) pointed out, there are key challenges in being an adult.

ERIKSON'S THEORY OF LIFELONG DEVELOPMENT

In Erikson's theory, as we enter early adulthood, our main psychosocial challenge is one of intimacy versus isolation. This is often the first time in our lives that we try to make a firm com-

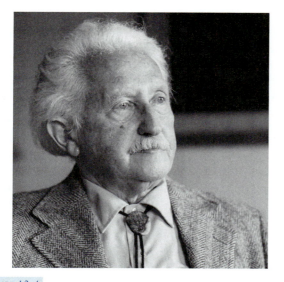

FIGURE 13-1   Erik H. Erikson (1902–1994). Erikson's theory of human growth and development emphasizes the impact of the psychosocial environment throughout the lifespan.

mitment to another person in an open, honest, loving relationship, and sexuality is often an element of this commitment. It is important that we do not feel that we have to change to please the other person, nor do we expect them to change to please us. It is widely believed that when a person has the ability and inclination to do this, he or she has left adolescence behind and has embarked upon the journey of early adulthood. This challenge often involves frustrations and disappointments, however. Erikson believed that when we have not yet cultivated the capacity for true intimacy we might feel alone, isolated, and self-absorbed. We might not be unhappy, but real equality in a relationship still eludes us. In particular, we do not yet understand what it really means to love another person or feel unconditionally loved by that person.

An optimistic aspect of Erikson's theory is that experiencing unhappy developmental outcomes at one stage in life doesn't necessarily mean that things will continue badly. Each stage presents its own risks and challenges for personal development and growth. When development is positive and productive in the intimacy versus isolation stage, we have cultivated a capacity for real, reciprocal love of another person and accept and respect them as they are.

Middle adulthood involves still another psychosocial challenge: generativity versus stagnation. As in other stages in Erikson's theory, these two terms represent a continuum rather than an "either-or" situation. It is not always clear exactly when middle adulthood begins. Some theorists (Levinson, 1978) believe that the mid-40s are the transition between early and middle adulthood, although there is no clear-cut line between these stages. Middle adulthood involves still another set of life choices and sometimes a need to rethink the usefulness of some of our values. Some people change jobs, divorce, remarry, or perhaps start another family at this stage. Mature adulthood involves exploring how to leave the world a better place than we found it.

Generativity involves efforts to help guide the generation that follows us, and there are many ways in which to do this. Having children and raising them well and lovingly is one, as are developing relationships in our jobs or professions. Teaching, social work, and other professional or volunteer activities offer the opportunity to be generative. While Erikson believed that generativity was the hallmark of healthy mid-life development, this is just one theorist's perception. and there are other ways also to experience positive development at this time in life.

Generative behaviors are characterized by altruism, generosity, and an authentic concern for the future of humankind. Generative adults are not self-absorbed. They are capable of real dedication and commitment to other people (Fig. 13-2).

A less attractive scenario occurs when a person does not develop a capacity for caring about the future or their children's tomorrows. Erikson calls this "stagnation." Sometimes, perhaps unfortunately, people are concerned only with themselves, and generosity, charity, and nurturance are lacking in their interactions with others. Words such as "selfish" and "narcissistic" are used to describe such individuals. The quality of a relationship with an intimate, generative person is quite different from that with an isolated, stagnant person.

HOW AND WHY PEOPLE GET TOGETHER

Most adults in virtually all cultures establish a long-term relationship with another person at some time in their lives, usually after adolescence. Several factors are involved in how peo-

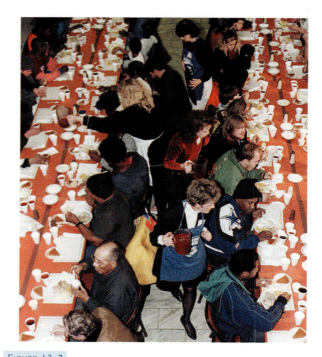

FIGURE 13-2   Generative adults are committed to the health and welfare of others. Here, a number of people volunteer at a shelter for the homeless.

ple perceive one another as appropriate and potential mates, as discussed in the following sections.

Assortative Mating

Assortative mating refers to the pairing of individuals based on similar characteristics (Buss, 1988). This means real similarity, not just how they think they might be alike. Opposites do not really attract, at least not for very long. Sexual attraction has a role in assortative mating, but in fact much more is also involved. Many demographic, social, psychological, and physical issues play a part in what evolutionary biologists call "pair bonding."

Much of the sexual experimentation that begins in adolescence develops into more consistent, longer-lasting, and often more nurturant relationships. Demographic and psychosocial issues often predict who finds whom interesting as relationships develop.

Age is a basic aspect of assortative grouping (Fig. 13-3). Other powerful predictors of who is appropriate for meaningful interpersonal relationships might include race, religion, ethnic background, socioeconomic status, and simple physical proximity; these are the obvious predictors of compatibility, according to Buss (1994). Subjective, interpersonal qualities are also highly important as people explore compatibility in relationships. For example, when asked what they seek in inti-

mate relationships, the characteristic that most college students list first is "kindness and understanding," with "intelligence," "exciting personality," "good health," and "adaptability" following in order of importance. When most young adults enter a meaningful interpersonal relationship in which sexuality is likely to be an important aspect, many attributes other than physical and sexual ones are important.

Physical attractiveness is also a significant factor predicting one's interest in another person, although even this situation is not simple. Although attractiveness is a great attention-getter, it is not always the best predictor of the success of a relationship— how rewarding the relationship is for two people. Simply put, attractiveness helps get a relationship off the ground but is less important in keeping it going. Psychologists sometimes use the term "functional autonomy" to describe how motives for behaviors change over time. The reasons we start doing something are often very different from the reasons we continue doing them. One of the best predictors of the enjoyment two people take in each other's company early in a relationship is the amount of time they spend together. This is largely determined by how near they are to each other. The term "propinquity" describes this proximity or closeness, as well as the frequency with which people interact socially. Although some elements of assortative mating may seem obvious, the importance of this issue has been established systematically and empirically.

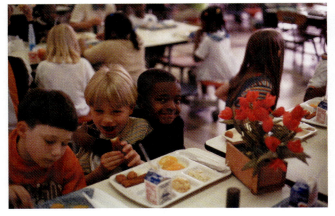

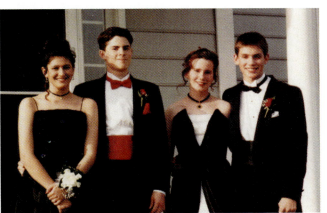

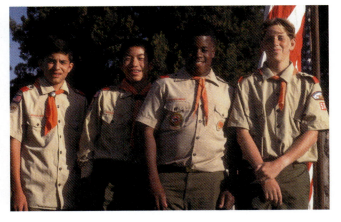

FIGURE 13-3 Our society creates many institutions in which children, adolescents, and young adults participate in groups with others of similar age. Potential partners for long-term relationships frequently meet in these groups.

Many of the topics in this chapter (marriage, extramarital relationships, divorce) will demonstrate the long-term implications of the fact that relationships often become very different from the way they began. This raises some very challenging questions for an individual's quality of life.

Courtship and Sexual Strategies Theory

Sociobiology (sometimes called evolutionary psychology) tries to explain the degree to which social behavior might be genetically determined and, therefore, influenced by the long, gradual process of evolution. Physical attributes are clearly affected by genetics, but the impact of genetics on social behavior also has intriguing implications for how and why people initiate and maintain long-term interpersonal relationships.

One way of thinking about how social behaviors evolve is to assume that genes have one key purpose: to get themselves into the next generation. Sociobiologists suggest that a variety of human social interactions serve the purpose of gene perpetuation. Interestingly, but not surprisingly, in this view women and men would have different goals in sexual interactions because they do not have the same thing at stake in the pregnancy and childbirth that might result from their union. Dawkins (1978) suggests that in this respect there is only one important difference between women and men: women have very few available fertilizable ova and men have very many sperm. Although a woman has far fewer chances in her lifetime to procreate and get her genes into the next generation, a man has no such limitations.

The implications of this simple difference are enormous. It may be the basic reason that women are generally far choosier about sexual interactions than men. With women having fewer opportunities for procreation but having to meet all the metabolic and physiological needs (and costs) of pregnancy and childbirth, a woman would do well to try to be sure that the man with whom she conceives a child will stay around to help provide for and protect the child and thereby enhance her opportunity to pass along her genes (Fig. 13-4). Men in contrast have no biological reason for selectivity or choosiness, beyond an attraction to younger (presumably fertile) women.

The sociobiological perspective offers an interesting explanation for an apparent difference between women and men in their readiness to engage in sexual behavior. Because evolutionary change takes place over very long time periods, it remains to be seen how the availability of convenient, reliable contraception may affect this situation. Apparently, courtship emerged in human civilizations to give females and their families an opportunity to evaluate a prospective mate as a provider and protector.

Although monogamy is recognized as a marital virtue in many societies, much has been written about whether humans are really "meant" to choose and stay with just one individual for their entire lives. The prevalence of sexual experimentation in adolescence and young adulthood and the common incidence of extramarital sexual affairs are good reasons to ask this question. Might there be genetic "biases" or "influences" that subtly make the prospect of multiple sexual partners attractive? Even if there is such a powerful biological imperative, equally powerful ethical, moral, and religious traditions have developed to oppose it.

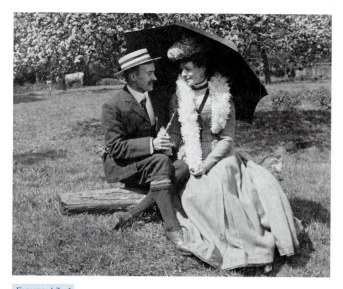

FIGURE 13-4   Courtship has always been a time when two people evaluate one another as potential spouses and assess the personality, potential, and priorities of the person they plan to live with for the rest of their lives.

Buss summarized much of thinking on this topic in *The Evolution of Desire* (1994) and in an excellent scholarly review article (Buss & Schmitt, 1993). He explains several hypotheses about **sexual strategies theory.** We present their hypotheses here to suggest how evolutionary, genetic, and psychological factors all may influence how people think about appropriate mates.

Hypothesis 1: Because of minimum parental investment incurred by men, short-term mating will represent a larger component of men's sexual strategy than of women's sexual strategy.

Hypothesis 2: Men have evolved a sexual psychology of short-term mating such that preferences for short-term mates will solve the problem of identifying which women are sexually accessible. Signs of promiscuity or sexual experience in women are valued by men interested in short-term but not long-term mates.

Hypothesis 3: Men have evolved a distinct sexual psychology of short-term mating such that preferences for short-term mates will solve, in part, the problem of minimizing commitment and investment when pursuing this strategy. This commitment would be desirable in long-term mating strategies.

Hypothesis 4: Men have evolved a distinct psychology of short-term mating such that preferences for short-term mates will solve, in part, the problems of identifying which women are fertile. Youth and physical attractiveness are consistently correlated with fertility, and these are especially important in short-term mating strategies.

Hypothesis 5: When men pursue a long-term mate, they will activate psychological mechanisms that solve the problem of paternity confidence (e.g., sexual jealousy and specific mate preferences.) Buss and Schmitt have demonstrated that sexual infidelity is more distressing to men, and emotional infidelity is more distressing to women.

Hypothesis 6: When men pursue a long-term mate, they will express preferences that solve the problem of identifying reproductively valuable women. Physical attractiveness offers indications of both youth and health.

Hypothesis 7: In short-term matings, women will seek men who are willing to impart immediate resources.

Hypothesis 8: Because women more than men use short-term matings to attract long-term prospective mates, they dislike characteristics in a potential mate that are detrimental to long-term prospects.

Hypothesis 9: Women seeking a long-term mate will value the ability of a man to provide economic and other resources that can be used to invest in her offspring.

—From Buss and Schmitt, 1993

These hypotheses describe interesting aspects of people's social interactions with potential mates and others to whom they feel some sexual attraction. Virtually all of these hypotheses are supported by questionnaire data in the research of David Buss and his colleagues; thus there is some support for the theory that sexual strategies are indeed genetically determined.

These hypotheses also reveal a speculative rationale for differences in how readily women and men engage in sexual intercourse outside marriage. Buss indicates that women require either immediate resources for sexual interaction (e.g., money through prostitution) or substantive long-term resources and commitments in exchange for sexual behaviors likely to lead to conception (a promise of marriage, and perhaps the symbol that she has been "taken"—an engagement ring). Furthermore, because of sociobiological motives to provide for and protect offspring, women and men would naturally want their partners to maintain sexual exclusivity. There may therefore be an evolutionary justification for jealousy and even the taboos against extramarital intercourse. People often react violently to learning of their partner's infidelity, perhaps because powerful pressures have emerged through human evolution to increase the likelihood of paternity and the supports it presumably promises.

BEING SINGLE

As noted earlier, most adults marry at some time in their lives, although obviously people are single before entering a more or less formal relationship. This section will discuss developmental, sexual, and intimacy issues as they relate to singlehood. At the outset we should note that neither singlehood nor being in a committed relationship automatically creates happiness or assuages loneliness. Anyone can maintain peace of mind and personal growth regardless of whether he or she is part of a long-term bond, just as having children isn't the only path to adult functioning and generativity. Still, from an early age most people see the eventuality of a long-term relationship as desirable or even "normal." Why?

Our feelings and thoughts about relationships begin to develop in later childhood, before reaching adolescence. The relationship we observe between our own caretakers gives us an early sense of what marriage is like—from loving, nurturant interactions to hostile, abusive ones. This initial impression develops and may change significantly over the course of subsequent years.

U.S. Census Bureau data reveal that after 1970 there has been a substantial increase in the number of individuals between the ages of 20 and 39 who have never been married. The desired freedom to make lifestyle and occupational choices independently may play an important role in this trend. Generally, the younger people are when they first marry, the greater is the probability that they will ultimately divorce. Deciding to marry at a later age might for many be an attempt to become more certain about what one seeks in a life partner.

Research by Cargan (1981) revealed that two of the most common stereotypes about single people are not supported by systematic data. First, the notion that single people are lonely is not generally true (Fig. 13-5). Similarly, most single people do not have many different sexual partners. Only about 20% of this sample of single people reported having multiple partners, and the remainder enjoyed monogamous relationships or were content with celibacy. This study was published in 1981, before widespread public concern about AIDS.

Interestingly enough, the stereotypes of loneliness and multiple partners may be more true of divorced people than of single people. Research in the Netherlands (Dykstra, 1995) indicates that marital status and age do not predict loneliness, but that the absence of a social support system might be associated with problems of reciprocity and mutuality in close relationships. In other words, it is not a lack of relationships (both sexual relationships and friendships) per se that predicts loneliness among single people, but rather a discrepancy between current relationships and their expectations of those relationships. Loneliness might mean that for some, friendship and social interactions seem inadequate, rather than reveal the lack of a relationship.

In our culture women might be at more of a disadvantage than men in adjusting to (or enjoying) being single. Chasteen (1994) interviewed single women and asked them about their experiences of singlehood. Interview data revealed that single women often have serious problems finding and affording adequate housing, access to convenient, economical transportation, and opportunities and choices of leisure activ-

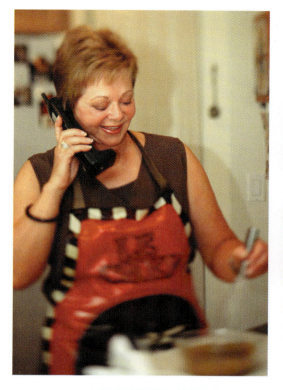

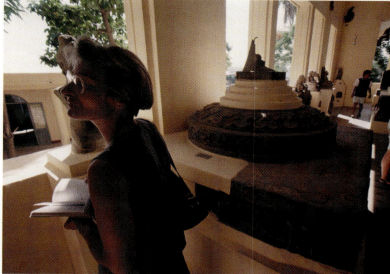

Figure 13-5 Stereotypes of single people as lonely and very sexually active are not supported by research. Many live diversified, interesting lives and genuinely enjoy their solitude.

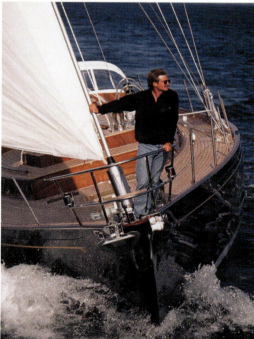

Cohabitation

Living together without being married is fairly common for many people in the United States. Almost half of the people in this country are estimated to have cohabited at some time by the time they reach their early thirties (Bumpass & Sweet, 1989). The reasons for choosing to cohabit are numerous and diverse. For an individual who is mature but not prepared to make a traditional marital commitment to a home, career, and family, cohabitation offers the choice of being very close to someone he or she wants to be with. Additionally, the current federal tax structure financially favors those who have two incomes and live together but are not married. The development of nurturance and friendship, as well as an exploration of a monogamous sexual relationship are important incentives for cohabitation.

The day-to-day problems encountered by cohabiting couples are very much like those of married individuals. Some encounter pressures to change their identity to please their partners. Others feel that they have lost their autonomy and become too dependent upon their partner. People in a cohabitation arrangement are just as likely to argue over money, jealousy, and who takes out the garbage as are married couples (Fig. 13-6). Many middle-aged, aging, and elderly couples also cohabit. Sometimes a pension or social security income that is lower for a married couple than for the same two people as singles is an incentive for seniors to maintain economic singlehood while living together.

Because couples are more likely to cohabit in their youthful years, their assumptions about love and intimacy often have a large role in their decision to enter this living arrangement. Larson (1992) discusses several unrealistic beliefs of many young people about finding a mate. People frequently believe

ities. These issues in a single woman's daily life are very different from those for single men. Gender powerfully affects the daily priorities, pressures, and activities of unmarried individuals. While these data reveal some problems single women may face, they by no means describe the lives of all single women.

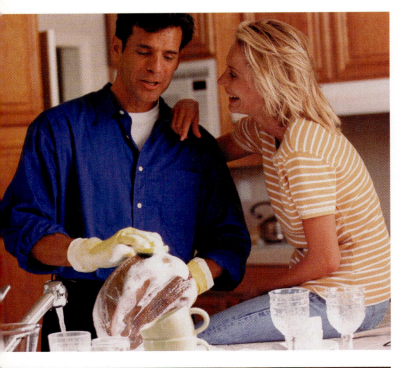

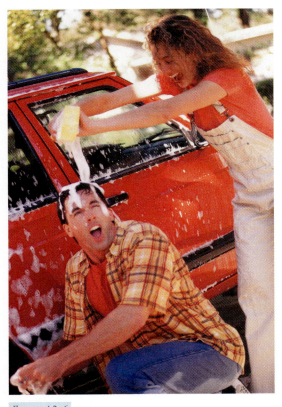

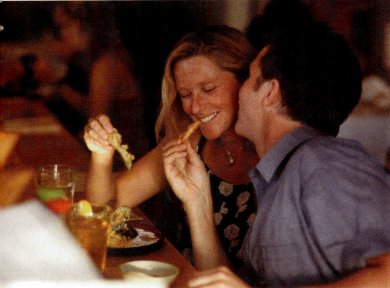

FIGURE 13-6   Cohabiting couples share a broad and varied range of activities while working to define the nature of their bond, its boundaries and understandings, and its course of development.

these myths without knowing it, and they would gain from confronting these ideas directly, especially if they are thinking about living with someone in a committed relationship or marriage. A prominent myth is that there is one perfect partner and that others are flawed or deficient and, therefore, unsuitable. A second is that the perfect partner is really "out there" and that all one needs to do is find him or her. A third is that one must be a perfect, developmentally mature individual before embarking on a long-term marital commitment. Fourth: perfect relationships can exist without tension, turmoil, or frustrations. A fifth unrealistic belief is that if an individual just "tries a little" harder, all serious relationship prob-

lems can be averted; all interpersonal problems can be solved. A sixth is that cohabiting with someone will teach you everything you need to know to live comfortably and happily with that person. Another unrealistic belief is that people with very different personalities will complement each other and form a compatible, comfortable relationship that somehow "neutralizes" their "extreme" attributes. Finally, a misconception about mate selection is that it should be easy and come naturally.

These misconceptions reveal a number of important concerns about how we consider the desirability and attractiveness of another person in relationships. Because many people see cohabitation as a prelude to a longer, more formal marital commitment, couples considering living together should talk with each other in depth about their beliefs and explore whether such myths influence their thinking, feeling, and behaving in a relationship.

Because many people decide to live together while thinking of getting married, sexual interaction in cohabitation relationships is important. Although there are few data on the overall quality of sexual relationships among cohabiting couples, a little is known about their frequency of intercourse. Regardless of whether the two people have been married to others before living together, cohabiting couples have intercourse more frequently than married couples. However, the longer they remain together without getting married, the more this frequency declines (Blumstein & Schwartz, 1983). This is also true of mar-

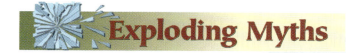

Exploding Myths

The "One and Only" Myth

There are a number of unrealistic beliefs that influence young adults thinking about the attributes of potential mates. One prevalent, enduring notion is that there is one perfect person "out there," and if we just take our time, keep our eyes and ears open, and stick to our standards, we will ultimately find him or her, fall in love, and live compatibly (emotionally, temperamentally, and sexually) forever after. This is a major theme in the fairy tales we grow up with, and it still exerts a powerful influence on our plans and expectations.

Research into the characteristics of successful marriages typically reveals an assortment of highly complex traits and attributes resulting from the interactions of two unique people—not an idealized set of qualities. Gottman and Krokoff (1989) describe some predictors of marital satisfaction. The quality of a couple's communication and the ease with which they can be honest, foresightful, and nonjudgmental when faced with difficult challenges and choices is basic to a harmonious relationship. Usually, however, the couple does not start out with these skills fully formed, as they emerge as the couple grows together over time and through sometimes trying circumstances.

Shared, equitable decision making is another common feature of a good relationship or marriage, although traditional socialization of women and men often does not foster such equality. In the past, men were raised to be leaders, guides, and "teachers" for their wives (especially sexually), and women were frequently raised to be somewhat passive, submissive, obedient "students" of their husbands. For women and men to accept one another as equals at the outset would be ideal, but often this equality has to develop.

Chapter 9 notes that homosexual couples have the same frustrations and challenges in their relationships as heterosexuals. Gays and lesbians too have problems with the equitable division of domestic labor, money decisions, and the use of alcohol and other drugs. They also have disagreements about how to raise children when they are present. Just as mythical beliefs color heterosexual relationships, they also affect homosexuals.

Finally, no matter how perfect the match, conflicts arise. Dealing with them effectively is a consistent attribute of long-lasting marriages in which both partners report a high degree of satisfaction. Solving a problem is very different from merely coping with it, however, which allows the problem to remain. Dealing with a problem requires problem solving, which is something a couple learns to do together.

---

riages. Interestingly, how the female thinks of the quality of the cohabitation arrangement is a good predictor of her willingness to initiate intercourse (Blumstein & Schwartz, 1983), as well as the overall *frequency* of intercourse (Rao & Demaris, 1995).

MARRIED PEOPLE AND SEX

Psychologists have discovered an interesting thing about perception: sometimes stimuli become so familiar that people stop noticing them. This can also affect how partners in a marriage feel about each other sexually. The number of books in the "Psychology" or "Sexuality" sections of bookstores about keeping marriage sexually stimulating suggests this is a common problem.

Basic to Erikson's theory is the notion that people change, grow, and develop throughout their lives. It may happen, however, that marriage partners do not change, grow, and develop together. What happens to sex when people change? The decrease in the frequency of intercourse over the years of a marriage has already been noted. Many couples also report that their physical intimacy becomes somewhat more routine and less adventurous the longer they are together. This section looks at how sexual aspects of marriages change over time and what such changes may reveal about the relationship overall.

The work of Lorna and Philip Sarrel (1984), based on many years of empirical investigation, is an informative analysis of how feelings and thoughts about sexuality change in adult development. This theory does not apply to all adults, and some of its features apply only to a few people. An interesting theory gets people asking questions and collecting data related to those questions, and in this respect the Sarrels' theory is fertile. It stimulates thinking about marital sexuality in a different way. Following are the stages of the Sarrels' theory.

Stage 1: Transition Through Adolescence. Chapter 12 discusses adolescence as a time of sexual growth, development, questioning, ambivalence, and experimentation. When things go well we usually emerge from this stage in our lives with positive feelings about physical intimacy in a supportive, nurturant relationship. We come to understand what we enjoy sexually. According to Erikson, these developmental challenges emerge as we try to formulate and clarify a coherent self-concept. To develop a sense of personal responsibility, we must become informed about contraception issues and avoiding sexually transmitted diseases.

Stage 2: Special Challenges of Young Adulthood. Earlier, this chapter discusses the challenges of establishing meaningful, intimate relationships. For many people this is an important aspect of being single. The meaning of intimacy, the advantages and disadvantages of singlehood, and the special challenges of cohabitation are all relevant at this stage.

Stage 3: Getting Into a Long-Term Relationship and Being in a Long-Term Relationship. In this stage two people have left their family of origin and are embarking together upon a life path they hope will be enjoyable, enriching, and sexually satisfying. Learning to be a full partner in a marriage can be a complicated task, one for which our family of origin does not always prepare us very well. Most people have observed only a limited number of marriages, which also may be very different from that in which they are now in. Sexual intercourse sometimes becomes predictable, routine, or boring and lacks the experimentation and excitement it once held when we were younger. This is a time when some people begin to have extramarital affairs. When one person in the couple has had an affair, the other person has probably thought of having one too.

Certainly, there are challenges and risks at this time in a relationship. Quality communication is important if a couple is to have mutuality, respect, and reciprocity in their relationship. Quality communication begins with an acknowledgment of the autonomy and integrity of the other person, but this isn't always easy to maintain.

Stage 4: New Babies Have a Big Impact on a Marriage. Ironically, the outcome of a couple's love, commitment, and passion, a baby, can change everything. Intimacy and intercourse during and after a pregnancy are often affected by fatigue, physical changes, and plans and preparations. There are some common pressures for a couple to have children. The attitude that having babies is a right and necessary part of adulthood is called pronatalism. Some people are comfortable with this idea and don't think much about it or raise serious questions about how suitable it might be for them. Others think very carefully about how children may affect their marriage, careers, and overall quality of life. Another serious challenge for many couples is infertility. About one in six couples who do not use contraceptives and have inter-

course once or twice a week will not conceive in a year. For some, this can be devastating and might force a reassessment of what their adulthood may be like without children (as discussed in Chapter 10).

Having a baby inevitably affects expressions of physical intimacy in new parents. Although some people experience physical discomfort during intercourse in later pregnancy, others do not. Taking care of a newborn, however, changes the distribution of affection in a marriage, and new fathers and mothers are usually overwhelmed by the demands of the child. How a couple deals with these demands may affect their sexual relationship for a long time.

Stage 5: Roles, Attitudes, Parenting, and Time Together. It is sometimes said that being a parent is the hardest job there is. One is expected to be attentive, affectionate, informed, informative, forgiving, and perhaps most important, available. Having and raising children is typically the central focus for people who decide to be parents. As noted earlier, these diverse activities reflect a person's generativity, a key challenge in adulthood. There is often too little time, too little money, too little privacy, and too little energy to rekindle the spontaneous, passionate intimacy of just a few years ago. When these demands and challenges grow very unpleasant or perhaps insurmountable, a couple may decide that their marriage can no longer be sustained.

Stage 6: To Split or Stay Put. Not everyone reaches this stage, but it may occur in a marriage of any duration. This stage begins before some couples have had children, or because a couple can't have children, or at any other time in the life of a family. Starting over can be an exciting adventure for many adults, especially sexually.

Divorces sometimes occur because of sexual incompatibility, extramarital affairs, or a growing sense of boredom. The transition to a new singlehood is sometimes exciting and sometimes very difficult, especially if a basic part of one's identity involved being part of a couple. Many people have never learned the pleasures of solitude and think of life only as being with another. Living alone may lead to anxiety-provoking questioning of one's attractiveness and desirability. We may ask, "Who would want me now?"

The Sarrels point out that this is a transition stage in which our stable, consistent characteristics are now suddenly blended with new people, relationships, and feelings about sexuality, intimacy, and commitment. The old and the new are happening at the same time. Although the Sarrels do not fully discuss it, another interesting development change occurs at this time involving the relationship between self-esteem and body image. If over the years we have gained weight through inactivity or unwise eating habits, for example, we might not like how we think we look to other people. Wanting to explore new relationships is often an incentive to want to look and feel better.

Stage 7: Staying Interested and Interesting. Middle age is not simply a matter of how old we are. In the past it was more common for a person to have one spouse, one family, one job, and one career, and then it was clearer what "middle" meant. Now many people have more than one spouse, perhaps

MESSAGE FROM DR. RUTH: HOW TO TALK TO YOUR PARTNER ABOUT WANTING TO STAY CELIBATE UNTIL THE WEDDING

*W*ith so many young people engaging in premarital sex, those who have made the decision to remain celibate until the wedding can feel a lot of pressure. This is especially true of college students who live away from their parents. A young person living at home can always say, "I can't, my folks would kill me if they found out," even if it's really their own choice. But when you're living away from home, you can't use that excuse.

If you want to communicate a personal belief like this, which could lead to future conflict, *when* you say it is as important as *what* you say. If you bring up the subject too soon, you may scare away a potential partner, but if you wait too long, you risk losing someone you may have fallen in love with. Unless that person also wants to wait until the wedding, I suggest that once you've reached the point of having real feelings for another person, look for an opportunity to make your position known at the first appropriate opportunity.

If there's a current movie that involves this subject, for example, see it together. Or ask a friend to start the ball rolling by bringing up the subject of virginity in a conversation. In any case, try to avoid suddenly finding yourself in a situation in which you have to tell someone that you won't have sex with them. Instead, make sure that anyone you are serious about understands that you intend to wait to have sex until you are married, no matter what, no matter who. This way, the other can't take it personally and they can decide whether they want to become that significant one or not.

Of course, not everyone will take no for an answer. You might find yourself involved with someone who continually presses the issue. And if you're already engaged to this person, the pressure may become even stronger. Tell this person that nobody has ever died from not having sex. You might also say that premarital sex does not make a marriage more successful, or sex more satisfying. If the person is feeling very frustrated, they can always masturbate. In my opinion, anyone who puts a lot of pressure on you to have sex, even if you are already engaged, should be carefully considered before you go ahead with those marriage vows.

Sex is important, but it is not the be-all and end-all of a relationship. That's why I support anyone's decision to remain a virgin until they are married. If you are one of these courageous people, you need to understand that you are bucking a trend. Because of that, you have a special responsibility to someone with whom you get emotionally involved. Take the initiative in bringing up this topic so that you don't hurt anyone else, and especially so that you don't wind up hurt yourself.

---

more than one family, and often more than one occupation or career. What used to be a period of stability, predictability, and relative comfort is often now a time of change, choice, risk, and new opportunity. Changes at this time are likely to affect the quality of marital intimacy and sexual expression.

Menopause involves a variety of physical symptoms and also sometimes emotional changes. Usually these are not too problematic, and most women deal with them well. Only one woman in five seeks medical or psychological assistance with menopause. Yet a woman with a traditional feminine socialization may question the focus of her life if she can no longer conceive and bear children. Lowered estrogen levels usually lead to some vaginal dryness, and a combination of physical and psychological factors can affect the enjoyment of sexual intercourse.

Another significant aspect of menopause can be the liberating feeling of not having to be concerned with contraception. Menopause offers some women relief from such worries, and this often leads to new sexual exploration and heightened responsiveness.

Men in middle age take longer to become erect but often enjoy a longer period of sexual stimulation before ejaculation occurs. Because of the changes of middle age in both men and women, communication issues grow in importance at this time. Age-related changes in sexual expression in later life are discussed in the next chapter.

Overall, the Sarrels' theory is a useful context to summarize changes that can occur within a marriage. Understanding such changes can be valuable, as Erikson points, out, because if people know something about the changes they are likely to go through during their lives, they are better prepared to deal with them when they happen.

Sexual Thinking, Feeling, and Behaving in Marriage

Marriage is generally a long-lasting, complex, and challenging relationship. Earlier in this chapter we described the evolutionary pressures for people to get together and stay together, at least long enough to conceive, bear, and raise offspring. Once the genetic female imperative to procreate has been met with children, what then do men and women do to enjoy their relationship, consolidate their interests and assets, and continue in a pattern of physical intimacy? Of course, women continue to live a long time after they are no longer fertile. Virtually all other female mammals, and most primates, die relatively soon after childbearing. The reality of sexual interaction beyond the goal of procreation is a relatively recent development in human evolution, as we now live far longer than the 30 or 40 years humans used to live. Now, many people are still living together as couples long after the fertile years are over, but still feeling pleasure and attachment through sexual contact.

Social scientists like to explore human *attitudes,* a term often used in different ways. Attitudes are complicated and have cognitive, emotional, and behavioral aspects. Our attitudes about women, men, and relationships, and the role of sexuality in those relationships, are basic to the enjoyment we feel as part of a couple. What is your attitude about marriage? What do you *think* about being a part of a couple? What are your *feelings* about the caring, sharing, arguing, lovemaking, childbearing, childrearing, and vulnerability in this kind of relationship? Finally, how do you *act* as a member of a couple planning to enjoy a lifelong partnership? With all of this complexity, how do you preserve that exciting, intimate sexual relationship that played a role in getting the two of you together? These are challenges that a couple faces over the course of their relationship.

The attitudes we bring to a relationship do not change easily. The same is true about the attitudes we formulate while married. Attitudes are important because they influence every aspect of our humanity, and understanding our own attitudes can result in interesting insights into our view of sexual relationships.

Sexual Satisfaction in the Early Years of Marriage

The transition between youth and adulthood doesn't just happen when young people get married. As noted earlier, many young couples are still dealing with the challenges of intimacy and isolation. How can you be a part of a couple and still preserve your personal tastes, preferences, and priorities? There is no simple answer to this, but researchers have looked at how people adjust in the first few years of their marriages. Henderson-King and Veroff (1994), using a carefully selected sample of respondents, studied the relationship among sexual satisfaction, adjustment to marriage, and other variables in a relatively large sample of Caucasian and African American couples in the first three years of their marriages. In this sample of respondents, sexual satisfaction was as important to women as it was to men. More interestingly, the degree to which the tasks and responsibilities of marriage were shared was an important predictor of sexual satisfaction in a marriage, especially for the women in this study. This is intriguing. These data tell us that it is difficult to assess how young people feel about being married without paying close attention to many significant aspects of their relationship. Apparently, when women and men consistently share domestic responsibilities, women report higher levels of sexual satisfaction. This is a good example of how the sexual arena of a marriage is interconnected with the relationship in general (Fig. 13-7).

An interesting question is whether people who are sexually compatible in a cohabitation relationship will have a similar sexual relationship if the couple eventually marries. In marriage many other factors may arise that sometimes are not present in a cohabitation arrangement: having children, establishing a quasi-permanent domicile, developing relationships with in-laws, sharing feelings about working, saving, and housekeeping tasks, and an explicit assumption of exclusivity of the sexual partnership.

Women and men often bring to marriage very different sexual backgrounds. In our culture, traditionally young men are considered the "sexual teachers" of their new wives. Young men often receive cultural messages that they should explore sexual experiences with numerous partners before

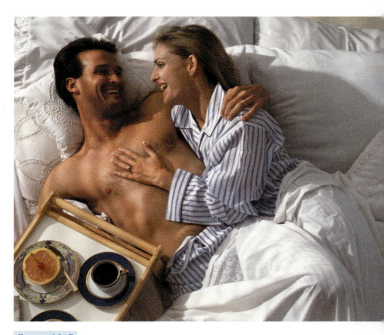

FIGURE 13-7   When newly married couples share their domestic responsibilities equally, they consistently report higher levels of satisfaction with the intimate and sexual aspects of their relationship. This is particularly true of women.

settling down with the "girl of their dreams." Although our society has considered this sexual adventurousness normal for men, the message to young women is that this kind of behavior is not right for them. For example, the word "promiscuous" is usually used to refer to the behavior of women, not men, and the use of this highly negative, judgmental word reflects the unacceptability of extensive premarital sexual experience among young women. Society used to see something faintly unsavory about women having intimate experience comparable to or perhaps exceeding that of their new husbands. In recent decades, of course, things have been changing, and many young women have a number and variety of premarital sexual experiences similar to those of their mates. Yet while female sexual independence has grown, society still generally doesn't promote full equality in such behaviors.

An interesting result of more women having broader sexual experience is the question that often arises: "Is it important for me to tell my new husband about my former lovers (boyfriends)? I don't want to think that I have been reckless, but I don't want him to think that I am naive either." Many men also ask themselves this question, but because this concern is voiced so often by women, it seems the old double standard is dying a slow death. Many young adults today still ask each other with great seriousness, "Do you want to marry a virgin?"

We return to the question with which we began: does sexual experience lead to greater sexual satisfaction in marriage? In fact, we have learned that the nature and number of premarital sexual experiences does not predict very much about the subsequent quality (or length) of a marriage.

The Characteristics of Marriages That Last a Long Time

Earlier we noted that often people get together for one set of reasons but stay together for different reasons. What do we know about people who have been married for a long time (Fig. 13-8)? Fenell (1993) explored this question in a large sample of couples who had been married over twenty years. This study examined what it takes for a couple to stay together for more than two decades in a society in which half of all marriages end in divorce long before that. Based on the responses to a carefully constructed questionnaire, following are the most important characteristics of a long-term, apparently successful marriage.

1. These individuals had an intellectual and emotional assumption that the person they married would be their one and only spouse.
2. They expected to give this person loyalty and friendship.

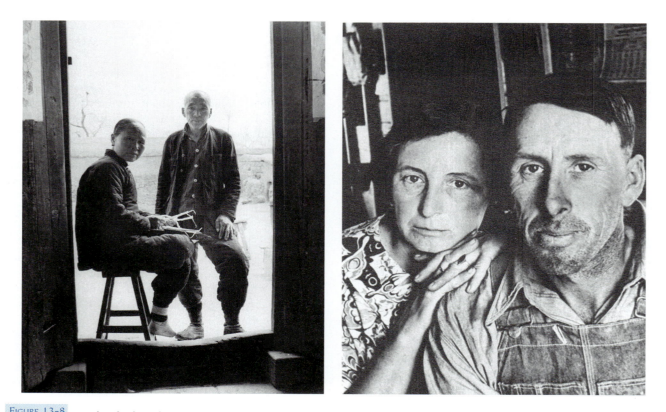

FIGURE 13-8   People who have been married to one another for a long time have made a loyal commitment and have worked together to create moral and spiritual compatibility. A concern for their spouse's happiness and being accepting of the other's shortcomings are important aspects of these relationships.

Other Countries, Cultures, and Customs

MARITAL SATISFACTION IN INDIA

Sexual satisfaction in marriage has been examined by many behavioral scientists. An interesting study was conducted in India, a patriarchal society (Fig. 13-9). Kumar and Makwana (1991) studied sexual satisfaction in this non-Western, highly traditional culture. Gender and the amount of time the couple had been married were examined, as well as the professional-vocational status of the wife. Regardless of an Indian woman's professional status, the amount of time a couple had been married significantly affected their reported level of sexual enjoyment in marriage. Couples married less than ten years seemed to enjoy their intimate relationship far more than couples married more than ten years. While this study may seem simplistic, it is important because there are very few cross-cultural data on this topic. These data indicate that mature marriages offer partners more diverse sources of satisfaction than younger marriages. Having children, raising them, and establishing and maintaining a home provide special pleasures that younger married people have not yet had the opportunity to enjoy. Nonetheless, based on this information, one cannot simply assume that people who have been together longer enjoy physical intimacy less than they did when they were younger.

3. Both individuals had strong moral and spiritual compatibility, and both had always thought that being a parent was a very important part of being married.
4. They expressed a consistent desire to make the other person happy.
5. They thought that it was very important to forgive their partner's fallibilities and similarly be forgiven.

Of course, marital success is not at all that simple, but the results of this research can guide and inform our thinking about marital satisfaction. It is noteworthy that

sexual pleasure is not on this list of predictors. Other data, which we will examine later in this chapter, does show, however, that sexual pleasure is an important factor in long-term relationships.

Sexual Frequency

In studies of the role of sexuality in marriage, the frequency of a couple's intercourse is usually included. Only rarely, however, do such studies ask about how much the couple enjoy their intimacy or the role of sexuality in their busy, changing lifestyles. It's important, however, to examine such quality and quantity issues together. One study (Hawton, Gath, & Day, 1994) found that women's feelings of sexual satisfaction with their marital relationships were not related to their age; both pre- and postmenopausal women reported similar frequencies of sexual intercourse and overall marital satisfaction. Frequency of intercourse does not necessarily mean both partners enjoy it, and non-intercourse physical pleasuring that they may enjoy is not often studied. Another issue is that the frequency of intercourse should not be equated with frequency of orgasm, especially in women. These are also important questions affecting how one interprets this research.

Doing research on this subject is also rather complicated, since this is a very personal, sensitive subject. Most people would find it intrusive if someone asked them how often they had sexual intercourse. Another methodological problem is that subtle social pressures encourage us to believe that it is "normal" to want to have intercourse very often, and that if we don't there might be something "wrong" with us. For all these reasons, one should critically examine

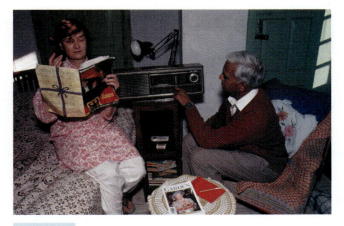

FIGURE 13-9 Indian couples report somewhat less sexual enjoyment in their marriages among couples married more than 10 years. This by no means implies any significant decline in the overall satisfaction of their relationship.

data about the frequency of sexual intercourse in any type of relationship.

Rao and Demaris (1995) studied the reported frequency with which cohabiting and married couples in the United States have sexual intercourse. The data in this study were collected in 1987-88 as part of the National Survey of Families and Households. Over 13,000 individuals were polled—a large, random, and representatively chosen group of respondents. Factors found to have an impact on reported coital frequency in cohabitation or marital relationships are the ages of the individuals, with younger people reporting higher coital frequencies; the length of the relationship, with lower frequencies reported in those of longer duration; and the male partner's perception of his overall health, better health being associated with higher frequency of intercourse. Additionally, the amount of satisfaction the female partner had in the relationship was also an important predictive variable of coital frequency.

The frequency of sexual intercourse in marriage has been reported in some valid, reliable studies. During young adulthood, most couples in long-term relationships have intercourse two to three times a week. By their late forties the figure has declined to about once a week. Again, these are only numbers; they do not describe the role of sexual intimacy in a marriage or the degree to which partners look forward to and enjoy making love. Several investigators have independently found about the same numerical data concerning the frequency of intercourse in marriage, beginning with the work of Kinsey in the 1930s and 1940s, and continuing with Hunt in 1972 and Westoff in 1970. A study by Blumstein and Schwartz (1983) explored frequency of intercourse as a function of how long the participants had been married. Forty-five percent of people married for two years or less reported having intercourse three or more times each week, while for those married two to ten years the comparable figure was 27%, and for those married more than ten years it was 18%. Yet these data do not really tell us the whole story. Without information about the range of frequencies and the specific numbers of people polled, we cannot determine whether we are dealing with a normal bell curve distribution, and we cannot determine what percentage of cases fall close to the mean and what percentage of cases are either very far below or very far above the mean. This is a problem of interpretation that can be solved only by a full reporting of all descriptive statistics in all research studies dealing with these questions. Measures of central tendency, such as the mean, mode, or median, also have informative value.

A final issue related to frequency involves alcohol abuse, a common problem in our and other societies. Alcoholism has been found to have a significant impact on the sexual quality of a marriage. O'Farrell, Choquette, and Birchler (1991) explored this subject in a group of couples seeking marriage counseling. In this study, 26 married couples in which the husband was an alcoholic were compared with two other groups of married couples, one experiencing marital problems and the other reporting no marital problems. These respondents an-swered several questions regarding the adequacy of their sexual interactions in their marriages. Interestingly, the couples with an alcoholic spouse and those experiencing marital conflicts were very similar on a number of factors related to their sexual satisfaction. Both groups reported less overall sexual satisfaction, less frequent sexual intercourse, a greater desire to increase the frequency of intercourse, greater misunderstanding about their spouses' desire to have intercourse, and more disagreements about sexual matters. These data suggest that marriages with an alcoholic spouse often experience serious conflicts that can undermine the enjoyment and sharing of intimacy.

Marriages With a Low Frequency of Sexual Intercourse

Social scientists have also studied sexual inactivity in a marriage. Family therapists, psychotherapists, counselors, and social workers often find that the sexual relationship in a marriage can be a microcosm of the relationship as a whole. If a marriage is reasonably harmonious and provides partners with a sense of emotional security, the sexual aspect of the relationship often reflects this. Similarly, when a marriage is characterized by conflict, mistrust, and volatile, angry emotional expression, such difficulties are more or less apparent in the sexual interactions between these two people.

Marriages in which the couple has little or no sex have been studied by Donnelly (1993). Caution is needed here in the interpretation of data, because people may not accurately answer questions having to do with why they don't have sexual intercourse. Behind this study was a reasonable question: are sexually inactive marriages characterized by unhappiness and a lack of predictable emotional support in the couple? The results revealed that people who were generally unhappy in their marriages tended to have sexual intercourse rarely. When it was likely that a couple was going to separate and when they enjoyed few shared activities, they were also more likely to have a sexually inactive marriage. Increased age, poor health status, and the presence of preschool children in the home are also highly correlated with sexual inactivity in marriage. Again, however, the frequency of sexual intercourse in a marriage is not as important as the enjoyment, trust, and fulfillment both people feel when they do have intercourse.

Blumstein and Schwartz (1983) offer some interesting insights into the issue of relative sexual inactivity in a marital relationship. Among their respondents who were married ten years or less, 6% reported having intercourse one time a month or less; for those who were married more than ten years, the comparable figure was 15%. There are some important things these data do not tell us. For example, they do not tell us the degree to which sexual intercourse occurs exclusively in the context of a monogamous marital relationship; they do not report how often a person has an orgasm during intercourse; and finally, they don't examine the relationship between frequency of sexual intercourse and frequency of masturbation independent of one's partner in marriage. Investigation of these issues would provide more information about sexual intercourse in marriage.

THE DIVERSITY OF SEXUAL EXPRESSION IN MARRIAGE

So far, the discussion has focused entirely on only one kind of sexual interaction in marriage: intercourse. Yet there is significant variety in erotic expression among married people, as social scientists have learned in the last two decades. Hunt's study of American sexuality in the 1970s revealed some very big changes since Kinsey's work first gave us a glimpse of the diversity of sexual expression in marriage in the 1930s and 40s. For example, there has been a big increase in the reported prevalence of oral-genital stimulation in marriage. Kinsey's early work (1948) reported that fewer than 10% of married individuals in his sample had participated in oral-genital stimulation during the month prior to their interview. He noted that there was a clear relationship between a person's level of education and their willingness to participate in oral-genital stimulation. It may be that greater exposure to education, particularly higher education, encourages broad thinking and possibly less conventional opinions about sometimes controversial topics.

Behaviors such as fellatio, cunnilingus, mutual masturbation, anal stimulation and intercourse, and a variety of extravaginal ejaculatory behaviors have become far more common before and within marriage. Activities that only a few decades ago were thought of as exotic are now practiced fairly frequently by a broad segment of the population, as discussed in Chapter 8. Clearly, less stigma is now associated with these non-intercourse avenues of sexual expression.

Fidelity and Trust

We began this chapter with a brief discussion of the psychosocial developmental aspects of youth and adulthood. Many marriages are built and maintained upon foundations of fidelity and trust. These are optimistic psychosocial aspects of adult development according to Erik Erikson. Janus and Janus (1993) reported that in a sample of 770 men and 802 women, 85% of the men and 82% of the women reported that their spouse or partner is also their best friend. But sometimes fidelity and trust erode over time. One possible cause or consequence of such a change is extramarital affairs.

Extramarital Affairs

As marriage evolved in most world civilizations, monogamy gradually came to be a primary model of a committed bond. Within such a sexually exclusive relationship, couples could provide for and protect their offspring in an emotionally supportive, nurturant nuclear family. Over time, shared labor, shared assets, and socialization training would promote the so-

ciobiological agenda discussed at the beginning of this chapter. Nonetheless, sexual behavior outside the marriage bond is common.

Chapter 2 discussed the Judeo-Christian antecedents of modern attitudes about sexual feelings, thoughts, and behaviors. These religious traditions discourage ambivalence in matters affecting faith and action. Judeo-Christian codes of morality and ethics, as well as the lengthy commentaries on those codes usually present good-bad, right-wrong dichotomies. Religious traditions influencing many people in the Western World proclaim that adultery, extramarital sexuality, sometimes called "fornication" are frankly wrong and sinful. There is little moral middle ground in this issue. Because extramarital sexual intercourse is incompatible with romantic, monogamous trust, such behaviors are often associated with historical conceptions of sin, and this topic is, therefore, difficult for people to talk about openly and honestly. We need to keep this in mind when we look at surveys that ask such questions.

RESEARCH ON EXTRAMARITAL SEXUALITY

Because extramarital sexual relations are not approved by traditional norms and mores in many societies, people often have difficulty being honest about their feelings about these liaisons. Even the term "cheating" shows that society frowns upon adulterous relationships. Because of the traditional historical double standard, men might find it easier to reveal their participation in sexual experiences outside traditional moral norms, but whether men actually have more extramarital affairs than women cannot be determined with certainty. Men do, however, report these experiences more frequently than women. The reporting of extramarital sexual experiences varies a lot becuase of historical, cultural, and gender-based reasons. Keeping in mind the problems of survey research, here are a few findings. Rates for the number of men who have ever had an extramarital sexual affair range from about 25% (Blumstein & Schwartz, 1983) to Kinsey's estimate of 50% (1948). Rates for women who have ever had an extramarital affair range from 18% (Hunt, 1974) to 69% (Wolfe, 1980).

A significant issue here is the degree to which extramarital sexuality is rare, situational, occasional, or habitual. The studies above do not clarify this issue, nor do they indicate anything about the motives involved in initiating, being receptive to, or continuing in an extramarital sexual relationship.

COMMON MOTIVES FOR EXTRAMARITAL AFFAIRS

Most extramarital affairs are secretive, although sometimes they may continue with the unspoken awareness of the person's spouse. Occasionally, although rarely, they do occur and continue with the full knowledge and consent of one's partner. Although these relationships are censured in most societies they are relatively common. Why do people initiate or feel receptive to a union that is so stigmatized? Apparently there are many different motives.

Even with the risks of discovery and the adverse impact on a marital relationship, as well as possible public humiliation, sexual curiosity can be a powerful factor motivating adulterous behavior. Here are other common motives:

1. Sudden infatuation and sometimes impulsive feelings
2. Dissatisfaction with the overall quality of the marital relationship
3. Dissatisfaction with the quality of sex in the marriage
4. Finding out that one's spouse has had an affair and desiring retribution
5. Expression of revenge for a nonsexual transgression of the spouse
6. A general and persistent desire to experiment with sexual encounters

While this list certainly isn't exhaustive, it includes the motives most frequently reported by people who acknowledge that they have had an affair or affairs (Glass & Wright, 1992). The last item on the list is an important one. Having a one-night stand is plainly different from having an affair that lasts longer or a lifestyle in which a person has serial sexual relationships outside of his or her marriage. There is a major qualitative difference between solitary, impulsive sexual couplings and persistent, habitual clandestine sexual relationships that are carefully maintained outside of one's marital relationship. While reason number 1 above suggests a one-night stand or a short-term affair, numbers 2 to 6 relate to a long-term affair.

Motivation for extramarital affairs has been researched in the social and behavioral sciences. Prins, Buunk, and VanYperen (1993) analyzed this issue based on anonymous questionnaire data in the Netherlands. In their sample of 82 married men and 132 married women between the ages of 22 and 92, 30% of the sample had engaged in an extramarital sexual relationship (Fig. 13-10). For both women and men, overall dissatisfaction with the quality of their marriage was a primary factor in becoming involved in such a relationship. Interestingly, anxieties about AIDS did not seem to dissuade these respondents from exploring extramarital sex, perhaps because they had been careful about protection. Nonetheless, this subject requires more systematic research before generalizations can be made about other populations and cultures. These researchers also revealed that a powerful factor among women who are receptive to extramarital relationships is their perceived lack of equality with their spouses in their marriages. As we have seen before, the sexual aspects of a marriage may reveal broader interpersonal problems in the relationship.

PATTERNS OF EXTRAMARITAL SEXUALITY IN MEN

Because there are higher reported rates of extramarital sexuality among men, more has been written about men than about women regarding behavior patterns. Trachtenberg's 1988 book *The Casanova Complex* discusses the motivations, implications, and lifestyles of both married and unmarried men

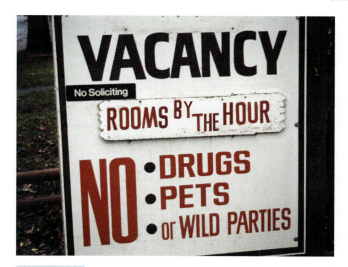

FIGURE 13-10 The motives for extramarital affairs are many and diverse. Women and men often have different reasons for exploring sexual relationships outside of their marriages. Cross-cultural perspectives on marriage may influence these decisions as well.

with a compulsive pattern of sexual involvements. Although this volume might be considered pop psychology, it summarizes well many aspects of apparently obsessional sexuality among many men.

Although questions can be asked about causes in any typology, here we are not examining possibly numerous, complex causes. Social and behavioral scientists are careful not to confuse a diagnostic label with its causes or explanations. Casanovas have a regular behavior pattern associated with a variety of interesting underlying personality traits. These men require constant female companionship. Without it, they become depressed and anxious and are likely to use and abuse alcohol and other drugs. Strong, exclusive attachments to one woman in traditional monogamous relationships do not last long before they initiate other liaisons. Their sexual attachments begin suddenly, passionately, and impulsively. Once these men begin sexual relationships, a highly routine sequence of progressively more "liberated" behaviors becomes their focus in intimate interactions. Casanovas are often attracted to total strangers and feel that with progressive closeness comes obligation and responsibility. They usually see women as "good girls" or "bad girls." When long-term attachments occur, they are always with the former type.

All Casanovas are not alike, however. The personality attributes described above exist in a range of variations. *Hitters* seek immediate satisfaction of their erotic feelings. They are utterly indiscriminate. Their "act" or "routine" may be incongruous with their occupational lifestyle. Women are their quest, and their preoccupation with control is total. They can't wait to leave once their conquest has been made. Hitters plan one-night stands. *Drifters* enter sexual relationships more patiently, seeing their erotic landscape as a "target rich" environment. They never hear or feel rejection and are optimistic that sooner or later someone will come along. Their lovemaking is highly routine and egocentric; there is an element of exploitation in these relationships. *Romantics* fall in love and have affairs often. Ultimately, every woman will prove inadequate, and they will find the need to leave her. Breakups occur often and are deeply felt. They are always hurting others or being hurt themselves. *Nesters* seem to want multifaceted affairs with their women, feel genuine affection and commitment, and initiate relationships with the intention of staying in them for a long time. But they will disengage with equal speed. The early commitment so deeply felt becomes very threatening over time. *Jugglers* have long-lasting relationships, but these are not stable or monogamous. They never know if their partner's love is offered unconditionally or is somehow coerced. They are fully and deeply enmeshed in the lives of their partners but never seem to feel that those who love them really mean it. Finally, *Tomcats* are promiscuous and inconsistent in their search for love and validation from women. Many are married and seem devoted to their families but cannot outgrow their pattern of promiscuous behavior that probably began before marriage. They are addicted to infidelity. Interestingly, each of these Casanova types can be sexually exclusive with his current love interest, while being ever sensitive to a new opportunity.

The characterizations of these different types of men apply both to those who are and are not married. Much less has been written about comparable issues among women.

PATTERNS OF EXTRAMARITAL SEXUALITY IN WOMEN

In the last generation, women have sought and gained greater sexual equality. The specific reasons for this are difficult to describe in simple cause-and-effect terms, but several explanations are common. More women are receiving higher education; in fact, since 1981 there have been more women than

Other Countries, Cultures, and Customs

A CROSS-CULTURAL PERSPECTIVE ON INFIDELITY

While the discovery of an extramarital affair is usually considered harmful to the future of a marriage, research has questioned whether this is so in all cultures. There are some interesting consistencies in the way infidelity contributes to the break-up of a marriage in other societies. In an excellent cross-cultural analysis of the reasons marriages end, Laura Betzig (1989) examined 186 different societies. By far, the most common reason for the dissolution of a marriage was the discovery (or in some cultures, even the suspicion) of an extramarital sexual encounter or relationship. In 88 societies, adulterous behavior plays a major, pivotal role in divorce. Infertility, incompatible personalities, and economic difficulties are less often the cause of divorce in most cultures. Betzig notes that divorce typically follows adultery by either spouse in 25 of these 88 societies, but in 54 of these it results only from adultery by the wife and in only 2 does it result from adultery by the husband. In those 2 cultures in which divorce follows the discovery of infidelity by the man, the woman does not go unpunished, however. Betzig notes that among the Huichol of western Mexico, an angry spouse, upon discovering that her husband has been with another woman, may leave him. This usually leaves this woman without economic support or the assistance of a large, extended kinship group, however. Among the Trobriand Islanders, the anthropologist Bronislaw Malinowski noted in 1929 that husbands have the tacit right to kill their wives upon discovering their infidelity but usually just "thrash" them.

This double standard is a consistent finding in cross-cultural studies of marriage and infidelity. In fact, Betzig notes that there is a powerful relationship between the divorce rate in the societies she studied and the frequency of female infidelity. In virtually all of the cultures investigated, an extramarital relationship can replace one social, economic, and reproductive relationship with another, and that may involve a huge change or reallocation of resources. She believes that sanctions against women may be more severe because even a single adulterous experience may result in pregnancy with a lifelong economic and parenting commitment to the offspring. Earlier we discussed sexual strategies theory and factors that are thought to promote and protect traditions of monogamy and the need of men to be certain of their paternity. Perhaps the common and disproportionate sanctions against women for adultery are another societal manifestation of this need.

men in college in the United States, and this enrollment gap between the genders continues to widen. This trend is also occurring in postgraduate training such as medical school, law school, and graduate school in many disciplines. With more women with degrees, more women are entering the workplace with advanced professional standing. These relatively recent changes have affected many aspects of women's sense of themselves, including sexual and reproductive freedoms.

According to Small (1992), increases in women's sexual autonomy have paralleled these broader societal trends. Further, women today are more comfortable with the physiological characteristics of their sexual responsiveness and have developed greater feelings of erotic reciprocity in their relationships with men. Women are less likely to see themselves as individuals to whom men do something but rather as full sexual partners with a basic right to safety, pleasure, and erotic sharing. Thus women today play a more assertive role in initiating extramarital sexual relationships and are also often more receptive when the opportunity is suggested by men. Small found that women engage in extramarital sexual relationships in virtually all cultures, especially in developed Western countries. Women today are exercising their sexual autonomy and assertiveness to a greater degree than ever before.

Women's motives for extramarital sexual affairs are similar to those expressed by many men (Glass & Wright, 1992; Grosskopf, 1983). Excitement, novelty, dissatisfaction with the marital relationship, and lack of feelings of marital sexual fulfillment are all common motives. For obvious reasons, most data on this issue come from anonymous questionnaires. Glass and Wright found that women are far more likely to participate in extramarital sex when they are in love with the other man; strictly sexual motives were less frequently reported as justification for extramarital sexuality among women than among men. Apparently, according to these writers, men find it easier to separate sexual expression and love than do women.

Interestingly, women often seem aware when other women they know are having an affair. Klassen, Williams, and Levitt (1989) report that when respondents were asked how many of their acquaintances had sexual intercourse with someone other than their husbands, 28.1% said "none" or "didn't know," 44.6% said "a few—less than 5," 9.3% said "several—5 to 9," 12.0% said "many—10 or more," and 6% replied "some, but don't know how many." These data come from a very large sample size (over 3000 respondents) and may be representative of the United States population as a whole.

As noted above, men may find it easier than women to separate the sexual and emotional aspects of affairs. If love plays an important role in the motivations for women, do they also end extramarital relationships for different reasons? Hurlbert (1992) addressed this question to a group of 59 women participating in an assertiveness training workshop. The findings are interesting in light of what most other data indicate about men's and women's different reasons for having affairs. Hurlbert found that the length of an extramarital sex-

ual relationship is predicted by the degree to which the woman enjoys positive attitudes about her own sexuality. More positive attitudes are associated with longer relationships. The degree to which these women fell in love with their extramarital partners and the extent to which they knew each other well before they became involved sexually were also predictive of longer affairs. These data indicate that in this sample of women, not only were affective and emotional issues involved in having an extramarital relationship, but sexual ones as well.

Influence of Social and Cultural Factors on Fidelity

Social and cultural influences have a big impact on many aspects of our growth and development, as well as our perceptions of our environment. For example, many young women's preoccupation with our culture's attitude toward thinness as an attribute of physical attractiveness is thought to contribute to eating disorders among adolescent and young adult females. Clearly, the social environment affects many of our beliefs. Is this true about extramarital affairs too? People of all racial, ethnic, religious, and socioeconomic groups have affairs. The forces of attraction are apparently powerful enough to transcend traditional mores about healthy marriage.

A number of years ago, actors Michael Douglas and Glen Close co-starred in the popular film *Fatal Attraction,* which depicts a wealthy, powerful, comfortable married man whose wife is out of town with their child (Fig. 13-11). The man has a one-night stand with a woman, as both are carried away with their passion and attraction. The woman is not only infatuated but becomes deeply obsessed with the man. Violence, assault, attempted murder, and exposure of the affair all ensue. The reaction of many men who saw the film, however, is very interesting. Throughout the country, literally thousands of men watching the movie abruptly left the theater. The scenario was apparently too real, too much like their own experiences—or at least their own fears and anxieties. But did

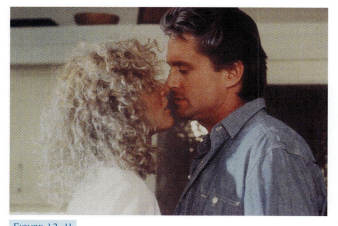

FIGURE 13-11 The film *Fatal Attraction* affected many men powerfully, highlighting some of the unanticipated and violent consequences of a volatile extramarital affair.

this movie scare anyone into maintaining marital fidelity? It would be difficult to establish a cause-and-effect relationship between media depictions of adultery and measurable changes in behavior.

Are people living in big cities more permissive about sex, as they seem to be more open to other novel experiences than those living in rural communities? Wilson (1995) wrote about the degree to which urbanism fosters sexual unconventionality in thought and action. Wilson found that urban lifestyles foster a more open, comfortable expression of homosexuality but do not seem to facilitate higher rates of premarital sexual experience, cohabitation, or extramarital affairs than rural lifestyles. People living in cities had more permissive attitudes about these issues, but they did not necessarily act more on these beliefs.

COMMON CONSEQUENCES OF THE DISCOVERY OF EXTRAMARITAL AFFAIRS

As noted above, some affairs remain clandestine for long periods of time, while others take place with some awareness on the part of the partner, even if this awareness is not acknowledged openly. When a spouse is discovered in a sup-posedly secret affair with someone else, the other partner almost always feels hurt, betrayed, inadequate, or angry. Some spouses forgive, but most never forget. Often, the entire emotional and familial fabric of the relationship is torn beyond repair. A couple must decide if the relationship is salvageable, which may be very difficult to discuss. If unspoken or poorly articulated marital problems played a role in precipitating the affair, it is unlikely that the couple has adequate communication skills to discuss putting the partnership back together.

A study of mostly married Dutch couples addresses many of these issues (Buunk, 1995). This investigation showed that women and men tended to respond somewhat differently to the discovery of their partner's infidelity. For example, women tended to report more feelings of self-doubt and disappointment but fewer feelings of betrayal and anger. This was especially true among women with low self-esteem. For both men and women, if the partner had been unfaithful before, feelings of disappointment were somewhat less. Nonetheless, there are not adequate empirical data on this subject to generalize about the effects of extramarital sexuality on a relationship. In a sample of 122 men and 127 women,

Dear Dr. Ruth

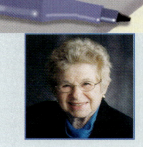

Questions:

I'm a 45-year-old woman. Six months ago I divorced my husband after 22 years. I'm still attractive and have been dating, but when it comes to sex, I feel like I was living on another planet all those years. I had sex with only one other guy before my husband, and sex with my husband was always of the plain vanilla variety. Now I meet men who seem to expect sex if not on the first date, then on the second, and the things they want to do, like oral sex, leave me aghast. On the one hand I want to have sex with them, but I really am having difficulties handling these men. What should I do?

Answer:

The problem may be the type of men that you are dating. There are many middle-aged men who are only looking for sexual conquests. Some have never married, but many of them are divorced. Apparently they can find enough women to satisfy their needs for one-night stands, so they maintain their habits. Having just been divorced, you may be vulnerable to these casanovas, but you have to learn to resist them. Other men out there are seeking a relationship, not just to hop in and out of bed, and you have to go out and find one of them. This man may also have a more varied sexual repertoire than your husband, but if it's in the context of a loving relationship, you may find yourself more open to things like other sexual activities. If you really don't want to do certain things, however, a man who cares for you is not going to leave you because of it.

Janus and Janus (1993) reported that 11% of divorced men indicated that discovery of an extramarital affair was the primary cause of their divorce, whereas 22% of divorced women indicated that this was the key factor in their decision to end their marriages.

In another study on the possible outcomes of infidelity, Weir (1992) studied the reactions of males and females to crimes of passion in hypothetical scenarios in which one spouse murders the other or the rival after learning about a marital infidelity. Weir found that female subjects recommended longer prison sentences than the male subjects—regardless of whether the murder victim was the rival or the spouse. Furthermore, married respondents and those with families considered murder following infidelity deserving of longer punishment than did subjects who were single and/or childless. Because violence occurs commonly after the discovery of an extramarital affair, these data reveal the depth of powerful feelings associated with this situation.

DIVORCE

Whether divorce results from the discovery of an extramarital relationship or other reasons, it is an event that typically requires social, emotional, and sexual readjustment. Many people are so socialized to think of their adult lives as a part of a couple that they have to get used to singlehood again. Being married involves learning to play the role of a married person. This role affects and in some cases determines our interpersonal relationships, our expressions of intimacy and affection, our activities in and outside of the home, and many economic aspects of our lives. Learning the role of a divorced person can be a perplexing and confusing process that may take a long time. Being divorced is not the same as being single again, however, as others often view singles and divorced individuals in different ways. Many people who divorce experience a period of guilt for their role in the failure of the relationship; this is a normal reaction.

The divorce rate has increased for both young and middle-aged adults. The United States has the highest rate of divorce in the world across all age groups. According to Burns (1992), when all age groups are considered, about two out of three first marriages are expected to end in divorce. Evidence suggests that 1 in 8 women in their first marriages will be divorced after reaching age 40, a particularly difficult time in one's life when generativity is an important psychological goal (Uhlenberg, Cooney, & Boyd, 1990). Generally, because of the lack of economic equality in most marriages, women experience a significant decline in their standard of living after a divorce at virtually any age, while men may actually experience an enhancement in their material comforts and financial security, in part because of discrepancies between what men and women earn in many cultures. People today are no longer as committed to staying together beyond midlife if they perceive problems in their marriages, particularly difficulties associated with poor communication and unrewarding physical intimacy.

Sometimes, people believe that a newly divorced person seeks and experiences a new sexual liberality. The stereotype of divorced individuals behaving permissively or promiscuously is not supported by research, however (Stack & Gundlach, 1992). Apparently personal values are a significant issue in postmarital decisions about sexual expression. One's level of formal education and spiritual values are correlated with the number of sexual partners a person will have after divorce, as well as the frequency of sexual intercourse. Almost all of the respondents in this study reinitiated sexual relations after their divorces. Both women and men reported having an average of 1 or 2 sexual partners during the year following their divorce. Apparently the stereotype noted above is not founded in fact. However, divorced women seemed more willing to explore non-intercourse avenues of sexual pleasuring more than when they were married.

Unrewarding sex is sometimes involved in a decision to separate or divorce. Sometimes a decline in quality is very gradual and may not even be apparent to one or both of the spouses (Vaughan, 1986). This is one reason why dating and exploring sexual opportunities after a divorce can seem so exciting. For some, there is a sense of exhilaration and relief in no longer having to keep an affair a secret. The outcomes of the split often depend on who wanted it, why, and for how long. In almost all cases, divorced people have to learn new social roles and sometimes new strategies for interpersonal relationships (Fig. 13-12). Society doesn't offer any "rules" about how to proceed, and it is often difficult to simply discard old ways of thinking, feeling, and behaving.

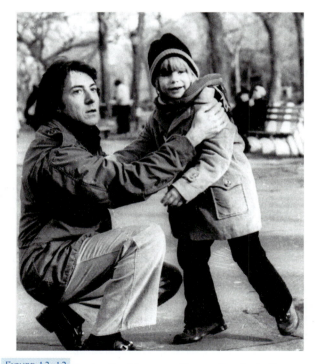

FIGURE 13-12   In the film *Kramer vs. Kramer*, Dustin Hoffman's character reveals some of the painful emotions of a man separated from his son after a divorce. A sense of failure and frustration accompanies divorce for many women and men.

Various factors affect the likelihood of remarriage after divorce. Generally, the younger a person is when divorced, the greater is the probability he or she will remarry. While 89% of people under the age of 25 who separate will remarry, the number falls to 31% of those over age 40. The shorter the duration of the first marriage, the greater are the chances that a person will remarry. Of those whose first marriage lasts less than a year, 89% will remarry. However, of those whose first marriage lasts ten or more years, 52% will remarry. Finally, the younger a person is at the time of the first marriage, the greater is the probability of remarriage. Of those who marry between 14 and 17 years of age, 84% will remarry if they divorce. Yet if a person does not marry until the age of 23 or later, 51% will remarry if they divorce. These data are from Bumpass, Sweet, and Martin (1990).

SEX IN LATER LIFE

The sexual issues and problems people confront change as they grow from adolescence into young adulthood and from young adulthood to middle age. These changes are a part of a person's overall growth and development and their functioning in social settings. Changes continue as we age into and through our later years. Our society has many beliefs and feelings about the place of sex in later life. Youth is equated with beauty, thinness, vitality, and sexiness. Older Americans are often portrayed as "cute," "darling," "wise," or "ornery"—anything but "sexy." Why? There is a common prejudice called **ageism,** which involves common perceptions of the aging and elderly that are much more negative than people are in reality.

Ageism is a prejudice no less troubling than racism or sexism. Although here we are referring to older people, ageism is also present in the stereotyping of teenagers, young mothers, and middle-aged men. Using age as a way to pigeon-hole people into categories lacks sensitivity to different characteristics of people and lumps them into categories they might not belong in. Ageism focuses attention on negative qualities in older people, and perhaps most troubling, it hurts an older person's self-esteem. An obvious problem with ageism is that it denies the existence and the normality of sexual feelings, thoughts, or behaviors in older people. For example, when teaching about sex in later life in our classes, we have often heard a student wryly comment, "Oh, please spare me the details!" (Fig. 13-13).

Let's first put this issue in a demographic and historical perspective. Segraves and Segraves (1995) remind us that in virtually every country in the world, older people are accounting for a progressively larger percentage of the population. For example, in 1900 in the United States, only 4% of the population was 65 years of age or older. However, in 1980, this segment of the population accounted for 12% of the population, and in the year 2000 20% of the American population were 65 or older. A person who turns age 65 today has a life expectancy of another 17 years (Bienenfeld, 1990). There is little reason why older people cannot enjoy their full vitality and humanity during this time, including sexual expression. Both women and men experience a gradual

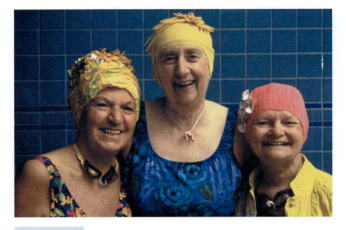

FIGURE 13-13   Ageism often makes it difficult to recognize the wholesome, vital, and energetic aspects of adults at mid-life and beyond. This prejudice colors our perceptions of the aging and elderly in unpleasant ways.

decrease in the frequency with which they have sexual intercourse through their 40s, and a more obvious decline after they have reached the age of 70 (Segraves & Segraves, 1995). This is not to say, however, that sexual expression and enjoyment have diminished importance in later life. It remains a basic source of feelings of well-being and self-esteem for many aging and elderly Americans.

Sexual changes in later life are closely related to other changes that accompany normal aging. Segraves and Segraves (1995) summarized these as follows:

1. Age is associated with an increased incidence of most disease states and many of these diseases or their treatment may interfere with sexual function.
2. The separation between normal aging and health problems often seems arbitrary.
3. Sexual functioning is quite variable among all age groups.
4. The definition of 'geriatric' needs to distinguish between 'young seniors' (65-70), a group who are more sexually active than 'old seniors' (80-90).
5. Sexual function is influenced by the availability of a partner, the relationship with that partner and that partner's general health.
6. Sexual function is multidetermined and a clear separation of biological from interpersonal and cultural factors is often impossible. (p. 89)

Aging and elderly people frequently have sexual thoughts and feelings and enjoy sharing sexual behaviors. In fact, one of the biggest problems for these populations is finding a regular, interested, interesting sexual partner. There is nothing at all wrong, abnormal, or unusual about wanting to have sexual intercourse well into old age. Maybe as older adults have a continuing large presence in our society, the stereotype of older people as asexual will diminish. There is nothing whatsoever unwholesome about eroticism in later life.

MYTHS ABOUT SEX IN LATER LIFE

Most stereotypes and prejudices involve false information, and the same is true with ageism. Felstein (1968) summarized a number of common misconceptions about sexuality in later life. Felstein's discussion of these myths is prefaced by an interesting fact in the history of geriatric medicine. (Geriatrics is the medical specialty, while gerontology is the social science that deals with psychological, sociological, and anthropological aspects of aging.) In 1948, *The Social Medicine of Old Age* by Dr. J. H. Sheldon identified some of the most common problems among old people and ways doctors could recognize these and assist their patients. Interestingly, this book entirely omitted any discussion of sexual expression among aging and elderly people. It almost seems that this well-known specialist had no interest in the place of sexuality in the lives of his older patients.

While social perceptions of the normality of sexual expression in later life have been slow to change, the fact that the population in the United States is getting older has stimulated an interest in sex in later life. One of the most popular books about sex written for the lay public, *The Joy of Sex* by Alex Comfort, was written by a specialist in medical, psychological, and social factors affecting older adults. One of his main messages is that nothing about shared sex is restricted to young people. This writer had an open, healthy attitude toward sexual behavior among members of the geriatric population. Although society now seems more receptive to such information, myths still abound regarding older people having (and enjoying) intercourse. Let's quickly review some of these myths described by Felstein (1968).

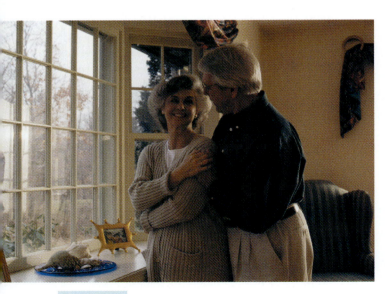

FIGURE 13-14 Aging adults often enjoy an active and varied sexuality. Declines in the frequency of sexual intercourse do not always reveal declines in sexual interest during these years.

Myth: Sex is Only for Procreation, Not Recreation

This is the common belief held that the only "appropriate" reason for having sexual intercourse is to make a baby. We explored this notion in Chapter 2 when discussing how historical, religious, and philosophical factors affect how people feel about sexuality. This belief implies that if intercourse cannot lead to pregnancy, then there is really no reason to be having sex in the first place. While men often continue to produce mature sperm throughout their lives, in some cases well into their 80s and 90s, a woman stops producing fertilizable eggs after menopause. Does this mean that this couple shouldn't be having sex? We disagree with this perspective and are certain that whether or not a couple can conceive a child, there is much love, intimacy, and nurturance to be shared during sex.

Myth: Feelings of Sexual Arousal are Built Primarily on Physical Attractiveness

As we discussed in an earlier chapter, physical attractiveness often gets people to notice each other and initiate a relationship, but the longer a couple stays together, the more obvious it is that many other factors help create and maintain good rapport, trust, communication, and affection. An obvious aspect of ageism is that older people are not perceived to be as attractive as young adults. Because many younger people do not perceive aging or elderly individuals as attractive, they find it hard to think about them having and enjoying sexual interactions. As we age, of course, our bodies change. But these changes do not usually diminish the devotion, freedom, and mutuality many older couples share, which can facilitate their enjoyable sexual sharing.

Myth: The Desire for Intercourse is Highest in Youth and Quickly Declines Afterwards

Although it is true that the frequency of intercourse usually declines with age, this is not a sudden loss of sexual interest or behavior (Fig. 13-14). Aging and elderly people still want to have intercourse, however, and often frequently. The most commonly reported reason for a decline in the frequency of sexual intercourse beyond age 65 is the lack of a regular partner, since 1 in 3 Americans over the age of 65 lives alone. Many of the elderly have sex just as frequently as their middle-aged counterparts.

Myth: Romantic, Passionate Love is Only for Young People

It is just plain wrong to think that romantic love occurs only among adolescents and young adults. Romantic love, feelings of infatuation, and sexual passion can be experienced and enjoyed throughout the lifespan. As we discussed in relation to Sternberg's Triangular Theory of love in Chapter 7, although passionate feelings are an important ingredient in feelings of love and affection, other attributes too maintain these strong, enjoyable feelings well into old age. Unfortunately, the public displays of affection we take for granted among teenagers and young adults (kissing, hugging, holding hands, walking arm-in-arm) may elicit thoughts of "Act your age!" when seniors are engaged in the same behaviors.

Myth: Our Sexual Anatomy "Deteriorates" as We Age

Although our bodies, including our sex organs, change as we get older, they certainly don't "deteriorate." This is just another misconception that contributes to ways old people are misperceived in our culture. Yes, a woman's breasts may sag. Yes, we lose some pubic hair just as we lose hair on our heads. Yes, we often put on a few pounds over the course of a lifetime. But there is nothing inherently unsavory, unhealthy, or impaired about our sexual anatomy just because we get old. There are some predictable changes in our sexual response cycle as we age into and through our later years, but these are not substantial organic declines. Most people remain healthy, vital, and energetic well into their 70s and often their 80s. People who take care of themselves can expect only insignificant declines in their ability to share sexual enjoyment. Lifestyle issues that contribute to good health in adolescence and during pregnancy are just as important at the other end of the lifespan.

Myth: Older People are Too Frail to Fully Participate in Sexual Intimacy

In addition to the myths described by Felstein, Schlesinger (1996) has added a few more, such as this one, which is plainly absurd for most older people. The emotional and physical enjoyment a couple experiences when they share sexual intimacy (whether or not it involves intercourse) has little to do with vigor. Changes in the sexual response cycle in later life might slow down arousal or lengthen the amount of time a person spends in the plateau stage, but this does not mean lessened delight in one's partner.

Myth: Older People Cannot Control Their Sexual Desires

Schlesinger (1996) includes this judgmental perspective among the myths that color people's thinking about sex in later life. It stems from the belief that older people are not desirable, desirous, or capable of enjoying guilt-free, undiluted pleasure when they share sexual intimacy. This myth is a manifestation of the belief that older people should "act their age." Additionally, this myth is behind phrases like "dirty old man" or "old fool," which are unfortunate ways of stereotyping men in later life. Some people also have trouble accepting the fact that older women may indeed also be very interested in enjoying shared sexual experiences.

All these myths distort reality. The simple truth, as described by Masters & Johnson (1966), is that a couple can continue to have an active, enriching sex life if they are in fairly good health and have an interested and interesting partner.

The Psychosocial Arena of Sex in Later Life

Erik Erikson's psychosocial theory of development is important and applicable in old age as in earlier life stages. The eighth and final stage in this theory explores the implications of integrity versus despair. Where an individual falls on a continuum between these two poles profoundly affects their adjustment to marriage in later life, as well as their friendship patterns. When a person arrives in late life with a sense of integrity, for Erikson this implies that this person can look back over the course of her or his entire life and feel that they have always tried to do the best they could with the resources available to them at the time. Winston Churchill once said, "Do the best you can with what you have where you are." When people can look back over the course of their lives and feel in all honesty that they have tried to do their best, they age with a sense of integrity and the sense of completeness that comes with it. In contrast, when someone approaches the end of his or her life feeling that at some point in time he or she gave up and stopped trying to do the best they could or be the best person they could be, they instead age with a sense of despair. They are often bitter, self-focused individuals with no real potential for intimacy and mutuality in later life.

How people feel about themselves and what they may (or may not) have achieved during their life can affect the ease with which they share true emotional and/or sexual intimacy. As we have discussed before in other contexts, sexual feeling and expression are a microcosm of one's wider social orientation to the world and significant people in it.

Social scientists have known for many years that one's level of sexual activity in later life often reflects one's earlier sexual behavior (Thienhaus, Conter, & Bosmann, 1986). Additionally, the degree to which a person understands the physical changes that normally accompany sexual aging is related to their resiliency and flexibility in adapting to these changes. Importantly, everyone is not equally susceptible to society's ageist messages, and how one thinks about one's own aging is extremely important in predicting how smoothly and happily a person will approach the changes in late life development. The old adage "You're only as old as you feel" has a lot of truth to it.

Knowing about normal sexual aging may help older women and men avoid falling into the trap of expecting or, even worse, trying to force the type of sexual behaviors and responsiveness they may have enjoyed as younger adults (Meston, 1997). Society's myths give older adults the idea that lessened sexual intimacy is inevitable as we get older. However, there are many important positive aspects of sexual expression in later life. Butler and Lewis (1973) summarized these succinctly:

1. The opportunity for the expression of passion, affection, admiration, loyalty, and other positive emotions.
2. The affirmation of one's body and its functions—reassurance that our bodies are still capable of working well and providing pleasure.
3. A way of maintaining a strong sense of identity, enhancing self-esteem, and feeling valued as a person.

4. A means of self-assertion—an outlet for expressing oneself when other outlets for doing so have been lost.
5. Protection from anxiety as 'the intimacy and the closeness of sexual union bring security and significance to people's lives, particularly when the outside world threatens them with hazzards and losses.'
6. Defiance of stereotypes of aging.
7. The pleasure of being touched and caressed.
8. A sense of romance
9. An affirmation of a life that has been worthwhile because of the quality of intimate relationships that have been developed.
10. An avenue for continued sensual growth and experience.

—After Schlesinger, 1996, 128–129

Following are some facts about the amount of sexual sharing common in later life (Schlesinger, 1996).

- People 65 and older are often having as much sex, and in some cases more, than people aged 18 to 26 (The Janus Report on Sexual Behaviour, 1993).
- Most older gays and lesbians prefer to associate with peers of a similar age and have active sex lives with same-age partners (Berger, 1982).
- Forty percent of the women and half of the men in their 60s masturbate. Two-thirds of the women are sexually active; half or more have sex at least once a week (Brecher, 1984).
- In old age, ignorance of the facts surrounding sex is the greatest single deterrent to the active enjoyment of sexuality (Masters & Johnson, 1966).

—After Schlesinger, 1996, 126-127

Steinke (1994) carried out two questionnaire studies to learn more about sexual attitudes and knowledge among aging women and men, as well as to explore their level of sexual activity and sexual satisfaction. Subjects in this study were between the ages of 60 and 83, with a mean age just over 70. Most subjects were married (70%); 19% were widowed. Two-thirds lived with their spouse, and 31% lived alone. In all, 308 respondents completed questionnaires. Their sample was relatively well-educated: 46% had attended or graduated from college, and 25% had attended graduate school or earned a postgraduate degree. Their questionnaire responses showed these subjects were liberal in their sexual beliefs. Sexual activity in these studies included having sexual intercourse, intimate fondling, and masturbatory behavior. The average sexual activity for the men in this sample was about 5 times a month and about 4 times a month for women. These subjects reported a wide variation in their sexual satisfaction or enjoyment. Generally the subjects who were most sexually active reported having more accurate information about sex, more permissive attitudes about sex, and a greater religiousness in their lives. Respondents who were married scored a bit higher on the sexual knowledge survey than subjects who were widowed, fol-lowed by those who were separated or divorced. Finally, many subjects were particularly interested in the impact of chronic ailments and the medications used to treat them on sexual behavior and enjoyment. Data like these emphasize the fact that aging and elderly people know a good deal about sex, remain sexually active, and are somewhat concerned about illnesses and medications with regard to their impact on sexual behavior. A later section in this chapter concerns sexual dysfunctions in later life.

MENOPAUSE

After menopause women can no longer conceive and bear children, at least not without some rather unusual assisted reproductive technologies. Menopause is often an important developmental event in a woman's life. Social scientists often use the term **climacteric** to refer to an important turning point during a person's life, and that term is frequently used for both women and men although in women only it is accompanied by a specific constellation of hormonal, anatomical, and physiological changes. Menopause is not a sudden cessation of menstruation and abrupt end of fertility, however. The process of menopause can take place over the course of a few years. It involves irregularities in menstruation for many months before a woman stops having periods, and during this time she may continue to ovulate occasionally. Menopause in women and the climacteric in men are often referred to as the "change of life," although there is no necessary diminished quality or life, lessened energy, or frequent unruly moods. Menarche and menopause are similar in that both are important developmental events in the life span of women. When women are well informed and prepared for these changes, they are far better able to understand and cope with them. Menopause often involves the re-emergence of a concern we discussed in regard to adolescent sexuality: the important relationship between self-esteem and body image. People often become concerned at midlife that they have gained weight, eaten unwisely, perhaps consumed too much alcohol, and have been too sedentary. This awareness at about the time of menopause often motivates people to explore more healthy lifestyles.

For women socialized to think of their primary role in terms of conceiving and bearing children, menopause may occasion a re-assessment of their values, identity, and roles within and outside of the family. Whether or not a woman has had a child or children, the simple awareness that she is no longer fertile can be troubling for some. For women who decided early in life not to have children, the onset of menopause is sometimes a reminder of how irrevocable that decision was and may provoke feelings of regret.

The changes accompanying menopause are hormonal, anatomical, and physiological. Additionally, menopause may cause some increased health risks for women, such as osteoporosis and coronary artery disease. In all, many aspects of a woman's life may be affected. Nonetheless, only 1 woman in 5 has enough difficulty to require medical assistance. Of course, women frequently do not go through menopause alone. The changes discussed below affect not only the woman but often her partner as well. Because some moodiness often occurs during menopause, men too need to be fully prepared for these changes.

Hormonal and Physiological Changes in Women During Menopause

Psychological, physiological, and anatomical changes accompanying menopause result from the gradual cessation and then the complete stoppage of ovarian function. A woman's ovaries stop producing hormones, the most important of which is estrogen. Historically, much was made about how this affects a woman's moods:

> . . . *Unfavorable news, slight mishaps, arguments, all manner of little occurrences that would not disturb a normal individual cause quite a nervous and mental flurry.*
> *These people are irritable and easily aggravated or excited to anger by deed or word. They are hard to please. Noises of playing children, the radio—almost anything stirs them to action. In fact, they need no special stimulus. They are simply hard to get along with. In many instances they acknowledge this condition but state that they cannot help being so.*

> —A. A. WERNER, IN FISBEIN AND BURGESS, 1947, 476

This statement provides an interesting perspective regarding the way the medical establishment used to view menopause. Happily, contemporary perspectives are less stereotyped and are far more optimistic.

Beginning at about the age of 40, the number of ovarian primary follicles in a woman's ovaries begins to decline more rapidly. Also at this time, the levels of FSH in a woman's bloodstream begin to fluctuate widely. Sometimes there are large increases in the amount of this hormone while the primary follicles are decreasing sharply in the ovary (Burger, 1994). Additionally, these changes are frequently accompanied by menstrual cycles of widely differing durations, from 28 days long to as long as 48 days. Yet even when these changes are happening, the woman may experience none of the traditional symptoms of menopause. Generally when women begin to experience the gradual onset of menopause, a number of symptoms begin to appear, including the following:

1. Women may begin to experience symptoms of premenstrual syndrome. These may occur for the first time, or, if a woman has experienced them in the past, the symptoms may grow more pronounced.
2. Regardless of PMS, mood swings become more common at this time.
3. Depression and/or anxiety may occur, often without obvious precipitating cause in the psychosocial environment.
4. Irritability and/or anger may occur in relationships when there is little apparent reason for these feelings.

5. Women may have difficulty concentrating on intellectual and/or motor tasks for prolonged periods of time.
6. Changes in one's normal sleep pattern may occur. Some women have a need for less sleep, while others feel they need much more. Some women have insomnia and the fatigue that usually accompanies it.
7. Changes in appetite. Although some women gain weight when they are going through menopause, others experience a noticeable loss of appetite.
8. Previously regular menstrual cycles begin to become irregular in both duration and amount of menstrual discharge. There may also be changes in the amount of discomfort accompanying menstrual cramps.
9. Diminished vaginal secretions. Lubrication accompanying sexual arousal is usually both reduced and delayed in onset after erotic stimulation begins.
10. "Hot flashes" begin to occur and sometimes wake women during the night when accompanied by night sweats. A hot flash is a sudden feeling of warmth that may involve excessive perspiration and itching of the skin.

Although this list does not describe all of the many symptoms that may accompany menopause, these are the most common. Despite the decreases in ovarian estrogens at this time, a woman can still become pregnant while going through these changes. The once small, smooth, pink ovaries of a younger

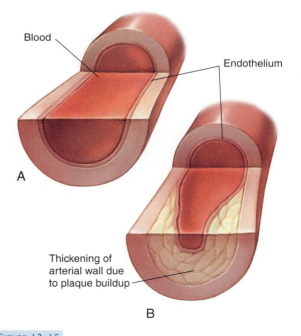

FIGURE 13-15   **A.** A healthy artery without any plaque deposits. **B.** An artery with plaque deposits. Narrowed brain and heart arteries, respectively, predispose individuals to strokes and heart attacks.

woman become tiny, shrunken, and gray. In the United States, most women reach menopause in their early 50s, with some variability, but this process can take many months or a few years. The term "perimenopausal" describes the months that immediately precede and follow the cessation of menstruation, and the term "postmenopausal" describes the years that follow this transition. We emphasize the fact that menopause takes place over a prolonged period of time because this is an important developmental challenge for women at mid-life, and while this is happening they are still wives, mothers, and workers with a number of important roles to play.

Health Problems Associated With Menopause

Decreasing amounts of estrogen in a woman's bloodstream predispose her to a number of health problems. For example, medical and social scientists have long known that estrogens offer women many protective effects against coronary artery disease. The "bad cholesterol," low-density lipoprotein (LDL), in a woman's bloodstream begins to rise, and the "good cholesterol," high density lipoprotein (HDL), begins to fall. Therefore, many of the protective effects of good cholesterol are diminished (Fig. 13-15). The risk of developing heart disease is magnified in women who smoke, drink, or are overweight. Later we'll discuss how an important benefit of hormone replacement therapy is a lowered risk of developing heart

disease. Many doctors encourage menopausal women to be cautious in their dietary habits, to give up smoking, and to get moderate exercise regularly.

Another consequence of lowered levels of estrogen in a woman's bloodstream is an increased risk of osteoporosis, a condition in which the loss of calcium from bones makes them more brittle and more likely to break in a fall or other injury (Fig. 13-16). This condition takes place gradually and may be affected by hereditary factors. According to Reinish (1990), women most likely to experience osteoporosis are:

1. Women who have a mother or sister with severe osteoporosis
2. Caucasian or Asian women
3. Slender women
4. Women who smoke cigarettes
5. Women who regularly consume alcohol
6. Those who do little or no weight-bearing exercise and are sedentary
7. Women who have consumed less than 1000 milligrams daily of calcium when they were younger (either as a part of their diets or in the form of supplements)
8. Women who have used cortisone over a number of years
9. Women with hormonal problems early in life that led to low levels of estrogen at that time

—After Reinish, 1990, 213

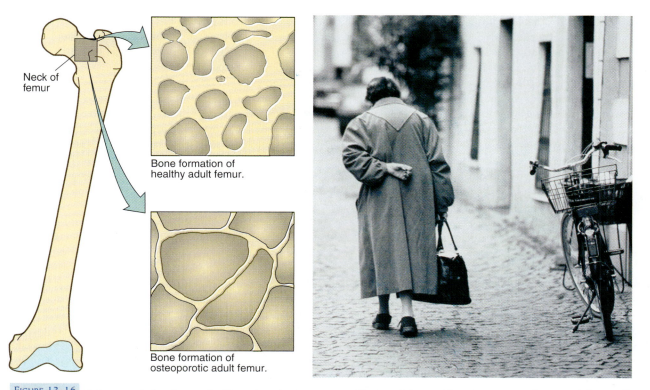

Neck of femur

Bone formation of healthy adult femur.

Bone formation of osteoporotic adult femur.

FIGURE 13-16 Osteoporosis involves a significant loss in the amount of bone calcium, with an increase in the size of the small pores normally found in healthy bone.

The most effective way to avoid osteoporosis in later life is to build and keep as much bone mass as possible during adolescence and early adulthood by eating a variety of foods rich in calcium (but ideally low in fat). Low-fat dairy products and leafy green vegetable are particularly rich in calcium and should be regularly incorporated in a woman's diet. Hopefully, these good eating habits continue throughout a woman's life.

Skin changes also result from declining amounts of estrogen in the bloodstream. One of the basic building blocks of skin tissue is collagen, which acts like an adhesive to keep skin smooth, soft, and taut. When estrogen levels fall, there is a breakdown in collagen in the skin, as well as in other body tissues. This may accelerate the normal wrinkling that accompanies the aging process. Smoking cigarettes further accelerates the breakdown of collagen in the skin, and the combination of menopause, smoking, and long-term exposure to the sun can cause some rather dramatic changes in the skin. Many women's face creams, especially the more expensive ones, contain synthetic estrogens because some think these agents keep skin tissues moist, soft, and taut.

Hot flashes are feelings of being flushed, warm, or itchy due to a sudden dilation of blood vessels in the skin. The physiological causes of hot flashes are not known. The head, face, and neck are frequently affected, although hot flashes can affect the entire body. They are often accompanied by heavy perspiration that, when occurring during sleep, is commonly called "night sweats." Neither heart rate nor blood pressure increase during these episodes, and skin temperature does not increase. As of this writing, we know of no specific hormone related to the incidence or severity of hot flashes, and there are no effective, reliable treatments. Hot flashes are often uncomfortable and highly distracting and may also cause embarrassment. Women are frequently distressed by them and can be upset if the men in their lives are not sympathetic or supportive about this normal aspect of menopause.

Breast changes are also common during the normal progression of menopause. Breast tissue responds to changing levels of estrogen and progesterone in the bloodstream, affecting the appearance of a woman's breasts, along with a loss of the elasticity of the connective tissues that support the breasts. Whether a woman has had and/or nursed babies is also thought to affect breast configuration. The impact of long-term use of oral contraceptives on breast changes in later life is not well understood. Breast appearance changes can be important at this time in the lifespan because of the relationship of body image and self-esteem.

Urinary system problems occur commonly with menopause but are seldom discussed. Because the tissues of the urinary system also require estrogen for proper health and functioning, the falling levels of estrogen at menopause also often affect a variety of urinary behaviors and may cause difficult or painful urination, feelings of needing to urinate frequently with little resulting volume, the need to get up frequently at night to urinate, an urgent need to urinate, and urinary incontinence. A variety of drug therapies are often effective for these uncomfortable and sometimes embarrassing problems.

Changes in the endometrium frequently accompany menopause, sometimes from its earliest signs. Because the thickness of the lining of the uterus changes during a woman's normal menstrual cycles due to the action of estrogen and progesterone, diminished secretions of these hormones during menopause affects the amount and regularity of menstruation at this time. Some women begin to have extremely heavy and uncomfortable periods at this time but can be helped by a variety of surgical and drug therapies.

Hormone Replacement Therapy

One of the most controversial aspects of medical treatments for menopause involves taking hormone pills to replace the hormones a woman's ovaries are no longer producing. Hormone replacement therapy (HRT) has stimulated an enormous amount of speculation, opinion, and research. Although some physicians are quietly and firmly supportive of the benefits of HRT, others have concerns and are more cautious. This is a very active area of research, and new drugs and drug combinations are being developed even as this is being written. Doctors take into account a number of factors when deciding whether HRT is appropriate for a patient, such as the seriousness of her symptoms accompanying falling levels of female hormones, her risks of developing coronary artery disease and osteoporosis, and her risks of breast cancer or other cancers of her reproductive system. Every woman has a somewhat unique situation to discuss with her doctor. As with any medical treatment, possible benefits must be weighed against potential risks. Physicians must also consider the patient's compliance or adherence, since gynecologists today estimate that one-third to one-half of women for whom HRT is prescribed either do not fill their prescription or stop taking the pills. Little is known about why patients do not follow medical recommendations that are likely to be beneficial.

Although HRT effectively minimizes the health problems discussed in the previous section, some women should avoid hormone replacement under most circumstances, including women who have a family history of ovarian, uterine, or breast cancer or who have large benign uterine tumors, blood clotting abnormalities, or gall bladder or liver disease. However, women who do not have these risks and who are likely to develop heart disease or osteoporosis after menopause may be very good candidates for these drugs. The earliest HRT agents used in the 1970s had rather large doses of estrogen and were implicated in a rise in the number of cases of endometrial cancer. Lower doses of estrogen significantly lowered the risks of this problem, and today many women use low-dose estrogen in combination with progestin or, in some cases, testosterone. The combination of estrogen and progestin essentially eliminated the suspected link between HRT and endometrial cancer. Even though the use of HRT is increasing in this country, most menopausal women do not take these hormones. Women who have had the uterus removed do not need HRT.

Synthetic hormones can be introduced into a woman's body in a number of safe, reliable ways. Hormone pills are the most common form of HRT. Oral hormones usually help raise a woman's level of HDL (the "good cholesterol" discussed earlier). Estrogen patches are another good way to introduce hormones into the bloodstream (Fig. 13-17), but estrogen patches do not raise good cholesterol levels. Another way to administer hormones is by injection, but this method requires monthly visits to the doctor and may also require expensive blood tests to assess hormone levels in the bloodstream. Also, these injections do not increase the amount of good cholesterol in the bloodstream. Although these alternatives introduce hormones into a woman's circulatory system, there are other forms of HRT as well.

With a topical application, hormone creams are applied directly on a woman's skin or vaginal tissues. Estrogen and progestin skin creams can be applied over the abdomen or on the arms or thighs. The same amount of cream should be applied each time, but this is not always easy to do, and many women report that this method is sloppy. Women using skin creams often have blood levels of these hormones much higher than in women taking hormone pills or using patches. Vaginal creams are especially useful, however, for women who are troubled only by vaginal changes during menopause, such as dryness, painful intercourse, and itching. The estrogen in vaginal creams does enter the woman's bloodstream, however, so care and consistency in applying them are important.

Despite the benefits of HRT pills, there are a number of annoying or troubling side effects. By some estimates, about half of the women using these pills will continue to experience vaginal bleeding for a number of months. The method of HRT administration depends on the individual's personal health situation and is generally decided in consultation with her physician.

BENEFITS OF HORMONE REPLACEMENT THERAPY

When menopause is accompanied by troubling, uncomfortable, or embarrassing symptoms, HRT is often highly effective in minimizing or eliminating these in addition to reducing the risks of developing more serious problems like heart disease and osteoporosis. Of women experiencing hot flashes, one-fourth to one-half will enjoy a significant relief when using HRT. This is especially important if a woman has been suffering from loss of sleep due to hot flashes at night and night sweats.

When estrogen levels in the bloodstream fall during menopause, there is also a loss in the elasticity, softness, and tone of vaginal tissues. This can cause burning, itching, and uncomfortable intercourse. Women using HRT are significantly helped with these problems, but a woman may need to wait several months before these benefits of HRT become obvious. Urinary incontinence can also be helped somewhat by HRT, but most physicians recommend Kegel exercises as well (described in Chapter 4). The combination of both approaches is often very effective in eliminating this problem.

Finally, many women experience periods of anxiety and depression during menopause and are often unprepared for the seriousness and persistence of these problems. These difficulties can be more troubling if the woman is having a hard time reevaluating her identity regarding the end of her fertility. For-

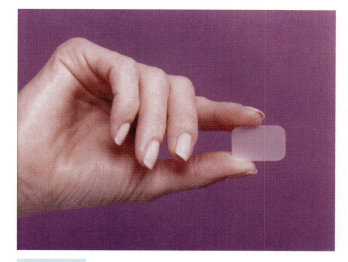

FIGURE 13-17 Skin patches impregnated with synthetic estrogens are one efficient means of administering hormone replacement therapy to women during and after menopause.

tunately, HRT can also help women regain a more calm, optimistic outlook on life.

THE RISKS OF HORMONE REPLACEMENT THERAPY

As with other medicines and medical treatments, there are some important risks women should be aware of before they and their doctors decide on HRT. These problems do not happen to most women who begin HRT, but again, the use of any medication must involve weighing the possible benefits against the potential problems. Medical investigators have long been worried about a possible link between HRT and reproductive system and breast cancers. The addition of progestin to estrogen replacement therapy seems to have significantly reduced the risks of these cancers, even though the suspicion of some risk continues. As of this writing, doctors believe that among women who have never had reproductive system or breast cancer, HRT for a period of 5 years or less seems to be medically advisable for women with troubling menopausal symptoms and is accompanied by relatively small risks (Burger & Kenemans, 1998). However, among women who have had these cancers, HRT should not be prescribed, even for women having a very difficult time with their menopausal symptoms.

Uterine cancer is the reproductive system cancer most likely to be related to HRT, especially when estrogen is used without progestin. The use of the latter agent, however, is thought to significantly reduce the risks of these cancers, but this is a complex issue with few clear answers or recommendations for every woman. The relationship between HRT and breast cancer has also been a concern for many years now, but the chances of developing this disease are affected by a number of fairly well-known risk factors. As with uterine cancer, it is not known precisely just how much the addition of progestin to estrogen will reduce the risk of developing breast cancer. Women with close relatives who have had breast cancer may not be good candidates for HRT, however, nor are women who smoke cigarettes and/or consume 2-3 alcoholic beverages each day (Zumoff, 1998). In fact, many doctors today recommend limiting alcohol consumption at this time and increasing the number of servings of antioxidant-rich vegetables (such as broccoli and cabbage) in one's diet. Still other scientists have found no increase in the development of breast cancer in women using HRT who have had a relative with breast cancer (Sellers, Mink, Cerhan, Zheng, Anderson, Kushi, & Folsom, 1997).

The potentially harmful risks associated with HRT may or may not affect any particular women, and overall the chances of developing these diseases is relatively low. There are, however, a number of side-effects that are far more common. Vaginal bleeding is probably the most common, troubling aspect of HRT and is most likely to occur when progestin is no longer a part of the treatment regimen. Vaginal bleeding will lessen in most women taken off progestin, but some women will continue to bleed as long as they are taking HRT. This side effect can be very difficult for some women to manage, and it is important to talk with one's doctor about different medications, different doses, and different timing of medication throughout the course of the month. In addition to vaginal bleeding, breast pain may also accompany HRT, and this is especially likely to occur when progestin is part of the management of menopausal symptoms.

MANAGING MENOPAUSE WITHOUT HORMONES

Many women choose not to use estrogen and/or progestin replacement after having discussed the matter thoroughly with their doctor, and there are a number of well-documented reasons they choose this alternative with a clear conscience (O'Leary Cobb, 1994). Here is a brief summary of some of these reasons.

1. **Many women view menopause as a natural life transition.** They feel that the discomforts and annoyances associated with the change of life are normal and can be tolerated with a little patience and guidance and reassurance from their doctor.

2. **All women do not see osteoporosis as a threat.** Women without a family history of this disease and those who have built bone mass through diet during their adolescence and young adult years do not feel that they are at risk for the development of osteoporosis.

3. **The side effects of HRT can be very annoying.** Earlier we noted that often women who are prescribed estrogen or estrogen and progestin combination drugs do not fill their prescriptions or do not continue to take them regularly if they do. Vaginal bleeding, weight gain, breast discomfort, and headaches may play a role. If a woman knows someone who is dealing with these problems, she may decide that HRT isn't for her.

4. **The distinction between prevention and treatment.** Women who have been careful to eat a good diet and get plenty of aerobic exercise do not feel that they need HRT as a prevention against the development of health problems later in life. After all, they have already been taking pretty good care of themselves and may not believe that medication can do what their lifestyles have already accomplished.

5. **Many women do not think estrogen is safe.** While a woman's doctor might tell her that HRT is safe, she is often skeptical when her blood pressure is checked, a cholesterol test is ordered, a mammogram is carried out, and a thorough medical and family history are taken. After all, if estrogen is supposed to be so safe, why do all these tests?

6. **Many women are aware of the suspected link between breast cancer and HRT.** Despite what her doctor may tell her, many women are very concerned about the development of breast cancer and the role HRT might play in this process. This is especially true of a woman who has had a friend who has or had breast cancer.

—After O'Leary Cobb, 1994, 526

These issues show there are several complex issues involved and that it is sometimes difficult to go against medical opinion for personal reasons. But there are a number of highly effective ways of managing menopause without using hormones.

Regular, moderate aerobic exercise will diminish the risks of developing both osteoporosis and coronary artery disease, and if exercise has been a lifelong part of a woman's lifestyle she can expect to enjoy substantial benefits. If, in addition, she has eaten a diet rich in calcium and low in both cholesterol and saturated fats, she can expect still additional protection against the development of these disorders. Additionally, data point to a lower frequency of hot flashes among women who are aerobically active, although more data are needed in order to learn more about this (Notelovitz, 1994). Finally, a number of herbal alternatives for menopausal symptoms have become more popular in recent years, and there has been a long tradition among Japanese women in using these remedies to lessen these symptoms. Some plants contain compounds that function like estrogen; called *phytoestrogens,* these have been clinically proven to diminish many of the more uncomfortable symptoms of menopause, such as hot flashes. These are present in soy products and isoflavones (Seidl & Stewart, 1998). Clearly, more research is needed in this area.

Psychosocial Aspects of Menopause

Women do not go through menopause alone. They live with husbands or partners, they interact with co-workers, they may be mothers, and of course they often have extended families as well. There is a relationship between the experience of menopausal symptoms and a woman's general adjustment in her entire psychosocial environment. Indeed, happiness and emotional well-being have long been the focus of studies on menopause. About 25 years ago physicians thought that depression was an almost inevitable accompaniment of menopause and even had a special name for it: "involutional melancholia." We know today that there is no causative relationship between menopause and clinical depression, and this rather old-fashioned term is no longer used. Although some investigations have pointed to an increase in the prevalence of psychological symptoms during menopause, others have found no such relationship. There has been very little research on feelings of well-being or happiness during menopause (Dennerstein, 1994).

In a large study carried out in Australia during 1991, 2000 women at mid-life were surveyed. These subjects were between the ages of 45 and 55, a period that includes the time window during which menopause occurs in most women. These women participated in a telephone interview that focused on feelings of well-being and happiness. Their names were drawn at random from the Melbourne White Pages. Perhaps the most obvious and important finding of this study is the fact that a very large percentage of these subjects used very positive adjectives to describe how they felt "most of the time." Here are some of the results of this study.

Positive Feelings	Percentage of Respondents
Satisfied	61.4
Relaxed	45.0
Clear-headed	72.0
Useful	68.4
Loving	55.5
Optimistic	51.4
Enthusiastic	43.5
Good-natured	70.5
Confident	57.8
Understood	60.4

Interestingly, a very low percentage of these subjects used very negative adjectives to describe how they felt "most of the time." Here are more results of this study.

Negative Feelings	Percentage of Respondents
Lonely	4.0
Helpless	2.9
Impatient	8.4
Depressed	3.9
Hopeless	15.4
Withdrawn	2.2
Discontented	4.6
Confused	3.6
Tense	11.4
Insignificant	4.2

—Data from Dennerstein, 1994

Clearly the women in this study did not generally describe their feelings in negative terms in this large, random, representative urban sample. Overall, subjects who reported fewer worries about aging and menopause described more positive feelings, and those who reported more worries about aging and menopause reported more negative feelings. Nonetheless, the relatively large percentage of subjects using very positive terms and the decidedly lower percentages of women using very negative ones is striking.

The relationship between menopause and depression is not easy to unravel. Medical researchers, sociologists, psychologists, and anthropologists often come to different conclusions because they are all working from somewhat different theoretical perspectives and use different techniques to study this problem. In two large studies carried out in Manitoba, Canada and Massachusetts, very similar data were collected regarding the prevalence of depression in women during menopause: somewhere between 9% and 11%. In both studies, a woman's menopausal status did not seem to be related to the presence or severity of depression. If lowered levels of estrogen are suspected of being implicated in depression, this association is seen in a very small number of women, and the depression does not seem to last very long (Kaufert, 1994). Kaufert has found that depression at or around the time of menopause seems to be more closely related to a woman's general health status. Longstanding health problems and overall poor health are the strongest predictors of depression among women at this time in their lives. Yet this author correctly points out that a large number of factors in a woman's wider psychosocial environment may also affect whether she experiences depression during menopause. Among these are:

> *. . . class, income or ethnicity, diet, whether a woman works, her type of work, whether she is married, has children, when these children were born and their number. In this model of menopause, a woman's response to the end of menses will have as much to do with social attitudes towards the menopausal woman as the impact of declining estrogens on sexual function.*

—Kaufert, 1994, 167

Although HRT is beneficial in lessening the seriousness or rate of development of osteoporosis and coronary artery disease, no similarly clear effect is yet clear with regard to depression. While overall well-being might be enhanced by taking estrogen during menopause, no cause-and-effect relationship has yet been demonstrated that HRT lessens a woman's chances of becoming depressed at this time (Hunter, 1994).

Sexual Experience and Expression During Menopause

Despite the normal physical changes that accompany menopause, this life transition need not mean the end of regular, enjoyable sexual interaction for women. Declining estrogens do indeed affect a woman's body, her sex drive, the ease with which she can experience orgasm, and the ease with which she can enjoy intercourse without discomfort. A woman's body changes during menopause, and sometimes these changes are marked. We have seen that declining levels of estrogen in the bloodstream alters skin softness and elasticity, breasts usually sag, there is a loss of muscular tone, and skeletal changes occur as well. For many women body image becomes a troubling preoccupation at this time of life. Often women who don't feel very good about their bodies become much less interested in sharing sexual intimacy (Bachmann, 1995). Therefore, lessened sexual desire is a result of both lower levels of estrogen and increased dissatisfaction with body image. When this scenario is coupled with the prejudices of ageism and the widely held myth that older women don't or shouldn't have any interest in enjoying sexuality, there are often some real psychological obstacles among women when it comes to fully enjoying sexuality in later life.

Surveys focusing on sexual activity among women at and after menopause all indicate a lower frequency of sexual intercourse and other avenues of sexual expression, although as we have already noted, the frequency of sexual expression in later life can be predicted by the frequency of sexual expression in young and middle-adulthood. Another important reason for this decline is the normal tissue changes in a woman's genital and urinary systems. Because of these factors and the increasing lack of availability of sexual partners, there are a number of unhappy sexual aspects about menopause for many women. One analysis of surveys concerning menopause and women's sexuality summarizes what is going on with most of the women studied at different times before, during, and after menopause (McCoy, 1994). These data reveal that vaginal dryness and diminished lubrication typically begin about two years before a woman's last menstrual cycle, with declining sexual interest and decreasing intercourse frequency occurring within a year of this point in time. Between one and two years after a woman's last period painful intercourse (dyspareunia) becomes more common, as do diminished sexual arousal and a lessened ability to have orgasms, and some women even stop having intercourse (McCoy, 1994, p. 586). These data are the summarized results of a number of different studies and may not predict or describe any particular woman's progress through menopause and its impact on her sexual experiences. Remember also that HRT has a beneficial effect on continued sexual expression in many women who use it.

"MALE MENOPAUSE"

There is no clear equivalent in men to menopause in women. Scientists have explored this question and have reported that male "andropause," as it has been called, is very different from menopause among women. Specifically, there is no clear end point to most men's fertility, nor any sudden fall in the level of male hormones, the two most obvious features of menopause in women (Fig. 13-18). At the same time, there is indeed diminished fertility among aging men, as well as gradually falling levels of sex hormones. Lowered androgen levels begin to become obvious in a number of ways. For example, there is a decrease in pubic hair, lessened muscle mass and muscular strength, diminished bone mass, decreased sex drive, and lowered frequency of sexual intercourse. These changes, however, may not be related entirely to falling levels of androgen in a man's bloodstream (Vermeulen, 1994). For

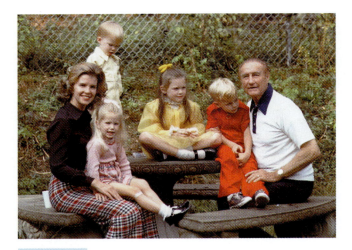

FIGURE 13-18   Senator Strom Thurmond of South Carolina with his wife Nancy and their children (clockwise): Paul, 20 months, Julia, 3, Strom Jr., 5, and Nancy Moore, 6. This picture was taken November 6, 1977. Senator Thurmond was born in 1902.

example, the build-up of fatty substances in the body's arteries may diminish the blood supply to the penis, making erection difficult. There are also the problems of unavailability of sexual partners, boredom with one's lifelong mate, long periods of sexual abstinence, and the fear of failure with respect to sexual performance. These psychosocial factors are also likely to play an important role in diminished sexual interest or performance among men in later life.

Between the ages of 20 and 80, most men undergo about a 35% decrease in the amount of testosterone in their bloodstream (Vermeulen & Kaufman, 1995; Tserotas & Marino, 1998). It is unclear whether the testes are making less of this hormone or are not being adequately stimulated by the pituitary gland. Very low levels of male sex hormones are seen in only a minority of men between the ages of 40 and 80. When these hormonal changes are coupled with fatigue and the common stresses of aging, lower levels of sexual interest and activity may be expected.

Can men just be given androgen to minimize or reverse these problems? As of this writing, there has not yet been a carefully controlled clinical investigation of the effects of male hormone supplementation on normal older men, so it would be premature to assume that this treatment would have beneficial or sexually restorative effects (Burns-Cox & Gingell, 1997). In addition, by some estimates (Vermeulen, 1994), about half of all men 70 and older have some cancerous cells in their prostate gland that are not causing any clinical, urinary, or sexual problems. This small number of cells usually doesn't cause any problems, and doctors often take a "watchful waiting" approach. However, male hormone supplements have the potential to accelerate the development of more obvious prostate cancer signs and symptoms, so their use is risky and many think unadvisable. Some research (de Lignieres, 1993) has demonstrated a beneficial effect of skin patches containing dihydrotestosterone without causing enlargement of the prostate in a sample of men

Other Countries, Cultures, and Customs

SEX IN LATER LIFE IN OTHER CULTURES

In 1982, Winn and Newton published a comparative study about the ways in which sexual feelings and expression in later life are viewed in 106 different cultures; much of the information was based entirely on oral reports, with no written record of the responses from these aging and elderly women and men. Despite the diminished sexual activity reported among American women, sexual behavior, inclination, and discussion among older people elsewhere is somewhat different from that seen in our own society. As of this writing, little is known about geriatric sexuality elsewhere in the world. Winn and Newton collected their data from the Human Relations Area Files (HRAF), which is a collection of data about different cultures, both "preindustrial" and "traditional." Cultures in Asia, Africa, Micronesia, the Middle East, and Native American Indians are included in this enormous sample.

Information from 293 different cultures is stored in these files, some of which include more "developed" cultures, but only 106 of these were used in their study of sexual behavior in later life. One interesting attribute of these data is that preliterate cultures do not normally assign a specific age or age range to "older" or "very old" members of their societies. However, oral reports from these people generally come from individuals in their 60s, 70s, and beyond. A person's *appearance*, not their chronological age, is what classifies them as an older member of society, according to local traditions. Among these 106 cultures, 28 provided data about sexual behavior in older men, and in 20 of these sexual behavior well into old age is normal and expected. Only at very "advanced" ages is there less expectancy of sexual interest or behavior. Because life expectancies among these preliterature cultures do not match those in more developed cultures, it is hard to say exactly what "advanced" means in this context. Data were collected from 26 societies regarding continued sexual interest and behavior among aging and elderly women, and 22 of these provide explicit accounts of sexual behavior in the majority of these women well into later life. Preliterate cultures referred to these subjects as "old women," or as being "many years after menopause." Indeed, in most places in the world where anthropologists have explored continued sexual interest and behavior in later life, they have found it.

Another consistent finding in this cross-cultural survey is the fact that as women and men become older, they are less inhibited about talking and joking around about sex. Indeed, among the older women in this study, overt "shamelessness" and sexual assertiveness were not uncommon. These older women were also likely to engage in sexual humor and banter. The exact reasons for the lessening of conversational and behavioral inhibitions about sex are unclear, but this is a rather prominent finding in about one-fourth of the societies surveyed in this research.

The final set of findings from these cultures concerns the consistency with which sexual feeling and behavior among the aging and elderly are viewed by younger members of their society as something unwholesome. Although these examples of ageism were relatively uniform in this group of cultures, only three (found in Taiwan, northern Greece, and the Philippines) were overly disapproving and suggested that sex among the aging and elderly openly violated cultural norms. In this sample of 106 cultures, older men were seen as sexually undesirable marriage partners for young women, and the attractiveness of older women as marriage partners was also viewed pessimistically. However, these writers note that there were "relatively few" reports that sexual expression in later life was inappropriate.

Data such as these are important if we are to avoid the ethnocentric biases mentioned earlier in this book. If your parents or grandparents came to this country from a different culture and customs, the traditions in which they were raised probably influenced your own home life to some degree whether or not you are aware of it.

between 55 and 70. It remains to be seen whether this kind of treatment will become more common in the future.

PHYSIOLOGICAL CHANGES IN SEXUAL RESPONSIVENESS IN LATER LIFE

Now let's examine biological aspects of sexual arousal and response among women and men as they grow through mid-life and into their later years. Such changes have been called "physiosexual." Because we have already discussed the anatomical changes in the genitourinary system in both sexes, the focus here is more on function than the changing structure of sexual anatomy. This information derives directly from laboratory investigations and is supported by questionnaire and interview data. Although there are indeed notable changes in sexual arousal and response among women and men, sexuality remains a high personal priority among many aging and older people even though their bodies are responding differently from how they did when they were much younger. Physical intimacy is still a richly rewarding experience and continues to help maintain good, loving relationships. Understanding these changes helps one more comfortably accept them in later life.

Physiosexual Changes in Aging Women

The Arousal Phase. The arousal phase involves feelings of growing sexual excitement and the beginnings of vaginal lubrication. There is an increase in overall muscular tension. Although these changes begin fairly soon after sexual stimulation in younger women, they are usually delayed, sometimes significantly, as women age through mid-life and into their later years. Some women are helped by vaginal suppositories that provide significant added lubrication promptly. These can be purchased over-the-counter. There is also a smaller increase in breast size during arousal as a woman ages.

The Plateau Phase. During the plateau phase sexual excitement continues to build, and in later life this too takes longer. Most women enjoy the noticeable but leisurely increase in sexual tension. In other words, the amount of time between initial sexual excitement and the feeling that orgasm will soon occur increases as we grow older. This is a wonderful time for sharing caresses and tender words while a woman becomes more and more excited.

Orgasm. While the first two stages of the sexual response cycle take longer as we get older, the remaining two stages are somewhat shorter. Orgasm, in particular, does not last as long and involves fewer vaginal and anal contractions. Additionally, if a woman has been multi-orgasmic in her younger years, she may have a somewhat lessened capacity for this in later life. Finally, many women report that their orgasms are not as intense as when they were younger. This doesn't mean they are unpleasant—only different.

The Resolution Phase. During the resolution phase, a person's body returns to its pre-arousal state, and in later life this takes place more rapidly than during youth and young adulthood. This does not imply that a woman no longer appreciates tender, prolonged after-play.

This is a rough outline of what most women can expect as they age. Individual differences are common. A woman with any specific concerns should talk with her gynecologist.

Physiosexual Changes in Aging Men

There is an important similarity in the physiosexual changes in women and men. Generally, the first two stages of the sexual response cycle take more time, and the second two stages take less time. If a man knows that these changes are normal, he will probably be less concerned about them when they occur.

The Arousal Phase. Erection in men is the physiological equivalent to vaginal lubrication in women. Just as it takes a woman longer to begin lubricating as she gets older, it takes a man longer to attain an erection. He may also notice that his erection is not as hard or large as it was in his younger years. While young men may attain erections in just a minute or two, older men may require several minutes. Older men need to know this so that they will not become impatient or frustrated. This phase of the sexual response cycle is adversely affected by erectile dysfunction, in which there is the loss of a man's capacity to attain and maintain an erection altogether (see Chapter 14).

The Plateau Phase. Just as with women, sexual excitement or tension takes longer to build during the plateau phase in men. Men often say that they like this feeling of growing excitement, because it often offers more time to enjoy foreplay without quickly proceeding to penetration. A man who was troubled by premature ejaculation in his younger years is much less likely to be bothered by this as he gets older. Men often report that they require more stimulation during the arousal and plateau phases to become erect and ready for orgasm.

Orgasm. During later life, a man's orgasms are briefer and involve fewer muscular contractions. The amount of semen leaving the penis is also diminished, and it leaves a man's body with less force as he ages. Also, most men report that their orgasms are not as intense as they were when they were younger, although are still highly enjoyable.

The Resolution Phase. As men age, their refractory periods last longer. They will not be able to attain another erection as soon as they could when younger. A man's body returns to its pre-arousal state much quicker than at an earlier age. The penis softens more quickly after orgasm. Again, this doesn't mean that men are disinterested in holding their partners or in being held after they have had intercourse.

Adapting to Changes in the Sexual Response Cycle

Although sexual changes usually accompany the aging process, a couple can take measures to adapt to or compensate for them. Hopefully, this couple has a good, open working sexual rapport and can comfortably communicate thoughts and feelings about a number of sexual issues. For example, the couple must learn to be more patient about the man getting an erection and about delayed lubrication in the woman. They need to understand the importance of prolonged tactile and/or oral stimulation of one another during foreplay. Working or trying to attain an erection can have exactly the opposite effect and further inhibit the process.

Couples usually don't need much guidance to adapt to a prolonged plateau phase. In fact, this stage can acquire a more relaxed, sensuous quality as the couple has more time to engage in unhurried intercourse or a variety of non-intercourse avenues of sexual pleasuring. Both women and men seem to need increasingly vigorous stimulation to have orgasms as they age, and the plateau phase takes longer to provide this stimulation. Again, trying to rapidly achieve orgasm can be very counterproductive. Because women experience a thinning of their vaginal tissues as they age and also have diminished vaginal lubrication, vigorous or prolonged intercourse may be painful. Additional lubricant in suppository form or in the form of sterile surgical lubricant from a tube can be very effective in minimizing this discomfort. Because the resolution phase does not last as long in later life, couples may find that their genitals suddenly lose sensitivity after orgasm. But this does not mean that they wouldn't enjoy some cuddling, hugging, and skin-to-skin time together afterwards.

Illness and Sexuality in Later Life

With increasing age comes a greater chance of becoming ill. Several ailments can diminish sexual interest or impair sexual responsiveness. In addition, the treatments for a number of these problems may in themselves affect sexual functioning. While some illnesses are very serious and life threatening, others are less so but still may affect sexual arousal and response. The following sections describe some of the more common health problems likely to affect the aging and elderly. Remember, these diseases affect many aspects of human behavior, not just sexual expression. Chapter 16 more thoroughly discusses sexuality and disability. The following sections are some of the most common ailments of later life.

CARDIOVASCULAR DISEASE

Diseases of the heart and blood vessels are among the most common health problems of older Americans, including heart disease, heart attack, and stroke. These common health problems may vary a great deal in their seriousness, and generally the more significant the ailment, the more pronounced will be its effects on sexual arousal and response. For people who have had strokes, sexual drive will generally decrease, but only somewhat and usually temporarily (Kellett, 1991). However, if a stroke results in weakness, loss of speech, or some degree of paralysis, sexual interest and activity are affected adversely. These effects may not be permanent, and with the recovery of normal functioning sexual interest typically returns. However, after a person has had a heart attack or other forms of impairment in the functioning of the heart muscle, lessened sexual desire is likely to be more prolonged. In addition to these problems, closure or constriction of the blood vessels supplying the pelvic area may contribute to problems in sexual arousal in both women and men.

Sometimes, drugs commonly used to treat heart and blood vessel disorders also diminish sexual interest and responsiveness. For example, many drugs used to treat high blood pressure significantly impair a man's ability to attain an erection and a woman's capacity to lubricate vaginally. Additionally, several of these agents also cause fatigue, which can make a person much less interested in sexual sharing. In fact, many people stop taking prescribed blood pressure lowering agents because of their adverse effects on sexual arousal and response. However, there are many different drugs used to treat hypertension, and often finding one with minimal or no effects on sexual functioning is just a matter of trial and error.

Finally, a person who has heart disease or has had a heart attack or stroke may be extremely anxious about having intercourse for fear of precipitating more problems. This hesitancy alone can dramatically reduce a person's interest in sharing physical intimacy, even if their doctor is approving or encouraging. Yet many people resume sexual functioning after heart attacks and strokes with little difficulty.

DIABETES

The effects of uncontrolled diabetes on blood vessels and nerves throughout the body can be devastating. Diabetes can lead to heart attacks, strokes, kidney failure, and blindness, to name only a few of the terrible outcomes of this chronic, degenerative disease. However, its effects on sexual functioning are equally problematic. When uncontrolled, diabetes often causes the destruction of the nerves responsible for erection in men, and as a consequence, many who suffer from this disease are impotent. This can be especially frustrating because feelings of sexual desire are unchanged while the capacity to respond with an erection is seriously impaired or eliminated. The effects of diabetes on women are not as severe, even though the disease may cause some deterioration of the uterus and ovaries.

CANCER

The effects of cancer on sexual functioning can be wide-ranging, powerfully affecting a person's body image, hormonal functioning, energy level, and overall sexual responsiveness. Depending on the site of the cancer, there may be a variety of different outcomes. Testicular and prostate cancers in men, depending on how early they are diagnosed and how they are treated, may or may not impair sexual functioning. Cervical, uterine, and ovarian cancers are pretty much the same. Generally speaking, early diagnosis and prompt, appropriate treatment leads to less loss of arousal and responsiveness. When sexual responsiveness is impaired or eliminated after cancer treatment, there may be over time some recovery of function.

In addition to the removal of various organs and diminished levels of the hormones they produce, another aspect of cancer's effects on sexual arousal and response involves feelings of disfigurement after surgery that substantially changes a person's body image. Women who have mastectomies often report that they no longer feel as sexual or as appealing to their partner.

DEMENTIA

The term dementia refers to substantial impairments in cognitive and emotional functioning that result from degenerative brain changes. Very often, those affected by this irreversible disorder become disinterested in sharing sexual intimacy, or in some cases they may become very assertive sexually, making unbecoming, forward gestures and demands. Examples of dementia include such disorders as Alzheimer's disease, Pick's disease, some cases of Parkinson's disease, as well as some others. Deficits in personal hygiene often accompany dementia, which may contribute substantially to a partner's undesirability. Another aspect of dementia affecting sexual feelings about one's partner is their new role as a dependent, helpless person. Sexual feelings are usually incompatible with these attitudes (Deacon, Minichiello, & Plummer, 1995). Sometimes, hypersexuality accompanies chronic degenerative changes of the central nervous system, and this often embarrasses the individual's family members although it may not be troubling to the person her or himself.

ARTHRITIS

Arthritis per se does not impair sexual functioning. But when stiffness and joint pain impair mobility and flexibility, some sexual positions can become distracting and uncomfortable, and vigorous intercourse might also present some problems. One's physician might recommend taking aspirin or a similar analgesic before intercourse, taking a long, leisurely warm bath, or even having sex on a warm electric blanket. These measures might diminish discomfort and make sexual sharing more enjoyable.

SEXUAL DYSFUNCTIONS IN LATER LIFE

Sexual dysfunctions involve physical and/or interpersonal problems that impair sexual arousal and/or response. Some stem from psychological factors, whereas others are biological in origin. Chapter 14 considers this subject in detail. In some dysfunctions, erection is significantly delayed or diminished or doesn't happen at all. Vaginal lubrication and other signs of excitement in women might be similarly absent. In other dysfunctions, arousal may be normal, but orgasm does not occur.

A recent study of several hundred respondents, most of whom were in their 50s, found that sexual dysfunctions are not uncommon among older Americans (Adams, Dubbert, Chupurdia, Jones, Lofland, & Leermakers, 1996). In many cases, the attitudes, beliefs, and misinformation held by these individuals are a major contributory factor in the development of these sexual problems. Not only might these factors contribute to the emergence of sexual dysfunctions, but they might also make it less likely that older individuals will seek help for these problems or be receptive to therapeutic strategies. When older people continue to think that the only appropriate avenue of sexual expression is having sexual intercourse, impaired erectile and arousal ability in men and women may discourage continued intimacy. Common misconceptions might also make people less interested in trying to have intercourse simply because of lack of knowledge or encouragement regarding other ways of sharing sexuality. It is, therefore, difficult to separate normal arousal and response changes in later life from the effects of inadequate level of sexual information so common in our culture, when examining the reasons people do or do not remain sexually active.

The role of psychosocial factors in the origin of sexual problems in later life is strong. Many older individuals have distinctly guilty or uncomfortable feelings about the "normality" of their continued sexual desires. Renshaw (1988), and Kaplan (1990) have suggested that small, normal sexual changes are often magnified a great deal in the minds of those experiencing them. The accompanying anxiety can further diminish sexual interest. Chapter 12 discussed a personality continuum with erotophilia and erotophobia as two extremes of an underlying interest in, and comfort with, sexual issues. Erotophilia is most obviously associated with comfortable feelings about sexuality, while erotophobia is more clearly related to negative, anxious, or fearful feelings. Erotophobia earlier in life is closely related to sexual problems in later life (Fisher, Byrne, White, & Kelley, 1988). But there are still other reasons for these difficulties. If a person believes that their partner's lack of arousal or delayed arousal is a reflection of their feelings of attraction, this can certainly decrease the likelihood of their initiating sexual sharing. Similarly, boring, predictable, routine sexual activities can diminish the desire for a variety of types of sexual interaction. Although these factors may be related to diminished sexual arousal, they would most certainly also lessen sexual response.

Are delayed or diminished erection in men and vaginal lubrication in women sexual dysfunctions? Probably not, since they are normal aspects of getting older. The same is true regarding the need for prolonged and perhaps more vigorous stimulation during the plateau stage in order to approach and enjoy orgasm. This is not dysfunctional. While there are changes in the quality of orgasms accompanying the aging process, the total lack of orgasmic response in healthy older individuals need not happen. Drugs, diseases, and a longstanding history of cigarette smoking may profoundly alter orgasmic responses. Generally speaking, healthy older adults with positive, flexible attitudes about sexual sharing usually find a variety of ways to share physical intimacy in keeping with the various limitations with which they might be coping.

Sex therapists want it to be known that their professional services are not just for younger individuals. These professionals help fulfill the same basic objectives as this book: education, motivation, and reassurance. Very often, however, the services of a sex therapist aren't needed. Gynecologists, urologists, internists, and family practice doctors can help many patients with normal, age-related concerns, as can many social workers and nurses.

CONTINUED SEXUAL EXPRESSION IN INSTITUTIONAL SETTINGS

As people live longer and longer, more people are spending some of their later years in some type of institution, such as nursing homes and assisted care facilities. In most cases, this has a powerful negative impact on shared sexuality. While everyone in this country has legal rights to privacy and freedom of association, the myths about sex in later life have adversely affected the ease with which the aging and elderly can enjoy shared intimacy without interference or interruption. In fact, frank prohibitions against sexual intercourse or other forms of sexual interaction among the residents of these facilities are not uncommon. Reprimands to "act your age" do nothing to enhance quality of life in a person's later years. When one member of a couple is living in one of these establishments and the other is not, it can be very frustrating to try to create and maintain privacy to enjoy sex. For those who are widowed and living in such a facility, staff often see sexual

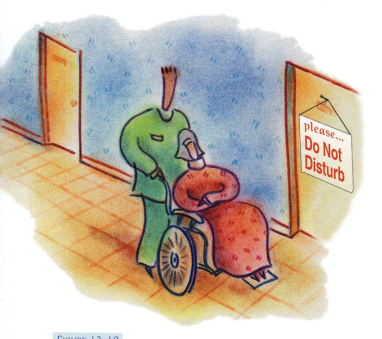

FIGURE 13-19 More frequently today, nursing homes and assisted living facilities provide privacy for their residents who wish to explore sexual intimacy with one another.

overtures among the aged unmarried as annoyances and nuisances. When a person moves into a nursing home, do they give up their right to be a sexual person? Absolutely not. In fact, many forward-thinking institutions have created policies and protocols to ensure the right to privacy when it is requested (Fig. 13-19).

A study carried out in the early 1980s (White, 1982) reported that among a sample of 84 men (average age 81) and 185 women (average age 83) in 15 Texas nursing homes, 91% reported that they had virtually no sexual activity. However, 17% of these people clearly indicated that they had a clear desire to engage in sexual activity while living in one of these facilities. This is a significant proportion of residents. In another study, Spector and Fremeth (1996) found that in general, male residents reported much higher levels of sexual desire than did females. The implications of findings like these are clear. If continued participation in sexual sharing is important to an older person, they or their children should explore policies regarding this issue before they move in. Remember, intimacy and sexual sharing are life-long needs. Deacon, Minichiello, and Plummer (1995) have reported that institutions often separate residents based on sex, and there is frequently little opportunity for married couples to share a room, much less a bed. While their research was carried out in Australia, American institutions aren't much different in these administrative policies. In addition to the problems older institutionalized individuals may have creating and preserving privacy, staff members may interpret sexual interest as a behavioral problem and sedate these patients (Brown, 1989). Although some children support their parents' rights to privacy and sexual expression, others may become quite angry at what they perceive as a "permissive" attitude on the part of hospital staff members (Deacon, Minichiello, & Plummer, 1995).

As discussed earlier, in later life a man's erectile functioning is somewhat diminished or impaired altogether. Although these changes are normal, the drug Viagra has beneficial effects for many men who have arousal problems. This puts doctors and nursing home administrators in an interesting position. Are they obliged to give this drug to the institutionalized aging and elderly who request it? When this drug was first made available in 1998, many adult children of nursing home residents were very uncomfortable about the prospect of their fathers getting Viagra on demand (Stenson, 1998). Ms. Rosemary McDonald, MSN, RN, coordinator of elderly care at a Veterans Affairs' Medical Center in Brockton, Massachusetts was chatting with a 101-year-old male patient who told her that, "If I had a sex partner, I'd be first in line" for Viagra. This drug may either help or hinder the development of more open, intelligent policies about sexual activity in nursing homes.

The American Association of Homes and Services for the Aging has formulated a white paper titled "Sexual Activity in an AAHSA Facility," in which are included a number of statements relevant to the interests of patients, staff, administrators, and corporate owners. Here is a selection of these, which were written to "stimulate conversation," as well as the considera-

Dear Dr. Ruth

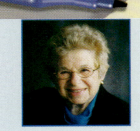

Questions:

I am a 70-year-old resident of a large nursing home. My wife died a long time ago. But Dr. Ruth, I still have some red blood in my veins! I want to make friends with some of the women here and many seem really interested, but feel ashamed that I still have such a strong sex drive at my age and don't know how to explore this possibility. On top of it all, this place is pretty careful about being sure we don't have too much privacy. I am in good health and am still pretty sharp mentally, but there is something very important missing from my life. Any suggestions?

Answer:

Any nursing home, and especially a large one, should have a room set aside where the residents can lock the door and find some privacy. Even at 90 years of age people are entitled to have sexual feelings and act on them, and especially so at your age, which these days seems almost young. So don't be ashamed of your sexual drive, and use that energy to find some warmth and companionship.

Don't be afraid to lead a campaign to urge the nursing home director to create some private space. It might be better to do this before you find someone, so that no one can accuse you of doing this just for your own personal pleasure. If you speak up for this cause, I'm sure it will lead several of the ladies to look up to you, and who knows where that might lead.

---

tion of ethics committees and other people who might be interested in this subject:

- As a general rule, all institutions bear some responsibility for the common good and for the well-being of individuals. The institution should respect the privacy and consciences of individuals.
- An individual's sexual activities are primarily a matter of personal conscience. They take on larger proportions in a long-term care or housing facility, however, when expressed in a public fashion. Concerns about the sexual activities of person's with limited capacity also arise in such facilities.
- There seem to be two main areas of administrative responsibility in this regard: monitoring the behavior of staff and judging the moral capacity of residents to engage in consensual sexual activity.
- Privacy and autonomy are important values and should generally be considered and observed when formulating any policy. However, proximity and intimacy in congregate settings may legitimately exclude some activities that could infringe either on the sensibilities of others or on the common good.

This organization emphasizes that it is especially important that every facility make its policies clear for all who live in them, who are considering becoming residents, family members, staff, and administrators and owners. While these policy statements might seem broad, they effectively define questions and concerns for residents and prospective residents and their families.

HOMOSEXUALITY AMONG THE AGING AND ELDERLY

While the impact of aging on the physiology of sexual arousal and response is the same for both heterosexuals and homosexuals, the psychosocial context in which these occur is often entirely different. The discussion here is limited to those women and men who came out during young adulthood or middle adulthood and have lived openly as gays. Common perceptions of a lonely, isolated life of gays are simply wrong. An important study published by Kelly (1977) essentially dismissed these beliefs. Prior to this investigation, many in the general public and many professionals believed that gay males became despondent over the loss of their youthful appearance, became reclusive and seldom went to bars any more, had few intimate friends, and were no longer sexually active (Pope & Schulz, 1990). Kelly's data indicated that in general, older gay men enjoy good quality of life and are still sexually attracted to men their own age and want to be physically intimate with them. However, after about the age of 55, longstanding partnerships are more rare, for two reasons: the death of a long-term partner and less appeal for a single life partner.

Another study by Kimmel (1977) indicated that most aging gay men are sexually active and still make sexual enjoyment a high priority in their lives. Interestingly, this study noted a number of benefits that might be enjoyed by the gay community that are less commonly found among aging heterosexuals: a keener sense of feeling responsible for oneself, not being dependent on family members and/or children, and not having to adjust to children leaving home (Pope & Schulz, 1990). Additionally, and very importantly, many gay males have lived alone for extended periods of their lives and so do not reach their later years devastated by the loss of a lifelong partner. These issues, coupled with the existence of a network of friends, describe a reasonably good quality of life for older gay men.

Pope & Schulz (1990) published an analysis of about 100 gay men between the ages of 40 and 77. Among respondents between 50 and 59, 34% reported having sex more than once a week. The comparable figure for subjects over 60, however, was only 5%. Collectively, almost 90% of the men over 50 reported that they were still sexually active to some degree. Even among men 60 and older, a "moderate degree" of sexual interest was common. Finally, among all the subjects in this study, 69% reported that there was "no change" in the amount of enjoyment they took in sexual behavior over the course of their adult lives. These studies offer strong support for the idea that sexual interest, feelings, and behavior continue to be an important part of the lives of gay men as they age.

Quam and Whitford (1992) studied the concerns of gay and lesbian individuals related to the aging process among 39 lesbians and 41 gay men over the age of 50 living in a large midwestern urban area. Almost 40% of this sample was over the age of 60. Among these respondents, 63% of the men and 41% of the women lived alone. About 48% of the men and 23% of the women had gone to a gay bar at least once during the last two months. When asked if they would consider living in a gay or lesbian retirement community, 62% of the men and about 80% of the women found this an attractive idea. Subjects believed that such an environment would be supportive and sensitive to the needs of aging gays and lesbians. In general, most respondents enjoyed feelings of life satisfaction and the clear majority (77%) were "somewhat" or "very accepting" of their own aging. When asked what special problems these women and men anticipated as they aged, about 1 respondent in 5 reported concern about being able to develop relationships in the future. Fewer subjects were concerned about their health (17.1%), making new friends (17.1%), and loneliness (13.2%). Many of the things that concern aging heterosexuals are also troubling for homosexu-

als, and strong interpersonal and community ties are viewed by both groups as very important in adjusting to the challenges of later life.

A questionnaire study of 50 lesbians between the ages of 65 and 85 found that most of the women in this sample had well-integrated personalities, were adapting well to the challenges of the normal aging process, and had outlived much of the prejudice and stigma so often associated with a homosexual gender orientation (Kehoe, 1986). Kehoe (1988) summarized many of the demographic characteristics of aging lesbians and found that they represent a cross-section of American society. They reside in both rural and urban areas, represent virtually all racial and religious groups, work in a wide diversity of occupations and professions, and have attained educational levels ranging from a high school diploma to doctoral degrees. As these women age, they report that the sexual aspects of their relationships grow progressively less important, but that feelings of companionship and connectedness grow more significant. Their most pressing worries concern loneliness and economic insecurity. A support group especially for gays and lesbians called "Gays and Lesbians Older and Wiser" (GLOW) has been formed in the Midwest to serve the special social support requirements of gay women and men in later life (Slusher, Mayer, & Dunkle, 1996).

CONCLUSION

This chapter along with the preceding chapter show that we are sexual beings from birth to death, although the ways in which we experience and express our eroticism changes throughout the life cycle. Once it was unbelievable to attribute sexual feelings to children and equally unsavory to do so with aging and elderly adults, but obviously sexual behavior and enjoyment aren't just for young, attractive people. While sexual arousal and response may change as we age, most people still report that sexuality is an important priority for their quality of life of their later years. Understanding that sexual feelings, thoughts, and behaviors will change as you age helps one avoid being overly disturbed or distressed when they do. This peace of mind is very important for aging and elderly people.

The focus here has been on normal or typical adult development and aging, but there are terrible, troubling, and traumatic events in some people's lives that profoundly alter their progression through the stages and events discussed in this chapter. The next chapter explores some of these difficulties and frustrations of sexual functioning.

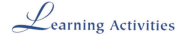

*L*earning Activities

1. This chapter discusses the "one and only" myth. You probably have a pretty good idea about the kind of man or woman with whom you could feel safe, compatible,

and passionate. You also likely have some feeling for the type of man or woman with whom you would not want to have a long-term relationship. Make two short lists, as you would to go shopping. On one write down the five most important favorable attributes, and on the other the five least desirable attributes, in a possible future spouse.

   a. Explain how the first list would enhance the chances of your experiencing intimacy instead of isolation and how the second would predispose you to isolation instead of intimacy, according to the theory of Erik H. Erikson.

   b. Discuss how the characteristics in the first list would become apparent in the first three stages of the Sarrels' theory of sexual change through adult development. Explain how the characteristics in the second list would become obvious in the same three stages.

2. Sexual strategies theory predicts that men with plentiful (financial) resources are likely to use them to acquire sexual partners who are young and physically attractive. Women who are young and physically attractive will extract immediate resources in short-term sexual liaisons.

   a. Collect a large number of personals ads and use them to test this hypothesis of the theory.

   b. Do men with abundant resources mention them in seeking young, attractive women?

   c. Do women who claim to be young and physically attractive seek contact with men who are affluent?

3. Some researchers have shown that in recent years, females under the age of 25 have shown markedly increased rates of infidelity, especially in comparison with women and men in other age groups. Speculate on reasons for this trend and the motives or justifications that may be involved.

4. There is a story about a man at mid-life who had a heart attack, and while visiting his doctor during recovery he asked if it was alright if he resumed sexual activity. His doctor replied, "Certainly, but only with your wife." What is the implication of the doctor's comment?

5. An old adage suggests that if, during the first year of marriage, a couple puts a dollar into a jar every time they have intercourse and after being married a year takes a dollar out of the jar every time they have intercourse, they will never retrieve all their money in their married life. What is the implication of this comment? Do you think it's true?

6. Imagine for a moment that you learned that the wife of a close family friend was having an affair, and that you had unmistakable evidence to this effect. What would you do, and what would be your justification for your action?

7. A colleague of ours teaching human sexuality in a university showed his class a film depicting a woman and man in their 70s sharing non-intercourse physical intimacy while nude. One student blurted out, "Oh, please spare me!" Comment on this student's behavior. Can you think of any other examples of ageism as it relates to sexual expression in later life?

8. Based on what you have learned about the risks and benefits of hormone replacement therapy, what would be your personal decision regarding the use of these drugs for yourself or your spouse? Explain your reasoning.

9. Now that you have had a chance to read about the rights and freedoms of women and men who live in nursing homes, what do you think would be the best way to sanction consensual intimacy between patients while trying to respect the rights of grown children and other residents?

$\mathcal{K}$ey Concepts

- Intimacy versus isolation is the sixth stage of Erikson's theory of psychosocial development. At this time, individuals develop the capacity for mutual, loving relationships or become more secluded and separated from close, affectionate bonds with others.

- Generativity versus stagnation is the seventh stage of Erikson's theory of psychosocial development. At this time, individuals express an authentic concern for the generation that will follow and enjoy a sense of generosity in their relationships with others. In contrast, stagnation involves a progressively narrowed circle of friendships, few love relationships, and a preoccupation with one's own comforts and possessions.

- The fact that people very often begin a behavior for one set of reasons but continue it for an entirely different set of reasons is referred to as functional autonomy.

- Attitudes are learned ways of thinking about, feeling about, and acting towards other people. Attitudes guide much human behavior and are typically highly resistant to change.

- Integrity versus despair is the eighth and final stage in Erikson's theory of psychosocial development. Individuals with integrity arrive at the end of their lives feeling that they have always "done their best," whether or not they were conspicuously successful. In contrast, despair involves feelings of wasted and lost opportunities or perhaps that the individual has given up at some point in life.

- Among women, the climacteric is accompanied by menopause, which involves irregularity and then cessation of menstruation. Menopause is accompanied by lowered levels of female hormone (estrogen) in the blood stream. Certain health problems, such as osteoporosis, heart disease, and hot flashes may occur at this time.

- Because of decreased levels of estrogen in a woman's bloodstream at and after menopause, some women elect hormone replacement therapy to minimize the health risks associated with menopause.

- The male andropause is very different from menopause in women. There is no clear end-point in most men's fertility, nor any sudden fall in their level of male hormones. Still, *diminished* fertility and *gradually* falling levels of male hormones do occur.

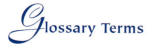

Glossary Terms

ageism

assortative
  mating

cohabitation

climacteric

menopause

sexual
  dysfunctions

sexual strategies
  theory

sociobiology

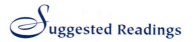

Suggested Readings

Butler, R. N., & Lewis, M. I. (1993). Love and sex after 60. New York: Ballantine Books.

Hammond, D. B. (1987). My parents never had sex: Myths and facts of sexual aging. Amherst, NY: Prometheus Books.

Jacobowitz, R. S., & Reinish, J. M. (1996). 150 most-asked questions about midlife sex, love, and intimacy: What women and their partners really want to know. New York: William Morrow & Co.

Kahn, R. L., & Rowe, J. W. (1998). Successful aging. New York: Pantheon Books.

Lee, J. A., & Kameny, F. E. (1991). Gay midlife and maturity. Binghamton, NY: Harrington Park Press.

Mason, F. B. (1989). To love again: Intimate relationships after 60. Oakland, CA: Gateway.

14

Sexual Dysfunctions: Incompatibility, Inadequacy, or Just Inappropriately Learned Responses

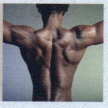

OBJECTIVES

When you finish reading and reviewing this chapter, you should be able to:

1. Define sexual dysfunction and discuss the impact of these disorders on an interpersonal relationship.

2. Explain how behaviorism has influenced theories about the origins of sexual dysfunctions and treatment strategies.

3. Analyze the usefulness of the *Diagnostic and Statistical Manual of Mental Disorders* for categorizing sexual dysfunctions.

4. Describe the characteristics of low sexual desire and the distinguishing features of hypoactive sexual desire disorder and sexual aversion disorder.

5. Describe the distinguishing characteristics of female sexual arousal disorder and male erectile disorder.

6. Describe the distinguishing characteristics of female orgasmic disorder, retarded ejaculation, and premature ejaculation.

7. Differentiate between sexual dysfunctions caused by psychosocial and organic factors, focusing on the specific effects of prescription and recreational drugs on sexual functioning.

8. Review societal factors that play a role in sexual dysfunctions, focusing on the importance of body image and myths that surround what "good sex" is supposed to be like.

9. Examine the role of religious orthodoxy in the development of a sexual dysfunction.

10. Comment on the influence of racial and ethnic traditions on how people learn to think of sexual behavior.

11. Discuss how interpersonal problems between two individuals can contribute to a sexual dysfunction in their relationship.

12. Discuss the role of prescription and recreational drugs in the development of a sexual dysfunction, explaining the specific inhibitory effects of each agent.

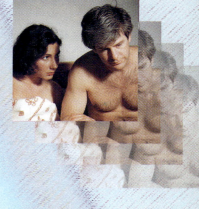

From Dr. Ruth

People are always asking me questions about their sexual dysfunctions, and that's great. Not that they have a sexual problem, but that admitting the problem and asking for help, even if it is only an e-mail question to an advice web site like drruth.com, is an important first step to fixing the problem. The biggest difficulty most people with sexual dysfunctions have is that they are unwilling to seek help. If these same people had a toothache, they'd not hesitate to see a dentist. Or if their eyesight was fading, they'd see an ophthalmologist. But if they are having some sexual difficulty, many people are ashamed of admitting to it themselves, much less to a family doctor, gynecologist, urologist, or sex therapist.

The other side of this coin is that many doctors too aren't very comfortable discussing sexual matters. They know that their patients are hesitant to ask them questions, and they don't try to initiate such conversations themselves by asking questions about their patients' sexual functioning, and so sexual problems remain under wraps.

Another piece of the blame has to go to the mass media. The media only now are beginning to show that problems with sexuality are common and for the most part treatable.

As you read through this chapter, if you encounter a description of a sexual dysfunction that you feel might apply to you, please don't become squeamish and quickly turn the page. Instead, vow you will try to learn as much about this problem as you can, and then seek help. I'm not trying to drum up business for my fellow sex therapists. My wish is for everybody to have the best sex possible, and that won't happen if people with a sexual dysfunction deny the importance of these difficulties.

The last two chapters explored sexual development throughout the lifespan. We are all sexual beings from birth to death, although the manifestations of sexual desire and response change as we age; however, people frequently encounter problems at various times in their lives having to do with sexual desire and response, and that is the subject of this chapter. If you know something about the problems and challenges you might encounter in the future, however, you will be better able to cope with them if and when they happen. It is in this optimistic spirit that we present the material in this chapter.

SEXUAL DYSFUNCTIONS

Generally speaking, sexual dysfunctions involve problems people experience in desiring sexual interaction, as well as physiological problems in the human sexual response cycle. Masters and Johnson have suggested (Personal Communication, 1978) that perhaps half of all marriages in the United States have a sexual dysfunction serious enough to lessen the quality of the relationship. These problems are often, although not always, accompanied by interpersonal conflicts between sexual partners. Sometimes, very strong feelings are associated with these

problems. Sexual dysfunctions involve problems in both sexual behaviors and the thoughts and emotions that accompany those behaviors. Some women and men become extremely distressed, frustrated, and even hostile about these difficulties. Sometimes the problems are caused by biological factors, while in other cases they result in psychological or psychosocial adjustment problems. Social, interpersonal, and individual factors all can cause or contribute to a sexual dysfunction.

People's different perceptions about sexual problems have a lot to do with whether they think they have a sexual dysfunction. For example, one woman might become quite frustrated with her partner's pattern of premature ejaculation, while another may view the same situation as proof that her partner finds her so sexually exciting that he just can't control himself. In such a case is there actually any sexual dysfunction at all, if neither individual is distressed about it? Yet when less than fully rewarding sexual interactions persist over prolonged periods of time, one or both partners are likely to feel that something's missing and may want to make changes in their pattern of physical intimacy to explore potentially more fulfilling avenues of sexual sharing. When two individuals consistently feel that their lovemaking is frustrating, uncomfortable, or in some way deficient over a prolonged period, then perhaps they need to candidly acknowledge their problem and begin to take the first steps toward better sexual communication and perhaps seek therapeutic assistance.

Sometimes sexual dysfunctions can make a person doubt their feelings about their partner or their partner's feelings about them. A man might say to himself, "If I really love her as much as I think I do, then why do I continue to have problems getting an erection when we want to have sex?" Or an individual might say to him or herself, "If she or he is really in love with me and claims to find me sexually exciting, why don't they seem interested in having intercourse more often?" Sexual dysfunctions can cause much doubt and inner questioning, often making people ask themselves "What's wrong with me?" Another troubling question is "Whose fault is this, anyway?" Concepts like "fault," "blame," and "guilt" are often involved in a person's thoughts and feelings about sexual problems. The terms used to refer to sexual dysfunctions have connotations of inadequacy, vulnerability, or even psychological difficulties. Terms such as "hang-ups," "disorders," or "problems" are commonly used to refer to sexual difficulties.

This chapter discusses fairly standard categories of sexual dysfunctions. Disorders of sexual desire, problems with sexual arousal, and difficulties in having orgasms are the most common dysfunctions, and these will receive much attention here. Also, many individuals also experience significant physical discomfort during intercourse that seems unrelated to any underlying medical condition. Finally, we will explore ways in which prescription and recreational drugs can impair sexual desire, arousal, or orgasmic capacity. In all, sexual dysfunctions exist in many forms. These disorders affect people of both sexes, all races, all levels of educational attainment, all religions, and all socioeconomic groups.

Self-Concept, Self-Esteem, and Sexual Dysfunctions

How we think of ourselves, the opinion we hold of ourselves, and our feelings of self-worth are described by terms such as self-concept and self-esteem in the social and behavioral sciences. How we think about ourselves has a big impact on how we form a relationship and how we behave in existing relationships. Because our sexuality is often a central part of our personality, any sexual problems or doubts we experience can lead to lowered feelings of self-esteem. It is difficult, therefore, to discuss sexual dysfunctions without acknowledging the relationship between sexual behavior or "performance" and how we feel about ourselves as sexual persons. In fact, people who are troubled by sexual dysfunctions often have lower feelings of self-esteem and adequacy. They often believe that they have some terrible, hidden "flaw" that makes them less desirable to others and, therefore, become hesitant to engage in intimate behaviors that are likely to be frustrating and unrewarding. The next chapter's discussion of therapies for sexual dysfunctions focuses on this type of self-sustaining problem.

Sexual dysfunctions affect the quality and longevity of important interpersonal relationships. A person who is dealing with a sexual dysfunction is often keenly aware of the mismatch between their apparent physical attractiveness and their

lack of sexual interest or impaired arousal or orgasmic capacity. Although sexual dysfunctions involve behavioral problems, they also involve the difficulties in the relationship between mind and body. The anxiety (and sometimes depression) that often accompany sexual dysfunctions can affect a person's whole outlook on life and members of the opposite sex.

> *"Sex is a natural function. You can't make it happen, but you can teach people to let it happen."*
> *William Masters, 1971*

Because everyone is unique, we are likely to handle our own or our partner's sexual dysfunctions in different ways. Some of us may just ignore the problem so long as we can enjoy sexual arousal and responsiveness through masturbation or some other avenue of non-intercourse sexual pleasuring. Others may begin to have less frequent intercourse or might even stop having intercourse altogether. Some of us may consult a clergyman, a family doctor, or perhaps a sex therapist, psychologist, or psychiatrist. In some cases, a "do it yourself" approach might be effective. But not everyone experiences pleasure, intimacy, or a capacity for cooperation in the same way (Levay & Kagle, 1977), and some people actually have less desire to experience these feelings than others. If so, the person may not want to do anything to improve the conditions that caused his or her sexual dysfunction but may just leave things as they are and hope that in time they will improve on their own.

Many of us grew up hearing that "Anything worth doing is worth doing well." This way of thinking often affects how a person approaches a sexual situation as something that has to be "completed" to the highest possible standards of excellence. In fact, these perfectionist thoughts have been implicated as psychological factors involved in sexual dysfunctions (DiBartolo & Barlow, 1996). Apparently, many people have trouble relaxing any high expectations of themselves about sexual performance, and this may lead to feelings of being an inadequate lover. Once a person begins to think in this way, she or he may become progressively less inclined to initiate intimacy when it is likely to lead to feelings of failure. Impossibly high standards of sexual performance can be inhibiting, and the effects of these expectations are sometimes related to erectile difficulties.

> *"If sex is such a natural phenomenon, how come there are so many books on how to do it?"*
> *Bette Midler*

The Sexual Response Cycle

You will recall from reading Chapter 6 that there are a number of models of human sexual response that have been important in stimulating research and explaining arousal, responsiveness, and orgasm. One of these was the result of the laboratory research of Masters and Johnson, first published in 1966, and the second derives from the clinical work of Kaplan and published in 1974. Because sexual dysfunctions affect a person's experiences and behavior during the various stages of sexual response when considered from the perspectives of these two models, it might be a good idea to just quickly review the basic characteristics of each of these.

The sexual response cycle described by Masters and Johnson includes four stages: excitement, plateau, orgasm, and resolution (see Chapter 6 for more detail). Kaplan's model includes three stages: desire, excitement, and orgasm. Kaplan's notion of desire emphasizes the role of thinking, perception, and emotion in a person's assessment of a sexual situation. Masters and Johnson's model tends to focus instead on genital changes, with less emphasis on a person's wishes or needs regarding sexual enjoyment. Remember that sexual arousal and response involves a *sequence* of changes. When responsiveness is absent or diminished in any one of these stages, an individual is likely to feel that the sexual tension or excitement has been stopped, diminished, or delayed. The discussion of the sexual response cycle in Chapter 6 did not explore what happens when this occurs, but these stages do not always unfold in a logical, inevitable pattern. When people encounter delays in sexual responsiveness or diminished physiological arousal, they often simply stop, even though they may have already reached some level of excitement. At these moments frustration is keenly felt, along with feelings of inadequacy and even guilt. These emotions can make continued sexual sharing even more difficult. Many sex therapists say that when couples experience sexual problems, they often find it especially difficult to be patient, caring, and supportive of one another. In fact, they often become sullen and prefer to be alone.

Origins of Sexual Dysfunctions

A later section in this chapter explores diverse factors involved in the development of sexual dysfunctions, but we'll briefly introduce main causes here. Often, organic factors are instrumental in the emergence of problems in sexual desire, responsiveness, and orgasm. These are typically biological, physiological, congenital, genetic, and hormonal issues and may result from illness, injury, aging, or the situational or chronic use of drugs. Additionally, many prescription drugs may contribute to the development of sexual dysfunctions. Even apparently normal conditions, such as pregnancy, may be involved in lessened sexual interest and diminished arousal and responsiveness. Psychosocial or sociocultural factors may also play a role, including a variety of issues: self-concept, faulty sexual learning, sexual assault, abuse, or trauma, inadequate sex education, or aloof, dysfunctional parenting styles. Certain psychological problems, such as anxiety, depression, fear, and guilt about sexual enjoyment, are also commonly involved (Halvorsen & Metz, 1992). Coupled with these factors are societal influences that may create expectations of sexual interest and performance with which a person is uncomfortable. For example, restrictive religious beliefs often adversely affect a person's potential to enjoy sexual feelings without conflict. Cultural norms for "appropriate" sexual behaviors by women and men may contribute to feelings of inadequacy as well. Because these etiological factors interact, the diagnosis and treatment of sex-

ual dysfunctions usually benefit from a multidisciplinary perspective. Nonbiological causes are often labeled as psychogenic factors.

The Influence of Behaviorism in the Social and Behavioral Sciences

In the early part of the 20th century, psychologists and other social scientists became uncomfortable relying only on personal reports about a person's thoughts and feelings and their relationship to human behavior. Bias, forgetfulness, prejudices, expectations, or lack of verbal or intellectual ability can distort an individual's account of what was happening in their mind. This lack of objectivity and rigor became a real and deeply felt concern among investigators, such as Wilhelm Wundt (1832-1920) and Edward Titchener (1867-1927). John B. Watson (1878-1958) (Fig. 14-1) brought a passionate conviction to changing the agenda and methods of modern psychology. Watson believed that psychology ought to deal only with *observable and measurable behaviors* and should avoid phenomena that couldn't be seen and quantified. This approach became the central paradigm of American psychology for many decades and only recently has been modified (but not replaced) by a renewed conviction in the importance of cognition and its many emotional facets.

When William Masters and Virginia Johnson published *Human Sexual Inadequacy,* their ground-breaking approach to sexual dysfunctions, in 1970, their basic approach was powerfully influenced by the behavioristic agenda of John B. Watson and the many like-minded psychologists who adhered to the simple, basic tenets of this approach. Masters and Johnson believed that if the behaviors involved in sexual dysfunctions could be lessened in severity or eliminated altogether, it really didn't matter much what was going on in the patient's mind or

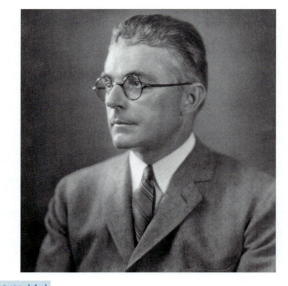

FIGURE 14-1   John B. Watson, founder of American behavioristic psychology. Watson believed that all behaviors are learned, including those thought to be problematic or maladaptive.

what had happened to her or him in the past. If you got rid of the behavior, you got rid of the problem. While this basic philosophical perspective has been useful for understanding the nature and cure of sexual dysfunctions, the issue isn't really as simple as it might seem. The distress that people with sexual dysfunctions experience is very real and persistent, and while the dysfunction may be improved or eliminated, it is too simplistic to say that the client's thoughts and feelings are unrelated to the problem. Therefore, while the application of the behavioristic approach to human sexual dysfunctions has some legitimate justifications, the "whole story" behind the dysfunction is important for a fuller understanding of the problem and its solution. The individual's thoughts and feelings are important when trying to understand causes of sexual difficulties.

Masters and Johnson proclaimed that sexual dysfunctions are not symptomatic of any "hidden" or "buried" psychological problems. If they were, they could probably not be helped substantially or cured in their intensive two-week approach to sex therapy. We discuss this therapeutic approach in greater length in the next chapter. Whether old, latent psychological issues are behind the development of sexual dysfunctions depends on one's theoretical perspective. For example, behaviorally based psychotherapists argue that dealing with symptoms is more worthwhile than exploring causes of these problems. In contrast, a psychiatrist may explore the historical development of sexual dysfunctions, as well as the reasons for their persistence. In general, most professionals today believe that sexual dysfunctions may in part be caused by a rather maladaptive learning process in which these behaviors endure because they are in some way reinforced in the client's psychosocial environment. For example, if a person had fears of intimacy, she or he might develop a sexual dysfunction in order to avoid fully experiencing the kind of closeness and affection that typically accompanies sexual intercourse. Similarly, if intercourse is accompanied by pain or the spastic contraction of the musculature at the opening to the vagina (vaginismus), a person would very likely avoid intimacy (and, therefore, be reinforced) by refraining from having or attempting coitus. Analogously, the embarrassment or humiliation that might accompany impotence may be avoided altogether if the person doesn't attempt intercourse. In each of these instances, avoiding sexual interaction allows a person to evade experiences that are unpleasant or be accompanied by feeling of shame, and the dysfunction is likely to continue because of these "rewarding" experiences. In fact, the term "negative reinforcement" is used to describe the good feelings we get when bad feelings stop (negative reinforcement is not the same thing as punishment).

The Diagnostic and Statistical Manual of Mental Disorders

There is an interesting paradox in the way many professionals think about sexual dysfunctions. On the one hand, these problems are not thought to represent latent, persistent problems in an individual's personality. On the other, sexual dysfunctions are described in the 4ᵗʰ edition of *The Diagnostic and Statistical Manual of Mental Disorders* (DSM), which cov-

ers a variety of fairly enduring psychological problems. Are sexual dysfunctions psychological disorders? We feel that sexual dysfunctions are not necessarily "mental disorders" but believe that a variety of thought patterns and mood states may contribute to the development and persistence of sexual problems. In general, when a person experiences significant subjective inner turmoil that hurts their ability to engage in rewarding interpersonal relationships or impairs their ability to work, they can be said to have a psychological problem. The DSM refers to a mental disorder as a condition that causes personal distress, impaired functioning in one or more areas of the individual's life, or a markedly increased risk of suffering death, pain, or disability.

Many problems included in the DSM-IV are so common that often people are surprised to hear them called "psychological disorders." For example, people who have persistent, troubling problems in adapting to social or job-related challenges or whose productivity is frequently impaired by high levels of stress are often diagnosed with "adjustment disorders," which are included in the DSM even though they are very common. Similarly, many of us will experience periods of anxiety, mild depression, or problems sleeping, which also are included in the DSM. All disorders described in the DSM are not equally serious or have the same potential to disrupt an individual's life. The fact that sexual dysfunctions are described in this volume does not necessarily mean they are "mental disorders" that profoundly impair an individual's day-to-day activities.

Here we will explore sexual dysfunctions from the perspective of both the individual and the relationship. Sexual dysfunctions are both intrapersonal, as well as interpersonal. We will consider both psychological and biological causes. Note also that an individual can have more than one sexual dysfunction at the same time, such as diminished sexual interest *and* problems in arousal *and* an inability to have orgasms reliably or at all. Although this chapter uses a descriptive classification scheme, not all difficulties fall into neat, mutually exclusive categories.

CLASSIFICATION OF SEXUAL DYSFUNCTIONS

This section introduces the most common sexual dysfunctions. There are varying degrees of seriousness in each, as well as in their impact on a relationship. Sometimes sexual dysfunctions cause tremendous distress and disruption, while in other cases it is relatively easy for a couple to adjust to their problem.

Problems With Low Sexual Desire

Not everyone wants to have sex as often as possible. There is much variability in a person's sex drive from one time to another and much variation among people. Some people have an extremely low inclination to share physical intimacy, and this low sexual interest may be a stable aspect of their personality. Others experience a frank dislike for or even repugnance at the thought of having any kind of sexual interaction.

HYPOACTIVE SEXUAL DESIRE DISORDER

Some individuals have a notable absence of desire to have sexual intercourse or engage in other forms of sexual activity and rarely if ever think or fantasize about sex. The word "frigid" is sometimes used to describe someone (unfortunately, typically a woman) who does not seem very interested in sharing physical intimacy. Professionals do not use the word frigidity but instead use more precise, less judgmental terminology. The circumstances of an individual's life must be taken into account when making a determination of **hypoactive sexual desire disorder**. This does not refer simply to a person who isn't in the mood for sex from time to time or to a loss of sexual interest attributable to more serious psychological problems, such as depression. Similarly this is not a lack of sexual interest occurring as a side-effect of a prescription or recreational drug or as a result of illness. Hypoactive sexual desire disorder is a consistent trait of an individual. This lack of sexual interest is likely to cause a person some unhappiness and may cause problems in their relationships.

Investigators believed that hypoactive sexual desire can be most meaningfully assessed by learning about how frequently people desire or think about sex, rather than simply noting how frequently they actually engage in sexual activity (Beck, 1995), since some people have sex when they really don't want to. A low level of sexual desire is the most frequently reported problem among people who visit sex therapy clinics, and more men are now being diagnosed with this difficulty. Many men experience low sexual desire, either briefly or for prolonged periods of time. Diminished sexual interest may affect all of a person's thoughts and fantasies about sex, or just certain behaviors (e.g., fellatio). Someone with this disorder rarely initiates sexual interaction with their partner, but they may comply with sexual requests in order to be held and feel loved. Someone with this condition generally scores low on tests that measure erotophilia (see Chapter 12). Hypoactive sexual desire may develop over a period of time for a number of reasons. Emotional problems, lack of sexual knowledge, low levels of sexual motivation, and interpersonal problems in a relationship may be involved in this dysfunction. It is difficult to precisely measure "sexual desire," and sex counselors and therapists might use different definitions of this term.

Desire is the first stage in Kaplan's model of sexual response. Anything that diminishes sexual desire is likely to similarly lessen responsiveness in the two other stages in this model (excitement and orgasm). A person who has problems experiencing and enjoying excitement and orgasm probably develops diminished initial sexual desire as well. Sexual desire may be hypoactive for one individual only or all possible partners. People with hypoactive sexual desire typically encounter problems cultivating sexual relationships and frequently experience a wide range of problems with their spouses when they are married. Hypoactive sexual desire disorder usually develops during one's adult years, rarely being present in adolescence or young adulthood. Additionally, it may emerge during particularly difficult or stressful times in a person's life and diminish or disappear completely when one's life circumstances improve.

All couples do not get together because they love one another and enjoy shared sexual attraction. Many couples marry for practical reasons unrelated to enjoying one another sexually. Family traditions and expectations, financial considerations, and religious and socioeconomic factors may all affect who gets together with whom. When such considerations impact on marital decisions in the absence of sexual interest or attraction, sexual attraction may simply not occur. Two individuals may be bound together by a large number of shared interests, but if they don't have any desire for one another sexually, they usually cannot just make it happen (Rosen & Leiblum, 1995).

"Some nights he said that he was tired, and some nights she said that she wanted to read, and other nights no one said anything."

"Play It As It Lays," Joan Didion

Some investigators have reported that low sexual desire is often symptomatic of marital adjustment problems and in these cases is frequently accompanied by moderate levels of anxiety and low levels of depression (Trudel, Landry, & Larose, 1997). Low sexual desire is perhaps best assessed within the context of the overall quality of a relationship and may not necessarily involve any significant incompatibilities. Therapists also explore the sexual behavior and sexual repertoire of couples who are dealing with hypoactive sexual desire. Trudel, Aubin, and Matte (1995) found that couples with a shared low level of sexual desire have a more limited, routine repertoire of sexual activities and report less pleasure in these behaviors than couples who do not have low levels of sexual desire, although having little interest in sexual experimentation is not the *cause* of low sexual desire. Couples with low sexual desire are generally not as likely to engage in novel sexual activities or experiment with a more diverse sexual repertoire.

"In sex one wants or one does not want. And the grief, the sorrow of life is that one can not make or coerce or persuade the wanting, cannot command it by mail order or finagle it through bureaucratic channels."

"Sita," Kate Millett, 1976

SEXUAL AVERSION DISORDER

Another sexual desire disorder is called **sexual aversion disorder**. The word "aversion" carries with it some strong connotations of dislike and repugnance. Individuals with sexual aversion disorder experience a strong dislike of shared sexual activity and avoid any physical contact or verbal interaction likely to lead to sexual interaction. These individuals report having very low or no sex drive whatsoever and feel very nervous about the prospect of becoming sexually aroused (Crenshaw, 1985). This sexual aversion can be present along with other sexual dysfunctions or may exist by itself. People who experience sexual aversion may become extremely upset at the prospect of sexual involvement and are likely to have a number of interpersonal problems with others because of their scrupulous avoidance of any sexual discussion, comments, or overt behavior.

Some people with sexual aversions are particularly repulsed by specific sexual stimuli or aspects of sexual interactions, while others experience a more generalized distaste for any and all cues with explicit or even implicit sexual meanings. These individuals sometimes go to great lengths to avoid encountering any stimuli with sexual connotations and are vigilant for the unexpected appearance of erotic stimuli.

"All this fuss about sleeping together. For physical pleasure I'd sooner go to my dentist any day."
"Vile Bodies," Evelyn Waugh, 1930

Sexual Arousal Disorders

Sexual arousal disorders are a very different kind of problem. In these disorders a person may indeed very much desire to share sexual intimacy with another, but their bodies do not go along with their inclinations. Both women and men experience arousal disorders.

FEMALE SEXUAL AROUSAL DISORDER

As women become aroused, they experience vaginal lubrication, as well as an internal swelling of the tissues at the opening to the vagina. While these changes can take more or less time, with continued foreplay, these will occur in most women, although they may be a little delayed and diminished in women in later life. In women who experience **female sexual arousal disorder,** these physiological events are absent or significantly reduced, making penetration awkward and/or uncomfortable due to a lack of adequate lubrication. Similarly, intercourse may be painful and is usually accompanied by tension between partners and feelings of anguish or anxiety in the woman. This woman may tell you that she feels sexually inadequate. Completing intercourse may be unreasonable and upsetting for the woman.

These diminished genital responses can occur if a woman feels she has had too little foreplay, doesn't particularly like, trust, or enjoy her partner, has a vaginal infection, or is affected by a medical condition or the side effects of a medication. Sexual arousal in women involves vasocongestion in her genital and lower pelvic area. These factors all can reduce this response, which is usually accompanied by significantly lower levels of vaginal lubrication as well. If a man tries to penetrate his partner before she has had time to experience sufficient arousal, she may have all the *symptoms* of female sexual arousal disorder when in fact all she needs is more time for her arousal response to occur.

Regardless of the causes or circumstances of diminished vasocongestion and lubrication, communication by the couple can help them make some adjustments in their lovemaking. Use of sterile, non-petroleum based lubricants or lubricating suppositories can also be helpful. But if a woman is experiencing problems becoming sexually aroused, the problem may lie in one of the desire phase dysfunctions already discussed.

MALE ERECTILE DISORDER

The inability or diminished ability of a man to attain and maintain an erection of sufficient firmness for a long enough period of time to enjoy sexual intercourse is the sexual dysfunction that has received the most attention in the popular press. It has also received significant scientific attention, with a journal devoted to the subject: the *International Journal of Impotence Research.* This condition was previously called impotence but is today usually called erectile dysfunction or **male erectile disorder.** Men with erectile dysfunction long term or situationally usually have normal fertility; erectile dysfunction and fertility are different things. While women with a sexual arousal disorder can use lubricants to facilitate comfortable intercourse, without an erection a man has no simple alternative. When men cannot attain and maintain erections on a repeated basis, or consistently lose their erection before they ejaculate and/or they and their partner have enjoyed some sense of sexual satisfaction, this situation is considered dysfunctional. The term dysfunction is used in circumstances in which men experience dismay and unhappiness about their situation. Biological, pathological, and drug-related factors may all play a role in the occurrence of impotence, as well as psychological causes. For example, longstanding, rigid religiosity may contribute to feelings of ambivalence about the pleasures of sexual intercourse, especially when conception is not being planned. Generally speaking, men who feel anxious about sexuality in general, and sexual intercourse in particular, are more likely to experience erectile difficulties. Similarly, men who worry a lot about how well they perform sexually and fear not satisfying their partners also commonly experience bouts of impotence.

"All it means, if you wilt that way with a lady, is that you haven't yet really met her. You're not trying to make love to a woman, you're trying not to miss an opportunity."
"Falling Towards England," Clive James, 1985

This sexual problem can create a vicious cycle in which the factors that contribute to the problem (such as marital distress and tension) are likely to make the condition worse, and the couple continues to find themselves experiencing more stress and anxiety that are even more likely to discourage regular, enjoyable intimate interactions (Fig. 14-2). Erectile difficulties often impair the quality of a sexual relationship over long periods of time. The *DSM-IV* describes them as playing a central role in unconsummated marriages.

While some men may experience a lifelong pattern of erectile dysfunction, most men will experience situational bouts of this problem from time to time through their adult years. Various risk factors have been described that are thought to play a role in the development of erectile dysfunction (Bortolotti, Parazzini, Colli, & Landoni, 1997). For example, men who smoke cigarettes, abuse alcohol regularly, and have high blood cholesterol seem to have disproportionately more erectile problems than those without these conditions. Additionally, Masters and Johnson (1978, personal communica-

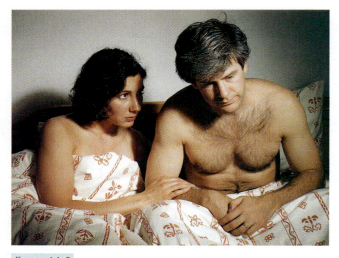

FIGURE 14-2   Male erectile disorder can create feelings of failure and frustration for men, as well as disappointment and distress in their partners.

tion) noted that when adolescents or young men have embarrassing or humiliating early sexual experiences in which they cannot attain an erection, or if they can, are unable to complete intercourse, or "get caught" having intercourse at this time in life, it can contribute to the occurrence of erectile dysfunction later. Sexual dysfunctions in general, and erectile dysfunction in particular, are also positively correlated with highly perfectionist personalities (Dibartolo & Barlow, 1996). Apparently, wanting to have "perfect" sex can create some significant pressures that adversely affect sexual responsiveness in men, as well as diminish their overall relationship satisfaction. Anything that increases pressures to perform well sexually can in fact have a very counterproductive effect.

Erectile dysfunction can result from various causes. Both biological and psychosocial factors can be involved. In about 4 out of 5 cases, erectile dysfunction has a biological, or organic, cause. A physician or counselor can discriminate between these two categories of causes. For example, nocturnal penile tumescence (NPT) can be determined in a sleep laboratory. Healthy men have an erection every 80 to 90 minutes in their sleep. When recording devices are applied to the base of the penis, sleep researchers can monitor the presence or absence of erections. If a man cannot attain an erection when attempting to have intercourse but *does* have erections in his sleep, this is a strong indicator that his erectile dysfunction has a primarily psychological cause. Very often, low blood levels of testosterone are found in men with erectile dysfunction, and administering doses of testosterone might have highly beneficial effects on sexual response. Finally, ultrasound studies of the pattern of blood flow in a man's penis also help reveal if his erectile dysfunction is due to a physical problem.

Nonetheless, it is often too simplistic to think that erectile dysfunction is exclusively *either* organic *or* psychological. It is often a combination of the two. For example, a man may experience problems attaining and maintaining an erection due to ill-

ness or a side effect of a medication. But even after he discontinues taking the medicine, he might still have a lot of self-doubt and nervousness, which are likely to continue to impair his erectile ability even though he is no longer ill or using medication.

> *"This is the monstruosity in love, lady—that the will is infinite and the execution confined; that the desire is boundless and the act a slave to limit."*
> *"Troilus and Cressida" Act 3, Scene 2*
> *William Shakespeare*

Orgasmic Disorders

Some people with sexual dysfunctions have a particularly frustrating situation. They have no problems experiencing sexual desire nor any difficulties in responding physically to erotic stimuli. They experience desire and arousal. But they just can't have orgasms. And if they do, their orgasms do not occur regularly and reliably under conditions that would foster a stable pattern of orgasmic response. While all sexual dysfunctions involve significant frustration, orgasmic disorders are particularly disheartening to those afflicted. People with orgasmic disorders often feel that something important is missing. Orgasm can be delayed, diminished, or absent altogether, and usually the person does not know what to do to improve the situation. Many people incorrectly assume that if a man enters a woman with an erect penis and the woman is also sexually aroused, all they have to do is engage in vigorous pelvic thrusting in order for both to have an orgasm. Sometimes this doesn't happen.

FEMALE ORGASMIC DISORDER

Most adolescent boys masturbate, sometimes quite often. By doing so they learn a lot about their bodies, their feelings of arousal, and the way those feelings grow in intensity, usually culminating in orgasm. Young males get a lot of "training," one might say, in their sexual response cycle. Society generally implicitly assumes that these masturbatory behaviors are a normal if not necessary aspect of their sexual development and socialization. For young women, however, a very different scenario often emerges. Fewer adolescent females masturbate, and thus fewer learn about their bodies and how they respond to erotic stimuli and genital stimulation. The subtle but significant message to many young women in our society has been to not touch themselves. Some even are told that sexual behavior is a "responsibility" of marriage and that it is a woman's obligation to meet the needs of her husband. While almost all boys have had orgasms and have ejaculated by the time they turn 13, only about a third of young women have had orgasms. Unless a young women learns to think differently about sexuality, lack of orgasmic response in early adulthood and later is not at all uncommon.

A **female orgasmic disorder** is usually referred to as *anorgasmia.* In the past many professionals in the medical, social, and behavioral sciences did not think that it was normal for women to have orgasms during sexual intercourse. As recently as 1957, a major gynecology textbook stated that women do

Dear Dr. Ruth

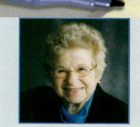

Question

My husband and I have been married for 2 years and everything seems to be going really nicely. We love each other, communicate very well, and have decided to put off starting a family for a few more years. But there is something that has been bothering me, and I'm not quite sure how to talk about it with my husband. Whenever we have sex, he is really concerned about me having an orgasm. It seems as if he doesn't feel he's been a good lover unless I've climaxed. And the problem is I never climax during intercourse. I can always climax when I masturbate and usually when my husband stimulates me orally. I am feeling that there is something wrong with me and the "pressure" to respond makes it even harder for me to relax. If I tell my husband this I am afraid he will feel terrible. Can you make any suggestions?

Answer

While it is possible that your husband will "feel terrible" when you tell him, though that is probably too strong a reaction, when you do tell him (and please note how I am putting this) the result will be that you are both going to have a much better sex life.

Many women share your sexual response and can have an orgasm only with direct clitoral stimulation that they cannot get during intercourse alone; however, that does not mean that they can't climax during intercourse, if they want to. By changing positions to one that allows the male to stimulate her clitoris during intercourse, such as the female on top or side by side positions, it is possible for many of those women to climax during intercourse.

Having said that, let me right away point out that this does not work for all women. These women need to enjoy their orgasms either before or after intercourse. There's nothing wrong with not being able to have an orgasm during intercourse, as long as you derive sexual satisfaction some other way. So explain all this to your husband and I'm sure he'll be very understanding.

---

not generally have any sexual feelings, sexual needs, or sexual desires, except in a few "unusual cases." In our contemporary perspective, this seems truly odd. Most segments of our society today are very comfortable with the idea that women are just as entitled to the enjoyments of sexual responsiveness as are men. However, when men think that women *have to have orgasms* to feel truly fulfilled sexually, this may cause some expectations that are unreasonable or even obstructions to relaxed lovemaking. Indeed, as we have noted earlier, *trying to* have an orgasm can make it actually more difficult to happen. Note also that orgasmic experiences vary much within a woman and may also vary much between different women. When women have the occasion to discuss their orgasms in structured interview settings, they say many different things about anticipating orgasms, as well as the intensity and duration of those orgasms. Coupled with this is the fact that some women believe that the only "appropriate" way to have an orgasm is during sexual intercourse (and in some cases, only when they are planning conception). For some women, orgasms experienced during masturbation or fantasizing are "second best" or don't really "count."

"Sex as I said, can be summed up in three P's: procreation, pleasure, and pride. From the long-range point of view, which we must always consider, procreation is by far the most important, since without procreation there could be no continuation of the race . . . So female orgasm is simply a nervous climax to sex relations . . . and as such it is a comparative luxury from nature's point of view. It may be thought of as a sort of pleasure-prize that comes with a box of cereal. It is all to the good if the prize is there, but the cereal is valuable and nourishing if it is not."

"The Normal Woman," Madeline Gray, 1967

Different types of anorgasmia have been described. **Primary anorgasmia** is a lack of orgasmic response in women who have *never* had an orgasm by any means, including masturbation, fantasizing, oral stimulation, or anal or vaginal penetration. As discussed in the next chapter in reference to sex therapies, semantic problems often make it difficult to determine whether a woman has in fact ever had an orgasm. While some women might think that they have not had an orgasm unless they could describe it as cosmic fireworks, they indeed may have had physiological orgasms but just didn't describe them as such. **Situational anorgasmia** is a condition in which women can have orgasms only by means of limited (and often highly stereotyped) patterns of stimulation. Unless everything is "just so" in terms of person, place, time, and method of stimulation, these women simply do not have orgasms. Feelings of safety and privacy and knowing that your partner knows how you like to be touched or caressed are very important, indeed necessary for some women to be orgasmic. A perplexing and frustrating problem of female sexual response is called **random anorgasmia,** in which orgasms do not occur regularly and dependably even when a woman feels sexual desire and arousal. Sometimes it happens and sometimes it doesn't, and it's hard to determine just exactly why. Random anorgasmia is not related to illness, prescription drugs, or the use of recreational drugs. Finally, some women have lost a previously reliable pattern of sexual responsiveness, a condition usually called **secondary anorgasmia.** While these women enter the plateau phase of the sexual response cycle, they don't reach the next stage of orgasm. Sometimes when women first begin taking birth control pills they experience secondary anorgasmia, at least for a little while. Additionally, many women who have been the victims of sexual assault experience painful intercourse, which can occur for a number of different reasons, or who are involved in unrewarding relationships may also lose their previously predictable pattern of orgasmic response.

Anorgasmia may also involve a pattern of *delayed* orgasmic response, although this delay can be difficult to define specifically. It could happen because of a change in foreplay behaviors, tension in a relationship, or boredom and monotony in a couple's style of lovemaking. When delayed orgasm seems unusual for a woman's age, life circumstances, and the effectiveness of foreplay stimulation, then her condition is similar to a lack of orgasmic response and is likely to cause the same kind of distress and interpersonal problems.

"Men always fall for frigid women because they put on the best show."

Fanny Brice

An interesting study compared questionnaire data collected from small groups of orgasmic and nonorgasmic women (Kelly, Strassberg, & Kircher, 1990). These focused on a woman's knowledge base about human sexuality, her susceptibility to sexual myths, and her overall sexual attitudes. Despite the fact that a relatively small number of women (10 women between the ages of 21 and 40) were studied, provocative data

emerged that described attitudes and experiences correlated with anorgasmia. Anorgasmic women had more difficulty and awkwardness talking with their partners about their enjoyment of direct clitoral stimulation. These women held negative attitudes about masturbation, were more likely to believe sexual myths, and experienced more guilt associated with sexual behavior.

MALE ORGASMIC DISORDER

Many men have no problems enjoying sexual desire and arousal, have no difficulty in attaining and maintaining an erection, find it easy to penetrate their partner and engage in pelvic thrusting, but do not ejaculate, or if they do, their ejaculation is long delayed and requires exceptionally vigorous, prolonged stimulation. Such stimulation may involve prolonged intercourse or manual or oral stimulation. If this condition occurs after a normal period of sexual excitement, it is called male orgasmic disorder, **retarded ejaculation,** or ejaculatory incompetence. When the vigorousness and duration of sexual stimulation seem adequate to precipitate orgasmic response, given the individual's age and health, a diagnosis of male orgasmic disorder is usually made. Like other conditions, this is not technically a sexual dysfunction unless the individual experiencing it and his partner are upset.

Sex therapists are often persuaded of the predominantly psychological origins of male orgasmic disorder because while these men do not generally ejaculate during sexual intercourse, they *do* ejaculate regularly during masturbation, when their partners masturbate them, or when their partners orally stimulate their penises. Something about intercourse and its associated intimacies is extremely inhibiting for these men. Men who have this orgasmic disorder can have orgasms during "wet dreams," so their physiological mechanism of orgasm is functional. Male orgasmic disorder is very rare. When Masters and Johnson published *Human Sexual Inadequacy* in 1970, with data based on 11 years of clinical experience, of 448 men who sought treatment for a variety of sexual difficulties, only 17 had this particular sexual dysfunction. In addition to the fact that these men require a great deal of penile stimulation in order to ejaculate, other factors may play a role in this dysfunction. Psychological factors, such as guilt, fear, resentment, and passivity, may also be involved (Munjack & Kanno, 1979). For example, if a man or his partner is very apprehensive about the possibility of a pregnancy and both are ambivalent or resistant to using contraceptives, these issues may contribute to the development of retarded ejaculation. A case study describing this situation has been published (Newell, 1978). When lack of ejaculation during intercourse occurs only occasionally, there is usually nothing to worry about, but when the pattern becomes persistent and distressing, consulting a sex therapist is a good idea. Interestingly, it has been reported that among men with retarded ejaculation, their consistent female sexual partner is *not* their main sexual interest, which instead is often another man (Munjack & Kanno, 1979).

PREMATURE EJACULATION

Earlier chapters discussed how the sexual response cycle varies in terms of how much time it takes men and women to progress through the stages of sexual arousal and response. Generally men (especially younger men) become aroused more quickly than women and spend less time in the plateau stage than their female partners. Similarly, often a man's orgasms do not last as long as a woman's. While many couples learn about these differences and find ways to negotiate them satisfactorily, others frequently have problems. The most common problem, **premature ejaculation**, involves a man's inability to withhold his ejaculation long enough for his partner to enjoy some significant sense of sexual satisfaction, which may or may not involve her having an orgasm. An earlier chapter has emphasized that sexual satisfaction does not require a couple to share simultaneous orgasms, and in fact, they often do not. Yet when a man enters his partner, engages in vigorous pelvic thrusting, and promptly ejaculates, he may leave her somewhat aroused when he is unable to continue pelvic stroking with an erection. This often leaves her unsatisfied. Premature ejaculation is the most common sexual dysfunction among men. One group of investigators estimated the prevalence of premature ejaculation to be about 29% (Laumann, Gagnon, Michael, & Michaels, 1994). Masters and Johnson (1970) arbitrarily defined premature ejaculation as a man's inability to withhold ejaculation about half the time he and his partner have intercourse. Other investigators have tried to define premature ejaculation more specifically. Grenier and Byers (1997) examined questionnaire responses from 112 undergraduate heterosexual males and found that four different ways of defining premature ejaculation were fairly similar in the ways these men described rapid ejaculation. These included how much control the man felt he had over the timing of his ejaculation, the amount of time that elapsed between vaginal penetration and ejaculation, perceived feelings of satisfaction and self-control over the timing of ejaculation, and how much concern or worry these men had about premature ejaculation. In essence, all of these ways of defining premature ejaculation were comparable, and none seemed to have better explanatory value than the others. According to the *DSM,* when a man is distressed over his lack of ejaculatory control and this problem contributes to interpersonal difficulties with his partner, premature ejaculation is a sexual dysfunction. But remember, if neither person is particularly bothered by it, this situation is not a dysfunction.

Nonetheless, this is a difficult subject. Knowing how long the "average" couple has intercourse may not tell us very much, since every couple is unique and has their own sexual style and preferences. What *is* important is whether both individuals feel satisfied after they share sexual intercourse, and this does not often happen with those who ejaculate prematurely.

The two broad categories of premature ejaculation are *primary* and *secondary.* In primary premature ejaculation, a man has always been a rapid ejaculator, often for a good reason. Many adolescents masturbate frequently, often once a day or more. Masturbation is a very private and often furtive behavior and is sometimes accompanied by guilt feelings. When teenagers masturbate alone, they obviously are not paying attention to a partner's sexual satisfaction. Adolescent masturbation among boys is often a very quick activity, sometimes tak-ing only a few minutes. But unfortunately, rapid ejaculation can become habitual and hard to unlearn; this is the problem that men with primary premature ejaculation confront. When these young men establish a relationship with a partner, this old, firmly established pattern of rapid ejaculation is still deeply set in their sexual thinking and responding. Because this behavior pattern was learned in the first place, however, it can be unlearned as well, as described in a later section. In secondary premature ejaculation, the man has typically enjoyed many years of intercourse in which he was able to control his orgasm so that his partner could also enjoy more prolonged sexual arousal and orgasm. But now he finds that he cannot withhold his orgasm as effectively as he had been able to.

Premature ejaculation can be caused by both psychological and biological factors. When rapid ejaculation results from the type of learning described above, it has an obvious psychological cause. Another common cause of premature ejaculation is performance anxiety. If a man is highly preoccupied with his skill as a lover, the tension and stress of his expectations often make it difficult for him to monitor his level of sexual arousal, and he is often unable to withhold his ejaculation. One of the most important things to teach men experiencing premature ejaculation is to pay attention to their growing sexual excitement and the rate at which they are approaching ejaculation. The point in time when a man is certain that he can no longer withhold ejaculation is called ejaculatory inevitability. The next chapter discusses effective techniques for men to better recognize the rate at which they are approaching this point and to learn ways to slow down and delay their orgasms.

Are There Dysfunctions of the Resolution Phase of the Sexual Response Cycle?

We have described sexual dysfunctions affecting sexual desire, arousal, and orgasm, corresponding to the three stages of the sexual response cycle. One might also wonder whether any sexual dysfunctions affect the last phase of the sexual response cycle, resolution. During resolution our bodies return to their pre-excitement level of arousal; we generally feel peaceful and calm and very close to the person with whom we just made love. But these serene and tranquil feelings don't happen to everyone. Some women and men treat one another indifferently rather than nurturantly after sexual intercourse. Is this a "sexual dysfunction"? Although sex researchers have not explored dysfunctions during the resolution phase, clearly bad feelings might become associated with this lack of warmth and affection, leaving one or both partners feeling isolated and alone.

Sexual Pain Disorders

Sometimes intercourse is uncomfortable. The woman may not have lubricated enough, or the man may attempt to insert a less-than-erect penis into an unlubricated vagina. Pelvic thrusting may also be so vigorous that the ligaments that support a woman's uterus can be suddenly stretched. Whatever the cause, when sexual intercourse is persistently and recurrently uncomfortable and a woman or man habitually experiences genital discomfort, this is a sexual dysfunction, especially if either party is distressed or their relationship suffers. Yet **sexual pain disorders** are not fully explained by lack of lubrication. The discomfort need not be associated only with vaginal penetration; it can occur even with the anticipation of vaginal penetration. These disorders can be caused by psychological factors or a combination of psychological and biological factors.

DYSPAREUNIA

Technically speaking, the term **dyspareunia** refers to pain that recurs during sexual intercourse in either women or men. This discomfort may be associated with vaginal penetration or the expectation of intercourse. It can be apparent after a couple has finished having sex. Women who complain of dyspareunia report that discomfort may accompany insertion and/or deep pelvic thrusting. Some people have experienced dyspareunia as long as they have been having intercourse, while others developed this disorder later in life, often in association with a particular situation or relationship. Different people use different language to describe their discomfort. Some speak of "sharp pains" while others report "twinges of hurting," and still others talk of "aching sensations" (Abarbanel, 1978).

Various factors may cause dyspareunia. Unusual anatomical variations may play a role. A small introitus, as well as a smaller-than-normal vagina, can contribute to this condition. Various health problems also can contribute to painful intercourse. In men, Peyronie's disease (in which there are irregularities in the curvature of the penis) can cause significant pain before, during, and after intercourse. In women, endometriosis (see Chapter 5) is related to substantial discomfort during penile penetration and especially during pelvic thrusting. Bacterial infections of the genitourinary systems of both women and men can cause serious pain during sexual intercourse. When the urethra and fallopian tubes are involved in women, or when the urethra, epididymis, or prostate is locally infected in men, the infection may cause or contribute to dyspareunia. Even benign growths of the lower colon and rectum may cause serious pain when a couple is having sex, regardless of the position they are using. Several bone and joint problems in the lower back and hips have been related to painful intercourse.

Sometimes the most perplexing causes of dyspareunia are psychological and/or psychosocial. If a person anticipates pain during intercourse because of a previous distressing experience, they may again anticipate this discomfort. In some people, this is such an aversive experience that they forego intercourse altogether. While in others, the anticipated suffering occurs because the individual *imagines* that they may actually be injured in the act of sexual intercourse. If an individual is feeling guilty or shameful about being in a sexual situation in the first place, they may avoid coitus. Finally, some people just don't know very much about the sexual response cycle and may proceed to vaginal penetration long before adequate lubrication has occurred. This factor, especially together with a clumsy, hurried partner, can create more than enough discomfort for a person

to develop a severe aversion to the prospect of intercourse and the expectation of pain that may accompany it.

A woman may also experience dyspareunia as a result of a surgical procedure. When scar tissue accumulates in the lower abdomen, after a hysterectomy for example, intercourse may be very uncomfortable, especially if a woman's partner is vigorous in his pelvic thrusting. When a painful scar remains after an episiotomy, this too may cause pain during sexual activity. In all, there are a number of causes of painful intercourse. But regardless of the cause of this often persistent, distressing discomfort, one thing is certain: people who have this kind of pain are much less likely to want to have intercourse, to enjoy it, or to feel like real partners when they are sharing intimacy. They often feel that a major aspect of their lives is missing.

VAGINISMUS

Since the writings of the French philosopher Rene Descartes (see Chapter 2) in the mid-1600s, thinkers have been very interested in the nature of the connection between the mind and the body. Descartes was among the first to wonder how something invisible and spiritual like the mind could exert such a powerful influence on the physical reality of the human body. Since his day, social and behavioral scientists, as well as neuroscientists, have been preoccupied with this basic issue. **Vaginismus** is a condition in which a woman experiences a spastic (highly uncoordinated) contraction of the musculature at the opening to her vagina and the outer one-third of the vagina. This usually makes penile penetration difficult if not impossible. These muscle contractions are completely involuntary: the woman can't control them, at least not until she learns special relaxation techniques, discussed in the next chapter. These involuntary muscle contractions occur in response to real attempts at penetration, as well as the expectation of intercourse. Vaginismus is one of the most common reasons for unconsummated marriages, and the feelings of frustration among women and men in this situation can be very troubling. Resistance to vaginal entry is so strong that not only is penile penetration impossible, but the attempted insertion of tampons or even a physician's finger or a speculum is often prevented. Interestingly, vaginismus occurs in all cultures in which sexual behavior and responsiveness have been studied.

In some cases, the muscular spasms in vaginismus are somewhat weak, while in others they are extremely strong. The *DSM* considers vaginismus a sexual dysfunction when its causes are primarily psychological or psychosocial, even though a number of biological conditions can contribute to it. For example, scarring caused by an episiotomy can make vaginal penetration very uncomfortable; the same is true of endometriosis, prolapsed uterus, or even low levels of female hormones that can cause chronic vaginal dryness. All of these can cause pain during intercourse, which in turn could lead to muscle spasms. Sometimes a history of sexual assault or abuse plays a powerful role in the etiology of vaginismus. In some cases, traumatic early experiences with a tampon can be involved in the development of this dysfunction. When many young girls begin menstruation, they are often told by their

Dear Dr. Ruth

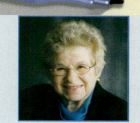

Question

When I was a little girl I was sexually abused by the father of one of my girl friends. Over the years I've come to terms with what happened to me and understand that I did not cause this, I did not ask for this, and there is nothing wrong or bad about me. Now I have a lot of trouble having intercourse. It's not that I don't want to, it's just that I tighten up so much that my partner cannot get his penis inside of me, at least not very far. It's very uncomfortable for me and frustrating for him and I just don't know what to do about it. Is there some medicine that can help me relax? Would a few glasses of wine help? Who should I talk to and what do you think they can do for me?

Answer

You have self-diagnosed your problem, and you might be right, but it's also possible that something else is causing you to tighten up. Since your history might lead to a psychological problem, such as vaginismus, which is the involuntary contraction of the vaginal muscles, I would urge you to consult with a sex therapist or counselor. It's a good thing that you know the potential source of your problem, but at this point, you need a professional's help to overcome the difficulties you are encountering.

---

mothers to use pads and to avoid tampons. But because of peer influence or just plain old curiosity, a girl may decide for herself to try a tampon. She may insert it too far, or in some cases forget it altogether. Often she and her mother have to make a rather embarrassing trip to the gynecologist. The feelings of shame, guilt, disobedience, embarrassment, and discomfort from this situation are often enough to cause vaginismus, even in a girl who may not be sexually active.

A recent study of vaginismus explored the marital dynamics of couples living with this problem (Tugrul & Kabakci, 1997). These investigators studied 40 married couples in Turkey; the women were between the ages of 19 and 35 and their husbands were between 19 and 42. The average length of their marriages was about 2¹/₂ years. A number of questionnaires were used to assess sexual satisfaction, family difficulties, anxiety, body image, sex roles, and personal information. In general, the women and men in this study reported low levels of sexual satisfaction in their marriages. While the men found intercourse manageable, the women reported that they did not enjoy having sex very often and did not feel especially sensual during sexual interactions. In fact, these women were quite candid about trying to avoid intercourse. They reported specific fears about pain, harm, and even physical injury during intercourse. While they were not averse to the idea of having sex, they were certainly concerned about the discomfort they often felt. The women in this study reported that they found their husbands highly au-

thoritarian and oppressive, as well as somewhat undependable, and these factors seemed to be highly correlated with vaginismus. Even though these data are from a small sample of subjects, there is reason to explore further the role of marital factors on the development of vaginismus. Treatments of this dysfunction are described in the next chapter.

Prevalence of Sexual Dysfunctions

Spector and Carey (1990) evaluated 23 studies that assessed the prevalence of sexual dysfunctions. While estimates were not available for all the dysfunctions discussed above, there was some consistency in these studies regarding the frequency with which these problems occur in the general population. Table 14-1 summarizes these data.

TABLE 14-1

Prevalence of Sexual Dysfunctions Based on a Review of 23 Clinical Studies

Inhibited female orgasm	5–10%
Male erectile disorder	4–9%
Inhibited male orgasm	4–10%
Premature ejaculation	36–38%

After Spector & Carey, 1990.)

Drugs and Sexual Dysfunctions

A wide variety of substances have been developed or adapted for the treatment of disease, and in all historical eras and all cultures, people have discovered and developed substances to alter consciousness. Of this wide variety of drug agents, both those used therapeutically and those used recreationally, many have a detrimental effect on sexual arousal and response. Because many people have access to powerful medications and illicit substances, the effects of these agents on sexual functioning are important.

Different drugs affect various stages of the sexual response cycle: desire, arousal, and orgasm. They can also play a role in discomfort during intercourse. Like other sexual dysfunctions, these impairments cause distress, as well as problems in interpersonal relationships. In cases involving some prescription drugs, a person does not experience any "intoxication" although a sexual problem becomes evident. In cases involving recreational drugs, intoxication is typically a prelude to a sexual dysfunction. This is an important distinction. When people are not performing up to their expectations because they have used a drug that significantly altered their consciousness, they generally do not feel any distress or frustration with this situational sexual inadequacy. This is usually the case with recreational agents. Substance-induced sexual dysfunctions in most cases become obvious while the individual is under the influence of the drug. At other times, their sexual feelings and functioning may be unimpaired. But when a person is taking their medication as prescribed by their doctor and finds that they are having problems with sexual desire, arousal, or orgasm, this distress occurs in an entirely different situation, which is more likely to be dysfunctional. Later sections in this chapter examine in detail the specific effects of prescription and recreational drugs on sexual functioning.

CAUSES OF SEXUAL DYSFUNCTIONS

Problems in desire, arousal, or orgasm may be caused by a number of factors in the wider psychosocial environment, in interpersonal relationships, or in connection with personal problems that stem from inadequate information, inappropriate learning, or a history of sexual abuse and/or assault. Often multiple factors are involved in the emergence of sexual dysfunctions, and in many cases it is difficult, if not impossible, to point with certainty to any single cause.

Bookstores stock dozens of titles about how to have "better sex," but few focus on sexual problems and solving them. In fact, sexual dysfunctions are relatively invisible in our society. Popular books and movies present images and stories of beautiful eroticism, uninhibited sexual expression, and attractive people enjoying wonderful, compatible, intimate relationships. It wasn't until the drug "Viagra" hit the market in the late 1990s that sexual dysfunctions became a part of the cultural discourse on quality of life in the United States. Although such problems are fairly common, only rarely are they depicted in the media, which represents the general climate of our psychosocial environment.

Societal Factors in the Development of Sexual Dysfunctions

Television, movies, and magazines are full of images of attractive people. Society's notions of "sexiness," "masculinity," and "femininity" are explicit or implicit in these depictions. Younger, impressionable adolescents often create a myth in their minds about all the wonderful (and sexual) things that will happen to them if they are physically attractive. But while they focus on external appearances, they are often beset by profound uncertainties and insecurities within. It might be easy to buy clothing that looks sexy, but being comfortable with your own sexual needs and knowing how to please your partner are entirely different matters.

"Outside every thin woman is a fat man trying to get in."

Katherine Whitehorn

Society's Myths About Sex

Common sexual myths and cultural beliefs may contribute to high, and sometimes unattainable, expectations about sexual behavior. These assumptions govern many people's expectations and self-perceptions. To the degree that one is aware of these, a person may be better able to understand variations in sexual interest or sex drive and to accept different sexual appetites. Consider these myths with respect to your own development and experience.

Myth Number 1: Everybody enjoys having sexual intercourse every chance they get.

This is simply incorrect. There are wide variations from time to time in a person's desire to have intercourse and wide variations among different people. Although some are very curious about many sexual matters, others prefer to refrain from sexual interactions. They are simply uncomfortable sharing physical intimacy, and that preference should be respected.

Myth Number 2: The frequency of sexual interaction is a good indication of the strength of a relationship.

Again, this is plainly false. Good relationships usually stem from two people sharing different activities together. In fact, an obsessive preoccupation with the sexual aspects of a relationship may leave a couple with a bond lacking vitality and diversity. In addition, when the couple wants to have sexual intercourse when they are well rested, free of stress, and free of interruption, they may find that there aren't too many times during the week when all these criteria are met.

Myth Number 3: Sexual intercourse isn't good unless both parties have an orgasm.

One can enjoy feelings of safety, intimacy, mutuality, love, and affection while sharing physical intimacy and not have an orgasm. While orgasm is often thought of as the goal of sexual intercourse, some very enjoyable, erotic experiences

Research Highlight

SOCIETY, OBESITY, AND SEXUALITY

Because of the powerful relationship between thinness, attractiveness, and sex appeal in our culture, research has examined the impact of obesity on sexual self-esteem and feelings of adequacy in interpersonal contexts. People often make inferences about the moods, impulse control, and erotic inclinations and behavior of overweight individuals. Many people are averse to imagining obese individuals sharing physical intimacy. This is a good example of the ways in which societal perceptions can influence feelings of sexual attractiveness and perhaps even sexual responsiveness.

Regan (1996) studied 96 undergraduates (48 females and 48 males) between the ages of 17 and 23. These subjects were presented with information about male or female obese and normal-weight individuals; they were given reports of age, height, and weight and told that they were participating in a study on "person perception." These respondents reported that they felt an obese man's sexual experiences would be similar to those of a normal-weight man. In contrast, they felt that obese women were less attractive sexually and less sexually responsive and had less sexual experience and mastery than their normal-weight counterparts. Further, obese women were thought to have diminished sexual desire and a more limited sexual repertoire than normal-weight women or obese men. Obese women in this study were a stigmatized minority viewed as less sexually inclined and responsive. There were no significant differences in the way male and female respondents replied to this questionnaire. Of course, these are reported beliefs that are more closely related to social perceptions of overweight individuals than to the reported behaviors of obese individuals themselves. Buss (1997) suggested that because obese people are often perceived to be unattractive according to social conventions of beauty, they may be "sexually maladjusted." Buss emphasized that any sexual problems obese individuals might have are more a function of a hostile social environment than any particular anatomical, physiological, or endocrine problems associated with being overweight. In the past, some social and behavioral scientists have suggested that people become obese as a defense against intimacy and their dislike of sexual behavior. As of this writing, however, there are no substantive, systematic data to support this suggestion.

Data have been reported that indicate that obese males may be somewhat less sexually inclined than their normal-weight counterparts. Jagstaidt, Golay, and Pasini (1997) studied sexual behavior and sexual dysfunctions in a group of 30 male obese individuals and compared them with 30 normal-weight individuals. These investigators found significantly diminished sexual desire, fewer sexual fantasies, and less inclination to pursue sexual experiences in the obese group compared than in subjects in the control group. It is unclear, however, whether obesity somehow causes diminished sexual interest or whether obesity and lowered sexual interest are only correlated. Importantly, these writers emphasize the importance of sexual counseling as a part of a multifaceted weight reduction program. In fact, other investigations have reported that weight loss may lead to increased sexual interest and activity. Werlinger, King, Clark, Pera, et al., (1997) studied sexual behavior in a sample of 32 middle-aged women who had lost significant amounts of weight in a medically supervised program and found notable improvements in body image, as well as increases in sexual behavior. Finally, Marshall and Neill (1977) noted that after intestinal by-pass surgery (which removes a large portion of small intestine so that less food is absorbed in the digestive tract), most of their patients reported an increased level of interest in sex and frequency of sexual activity. Apparently, when people lose weight and more closely resemble social conventions of attractiveness, they are more likely to experience sexual desire and increased levels of sexual behavior as well. But someone who is obese should not be presumed to necessarily have less sexual interest or responsiveness.

Other Countries, Cultures, and Customs

SEXUAL DYSFUNCTIONS IN CHINA

It is often instructive to examine sexual dysfunctions within their psychosocial context. The cultural and historical traditions of the Chinese, of course, influence the manifestations, diagnosis, and treatment of sexual dysfunctions in this enormous nation. For example, Liu and Ng (1995) have reported that Chinese beliefs in the essential significance of semen and various relatively ineffective folk remedies for sexual problems commonly lead to long delays in seeking assistance for sexual dysfunctions. Additionally, because of its patriarchal, male-dominant culture, women often feel very hesitant to ask for help when they feel they are not fully enjoying physical intimacy with their partners. In the mid-1980s, there were virtually no clinics for the treatment of sexual dysfunctions in the entire country, although by the mid-1990s there were 34. As in the United States, there is little uniformity in the credentials of those who staff these establishments, and their therapies ranged from Chinese herbal agents to cognitive-behavioral techniques. This number of clinics is very small relative to the number of people who live in China but at least is an important acknowledgment of the problem facing many Chinese women and men.

Cultural traditions affect the commonness of sexual dysfunctions in China and the enormous differential in the gender of those who seek treatment. For example, retarded ejaculation is the most common problem in Chinese clinics, and the reasons for this may be difficult for people in other countries to understand. For centuries in China, mystical properties have been attributed to semen; in fact, many Chinese men are socialized to believe that "one drop of semen is as valuable as ten drops of blood" (Liu & Ng, 1995, p. 729) and, therefore, make every reasonable effort to avoid wasting it. Semen is a fundamental part of the *yang* element, which represents an amalgam of heaven and earth. Throughout history, books about sex in China have offered lessons on how to withhold semen to avoid its inappropriate dissipation. Careful instruction is offered on how to have intercourse without ejaculation because each dispensing of semen causes a loss of spiritual energy for the man. This is still a powerful idea for many men in China, and many Chinese youth practice masturbating and having intercourse without ejaculating. In the same vein, women who want to have intercourse "too frequently" are seen as a threat to preserving this precious fluid; therefore, retarded ejaculation is not a surprising consequence of this tradition. The discussion of sex therapies in the next chapter describes how it is hard to unlearn a message that has been a big part of a person's sexual value system for a long time.

Another interesting aspect of sexual dysfunctions in China is the extremely small percentage of female patients who seek the services of sex clinics. During the 1970s in the United States, 43.3% of those seeking sex therapy were women. The comparable figure during the 1980s in the Soviet Union was 39.4%. In Liu and Ng's study, the percentage of women seeking sex therapy in China ranged from 2.7% in Harbin to 6.9% in Beijing. For many women in China, sexual intercourse is a wife's duty, and whether she enjoys it or responds to her husband physically is often a matter of little concern to men. In fact, Liu and Ng point out that if a woman seems absorbed in sexual issues, "she would be accused of indecency and breaching her female role, or even considered to be obscene" (p. 729). For these reasons, many Chinese women are embarrassed about sexual intercourse, are hesitant to initiate intimacy with their husbands, and are frequently coerced into having sex. Not surprisingly, many Chinese women report highly unsatisfactory feelings about sexual activity within the context of their marriages. Most Chinese women behave as if they have few marital rights regarding sex.

These authors point out that lack of authoritative sexual information also contributes to the prevalence of sexual dysfunctions in China, although this fact is by no means specific to that country. In particular, couples seem unaware of the importance of foreplay in facilitating comfortable intercourse, often spending less than one minute in intimate sharing before penetration. Because of this, many women report significant discomfort, nervousness, and disappointment in connection with coitus.

More so than in most other countries, in China there are rather explicit prohibitions against intercourse among the aging and elderly, contributing to the prevalence of sexual dysfunctions among those at mid-life and later. Physical intimacy may cease long before later life. In a study of 20,000 Chinese women and men, Liu, Ng, and Chou (1992) reported that about 35% of the women had already stopped having intercourse between the ages of 41 and 50, and 38% of women over the age of 50. Among men, almost 20% had stopped having intercourse between 41 and 50, with the number rising to 60% among men over the age of 50. This disparity between women and men may be accounted for by differences in how willing the two sexes are to *report* that they have stopped having sex, when in fact they may continue to do so. Because of these powerful cultural beliefs, it is not surprising that sexual difficulties are different in both nature and scope in China from in North America and other countries. The point is not, of course, that the Chinese should change their traditions, but that traditions have powerful influences on people.

can be shared without any pressure to "perform" and have an orgasm or "make" one's partner have an orgasm.

Myth Number 4: Men are sexual leaders and teachers and women are supposed to be sexual learners and take a more passive attitude during sexual sharing.

Unfortunately, this myth has been slow to die. In reality, women and men today enter marriages with similar sexual backgrounds in terms of number of partners and diversity of sexual behaviors. Much performance anxiety can be eliminated when couples communicate more clearly and completely about their level of sexual knowledge and their expectations for their partner. With the decline in the sexual double standard previously discussed, there is little reason to assume that men are more knowledgeable about sex or more experienced than their female counterparts.

Myth Number 5: After sexual intercourse, people are always satisfied, happy, and peaceful.

We wish this were the case. In fact, many people feel unsatisfied, detached from their partners, neglected, or even exploited after intercourse. Because these feelings are often not openly discussed, further sexual interactions are not likely to be any more satisfactory. Society's perspective, however, is often at odds with the realities of this unrewarding situation. Many people assume that shared intimacy will always be enjoyable and satisfying and are often quite distressed, although often quietly so, to discover that sexual intercourse may reveal more serious, pervasive problems in a relationship.

Interpretation of Religious Traditions and Sexual Dysfunctions

Chapter 2 discussed how our sexual thoughts, feelings, and behaviors have been powerfully influenced by many of the religious traditions of Judeo-Christian cultures. For example, the heritage of male dominance and the inappropriateness of sexual intercourse before marriage has its roots in the doctrines of an-

cient Jews and Christians. Similarly, the idea that sexual intercourse is appropriate only if a couple is planning to conceive is another very powerful notion with old religious roots. Many of our culture's more somber and serious attitudes about human sexual expression have their origins in old spiritual texts, teachings, and customs. How people interpret the religious traditions in which they have been raised often has a clear, and often inhibiting, influence on the ways they think, feel, and act sexually.

"Marital intercourse is certainly holy, lawful and praiseworthy in itself and profitable to society, yet in certain circumstances it can prove dangerous, as when through excess the soul is made sick with venial sin, or through the violation and perversion of its primary end, killed by mortal sin; such perversion, detestable in proportion to its departure from the true order, being always mortal sin, for it is never lawful to exclude the primary end of marriage which is the procreation of children."

"Introduction to the Devout Life,"
St. Francis DeSales, 1609

Historically, and still to some extent true today, religious groups have enforced conformity with belief systems by creating guilt among those who do not comply with the behavioral requirements of the faith. Not all religions do this, of course, but some certainly do. The guilt many people feel because of their thoughts or actions that diverge from religious expectations often fosters anxiety, and anxiety frequently impairs sexual interest, arousal, and response, as we have already seen. In fact, sexual pleasure itself is often considered bad or wicked in many Christian religions (Runkel, 1998). Generally this is not the view of Judaism or several Eastern religions, such as Buddhism, Shinto, or Hindu. Even at the beginning of the new millennium little has changed in some religions.

When people feel guilty about masturbating, oral sex, or intercourse without planning conception, remorse and shame often come to be associated with one of the most basic and important aspects of our humanity. We encourage everyone to learn as much as they can about sex so that myths and misinformation cannot diminish the healthy expression of sexuality. People do not all experience guilt for the same reasons, and anxiety often manifests itself differently. Masters and Johnson (1970) noted that sexuality is the only human drive that can be molded and manipulated by culture in such a way that it can be delayed or denied outright or its onset postponed almost indefinitely, and religious values are often involved in this teaching. For delay of sexual gratification to take place, an individual must see the religious teaching as valid and valued codes of human conduct and must be willing to endure sexual feelings without acting on them for prolonged periods of time. This is not always practical or easy. While a person's perspectives on religious teachings might involve sexual abstinence outside marriage, desire and arousal may occur when there is no intention of participating in intercourse. This situation commonly causes the type of guilt and anxiety noted above. In fact, sex therapists have long recognized the fact that religious factors may interfere with all stages of the sexual response cycle.

One last point: in cultures dominated by males, especially in the domestic arena, female desire, arousal, and response may be seen as secondary to the pleasures her husband derives from the act of intercourse. This is certainly the case in China (see Other Countries, Cultures, and Customs sidebar). To the degree that women are not accepted as full partners in a marital relationship, whether due to religious or other reasons, they are more likely to experience ambivalence and guilt about their sexual feelings, which would further complicate their sexual value system and the recognition of themselves as healthy sexual beings.

Sexual Dysfunctions in Later Life

Because many in our society are hesitant to accept the normality of sexual expression throughout the life span, acknowledging sexual dysfunctions among aging and elderly people is even more uncommon. A society that doesn't want to accept the fact that old people have sex is not very interested in why older adults may be having trouble with sex. There is a basic difference between the sexual dysfunctions discussed thus far and the inability to adapt to normal age-related changes in sexual functioning discussed in the previous chapter. If one's psychosocial environment does not accept or encourage lifelong sexual expression, adapting to normal biological changes becomes more complicated. For example, if an individual experiences diminished sexual desire or delayed arousal, does this necessarily mean that they have a dysfunction of desire or arousal? We don't think so. Most of the problems that in later life are associated with dysfunctions of desire, arousal, or orgasm are more clearly related to the health status of the individual and/or any medications they may be taking than to a sexual dysfunction *per se* (Sbrocco, Weisberg, & Barlow, 1995). Sbrocco, Weisberg, and Barlow (1995) suggested that

sexual dysfunctions in later life are more a function of an individual having problems attentively focusing on erotic stimuli in their immediate environment. Some might call this "increased distractibility."

Some social and behavioral scientists think that aging and elderly adults might feel a little guilty about their interest in remaining sexually active, as if these feelings were somehow "abnormal." Even though this isn't true, if someone *thinks it's true* they will be just as uncomfortable about their continued erotic interests. When this happens, small changes in sexual desire, arousal, and orgasm may be magnified out of proportion in a person's mind, and this in turn fosters the development of anxiety in connection with the prospect of having sexual intercourse. People who were somewhat erotophobic earlier in life become progressively more erotophobic as they age, and this then plays an important role in the development of a sexual dysfunction. Older people's self-concept may not include the prominent sexual component it once did when they were younger.

"Older women are best because they always think they may be doing it for the last time."

Ian Fleming

Race and Ethnicity

Just as ageism as a prejudice distorts our thoughts and perceptions about older adults, other prejudices often affect how one thinks about the sexual behaviors and "abilities" of various racial and ethnic groups. Almost every culture has some preconceptions that some other culture has sexual customs and traditions that include very high levels of sexual desire and responsiveness and an unlimited capacity for orgasms. These beliefs often include notions about the size of the male genitalia of these peoples, as well as the phenomenal beauty and sexual readiness of the women. While there indeed are interesting and important sexual differences among many of the world's cultures, the ideas described above are mostly mythical and involve very little substantive truth. Sexual dysfunctions occur in virtually every society cultural anthropologists have studied.

The meaning of sexuality itself, ideas of "normal" sexual relationships, and the nature of sexual dysfunctions are *all* affected by cultural norms and traditions (Lavee, 1991). Although there are genuine culture-specific anxieties about sexual behavior, no culture is characterized by sexual "supermen" and "superwomen," and no racial or ethnic group has "incredible sex" all the time. The dysfunctions that trouble one group of people most assuredly trouble others.

Interpersonal Problems and Sexual Dysfunctions

Problems two people have between themselves are no less important than cultural and societal factors in the development of sexual dysfunctions. Openly and clearly expressing one's feelings and desires is not always easy, but the better you know your partner and the more complete your knowledge about sex

Other Countries, Cultures, and Customs

SEXUAL DYSFUNCTIONS AND ARAB MEN

Sexual dysfunctions occur in every culture. But think for a moment of the stereotype of the romantic, adventurous men of the Middle East. For decades, movies have depicted proud, assertive male Arabs with harems, horses, and power. Yet this is another example of how things are never perfect in paradise. Osman and Al-Sawaf (1995) reported the results of some serious exploratory research concerning anxieties about sexuality and sexual dysfunctions in the Middle East. Over the course of 1 year, 38 men and 5 women were studied. Although this is not a very large sample, early investigative research is often limited in scope. All of these subjects consulted professionals in a hospital specializing in the treatment of psychiatric disorders.

These investigators found that among these patients from Saudi Arabia, Yemen, the Sudan, and other neighboring Arab countries, guilt and anxiety were commonly associated with an inability to conform to common social conceptions of potent, fertile men and submissive, willing women. Indeed, in these countries the "success" of a marriage is judged on two straightforward characteristics: frequent sexual intercourse and having many children. If anything interferes with these two simple objectives, both women and men feel serious distress and apprehension. Osman and Al-Sawaf believe that Arab men are powerfully motivated to create and maintain their dominant roles sexually in their marriages (and many of their male subjects had more than one wife) and become extremely troubled and fearful when they feel that there are problems or inadequacies in their sexual performance. In fact, many young Arab men have grown up believing that it is normal to have intercourse with their wives 3 to 5 times each day. With such high expectations, it is no wonder that some men have very persistent and distracting sexual anxieties that affect their erectile ability and sexual behavior.

Many of the men in this sample believed that they had been "bewitched" by an ex-wife, co-wife, ex-fiancé, or an envious neighbor and had initially sought advice and assistance from a traditional Arab advisor before seeking professional assistance. Twenty-one of these men experienced erectile difficulties after having already had normal intercourse that same day, while another 18 reported a complete inability to attain and maintain an erection sufficient to allow comfortable intercourse. Of these subjects, 3 men were impotent with their wives but not with other women. These researchers described these men as "extremely anxious, agitated, and depressed." In addition, 10 men developed premature ejaculation after having had a normal pattern of controlled ejaculation, and 3 others had been men who prematurely ejaculate as long as they had been having intercourse. The 5 women in this study reported difficulties associated with the physical act of intercourse itself, specifically, vaginismus and dyspareunia.

Osman and Al-Sawaf noted the large discrepancy between the number of women in Arab countries and the number of women in Western countries who seek assistance from sex therapy clinics. Of course, in the West, more women than men explore these therapeutic opportunities, the opposite of these Arab cultures.

A culture's traditions concerning sex roles and the behaviors associated with them play a major role in the etiology and manifestations of some sexual dysfunctions.

in general, the better are the chances of mutually enjoyable physical sharing. Masters and Johnson wrote about the importance of something called "I" language. This is a type of communication in which people can comfortably convey what they desire sexually without feeling guilty about it. Their statements begin with "I," as in "I would like you to fondle my breasts more tenderly," or "I would enjoy it if you would stimulate my penis more vigorously," or "I would like to take a long time to enjoy you tonight." Many of us have been taught that it is never right to put yourself first, yet to fully enjoy sexual intimacy it's a good idea for two people to know exactly what the other enjoys. "I" language seems to be a very effective way to do this; however, many people have to learn how to put themselves first, at least sometimes, in order to do this. Many adults have difficulty learning to use "I" language unselfconsciously. When people don't express their preferences and desires, however, often less than enjoyable sexual encounters will result, and these problems in sexual communication can play a role in the development of sexual dysfunctions.

Just as sexual dysfunctions frequently develop without people talking about the emergence of these problems, these difficulties often continue for long periods of time without the couple ever talking seriously and candidly about how to solve them. Sexual problems can develop a momentum of their own, and after a while each partner doesn't quite know what to say or do about them. The frustration leads to silence, and silence doesn't lead to any solution, and the initial frustration gets worse, and before they know it, virtually all meaningful communication in the relationship suffers. Because sexual dysfunctions do not usually get better on their own, someone has to take the first step to initiate a dialogue, and this is rarely an easy thing to do. For these reasons, a counselor or sex therapist is often very helpful in opening up the issues that may have led to the dysfunction and in helping a couple explore alternatives

to improve things. The next chapter discusses a variety of approaches used by sex therapists.

LONGSTANDING, UNSETTLED RELATIONSHIP PROBLEMS

As a couple lives together over time, inevitable incompatibilities become obvious. While some of these are trivial, others are more important and distracting and have the potential to diminish the quality of the bond. One of the more persistent conflicts couples have is about "power." The power to do what one wants. The power to make your partner do what you want them to. The power to plan problem-solving strategies and work to carry them out. Even the power *not* to engage in productive problem solving. Perhaps you have heard about how a couple has "power struggles" as they try to decide how to use their time, money, space, or participate in raising children. These aren't arguments with clear, unambiguous solutions; they are generally longstanding "battles" for the upper hand in a relationship. These conflicts often emerge for a number of reasons: differences in the maturity levels of the partners, problems discarding problematic influences of one's family of origin, or perhaps even a lack of mutual respect. When a couple frequently has disputes over autonomy or authority, sooner or later this affects their sex life too. If you spend a lot of time battling for control and respect and influence during most of the

MESSAGE FROM DR. RUTH: IT MIGHT JUST BE FATIGUE

Since women began entering the workplace in greater numbers, a new phrase has entered the lexicon: "too tired for sex." In the not-so-distant past, some women might have faked a headache when they did not feel like having sex, but these days either partner might simply be too exhausted. Not only are people working longer hours, but with both fathers and mothers sharing in child care (even though, I realize, many moms still bear more of the brunt of this burden), sometimes one or both partners just don't have enough energy to maintain an active sex life.

Notice my use of the word "active." My first advice is to be careful that your relationship doesn't become platonic just because you have children. That can be a recipe for lost intimacy in a marriage. Yes, you have to make allowances for fatigue, but it's still important to acknowledge your sexuality and maybe take steps to ensure that you make the time and save the energy to keep your sexual relationship alive. A marriage in which the sexual fires have dimmed is not as likely to be fulfilling to both partners and may not last very long. This isn't to say those fires can't be rekindled!

Even though you may go for certain periods with minimal sex, if a conflict develops because one partner desires sex more than the other, you need to work out a solution together. Remember: a low frequency of sexual intercourse does not automatically mean either of you has less desire for the other or has a sexual problem—it may be plain old fatigue. There are things you can do to avoid fatigue and renew your relationship. Go for a mini-vacation together, or hire a babysitter and rent a motel room for the evening. Take the time to plan for such occasions, so that both of you can become as aroused as possible, and let yourselves go. Not only are sexual energies released on such occasions, but you and your partner can work this way to achieve a balance between your "regular" fatigue-filled lives and these special moments that help keep your relationship strong.

waking day, things don't change a lot when you go to bed at night.

"Sex is a conversation carried out by other means. If you get on well out of bed, half the problems of bed are solved."

Peter Ustinov

Learning to live with interpersonal problems and learning to solve them together are two very different things. Living with someone almost inevitably involves disputes and disagreements. Some inescapable aspects of all relationships have the potential to hurt the quality of that relationship, including its sexual aspects. Couples often argue about the conflicting demands of their careers and families. Women are frequently distressed about the inequitable distribution of housekeeping tasks and often complain that the person in a relationship who earns the most money "buys" their way out of cleaning and other home maintenance chores (this is usually the man). Couples must also contend with their feelings about changing sex roles. If a man has been raised to believe that his wife is his obedient servant, conflict is inevitable when he discovers that she is an independent, assertive person in her own right. In fact, many men still think of their spouses in the same way they think about their children: dependent, unskilled, passive, and obedient. While these stereotypes are dying slowly, they are still prevalent in our society. Distressing interactions are likely in households like these. In addition, the emotional and time demands of raising children can diminish quality communication, especially when children are very young. Again, a couple's sexual relationship is a microcosm of the characteristics of the marriage in general. If tensions and stresses diminish the quality of a couple's communication and interaction, their sexual intimacy will likely be similarly affected.

These issues and others often contribute to conflicts in a relationship. But the sexual arena seems especially vulnerable to the negative effects of these problems. In many cases, a couple simply has less sexual desire, interest, or energy and therefore has intercourse much less frequently. As we get older, however, there is also a general decline in sexual frequency that may be wholly unrelated to problems in a relationship. These changes can begin when individuals are in their 30s and 40s. Beck (1988) has emphasized that couples often have different preferences for when it is appropriate to have sex, where, how often, and the behaviors involved. These differences sometimes create anxieties, resentment, or even guilt (p. 358). Often these emotions substantially diminish sexual desire. Strong feelings can cause some very distracting, intrusive thoughts, and these can lessen sexual pleasure and make orgasms unlikely. Beck believes that these "negative automatic thoughts" can reduce sexual interest and responsiveness. Here are some examples of these distracting ideas:

- I'm not good at this.
- I won't reach a climax.

- I won't satisfy my partner.
- You're too mechanical.
- I'm bothered that you're not turned on.
- That doesn't feel good but I'm afraid to tell you.
- I feel I have to do whatever you want.
- I feel obliged to give you an orgasm.
- I might as well give up.
- I'm going through the motions but it means nothing to me.
- I'll be damned if I'll give in to your desire.

—Beck, 1988, 360–361

These are just some of the thoughts people may have during sex when other aspects of their relationship are not rewarding. As long as a couple is having interpersonal problems, it's not likely that these negative, inhibiting thoughts will go away. Many people who have relationship difficulties and fight frequently, however, often use sex as a way of making-up. In this case, having intercourse can actually distract a person from the problems that caused the fight in the first place.

LACK OF SEXUAL INFORMATION

Another interpersonal problem that frequently contributes to sexual dysfunctions is a lack of sexual information about anatomy and the sexual response cycle. As described in this book, certain parts of our bodies are sensitive to erotic stimulation and some are extremely sensitive. Women and men progress through four stages of the sexual response cycle, and generally women take longer to do so than men. When women and men do not understand these basic realities and do not know how and where and how long their partner likes to be stimulated, they are likely to have two entirely different sexual experiences. For example, men need to remember that it is often best to begin foreplay by focusing on the less sensitive areas of a woman's body and gradually proceed to the more sensitive areas, perhaps eventually involving prolonged manual stimulation of the clitoris. Similarly, women need to remember that the glans and frenulum of the penis are especially sensitive and that directly stimulating these areas vigorously early during foreplay may precipitate premature ejaculation. It is especially important for men to remember that arousal takes much longer in a woman than in themselves and that a sensitive, caring lover will spend enough time tenderly touching, kissing, and perhaps orally stimulating his partner before he penetrates her vaginally.

"Good lovers have known for centuries that the hand is probably the primary sex organ."

Eleanor Hamilton

When sexual interactions are unskilled, tactless, and selfish, one person likely feels short-changed, and it is usually the woman. If a man is only paying attention to his own feelings, his self-centered attitude gives his partner a very clear message: My feeling good is more important than your feeling good. In such circumstances, a woman is still in the arousal or plateau stage when her partner ejaculates, essentially ending intercourse. A man in such a hurry isn't likely to be interested in continuing to stimulate his partner afterwards, leaving her feeling somewhat aroused and perhaps experiencing some pelvic vasocongestion but not having had an orgasm, which would relieve these feelings. In such a case one could ask which partner has the sexual dysfunction. Does the problem lie in the hurried, egocentric behaviors of the man or in the fact that the woman has "failed" to have an orgasm?

"Skill makes love unending."
Ovid, Roman Poet, 43 BC—17 AD

THE GROWING FAMILY

Households and families are dynamic systems. This means that they are always changing, and each individual affects all the others. Sometimes these changes require big adjustments, and at other times hardly anyone notices that things are not quite the same. However, certain domestic events are likely to have a ripple effect and may influence the communication patterns and sexual style of a couple. One big change is the arrival of a new baby. Nine months of optimistic anticipation are followed by the realities of dirty diapers and sleep deprivation. As discussed in Chapter 10, a couple should not have sexual intercourse for about 6 weeks after the birth of a baby, and during this time the woman often has mood swings and may become depressed. All these changes happening at the same time can have a big impact on a couple's sex life, and many men feel that the new baby has taken their wife away from them. Resuming rewarding sexual relations may take some time, patience, and good communication. While these changes can occur after the birth of any child, it is usually after the birth of a couple's first baby that these concerns become most apparent. Some women lose interest in sex altogether for some time after their baby has arrived. Of course, things usually return to normal.

CHANGING SEX ROLES

When Masters and Johnson published *Human Sexual Inadequacy* in 1970, they reported that for the previous two decades there was a subtle but very important change in male/female relationships that seemed to affect the prevalence of sexual dysfunctions. Those changes have grown even more dramatic since the publication of their book. Since the late 1940s and early 1950s, men gradually began to understand that sexually, a woman is not someone you do something *to*, but instead a partner you do something *with or for*. A sense of defensiveness and anxiety began to emerge among many men, leading to"performance anxiety" or "spectator anxiety." The term "spectator anxiety" refers to the awareness that one is being observed by one's partner during sexual in-

teractions. For the first time, men began to feel that they were being evaluated or "graded" by their female partners, and this made many men very nervous. A common consequence of this nervousness was increased reports of premature ejaculation and erectile dysfunctions, which in turn played a role in more reports of female difficulties in arousal and response as well. Even college and university counseling centers noticed an increased number of young men reporting problems in attaining and maintaining an erection. For men in their late teens and early 20s, this was very unusual. What was behind it?

For one thing, some men have problems with assertive women, and even more problems with *sexually* assertive women. Historically, women were more passive and subservient in their relationships with men. As "women's liberation" and other feminist agendas entered the American social terrain, how women and men began to interact with each other changed in marked ways. For example, women began to ask men out on dates. Some women became more comfortable in initiating sex with their partners instead of waiting for the man to "make the first move." Once foreplay began, women were no longer so shy about being more directive in bed, making their likes and dislikes known. These changes in the ways women and men communicate with each other are threatening for some men, and the development of sexual dysfunctions is one common consequence. (Other men report that they especially enjoy making love to sexually assertive women.) Even in contemporary times many men have been socialized to be sexual "teachers" and assume that their wives are untutored, naive, and in need of directive erotic instructions. Such men are therefore extremely distressed to find out that their partners are indeed sexually skilled and might even have a more diversified erotic repertoire than they. This is just another example of the results of the sexual double standard and the ways in which people have tried to cope with it.

"When modern woman discovered the orgasm it was (combined with birth control) perhaps the biggest single nail in the coffin of male dominance."
Eva Figes

LACK OF DOMESTIC PRIVACY

Most people believe that sexual behaviors are very private and appropriate when they are alone in a quiet place free of potential interruptions. Yet for many, the presence of small children, roommates, or family members make it hard to have privacy and ensure that sexual enjoyment won't be overheard by the whole household. These concerns can have a very inhibiting impact on sexual desire and arousal. With the growing number of multigenerational households in this country, many couples are living in the same house with their parents and their children. When a couple is anxious about their lovemaking being overheard, much of the spontaneity and freedom associated with sexual arousal and response are suppressed. The

Dear Dr. Ruth

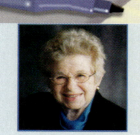

Question

Before my wife and I had our two children, we enjoyed a very spontaneous sex life. We had sex everywhere in the house at all times of day and night. She and I both were very comfortable initiating intercourse. Well! Now that the kids have arrived there's been a big chill on our sexuality. My wife won't even consider having sex unless it's late at night and our bedroom door is tightly locked. Even then, she shushes me for being too loud or vigorous. I feel my own sex drive is beginning to decline because of this. Do you have any ideas that might be helpful for us?

Answer

When the kids are asleep, do you ever watch television or listen to music or talk on the telephone? I'm sure you do, and you never think twice that it might wake the children. As long as you are not screaming at the top of your lungs, and as long as the door is locked, you really shouldn't have to worry about the children. Even if they wake up with a nightmare, they're not going to be concerned about what you were doing but only with their own fears.

Now it's true that once you have children, spontaneous sex does become more difficult. To compensate, make your planned sex life as exciting as possible. By building up your anticipation of a planned sexual evening you can make it just as or even more satisfying than a spontaneous one. When you lock the door after the kids are asleep, don't rush into it, but take some time to slowly get more and more aroused. Maybe you could give each other massages. Those don't make a lot of noise.

---

anxiety of this situation can impair sexual arousal in both women and men, and the perceived need for haste may encourage premature ejaculation.

"Personally I know nothing about sex because I have always been married."

Zsa Zsa Gabor

Personal Problems and the Development of Sexual Dysfunctions

In addition to societal and interpersonal issues involved in the development of sexual dysfunctions, other factors exist within the individual. Such factors are difficult to isolate and study apart from the wider psychosocial network, a number of personal psychological issues may impair any individual's sexual functioning. These involve a person's own developmental experiences, learning, and possibly subtle or obvious psychological disorders. We intend not to attempt a complete outline of psychological problems and their impact on sexual functioning but to point out some of the

more common individual factors related to problems in sexual functioning.

PROBLEMS IN PSYCHOLOGICAL AND PSYCHOSOCIAL FUNCTIONING

One of the most common psychological problems is anxiety. This mood state is associated with a diffuse, pervasive feeling of apprehension or dread. It is not always associated consistently with any specific stimulus or stimuli or person. Its onset can be very unpredictable and its physiological and psychological effects devastating. Anxiety is experienced on a continuum ranging from very mild to debilitating and severe. Experiencing anxiety while taking a test is one thing, but a panic attack is something entirely different. Anxiety can be an adaptive emotion, a sort of "watch out" mechanism to keep us aware of potential threats in our environment. But some people have disturbing amounts of anxiety almost daily, and this can get in the way of productivity and personal relationships. Because anxiety is commonly experienced in situations in which we don't know what is going to happen or how we're going to deal with it, many people experience anxiety when they think about or find themselves in sexual situations. People are sometimes apprehensive about being clumsy or doing the wrong thing, or even doing something we were taught as children is wrong or sinful. Anxiety can affect the balance in the functioning of the two parts of the autonomic nervous system: the parasympathetic and sympathetic branches, which are involved in sexual arousal and orgasm. If a person is experiencing a lot of anxiety, these feelings will affect the autonomic nervous system in such a way that arousal or orgasm may be significantly diminished or absent altogether.

"People will insist in treating the mons veneris as though it were Mount Everest. Too silly!"

Aldous Huxley

In addition to anxiety, anger is another emotion that can affect sexual arousal and response. Hostility and indignation not only diminish the affection and love we feel for our partner, but they also may directly suppress sexual arousal. In an interesting experimental investigation, Bozman and Beck (1991) presented 24 male undergraduates with tape recordings that included sexual content and statements that were supposed to elicit anger or anxiety; the control group instead heard statements of feelings one would expect in a sexual situation. Subjects were asked to report their feelings of sexual arousal, and their penile tumescence was monitored with electrical recording devices while they were listening to these tapes. Measures of sexual arousal were highest in the control group, with less sexual arousal reported in connection with the tapes that elicited anxiety. Tapes that evoked angry responses were associated with the lowest reported levels of sexual arousal. When these investigators reviewed the physiological data on penile enlargement, they found that angry feelings have the most powerful effect in decreasing tumescence, with the control and anxiety groups showing somewhat lessened effects. Apparently, anger and anxiety both diminish sexual arousal, and anger had the stronger impact. This makes intuitive sense, since people seldom fight and share sexual intimacy at the same time.

Depression is another common psychological problem. Depression can adversely affect sexual functioning, as can the medications used to treat it (Baldwin, 1996). Depression has been associated with reduced sexual desire and diminished arousal. Additionally, depressed individuals have reported delayed orgasm and lessened enjoyment associated with orgasm. Investigators have reported rates of sexual dysfunction associated with depression that range from 35% to 47% of the individuals affected by this psychological disorder. Several drugs are effective in the treatment of depression, but sexual dysfunction is a common side effect of these agents in a sizable number of the people who use them; however, all antidepressants do not have these effects. When these side effects become troubling, reducing the dose or changing the medication often lessens these sexual problems.

When people are anxious, angry, or depressed, they often don't feel very good, and this can have a negative impact on their interpersonal relationships. Even more problematic are a family of psychological problems called **personality disorders.** These are long-lasting patterns of thinking, feeling, and behaving that are at odds with common social expectations. In addition to these people being unhappy, their personal and professional relationships are frequently disturbed; they aren't much fun to be with or work with. While some personality disorders are extremely serious and are likely to get a person in trouble with the law, others are less socially disturbing. Following are personality disorders likely to be associated with serious relationship difficulties that may also involve sexual problems.

Paranoid Personality Disorder. These individuals are deeply mistrustful of others and worry constantly about whether others are trying to hurt, use, or lie to them. They constantly question the motives of other people.

Schizoid Personality Disorder. This personality disorder is characterized by an aloof, detached attitude toward relationships with other people. These individuals enjoy being alone and don't want much part of close, intimate relationships.

Borderline Personality Disorder. Someone with a borderline personality disorder may have many unstable, intimate relationships with others, and these tend to swing from intense feelings of idealization to similarly intense hatred. These are often very impulsive individuals who may engage in behaviors that are potentially very self-destructive.

Narcissistic Personality Disorder. These individuals have a magnified, unrealistic sense of their own importance and find it very difficult to empathize with others. They believe that they are truly unique and special and are entitled to special privileges and allowances. They commonly exploit others for their own ends and are arrogant and condescending.

This is not a complete list of personality disorders described in the DSM-IV, but these examples show how it would be difficult to initiate and maintain a long-term, rewarding sexual relationship with people having these problems. Unfortunately, psychological counseling is not always effective in substantially improving these personality disorders.

SEXUAL ASSAULT AND/OR ABUSE

Sexual assault and abuse are horrible experiences and may affect the way a person responds to sexual stimuli or circumstances afterwards, but the victims of these incidents often get over them and go on to have a normal sex life. Adjustment might be difficult, but it can be done. There is no simple cause-and-effect relationship between being a victim of such a crime and later sexual interest or responsiveness. In a study of 202 female university students, Kinzl, Traweger, and Biebl (1995) found that childhood sexual abuse was related to sexual dysfunctions in adulthood. Approximately 22% of these respondents reported at least one incident of childhood sexual assault. Subjects' responses on questionnaires revealed that when children experienced many episodes of childhood sexual abuse, they were more likely to report disorders of sexual desire and orgasm than respondents who had only a single abusive experience. The data reported in this study revealed that orgasmic dysfunctions were especially likely to occur in later life among women who had been abused sexually as children. Since this was a relatively small sample of subjects, further large-scale studies are needed to validate these results. Another study (Bartoi & Kinder, 1998) involved the questionnaire responses of over 200 university students and found that when women were sexually abused during childhood or adulthood, they were far less likely to feel fulfilled in their current or most recent sexual relationship and had unsafe sex with more partners than subjects who did not report incidents of sexual abuse.

The impact of childhood sexual abuse on the development of sexual dysfunctions in a sample of 301 men was studied by Kinzl, Mangweth, Traweger, and Biebl (1996). About 10% of these subjects reported at least one incident of childhood sexual abuse, with 4% having especially harsh and prolonged incidents. This investigation revealed that male subjects were more likely to develop sexual dysfunctions as a consequence of prolonged negative family experiences with their parents than as a result of isolated episodes of childhood sexual abuse. But in this sample of subjects it was not possible to establish a cause-and-effect relationship between childhood sexual abuse and adult sexual dysfunctions in males.

Some individuals seem to be especially vulnerable to the long-term impact of childhood sexual abuse, while others seem to find it easier to put the experience behind them. It can be very difficult to feel close and trusting in a sexual relationship after having been victimized and exploited in one's past. As more people become comfortable about acknowledging sexual abuse in their past, research concerning this troubling issue will grow progressively more complete.

PRESCRIPTION AND RECREATIONAL DRUGS IN THE ETIOLOGY OF SEXUAL DYSFUNCTIONS

Many prescription and recreational drugs can impair sexual functioning, even if sometimes a person continues to enjoy highly erotic feelings. Following is a brief list of the drugs most likely to have some adverse effects on sexual desire, arousal, or orgasm. This list is not complete but demonstrates the number and diversity of chemical agents that can be implicated in sexual dysfunctions. Some of these agents are legal while others are not.

1. Alcohol and other addictive central nervous system-depressing drugs, especially opiates
2. Amphetamines ("speed")
3. Amyl nitrate ("poppers")
4. Anti-anxiety agents ("tranquilizers")
5. Antidepressants
6. Antihypertensives (drugs which lower high blood pressure)
7. Barbiturates ("downers")
8. Cocaine
9. Hallucinogens (e.g., LSD)
10. Marijuana

Alcohol

In small or moderate amounts, alcohol has been considered an aphrodisiac. It can lessen inhibitions and enhance relaxation, which can prolong intercourse and lessen the incidence of premature ejaculation. One study has reported that two-thirds of alcoholics say they have enhanced sexual feeling while they are "under the influence" (Smith, Wesson, & Apter-Marsh, 1984), although "enhanced sexual feeling" may not always be reflected in enhanced sexual performance. In fact, alcohol, even in moderate amounts, may be associated with problems in sexual arousal. When alcohol is consumed in large amounts on a regular basis, sexual responsiveness may be significantly impaired, as is the individual's general awareness of their immediate circumstances. Additionally, alcohol dependency is often accompanied by a lack of sexual interest. Female alcoholics often report lessened pleasure during orgasm, and male alcoholics report frequent episodes of erectile dysfunction. Masters and Johnson have noted that heavy drinking is the most common cause of secondary impotence in men at mid-life (1970).

Lemere and Smith (1973) reported that long-standing heavy drinking may play a role in the development of permanent erectile dysfunction. Interestingly, the men in this study were unable to regain erectile ability even after years of abstaining from alcohol. In another study of 20 alcoholic men who were not drinking at the time of the investigation, with a duration of sobriety between 2 months and 3 years, there were no differences in sexual functioning compared with a control group of men who had never been alcohol-dependent; however, the spouses of these recovering alcoholics reported serious marital dissatisfaction despite the fact that their sexual relationship was normal (Schiavi, Stimmel, Mandeli, & White, 1995). The relationship between alcohol consumption and sexual and marital functioning is complex and requires further investigation.

Opiates

Opium comes from the opium poppy, which is found throughout the world. Opium is a resin derived from this flower. Examples of opiates include morphine, codeine, and heroin. Heroin's impact on sexual functioning has been studied extensively. Because of its powerful sedative effects, users often become disinterested in sex and infrequently masturbate, fantasize, or have intercourse. This is just one aspect of their diminished interest in human interactions in general. Delayed orgasm is common when heroin users do have intercourse, and they frequently report that orgasms lose much of their enjoyability (Winick, 1992). As a heroin user's tolerance to the drug increases, sexual interest and activity decline sharply. The euphoric effects of opiates seem far more pleasurable and rewarding than sex. Opiates significantly impair desire, arousal, and orgasmic response in those addicted to them. Until the 1990s, heroin was used mostly by "back alley" addicts who injected themselves in isolated, secretive circumstances; however, today heroin is inhaled and smoked, as well as injected, and is used by individuals of all socioeconomic and occupational levels. Unfortunately, this terrible drug is being more widely and commonly used now. While only a generation ago prostitutes sold sex to buy heroin, today high school students in affluent suburbs are using the same drug to get high in a variety of social settings.

Amphetamines

Prescription use of amphetamines, especially to reduce a person's appetite and help them lose weight, has been dramatically reduced in recent years. A problem with this group of drugs, which includes benzedrine and Dexedrine, is that a person needs to take progressively larger doses for the same appetite suppressant effect. After only a few weeks, a person's system has difficulty metabolizing the drug and its effects become extremely toxic. People also use illicit forms of this drug, including methedrine and methamphetamine, recreationally as a stimulant for the euphoria they experience. Its effects on sexual functioning can be somewhat unpredictable. For example, when men are injected with amphetamines, spontaneous erection sometimes occurs (Winick, 1992). People who use amphetamines may experience acute episodes of sexual desire, often accompanied by vivid fantasies and feelings of sexual urgency. Many report feeling sexually adventurous and assertive. Those who use amphetamines habitually and excessively may become totally disinterested in sexual behavior, however. Long-standing use of this family of drugs may significantly reduce a person's sex drive and play a role in impaired ejaculation in men.

Many people use amphetamines because they believe they have aphrodisiac qualities, making them more sexually inclined and adventurous. These are agents of abuse, however, and can cause profound dependency and impairment in everyday functioning. Many amphetamines on the street are not made to known standards of potency and purity, a common problem with many illicit drugs, and dangerous side effects may occur.

Amyl Nitrate

A number of substances, when inhaled, intensify the pleasure associated with orgasm and increase the amount of blood flowing to the brain, as well as the genitalia. Amyl nitrate is an inhalant most commonly used for the intensification of sexual pleasure. In everyday language, the term "poppers" is used to describe the use of this agent because it is distributed in glass vials that "pop" when they are broken for the drug within to be inhaled. This agent is used most frequently by men who find that their ejaculations can be delayed and intercourse and orgasm prolonged if they are inhaled just before orgasm (Winick, 1992). There have been reported cases of heart attacks with use of this agent. Although amyl nitrate often enhances sexual pleasure, it does nothing to enhance sexual communication and intimate sharing, and some individuals eventually come to believe that they cannot have a satisfactory, enjoyable sexual experience without using it. In that respect, habitual use of amyl nitrate may contribute to dysfunctional patterns of sexual desire, arousal, and response.

Antianxiety Drugs

Here we'll discuss only those antianxiety drugs that are commonly called minor tranquilizers. Some tranquilizers cause profound sedation (such as Thorazine). Many people daily take more common minor tranquilizers to manage fears and apprehensions, such as Valium, Librium, Ativan, Xanax, and BuSpar. New drugs are developed often. The good news is that these agents rarely if ever cause diminished sex drive or problems with ejaculation or orgasm. In fact, improved feelings of relaxation frequently contribute to sexual reassurance and interest. On the other hand, some people who use these agents (especially at higher doses) seem to lose emotional "highs" along with the "lows" and may become disinterested in sharing sexual intimacy.

Age and health factors must be taken into account in assessing the impact of these drugs on sexual functioning. While a young adult might not have any impairments in sexual functioning attributable to minor tranquilizers, older individuals might develop some problems. For example, men in later life who use these agents sometimes develop retarded ejaculation, which is reversible if they discontinue taking the drug for a day or two.

Antidepressants

Depression is a very common problem in the United States. Some psychologists believe that as much as 20% of the population in North America and Europe may be affected by this psychological disorder, and 5% may be severely affected. Although changing lifestyle, reducing stress, and counseling frequently help, antidepressant medications are prescribed for many people and are frequently very effective. But as with any medication, the benefits have to be weighed against the side effects. Different types of drugs have been used to treat depression, and all have been implicated in lowered sexual desire and arousal. One family of antidepressants prescribed less often by doctors because of sometimes unpredictable side effects are the monoamine oxidase (MAO) inhibitors, such as Parnate. These are known to be related to diminished orgasmic capacity (Jacobson, 1987). Another family of antidepressants, the tricyclic antidepressants, too are associated with lowered sex drive and erectile ability in men (Wein & Van Arsdalen, 1988).

Another group of antidepressants, which are perhaps the most popular and effective of all, act more promptly and have fewer side effects than the others. These are selective serotonin reuptake inhibitors (SSRI agents), which include drugs like Prozac, Zoloft, and Paxil. In both women and men using these drugs, delayed orgasm and lowered enjoyability of orgasm have both been reported with some consistency in the literature

(Rothschild, 1995; Hsu & Shen, 1995; Labbate, Grimes, & Arana, 1998). Sometimes these difficulties become less obvious the longer a person takes the drug, but if they continue, another antidepressant agent may be prescribed that has fewer sexual side effects. Briefly discontinuing the medication often allows a return to normal sexual functioning without a recurrence of serious depression.

Antihypertensives

An estimated 54 million Americans have high blood pressure. As American lifestyles become progressively more stressful (and sedentary), high blood pressure is apparently a consequence. Fortunately, a number of drugs are often effective in treating this serious health problem. Unfortunately, many of them significantly diminish sexual arousal, although not all antihypertensives have this side effect. A patient's not taking a medicine as prescribed by their doctor is called *nonadherence,* and of all prescription drugs, Americans are more likely to be nonadherent with antihypertensives than with any other category of medication. The reason is simple: they experience delayed or absent sexual arousal. Nonadherence may also stem from the fact that there is typically no discomfort associated with high blood pressure, so the patient doesn't feel much different whether they are or are not taking their medication. So, they usually just stop taking their medication (and tend to go back to their doctors less often for blood pressure checks). But dozens of drugs are available that can lower high blood pressure, and very often changing medications restores normal sexual arousal.

Barbiturates

This family of drugs is often called "downers" because they are powerful sedatives, although they are also used for other medical indications, such as the management of epilepsy. A commonly used barbiturate is phenobarbital. Used recreationally, it has a powerful sedative effect that people use to diminish bad feelings associated with being in difficult or intolerable situations. These drugs often cause a significant decline in sexual interest, powerfully impairing desire and arousal. This is especially true when large quantities are used. On the other hand, for some individuals, the relaxation and lack of anxiety associated with moderate barbiturate use sometimes helps them more comfortably explore sexual intimacy and therefore enhances feelings of sexual enjoyment. The impact of this drug depends on how much a person uses and the reason for using it. Barbiturates and alcohol potentiate each other; that is, they magnify one another's effects. When consumed together, their combined sedative effects can be extremely pronounced and even dangerous, sometimes causing a person to stop breathing.

Cocaine

Derived from the leaves of the coca plant, cocaine can be snorted, smoked in crystalline form, or injected intravenously. It is powerfully addictive and may profoundly affect an individual's lifestyle and productivity. Addiction involves powerful cravings for the drug and compulsive use of it, while *abuse*

refers more generally to the compulsive use of agents that are not socially or culturally sanctioned.

People who use cocaine commonly report that the "rush" they get from it is very much like a sexual orgasm and that it can prolong sexual sharing and enhance the strength of an orgasm. For these reasons, many use this agent regularly in conjunction with sexual activity. Women using cocaine may report that they experience multiple orgasms under its influence. Cocaine is also a topical anesthetic, and men who apply cocaine to the glans of their penis lose a little sensitivity and find that they can engage in more prolonged sexual intercourse. Similarly, women who apply it to their vaginal tissues or douche with it also report significantly magnified orgasmic response (Winick, 1992). While these "aphrodisiac" properties of this substance are well known, the overall picture is much less rosy.

Heavy and habitual cocaine use has an unfortunate and unpredictable impact on sexual behavior. For example, low sperm count, menstrual problems, low sex drive, and temporary infertility have all been reported with prolonged cocaine abuse. Additionally, the use of large quantities of cocaine for long periods of time can foster an indiscriminate, promiscuous approach to sexual interactions, sometimes associated with a compelling desire to masturbate frequently or engage in group sex. Sexual inhibitions are further compromised when cocaine and alcohol are used together. As with opiates, cocaine users find drug-related euphoria a more compelling experience than the safety, intimacy, and pleasure of sexual intercourse. Despite its aphrodisiac qualities, disturbances in sexual desire and response, as well as confusion about the role and meaning of sexuality in a person's life may accompany its use.

Lysergic Acid Diethylamide (LSD)

LSD is an hallucinogen, meaning that its use causes hallucinations, or altered perceptions. While under its influence, people see, hear, and feel things that are not there. Hallucinations can be interesting, entertaining, or terrifying. Using LSD is often referred to as taking a "trip." The effects of LSD on sexual functioning depend on the interpersonal and social context in which it is used. If an individual is with someone they know and trust, a rewarding, interesting sexual interaction might happen. But if a person has a negative or frightening reaction, enjoyable sexual desire, arousal, and orgasm are not all likely to occur. Frequent users are often not as interested in having sex.

Marijuana

Marijuana is the most commonly used illegal recreational drug. (Alcohol is the most commonly used drug). For decades professionals have known that marijuana use is frequently associated with increased sexual desire, magnified perceptions of sexual arousal, and prolonged, intense orgasms. While these are the perceptions of some using this drug, there are no correlative physiological data to support these reports. The person's perceptions and bodily responses may not be completely in line with each other. Marijuana on the street varies considerably in its concentration of the active ingredient tetrahydrocannabinol (THC), and it is difficult for a person to be sure about the potency of the marijuana he or she consumes. It is usually smoked, although it can also be put into various foods, such as brownies or spaghetti sauce. As with any street drug, there is no easy way to determine its purity.

Despite its effects in enhancing sexual desire, arousal, and orgasm, one important investigation revealed that habitual, heavy use of marijuana may have temporary effects on a person's arousability and fertility. Cohen (1976) studied a group of men who smoked 5 marijuana cigarettes every day for a period of 9 weeks. At the end of this period, the testosterone level of these subjects had fallen by about one-third. Decreases in testosterone of this magnitude are often related to temporary erectile difficulties and lowered sperm count. Still, young adults are more likely to report that marijuana enhances sexual pleasure than any other agent. Because marijuana tends to promote feelings of "time expansion" (things seem to take longer), as well as enhanced sensory acuity, many incorporate it in their sexual interactions.

Yet problems may occur with the habitual use of marijuana for sexual activity. People may come to the conclusion that the "best" sex happens only when they are using marijuana, and that intimacy without this agent is somehow "second best." This may create a psychological dependency on marijuana that could limit a person's perspectives on sexual sharing.

Drugs and Sex in Perspective

In all, some prescription and recreational drugs can enhance or stimulate sexual pleasure while others impair sexual desire, arousal, or orgasm, but both types can contribute to sexual dysfunctions. Feelings of dependency on stimulants can cause problems, especially if a person gradually comes to think that they cannot enjoy satisfactory sexual sharing without them. We may be considered old-fashioned for thinking that relaxed, clear-headed people can communicate best and enjoy sexual mutuality when they are unimpaired by controlled substances, even those supposed to "enhance" sexual pleasure. Even though alcohol is not a controlled substance, its use in conjunction with sexual sharing has similar results. Chapter 17 will further discuss how people under the influence of various substances are more likely to engage in behaviors that put them at a higher risk for AIDS and other sexually transmitted diseases.

CONCLUSION

This chapter has discussed the nature of sexual dysfunctions and the societal, interpersonal, and individual factors that may work together to cause them. A sexual problem isn't necessarily a deep psychological problem, as the person experiencing the problem has likely instead learned a number of emotional and physical responses that inhibit or diminish sexual desire, arousal, and orgasm. Just as these bad habits can be learned, they can be unlearned too. The next chapter will discuss approaches commonly used in sex therapy for sexual dysfunctions. There is a real cause for optimism when two people are fully informed as to the nature of their problem and are motivated to do something about it.

Learning Activities

1. It sometimes happens that couples who separate or divorce enjoy fulfilling sexual intimacy right up until the time their relationship dissolves. Speculate on how people can continue to have good sex when their relationship seems to have serious problems.

2. You read in this chapter about hypoactive sexual desire, which is an increasingly common problem encountered by sex counselors and therapists. Speculate about what kinds of sexual behaviors could be a compromise when one partner has low or no sexual desire and the other has a normal sex drive.

3. When a couple has intercourse and the woman becomes sexually aroused but does not have an orgasm, she may feel unsatisfied. How might she approach her partner about manual-clitoral or oral-clitoral stimulation after intercourse so that she too can enjoy an orgasm? Would this be conveyed most clearly verbally or with nonverbal gestures?

4. An unconsummated marriage is one in which the couple has not had sexual intercourse. Describe your impressions of the nature of sexual communication in these relationships. Speculate on the nature of any premarital sexual interactions these couples may have shared.

5. Because the roots of a sexual dysfunction sometimes come from childhood experiences, what can a parent do to foster healthy, open, and wholesome attitudes about a child's genitals and the good feelings elicited by touching them?

6. People in relationships sometimes try to change their partner into someone or something they aren't. How might this affect sexual intimacy between two people? Has anyone ever tried to change something about you? Speculate on why they might try to do this.

7. Various estimates have been made of the incidence and prevalence of sexual dysfunctions in the general population. Masters and Johnson have suggested that 50% of all marriages have a sexual problem serious enough to hurt the quality of the couple's overall relationship. In the literature more precise figures have been published. We have noted earlier in this chapter that Spector and Carey (1990) reviewed 23 clinical studies and reported the prevalence of a number of sexual dysfunctions (see Table 14-1). Because sexual dysfunctions are common, people often approach their clergyman or physician first when they don't know what to do. Please respond to the following questions:

   a. Do you have a family doctor whom you have known for a long time and with whom you can discuss your sexuality?

   b. (For women:) Does your gynecologist seem interested, patient, and prepared to talk with you about sexual issues and problems? If your gynecologist is male, does this in any way inhibit you from asking for information or assistance?

c. (For men:) Does your physician or urologist seem interested, patient, and prepared to talk with you about sexual issues and problems? If your physician is female, does this in any way inhibit you from asking for information or assistance?

d. Do you feel that your clergyman is likely to be knowledgeable about sexual problems and skilled at counseling members of his or her congregation in this area?

e. Many individuals discuss their sexual dysfunction with an attorney if it is pertinent to divorce proceedings. Comment.

8. In her report on male sexuality, Shere Hite (1981) describes several anxieties that men frequently experience regarding the adequacy of their sexual techniques. Because women have been "sexual students" and men have been "sexual teachers" in the historical double standard, concerns about female responsiveness preoccupy men and often create doubt about their sexual skills. Here are a few quotations that summarize some of these frustrations and concerns:

"The main demands made of me during sex are to hold off ejaculation and to stimulate the right 'spots' on my partner without much trying on her part. I feel a woman has to concentrate on stimulation and learn to receive it, as well as the man performing it. If a woman doesn't try, then she blames the man for failure, he is going to have guilt feelings and then shy away from sex because he thinks he will fail next time." (p. 368)

"Since I'm currently having problems sustaining erection, I am quite aware of 'performance' pressures. I lay the blame for the woman's lack of orgasm with me. But I've tried everything, what else can I do?" (p. 369)

"Unless I feel capable of imparting some satisfaction to my partner, I'd rather abstain." (p. 372)

a. What "demands" do you feel men experience from women during sexual intercourse?

b. How might a woman learn to "receive" sexual stimulation? What connotations does the word "receive" have?

c. Do you think it is normal for guilt feelings to accompany sexual intercourse?

d. How does a man go about sustaining an erection?

e. Is "blame" too strong a word for how men should feel about their partner's lack of consistent sexual responsiveness?

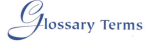ey Concepts

- Sexual dysfunctions involve problems people experience in desiring sexual interaction, as well as in the physiological

aspects of sexual arousal and orgasm. They also include pain associated with sexual intercourse.

- Among the various causes of sexual dysfunctions, organic factors involve biological, physiological, or hormonal causes and may result from illness, injury, normal aging, or the situational or chronic use of prescription or recreational drugs.

- Psychosocial factors may also contribute to the development of a sexual dysfunction. These involve issues such as self-concept, faulty sexual learning, sexual assault, sexual abuse, or inadequate sex education. Even a distant, cold parenting style may contribute to sexual difficulties.

- Behaviorism is a perspective in the social and behavioral sciences that emphasizes studying only observable, measurable behaviors and de-emphasizes what cannot be seen or quantified. Behavioristic thinkers minimize the significance of thoughts and emotions because they are unobservable. Behavioral approaches to sexual problems focus on the current manifestations of the issue, rather than its history or the feelings associated with it.

*G*lossary Terms

dyspareunia	personality	secondary
female orgasmic	disorders	anorgasmia
disorder	premature	sexual aversion
female sexual	ejaculation	disorder
arousal	primary	sexual pain
disorder	anorgasmia	disorder
hypoactive sexual	random	situational
desire disorder	anorgasmia	anorgasmia
male erectile	retarded	vaginismus
disorder	ejaculation	

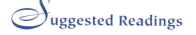uggested Readings

Bancroft, J. (1991). *Human sexuality and its problems.* New York: Churchill Livingstone.

Crenshaw, T. L., & Goldberg, J. P. (1996). *Sexual pharmacology: Drugs that affect sexual function.* New York: W. W. Norton.

Forrest, G. G. (1995). *Alcohol and human sexuality.* Northvale, NJ: Jason Aronson.

Kaplan, H. S. (1995). *The sexual desire disorders: Dysfunctional regulation of sexual motivation.* New York: Brunner/Mazel.

Kaplan, H. S. (1989). *How to overcome premature ejaculation.* New York: Brunner/Mazel.

Kaplan, H. S. (1988). *Illustrated manual of sex therapy.* New York: Brunner/Mazel.

Kaplan, H. S., & Klein, D. F. (1987). *Sexual aversion, sexual phobias, and panic disorder.* New York: Brunner/Mazel.

Montague, D. K. (1988). *Disorders of male sexual function.* Chicago: Year Book Medical.

Pillari, V. (1997). *Shadows of pain: Intimacy and sexual problems in family life.* Northvale, NJ: Jason Aronson.

Zoldbrod, A. P. (1998). *Sex smart: How your childhood shaped your sexual life and what to do about it.* Oakland, CA: New Harbinger.

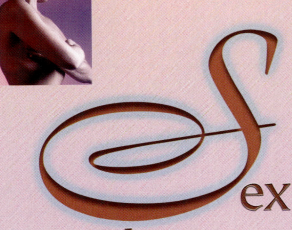

15

Sex Therapy: "Helping People to Help Themselves"

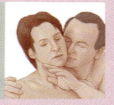

OBJECTIVES

When you finish reading and reviewing this chapter, you should be able to:

1. Discriminate between problems in a relationship and difficulties specific to the sexual aspects of that relationship.

2. List issues people need to consider when they seek the services of a professional for a sexual problem, and describe the types of professionals who assist with sexual problems.

3. Weigh the pros and cons of the cotherapist approach pioneered by Masters and Johnson and summarize the effectiveness of this strategy compared to individual therapy or group therapy.

4. Summarize the theoretical foundations of the cognitive-behavioral approach to the treatment of sexual dysfunctions.

5. Describe sensate focus techniques and explain why they are often extremely effective in sex therapy for many different problems.

6. Define the elements of the PLISSIT approach to the treatment of sexual dysfunctions, and give an example of each.

7. Explain the importance of positive reinforcement, negative reinforcement, and successive approximation in the treatment of each of the sexual dysfunctions described in this chapter.

8. Explain why masturbation and mutual masturbation can help a couple learn more about each other's sexual difficulties.

9. Explain what "vasodilators" are and why they are used in the treatment of impotence. Give three examples and describe the different ways in which they are introduced into the body.

10. Summarize reasons people with sexual problems approach their family doctor, gynecologist, or clergyman first.

11. Discuss reasons gays and lesbians might have problems finding a sex therapist willing to work with them in the treatment of a sexual problem.

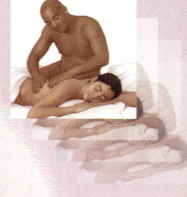

From Dr. Ruth

It surprises people that I maintain a private practice in sex therapy in Manhattan. I do it for many reasons, the most important being that I enjoy helping people to become terrific lovers. As you will learn in this chapter, sex therapy is usually a short-term treatment. You may have heard of people who see their "shrink" for years and years, but either I can help somebody in a matter of weeks or their problems require a different therapeutic approach. With this type of treatment, my clients quickly get what they are seeking, and I get the satisfaction of those results too.

My advice is not to choose a sex therapist blindly. Everyone has their own style, and while they may be very good at what they do, their style or personality may not be right for you. If you ever feel the need to see a sex therapist, make your first visit a trial, and if you don't feel comfortable, don't hesitate to look around some more.

If you ever think about seeing a sex therapist, you may wonder how the therapist is affected by hearing the most intimate details of your sexual habits. Though certainly I've "heard it all," it's impossible to be completely detached. I have to picture in my mind's eye what my clients are doing in their bedroom, and that's why I won't treat people with certain problems, like bestiality. I don't want to picture such goings on because I would be affected by it. On the other hand, the fact that I do have feelings for my clients makes me a better therapist. I remember the joy I felt when I helped a man in his 80s, who had given up on ever having sex again, to resume sexual relations with his wife. It's for moments like those that I continue my private practice, and I believe it is my enthusiasm that makes me a good sex therapist. And I believe that if you go to a sex therapist, you should bring your enthusiasm also. If you go in with the attitude that you can't be helped, it's going to be a lot harder and maybe impossible. But if you take a positive outlook, then I'll almost guarantee you that you can make the necessary improvements in your sex life.

The previous chapter described various sexual dysfunctions and the societal, interpersonal, and intrapersonal factors that often play a role in them. This chapter looks at what can be done about these disorders. The effectiveness of various treatments for sexual dysfunctions presents an optimistic picture. The "right" treatment, however, is rarely a matter of simply applying therapeutic techniques to known disorders. Personal characteristics, gender, developmental events, and the background and training of the therapist must all be taken into account when deciding upon a strategy to treat a sexual problem. Sex therapy is very much an art, even though it involves effective counseling techniques and a variety of exercises by the couple.

When people have a less than satisfactory sex life, they often wonder how bad it has to get before they seek treatment. This is a personal decision, of course, but the person or couple should consider questions like these:

1. Has the role of sexual expression as an aspect of your relationship diminished significantly?

2. Do you find that you no longer look forward to making love?
3. Do you experience notably delayed or diminished sexual arousal, even with what you feel is ample foreplay?
4. If you used to have orgasms regularly and reliably, do you no longer do so?
5. After having sex, do you frequently feel frustrated, angry, or perplexed by your lack of responsiveness?
6. Have changes in your relationship with your partner diminished the enjoyment of your shared sexual expression?
7. Does sexual intercourse cause you significant physical discomfort?
8. Has the use of prescription or recreational drugs lessened your capacity to become sexually aroused and to have orgasms?

These questions might help one focus on changes in their sex life that are distressing. If these or other sexual difficulties seem to hurt one's self-esteem or diminish the quality of their relationship with their significant other, then they might benefit by talking things over with a sex counselor or sex therapist.

The media frequently present images and information that give the impression that "real men" and "real women" are always ready to have sex, become wildly aroused in moments, and have great orgasms. In fact, sex drive varies considerably among people and in any one person from time to time. Many people don't put sex at the top of the list of their favorite things to do, and this doesn't mean that they have a serious psychological problem. Instead of asking ourselves how rewarding our sexual expression *is*, we instead wonder how rewarding it *should be*, based on these idealized and often inaccurate media messages. Data from the Kinsey Institute collected between 1938 and 1963 (Gebhard & Johnson, 1979) revealed some interesting facts about the role of orgasm in female sexual behavior.

- Among unmarried women not living with a man, 40.3% of their sample had never had an orgasm during sexual intercourse, and 54.6% had orgasms less than half the time they had intercourse.
- Among married women, 13% had never had an orgasm during sexual intercourse, with 47.3% having orgasms less than half the time they had intercourse.
- Among married women, about one-third reported having orgasms every time they had sexual intercourse.

Men, on the other hand, have orgasms most of the time, if not every time they have intercourse. Therefore, women are more likely to seek the services of a sex therapist, although men too have their difficulties, such as inhibited sexual desire, retarded ejaculation, and premature ejaculation. The Kinsey data suggest that as women age through early adulthood, their capacity to have orgasms on a regular basis increases.

When a couple is experiencing a sexual problem, the first thing they should do is *talk about it*. "Talk" is a healthy four-letter word. Yet because many people are hesitant to discuss sexual subjects (especially those related to one's own sexual behavior), individuals with sexual dysfunctions often say little or nothing about them, sometimes for quite a while. But if the relationship is important and the place of sexuality in the relationship is important, then sooner or later the couple is going to have to talk about the problem. If one person in a relationship has a sexual dysfunction, often the other does too. For example, if a man has retarded ejaculation and requires vigorous, prolonged thrusting to ejaculate, his partner may experience dyspareunia as a result of this extended lovemaking. The couple needs to discuss any incompatibilities that contribute to sexual dysfunctions as a first step.

SEX THERAPY

How Common Are Sexual Dysfunctions?

It is not precisely known how many people have sexual dysfunctions. Remember that the term "prevalence" describes the number of people at any specific point in time who have a problem or characteristic. A key issue regarding the prevalence of sexual dysfunctions is the need for clear descriptions and an unambiguous classification scheme (O'Donohue & Geer, 1993). The

DSM offers a useful scheme for categorizing and analyzing data on sexual dysfunctions. Spector and Carey (1990) summarized the results of 23 investigations concerning the prevalence of sexual dysfunctions and concluded that it is simply not known how common female sexual arousal disorders, vaginismus, and dyspareunia are in the general population. Reported prevalence rates may be very low, inconsistent, or based on samples of subjects that are not comparable. These researchers reported that the prevalence of female anorgasmia is between 5 and 10%. As we saw in the last chapter, prevalence rates for male erectile disorder were 4 to 9%, 4 to 10% for retarded ejaculation, and 36 to 38% for premature ejaculation. These data vary depending on the techniques used to sample respondents, the size of the sample studied, and whether the investigation involves the random selection of subjects and the degree to which those subjects are representative of the general population.

Relationship Problems Versus Sex Problems

Because the sexual aspect of a relationship can reveal problems that occur outside the bedroom, counselors and therapists cannot always clearly distinguish between the need for couple therapy and the need for sex therapy. Borelli-Kerner and Bernell (1997) made some suggestions about this issue. They recommend that a couple having a sexual problem is probably best treated with couple therapy when they seem to need more than short-term treatment to deal with a number of nonsexual marital issues. In this approach, a male and female client are counseled by a male and female therapist, sometimes together as a group and sometimes individually with one therapist working with one client. In particular, couple therapy seems the best alternative when:

- One or both members have significant psychopathology but are still able to work on their relationship
- The commitment to the relationship is a significant and immediate issue
- Resentment, distance, mistrust, and inability to communicate indicate that brief sexual therapy would be impossible or unsuccessful
- The sexual issues or disorders are mild or peripheral to the immediate conflicts facing the couple
- The couple has tried and failed a course of focused sex therapy (Borelli-Kerner & Bernell, 1997, p. 169)

These authors recommend sex therapy instead for a specific sexual disorder when the couple is willing to try a brief, focused therapeutic approach. These couples typically have:

- A committed relationship
- Motivation to work specifically on the sexual problems
- A willingness to interact sexually
- A lack of significant individual psychopathology
- A level of nonsexual conflict that is not disruptive to sexual interaction (Borelli-Kerner & Bernell, 1997, p. 168)

In other words, the issue is whether to work on the relationship or the sexual problem first. Every couple is unique, however, and these recommendations may not apply to everyone.

It is sometimes difficult to determine whether problems in a relationship cause sexual dysfunctions or whether sexual dysfunctions cause problems in a relationship. Both can occur. It can be difficult to describe the impact of a sexual dysfunction on a relationship, which depends on how distressed one or both individuals are by their intimate problems. Many people have sexual dysfunctions and don't think very much about whether the situation can be improved. Others may have a sense of real urgency about trying to improve their situation. Sex therapists don't know as much as they would like about factors that eventually motivate an individual or a couple to seek clinical assistance. Additionally, not very much is known about how long a couple grapples with a sexual problem before they finally do something about it. Finally, social and behavioral scientists would like to know more about the role of sexual dysfunctions in the dissolution of marriages. Recall that the *DSM* defines a sexual problem as a "dysfunction" only when it causes personal or interpersonal distress for an individual or a couple.

Unmarried Couples and Sexual Dysfunctions

As discussed in Chapter 7, there are many kinds of loving relationships that do not involve marriage. Cohabitation is an arrangement in which unmarried individuals live together. Because regular sexual activity is often a characteristic of these relationships, sexual problems are likely to occur as in marriage. In-

terestingly, a reason people commonly give for deciding to live together is that they want to find out if they are compatible, including sexual matters, as well as other aspects of the relationship. We are aware of no data, however, that indicate that couples who have lived together before getting married are any more or less likely to experience a sexual dysfunction at some point in their lives. We are also unaware of any evidence that suggests that couples who are virgins when they marry are any more or less likely to develop a sexual dysfunction at some later time.

The causes of sexual dysfunctions discussed in Chapter 14 apply just as much to unmarried people living together as to married couples. What might be most important for cohabiting couples in terms of their sexual compatibility are their sexual value systems. To the degree that these are congruent or complementary they might experience sexual accord, yet to the extent that they differ the couple might experience problems in their shared sexual intimacy. Getting to know someone sexually takes time, good communication, and trust. If these are present in an unmarried couple, they will likely develop their own, mutually rewarding sexual style; however, if these elements are absent, even in a marriage, then there will be a risk of sexual incompatibility.

WHO DOES SEX THERAPY?

Professionals who become sex therapists and counselors generally have a keen curiosity about human nature, interpersonal relationships, and the role of human sexuality in the quality of life. Psychiatrists, psychologists, sociologists, endocrinologists, nurses, clergy, and licensed clinical social workers all become

---

MESSAGE FROM DR RUTH: DON'T TAKE SEXUAL QUESTIONS AND PROBLEMS TO A PSYCHIC HOTLINE

I'm often asked how I became so well known for dispensing sexual advice. Part of the answer may be my appearance, which I'm told is reassuring and nonthreatening, and so I've been allowed to say things on radio and television that had not been said before. My accent, which some people say sounds like a cross between a Viennese psychoanalyst and a Jewish grandmother, may also have helped. On the other hand, I am also a trained sex therapist, and I only offer advice that is based on scientific knowledge and clinical experience, and I have always maintained a private practice seeing clients.

But not everyone who dispenses advice has legitimate training. Someone hiding behind an anonymous phone service is likely to have no relevant training or expertise at all. "Advisors" who charge callers by the minute may even ask highly personal questions and offer inappropriate suggestions just to keep the meter running.

So here's some advice. If you have a question about sex or relationships, don't waste your time or your money on a telephone advisor or a psychic hotline. There are lots of better ways to get information. Start by looking at books or reputable web sites, and see if they offer good advice for a situation similar to your own. You may find advice that helps you. Or you could see a counselor for personal attention.

If you broke a leg or had a high fever, you wouldn't consult a psychic hotline, so don't pick up the phone for a broken heart or a feverish sex question either.

sex therapists. Some practice sex therapy within a highly diversified clinical practice (group therapy, individual therapy, marriage counseling, personal growth issues, etc.), while others focus exclusively on sexual concerns.

The settings in which sex therapy takes place are similarly diverse. Because sex therapists generally never observe their clients being intimate, most sex therapy takes place in an office. This allows comfort and privacy for talking, examining illustrations and anatomical models, and perhaps viewing sexually related instructional materials and perhaps erotic videos. Any needed medical tests are usually done in a medical facility with which the sex therapist is affiliated. Sex therapy is not a part of the standard curriculum of psychologists, psychiatrists and other physicians, or social workers, however, and those who specialize in this area must have additional, specialized training.

The American Association of Sex Educators, Counselors, and Therapists (AASECT)

The American Association of Sex Educators, Counselors and Therapists (**AASECT**), with headquarters in Richmond, Virginia, ensures that those who work in this area meet uniform standards of training and performance. AASECT has a simple but important mission: to certify professionals who meet their standards for academic training, ethical conduct, and clinical ability; to promote sexual health; and to set the highest standards for work in this complex discipline. This mission helps create personal accountability among sex counselors and therapists, current levels of competence and integrity, clear moral, ethical, and legal standards, and the welfare of consumers, students, trainees, and research subjects.

AASECT certifies professionals in three areas: Sex Educator, Sex Counselor, and Sex Therapist. For each of these certifications, specific academic and sex education is required, along with work experience, supervised clinical experience, and the documentation of all of these. Supervised training as a sex counselor or sex therapist is also required. Requirements for Sex Therapist are more extensive than those for Sex Counselor. Still, it is extremely important to remember that there are many highly competent sex counselors and therapists who are not AASECT certified. An individual's background and training may make such certification more or less necessary.

Many states have few or no legal requirements for a person to designate or advertise themselves as a sex counselor or sex therapist. In fact, some unqualified people have done just that. Therefore, it is *always* appropriate when contacting a potential therapist to ask specific questions about his or her educational background, training, supervised clinical experience, certification, and licensure.

If a couple would benefit from seeing a sex therapist or counselor, the best place to begin the search is often their primary care physician. Many women and their insurance companies consider their gynecologist their primary care physician. One's physician is in a good position to know the resources available locally and may be trained to ask prelimi-

nary questions and make some suggestions before proceeding further. A recent study (Read, King, & Watson, 1997) based on the prevalence of sexual dysfunctions among 170 patients visiting their general practitioners in England revealed that 35% of the men reported some type of sexual dysfunction. Premature ejaculation was reported by 31% of these subjects, and 17% reported erectile dysfunctions, in most cases related to the medications they were taking and advanced age. Among the women in this sample, 42% reported some form of sexual dysfunction, with 30% reporting vaginismus and 23% anorgasmia. A study in the United States (Bachmann, Leiblum, & Grill, 1989) reported the results of almost 900 visits women made to their gynecologists. Only 3% of this sample reported sexual problems without being asked directly, yet when questioned more specifically, 29% said that they had experienced sexual dysfunctions of one type or another. Dyspareunia was the most common complaint (48% of the sample), with diminished sexual desire (21%) the next most common. Among this group of respondents, vaginismus and anorgasmia were relatively uncommon, each accounting for less than 10%. Importantly, most of the complaints raised by these women could be helped by their gynecologist.

Physicians who teach in medical schools are generally aware of trained, trusted sex therapists in the area and often will make referrals. However, the professional most likely to be consulted first when it comes to marital and/or sexual problems is one's clergyman. Although many members of the clergy engage in marriage and family counseling, little is known about their preparation for sex therapy. Recent information (Conklin, 1997) emphasizes the need for a more comprehensive, systematic sex education and counseling component in the training of clergy in many different faiths. Additionally, very little discussion has been given to the ways in which members of the clergy and sex and marriage counselors can work together to help those who seek their counsel (Weaver, Koenic, & Larson, 1997). Individuals at mid-life and older are somewhat more likely to seek the counseling services of their clergyman than are younger members of a church or synagogue.

BASIC ISSUES IN SEX THERAPY

Before we discuss a variety of specific techniques that are employed in the treatment of sexual dysfunctions, it is important to examine a number of basic issues that lie behind therapy and the different approaches to sexual disorders.

Lack of Attentiveness to One's Partner's Desires and Preferences. Knowing about the sexual response cycle can be extremely important for avoiding poor sexual communication and understanding the basic differences between women and men in sexual arousal and response. Often, however, there are fundamental incompatibilities between sexual partners. For example, many men seem unconcerned that their female partners take much longer to become aroused and don't attend

USING THE INTERNET TO LEARN ABOUT SEXUAL ISSUES

With so much information available on the Internet, it is risky to assume that it is all correct, useful, and helpful. Much on the web can provide information, help, and reassurance, but unfortunately there is much that is wrong or even harmful. A number of organizations deal with a wide variety of sexually related issues, however, and virtually all of them have websites. Some of the better ones are listed below, but we'll not provide telephone numbers, addresses, and website addresses since these change frequently. Call the directory of toll-free numbers at 1-800-555-1212 to obtain the telephone number of a group listed here, or use an Internet search engine to find their website address. There are many other reputable organizations in addition to those listed here.

American College of Obstetricians and Gynecologists
National Abortion Rights Action League
National Right to Life Committee
Planned Parenthood Federation of America
Alan Guttmacher Institute (a research organization for women's sexual health and reproductive concerns)
American Association of Sex Educators, Counselors, and Therapists (AASECT)
Sex Information and Education Counsel of the United States (SIECUS)
STD National Hotline
National AIDS Hotline
National Gay and Lesbian Task Force
Resolve (a support organization for couples having problems with infertility)
National Center on Child Abuse and Neglect
National Directory: Rape Prevention and Treatment
U.S. Department of Health and Human Services
National Center for the Prevention and Control of Rape

Think critically about anything you read on the Internet. The Internet offers anonymity and immediate information that in many cases is current and authoritative. Following are a few tips when using the Internet to learn about sexual issues.

1. Avoid websites that include photographs of nude women and/or men.
2. Avoid websites that use inappropriate language.
3. Avoid websites where you are asked for identification and credit card information. Good information is *always* free on the Internet.
4. Seek websites affiliated with medical schools, reputable research institutions, colleges and universities, and government agencies. These typically have ".org," ".edu," or ".gov" in their addresses.
5. Be skeptical of websites that offer self-help therapies without encouraging you to speak to your family physician, gynecologist, or a urologist.
6. Avoid websites that discourage parental involvement in sexual issues.
7. Use wire service and newspaper websites for current information about sexual and reproductive issues in the news.

Remember you shouldn't believe everything you read, no matter where you read it. If you don't fully understand everything you read on the Internet, check your public library for a medical dictionary or resource handbooks in the social and behavioral sciences. It is important to be a critical consumer of information, and sometimes this takes time and patience. Consult the list of suggested readings at the end of this chapter as well.

closely to their partner's needs and desires during foreplay and intercourse. Many women have been socialized to believe that they are supposed to subordinate their own sexual inclinations and pleasures to their male partners and often do not assert themselves or make their preferences known. These differences of perspective are not always easy to discuss, even though they involve simple information (Fig. 15-1).

The Distinction Between Organic and Psychosocial Causes of Sexual Dysfunctions. How different sexual dysfunctions are treated depends on whether they have a primarily organic or psychosocial cause. Possible physiological and medical problems are often ruled out before cognitive-behavioral counseling can begin. Physical examinations and blood tests or sophisticated diagnostic procedures may be necessary to be sure that there isn't a medical problem to address before more psychosocial avenues are explored.

TREATING SEXUAL DYSFUNCTIONS

Various theoretical approaches have been useful in treating sexual dysfunctions, although psychosocial and biological considerations are fundamental in all. The specific approach used by any one sex counselor or therapist depends on their educational background, training, and clinical experience and the unique characteristics of the couple.

Cognitive-Behavioral Therapies

The term "cognitive-behavioral" involves the relationship between behavior and how we think and feel. This model focuses on how our feelings and thoughts about sexuality and sexual issues directly affect how we will experience (or not experience) sexual arousal and response. This approach de-emphasizes developmental events in our lives and most but not necessarily all past experiences. This theoretical perspective focuses on what is going on in the client's present life rather than what happened to them while growing up or in past romantic or intimate relationships. This approach focuses on the nature of the problem and what can be done immediately to diminish the severity of its symptoms or eliminate them altogether. The therapist won't ask the client about dreams or early family life unless this information has a direct and immediate influence on a sexual dysfunction. The cognitive-behavioral perspective suggests that if the problem behaviors are eliminated, then the problem is eliminated. Of course, all sex therapists do not take the cognitive-behavioral perspective, but many do. This was the approach pioneered by Masters and Johnson. This approach does not say that a better understanding of one's past is useless, only that time and energy are better spent looking at the problem today and working to solve its current manifestations. The assumption here is that if sexual behaviors change, the thoughts and emotions associated with those behaviors will change too. Traditional Freudian psychoanalysis, dream interpretation, slips of the tongue, and one's relationships with parents, peers, and siblings are not important in this approach.

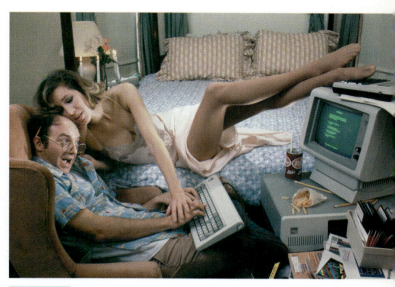

FIGURE 15-1 Women have become more sexually assertive in their relationships during the last generation. Sometimes a person becomes too preoccupied with their job to fully enjoy sharing sexual intimacy.

SENSATE FOCUS

Sexual pleasure involves all the major senses: vision, hearing, taste, touch, and smell. Our sexual value system includes visual images and sounds we interpret as erotic. Certain tastes and odors also often have sexual associations. The sense of touch is often most important for how we experience and express our sexuality, although many people find it hard to "tune out" other sensory inputs and focus intently and exclusively on tactile experiences during foreplay or intercourse. Indeed, cognitive-behavioral therapists believe that many people have to be taught how to do this. To focus on these tactile sensations, Masters and Johnson developed a number of "sensate focus" techniques for their clients to incorporate in their "homework" assignments at the end of each day of sex therapy. These exercises can help clients with virtually any sexual dysfunction and involve one person touching the other in a tender, caressing fashion but not stimulating their genitalia or the woman's breasts (Fig. 15-2). This nondemand, nonintercourse sexual pleasuring helps people relax and learn more about what they find exciting and how their body responds to this kind of stimulation. The exercises do not take much time; but to feel sexual without any expectation of intercourse or having to achieve an erection or to lubricate can be quite liberating for people who have been very performance-oriented in their lovemaking. For many, this is the first time they have been undressed and enjoying touching and being touched *with the lights on.* The couple takes turns. The person who was doing the touching now becomes the person who is being touched. For a few days the couple is discouraged from stimulating one another's genitalia or the woman's breasts.

As the couple becomes progressively more comfortable with sensate focus exercises, they are encouraged to touch their partner's genitalia and the woman's breasts, but to continue to

FIGURE 15-2   Sensate focus exercises involve touching and caressing one's partner in a tender, nurturant way without any expectation of having sexual intercourse immediately. This diminishes anxiety and performance expectations and help, a couple relax.

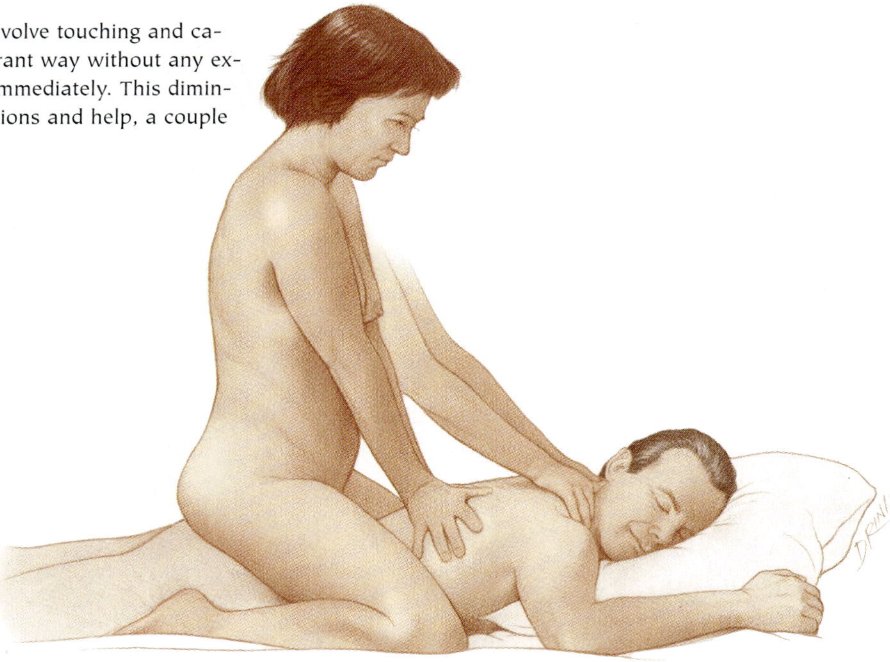

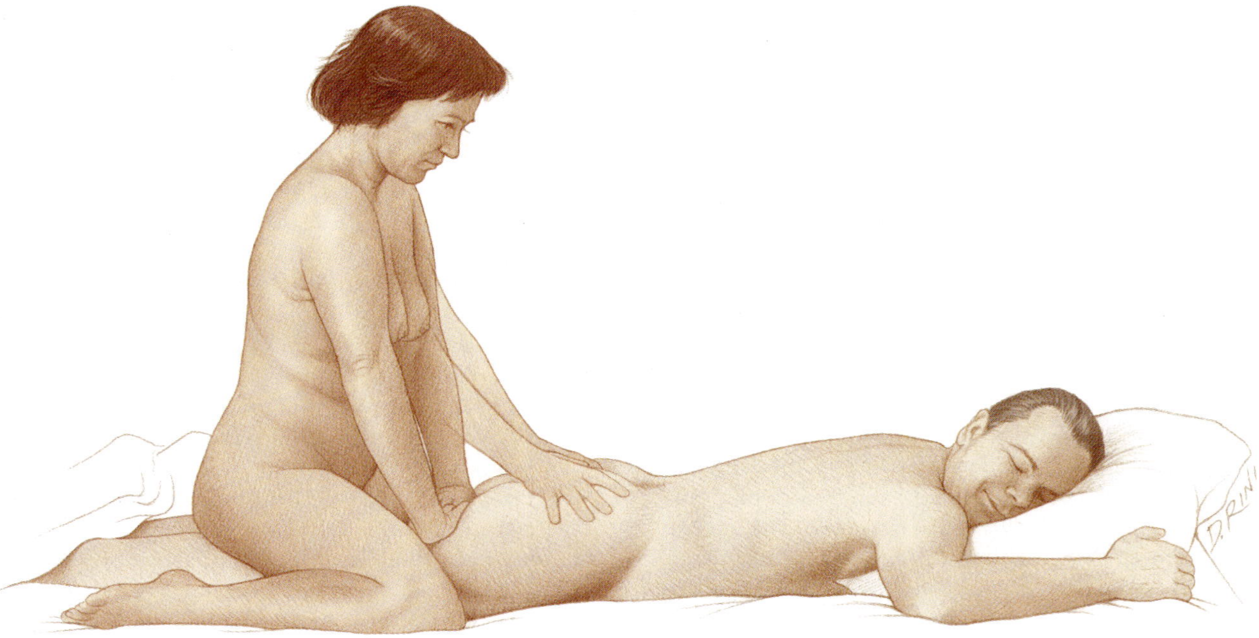

postpone intercourse. Most people find that when the expectation of sexual arousal has been removed and there are no pressures to perform, they often begin to enjoy the aspects of sexual arousal they were initially worried about. These feelings can be tremendously rewarding and create much confidence in both women and men. Eventually, this self-assurance makes it easy for a couple to proceed to sexual intercourse fully aroused. Single "successful" experiences can be wonderfully reassuring and give a couple a whole new confidence about themselves and their ability to be responsive and please their partners as well.

These exercises help a couple attend more closely, nonjudgmentally, and noncompetitively to their own and their partner's sexual and erotic arousal and pleasure. This couple is advised not to compare their feelings and activities to what they once thought was "great sex" but to attend instead to the full, focused experience of one's intimate enjoyment. In an orgasm-focused culture this can be hard for some couples to learn.

Sensate focus exercises emphasize not proceeding promptly to vaginal penetration but attending instead to erotic pleasures in and of themselves. Many of the behaviors a couple enjoys during these exercises can be enjoyed without any imperative to have intercourse. A couple learns more from sensate focus exercises when they already have a relationship, a foundation they together share upon which they can build an enhanced sexual communication and shared erotic enjoyments. Casual sex, on the other hand, generally involves impatient feelings that afford a couple little time to savor one another sexually.

THE PLISSIT APPROACH

Helping a couple try to deal with a sexual dysfunction can involve progressively more complex, directive strategies, and as in other kinds of counseling, sex therapists typically take a gradual approach to the diagnosis and treatment of these disorders. Annon (1976) devised a paradigm for proceeding in small steps. Although every couple is unique, there is much agreement about the usefulness of this approach in treating sexual dysfunctions. PLISSIT stands for "permission," "limited information," "specific suggestions," and "intensive therapy." This model incorporates the strengths of many approaches to sex therapy and reflects the research and writing of many investigators.

Permission involves validating the client's thoughts, emotions, and sexual activities. Often this involves "undoing" things the individual was taught long ago. Permission may justify a person's dislike for a particular form of sexual expression and reassure them that everyone has different sexual inclinations and preferences. This permission is granted with the therapist acting as a nonjudgmental helper rather than a cold, objective clinician. Permission is most meaningful if it comes from someone who is informed, authentic, and understanding.

Once the clients begin to feel more comfortable knowing that many people have sexual problems and that their problem is common, they are often very receptive to learning more about their difficulties, factors that may have caused them, and what can be done about them. At this point, *limited information* can be very helpful and reassuring. Information about the sexual response cycle and how it is different in women and men can be very important. Helpful facts can eliminate some sexual myths people have held for years that may have had an effect on their sexual functioning. The therapist offers the client only information that they can use to gain a better understanding of their problem.

Now that the client or couple is better informed, *specific suggestions* for helping their particular problem are offered, sometimes in a very structured manner. These suggestions usually involve sexual activities the couple can try at home, hopefully when they are well rested, free of stress, and free of interruptions. The sensate focus exercises described earlier are one example of specific suggestions that can be of some help to a couple. Additionally, the couple might be encouraged to engage in mutual masturbation to learn more directly how their partner's body changes during increasing sexual excitement. Specific suggestions are intended to help the couple feel more confident and in control of their shared intimacy and to be active rather than reactive in interacting with their partner. These experiences can also help build confidence.

At the deepest level of the PLISSIT format is the *intensive therapy*. Here, the client explores any psychological or social difficulties they may be having that impact adversely on their sexual expression or feelings. Anxiety disorders, depression, or personality disorders often hold clues to the cause of sexual dysfunctions, and discussing these in counseling can often teach the client about inappropriate ways in which they may have been relating to their partner. Sometimes it might be necessary to talk about the client's childhood or adolescent development and any traumatic sexual experiences they had in the past. The therapist might learn, for example, that the client grew up in a very sexually repressive environment that contributed to their current difficulties.

All clients in sex counseling or therapy do not necessarily need to go through all four levels of this model, but this technique is useful in the treatment of virtually all dysfunctions of sexual arousal and response. It can be tailored to meet the needs of any particular person or couple. The benefit of this approach is that it is organized and systematic but still flexible for the unique situation of any client.

Cognitive-Behavioral Approaches to Treatment

The following sections explore how this treatment model is applied to the sexual dysfunctions outlined in Chapter 14. New therapeutic techniques are often developed, and usually there are a number of successful approaches to the treatment of these problems.

SEXUAL DESIRE DISORDERS

This category of sexual dysfunctions includes hypoactive sexual desire disorder and sexual aversion disorder (see Table 14-1). The formidable challenge facing the sex counselor or therapist is to try to help the client find pleasure in their sexual feelings, where in the past those feelings may have been absent, diminished, or ambivalent. This is an increasingly common disorder, but to date, counselors and therapists have not been highly successful in quickly improving it. A big change in the client's sexual value system is necessary to change how they look at the desirability of sexual interaction. The basic task of the sex therapist is to help the client pursue sexual pleasure in a safe counseling setting. Beck (1995) noted that current therapies often operate under the assumption that if the client's sexual arousal and the pleasure they enjoy in orgasm is increased first, *then* sexual desire will gradually increase over time. Rosen and Leiblum (1995) reported that therapy for secondary or situational sexual desire disorders (those acquired later in adulthood) seems notably more effective than therapy for primary sexual desire disorders (those with a lifelong pattern of sexual disinterest). Additional research (MacPhee, Johnson, & Van der Veer, 1995) has shown that women with low sexual desire experience more marital problems than women who do not have sexual desire disorders, and that marital therapy is often helpful in increasing sexual desire in these subjects.

Couples in which one partner has a sexual desire disorder should first try to determine what kind of sexual interaction is pleasurable, how often they would enjoy it, and under what circumstances (Charlton, 1997). With sexual aversion disorder, some people react to the prospect of sexual interaction with severe anxiety and sometimes even panic; they may even have serious psychosomatic reactions including irregular heartbeat, dizziness, and trouble breathing. Until these issues are clarified, it is difficult to choose the appropriate therapeutic strategy. Similarly, other aspects of the couple's relationship are examined to determine whether interpersonal and/or emotional difficulties make sex seem unfulfilling. Individuals with a sexual desire disorder often experience significant performance anxiety and frequently are averse to certain sexual behaviors. Because of this, they should stop participating in those behaviors that cause distress. Because intercourse is usually the activity that causes the most distress, discontinuing this form of sexual activity for a while frees the couple to explore other avenues of physical intimacy without anxiety, fear, or perhaps even revulsion. This can be a big relief. Therapists encourage the couple to avoid intercourse for a significant time, such as 2 months or so. Having sex without having intercourse may actually make the initially unpleasant activity seem more interesting and positive.

Because the roots of sexual desire disorders often reach back to early developmental experiences, some sex therapists believe that the distinction between sex therapy and psychotherapy here are blurred (Rosen & Leiblum, 1989). Behavioral approaches are unlikely to be as effective in the treatment of these disorders. Again, the basic assumption behind this approach is that the couple's sexual relationship is affected by their overall relationship. These writers suggest that a common problem behind sexual desire disorders is the fact that women and men seem to have lost the inclination to gently and romantically seduce one another—to make erotic overtures with the intention of arousing sexual desire in their partner. Fortunately, a number of simple maneuvers can accomplish just this end.

Yet when all is said and done in the context of talk therapies, a "hands on" approach can still be extremely effective. Charlton (1997) recommends that people with low sexual desire learn to enjoy the pleasures that derive from masturbation, in a sense rehearsing for interpersonal intimacy. Often people appreciate being given permission to use vibrators in these self-exploratory exercises and gradually come to enjoy an enhanced sense of sensitivity to physical and interpersonal sexual stimuli. In addition to masturbation, massage offers a couple the chance to share sexual interaction in a nondemand, nonintercourse situation. As in sensate focus exercises, a couple can take turns caressing one another while talking about their feelings and perhaps giving their partner gentle suggestions and encouragement. The couple should understand at the outset that there is no "right" or "wrong" way to share these physically intimate, nonintercourse moments, and their former performance anxiety often diminishes significantly.

Trudel, Aubin, and Matte (1995) have reported that in working with clients with low sexual desire, they found much less openness to sexual experimentation and participation in far fewer sexual activities than among respondents who did not have sexual desire problems. When their clients with low sexual desire did participate in a diversified sexual repertoire, they reported much less enjoyment of various sexual activities.

SEXUAL AROUSAL DISORDERS

Sexual desire and sexual arousal are not the same thing, and the work of Helen Singer Kaplan has shown that desire does not always lead to arousal. Disorders of arousal in women involve delayed, diminished, or absent vaginal lubrication with little or no vasocongestion in the pelvic region, and men with arousal disorders cannot attain and maintain an erection of sufficient firmness to facilitate comfortable vaginal penetration. Clients with arousal disorders express a deep and consistent sense of frustration about their inability to respond to sexual stimuli. The key to treating sexual arousal disorders often involves first learning enough about the client's sexual value system that the counselor or therapist can help her or him discover what is sexually arousing for them and to feel comfortable about it. Once a person has discovered or acknowledged what they find sexy, the next step is to approach those goals in small steps, each of which is likely to be rewarding and enjoyable to the client. Sensate focus exercises are an excellent method. A couple begins with caressing or massage not involving their genitals or the woman's breasts. They then progress to genital and breast touching (Fig. 15-3), eventually engaging in intercourse, although the couple is encouraged to enjoy the feeling of the penis being contained in the woman without any pelvic thrusting. This is difficult for some people, especially if they have always been anxious about being a good lover. For a man to enter his partner and then hold still may feel very unusual. The couple then progresses to intercourse without orgasm. Mutual gentle pelvic thrusting is recommended, but the couple is told that orgasm is not a part of this exercise. People often find that they want what they have been told they can't have. These exercises promote sexual self-confidence and significantly lessen performance anxiety.

Often erotic literature, illustrations, or videotapes are incorporated in the treatment of sexual arousal disorders, as are vibrators (Fig. 15-4). These are not substitutes for intimate interpersonal sexual enjoyment; they are only ice-breakers to help a person learn more about their sexual response cycle and begin to become comfortable with images and thought patterns associated with excitement. Most sex counselors and therapists encourage their clients to learn to enjoy masturbation in association with these depictions of sexual behavior and to develop a capacity for vivid sexual fantasies. These fantasies can often be extremely effective in helping a woman or man become aroused, but the images in these fantasies do *not* generally take anything away from the real sexual relationship. They only facilitate arousal so that genuine sexual communication and sharing can be more enjoyable. As well, the activities people enjoy as foreplay can be the focus of their sexual sharing without any expectation of intercourse.

People who experience sexual arousal disorders can often be treated successfully over a number of therapy sessions, each with a homework assignment involving progressively closer, more intimate interactions with their partner. The steps should be small ones, with no anxiety about performance, and should not progress too quickly. Following is an example of how this works for a 26-year-old client named Amelia who experienced a virtual absence of sexual arousal. Each act is a small step toward an intimate interaction, intended to help this couple pay attention to the way sexual arousal can build gradually.

1. Husband in the other room, door closed; Amelia on the bed in bra and panties
2. Husband in the other room, door open
3. Husband, dressed, in the room with Amelia in her bra and panties, lights off
4. Husband, dressed, across the room; Amelia naked but covered by a towel, in candlelight
5. Husband, dressed, across the room; Amelia lowers the towel when she feels safe, in candlelight
6. Husband, naked, across the room, towel as needed, in candlelight
7. Husband, naked, lying on the bed next to Amelia, towel as needed, in candlelight
8. Amelia and her husband on the bed together, towel as needed, begin Masters and Johnson sensate focus exercises with nongenital caressing (Charlton & Brigel, 1997, pp. 260–261)

When each of these steps is preceded and followed by a therapy session, the client and her therapist have the opportunity to

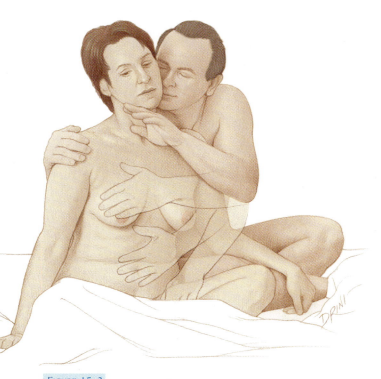

FIGURE 15-3 As sensate focus exercises progress over a number of sessions, caressing and touching of the breasts and genitalia increase arousal for the gradual advancement to vaginal penetration.

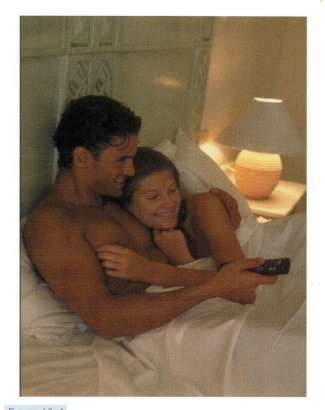

FIGURE 15-4 Some couples find watching erotic videos highly arousing and this can facilitate excitement among those who experience sexual arousal disorders.

fully discuss her thoughts and feelings throughout this sequence of progressively more intimate steps. She gradually feels safer and more comfortable and also receives the praise and encouragement of her therapist, an important combination.

As in women, arousal disorders in men sometimes have an organic basis but often have psychosocial causes too. Because a number of drugs have been helpful in treating impotence, the public has heard much more about erectile disorders and their prevalence than in the past; some of those drugs are discussed later in the chapter. Cognitive-behavioral strategies also are used in the treatment of erectile disorders. Generally sex counselors and therapists have a better success rate with secondary impotence than primary impotence. A man with primary impotence has never penetrated anyone orally, rectally, or vaginally with an erection. A man with secondary impotence has done so but has lost the capacity to have an erection, either consistently or situationally. In evaluating impotence, the therapist first determines whether the problem has to do with an endocrine or physiological disorder, or whether psychosocial factors seem responsible. The sex counselor or therapist also discusses the client's sexual value system to learn what this particular individual finds erotic and arousing. Many men who are impotent become anxious about initiating intimacy because they fear it will lead to a "failure." Arousal problems are difficult to cope with for both women and men, but the situation is particularly apparent with men because vaginal penetration is not possible unless the man is at least somewhat erect.

If diagnostic tests have ruled out biological factors as a cause of impotence, cognitive-behavioral approaches to therapy are generally used. Of the various types of sexual dysfunction treated by Masters and Johnson, their rates in "curing" impotence were not very reassuring. In fact, they reported a 40.6% failure rate with primary impotence and 26.2% with secondary impotence. These data pre-date the development of drugs that are often very helpful in the treatment of erectile dysfunction. In the absence of organic pathology, however, the client's thoughts, feelings, and memories are the primary cause of the difficulty. Most sex counselors and therapists use a number of different approaches to treat male erectile disorder, exploring the couple's communication style, daily stressors, and level of knowledge about the sexual response cycle. In many cases, the female partner is offered explicit instructions for stimulating her partner's penis, perhaps using manual and oral methods. This first step focuses on the psychosocial aspect of the relationship and level of awareness regarding erotic response. Since Masters and Johnson first described their treatment for impotence, other investigators have typically made only minor variations on their approach.

Cognitive-behavioral therapies have demonstrated that in those cases where sensate focus exercises and enhanced relationship communication lead to some erectile response, this is enormously reinforcing and encourages the couple to continue these exercises. These "success experiences" are more likely to occur when a man can tell and show his partner which parts of his penis are particularly sensitive, how firmly he likes to be grasped, and how rapidly his partner should stroke his penis. When a man experiences some degree of erection, his partner then assumes the female-on-top position and helps insert his penis into her vagina (Fig. 15-5). This "penile containment" shows the man that he *can* become sufficiently erect to engage in vaginal penetration. His partner has been told that she should make no vigorous pelvic movements at this time but simply allow them to mutually enjoy the feeling of penile containment. This almost always leads to feelings of "success" and enhanced sexual self-confidence. Effective, clear communication is necessary for the couple to use this approach to therapy. Once the man has penetrated his partner this way, they are told to discontinue their intimacy for a while and to resume their sensate-focus exercises later during the same session. This shows a man that "what goes up comes down" but that "it can always go up again." Again, the feelings of control and self-confidence are very rewarding and usually motivate the couple to continue their therapy. Once the period of formal therapy has ended, it is very important that the couple periodically continue their new habits of communication and sensate focus exercises.

ORGASMIC DISORDERS
Anorgasmia
Chapter 14 describes four types of anorgasmia: primary, secondary, random, and situational. In addition to the lack of regular or reliable orgasmic response, each generally causes feelings of distress and sometimes inadequacy. In the past, the rather unfortunate label "frigid" was used to describe women who did-

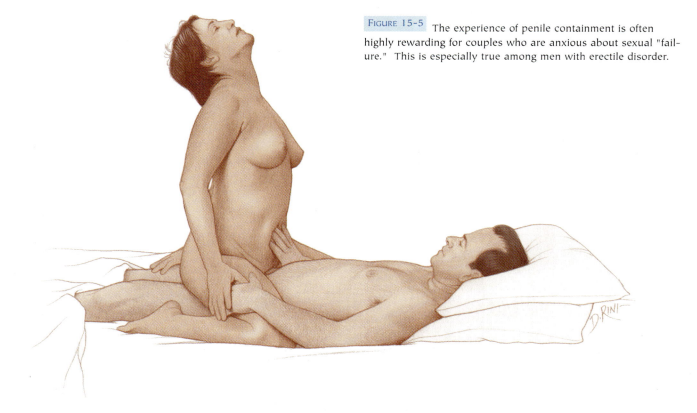

FIGURE 15-5   The experience of penile containment is often highly rewarding for couples who are anxious about sexual "failure." This is especially true among men with erectile disorder.

n't have orgasms. This term had damaging connotations; women who were sexually unresponsive were thought to be cold, aloof, or icy. Today professionals are far more enlightened, informed, and sympathetic about this problem. As with treating other sexual dysfunctions, the first step is to examine the woman's sexual value system to determine what she finds sexy and exciting. Often visual or prose erotica or videotapes are used to stimulate sexual thoughts and feelings, and anorgasmic women are frequently encouraged to develop their capacity for sexual fantasies and to enjoy these during masturbation or intercourse. Sex counselors and therapists also encourage their clients to use vibrators to stimulate the clitoral area during masturbation or even intercourse to increase the intensity, consistency, and controllability of sexual stimulation. A problem encountered by sex counselors and therapists is the fact that women use very different words to describe their orgasms, and it is difficult to determine whether one woman's orgasmic experience is in any way comparable to another's based on their descriptions. While one woman might say that her orgasms are like fireworks and bells ringing, another might describe a warm, gentle throbbing. Therefore, it is important for the client and therapist to learn to appreciate the nature of the orgasmic experience based on the words used to describe it. Additionally, it is difficult for some women to become relaxed enough about their sexuality so that they can be taught how to use a vibrator by their therapist. The combination of enhanced sexual mental imagery with vibratory stimulation can be very effective for teaching women about the way they respond to erotic cues and the amount of time it takes them to become aroused.

Nairne and Hemsley (1983) summarized the literature on masturbation training for women with primary anorgasmia (women who had never had an orgasm by any means). Because women can more easily and regularly have orgasms during masturbation than during sexual intercourse, some researchers have suggested using the former as a teaching tool to enhance the potential for having an orgasm during the latter. Nairne and Hemsley described "masturbation training" as a combination of relaxation techniques and self-stimulation homework assignments. Counseling, sex education, and improved body awareness are also elements of this treatment strategy. Based on an analysis of 10 published reports, Nairne and Hemsley stated that women who had undergone masturbation training were ultimately far more likely to have orgasms during sexual interaction with a partner. This was true whether or not the women undertook masturbation training alone or with the assistance of their partner. Success rates were about the same among women who distributed their training over the course of a number of weeks with one session per week as among women who condensed their training with more sessions per week over fewer weeks. Women who were shown instructional videotapes were just as successful as those who had received written instructions concerning relaxation and masturbation techniques.

Sex counselors and therapists have had some success treating anorgasmia with another method called the **coital alignment technique**. This is an intercourse position that is a slight variation on the man-on-top, "missionary" position. One of the rea-

sons that many women do not have orgasms during intercourse is that their clitoris doesn't receive much stimulation in most of the more common intercourse positions (see Chapter 8). In the coital alignment technique a woman lies on her back and her partner enters her in the traditional man-on-top position, but he now moves his entire body forward so that each time his penis enters her vagina it also directly stimulates her clitoris (Fig. 15-6). Together, their pelvic thrusts create far more contact with the clitoris, and because of the positions of their bodies their lovemaking involves rocking movements. In one study involving 36 married women and their partners (Hurlbert & Apt, 1995), 56% of the female subjects using the coital alignment technique increased the regularity of orgasms during intercourse and the perceived strength of orgasms. These data were compared to another group of subjects who received instruction in directed masturbation, 27% of whom had similar changes.

In sum, a number of effective techniques can be used in the treatment of anorgasmia. While the therapy seems relatively straightforward, encouraging women to seek assistance is an entirely different matter. If more women sought help, more women would begin to enjoy orgasm more regularly during shared intimacy with their partners.

Premature Ejaculation

Like female orgasmic disorders, male orgasmic disorders take time and careful professional attention to remedy. These include premature ejaculation and retarded ejaculation. Premature ejaculation is the most frequently reported sexual dysfunction. Fortunately, the therapeutic strategies for these problems are simple and straightforward and have an excellent record of success. As with the treatment of anorgasmia, sensate focus exercises are important in helping men to learn more about how quickly they are or are not becoming aroused during erotic stimulation.

An important contribution from Masters and Johnson's book, *Human Sexual Inadequacy,* was the popularization of a simple, efficient technique for treating premature ejaculation. This method was first described by James Semans in 1956. While a couple is participating in sensate focus exercises, both partners learn how quickly the man becomes erect and ready to ejaculate. They learn to proceed slowly, stopping frequently when the man reports that he feels ejaculation is imminent. This is sometimes called the start-stop technique. This feeling, called **ejaculatory inevitability,** occurs when a man is sure that there is nothing he can do to delay his ejaculation. Sensate focus exercises involve genital stimulation until a man becomes erect, then interruption during which he begins to lose his erection, and then continued stimulation with the recurrence of his erection. These exercises teach a man the feelings associated with building sexual tension, and also that he can lose and quickly regain his erection. These feelings lead to greater sexual self-confidence, as well as self-control. Ejaculating too quickly makes many men feel that they have lost their sexual self-control and have left their partner unsatisfied.

The **coronal squeeze technique** is a variation on sensate focus exercises. The man lies on his back with legs spread apart, his

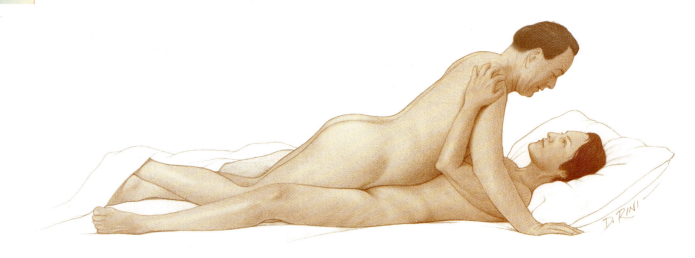

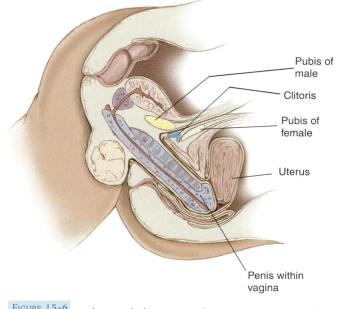

Pubis of male

Clitoris

Pubis of female

Uterus

Penis within vagina

FIGURE 15-6   In the coital alignment technique, a man on top of his partner moves his entire body forward so that the top of his penis may more directly stimulate his partner's clitoris during pelvic thrusts.

pelvis more or less in his partner's lap, who is facing him. She initiates manual genital stimulation until he attains a firm, full erection. At that point she grasps his penis in a special way, putting her thumb on the frenulum (on the underside of the penis) and her first and second fingers on both sides of the coronal ridge. (The coronal ridge is easy to feel in men who have not been circumcised.) She now applies firm pressure for 3 or 4 seconds. If a man didn't have an erection, this might be somewhat uncomfortable, but with an erection there is little if any discomfort associated with the squeeze technique. This pressure leads to an immediate loss of the desire to ejaculate and a temporary decrease in the firmness of the man's erection. The woman then again manually stimulates the penis until he attains a full erection, and again applies the squeeze technique. In this

way, a couple can engage in prolonged stimulation of a man's penis without ejaculation occurring. These "success" experiences are very rewarding for the man, increasing his feelings of control.

Applying pressure to the base of the penis as a man approaches ejaculatory inevitability can have similar results. This is called the **basilar squeeze technique** and is also quite effective in treating premature ejaculation. With this technique the man's partner or the man himself applies firm manual pressure to the base of the penis, just at the point where it joins his body. This variation has two advantages that the coronal squeeze technique does not. The man can more easily do it himself, and he can apply pressure to the base of the penis during intercourse, therefore, giving him more control over the timing of his ejaculation. Figure 15-7 illustrates these techniques.

Once the couple has learned the basics of the squeeze technique, they are ready to move to the next step in the treatment of premature ejaculation. They use the same stimulation techniques until the man attains an erection, repeating the process a few times to remind the man how it feels to become erect without ejaculating. Then the woman stimulates him until he becomes erect, but this time she slowly and gently assumes the female-on-top intercourse position, gradually inserting his penis inside her vagina and then holding completely still. This allows the man to experience the feelings of penile containment without the immediate desire to ejaculate. This is another "success" experience for him, increasing his feelings of control and confidence. This may take a long time, since most men with this problem still feel a desire to ejaculate soon after they have entered their partner. At this point, by word or gesture, he communicates this to her, she raises herself so that his penis is no longer inside of her and applies the squeeze technique. This again eliminates the desire to ejaculate. Before her partner's penis becomes too soft, she again inserts it into her vagina and engages in slow, gentle pelvic thrusting. Over a number of days, the couple begins to enjoy a feeling of control and mastery they had not previously enjoyed. Masters and Johnson noted that the ejaculatory control the man acquires in the female-on-top position generalizes to other intercourse positions as well.

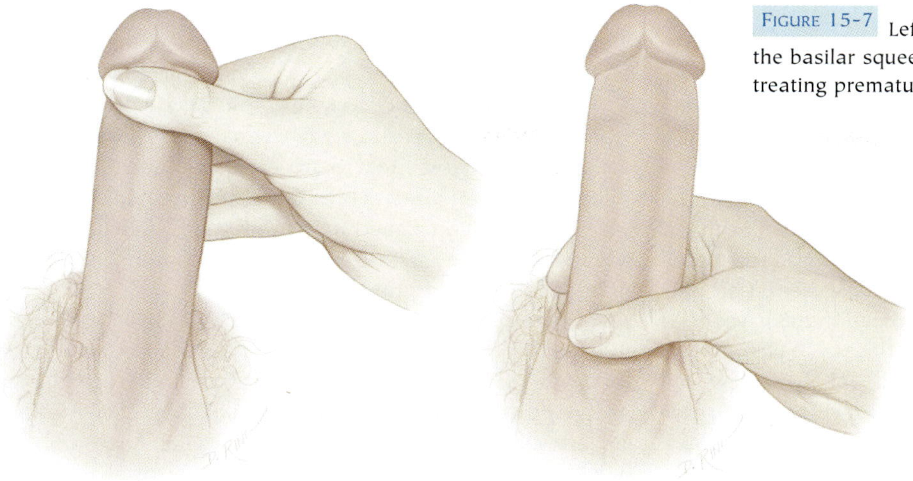

FIGURE 15-7 Left: the coronal squeeze technique. Right: the basilar squeeze technique. Both are effective for treating premature ejaculation.

A third technique called the "start-stop" method involves a woman manually stimulating a man's penis until he becomes erect, then stopping her stimulation until her partner's erection begins to soften and then resuming her stroking hand movements (Fig. 15-8). This technique also teaches men that once an erection begins to soften it can return fairly quickly.

A female partner of premature ejaculators is often anorgasmic because their partner's erection does not last long enough for her to enjoy prolonged pelvic thrusting and the orgasms that sometimes accompany this kind of stimulation. Both partners are then somewhat frustrated or even angry. Since the therapeutic techniques for helping premature ejaculators completely focus on the man, this typically continues to leave the woman unsatisfied. Therefore, it is important for the female partner to begin to engage in gentle pelvic thrusting to enhance her own pleasure as soon as her partner gains some control over ejaculation. Solving the man's sexual dysfunction meets only half the goal if his partner continues to be troubled by her own lack of response.

Retarded Ejaculation

The other common male orgasmic disorder is retarded ejaculation, also sometimes called "ejaculatory incompetence." This does not involve problems with desire or erection, but for men with this disorder even vigorous, prolonged pelvic thrusting does not easily precipitate ejaculation. As with the treatment of other sexual dysfunctions, it is important for the counselor or therapist to find out as much as possible about the man's sex-

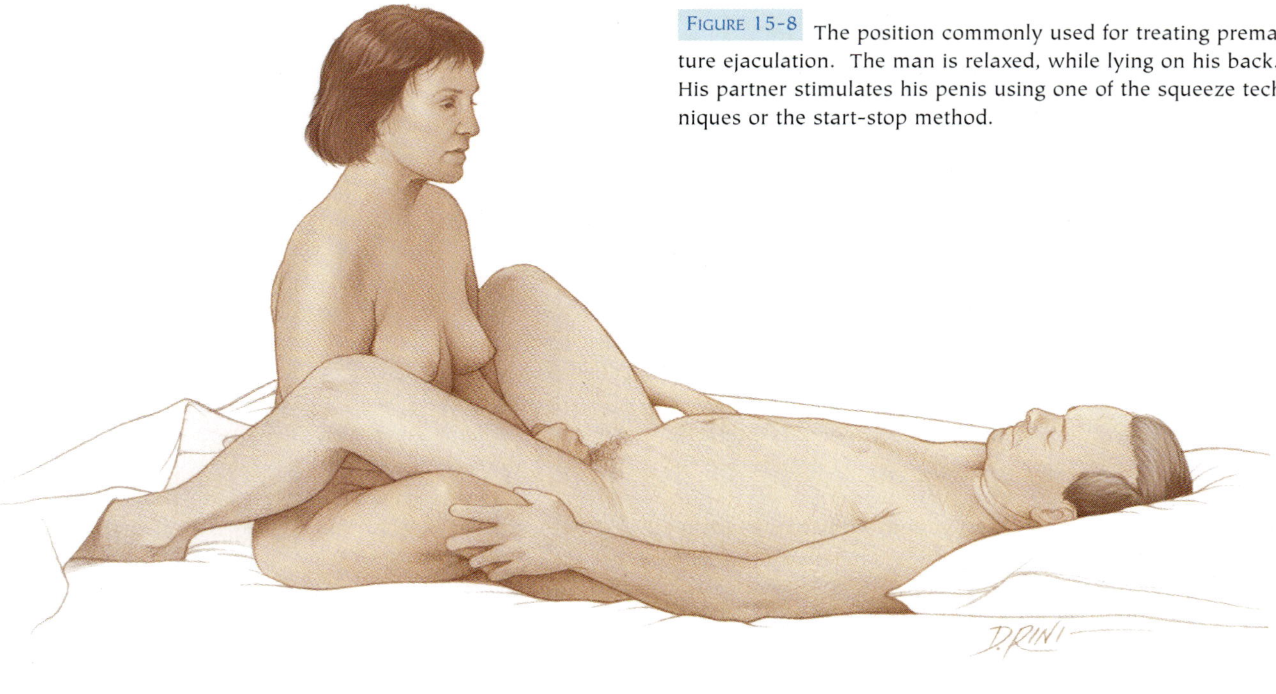

FIGURE 15-8 The position commonly used for treating premature ejaculation. The man is relaxed, while lying on his back. His partner stimulates his penis using one of the squeeze techniques or the start-stop method.

ual value system to determine what he finds erotic and sexy. Before therapeutic techniques are directed toward facilitating ejaculation during intercourse, the first step in the treatment of retarded ejaculation is for the female partner to use manual stimulation to elicit this response (Fig. 15-8). This is a rewarding first step in a chain of events that eventually leads to ejaculation during intercourse.

Once a woman has manually stimulated her partner's penis until he attains an erection, the next important thing to do is straddle him in the female-on-top position and insert his penis into her vagina. At this point, the woman immediately begins vigorous pelvic movements. Often, this is sufficient to facilitate her partner's ejaculation, but at the beginning of therapy this may not happen. He should then withdraw his penis so that his partner can again vigorously stimulate it manually until he reaches ejaculatory inevitability, at which time she again straddles him and puts his penis into her vagina. She then again resumes vigorous pelvic thrusting. With this method of treating retarded ejaculation, as soon as a man ejaculates inside of his partner once, the experience builds tremendous feelings of self-confidence almost immediately. Only a few additional experiences like this are necessary for the couple to begin to more consistently enjoy intercourse involving intravaginal ejaculation.

Often women don't mind it if their partner can engage in prolonged, vigorous intercourse with a full, hard erection, whether or not he ejaculates. This often gives the woman the opportunity to enjoy a lengthened plateau stage in her sexual response cycle and perhaps to have orgasms consistently during intercourse. But sexual intercourse is a shared experience, and when one partner, female or male, isn't having fulfilling, pleasurable feelings, then the couple's relationship would be enhanced by resolving the problem.

SEXUAL PAIN DISORDERS

In treating sexual pain disorders, the most important thing to do at the outset is determine whether the problem results from some medical or physiological abnormality. The descriptions of dyspareunia and vaginismus in Chapter 14 noted a number of health problems that could contribute to these dysfunctions, and in such cases medical treatments are used first for medical problems. Here we focus on cognitive-behavioral strategies for treating these disorders when they are caused by psychosocial factors. Regardless of the initial reason for discomfort during intercourse, the continued combination of pain and sex can leave a person anxious and uncomfortable long after the original cause has been successfully treated.

Dyspareunia refers to painful intercourse in either a woman or man. Additionally, the *DSM* notes that the problem is not entirely attributable to a lack of vaginal lubrication. It occurs far more often in women than men and is also more likely to involve psychosocial causes in women than men. Dyspareunia and vaginismus are often interrelated because prolonged, persistent painful intercourse often leads to vaginismus, the spastic, uncontrollable contraction of the musculature at the opening to the vagina. A woman with vaginismus will inevitably have dyspareunia, but the woman is not given a double diagnosis because, by definition, vaginismus involves discomfort during attempts at penile penetration. Brant (1978) distinguished between *superficial* dyspareunia felt at the opening to the vagina and *deep* dyspareunia perceived closer to the cervix or even in the woman's lower abdominal area. Additionally, the term *primary* is used if it has occurred throughout the woman's lifetime and the term *secondary* is used if the discomfort develops after a woman has had pain-free intercourse for a long period of time.

In treating dyspareunia, it is difficult to make a clear distinction between vaginismus and painful intercourse that occurs without an organic basis. When a woman has scarring due to a poorly repaired episiotomy, some type of vaginal lesion, or an estrogen deficiency, these are clearly physical problems whose treatment can lead to the elimination of painful intercourse. In general, women who have hysterectomies experience improvement or no changes at all in their sexual functioning (Carlson, 1997). Cognitive-behavioral approaches to the treatment of this dysfunction often involve the use of surgical lubricant to make vaginal penetration more comfortable. Additionally, a woman with dyspareunia may find some relief by assuming the female-on-top position during intercourse, thus allowing her to control the angle, rate, and depth of penile penetration. Apart from these relatively simple remedies, many women experience dyspareunia because of anxiety surrounding sexual intercourse, and in this instance relaxation exercises and sometimes hypnosis have been of some benefit. Diminished anxiety along with the use of lubrication and a change in intercourse position can be very helpful in minimizing or eliminating pain associated with sexual intercourse (Quevillon, 1993).

Diagnosing and treating vaginismus can be somewhat more complex. Because vaginismus is often associated with a history of sexual abuse and/or assault, psychological therapies are often needed to address these terrible events and to help the client try to put them behind her. One of the basic tenets of the cognitive-behavioral approach, however, is that the causes of sexual dysfunctions are not as important as their current manifestations, and that the focus of therapy should be eliminating the problem in the present rather than trying to understand its historical roots. Masters and Johnson have recommended that the woman's partner be brought into the gynecological examination so that he can attempt to insert his gloved finger in his partner's vagina. In this way he perceives the nature of the spastic, uncoordinated muscular contractions that have made penile penetration difficult or impossible. They then recommend that a woman use a set of vaginal "dilators" of progressively larger circumference to gain practice in vaginally accommodating a highly lubricated penis-shaped object. Technically speaking, a dildo is any object shaped like an erect penis. Sometimes, a dildo is also a vibrator, but not all vibrators used for genital stimulation are shaped like erect penises. The woman uses a set of these (Fig. 15-9) to gradually grow more comfortable with the experience of vaginal penetration. She first lubricates the smallest circumference dilator and gradually inserts it into her vagina and then, ideally, sleeps

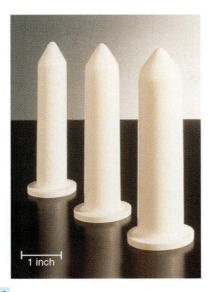

1 inch

FIGURE 15-9 Progressively larger vaginal dilators are used in the treatment of vaginismus.

through the night with it inside of her. Over a number of weeks, she then uses increasingly larger circumference dilators. These exercises eliminate the involuntary vaginal spasms that once made intercourse very uncomfortable or impossible. Through this process the woman's partner must be as patient and cooperative as possible (Beck, 1993).

BEHAVIORAL PRINCIPLES IN SEX THERAPY

Short-term, intensive cognitive-behavioral approaches to the treatment of sexual dysfunctions are often quite successful, and focusing on the problem and its current manifestations is usually more fruitful than long-term, in-depth psychotherapy. Some sexual dysfunctions, however, may benefit from a thorough, systematic, prolonged period of counseling or psychotherapy. But why do cognitive-behavioral approaches work so well? The answer involves concepts basic to behavioral approaches to how people change their actions over a period of time. These principles, explained in the following sections, are by no means exclusive to sex therapy.

Positive Reinforcement

One way behavioral theorists conceptualize positive reinforcement is as a stimulus that increases the probability of a response recurring. It can be food if you are hungry, cold lemonade if you are thirsty, sleep if you're tired, or your paycheck. These rewards increase the chances of the behavior that preceded them of happening again, and they always get the person's attention. An orgasm following sexual interaction is a good example of positive reinforcement.

Negative Reinforcement

Negative reinforcement is often confused with punishment, which in fact is very different. Negative reinforcement can be just as powerful as positive reinforcement for learning and maintaining learned behaviors. Negative reinforcement is the good feeling you get when a bad feeling stops. This cessation of discomfort, pain, or even nervousness and embarrassment can be very pleasant. When a man gains some control over the timing of ejaculation or a woman begins to have orgasms regularly and reliably when in the past she had none, feelings of failure and anxiety are replaced by feelings of pleasure and self-confidence. These are examples of negative reinforcement in sex therapy.

Successive Approximation

The term successive approximation, also called "shaping" in behavioral literature, is a basic concept of learning in this theoretical perspective. Successive approximation means that learning takes place in small steps, each of which is reinforced as it gets closer to a goal. In this way responses are connected to one another by reinforcements, and behavior is accordingly shaped. This perspective emphasizes that learning is a gradual process, rather than a sudden, permanent change in behavior. If you know which behaviors to change and which reinforcements are rewarding to the particular person, then permanent adjustments in thinking, feeling, and acting can be learned efficiently.

Successive approximation is fundamental to cognitive-behavioral approaches to sex therapy. If the goal of sex therapy for a man is ejaculatory control or intravaginal ejaculation, or for women the occurrence of orgasms during sexual interaction, then sex therapy will likely be effective if the therapist sets up a sequence of exercises that get closer and closer to these goals and are reinforced. This is what sensate focus exercises do. They begin with shared intimacy that doesn't involve immediately confronting the problem and gently and gradually create rewarding experiences for behaviors that are "successful." As problem behaviors are slowly eliminated, along with the anxiety that often accompanies them, they are replaced by other, more rewarding behaviors. This is sometimes also called systematic desensitization because the client gradually becomes less sensitive to the anxiety that once accompanied their sexual dysfunction.

Sex "Aids" in the Treatment of Sexual Dysfunctions

This chapter has already noted that the use of vibrators and/or dildos can be very helpful in assisting women and men to learn more about their sexual response cycle, to have orgasms regularly, and to learn to relax the musculature at the opening to the vagina (Fig. 15-10). Yet many people feel nervous, guilty, or ashamed about using these adjuncts to therapy and think of them as "sex toys." These tools are not a substitute for a partner or the feelings a partner can provide, but they often serve a function as tools. Most counseling or therapy involves improved self-awareness, behavioral changes, and diminished bad feelings of many kinds. In addition, sex therapy can use exercises and tools to assist clients confront and eliminate their sexual dysfunctions.

Dear Dr. Ruth

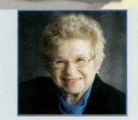

Question:

I was raised in a very strict religious home and it took me years to become comfortable with my own sexuality. By now (I'm 30) I understand that people have sex for many good reasons, not just planning to have babies, and that sexual expression is an important part of a marital relationship. I just wish I had a freer attitude about my own orgasms. Based on what I've read, a vibrator might help me learn more about how I respond, but I would feel really embarrassed buying a vibrator. I don't think it would bother me to use one, but getting one is another matter. Am I normal? How can I discreetly get a vibrator?

Answer:

Many people are embarrassed to buy vibrators and other items that are sometimes called sex toys, but these can really be important enhancements to a couple's sex life. Luckily you don't have to find a sex shop to purchase a vibrator but can do so from the privacy of your own home by computer or by mail.

Two vendors that I can recommend are Good Vibrations and Eve's Garden. The address for Good Vibrations is 938 Howard Street, San Francisco, CA 94103 and their web site is www.goodvibes.com. Eve's Garden's address is 119 West 57th Street, New York NY 10019, and they'll send you a catalogue if you call 1-800-848-3837.

Many people's sexual value system makes it difficult for them to incorporate sex aids into their treatment. These might include vibrators, sexually explicit prose or photographs, and home videos. Therapists sometimes call these "ice-breakers."

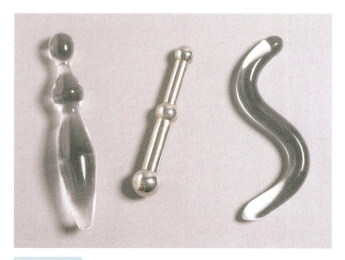

FIGURE 15-10 The plastic sex aids at left and right can stimulate various areas inside a woman's vagina. The metal device in the center is weighted and used during Kegel exercises to improve tone in the vaginal muscles.

For many people, these can effectively increase sexual desire and arousal, especially if use of such items is tailored to the client's sexual value system. The therapist must be thoroughly familiar with the client's sexual value system to select the right avenues of exploration. When these tools do increase the client's desire and arousal, actually incorporating them into lovemaking itself can be an additional challenge.

Only a counselor or therapist who is thoroughly familiar with a couple and their sexual difficulties is in a position to recommend the use of these tools, but many people own and enjoy using vibrators of various types and have learned much about themselves and their partner by using them. There is nothing "dirty" or dehumanizing about these sex aids; using them is a matter of personal preference. Over the last three decades, sex counselors and therapists have recognized that vibratory stimulation is extremely effective in the treatment of anorgasmia in women and may also help treat retarded ejaculation in men. Still, some couples believe that the use of a vibrator indicates they have a sexual deficiency and, therefore, hesitate to use one (Hawton, 1985).

Sex aids have a clear role for people with trouble having orgasms. But what about people who for years had no trouble at all? Secondary sexual dysfunctions are those that occur after sometimes years of normal, problem-free sexual functioning. The counselor or therapist carefully assesses the needs of these

Research Highlight

COMBINING COUPLE THERAPY AND SEX THERAPY

One of Masters and Johnson's most important contributions is the understanding that people with sexual problems don't necessarily have any deeper psychological problems. Sexual dysfunctions can result from inappropriately learned behaviors rather than major anxiety, depression, or personality disorders. Still, sexual problems are often in some way tied into a couple's relationship and their interpersonal communication styles. In 1997, Kevan R. Wylie, a British sex therapist, published a study evaluating the effectiveness of combined couple therapy and sex therapy. His aim was to give his clients a brief, structured blend of the two therapeutic strategies. In addition to focusing on the couple's sexual problem, which in this case was psychogenic male erectile disorder, he explored the behavioral, cognitive, and interpersonal aspects of this problem on their relationship.

His patients were referred by their general practitioner, psychiatrist, or urologist. Using paper-and-pencil tests he assessed the couple's relationship satisfaction and sexual satisfaction. The males in his sample had been unable to attain and maintain an erection in at least 50% of their attempts at intercourse in the last 3 months. Couples attended six therapy sessions, one every other week. In addition to working on a number of relationship issues, the couple was given instruction in sensate focus exercises with specific guidance for dealing with male erectile disorder.

Twenty-three couples completed the treatment; 10 had an "excellent" outcome, 4 had a "moderate" outcome, and 6 had a "mild" outcome. Three couples showed no change from their preliminary relationship and sexual evaluations. Because of the small sample size, it is difficult to compare the effectiveness of this method with that used by Masters and Johnson. On average, couples reported an increase in the frequency with which they shared sexual intimacy and improvements in sexual communication. Importantly, fewer couples reported avoiding sexual activity. Most couples described more pleasurable feelings associated with sexual interaction and fewer unpleasant feelings. While it is difficult to precisely define what constitutes "successful" therapy, these data are encouraging. Unfortunately, too few subjects came to their 6-month follow-up visit, so it was difficult to assess the permanence of the therapeutic gains.

The importance of this study lies in Wylie's attempt to combine relationship and sexual therapy for a single, specific sexual dysfunction. His systematic approach makes efficient use of time. Finally, his data revealed genuine gains in sexual functioning and relationship communication.

---

clients and the therapies with which they would be most comfortable. As Hawton (1985) has noted, suggesting that a 55-year-old woman buy a vibrator to help her regain some of her former responsiveness may be a shocking recommendation. Personal rapport and trust between therapist and client is especially important.

Although vibratory aids are used more for women, this type of stimulation is effective for some men too. Vacuum constriction devices have been shown very effective in the treatment of erectile dysfunction that is organic or psychosocial in nature. The man inserts his penis into a plastic tube a few inches in diameter, and the air is drawn out through the use of a hand pump. The vacuum created inside the tube pulls blood into the corpora cavernosa, causing an increase in the length, circumference, and hardness of the penis. A tight band of rubber is then placed around the base of the penis, essentially trapping the blood inside it, and this allows the man to maintain his erection long enough to comfortably penetrate his partner, engage in pelvic thrusting, and often ejaculate as well. This device has been used in one form or another for over 80 years (Tiefer & Melman, 1989). Vacuum constriction devices are still popular and are a simple treatment for erectile dysfunction that does not involve drugs or surgery (discussed later). Not much is known about the long-term use of vacuum constriction devices. A report by Ganem, Lucey, Janosko, and Carson (1998) described a few instances of urethral bleeding, mild bruising, and damage to the membranes surrounding the corpora cavernosa when the ring at the base of the penis is applied too tightly. In most cases, these devices do not cause harm, discomfort, or injury.

MESSAGE FROM DR. RUTH: A COMMENT ON USING VIBRATORS

Vibrators are often considered sex toys, and for some people that's appropriate because they use a vibrator merely to enhance sexual pleasure from time to time. Some women, however, are reluctant to use a vibrator because it doesn't seem natural to them. And that's fine—I'd never urge a woman, or a couple, to experiment with a vibrator if they were uncomfortable doing so. On the other hand, for some women, a vibrator is the only way they can have an orgasm.

Some women first use a vibrator to learn how to have an orgasm. Then they can show their partner how to provide the right stimulation to lead to an orgasm, or they may learn how to use their own hand to have an orgasm without using a vibrator. For some other women, the strong sensations provided by a vibrator remain the only way to achieve orgasm, and integrating a vibrator into their love life can thus be important for achieving sexual satisfaction. There is nothing wrong with these women—it's like using glasses for reading. That vibrators can't be purchased at the corner drug store is a pity. I get lots of letters from women who need a vibrator but haven't the slightest idea where to get one, or they know of a sex shop but are ashamed to go inside. What's important is that if you feel a vibrator may help provide a sensation you are missing, don't be reluctant to seek it.

I hope that one day people won't snicker at the mention of vibrators, but whether society's attitudes change or not, anyone who feels that a vibrator is what she needs to fully enjoy sex should not hesitate for a moment in purchasing one.

MASTURBATION AND MUTUAL MASTURBATION IN THE TREATMENT OF SEXUAL DYSFUNCTIONS

Most sex counselors and sex therapists agree that masturbation can teach us a lot about our own sexual responsiveness and we can use this information in sexual interactions with others. Interestingly, the psychosocial factors that inhibit a person from being fully aroused and responsive during sexual intercourse are the same factors that discourage a person from masturbating. As noted earlier, a person's interpretation of religious orthodoxy can suppress their independent or mutual sexual exploration. Yet when a person knows how to touch themselves in a way that elicits arousal, they can tell or show their partner how they like to be stimulated (Fig. 15-11).

Leff and Israel (1983) found that there was no relationship in a sample of 117 middle-class women between the ability to masturbate or the preferred way of masturbating and the capacity for orgasms during intercourse. Most of the respondents reported that direct clitoral stimulation was the most common method of masturbation. Among the women who reported masturbating, clitoral stimulation during intercourse was often effective in precipitating an orgasm. Masturbation and mutual masturbation within the context of sex therapy are often very satisfying first steps that may lead to enhanced responsiveness during intercourse and are a good example of successive approximation. Some individuals enjoy their strongest orgasms during masturbation

and/or the use of a vibrator but also often enjoy the intimacy of intercourse.

Clients Without Partners

A challenge facing sex counselors and therapists is clients who seek sex therapy but who do not have a partner. These individuals are unmarried and do not have regular sexual relations with a steady partner. Without a consistent partner, these individuals are not having intercourse, not having intercourse very often, or not having intercourse with someone they can get to know well enough to begin to explore their real sexual needs and preferences. When a client is not having regular intercourse over an extended period of time with one partner, it is not likely that they can work though their sexual difficulties in a warm, nurturant climate of psychological safety with someone they have come to know very well and fully trust. This situation leads to a basic question about sex therapy: How can a client without a regular partner get help with her or his sexual dysfunction (Fig. 15-12)?

From the beginning, Masters and Johnson encouraged unmarried clients to bring partners with them, and these spouse substitutes were called replacement partners. When their therapy program began in 1959, this was still somewhat controversial. The most controversial aspect of their institutional policy was to provide unmarried men with partner surrogates during their intensive, 2-week therapy. Over the 11 years during which this policy was in place, Masters and

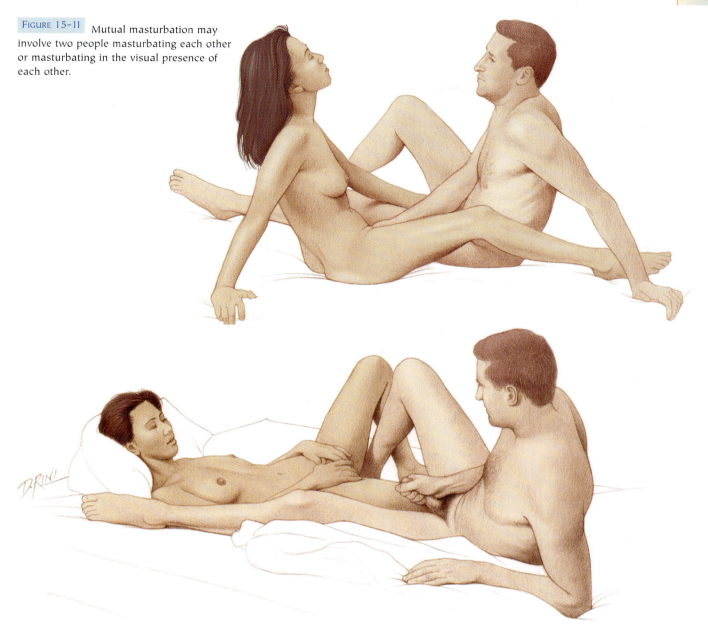

FIGURE 15-11 Mutual masturbation may involve two people masturbating each other or masturbating in the visual presence of each other.

Johnson provided 41 men with partner surrogates. These individuals engaged in all the homework assignments prescribed by the therapists, including sensate focus exercises and sexual intercourse. Partner surrogates were not used in the treatment of single women who came to their facility for the treatment of sexual dysfunctions. Partner surrogates were all volunteers between the ages of 24 and 43. Masters and Johnson selected 13 from an initial pool of 31. Eleven of these women had been previously married, but none of them was married at the time they worked as partner surrogates. For a number of years Masters and Johnson had a quiet understanding with the press in St. Louis, and reports of the

partner surrogate program didn't become public until one of these women accepted a monetary offer to write a book about her experiences. The partner surrogate program then abruptly ended.

Today, a number of effective, noncontroversial alternatives can be used in treating individuals who request sex therapy. Often short-term individual counseling along with sex education can effectively help clients without partners. Sometimes these clients do have partners who are unwilling or unable to participate in the treatment program, counseling, or marital therapy. Additionally, when psychological or medical problems are the prime causes of a sexual dysfunc-

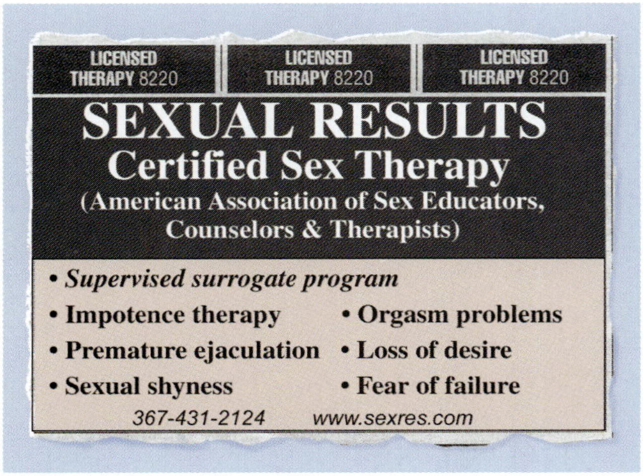

LICENSED THERAPY 8220   LICENSED THERAPY 8220   LICENSED THERAPY 8220

SEXUAL RESULTS
Certified Sex Therapy
(American Association of Sex Educators,
Counselors & Therapists)

- *Supervised surrogate program*
- **Impotence therapy**   • **Orgasm problems**
- **Premature ejaculation** • **Loss of desire**
- **Sexual shyness**   • **Fear of failure**

367-431-2124   www.sexres.com

FIGURE 15-12   Reputable sex therapy clinics sometimes offer surrogate programs for clients without partners.

tion, individual therapy may actually be a preferred type of approach.

Anorgasmic women, for example, can begin to explore their erotic responsiveness with the aid of a vibrator and can learn more about their bodies through genital self-examination without the aid of a partner (Hawton, 1985). Similarly, a woman with vaginismus can use a series of vaginal dilators without the assistance or support of a partner. Some types of female sexual dysfunctions do respond well to individual therapy. Likewise, men who are premature ejaculators can engage in solo masturbation, learning to progressively prolong the time before they ejaculate. Additionally, a man can use the start-stop technique, engaging in self-stimulation until he becomes aroused and erect, pausing until he begins to lose his erection, and then resuming his masturbatory stimulation. These exercises, along with the basilar squeeze technique, can help men with this problem who don't have a partner. Finally, men with retarded ejaculation can use a combination of masturbation, vibratory stimulation, and perhaps erotic pictures or videotapes to develop a regular pattern of ejaculatory response.

SEXUAL DYSFUNCTIONS IN DEVELOPMENTAL CONTEXT

We would like to close this section on a reassuring note. It is generally the rule rather than the exception for young people just beginning to have sexual intercourse to experience frustrations and problems that in older individuals would be termed dysfunctional. For example, when adolescents and young men first begin having sex, they are very likely to ejaculate long before their partner has experienced any significant sexual satisfaction, but this does not necessarily mean that they are premature ejaculators. The same is true of women who may have sex for quite a long time before they eventually have an orgasm during intercourse, but this doesn't mean that they are anorgasmic. Like men, they will learn from their experience. Therefore, the term sexual dysfunction should be reserved for adults with more than a little sexual experience, who are troubled and

frustrated by their problem, and who continually and consistently experience the problem.

MEDICAL APPROACHES TO THE TREATMENT OF SEXUAL DYSFUNCTIONS

The discussion thus far has focused on the cognitive-behavioral approach to treat sexual dysfunctions that are primarily psychosocial in origin. It is essential to rule out physiological, endocrine, or medical causes before proceeding with cognitive-behavioral therapies. Yet many disorders do have a clear biological basis and, therefore, require very different, and sometimes quite radical, therapies. Physicians provide medical treatment for sexual dysfunctions. These might include gynecologists, urologists, endocrinologists, internists, and surgeons. Medical interventions include drugs and sometimes surgery to enhance sexual arousal or facilitate its overt physiological manifestations, such as erection. While medical approaches to treatment seem more clear-cut, these measures are ideally undertaken within the context of a good interpersonal relationship. Sex therapy without a consistent, trusted partner does not often provide optimistic results.

Americans frequently seek the quickest, easiest solutions for problems of many kinds, including sexual dysfunctions. Individual and group therapy approaches take commitment, time, and considerable personal and interpersonal work to succeed, however. In contrast, medical approaches seem quick and effective, even when not painless or inexpensive. Nonetheless, a person who has a sexual dysfunction generally should consider the more conservative and least physically invasive strategies first, and only later on more radical and sometimes irreversible tactics.

Sex Hormones in the Bloodstream

In some cases testosterone supplements may help men with an erectile disorder. Because of the cyclic changes in female hormones throughout a woman's menstrual cycle, however, it is more difficult to predict possible benefits of hormone supplements for women. Still, when levels of estrogen are very low, increasing them through the use of oral tablets can make a difference in a woman's sexual arousal and responsiveness. Because the connection between hormone levels and sexual arousal is not as clear in women as it is in men, this section focuses on the use of testosterone supplements in the treatment of erectile dysfunction.

The term **hypogonadism** is a condition of diminished secretion of testosterone from the testes. This can occur because the pituitary gland is not stimulating the testes to make testosterone or because the testes simply stop manufacturing testosterone. Certain diseases, such as mumps, infections, trauma, and genetic disorders may also cause this problem. Doctors, however, sometimes find low testosterone levels in otherwise healthy, normal men. There are a number of different estimates, but conservatively speaking, about 20 million men in the United States experience erectile dysfunction some or all of the time they attempt intercourse. When low testosterone is a factor, this hormone can be introduced into a man's bloodstream in several ways. The relationship between testosterone levels in the bloodstream and erectile dysfunction is not completely clear, however. Govier, McClure, and Kramer-Levien (1996) studied over 250 men who reported bouts of erectile dysfunction. Of this number, 16% were diagnosed with hypogonadism. These investigators noted that other studies, however, report that between 1% and 45% of men with low testosterone levels have erectile dysfunction. Testosterone levels in the bloodstream may not be the most important biological factor in erectile dysfunction.

When hypogonadism is indeed the primary reason for impotence, giving testosterone is often effective. Testosterone can be injected, taken in oral tablet form, or administered through a transdermal (skin) patch, similar to nicotine patches used by people who are trying to stop smoking cigarettes. A new testosterone gel that can be rubbed on the skin daily is also available. The Testoderm patch is applied directly to a man's scrotum (Fig. 15-13), which must be shaved once a week to ensure that there is good contact between skin and the patch. With another patch called Androderm, two patches are placed symmetrically on the sides of a man's body. Patches are generally more expensive than other forms of testosterone administration. There may be some troubling side-effects associated with this patch, including rapid heart beat, nervousness, irregular heart rate, an increased PSA level (prostate-specific

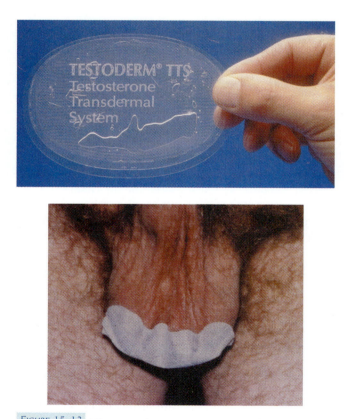

FIGURE 15-13 Like many drugs, testosterone can be absorbed into the bloodstream directly through the skin. Above is the patch before application and below it is affixed to the scrotum.

antigen, which is one indicator of prostate cancer), and unpredictable sexual arousal. These side effects are rare and not often serious. Men who receive testosterone injections every two weeks report increased sex drive, as well as irritability and aggressiveness for the first few days afterwards, but these effects diminish until it is time for the next injection. Overall, when hypogonadism is the cause of erectile dysfunction, testosterone replacement therapy is often a very effective treatment. This drug is most effective when used in the context of a good, trusting relationship.

Nonhormonal Drugs in Treatment

In addition to the use of sex hormones, other drugs are used for the treatment of sexual dysfunctions. These agents are *not* aphrodisiacs, however. Aphrodisiacs are substances that produce or increase sexual *desire*. Often people with sexual dysfunctions have problems not with sexual desire but with *sexual arousal*. One drug, however, that has received some attention for its aphrodisiac properties has been found useful in the treatment of erectile disorders in men. *Yohimbine,* derived from the bark of the yohimbine tree in Central Africa, increases blood flow to the penis. For a long time its aphrodisiac properties have been debated, and in 1996 the American Urological Association issued a report that indicated that yohimbine may not be reliably effective in the treatment of erectile dysfunction (Montagne, Barada, Belker, et al., 1996). A recent review of the clinical research indicates that yohimbine works significantly better than a placebo in the treatment of this sexual disorder. Any side effects of this drug were typically mild and went away as soon as it was discontinued. Because it is inexpensive (less than $ .50 per day as of this writing) and does not involve injections or surgery, yohimbine may be an important medical treatment for erectile dysfunction (Witt, 1998). Further testing of this agent is needed.

One effective treatment for erectile dysfunction, introduced in the mid-1990s, uses a thin tubular applicator to insert a tiny pill directly inside a man's urethra. The drug Aprostadil has had mixed success in the treatment of this sexual disorder. Aprostadil is a synthetic version of the hormone prostaglandin E_1. Williams, Abbou, Amar, et al. (1998) administered this drug to 249 patients and found that 64% of them were able to attain an erection of sufficient firmness that they could have intercourse. A small percentage of patients (about 7%) experienced some pain or burning inside their urethra, but most subjects in this experiment had only slight discomfort or none at all. Other research (Werthman & Rajfer, 1997), however, found this treatment approach less effective, with only 7% of a sample of 100 patients attaining rigid erections, 30% having partial erections, and fully 63% not having erections at all. It is often difficult to compare clinical studies, and it was not clear whether all the men in these investigations had impotence with an organic basis; as well, the general overall health of the subjects in the two studies was not reported. Insertion of Aprostadil tablets into the urethra is called MUSE therapy, which stands for medicated urethral system for erection.

A variety of other chemical agents make blood vessels expand, called **vasodilators**. These agents can be of benefit in treating erectile dysfunction by facilitating the dilation of blood vessels in the penis and thereby creating an erection. By the time you read this, other new drugs for the treatment of erectile dysfunction will have been released on the market, including one that acts directly on the brain. Until recently, sex therapists and physicians had few reliable, effective drugs of this type as oral medications. For many years, however, effective penile vasodilators have been available in injectable form, and as much as many men wanted to have erections, having to inject a substance into their own penises was a difficult decision. Prostaglandin E_1 in injectable form is one of these alternatives. These injections have been an effective, predictable treatment for organic erectile difficulties. Because these drugs are injected into the corpora cavernosa of the penis, this form of treatment is called intracavernous pharmacotherapy. Several different agents have been used with some success.

While the effectiveness of prostaglandin E_1 administered inside the urethra has been debatable, when the same drug is injected into the penis it seems to be far more effective. This way of administering drugs to enhance erectile ability has been used since the early 1980s. In one study involving 103 impotent men (Porst, 1997), this agent was effective in facilitating an erection in 10% of the sample when used urethrally, but 48% of the sample attained an erection when the drug was injected into the penis. Many men who have erectile dysfunction for organic reasons have been satisfied with the effects of these drugs. In addition to prostaglandin E_1, other agents, such as papaverine, have demonstrated effectiveness in stimulating erection. All of these substances act locally to dilate blood vessels in the penis without having an effect in other parts of the body. In some men these injections are not effective, although they do respond well to the urethral administration of prostaglandin E_1 (Engel & McVary, 1998). In other words, if one route of administration doesn't work very well the other might be effective. Since not everyone can use a drug like Viagra because of its side effects, these other treatment alternatives remain important.

These therapies for erectile dysfunction have been used for several years. There are advantages and drawbacks to each, and all patients do not respond in the same way to these drugs. In recent years there has been a remarkable advance in the treatment of erectile dysfunction with the drug Viagra (sildenafil), which facilitates vasodilation in the penis. Although expensive (about $10 per pill), Viagra seems effective for many men with organic impotence (Fig. 15-14). It too acts as a local vasodilator to facilitate erection. Remember, a man who has an organic erectile dysfunction has generally not lost his capacity for ejaculation. This is one of the most frustrating things about erectile dysfunction. Drugs like Viagra restore the capacity for erection and frequently lead to an enhanced quality of life. It is often effective for men who have lost erectile ability because of surgery

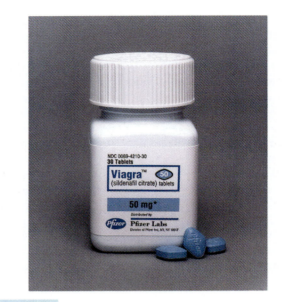

FIGURE 15-14   Viagra is an effective drug for the treatment of erectile dysfunction. This agent dilates blood vessels in the penis and facilitates erection.

to remove a cancerous prostate and for those whose erectile dysfunction results from uncontrolled diabetes and the destruction of nerves along the floor of the pelvis that often results. Viagra is rapidly absorbed after oral administration, acts fairly promptly (men are instructed to take Viagra about an hour before planned intercourse), and has very little effect on heart rate and blood pressure. One study (Goldstein, Lue, Padma-Nathan, et al., 1998), however, found that 6% to 18% of over 500 subjects they studied complained of headache, flushing, and indigestion when using Viagra. Importantly, this drug is metabolized fairly rapidly and does not accumulate in a man's body with repeated administration. It has also been tested on men with erectile dysfunction without an organic basis and has been found to enhance erectile response to visual erotic stimuli (Boolell, Allen, Ballard et al., 1996). When Viagra first became available, unfortunate and even fatal side effects occurred in men who were taking other medications containing nitrites. Probably the most common drug to cause problems for men taking Viagra is nitroglycerin, which is used for chest pain that results from heart disease. The combination of Viagra and nitroglycerin is potentially fatal, and patients who use nitroglycerin should not use Viagra.

As noted earlier, treatments for erectile dysfunction are undertaken within the context of a strong, trusting relationship. Viagra has had some rather unfortunate consequences for relationships. Some men who were impotent in their marriages or longstanding cohabitation arrangements left their wives or partners (taking their Viagra with them) and aggressively began to explore sexual relationships in their new single lifestyle. In other cases, couples adjusted to the man's impotence and

Other Countries, Cultures, and Customs

VIAGRA USE AROUND THE WORLD

The impact of Viagra in the United States has been huge. It is a treatment for impotence in keeping with the American attitude toward health problems: just take a pill. For the first time there is an effective oral medication that can be of some real help to many men with erectile difficulties. When Viagra was first released by the Pfizer Pharmaceutical Company, there were literally hundreds of articles about it in newspapers and magazines, and many jokes were told involving the new drug. But American society is more open to public discussion of sexual issues than many other cultures around the world, in which many men have erectile dysfunctions. Viagra has been smuggled into countries where it has not been approved for usage, and men are paying astonishing amounts of money for only a single pill. Following are a few news items from other cultures that reveal reactions to the drug around the world:

Mumbai [a city in India], May 7 [1998]: "There's good news and bad news for the impotent Indian male drooling over the new wonder drug Viagra. The good news is that the tiny but expensive pill, which promises to enhance sexual performance, will hit Mumbai in about 4 days. Hawked at an exorbitant Rs 600 [600 rupees is approximately $14] per tablet, drugstores will not demand a prescription—or issue a receipt. Every male's ultimate fantasy can be fulfilled only under the counter as across-the-board dealings could also activate the legal machinery."

The Indian Express—May 8, 1998. This article goes on to note the men who want to buy Viagra have deposited as much as 3000 rupees (about $70) with their local pharmacy, the owners of which are demanding payment in advance. These sums of money are very large amounts for many poor Indians.

Mumbai, July 22 [1998]: "Till two months back Deepak Lalwani introduced himself to people as a chemical exporter. Today he runs a flourishing business in the sale of the wonder pill Viagra, but doesn't tell anybody about it. Only eight more people and a few contacts at the airport and in the market know about it. Together they form the Viagra cartel in Mumbai, which in its precision of operation and brutality in dealing with 'irritants' could beat any of the underworld gangs."

The Indian Express—July 22, 1998. This article goes on to note that the cartel spends more than 3,000,000 rupees every week keeping people quiet at the airport. On May 17, 1998 Viagra became available in Saudi Arabia at the price of $80 per pill, roughly eight times its cost in the United States. These pills were being smuggled from Britain and Taiwan and through Egypt. "According to pharmacy sources quantities of Viagra are brought in by travelers from Cairo and sold at 200 to 300 riyals ($53–$80) a pill."

ArabiaLiving—May 17, 1998. While diet pills and abortion pills (e.g., RU486) have been smuggled into the Middle East before, it was just a matter of time before Viagra was added to the list of these agents.

The Korea Herald—May 6, 1998. "Smuggled into the country mostly by vendors and travelers, the medicine is selling at around 30,000 won (some $22) a pill at Itaewon and Namdaemun markets in Seoul . . . As the demand for the drug soared, some Koreans returning home from their U. S. trips were found hiding the bottles in their bags, disguising them as vitamins or dietary supplements. According to reports, post offices found about 40 bottles shipped illegally into the country in just one week, last month."

Cairo, May 19 [1998]: "Egyptian police and health ministry officials are confiscating illegally imported bottles of the impotence drug Viagra from the drug stores, the Associated Press said . . .

Until this happens [approval from the health minister], health inspectors and police will continue raiding pharmacies and confiscating the drug, which has been smuggled into Egypt and has been illegally sold on the streets and in clinics."

ArabiaLiving—May 19, 1998. *"Viagra In Lebanon, Terrorizes Woman."* Beirut. "A 35-year-old wife, terrorized by her husband's sudden 'savage' behavior, rushed to the police, complaining that he attempted to kill her . . . According to An Nahar newspaper today, the wife, identified only by her first name Beatrice, said her 59-year-old husband Antoine, who recently returned from the United States, wanted to make love to her 'while he was in a state of extreme excitement never seen before.' Beatrice said he treated her 'savagely' to the extent that she had to go to the hospital to treat 'wounds in her breast.'"

ArabiaLiving—June 25, 1998. *"Kuwaiti Died, Viagra Overdose."* Kuwait. "A Kuwaiti national has died from an overdose of the anti-impotence pill Viagra in what was the Gulf's first recorded death from the US wonder drug, a newspaper said Sunday. The unidentified man was found dead at his home lying next to a box of the pills, the Al-rai Al-aam Daily said."

ArabiaLiving—August 23, 1998. Different cultures attribute different meanings to masculine sexual performance. When Viagra became available, it had important repercussions throughout much of the world.

had fulfilling experiences exploring other avenues of intimacy. With Viagra available, still other couples are again considering the place of intercourse in their relationship, sometimes after a number of years (Steinhauer, 1998). As discussed throughout this book, good sex and good relationships require more than quick arousal and good orgasms.

Because a woman's clitoris becomes engorged with blood during sexual arousal just like a man's penis, researchers have considered whether Viagra might benefit women with disorders of arousal. Anatomical similarity between these two structures doesn't necessarily mean that this drug will act in the same way for women and men. As of this writing, no large-scale, systematic investigations of this question have supported the effectiveness for women.

Surgical Treatments for Erectile Dysfunction

The most radical and irreversible treatments for erectile dysfunction involve the insertion of semi-rigid rods or expandable plastic cylinders inside a man's penis (Fig. 15-15). These are referred to as **penile implants.** This surgery cannot be reversed, so it is important to try all other approaches to therapy before proceeding. Some urologists recommend that a man considering one of these procedures consult with a sex therapist, and ideally with his partner, before deciding to have the operation. When impotence is due to the removal of the prostate gland or the destruction of nerves along the floor of the pelvis due to the effects of uncontrolled diabetes, these surgical alternatives often offer the patient excellent enhancement in quality of life, good erectile ability, and enjoyable sexual intercourse. With the availability of drugs like Viagra, however, these procedures are being performed less often.

Semi-rigid rods made of silicone take the place of both corpora cavernosa. They are manufactured in different lengths and diameters. It is unusual for a man to have any problems with this approach once the rods have been implanted, however, because these rods never get shorter or smaller, it is difficult for some men to conceal their presence. A more natural alternative is the inflatable penile prosthesis. Two expandable cylinders made of polyurethane or silicone replace the corpora cavernosa. A reservoir of fluid is im-

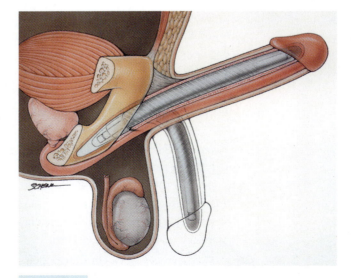

FIGURE 15-15   Semi-rigid silicone rods are one type of penile implant used in the surgical treatment of erectile dysfunction.

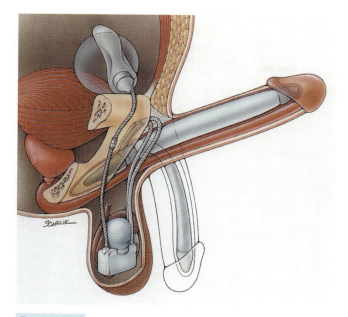

<figure>FIGURE 15-16 The inflatable penile prosthesis. Note the pump located in the scrotum and the fluid reservoir behind the pubic bone.</figure>

planted near the bladder, and a pump to transfer the fluid back and forth between the cylinders and the reservoir is placed in the scrotum. Figure 15-16 illustrates these components and their location in the body. Different designs have been manufactured, most with a record of high reliability. By gently grasping the pump inside his scrotum, the man can pump fluid from the reservoir into the cylinders, making them expand and causing his penis to become erect. He can then close a valve in this pump, causing the fluid in the cylinders to stay there. This causes an erection adequate for intercourse. After intercourse, the man releases the valve, allowing fluid to flow out of the cylinders and back into the reservoir. One recent report notes that after being in place for a period of 5 years, only 5% of such devices have a mechanical failure. The overwhelming majority of patients who receive this type of penile prosthesis are completely satisfied with it (Lewis, 1995).

OTHER PSYCHOTHERAPEUTIC APPROACHES TO SEX THERAPY

In addition to cognitive-behavioral and medical approaches to the treatment of sexual dysfunctions, many different kinds of professionals do sex therapy and use a variety of techniques and approaches. The two-therapist strategy is no longer very popular. Psychiatrists, clinical psychologists, licensed clinical social workers, licensed professional counselors, nurses, the clergy, and even primary care physicians provide treatment as

well. All of these professions recognize the importance of good sex education and a focus on behavioral change rather than deep emotional restructuring. Virtually none of these professionals observes the couple sharing sexual intimacy, and all rely on the client's verbal reports of their behaviors, thoughts, and feelings about this area of their lives.

Additionally, all professionals doing sex therapy today recognize the importance of evaluating the client and her or his problems within a wider psychosocial context. Since the introduction of Masters and Johnson's dual therapist approach, a number of effective alternatives have emerged through the years. One-on-one individual therapy, group therapy, and even hypnosis have been used in the treatment of sexual dysfunctions, in addition to more traditional couple therapies. These may be used alone, in conjunction with cognitive-behavioral methods, or as a prelude or epilogue to them. The only therapeutic method rarely used anymore is the long-term depth approach known as Freudian psychoanalysis, which was virtually the only psychotherapeutic approach used for sexual dysfunctions before the publication of *Human Sexual Inadequacy* in 1970. It was highly ineffective, very expensive, and time consuming.

The Family Doctor

Many people turn with sexual concerns to their family doctor or gynecologist. Often, a few reassuring words from a health care professional go a long way toward putting someone at ease about situational or temporary sexual difficulties they might be having. Increasingly often, doctors are being trained in the basic facts of sexual dysfunctions and in home exercises couples can try to alleviate their problems or at least make them less troubling. For example, secondary impotence is often helped by telling the patient how common this problem is and by encouraging the patient to engage in foreplay without having intercourse for a period (Levitt, 1975). Similarly, the squeeze technique for premature ejaculation and the sensate-focus exercises used for it are easy to explain in a short period of time and offer the individual a place to start in trying to understand and deal with this particular sexual disorder. Anorgasmic women may also receive some authoritative encouragement to explore their sexual response cycle through masturbation and the use of a vibrator. Very often the *source* of information about sex is just as important as the information itself.

The Clergy

After the family doctor, the person someone with a sexual problem is most likely to consult is a clergyman. As Conklin (1997) writes, people often hear others say about personal problems, "Go talk to your minister" or "The priest may have a suggestion" or "Ask the rabbi" or "The chaplain can help" (p. 144). Yet these religious leaders usually did not receive in-depth, systematic training in human sexuality when they were preparing for their roles of spiritual leadership. Students in seminaries and theological schools may not know how much they need training in this area until after they have completed

Dear Dr. Ruth

Question:

When I was growing up, my parents told me that if I ever had a really troubling problem that I should discuss it with my minister. Well, I do have a big problem but doubt that my minister could help. My problem is that I do not always enjoy intercourse when my husband wants to make love. I am extremely doubtful that my minister could be helpful. In fact, he's an extremely moralistic man who doesn't seem to see much good in sex at all. Do you think I should go to him with my concern?

Answer:

I know that you are looking at your problem as a sexual one, but it actually may be a relationship issue that you are having with your husband. He may not be paying enough attention to your needs. Now let's say that instead of playing itself out in the sexual arena, the conflict that you may be having with your husband involved taking care of the children. That's something you could talk about with a minister. Well, your situation is really not much different.

But while your minister could probably help you with this issue, that's not to say that he's the best person to whom you should turn. If you see a sex therapist, once the problem is cured, you'll never see that therapist again, while your minister you will continue to see regularly, and perhaps you'd be uncomfortable with his knowing intimate details about your sex life. As well, just as not every sex therapist is right for every couple, some ministers may be able to handle some situations better than others.

I recommend that people see their religious leader for relationship issues. When a problem is purely sexual, then I recommend a sex therapist. Your problem falls somewhere in between, so it's really up to you.

their training. This means that when members of the congregation approach their religious leader with a sexual concern, the facts and counseling they receive may not be based on current, thorough, factually correct information or accepted counseling techniques. Hopefully, the clergy do not hesitate to refer members of their congregations to well-trained, licensed professionals. A sexually explicit curriculum for clerical students may be controversial in some instances while welcomed in others. Yet the clergy is more aware than ever before that their congregations are likely to approach them with concerns about sexual assault, abuse, AIDS, premarital intercourse, contraception, and infidelity. Faculties in seminaries and theological schools generally support curricula that include a sexual component (Conklin, 1997), while still acknowledging the spiritual, mystical aspects of this domain of human nature.

Group and Couple Therapy

Social and behavioral scientists have long known that some kinds of problems are effectively confronted and dealt with in a group format. Individuals with the same or similar problems meet to discuss their feelings and share their thoughts under the guidance of a therapist or facilitator. Group therapy is as effective as couple therapy in the treatment of certain sexual dysfunctions. Members of a group with the same or similar problems learn that they are not unique in their distress and feel less "abnormal." They are often reassured to find out that other people have the same problems they have. Golden, Price, Heinrich, and Lobitz (1978) compared two groups of couples in which the men were premature ejaculators and the women were anorgasmic. In the first group, the couple worked with a male and female cotherapist once each week for 3 months. In the second group, three or four couples were treated together in a group context led by the male and female cotherapist once each week for 3 months. Both groups of subjects showed significant improvement in dealing with their dysfunctions, and 2 months after the study ended there were no differences in progress made by the couples in the two groups. This is an important finding because group therapy is less expensive than couple therapy.

In another study, men with primary and secondary erectile dysfunctions were treated in two groups of 6 individuals. These men did not have a regular sexual partner when they participated in this study, which sought to improve their sexual self-confidence with women and to teach them skills in self-control that would allow them to attain and maintain an erection and participate in heterosexual intercourse (Lobitz & Baker, 1979). These subjects met for 90 minutes on 12 separate occasions. During these sessions the subjects were taught relaxation skills, were given homework assignments to be carried out with or without a partner depending on the subject's circumstances, saw films about treating premature ejaculation, and had the opportunity to discuss their dysfunction with a female therapist and receive feedback from her. Additionally, group sessions afforded the participants the chance to talk about their overall feelings about sexual issues. The therapeutic format in this study helped 5 men with secondary impotence and 1 man with primary impotence attain erections. The subjects in this study enjoyed improved sexual functioning. Again, data indicate that group therapy might be more cost-effective than couple therapy in the treatment of sexual dysfunctions. For several reasons, however, we cannot be fully certain about the effectiveness of group therapy for sexual problems (Shah, 1996). Rarely are all participants in groups similar at the beginning of the therapeutic intervention, so it is difficult to know whether all subjects benefit equally by taking part in the sessions. Further, it is unwise to make broad generalizations about the effectiveness of this treatment approach when sample sizes are so small. Finally, there just haven't been enough studies done on group therapies for sexual dysfunctions to state with certainty the benefits and inadequacies of this technique.

DOES SEX THERAPY WORK?

This chapter has described several different methods used in the treatment of sexual dysfunctions. Potential consumers should ask which work best, and someone considering going to a sex counselor or therapist should consider issues such as the following. With any social/behavioral/medical issue, however, what is right for *most people* may not be right for *all people.*

- Whether it's a man or a woman who has the dysfunction, most sexual disorders are best treated in the context of the couple's relationship, and if at all possible,

it's best to involve one's partner in treatment. If one's partner is unable to participate or refuses to do so, one person getting help is better than no one getting help. Therapy still can be effective in making the individual more aware of the causes, manifestations, and consequences of the sexual dysfunction.

- Except for those seeing two co-therapists who practice the Masters and Johnson method of sex therapy, most people likely are helped by a single therapist. Research indicates that working with a single therapist is no less effective in the long run than working with two co-therapists (Clement & Schmidt, 1983).

- Sexual problems often take quite some time to develop, so one shouldn't anticipate quick, easy cures, even though cognitive-behavioral approaches are often successful in brief, intensive formats. After beginning to enjoy improved sexual functioning, the couple should continue to practice the cognitive and behavioral strategies that helped them to make these gains.

- One should check the credentials and experience of a sex counselor or therapist. For extremely troubling and persistent sexual problems, a specialist in the area of human sexuality may be best. For brief, situational problems, however, a variety of competent professionals who do not specialize in the treatment of sexual dysfunctions may offer some good counsel and helpful homework assignments.

- When starting sex therapy, the physician or sex therapist should determine as quickly as possible whether the problem is organic or psychosocial. This will help determine the best treatment most quickly.

- Often sexual problems reflect difficulties in a relationship. A sex counselor or therapist may recommend some type of marriage or relationship counseling as a prelude to sex therapy or as an aspect of the therapy itself.

The Masters and Johnson model of sex therapy requires daily sessions over the course of two intensive weeks. Of course, most people with a sexual problem can't just drop everything for two weeks, so sex counselors and therapists have tried to determine whether weekly or even monthly sessions can help people improve sexual functioning. Generally speaking, weekly and sometimes monthly sessions are just as effective as the Masters and Johnson model in the long run. This is especially true when a number of relationship problems have to be worked through as part of the sex therapy (Carney, Bancroft, & Mathews, 1978).

The approaches described so far all involve the assistance of professionals, but many people also try self-help approaches. Men who are premature ejaculators have been helped significantly by written instructions used in conjunction with periodic telephone conversations with their therapist (Lowe & Mikulas, 1975). Similarly, anorgasmic women

TABLE 15-1

Reported Success Rates for the Treatment of Sexual Dysfunctions

Type of Sexual Dysfunction	Number of Cases	Failures	Successes	Success Rate
Primary impotence	51	17	34	66.7%
Secondary impotence	501	108	393	78.4%
Premature ejaculation	432	17	415	96.1%
Ejaculatory incompetence	75	18	57	76 %
Male Totals	1059	160	899	84.9%
Primary anorgasmia	399	84	315	79.0%
Situational anorgasmia	331	96	235	71.0%
Vaginismus	83	1	82	98.8%
Female Totals	813	181	632	77.7%
Combined Totals	1872	341	1531	81.8%

These data were compiled by Dr. Robert C. Kolodny (1981), a colleague of Masters and Johnson and were reprinted in O'Donohue, W., & Geer, J.H. (Eds.) (1993). Handbook of sexual dysfunctions. Assessment and treatment. Boston: Allyn and Bacon.

have shown some treatment benefits through the use of guided instruction in masturbation (McMullen & Rosen, 1979). Improvements in sexual functioning through self-help approaches support the premise that enhanced sexual functioning can result from therapies that do not explore the client's deep psychological issues but focus on the troubling symptoms themselves.

Because of the thoroughness of Masters and Johnson's research and their concern for effectiveness, the results of their work from 1959 to 1977 are significant (Table 15-1). These data are all based on the co-therapist approach applied in a 2-week intensive therapeutic format.

The data in Table 15-1 are specific to one method of sex therapy and one sample of subjects. Further, the criteria used by Masters and Johnson to diagnose these sexual dysfunctions may not be the same as those used by other investigators. For these and other reasons, different success rates might result with other diagnostic procedures, other samples, and other methods. Still, these data clearly reveal that most people who have a sexual dysfunction don't have to live with it if they seek some clinical assistance for their problem. Most can be helped.

SPECIAL CHALLENGES FACING GAYS AND LESBIANS WITH SEXUAL DYSFUNCTIONS

Anyone, regardless of sexual orientation, can develop a sexual dysfunction or incompatibility in the expression of intimacy. Although the therapeutic approaches for treating heterosexuals with these problems should theoretically be just as effective in therapy for gays, many homosexuals perceive a lack of access to sex therapy. Homosexual dysfunctions have not been explored as extensively as heterosexual dysfunctions, and it is difficult to know precisely how prevalent homosexual sexual disorders are. Additionally, much less is known about sexual dysfunctions among lesbians than among gay men. Various responses have been reported associated with desire, arousal, and orgasm phase difficulties in gay men, but the use of different research methods makes it difficult to compare findings across the few studies that have been done (Reece, 1988). Secondary erectile disorders are the most commonly reported sexual dysfunction among gay men, and retarded ejaculation might be more prevalent among gay men than among heterosexuals.

Reece (1988) describes two desire stage problems that have been reported by gay men. Anal spasm is involuntary contractions of the anal musculature that makes penetration uncomfortable. In the other, disinterest in fellatio results from discomfort with semen and the odors associated with oral sex. Men who are averse to fellatio are also more likely to experience gagging. With both problems, the sex therapist can offer reassurance that the more frequently a person engages in these behaviors, the less unappealing they become. Reece also notes that the most commonly reported arousal stage dysfunction is men losing their erection when trying to penetrate their partner anally. Other men note that they lose erections while being stimulated orally or manually. In a casual sexual encounter a man who experiences delay in attaining an erection may be rebuffed by his prospective partner. Another factor that may contribute to the loss of an erection during attempted anal penetration is a concern about possibly hurting one's partner. Finally, because of the AIDS epidemic and the perceived imperative to practice safe sex, some gays intend to use condoms but have little experience with them. During the interruption in intimacy that is required to apply a condom, many gays lose their erections (as sometimes happens with heterosexuals too). With all these difficulties the couple would benefit from a more patient approach to sexual intimacy and knowing one's partner well.

The techniques used to treat these dysfunctions in heterosexuals should be as effective when used with gays. The squeeze technique is effective for gay men too. Reece notes that sexual inexperience may be a significant problem occurring more commonly in gay men than heterosexual men. When a man comes out of the closet he may be well into early or even middle adulthood and have little or no experience with other men. These individuals may be dealing with ambivalence, anxiety, or even shame during their homosexual encounters. This awkwardness may become obvious in desire, arousal, or orgasm stage interactions with another man.

Treating sexual dysfunctions in gay men requires that the counselor or therapist take account of the client's sexual value system, just as with heterosexual men. For men who experience anal spasms during penetration, therapists recommend the insertion of dildos progressively larger in circumference as is done in treating women for vaginismus. Similarly, in treating men who are averse to fellatio, the behavior most commonly engaged in by gay men, the client often needs to give himself permission to participate in these activities and try to minimize any guilt that may be behind his dislike for this avenue of sexual expression and sharing. In treating arousal phase problems in gay men, sensate focus exercises are also appropriate and are frequently effective in restoring erectile ability for men who have been diagnosed with secondary erectile disorder. Reece also recommends that men who lose their erection while trying to apply a condom might benefit by experimenting with condoms during masturbation. This is another use of the process of successive approximation described earlier. Finally, orgasm stage dysfunctions in gay men seem especially difficult to treat successfully. While these men respond well to guidance for dealing with premature ejaculation, a longer period of patient therapy is often required for retarded ejaculation. Non-demand intimate pleasuring followed later on by vigorous manual stimulation of the penis often helps with this problem.

Much less is known about sexual dysfunctions among lesbians than among gay men; however, Nichols (1988) raised some interesting issues concerning a common sexual problem in lesbians: low sexual desire. This writer suggests that females are more likely to be sexually abused than males and that because of this, the likelihood of one person in a lesbian relationship having been abused is substantially larger than in heterosexual relationships (Becker, 1993). Lesbian women who have been sexually abused are most likely to report low sexual desire in adulthood. For them, cognitive-behavioral approaches may be less important than helping the client better understand the impact of the abuse on the development of her sexuality and its effects on her current sexual functioning. The term "lesbian bed death" has been used to describe long-term lesbian relationships in which both partners have apparently stopped having sexual interactions and seem to be comfortable with this (Hill, 1996). In cases like these, the sex therapist should ascertain whether the asexual bond causes either partner distress and should not advocate a return to physical intimacy if the couple is comfortable the way they are.

Those who have studied sexual dysfunctions in gays and lesbians have noted that homophobia may contribute to a diminished capacity for desire, arousal, or orgasm. Homophobia includes self-loathing with regard to one's own homosexuality. This can certainly contribute to feelings of anxiety and ambivalence in same-sex intimate interactions. This element is not likely to be resolved through cognitive-behavioral approaches to sex therapy but probably requires more in-depth psychotherapeutic evaluation. As discussed in Chapter 9, lesbians are more likely than gay men to initiate and maintain long-term, exclusive sexual relationships, and gay men are more likely to have more partners in transient sexual encounters. This difference may impact the effectiveness of sex counseling or therapy for these populations.

CONCLUSION

From time to time, depending on one's life, everyone may experience a sexual dysfunction. One's health and personal circumstances may contribute to the development of such problems. Premature ejaculation happens to virtually all men at one time or another, as does situational erectile dysfunction. Most women do not regularly and reliably have orgasms, even when they are with someone whom they love, trust, and know very well. Additionally, a variety of drugs and medications can foster the development of sexual dysfunctions. Nonetheless, few people overall need to receive sex therapy or even talk to a professional about a sexual problem. But when these problems become persistent and significantly impair a person's self-esteem and/or the quality of a relationship, seeking the services of an experienced sex counselor or therapist is often a good idea.

The next chapter addresses the impact of organic illnesses, mental retardation, trauma, and disability on sexual functioning. While the problems discussed in this and the previous chapter are usually reversible and people who receive sex therapy can expect some improvement in sexual arousal and response, those with more serious psychological or medical problems cannot always expect similarly optimistic outcomes. *There is still much that can be done,* however, as we will see in the next chapter.

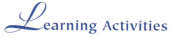

*L*earning Activities

1. Speculate as to how long a person might experience a sexual dysfunction before she or he seeks professional assistance. How bad or disruptive do you think the problem has to get before the individual is motivated

to explore therapeutic options? Why do you think some people never try to do something about a sexual dysfunction?

2. Suggest ways that a sex counselor or therapist might put a client or clients at ease during a first visit. What professional behaviors strike a balance between being too formal and too informal?

3. If you have ever seen an X-rated movie, do you think it creates expectations of sexual performance that may be difficult or impossible to meet and, therefore, foster feelings of sexual inadequacy? If so, how? On the other hand, do you think that viewing these can serve as an ice-breaker for couples who are hesitant to experiment and explore sexual behaviors?

4. Based on what you have observed about female and male gender differences, would the female or male member of a couple be more influential in the decision to seek professional assistance for sexual problems? Why?

5. What might be some reasons that sensate-focus exercises are so helpful in assisting a couple to attend selectively to their bodies and their feelings during physical stimulation? Explain how these exercises are an example of successive approximation.

6. People receiving counseling or therapy for some psychological disorders frequently find it difficult to terminate treatment when their therapist thinks it is time to do so. Do you think this also occurs with sex therapy? Why or why not?

7. We discussed the controversial practice of partner surrogates in sex therapy. Under what circumstances might partner surrogates serve an important function in sex therapy? How do you think *your* community would react if it became known that a local sex therapy clinic was using partner surrogates? Why?

8. Recall that a person's sexual value system (SVS) is the sum of all things that have erotic meaning for that individual. Because our SVS is such an important part of our self-concept, it is important to try to learn more about it. Here are some open-ended questions to help you to clarify the elements of your SVS. Remember, there are no "right" or "wrong" answers.

   a. What developmental experiences during your childhood and/or adolescence do you feel influenced the development of your SVS?

   b. Give some of examples of how social and cultural factors have affirmed or repudiated the normality of your SVS?

   c. Do you think a person can change their SVS? Should this be one of the goals of sex therapy?

9. If one person in a couple was having an extramarital affair because of unsatisfactory intimacy within their marriage, should a sex counselor or therapist require that the individual reveal the relationship as a condition of con-

tinuing with therapy? Why or why not?

10. Much has been written in the popular press about drugs for the treatment of erectile dysfunction. We have emphasized that these drugs are ideally used in the context of a committed, loving relationship. Under what circumstances would you see some usefulness for these agents when a person is not involved in such a relationship?

11. Of the sexual dysfunctions we have discussed, hypoactive sexual desire and sexual aversion are the most difficult to treat. Why do you think this is so?

Key Concepts

- The dual sex therapist approach developed by Masters and Johnson involves male and female co-therapists working with a client couple.

- Cognitive-behavioral approaches to sex therapy emphasize the importance of the client's thoughts and feelings and the impact they have on sexual behavior. This strategy de-emphasizes old, possibly repressed memories and their potential impact on sexual desire, arousal, and response.

- Masters and Johnson developed a number of sensate focus techniques in which couples engage in nonintercourse, nondemand physical pleasuring. These exercises encourage a couple to approach intercourse gradually, in small, rewarding steps, without feeling they have to proceed promptly to penetration and pelvic thrusting. Sensate focus exercises create a relaxed, intimate sexual climate.

- The PLISSIT approach to sex therapy includes the main common ingredients of different strategies of treating dysfunctions. P stands for *permission,* which involves validating the client's thoughts, emotions, and sexual activities. LI refers to *limited information,* which involves the provision of simple facts. SS stands for *specific suggestions,* which usually involves homework assignments the couple can work on privately. And IT stands for *intensive therapy,* which involves a more systematic and prolonged approach to the dysfunction and ways of treating it.

- Positive reinforcement strengthens the behavior that follows it. These events are often interpreted as rewards.

- In contrast to positive reinforcement, negative reinforcement is the good feeling one has when a bad feeling stops. This cessation of discomfort, anxiety, or embarrassment can be very rewarding.

- Successive approximation means that learning takes place in small steps, each of which is reinforced, and each of which gets closer to some goal. This is sometimes referred to as systematic desensitization, in the context of psychological therapies in which an individual experiences diminished arousal to an anxiety-provoking stimulus over time.

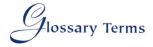lossary Terms

AASECT

basilar squeeze
  technique

coital alignment
  technique

coronal squeeze
  technique

ejaculatory
  inevitability

hypogonadism

penile implants

vasodilators

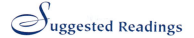uggested Readings

Barbach, L. (1976). For yourself: The fulfillment of female sexuality. Garden City, New York: Anchor.

Charlton, R. S., & Yalom, I. D. (Eds.) (1996). Treating sexual disorders. San Francisco: Jossey-Bass.

Crowe, M., & Ridley, J. (1990). Therapy with couples: A behavioural systems approach to marital and sexual problems. Maldon, MA: Blackwell Science Inc.

Kaplan, H. S. (1989). How to overcome premature ejaculation. New York: Brunner/Mazel.

Kaplan, H. S., & Passalacqua, D. (1988). Illustrated manual of sex therapy. New York: Brunner/Mazel.

Rosen, R. C., & Leiblum, S. R. (1995). Case studies in sex therapy. New York: Guilford Press.

Spence, S. H. (1991). Psychosexual therapy: A cognitive-behavioral approach. New York: Chapman & Hall.

Wincze, J. P., & Carey, M. P. (1991). Sexual dysfunction: A guide for assessment and treatment. New York: Guilford Press.

Wylie, K. R. (1997). Treatment outcome of brief couple therapy in psychogenic male erectile disorder. Archives of Sexual Behavior, 26, 527–545.

16

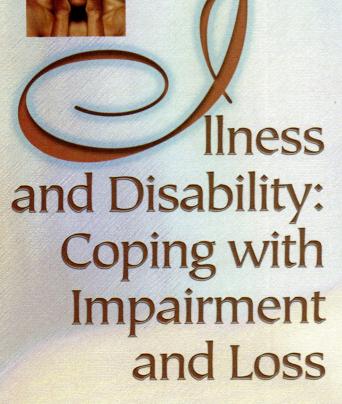

Illness and Disability: Coping with Impairment and Loss

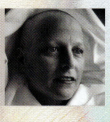

OBJECTIVES

When you finish reading and reviewing this chapter, you should be able to:

1. Describe the medical model and discuss its limitations in the study of sexual expression by people who are ill or disabled.

2. Summarize the characteristics of the "sick person" role and explain how it affects a person's ability and inclination to deal with limitations imposed by their illness.

3. Review the effects of illness and disability on close personal relationships and a person's self-concept and self-esteem.

4. Explain the link between the cognitive and emotional effects of illness and note the impact of these on the desire to remain sexually active.

5. Summarize ways in which individuals can continue to enjoy sexual expression when afflicted with heart disease, stroke, cancer, diabetes, kidney diseases, arthritis, ostomy surgery, amputation, spinal cord injuries, cerebral palsy, multiple sclerosis, or Alzheimer's disease.

6. Summarize the cognitive, emotional, and behavioral manifestations of mental retardation and discuss their impact on a person's desire to engage in consensual sexual activity.

7. Enumerate the educational, interpersonal, and legal challenges in teaching the mentally retarded about contraception and in facilitating their consistent compliance with recommendations.

8. Discuss some of the unique challenges facing visually impaired and hearing impaired people who wish to establish intimate relationships and engage in sexual activities.

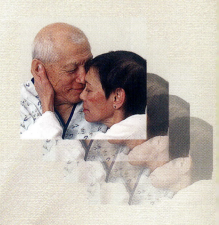

From Dr. Ruth

You can't have gotten this far in our book without knowing we believe sexual enjoyment isn't just for thin, young, attractive people. Sexual enjoyment and responsiveness are a birthright for all of us. But illness, injuries, and disabilities can affect a person's desire and ability to be a sexual being.

Even when they are healthy, most people have trouble talking about their sexual desires and the sexual behaviors they enjoy. When people are sick, injured, or disabled they are often even more hesitant to ask about how they can still enjoy a rich sex life. Society doesn't think much about a person's strong desire to remain sexual when these things happen. Heart disease, cancer, and diabetes are very common, but do people with these conditions just quit thinking about sex? Absolutely not! The same is true for people with many other health problems.

Although this chapter describes some unfortunate illnesses and disabilities, the emphasis will be on how people can continue to enjoy an interesting and exciting sex life despite health problems. If you ever have any of these conditions, we hope you'll find this book in your family library for the inspiration and advice you might need then.

It's a simple fact of life that people often become ill and sometimes incapacitated, sometimes later in life and sometimes earlier. The central point of this chapter is that the problems associated with chronic illness, short-term illness, and disability need not end the sexual dimension of one's life. Many people continue to place a very high premium on their sexuality when they are ill and infirm. When a person is sick and frightened and feels bad, there is nothing like the intimate, caring touch and support of a loved one. Sharing sexual intimacy is just one way in which sick and disabled people maintain a feeling of connection to their spouses or partners, and indeed to the entire human race.

This chapter begins by examining the medical model of illness and disability. The **medical model** generally views illness and abnormality as amenable to diagnosis and treatment by physicians using the many interventions at her or his disposal: medication, surgery, physical therapy, and so on. Yet this perspective may not be the most useful for understanding continued sexual expression among sick and disabled people. We will also examine some of the confining characteristics of the "sick role" people often feel they must play when they are unwell. The first part of this chapter focuses on many psychological and sociological aspects of being sick and resisting the negative stereotypes of sick people. Then we examine a number of physiological and developmental illnesses and disabilities and ways in which people manage to stay active sexually despite their infirmities. Some of these are serious or life-threatening conditions, while others are more easily treated and cured. Some, unfortunately, are incurable,

and the best one can hope for is the best possible adaptation to the limitations caused by the ailment. We will also consider mental retardation and sexual expression and explore the rights of these individuals to enjoy their sexuality. This discussion will lead us to some of the challenges regarding contraception and sexual consent among people who might not have the psychological capacity to make foresightful judgments for themselves.

One should be optimistic and open-minded about all these topics. The study of sexual expression among the ill and disabled is a large, active area of research, and many scientists and professionals are actively studying these challenges and devising ways to restore sexual functioning as much as possible under many different circumstances. Although students in a course in human sexuality seldom expect to consider these types of topics, they are an intrinsic aspect of sexuality for human beings.

THE MEDICAL MODEL OF ILLNESS AND DISABILITY

Because illness and disability are by their very nature medical problems, people often focus too closely on physiological issues and neglect the functioning of the affected individual in their wider psychosocial environment and ongoing intimate relationships. Although the medical model is useful in the health care professions, the focus on symptoms, syndromes, diseases, diagnosis, authoritative physicians, passive patients, and physical impairments might lead to overlooking crucial issues of the patient's *quality of life*. This is a central challenge in the disciplines of rehabilitative medicine and physical therapy. While health care professionals often talk about getting the patient "back on their feet," they frequently do not mention anything about resumed sexual intimacy with their spouse or significant other. Healing the body while neglecting the psyche does not generally promote such restoration.

The Role of the "Sick Person" in our Culture

We often behave towards others on the basis of the characteristics we think they have rather than on the basis of characteristics they might *really have*. Many of us attribute passivity, lack of interest, slow movement, and an inability to enjoy life to people who are sick or disabled. Similarly, we often assume that sick people cannot take care of their responsibilities while they are ill or in treatment. These attributions can be especially apparent when a person is ill for a long time and there is little hope for substantial recovery. Yet often these attributions are wrong, and we need to examine carefully the person's thoughts, feelings, and actions in the psychosocial networks in which they live and work.

The term "sexual self-schema" has been used to describe a person's sexual self-concept (Anderson, Woods, & Cyranowski, 1994). The term schema means something like "image" or "general type." This term is used to summarize a person's thoughts about their sexuality and variables (e.g., physical attractiveness) that contribute to it. These writers emphasize that events in a person's past often affect how they view their sexuality and how they evaluate sexual information in their psychosocial environment. Anderson, Woods, and Cyranowski developed a paper-and-pencil test to evaluate subjects' sexual self-schemas. In general, one's sexual self-schema has two positive aspects and a negative one. The two positive aspects include the individual's desire to explore romantic and/or passionate feelings and an interest in venturing into different sexual behaviors and relationships in which they are likely to occur. The negative aspect is a person's feelings of embarrassment and hesitancy or shame related to sexual experience and expression. They explored responses among young, healthy women and the impact of cancer on a woman's sexual self-schema. They predicted that when a woman's sexual self-schema was more negative before she was diagnosed with cancer, she would be at a high risk for developing sexual problems after the diagnosis and during treatment. That is just what they found (Anderson, Woods, & Copeland, 1997).

When we see individuals who do not conform to our own sexual self-schema, we sometimes make the attribution of illness or disability when in fact the afflicted individual may be functioning quite well in many spheres of their life (Fig. 16-1). The Independent Living Movement, however, has changed people's attitudes about the medical model and the "sick role." Centers for Independent Living began in California in the late 1960s and early 1970s and are found all over the United States today. The Independent Living Movement is a product of the civil rights movement, self-help movements, holistic approaches to health care, and growing consumer activism in the United States. These organizations have described the unattractive attributes of the sick role. Note that the phrase "sick people" can refer to highly variable degrees of impaired health and physical functioning. Following are attributions common in our society:

1. "Sick" people don't have to engage in everyday social activities because they are ill. They don't have to meet their responsibilities or obligations.
2. "Sick" people have had nothing at all to do with becoming ill, nor are they accountable for any behaviors that may have contributed to their ailment. Sick people are not expected to "pull themselves together" and get well.
3. "Sick" people are supposed to accept the idea that being ill is abnormal and unacceptable and to do everything they can to recover. Refusing recommended treatments are always considered to be unacceptable patient noncompliance.
4. "Sick" people *need* the assistance and technical expertise of medical professionals to recover.
5. "Disabled" individuals are expected to accept the permanence of their impairments and accept unquestioningly the dependency characteristic of all disabilities.

Centers for Independent Living were founded because of the perceived dehumanization of the medical model and confining characteristics of the sick and disabled roles that people are expected to play. Yet consider how difficult it would be for a person to maintain a positive sexual self-concept if they subscribed to the five beliefs above.

Although many sick people are genuinely incapacitated or disabled by their ailments, this situation doesn't always last for very long, and many people work hard to make the best recovery they can in their circumstances. Recovery, cure, and improvement are all powerfully affected by a person's state of mind and their thoughts when they are sick or incapacitated.

Who supports people in their efforts to retain or regain their capacity for sexual expression? Hopefully, a wide variety of friends, family, and professionals. However, restoring sexual functioning after illness or disability is not always part of the training of doctors, nurses, psychologists and other behavioral scientists, and social workers. What a person thinks about their predicament and what they can do to get well or better as soon as possible involves a private internal dialogue that might be extremely important for the individual's recovery. All avenues of treatment and rehabilitation take place against the background of these thoughts and emotions. While people cannot be told how to "think themselves well," the more information they have about their circumstances, the more likely they will be to make the most of a bad situation.

The Restoration of Sexual Expression

Health care providers and family members need to know about several issues when working with people who are sick or disabled. These broad perspectives concern both those affected by

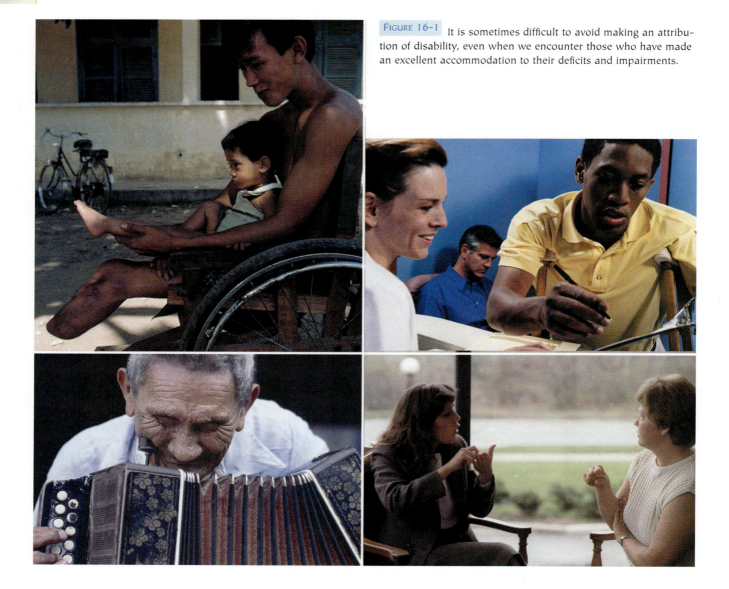

FIGURE 16-1   It is sometimes difficult to avoid making an attribution of disability, even when we encounter those who have made an excellent accommodation to their deficits and impairments.

illness and those who care for them. Woods (1984) summarized these issues in terms of the many different roles family members and health care professionals must play.

Facilitating a Milieu Conducive to Sexual Health. This refers to the general psychosocial environment in which the patient lives, comprised of their private thoughts, as well as the influence of their family, friends, and wider social networks. It is important for the client to experience as little guilt or anxiety as possible in connection with their changed health status. Ironically, for some people this might involve their first really candid exploration of their sexuality. The nature of the patient's lifestyle and sexual value system prior to their injury or illness is the baseline against which future plans and recommendations are made.

Providing Anticipatory Guidance. Recovery, even if limited, usually involves a series of stages of which the patient should be aware. These depend somewhat on the age of the

patient. Adolescents may be curious about the impact of their circumstances on their menstrual cycle, masturbation, or wet dreams, while people at mid-life generally have entirely different concerns and anxieties. Continued sexual expression, delayed sexual arousal, and menopause are different clusters of issues that may make older patients uncertain or apprehensive.

Reassuring Patients That They Are Normal Under the Circumstances. A person's perspective on what is "normal" changes when they are seriously ill or disabled. A new lifestyle is hard to get used to, especially when it affects the way we feel or act sexually. This involves two somewhat different agendas. Appropriate treatments must be initiated promptly, but helping the patient function optimally in their current circumstances is essential as well. Discomfort, moodiness, anxiety, and feelings of helplessness and vulnerability are never easy to deal with but are normal for people who are sick or disabled. Family members may discount the patient's sexual thoughts and desires as "unwholesome" for a sick or disabled person. Patients often want to talk about new avenues of sexual behavior as a result of their condition and need to be reassured that they are entirely normal.

Education Always Helps. Good teaching involves much more than conveying information. A person who is being treated for an illness or disability or is recovering usually appreciates it when others share facts, concepts, and principles related to their circumstances, especially when this information is offered in an encouraging, optimistic way that motivates the individual to learn more and be personally involved in their own recovery. This can be especially challenging when the patient has an unrealistic perspective about the progress they expect to make.

Woods (1984) emphasized that it is often beneficial to discuss possible changes in sexual functioning *before* therapeutic procedures, such as surgery. Under most circumstances, doctors will not withhold information about a patient's health, and candid professional opinion sensitively offered is in the highest traditions of ethical medical practice.

Counseling Patients Can Be Very Helpful. In addition to giving a patient information about their illness or disability, often counseling helps a person come to grips with future limitations in their sexual expression. Good counseling begins with a patient feeling comfortable admitting that they want help and setting objectives with their counselor (Fig. 16-2). Without these goals, counseling may not have a purpose or direction. A benefit of counseling is that it usually gives patients an arena in which they can express their deepest fears, anxieties, and worries without feeling that they are being judged or thought to be weak.

Overall, a number of important issues related to a patient's recovery and continued sexual expression are considered by health care providers. It isn't enough to just treat the body, and psychosocial support is often necessary and highly beneficial for the patient.

The Impact of Illness and Disability on Relationships

Any interruption, change, or permanent loss in the ability to become sexually aroused and responsive adds a depressing dimension to one's illness or disability. Many important interpersonal changes inevitably occur to some degree in sickness or disability.

Changes in Interpersonal Communication. When one isn't feeling well or can't get around as they used to, they frequently don't work as hard to be a good friend, spouse, or listener. Many people keep to themselves and may act like they're feeling sorry for themselves. But others find it difficult to help someone who is acting this way, much less reach out to talk about their deeper feelings and fears.

Expressing Emotions. Not everyone has the ability to express their emotions with equal ease. Some people feel ashamed of saying that they're scared about something or worried about what might happen or how they'll adjust to some discomfort or loss. Freud taught us that people often feel better about their fears and anxieties if they have the chance to

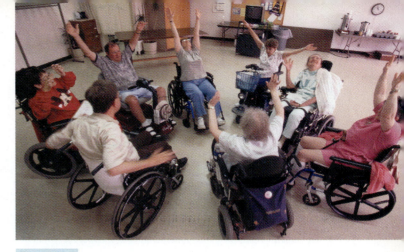

FIGURE 16-2 Counseling and support groups often help those with disabilities make a positive, productive accommodation to their handicap. Social support, emotional encouragement, and physical activity are all aspects of this type of care.

talk about them. The loss or interruption of sexual activity deserves this opportunity for good communication with one's doctor or spouse.

Feelings of Dependency. Not very many people feel good about having to depend on someone else to meet some or all of their most basic needs in life. This can be a very helpless feeling. Independence is an important value in our culture, developed through most of our childhood and adolescent years. One of the hardest things about getting old or becoming ill is sometimes suddenly finding oneself in a situation in which one is as reliant on others as when an infant or child.

Changes in Body Image. This book has often referred to the important relationship between self-esteem and body image. For many people, feelings of self-worth and attractiveness depend on how they think they look to other people. Our body image changes throughout our lives (Fig. 16-3). Being sick or disabled changes one's body image, and disfigurement may permanently affect one's self-perceptions.

Initiating Physical Intimacy. Many people have difficulty making sexual gestures when so many emotional and physical changes are occurring. Problems in communication, having trouble expressing emotions, feeling reliant on others, and a poor perception of one's attractiveness make it difficult for a person to feel spontaneous and self-confident about initiating sex.

Separating the Mental From the Emotional

When trying to cope and deal with illness and disability, our thoughts may be powerfully affected by our emotions. People who are ill need to understand this and make some allowances. How we deal with the facts and day-to-day physical realities of our illness does not always involve rational, clear thinking. Anxiety and fear powerfully distort a person's ability to see things as they are instead of the way they want them to be.

In the best circumstances, sexual information and recommendations and new approaches to sexual expression should be presented in a way that their emotional meaning is both

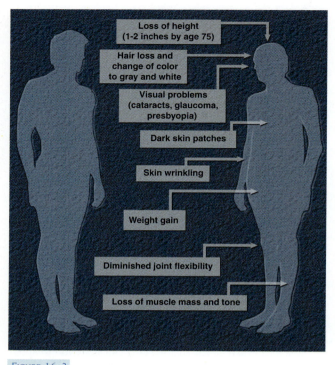

FIGURE 16-3   Inevitable physical changes accompany the normal aging process, although these are not all equally apparent in all aging and elderly individuals.

convincing and direct. Many sick people need "permission" to continue to feel that sex is important in their lives. But if this encouragement is too clinical, formal, or objective, it doesn't seem very real, especially when the patient has trouble communicating about sex in the first place.

Illness and Sexuality in Development

Just as sexual behavior in later life can be predicted by sexual behavior earlier in life (as discussed in Chapter 13), sexual behavior during or after the onset of illness or disability is related to and must be assessed in terms of the patient's sexual behavior before the illness or disability.

Many people later in life have lost some of their youthful interest in sex long before they became ill or disabled. Until health care professionals fully understand the patient's baseline of sexual behavior, it is difficult to talk about what would be an improvement or restoration of a previously established pattern and frequency of sexual behavior. Furthermore, health problems might actually give some people a justification for diminishing the place of sexuality in their marriage or relationship. Before talking about adjusting to illness and disability and finding avenues of sexual expression, helpers must first understand the place of sex in the person's earlier life.

When people become ill or disabled, they typically become depressed. A common symptom of depression is a loss of sexual interest, which happens even when people are not physically ill or debilitated. Depression often involves emo-

tional isolation, lack of initiative, and a loss of enjoyment in doing the things the person used to like to do. Together with the fact that the friends and family of the afflicted individual are also frequently depressed, the psychosocial context of illness is anything but conducive to continued, enjoyable sexual expression. Depression can be brief and transient or prolonged and debilitating. Depressed people usually have problems with motivation and energy that may make it difficult for the person to even consider exploring ways to adjust to illness or disability and restore some sexual functioning. Depression can be treated with medication, but this does not restore the loss that led to the depression in the first place, and sometimes side effects of antidepressants can cause sexual dysfunctions. Depression can also seem like a contagious disease; when one person is depressed, those close to that individual often become depressed too.

Balancing Benefits and Losses

The patient's personal evaluation of the gains and losses associated with various treatment strategies involves decision making with long-term or even permanent consequences. Discussions with one's physician, spouse, partner, and family often involve an open analysis of the drawbacks of medical intervention in terms of the person's body image, self-esteem, and sexual functioning. Often, patients select treatments for diseases in consultation with their doctor even though they may not be as immediately effective as more radical, invasive approaches. For example, men with prostate cancer may be offered a number of treatments depending on the size and location of the tumor and how quickly it is growing. "Watchful waiting" involves only monitoring the disease closely at regular intervals. This approach is often taken with men in their 70s or with tumors that do not appear to be growing very rapidly. Other treatments are radiation treatments or the implanting of radioactive particles in the prostate gland. Generally these alternatives do not significantly impair sexual functioning. Finally surgery may spare the nerves responsible for erection or may involve the removal of the entire gland and all the nerves running through it, thus eliminating a man's capacity to attain an erection without a penile prosthesis or using a drug, such as Viagra. This patient must make a difficult decision. He may have to choose between a few years of a higher quality of sexual functioning or a potentially shortened lifespan.

Women often face similar dilemmas. With a diagnosis of breast cancer, for example, the tumor may be one centimeter or less in diameter, and removing just the tumor (lumpectomy) may be as effective as a complete mastectomy in terms of the risk of the cancer recurring, especially if this procedure also includes chemotherapy. But what should a woman choose if her tumor is larger than one centimeter? A lumpectomy will leave her with normal appearing breasts and is not likely to affect her body image or sexual self-concept, but the decision not to have a mastectomy will increase the risk of the cancer coming back, even if she does have chemotherapy. Much depends upon the size of the tumor, whether it has spread to the lymph nodes, and the specific type of cancer.

Such decisions are difficult and irrevocable. A person's sexual value system affects much more than just treatment of sexual dysfunctions but is also involved in decisions they make regarding treatments for other serious illnesses. For the patient to be a full partner in exploring and discussing various therapies, the doctor must sometimes be prepared to manage treatment strategies with which they might disagree. Disease or treatment may leave the patient disabled, disfigured, or feeling that they have lost much of their sexual attractiveness, and in such cases the person may fear that they will be sexually rejected by their partner. Some patients report that they feel like something less than a complete human being. Support groups offer the opportunity to share their ideas and worries with other people who have the same or similar health problems, and this can be very helpful in fostering a sense of optimism and normality.

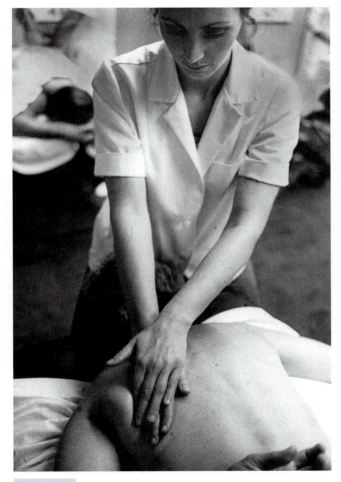

Figure 16-4 Therapeutic massage for those with spinal cord injuries is sometimes associated with sensual pleasure and relaxation. Here, a therapist applies tactile stimulation and pressure in order to foster restfulness and enhance well-being.

Enhancing Sexual Pleasure When Ill or Disabled

There are many interesting ways in which sexual awareness and pleasure can be enhanced or restored to some degree even in those who are severely incapacitated. For example, Chapter 15 describes sensate focus exercises, which involve sharing non-intercourse physical intimacy. Over a number of sessions couples gradually focus erotic touching and kissing on more sensitive areas of the body, including the genitals, breasts, and buttocks, beginning with less sensitive parts of the body. Even gentle touching and massage of less sensitive areas can yield erotic pleasure. If a person has lost some or all sensation in their genitals because of illness or disability, they can still enjoy the erotic feelings associated with touching or massaging other parts of their bodies (Fig. 16-4). About half of all people with spinal cord injuries report sexual arousal and sometimes orgasms when they are touched or massaged above the level of spinal injury even though they cannot feel genital stimulation. As discussed later, fantasy also can help precipitate orgasm in people with spinal cord injuries.

When genital feelings are diminished or eliminated altogether, patients can learn to "map" the non-genital areas of their bodies. They often find that stimulation of the neck and shoulders, ears, and breasts yields sexual pleasure and occasionally feelings similar to orgasm. Everyone has a personal erotic map based on their own, unique sexual experiences. For example, some people might find a gentle caress of their neck or gentle fondling of their thighs extremely exciting and arousing (Fig. 16-5). This book has emphasized throughout that there is much more to sex than having orgasms, and the ways in which sick and disabled individuals conceptualize their body surface shows the merit of this perspective.

Resistance to Reading About Sex in Illness and Disability

Many people think that the topics in this chapter have little to do with them. Perhaps life would be too depressing if we were preoccupied with all the bad things that *might* happen to us. Indeed, some social and behavioral scientists believe good mental health may include having false beliefs in our invincibility or assuming that we are healthier, happier, and more able than we might actually be. In fact, A book by Dr. Shelley Taylor, *"Positive Illusions: Creative Self-Deception and the Healthy Mind"* (1989), describes strategies we employ to see our world as rosier and safer than it is; in a very real sense we lie to ourselves about our vulnerabilities and inadequacies and the risks we run on a daily basis. According to Taylor and Armor (1996), our positive illusions usually involve having an enhanced self-image, being unrealistically optimistic, and feeling that we have more control over things than we really do. Nonetheless, cardiovascular disease, cancer, strokes, diabetes, kidney disease, arthritis, spinal cord injuries, disfiguring surgeries, amputation, multiple sclerosis, and Alzheimer's disease are all facts of life and part of the human condition. Even if we do not recognize our own potential to develop such problems, with some information about

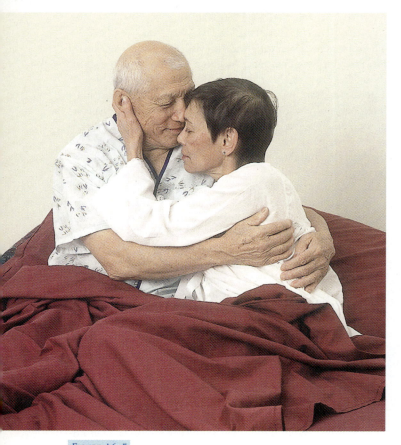

FIGURE 16-5   Many avenues of non-genital sensual pleasuring afford intimacy and nurturance to those who are ill, aging, or disabled.

them we can better understand the unspoken concerns of our friends, parents, and family members.

IMPACT OF ILLNESS AND DISABILITIES ON SEXUAL AROUSAL AND RESPONSE

Chapter 5 described some conditions and illnesses that may affect sexual arousal and response, as well as the important relationship between self-esteem and body image. In this chapter we examine adjustments that can be made in illness and disability to allow some degree of sexual functioning and enjoyment.

Young people generally view illness as *reversible:* we get sick, and then we get well. As people get older, however, illness takes a progressively *irreversible* toll, and with many illnesses we can no longer expect a full recovery to our pre-illness health status. Similarly, disabilities resulting from accidents may be permanent. Therefore, the following sections on diseases and disabilities also focus on how we can learn to live with health problems that may not be entirely curable or even amenable to medical or rehabilitative treatments.

Heart Disease

Heart disease is the number 1 cause of death in the United States. But not all people who have heart disease die from it. With early diagnosis and treatment a person can have a reasonably normal life. There are different forms of heart disease, with differing effects on sexual functioning. Because heart disease usually weakens a person's heart, exertion, sometimes even minor physical effort, can cause discomfort, weakness, shortness of breath, or other symptoms. People with heart disease often worry whether the physical effort involved in sexual intercourse can hurt their hearts or even cause a heart attack. In most instances, these worries are unfounded. People can make adjustments and still enjoy sexual activity.

For many decades physicians and physical therapists have known that heart rate, blood pressure, and breathing rate all increase during sexual activity. In healthy individuals, these measures return to normal relatively quickly after orgasm. Intercourse position also affects how physically demanding sexual intercourse is. Generally lying on one's back (the woman in the man-on-top position or the man in the woman-on-top position) involves less exertion and presumably less of an increase in heart rate, blood pressure, and breathing rate. These are important factors for people recovering from a heart attack or heart surgery.

PHYSICAL EFFECTS AND MANIFESTATIONS

The heart is a remarkably durable muscle that pumps blood, oxygen, and nutrients to every part of the body. Heart problems lead sooner or later to abnormalities in the workings of other organs. Heart disease is also associated with shortness of breath, chest pain, irregular heart rhythm, fatigue, and sometimes pain in other parts of the body, such as the upper arm, wrist, or jaw (called "referred pain"). Heart patients often tire easily and have low levels of energy and strength.

A common symptom of heart disease is an irregular heart beat, called an arrhythmia, which literally means "without rhythm." When the top chambers of the heart, the auricles, beat irregularly, one feels a fluttering sensation in our chest. A potentially more serious arrhythmia involves the lower chambers of the heart, the ventricles. Because sexual intercourse often involves physical exertion, people with heart disease often worry about an irregular heart rhythm. However, in a study of almost 90 men who had been diagnosed with coronary artery disease, none of whom were hospitalized, Drory, Fisman, Shapira, and Pines (1996) found that ventricular arrhythmias were not made worse during sexual intercourse but were usually very mild and similar to what occurs when the patient went about his daily activities. In fact, worrying about sex after a heart attack is a more significant factor in a patient losing interest in sex than medications they take or any lack of information about the safety of continued sexual expression (Rosal, Downing, Littman, & Ahern, 1994).

Advanced heart disease is associated with a marked drop in sexual interest and pronounced decrease in the frequency of sexual intercourse (Jaarsma, Dracup, Walden, & Stevenson,

Research Highlight

SEXUAL FANTASIES AND ORGASMS IN WOMEN

We have commented on the importance of a person's thought processes for sexual arousal and response. Some women can have orgasms without any genital physical stimulation at all. Touching other parts of the body, such as the breasts, or even fantasy alone may precipitate orgasms. An interesting research study explored the physiological measures of orgasms caused entirely through mental imagery. These data offer promise to those who for one reason or another cannot experience the sensations of genital stimulation. Whipple, Ogden, and Komisaruk (1992) studied 10 women between the ages of 32 and 67 who had reported in an interview that they were able to have orgasms without genital or other physical stimulation. The average age of the subjects in this study was just under 45 years. Seven of these women had regular periods, one had had a hysterectomy, and had gone through menopause. All had graduated from college or had some college experience.

A number of physiological measures were recorded during a period of self-induced sexual fantasies (during which they engaged in no physical self-stimulation at all) and a later period of genital self-stimulation. The subjects' heart rate, blood pressure, pupil diameter, pain detection threshold, and pain tolerance threshold were recorded and compared in the two experimental conditions. Between periods of mental imagery or self-stimulation the subjects rested for 5 minute periods, during which they did not engage in genital self-stimulation or sexual fantasies. During the self-stimulation periods women used manual genital touching, vibratory stimulation, or both together.

The women who engaged in sexual imagery and reported orgasm showed blood pressure increases similar to that seen during genital self-stimulation. Heart rate increases were comparable during self-induced sexual imagery and genital self-stimulation, and pupil dilation during orgasm was similar in the imagery and self-stimulation conditions. The detection of discomfort or tolerance for pain during orgasm was also similar in the imagery and genital self-stimulation conditions. Overall, the physiological aspects of orgasm are highly similar with self-induced erotic imagery and genital self-stimulation. This capacity to have orgasms without direct genital stimulation challenges the notion that the sexual response cycle requires this precipitating action.

1996). One-fourth of a sample of Dutch patients with advanced heart disease stopped having sexual relations altogether, and half of the 62 patients reported a notable decrease in the pleasure they took in sexual activity. Despite these changes in the intimacy patterns of these couples, however, few subjects reported any overall decline in the quality of their marriage. As with many other diseases, the more advanced the heart disease, the more disruptive are its effects on the patient's lifestyle.

COPING WITH HEART DISEASE
IN THE PSYCHOSOCIAL SETTING

Heart bypass surgery is a common treatment for patients with coronary arteries that have become narrowed with fatty deposits. If the heart is deprived of blood and oxygen, it cannot work very efficiently, and if one or more of these arteries closes completely, the patient might have a heart attack. A heart attack is permanent damage to the heart muscle that occurs because it was deprived of oxygen. In heart bypass surgery, healthy blood vessels from elsewhere in the patient's body are used to bypass blockages in the coronary arteries and keep the heart supplied with blood and oxygen. While many people say that they feel "good as new" after the surgery, others are nervous about resuming any activities that require exertion, including sexual intercourse (Fig. 16-6).

Today, more medical, social, and behavioral scientists recommend that doctors be more open and encouraging about resuming sexual activity after heart bypass surgery when they feel the patient is ready. While a patient is recovering from a heart attack or heart bypass surgery, the doctor can make a few suggestions or recommendations about resuming sexual activity while telling the patient about other issues, such as diet and exercise. Renshaw and Karstaedt (1988) suggested the following guidance for these patients:

1. Do not drink large amounts of alcohol or eat a big meal before intercourse.
2. Upon waking in the morning is a good time for sexual intimacy or intercourse because people often have more energy then.

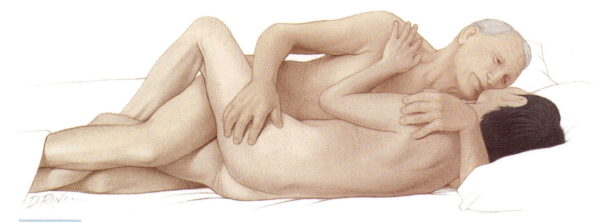

FIGURE 16-6 Patients who have had coronary bypass surgery are rarely discouraged from continuing to enjoy sexual sharing with their partners after they have fully recovered from the procedure.

3. The room shouldn't be too hot or too cold.
4. Intercourse positions should be comfortable and involve a minimum of muscular tension or exertion.
5. Patients should have their medications available and use them if they experience chest discomfort or an irregular heart beat.

Albarran and Bridger (1997) published recommendations about resuming sexual activity after a heart attack, which are also useful for patients after bypass surgery. Their advice focuses on the following questions and issues:

Q: When is it OK to start making love again?
A: When you feel ready. When you can climb stairs and walk briskly. Two weeks after you have left the hospital.
Q: Does sexual intercourse put a strain on the heart?
A: About as much as climbing two flights of stairs or driving to work.
Q: I don't feel like making love any more.
A: This is normal. People usually feel a little depressed at a time like this. When you feel better you will probably become interested in sex again.
Q: My partner doesn't seem very keen to make love.
A: Your partner may worry that you will have more health problems if you have sex. She or he will usually feel differently as time passes.
Q: Which position is the safest?
A: Any one comfortable for you. You might want to try the side-to-side position. Oral sex presents no special risks, although anal sex might cause an irregular heart beat.
Q: What should I do if I get chest pain during sex?
A: Stop and rest. Call your doctor if the pain continues. Taking nitroglycerine before having sex may help some people.
Q: Could the tablets I am taking affect my sex life?
A: Some medications can do this; don't stop taking them. Talk to your doctor.

Q: Should I ever avoid sexual intercourse?
A: When you have had too much to eat or drink, when the room is too hot or too cold, when you are wearing tight clothing.
— From Albarran and Bridger, 1997, 5

The patient's spouse can play a big role in recovery from a heart attack or heart bypass surgery (Fig. 16-7). Spousal support can take many forms. Beach, Maloney, Plocica, Sherry, Weaver, Luthringer, and Utz (1992) studied aspects of marital interaction after one spouse had a first, sudden heart attack. Seventeen married couples were studied over 6 months following the heart attack, including the spouse's social support, levels of family stress, reported levels of marital satisfaction, and the level of sexual activity and physical comfort associated with various intimate behaviors. These researchers considered it important to study forms of physical intimacy that do not involve sexual intercourse; during recovery from any serious, sudden illness this is often a good approach to take. Patients responded to questionnaires on three occasions during the six months following their heart attack. The study found that patients' spouses who enjoyed higher levels of social support, less family stress, and greater feelings of satisfaction with their marriages seemed to play a big part in the recovery of the patient. In addition, the more comfortable the patient's spouse was with a variety of sexual behaviors, the better was the patient's pace of improvement.

Until recently, most Americans mistakenly believed that heart disease is far more common in men than in women. We now know this is not necessarily true, and women and their doctors have begun to take symptoms of heart disease far more seriously than they used to. Still, specialists in rehabilitative medicine don't know as much as they would like to about women's recovery from a heart attack. A study by Hamilton (1990) revealed that compared with men who had had heart attacks, women were less likely to participate in cardiac rehabilitation programs and, when they did, tended to drop out at a higher rate. Women resume sexual intimacy later after heart

FIGURE 16-7 Following recovery from coronary bypass surgery, the patient's spouse can offer emotional support, appreciation, encouragement, and companionship, as well as share sexual intimacy.

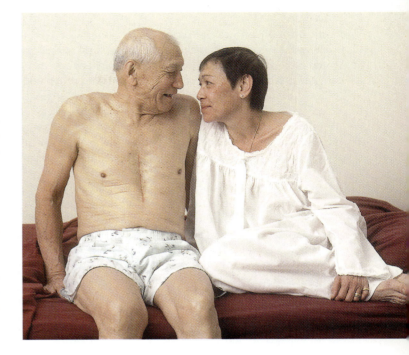

attacks than men and tend to report more discomfort and apprehension about intercourse. However, a study involving over 250 female and male patients (Froelicher, Kee, Newton, Lindskog, & Livingston, 1994) revealed that most patients had resumed some degree of sexual interaction, if not intercourse, by 12 weeks after their heart attack.

Cultural factors may also affect a person's adjustment to resuming sexual activity after a heart attack. For example, in a study of 300 men in India who had had heart attacks, almost one-third reported a decline in the quality of their sexual experiences because their doctors encouraged their partners to adopt the female-on-top position. In a society in which male dominance is common, a change of this nature could be expected to have adverse psychological consequences for men.

Dear Dr. Ruth

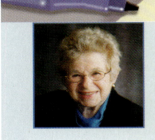

Question:

I am a 56-year-old man who just had successful heart by-pass surgery. My doctor says I am making an excellent recovery, and I feel great. No more chest discomfort or shortness of breath. I'm eager to resume sexual relations with my wife, and my doctor says that it shouldn't cause any problems. But my wife is extremely anxious about this and is afraid that our having sex will cause serious health problems for me. She has been withdrawn and very unresponsive to my sexual overtures. What can I do to reassure her that I'm fine?

Answer

The first step you must take is to make an appointment for your wife to see your doctor. I think hearing him give permission to have sex, and getting to ask any questions she may have, would help build her confidence.

My other suggestion is to start integrating sex back into your marriage gradually. Instead of having intercourse right away, the first few times you have sex, agree ahead of time that you will only masturbate each other. That will be a lot less physically taxing, so your wife shouldn't worry about your health. Once she has reached a stage where she can have an orgasm and is more comfortable with you having one too, it will be easier to graduate to intercourse.

If your wife is still having problems, ask your doctor for a referral to a sex therapist who works with couples with similar problems. It may take some time to calm her fears, but if you show some patience and get the help you both need, I'm sure you'll be able to overcome this hurdle.

Stroke

A stroke, or **cerebrovascular accident,** is an abnormal event involving the circulatory system of the brain. Strokes are very common in the United States. Many of the underlying conditions that contribute to heart disease also increase the probability of having a stroke. Because the brain is affected, strokes affect cognitive processes, the experience and expression of emotion, and motor behaviors as well, all to varying degrees depending on the amount and location of the brain tissue affected. When heart muscle cells or brain cells die from being deprived of oxygen during a heart attack or stroke, these types of cells do not regenerate or repair themselves. If many cells die in large portions of the heart or brain, the heart will stop working or the brain will cease to function and the person will die.

High blood pressure and obesity are common predisposing conditions for having a stroke. The prevalence of stroke for women is 759 per 100,000, and for men 917 per 100,000 (Brown, Whisnant, Sicks, et al., 1996). Stroke ranks third in the United States as a cause of death and 11th as a cause of disability. When the extent of brain damage is large, a person may survive the stroke but be left with disabilities in thinking, emotional expression, and movement, such as temporary or permanent paralysis.

PHYSICAL EFFECTS AND MANIFESTATIONS

There are three types of strokes (two are shown in Fig. 16-8). In the most common type, a blood clot lodges in a blood vessel in the brain causing brain cells supplied with blood and oxygen through that vessel to die. A second type of stroke involves the rupture of a blood vessel in the brain, with the brain cells supplied by that vessel rapidly dying. The third, rare type of stroke involves bleeding beneath the membranes that surround the surface of the brain, causing deficits that depend on the location and extent of brain damage. Some people become paralyzed temporarily, usually on one side of their body, and also may temporarily lose the ability to speak. The length of time it takes to recover from a stroke depends on the location and extent of brain damage, as well as resources for rehabilitation and the patient's motivation to recover.

COPING WITH STROKE IN THE PSYCHOSOCIAL SETTING

When a person's thoughts, emotions, and actions are altered, sexual experience and expression are likely to be affected. The term *hemiparesis* describes paralysis on one side of the body. In a study of people who were hemiparetic after a stroke, Boldrini, Basaglia, and Calanca (1991) reported that both women and men reported a significant decline in sexual interest and activity. Men claimed a more profound loss of sexual inclination after their stroke than women. The spouses of these patients consistently noted a marked change in their previously established pattern of sexual intimacy; however, these researchers noted that the patient's psychological adjustment to her or his illness and the nature of their marital relationship were more important factors in the patient's sexual adjustment.

In a study carried out in Sweden (Sjogren, Damber, & Liliequist, 1983), 51 female and male patients were interviewed about their sexual functioning after a stroke. Both female and male patients reported that the duration of foreplay and intercourse decreased significantly, and the frequency of intercourse declined as well. Among the women in this sample, 75% experienced anorgasmia after their stroke, but many had experienced this dysfunction before they became ill. This study included monitoring sex hormone levels in all subjects, which were found to be normal in both the women and men. Monga, Lawson, and Inglis (1986) also reported that their female patients reported marked decreases in vaginal lubrication after a stroke. Sjogren (1983) suggested that these sexual problems may also stem from inadequate sexual information and lack of opportunities for marital counseling regarding these issues. Overall, a decline in the quality of sexual expression is common after a stroke. Hawton (1984) reported that when and whether a couple resumed sexual activity after a man had a stroke could be predicted by the frequency with which the couple had intercourse before the stroke, a factor that seemed more important than the man's age or the seriousness of the stroke. Also, Monga, Lawson, and Inglis (1986) found that the most pressing concern stroke patients and their partners shared was whether having intercourse would cause a sudden rise in

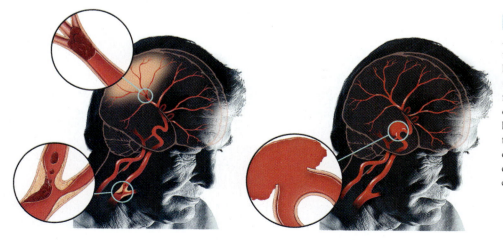

FIGURE 16-8 Two types of stroke. At lower left, a blood clot detaches from the inside of an artery and becomes lodged in a blood vessel (upper left). This interrupts the flow of blood and oxygen to brain cells. At right, a blood vessel in the brain ruptures, again with disruption in blood and oxygen to brain cells. Strokes vary in severity and degree of loss of perceptual, motor, cognitive, and emotional functions.

blood pressure that would cause another stroke. In fact, this rarely happens.

While most patients report diminished sexual interest and activity after a stroke, in some cases the opposite happens. Monga, Monga, Raina, and Hardjasudarma (1986) reported three case histories of patients who became hypersexual after a stroke and began to engage in sexual behaviors that were very different from their sexual repertoire before they became ill. One 53-year-old man reported a marked increase in the frequency with which he and his spouse had intercourse and also had notable mood changes. This subject also began to experience a persistent erection in the absence of any sexual stimulation, a condition called priapism. The two women described in this study had a dramatically increased inclination to explore a wide variety of sexual activities they had never engaged in previously. It has been estimated that more than 7% of aging and elderly people who have had a stroke have a pronounced lessening of sexual inhibitions after having a stroke or other age-related cognitive deficits (Lothstein, Fogg-Waberski, & Reynolds, 1997).

Cancer

There are more than 100 different kinds of **cancer,** which have one thing in common: the uncontrolled division of some of the body's cells and the tendency for these cells to spread to other parts of the body. These are malignant cancers. Sometimes the body's cell growth becomes abnormal but not cancerous; these are benign tumors. Cancers may involve malignancies of the blood or grow as solid tumors. Generally a person's risk of developing cancer increases with age. Some estimates are that up to one in three Americans will develop cancer at some time in their lives. Some cancers are clearly related to factors in the environment, such as irradiation, excessive sun, exposure to toxic chemicals, and the use of tobacco. Other cancers seem to happen for no known reason. Cancer can be treated with varying degrees of success depending on the type of cancer, how early it is diagnosed, and the age and overall health of the individual. Cancer like other serious health problems affects sexual behavior. While the disease itself can affect a patient's interest in having sex, many of the treatments for cancer have a similarly inhibiting effect on sexual expression and experience.

In adults in the United States, lung cancer is the most common cancer, with breast, prostate, and colorectal cancers ranking next. Of course, all cancers do not directly affect sexual arousal or response or reproductive potential, but cancer treatments may affect the person's overall feelings of wellness and attractiveness, and some treatments may affect interest in sex. In some cases, treatments for cancer may cause infertility, such as chemotherapy in women who are still ovulating.

PHYSICAL EFFECTS AND MANIFESTATIONS

The physical effects of cancer depend on the organ or organ system affected. In many cases, cancer does not involve any physical discomfort in its early stages. If cancer affects the body's endocrine glands, there may be increases or decreases in hormone levels accompanied by physical or emotional changes. Sometimes these hormone changes affect a person's sexual responsiveness. Brain cancer may affect cognitive abilities, emotional responsiveness, or motor skills, depending on the location of the tumor and its size.

COPING WITH CANCER IN THE PSYCHOSOCIAL SETTING

Robinson, Scott, and Faris (1994) worked with over 80 women between the ages of 19 and 81 who had been diagnosed with endometrial, cervical, or ovarian cancer. They wanted to find out if their patients were helped by reading a book about the sexual concerns of women with cancer of their reproductive system. This book described the impact of the disease on sexual responsiveness, as well as the effects of different therapies used to treat these cancers. Before being given the book, these subjects filled out a questionnaire in which they were asked to describe their sexual behaviors, communication style, body image, and general anxieties about having cancer. Most women reported that they appreciated the opportunity to read the book and had learned much about cancer and the effects of the disease on sexual behavior. Yet these subjects said they still had many serious concerns about their sexuality and the impact of treatment on their continued sexual functioning.

Prostate cancer has particularly disruptive effects on a man's sexual functioning, as described in Chapter 5. Urinary incontinence and impotence are common consequences of surgical treatments for prostate cancer. In some cases the patient can choose between continuing to enjoy their current level of sexual functioning or giving it up in exchange for a better long-term survival rate. This question has been studied in a sample of 163 men between the ages of 35 and 84 (Mazur & Merz, 1995). The average age of the participants in this study was just over 65 years. These individuals did not have prostate cancer at the time they were questioned about possible consequences of surgical treatment but were simply asked their personal feelings about losses in sexual functioning versus the chances of living longer. Ninety-four percent of the men in this study said that they would choose the treatment strategy that might leave them incontinent and impotent in exchange for a higher probability of living at least five more years. These subjects said that they would choose surgery and the problems likely to result even if for only a 10% chance of living another five years.

In a study on the impact of breast cancer on sexual functioning in women, Ghizzani, Pirtoli, Bellezza, and Velicogna (1995) interviewed 50 Italian women who had been diagnosed with breast cancer and had had the tumor removed surgically. Of these women, 28 were still menstruating and 22 were menopausal. The average age of the women in the first group was 43, and in the second, 59. These researchers were especially interested in these women's emotional reaction to being diagnosed with breast cancer, the nature of the family support she enjoyed when she learned she was ill, her emotional reactions to the scars left by the surgery (all subjects had modified mastectomies and removal of lymph nodes in the arm pit), and her inclination to resume sexual activity after her operation. Virtually all of the subjects reported extreme levels of anxiety upon learning they had breast cancer, and many found it hard to accept the reality of their diagnosis. Generally, younger women depended more on their husbands in coming to terms with the cancer, while the older women relied more on their extended families for support. This relationship was very strong in the younger women who enjoyed good marriages, but among older subjects there was no clear relationship between reported quality of the marital relationship and the later resumption of sexual activity. Because of the common sexual connotations of breast size and appearance, many women with breast cancer have deep worries about their body image and continued sexual activity.

Surgery, of course, is only one treatment for breast cancer. Kaplan (1994) reported that different therapies for this disease may each be associated with problems in resuming sexual relations or with the patient's overall attitude about feelings of physical attractiveness. Treatments for breast cancer can have some specific sexual side effects. Kaplan emphasizes that some doctors, nurses, or social workers are less willing to talk with women about resuming sexual relations after surgery and that some women feel uneasy about raising the subject because they feel they are supposed to be "happy just to be alive" and, therefore, shouldn't be concerned with reclaiming their sexuality. Plastic surgical techniques for rebuilding a woman's breast include realistic looking nipples. For women who find these procedures unappealing, highly realistic breast prostheses can be worn in a bra, giving a woman the appearance of two normal breasts.

Chemotherapy after surgery for breast cancer can leave a woman tired and depressed. She may experience nausea and vomiting and lose her hair (Fig. 16-9). Sleep loss is common, as is weight loss. She may become more vulnerable to infection during her course of treatment. The type and duration of chemotherapy depend on how large the tumor was and whether cancer cells were found in adjacent lymph nodes. Kaplan emphasizes that medical, social, and behavioral researchers still do not know enough about the impact of chemotherapy on a woman's sexual self-concept, which remains an important research question deserving further investigation. Another drug, Tamoxifen, is also used as a follow-up treatment for breast cancer. This drug is administered orally and may be taken for years after diagnosis and surgical treatment for breast cancer. An extremely small number of women taking Tamoxifen discontinue it because of unwanted side effects. However, some women using Tamoxifen report vaginal shrinkage, soreness, and dryness, as well as loss of sexual interest and loss of orgasmic response (Kaplan, 1994). Since a large number of women are taking Tamoxifen, more research is needed to better understand the prevalence of sexual side effects and their seriousness.

Gynecologic cancers directly affect a woman's sexual and reproductive organs and, therefore, these ailments normally affect her sexual self-schema and the relationship between her self-esteem and body image.

Other cancers also, including those unrelated to sexual and reproductive organs, may impact powerfully on an indi-

vidual's desire to continue to enjoy sexual behaviors. Surgery or radiation treatments may lead to physical disfigurement. Siston, List, Schleser, and Vokes (1997) studied the impact of head and neck cancers on sexual functioning in a sample of 36 patients who had completed treatment at least one year prior to their investigation. An estimated 40,000 cases of head and neck cancer are reported annually in the United States (Wingo, Tong, & Bolden, 1995). Smoking- and alcohol-

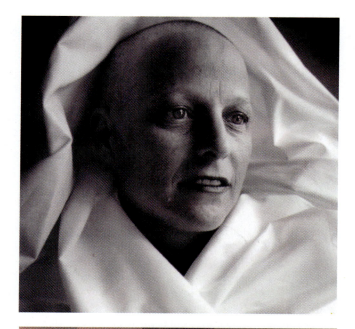

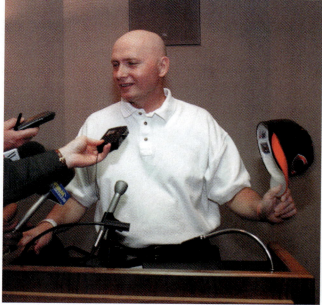

FIGURE 16-9   Top: While many patients undergoing chemotherapy lose their hair, many retain a positive body image and sense of their own attractiveness. Bottom: Illinois Attorney General Jim Ryan leaves the hospital in good spirits after 18 days of chemotherapy and radiation treatments for cancer.

Other Countries, Cultures, and Customs

CHINESE WOMEN ADJUST TO GYNECOLOGIC CANCER

An interesting and important difference among diverse cultures involves how they react to illness. People in other societies may indeed react very differently than we do to certain ailments. Because effective cancer treatment usually requires sophisticated medical technology, access to the most up-to-date surgical techniques, and expensive medications, one would expect some interesting differences in ways in which people elsewhere in the world adjust to cancers that might be treated very differently than in this country.

Tang, Siu, Lai, and Chung (1996) give an interesting glimpse of ways in which Chinese women in Hong Kong make sexual adjustments after surgery for gynecologic cancer. They note that Westerners don't know very much about sexual behavior in China, with very few rigorous investigations having been conducted. Chinese sexuality may best be understood within the Confucian and Taoist religious traditions that affect many behaviors in that country. Sex within the Confucian tradition in China takes place in an explicitly patriarchal culture: women are expected to be subservient, passive, and submissive sexually. Procreational sex is a fundamental religious value; recreational sex and extramarital sex are explicitly prohibited or actively discouraged. In contrast, the Taoist tradition views sexual expression as a basic source of creative energy deriving from the physical interaction between men (Yang) and women (Yin). The balance between these two life forces is basic to the Taoist perspective on human sexuality.

These two religious perspectives strongly influence how Chinese women react to a diagnosis of cancer and their sexual lifestyle adjustments after treatment. Tang, Siu, Lai, and Chung reported that cancer among Chinese women often leads to a reduction or cessation of sexual relations between the woman and her partner to aid in the recovery process. Couples with Confucian beliefs are likely to think about resuming sexual activity for the purpose of having children rather than enjoying sexual pleasure. If these couples do not plan to have any more children, they will probably not be very concerned about resuming sexual activity after cancer treatment, nor are they likely to approach their doctors with their concerns about continued physical intimacy.

These cultural beliefs affect the reasons Chinese women gave for reducing the frequency of sexual intercourse with their partners or stopping altogether. Some women reported that sexual relations before treatment began would "traumatize" their genitals (p. 192). Interestingly, folk myths also influenced these women's sexual decisions; some believed that their partners would contract the disease if they had intercourse with them. Still others believed that their postoperative recovery would be prolonged if they had sex before surgery. In fact, 70% of the women studied reported that they were unsure whether they could have sexual intercourse if their internal reproductive organs had been removed. Even though the women who were studied were between the ages of 43 and 53, some said that they were getting too old to even consider the desirability of resuming sexual activity. Because of the patriarchal family structure in China, women whose partners did not initiate sexual relations simply refrained from having intercourse.

Overall, cultural influences and traditions can have an enormous impact on whether or when a woman continues to have sexual relations after having been diagnosed with and treated for cancer.

related cancers affecting the mouth and throat are common cancers of this type. When Siston and her colleagues approached a number of these patients for their study, they found that about a third of them declined to participate. Apparently, many found it difficult to discuss or report their sexuality. The subjects who became part of the study filled out questionnaires addressing personal characteristics and the nature of their cancer and its treatment. Other questionnaires addressed the patient's sexual activity and responsiveness, the quality of their marriages, and their overall capacity to take care of themselves and engage in daily activities. More than three-fourths of the patients in this study reported that sexual expression occupied a "somewhat" or "very important" place in their lives. However, about half of the subjects in this sample reported problems becoming sexually aroused, with about 40% noting a decrease in sexual activity and a loss of sexual interest. In fact, 55% of these respondents said that they rarely if ever had sexual intercourse with their partner anymore, presumably because of the disfigurement that sometimes results from surgery. This is another example of ways in which cancer can adversely affect a person's sexual self-schema.

In summary, data consistently reveal that cancer powerfully affects the way a person perceives the attractiveness of their body and their sexual self-schema, although many studies reveal that subjects often still report a generally satisfactory level of sexual responsiveness and sexual activity (Kurtz, Wyatt, & Kurtz, 1995). As health care providers come to better understand factors that help a person resume sexual activity after they have been treated for cancer, doctors and rehabilitation specialists will be in a better position to explore this often sensitive subject with their patients.

Diabetes

The impact of diabetes on sexual functioning is described in other chapters, and this section only briefly reviews the impact of chronic diabetes on peripheral blood vessels and nerves. One type of diabetes has an onset in childhood and adolescence, and the other develops during adulthood. This disease involves the body's inability to metabolize carbohydrates in the form of glucose into energy.

PHYSICAL EFFECTS AND MANIFESTATIONS

For our bodies to break foods down into usable glucose, one of our endocrine glands, the pancreas, has to secrete the hormone insulin. Insulin allows glucose to enter the body's cells where it can be used. In diabetes, either the body doesn't make enough insulin or the body can't use this insulin efficiently. In either case, glucose builds up in the bloodstream. The Centers for Disease Control notes that blindness, kidney failure, heart disease, and the need for amputations of the lower extremities are common effects of diabetes. Diabetes is the 7th leading cause of death in our country. Depending on the type of diabetes, it can be controlled with dietary changes, exercise, and oral or injectable insulin. As of this writing, there is no cure for diabetes. It is a chronic disease that can be effectively treated, but patients must be compliant with *all* of their doctor's recommendations.

Both types of diabetes are often accompanied by abnormal functioning of the testes in men and the ovaries in women (Morley, 1998) although in juvenile onset diabetes, these may not be apparent for many years. Men with diabetes often have low levels of testosterone in their bloodstream. In women, diabetes is associated with changes in the function of ovaries, as well as changes in their secretion of sex hormones. In both sexes, diabetes may be accompanied by a decline in sexual interest. As described in Chapter 14 on sexual dysfunctions, erectile dysfunction is common in men with diabetes, affecting 50–75% (Vinik & Richardson, 1998). Gener-

ally, older diabetic men are more frequently affected than younger diabetic men. The effects of diabetes on female sexual functioning are less well understood. Diabetes is known to be frequently associated with vaginal dryness, but less is known about the impact of diabetes on menstruation, pregnancy, the effectiveness of chemical contraceptive alternatives, fertility, and the prevalence of sexual dysfunctions (de Veciana, 1998). There remains a huge discrepancy between the number of research studies done on the impact of diabetes on male sexual functioning compared to female sexual functioning (Jovanovic, 1998).

COPING WITH DIABETES IN THE PSYCHOSOCIAL SETTING

Because diabetes is frequently accompanied by less interest in sex, as well as erectile dysfunction in men and vaginal dryness and other genital changes in women, a couple is often challenged to explore ways of managing these problems. Women and men with diabetes may have very different levels of sex drive, and both may rarely feel like having sex at the same time. Good communication is often needed if the couple is to explore and enjoy various non-intercourse avenues of sexual pleasuring. Men with erectile dysfunction have a number of alternatives they and their partners can try to improve sexual functioning. Chapter 15 discusses oral medications, urethral suppositories, vacuum-erection devices, intracavernosal injections, and penile implants (Levine & Fones, 1998)—which of these a man chooses often depends on serious discussion with his partner and an awareness of her needs as well.

While these treatments for diabetes focus on organic factors, many psychological issues require attention too, reinforcing the importance of evaluating this disease psychosocially. Some of the following issues can be fruitfully approached within the context of the couple's communication, but others may require a counselor to facilitate a more open conversation and problem-solving tactics. Levine and Fones (1998) discuss many of these concerns. Five issues seem most important. First, the couple needs to examine their level of sexual desire and the way it has changed, if it has, due to diabetes. It doesn't make much sense to encourage two people to find new ways of sharing sex if they've lost interest over the years. Second, the nature of the couple's relationship is basic to any recommendations regarding shared sexual intimacy. If the relationship is fraught with conflict, tension, and big differences in values, better sex might be the last thing on their minds. Third, the nature and time frame over which sexual problems develop is relevant to any sexual dysfunctions. We shouldn't assume that diabetes impairs sexual relationships that were perfect from the outset! Fourth, and perhaps most important, is the couple's interest in asking for professional help. For some this is very difficult; not everyone feels comfortable talking about sex with a stranger, even if that stranger is a counselor or therapist. For a professional to help, the couple needs an expectation of help at the beginning and an openness to sharing the details of their sexuality with a counselor or therapist. Finally, just going to a counselor or therapist isn't enough; the couple really must be motivated to follow the guidance and suggestions suited to their personal circumstances.

Overall, effective psychosocial approaches to coping with diabetes require attention to both organic and interpersonal factors for any specific couple's needs.

Kidney Disease and Transplantation

Although everyone urinates several times a day, few people give much thought to their kidneys, where they are, or what they do—until a problem develops. The many kinds of kidney disease all have one thing in common: the kidneys are not functioning well, or at all, in filtering the blood and forming urine to remove wastes from the body. The kidneys also regulate the amount of water in the blood and the amounts of various trace minerals in the bloodstream and are essential to the maintenance of normal blood pressure. Chronic renal failure (renal refers to the kidneys) can result from diabetes, drug side effects, cancer, high blood pressure, prostate disease, the formation of stones in the kidneys, and hereditary factors. Kidney disease, kidney transplantation, and dialysis all can have an impact on sexual functioning. **Dialysis** is a medical procedure in which wastes in the blood are filtered by a machine rather than the kidneys.

Kidney disease is common. According to the Thornton Kidney Research Foundation at the University of Southern California, more than 30 different kinds of kidney disease affect more than 13 million people in the United States. An estimated 100,000 people will need dialysis or a kidney transplant in order to live. Additionally, 12% of all men and 5% of all women will have symptoms of a kidney stone at some time in their lives. In addition, over 60 million Americans have high blood pressure, the most common cause of kidney failure.

PHYSICAL EFFECTS AND MANIFESTATIONS

High blood pressure is a common symptom of kidney disease. Other symptoms include extreme fatigue, loss of appetite, and often nausea and vomiting. As discussed earlier, many of the medications used to treat high blood pressure impair sexual arousal in both women and men. Even if people with kidney disease get prompt, appropriate treatment the disease does not always improve. When kidney function is severely diminished, dialysis and/or a kidney transplant are the only effective treatments.

COPING WITH KIDNEY DISEASE
IN THE PSYCHOSOCIAL SETTING

Kidney disease like most chronic illnesses frequently affects sexual functioning. Berkman, Katz, and Weissman (1982) interviewed 32 men receiving dialysis and 14 of their wives. The degree to which kidney disease affected their sexual functioning depended on the seriousness of the disease and its impact on the nerves and blood vessels of the patient's pelvic area. In this sample, 9 patients reported being fully functional sexually, 7 reported "moderate" sexual problems, and 16 reported "severe" sexual dysfunction. Another study (Milde, Hart, & Fearing, 1996) evaluated questionnaire re-

sponses from 135 subjects in 7 hospital-based dialysis centers in Iowa about sexual satisfaction, patterns of intimacy, and frequency of sexual intercourse. In this sample of dialysis patients, 65% reported that they were "dissatisfied" with their sexual interaction, and 40% had stopped having sexual intercourse or any other form of sexual sharing. Only 25% of these subjects had received any information from health care professionals concerning the impact of kidney disease and dialysis on sexual functioning.

In another study, Procci and Martin (1985) evaluated the impact on sexual functioning of advanced kidney disease without dialysis in 23 subjects and a regular program of dialysis in 23 subjects. Although men in both groups continued to have erections in their sleep as measured in a sleep laboratory, men who had advanced kidney disease reported a significant increase in the frequency of intercourse after beginning dialysis. While dialysis might not make much physiological difference in a man's ability to have an erection, it apparently improves his overall health and energy level, making him more inclined to initiate sexual intercourse or be receptive to his partner's sexual overtures.

Holley, Schmidt, Bender, Dumler, and Schiff (1997) studied a sample of women on dialysis and questioned them about a number of gynecologic and fertility issues. They studied the responses from 191 women, 76 of whom were 55 years old or younger and 115 of whom were older than 55. Because women on dialysis frequently stop having periods and stop ovulating, these investigators were especially interested in learning about the impact of dialysis on female sexual issues. Of the women in this sample, about half reported that they were still sexually active. Women receiving dialysis seem not to have thorough discussions about gynecologic and fertility issues with their doctors.

Little is known about the impact of kidney transplants on sexual functioning. One small study (Slavis, Novick, Steinmuller, Streem, Straffon, Mastroianni, & Graneto, 1990) evaluated a variety of quality of life issues among 14 subjects with a functioning kidney transplant after 20 or more years. In 13 of these 14 subjects, overall quality of life was excellent, and all of these individuals reported that they continued to enjoy sexual activity.

Arthritis

Approximately 15% of all Americans develop some form of arthritis, or roughly 37 million people, as they get older. To date, there is no cure. It is a painful disease that can limit a person's flexibility and mobility. Chapter 13 noted that using non-steroidal anti-inflammatory drugs before intercourse, a warm bath, or making love on an electric blanket can all help ease its symptoms, minimize discomfort, and improve ease of movement.

PHYSICAL EFFECTS AND MANIFESTATIONS

The most common form of arthritis is **osteoarthritis.** This disorder affects the cartilage in joints, causing it to wear out or completely disappear. This leaves little or no cushioning between bones, resulting in pain, stiffness, and restricted movement. A more serious condition, **rheumatoid arthritis,** affects several joints; about two-thirds of the people with this condition are women. Joints become inflamed, swollen, and very sore. Like osteoarthritis, rheumatoid arthritis is a chronic disease, but the latter may have flare-ups during which symptoms are especially uncomfortable. Medications, rest, and special exercises are generally used to treat these ailments.

COPING WITH ARTHRITIS IN THE PSYCHOSOCIAL SETTING

Although many people are adamant about taking care of themselves, arthritis should definitely be treated by a physician; the earlier the condition is diagnosed and treatment begun, the better. Because osteoarthritis affects flexibility and mobility, it can significantly affect the ease with which a person can enjoy intercourse. Rheumatoid arthritis has similar effects. Kraaimaat, Bakker, Janssen, and Bijlsma (1996) studied over 200 women and men with this disorder to learn more about the impact of rheumatoid arthritis on sexual expression. Patients who experienced the most pain and depression due to this illness also experienced the greatest disruption in sexual intimacy. The women in this study reported that the disease impaired their mobility more than the men did.

When osteoarthritis or rheumatoid arthritis causes significant joint damage, orthopedic surgeons often recommend joint replacement surgery. Many people have had a hip or knee replacement, which involves implanting an artificial bone segment in the joint to replace old, worn bone. The surgery is serious, and recovery can take a long time. Stern, Fuchs, Ganz, Classi, Sculco, and Salvati (1991) studied the impact of hip replacement on sexual activity after surgery. In their sample of 86 patients, 46% before surgery reported that their hip problems significantly disrupted their sexual activity.

Only 1% of these subjects, however, encountered similar problems after the surgery. About 55% of these patients were able to comfortably resume sexual intercourse one or two months after their operation (Fig. 16-10). The overwhelming majority of these patients (89%) said that they wanted more information about the impact of this surgical procedure on sexual activity.

Ostomy Surgery

With some diseases, such as cancer, surgical procedures remove affected tissue making the need for an opening in the body called a **stoma** through which bodily fluids leave the body and are collected. Patients wear a bag to catch these gastrointestinal contents (Fig. 16-11). Some cases of colon cancer or ulcerative colitis require a colostomy, through which the contents of the large intestine are collected. If a cancerous bladder must be removed, a similar opening is made to collect urine. The impact of such an operation on a person's body image can be devastating, and their sexual self-concept is similarly affected in most cases. Finding a way to resume sexual activity is often a high priority for these patients and their partners. This is another situation in which sexuality can continue to have a prominent place in our lives, even when we are recovering from serious diseases and the sometimes radical surgery necessary to treat them. The body image issue here is similar to that of women recovering from breast surgery.

COPING WITH OSTOMY SURGERY IN THE PSYCHOSOCIAL SETTING

People who need ostomy surgery often fear rejection by their partner. They worry about how the wound and the bag will look and smell and any sounds of bodily fluids entering the

FIGURE 16-10   Some intercourse positions are more comfortable for those who have just had hip replacement surgery. Minimizing pressure and muscular tension, as well as excessive exertion, all help to create a more comfortable intimate experience.

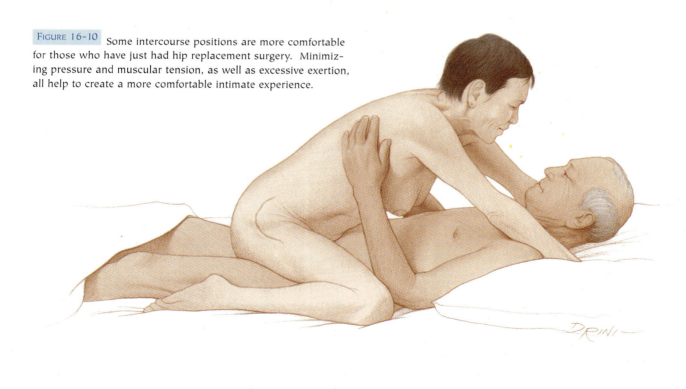

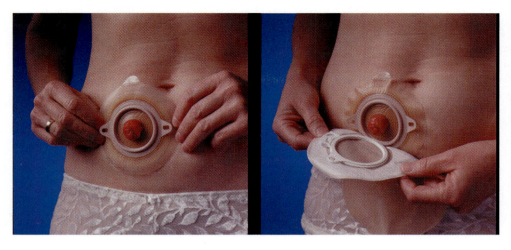

FIGURE 16-11   A stoma is an opening surgically created in the abdomen through which gastrointestinal contents may be collected in a bag. Those who have had this procedure often find ways to resume sexual intimacy with a minimum of self-consciousness or embarrassment.

pouch. They worry whether it will be possible to continue having sexual relations (Young, 1982). Men often experience impotence, and women report a significant loss in sex drive. Women also note diminished lubrication after surgery and worry about whether having sex will hurt. Specialists in rehabilitation medicine recommend that the patient and their partner be counseled before surgery and learn about the scar, the opening itself, and the pouch that will be worn. Sexual problems that develop after the surgery can be treated effectively with the approaches outlined in Chapter 15.

When the pouch fits well, it can be changed quickly and efficiently when the individual wishes to engage in athletic activities or sexual intercourse, and this usually helps the person feel more confident and comfortable (Salter, 1992). Depending on the location of the stoma, the individual can wear a money-belt type waistband to hide the pouch. An appliance that fits well will generally stay in place during a wide variety of physical activities, including sexual intercourse. Some people with a stoma skip meals to ensure that fluids are not expelled during intercourse, but most physicians recommend regular meals so that the individual can learn the regularity with which materials leave their body. The couple needs to find the intercourse position that suits them best and allows for the presence of the pouch.

Golis (1996) has suggestions for ostomy patients concerned about having sex. These can help minimize any embarrassment and prepare patients to handle the accidents that sometimes happen:

- Wear cover-up clothing, such as a T-shirt or special cover-up garments
- Empty bag before intimate moments
- Irrigate before intimate moments if irrigation is part of normal care
- Wear money belt-type waistband
- Tape the bag down to stabilize it
- Eat at regular times
- Minimize the intake of gas-forming foods
- Use deodorants and perfumes

- Experiment with options, positions
- Play music as cover-up for embarrassing sounds
  —After Golis, 1996, 34

Among married individuals with colostomies, sexual practices and frequency of intercourse in a group of 178 subjects did not differ compared with the general population in Sweden (Gruner, Naas, Fretheim, & Gjone, 1977). Apparently, couples can adjust to wearing a pouch and continue to enjoy sexual expression in their marriage. This suggests, again, that the desire to share sexual intimacy is very powerful and people can find their way around many frustrations and obstacles to enjoy it.

Amputation

Many people have had a limb amputated because of a traumatic accident or disease (Fig. 16-12). Some people are born

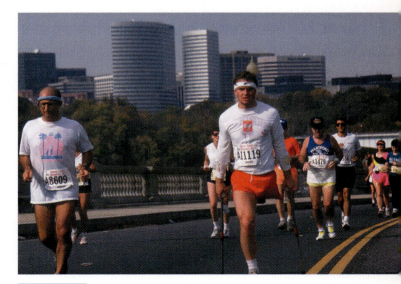

FIGURE 16-12   Amputees frequently enjoy an active, vital lifestyle and often perceive no limitations on their interests and activities.

without a limb as a birth defect. Land mines remaining after armed conflicts throughout the world are another major cause of amputations. Amputation of a lower extremity is also an unfortunate consequence of uncontrolled diabetes; according to the Center for Podiatric Information, 5% to 15% of diabetics will have an amputation. Altogether, the *Amputee Website* reports that there about 3 million amputees living in the United States today. The Centers for Disease Control and Prevention report that there are approximately 54,000 amputations in this country each year, about three-fourths because of the complications of diabetes and heart disease. Because of the close relationship between a person's self-esteem and body image, disfigurement powerfully affects the way we feel about ourselves and our attractiveness to others.

PHYSICAL EFFECTS AND MANIFESTATIONS

Most diabetes-related amputations involve removing a portion of the leg below the knee. The patient is usually fitted with a prosthesis (artificial limb) custom-made to fit the patient's physical dimensions, which can perform many of the functions of the natural limb. New technology has developed better-fitting limb prostheses made of strong, flexible, lightweight materials. Rehabilitation can take a long time, however, and usually involves physical therapists and occupational therapists, as well as physicians.

COPING WITH AMPUTATION IN THE PSYCHOSOCIAL SETTING

Reinstein, Ashley, and Miller (1978) studied the impact of amputation on sexual activity. They studied 39 men and 21 women after they had received their prostheses. Among the male subjects, 77% reported a significant decrease in the frequency of sexual relations, while 38% of the women reported a similar change. Sexual activity was more adversely affected when the amputation was above the knee and was more marked in unmarried men. These researchers found that other aspects of the patient's sexuality were not affected by amputation, in particular, continued oral-genital stimulation, masturbation, extramarital sex, and homosexual intimate behaviors. A more recent study (Williamson & Walters, 1996) reported somewhat similar data. About 75% of a sample of 76 subjects between the ages of 29 and 84 years reported decreased frequency of sexual intercourse, yet these researchers emphasized that feelings of depression were largely responsible for the decline in sexual activity in these subjects. Akesode and Iyang (1981) reported on the impact of amputation on sexual functioning in a group of 100 Nigerians, most of whom had lost a limb because of war-related (land mine) injuries. Diminished social interaction and sexual activity also occurred in these subjects and continued for an extended period of time after the injury. Yet, as with other diseases and injuries, couples often make positive, comfortable adjustments to maintain a rewarding pattern of sexual intimacy.

Spinal Cord Injuries

Nerve cells in the brain and spinal cord when injured cannot repair themselves or regenerate, and their functions are no longer a part of one's cognitive, emotional, or motor activities. The spinal cord is approximately 18 inches long, extending from the base of the skull to about the lower mid-section of the back. The spinal cord does not extend to the bottom of the spinal column. Sensory messages from the body travel through the spinal cord to the brain, and motor (movement) messages from the brain travel through the spinal cord to the muscles of the body. These messages initiate and guide all of our movements. If the spinal cord is seriously injured, messages from the brain can no longer get to spinal nerve cells below the injury, and some degree of paralysis results.

An estimated 8,000 to 10,000 cases of spinal cord injury occur in the United States each year. Almost a quarter million people in the United States have varying degrees of spinal cord injury. Automobile accidents account for 44% of spinal cord injuries in this country, with violence, sports injuries, and falls accounting for the rest. In all, 82% of all spinal cord injuries occur in men.

PHYSICAL EFFECTS AND MANIFESTATIONS

Spinal cord injury (SCI) is any injury affecting the spinal cord within the spinal column (Fig. 16-13). Most spinal cord injuries are caused by accidents (trauma), but some diseases also damage and kill spinal nerve cells. Whenever the bones of the spinal column sustain an injury, there is a chance that the spinal cord within it is damaged. Then sensory information from the body may not reach the brain, and motor messages from the brain may not reach the muscles that move the body. The outcome of SCI depends on the location and extent of the injury or damage. Generally, nerves above the site of injury continue to function normally, but nerve cells below the site of injury may stop functioning normally or stop functioning completely. An injured person who has lost the use of their legs but still has normal feeling and movement in their arms has *paraplegia*. An injured person who has lost normal sensation and movement in their arms and legs has *tetraplegia* (which used to be called *quadriplegia*). When SCI is not severe and the spinal cord is only bruised or swollen after an injury, the person normally regains sensory and motor functions, but it is difficult to predict which functions will be affected, how severely, or how long recovery may take. In addition to sensory and motor functions, SCI may also affect breathing, bowel function, bladder control, and sexual arousal and response.

COPING WITH SPINAL CORD INJURIES IN THE PSYCHOSOCIAL SETTING

Partial or complete paralysis requires an enormous and for some insurmountable challenge. Everything in the person's life changes dramatically and instantly. People with spinal cord injuries that may involve a need for mechanical assistance to breathe and the loss of bowel and bladder control always report feelings of profound helplessness, depression, and total dependency. The person may also be grieving the loss of the sexual part of their personhood. Yet restoration of some sexual responsiveness and enjoyment is often feasible.

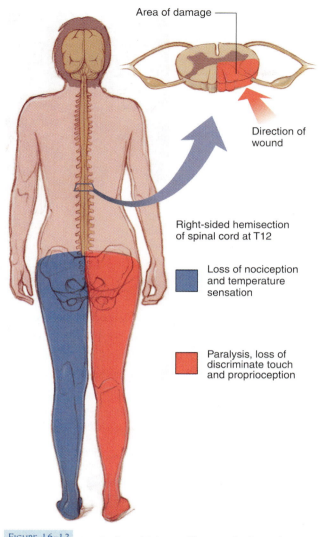

Area of damage

Direction of wound

Right-sided hemisection of spinal cord at T12

■ Loss of nociception and temperature sensation

■ Paralysis, loss of discriminate touch and proprioception

FIGURE 16-13   A spinal cord injury will cause the loss of various perceptual and motor abilities depending on the location and severity of the trauma. Shown here are the deficits that often accompany damage in the thoracic region of the spinal cord.

While in the past most research on sexual functioning in SCI focused on males, from the early 1990s, more attention was given to women with these injuries. Marca Sipski (Fig. 16-14), perhaps this country's leading expert on the impact of illness and disability on sexual functioning, reviewed the literature on the impact of SCI on women (1991). She notes that while some women stop having periods temporarily after their injury, most resume their previous pattern of menstruation within a few months. We are not aware of any studies that systematically evaluated different contraceptive methods for this population of women, but of course the appropriate method might depend somewhat on whether a woman had the use of her hands. Birth control pills may be a poor alternative because they would increase any tendency to develop blood clots in the legs if a woman could not regularly use her legs. Sipski notes that Norplant may be an attractive alternative for these women.

Women who are pregnant at the time of their injury have a high risk of miscarriage because of the trauma. When women become pregnant after their injury, there is an increased risk of premature labor and a tendency toward low–birth-weight babies. SCI women deliver their babies by Cesarean more often than women in the general, non-SCI population. Many doctors recommend that the woman be hospitalized as soon as her cervix begins to dilate. Women with SCI can breast-feed their babies, but patients with damage high in the spinal cord often produce less milk.

Sexual activity and the importance the injured woman attributes to it have been studied by a number of researchers. Westgren, Hulting, Levi, Seiger, and Westgren (1997) reported that regardless of the point of spinal injury or its degree of seriousness, many women attribute less importance to sexual activity after their injury. When asked what they found most disturbing about sex, these women reported that lack of coordinated motor activity, leakage of urine, discomfort, and problems assuming a comfortable position were particularly troubling. These investigators found that women who were younger at the time of their injury (under age 15) were more likely to have sexual activity than were older women (those over 30) in this sample of patients. With the exception of women whose injuries were very low in the spinal cord, all respondents reported that they became sexually aroused by different types of stimulation, including masturbation, vibratory aids, erotic literature or films, general body massage, genital touching, and sexual intercourse. Astonishingly, of the 62 women in this study, *only 6* had been counseled about sexual issues before they left the hospital.

Because spinal cord injuries often result in a loss of skin sensations below the level of spinal injury, investigators have explored whether psychological, nonphysical stimuli could lead to feelings of sexual arousal in these subjects. Sipski,

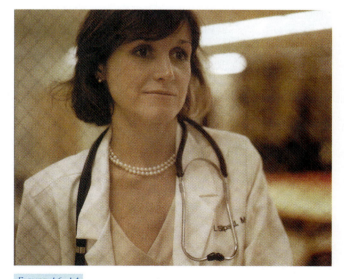

FIGURE 16-14   Dr. Marca Sipski is one of the foremost experts in the study of the effects of illness and disability on sexual functioning.

Alexander, and Rosen (1995a) compared the psychological and physiological responses of SCI women with normal women when presented with erotic audiovisual stimuli or erotic audiovisual stimuli combined with manual stimulation of the genitalia. Responses from 13 SCI subjects were compared to data from 8 normal women. The physiological measures recorded included increased blood flow to the vagina, heart rate, blood pressure, and breathing rate. The degree of subjective arousal was also assessed. The results showed that women in both groups experienced subjective sexual arousal, increased heart rate, increased blood pressure, and increased breathing rate. However, SCI women did not show signs of increased vaginal blood flow because the nerve pathways responsible for this response are located below the point of spinal cord injury. Interestingly, SCI women *did* show an increased blood flow to the vagina as a reflex to manual stimulation, even when they did not report subjective sexual arousal.

Researchers have also studied whether SCI women experience orgasms. In a separate study, Sipski, Alexander, and Rosen (1995b) used procedures similar to those described above but focused on whether the SCI subjects reported having orgasms. Data were collected from 25 women with SCI

Dear Dr. Ruth

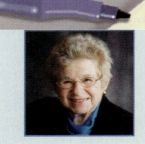

Question:

My husband and I have a beautiful daughter who is now 25. She was born with cerebral palsy and is moderately mentally retarded but normal physically. Recently, a young man at the special school she attends has begun to show interest in her, and she is very receptive to his attentions. I am concerned that they will become sexually involved and I don't know how to talk with her about birth control and sexually transmitted diseases, or even how to set limits on his advances. Can you tell me what to tell her, or can you recommend someone who specializes in situations like this? She doesn't always remember important things, so we are especially worried over all of this.

Answer:

I assume that your daughter and this young man are always supervised and do not have opportunities to engage in sex without your knowledge. If that's not true, if you think that they can find time to be alone and might engage in sexual intercourse, then I would suggest you not waste any time but take her to a gynecologist. The pill may be fine if you can be sure that she'll take it every day, or she can use an injectable form of birth control. But remember, these types of birth control offer no protection against STDs.

Once the contraceptive situation is under control, you still have to face other issues involved in their budding romance. Since they may already be missing out on much of what life has to offer, they should not be denied the right to feel love and have a romantic relationship. Although all parents worry when their children first start to date, you also have the main job of not letting go. You will continue to have responsibilities as she grows older, and so you have to be intimately involved in her life. You must make sure that no unintended pregnancy takes place. You will also have to teach her how to exercise self-control and understand when it is appropriate to be physically intimate and when it is not. They may decide they want to marry and have children, and that will certainly add complications.

While your child may never have what others may call a "normal" life, you can help her to partake in as many of life's joys as possible, and if appropriate, falling in love and having sex should be part of it. It will be difficult, but I believe that both you and your daughter will find that the rewards justify overcoming these difficulties. Talk to her doctor to find professional help if you feel you need it.

and 10 normal subjects. All of the normal women reported having orgasms, and 52% of the SCI subjects reported orgasms. Whether an SCI subject reported having an orgasm could *not* be predicted on the basis of the location and extent of her spinal cord injury, however. Subjects with no functions at all in the lower parts of their bodies took much longer to have an orgasm than did the control group of normal women. This may be due in part to the fact that many SCI patients lack good hand coordination, making genital self-stimulation less coordinated (Sipski, Alexander, & Rosen, 1997).

Because erection in men is a more obvious sign of sexual arousal than vaginal lubrication in women, the study of sexual functioning in SCI men involves somewhat different issues. Because many men find it hard to think of being sexual without having an erection, sexual activity after spinal cord injury in men presents specialists in rehabilitation medicine with a different set of challenges. Alexander, Sipski, and Findley (1993) evaluated the sexual activities in a group of 38 SCI males with a median age of 26 years before and after their injury. Among these subjects, the frequency of shared sexual behavior decreased after the injury, with a significant reduction in the frequency of sexual intercourse and a greater interest in avenues of non-intercourse sexual pleasuring. Even among the tetraplegic subjects in this sample, 38% reported having orgasms and ejaculating. In most cases, sexual desire was significantly diminished after the injury.

Problems in sexual responsiveness are not easy to diagnose promptly and accurately in SCI men, however. Courtois, Charvier, Leriche, and Raymond (1993) emphasize that sexual advice is often given to SCI men without a full clinical understanding of exactly how much sexual responsiveness remains after spinal cord injuries. These researchers recommend a full physiological assessment before any medical recommendations or interventions are begun. Their research reveals that 100% of men with high spinal cord injuries and 90% of those with damage lower in the spinal cord are still able to have an erection elicited reflexively by genital stimulation. Almost all of the men in their sample were able to ejaculate. These writers believe that because SCI men almost always underestimate their sexual responsiveness, laboratory testing procedures may be helpful in encouraging some men to explore a variety of erotic activities with their partners and find out that in fact they may still enjoy a notable degree of sexual responsiveness. In another study, White, Rintala, Hart, Young, and Fuhrer (1992) asked a group of 79 SCI men about their most pressing sexual concerns. The men in their sample reported three specific issues of particular importance: exploring new ways of enjoying sex, finding a way to help their partner adjust to their diminished sexual responsiveness, and exploring different ways to have children. While vacuum erection devices are not chosen by all men with spinal cord injuries, they are an effective, inexpensive, and reliable way to attain erections in SCI men (Denil, Ohl, & Smythe, 1996).

We have focused on the person with the spinal cord injury, but their partner's sexual experience is important also. Kreuter, Sullivan, and Siosteen (1994) administered a questionnaire to 49 partners of SCI patients in Sweden, 39 women and 10 men. In all, 84% of these partners reported that their overall relationship was satisfactory, and 50% of these couples had sex (which may or may not have involved intercourse) at least once a week. Over half of these subjects were satisfied with their frequency of sexual interaction, while one-third reported that they would like to have sexual relations more frequently. Almost half of these subjects were very clear in noting that their current sexual activity was as enjoyable as it was before the injury. While these injuries can be devastating to some people and their relationships, informed, motivated, and creative individuals continue to explore new sexual activities and find them highly rewarding.

Cerebral Palsy

Brain injury at or around the time of birth often causes a condition called **cerebral palsy**. "Cerebral" refers to the brain, and "palsy" refers to a lack of motor control. This condition is not inherited, contagious, or fatal. It is not a progressive, degenerative disease; it does not get worse, but it also does not improve. The United Cerebral Palsy Associations, Inc. has estimated that roughly 3000 infants are affected by this disorder each year, and that between 500,000 and 700,000 Americans have cerebral palsy. As these individuals approach adolescence and young adulthood, many begin to explore sexual behavior. Continued sexual expression is their right, despite personal and societal obstacles.

PHYSICAL EFFECTS AND MANIFESTATIONS

The more extensive the brain damage, the more marked are problems of muscular control. In some cases, cerebral palsy may involve varying degrees of mental retardation. Anything that blocks or interrupts the supply of oxygen reaching the baby's brain before, during, or after birth can cause some degree of cerebral palsy. Fragile brain blood vessels that leak or break before, during, or after birth may also cause cerebral palsy. Infants born prematurely or very prematurely have an increased risk of developing disorders of movement, including cerebral palsy.

COPING WITH CEREBRAL PALSY IN THE PSYCHOSOCIAL SETTING

Children and adolescents with cerebral palsy need sex education programs tailored for their impaired motor ability and perhaps some degree of mental retardation. Issues such as birth control, menstruation, masturbation, and sexual intercourse must be introduced in a way that is clear and understandable and easily remembered (Ziff, 1981). Masturbation requires some degree of manual coordination, which may be an obstacle for individuals with cerebral palsy. Often parents are highly protective of a child or teenager with cerebral palsy, yet encouraging self-reliance in a climate of trust and love are extremely important for developing independence. An issue of special importance is the parents' preparing a daughter for her first pelvic examination and what the doctor will do while she is being examined. Contraception can be especially problematic with impaired motor ability, although taking oral contraceptives generally poses no real obstacles except remembering to take them. Sexually active women with cerebral palsy may benefit from Norplant, although little is known about the use of this contraceptive in these patients.

Adults with cerebral palsy may need assistance from trusted others in positioning themselves so to enjoy sexual sharing or intercourse. In addition to possible intellectual and motor disabilities, many people with cerebral palsy have impaired verbal communication and are not easily understood. They may not easily describe their sexual intentions, desires, or dislikes. Specialists in rehabilitation medicine are an essential resource in this process. Facilitating sexual expression among those with cerebral palsy is a multidisciplinary challenge, involving the guidance of physicians, physical therapists, and perhaps sex counselors and therapists as well (Fig. 16-15).

Multiple Sclerosis

Multiple sclerosis (MS) is a disease of the nervous system with a highly unpredictable progression. It is incurable, debilitating,

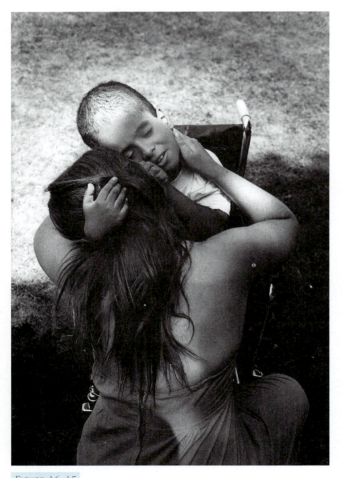

FIGURE 16-15   Like everyone else, intimate emotional and physical expression are very important for the psychological wellbeing of those with cerebral palsy.

and progressive. Approximately 300,000 people have MS in North America, with most people developing the disease between the ages of 21 and 40. For unknown reasons more women than men are affected. Genetic factors may be involved in MS. This disease has active and inactive periods: symptoms may be especially severe at some times and then diminish significantly for long intervals.

PHYSICAL EFFECTS AND MANIFESTATIONS
The symptoms of MS are many and diverse. Not everyone with MS has all, or even most symptoms. The most common are muscular weakness and spasticity, problems keeping one's balance and walking, tremor, visual difficulties, bladder and/or bowel problems, depression, pain, and impaired temperature sensitivity. Symptoms may come and go unpredictably. Perceptual and motor skills are both affected. There is no single diagnostic test for MS, and a definitive diagnosis can take months or even years.

COPING WITH MULTIPLE SCLEROSIS IN THE PSYCHOSOCIAL SETTING
Barak, Achiron, Elizur, Gabbay, Noy, and Sarova-Pinhas (1996) studied 41 individuals with MS, 32 women and 9 men. Of these, 16 women and 5 men reported problems with lowered sex drive, impotence, problems with sexual arousal, anorgasmia, or premature ejaculation. About one-fourth of this sample noted a significant loss of libido, and about 20% noted problems with arousal. Generally the women described their symptoms as more severe than the men. Another study (Dupont, 1996) confirmed that women and men with MS reported that their sexual intimacy was powerfully affected by their disease. About one-third of the 72 women and 44 men in Dupont's study noted serious relationship problems connected with their disability, with women generally being somewhat more dissatisfied with their sexual activities. Finally, Stenager, Stenager, and Jensen (1995) studied a group of 27 women and 22 men with MS and found that sexual dysfunctions increased significantly through a 5-year period, with both sexes being equally affected.

Just as with cerebral palsy, motor deficits and communication difficulties can contribute significantly to sexual problems among women and men with MS. Although cerebral palsy doesn't get worse, there is no way to predict whether or when MS will cause a decline in motor or perceptual functioning.

Alzheimer's Disease
The term *dementia* refers to diminished intellectual functioning and behavioral deficits associated with degenerative brain disorders that sometimes accompany aging. The most common kind of dementia is Alzheimer's disease, which is accompanied by specific, microscopic changes in brain tissue. Alzheimer's disease is found in about 10% of people over the age of 65, and almost 50% of those over the age of 85. It appears in individuals as young as their 40s in 10% of cases. Generally, the earlier the onset, the more rapidly the disease progresses. Because many people remain sexual beings until the end of their lives, this disorder can profoundly affect a person's sexual expression.

PHYSICAL EFFECTS AND MANIFESTATIONS

The microscopic changes in brain tissue are progressive and irreversible. These degenerative alterations in the brain cause dramatic behavioral, cognitive, and emotional changes in the person as the disease advances. In its earliest stages, Alzheimer's disease is characterized by problems in concentration, irritability, and short-term memory loss. There is no way to predict how rapidly this disease will progress, but as it does, people begin to neglect their appearance and personal hygiene and may behave impulsively. In its more severe manifestations, people begin to engage in involuntary movements and may have convulsions; they may engage in acts of unprovoked physical aggression and have delusions and hallucinations. Eventually, language functions are profoundly affected. People over the age of 65 who are diagnosed with Alzheimer's disease usually die within five years. In a sense, Alzheimer's disease robs an individual of their personality; they become someone who lacks appropriate cognitive and emotional capacities and may eventually lose the ability to initiate all voluntary movements. These individuals become totally dependent on others for all of their needs.

COPING WITH ALZHEIMER'S DISEASE IN THE PSYCHOSOCIAL SETTING

This disease dramatically affects the marital relationship, which in many cases still involves regular sexual activity. Wright (1991) found that 27% of the 29 couples in this sample continued to remain sexually active (although not at the more advanced stages of the disease), and found a very high level of sexual expression in 14% of the couples in which the male was afflicted with the disease. This presented a problem for most of the female spouses, who reported that they had tried to adjust to their husband's changed behavior while still trying to exercise some personal control. Unfortunately, their husbands no longer had a clear understanding of their behavior or their interactions with their wives. Some caregivers continue to have intercourse with their spouses and report that they are satisfied with their sexual relationship, yet some reveal that they are dissatisfied with the absence of any sexual sharing at all (Ballard, Solis, Gahir, Cullen, George, Oyebode, & Wilcock, 1997).

In a study carried out in France, 135 individuals with Alzheimer's disease were evaluated in terms of their continued sexual activity. The spouses of these patients filled out a questionnaire about their relationship. Seventy percent of the spouses reported that they had become unconcerned with continuing the sexual aspect of their relationship, yet half of these partners acknowledged that they had made lifestyle changes to meet their spouses' sexual needs (Derouesne, Guigot, Chermat, Winchester, & Lacomblez, 1996). Inappropriate sexual advances or touching are not common among people with Alzheimer's disease, but when they occur they are extremely upsetting to family members and health care practitioners (Davies, Zeiss, & Tinklenberg, 1992). With more people living into older age, the number of cases of Alzheimer's disease will increase, and more research will explore the impact of this terrible affliction on sexual functioning.

MENTAL RETARDATION

The subject of **mental retardation** is large and complex, and consideration of all the causes and manifestations of this large family of disorders is beyond the scope of this book. We will only describe some of the behaviors and thought processes associated with mental retardation and explore the importance of sexuality in mentally retarded individuals, their interpersonal behavior patterns, and their legal rights regarding fertility, contraception, and protection from exploitation.

The most obvious characteristic of mental retardation is below-average intelligence as measured by various psychological tests. Additionally, mentally retarded individuals do not adapt quickly and appropriately to the normal demands of an ever-changing environment. There are many degrees of mental retardation. The *Diagnostic and Statistical Manual of Mental Disorders* (4th edition, 1994) describes the attributes of mild, moderate, severe, and profound mental retardation. Mental retardation is usually obvious before the age of 18, and the different degrees of mental retardation involve an increasing inability in various areas of life: caring for oneself, verbal communication, social and interpersonal skills, the ability to take advantage of community resources, the capacity for self-direction, and the ability to work, participate in leisure activities, engage in health-enhancing behaviors, and remain safe from harm or threats of harm (p. 39). Mentally retarded individuals often have trouble expressing affection and their sexual feelings, responding to affectionate and sexual gestures of others, and anticipating the consequences of sexual behaviors.

Individuals with mild mental retardation do not typically require institutionalization, nor in most cases do those with moderate mental retardation. However, in severe or profound mental retardation, both the individual and the community often benefit by the individual being placed in a group home or the close, constant supervision of their families. In its most profound forms, specialized nursing care in closely supervised institutional settings is usually necessary. Most mentally retarded individuals enjoy the pleasures of masturbation and also desire to share physical intimacy with others. Health care professionals face many challenges as they try to acknowledge the independence and personhood of the mentally retarded and teach basic skills in impulse control and delay of gratification.

Social and Educational Issues and Sexuality

People with mental disabilities may encounter problems forming intimate relationships (Bhui & Puffett, 1994). Over the past three decades, professionals have sought to create as "normal" a life as possible for those with mental disabilities and to assimilate these individuals as fully as possible in the mainstream of society. With mild or even some moderate forms of mental retardation, marriage is feasible and mutually rewarding to both people (Fig. 16-16); however, it is essential to meet the challenges of providing accurate, understandable information about birth control and the significant stresses of parent-

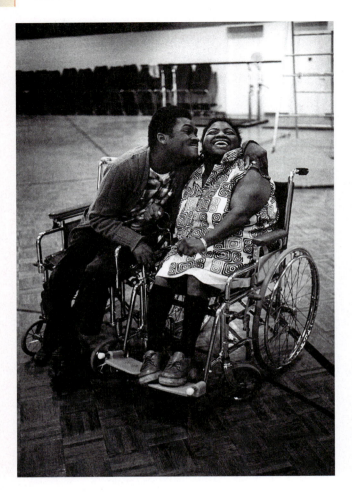

FIGURE 16-16 Those with physical and mental abilities often require social guidance and support in establishing relationships. Sexual health and wellness, as well as contraceptive issues, are all important to these populations and must be presented in lucid, understandable ways.

members of the other sex and decreased the number of same-sex interactions.

Social and behavioral researchers have known for decades that mentally retarded adolescents masturbate just like those of normal intelligence but tend to engage in homosexual exploration very often (Simonds, 1980). Parents of these youngsters are typically quite anxious about their child's developing heterosexual interests also. Simmonds emphasizes that these adolescents may be highly susceptible to inappropriate sexual advances, may use poor judgement in responding to these overtures, and may fail to fully understand the outcomes of their actions. Because the parents of mentally retarded adolescents may be very upset about these matters, youngsters may get the idea that all sex is "bad" and that they are "bad" for having sexual interests and feelings.

Varying degrees of mental retardation accompany Down syndrome, a congenital, genetic abnormality that also results in a characteristic facial appearance, shortened height, and other distinguishing physical characteristics. Despite a somewhat shorter life expectancy, most individuals with Down syndrome grow into adulthood. Sexual expression among these teenagers has been a concern for their parents and caretakers, as well as health care professionals for many decades. Shepperdson (1995) pointed out an interesting facet of raising youngsters with Down syndrome. Although many parents and caretakers proclaim the rights of retarded individuals to explore their sexuality and eventually marry, they did *not* necessarily believe this about their own mentally retarded child. Parents and caretakers of 78 children with Down syndrome born in the 1960s and 1970s seldom supported the idea of their child becoming a parent, and over half of them believed that in some cases sterilization might be appropriate for their child. Still, most parents and caretakers believed that sex education was important for their child, and that ideally such information would be offered in the home, by professionals, or both. While these youngsters knew something about pregnancy and childbirth, few were fully aware of sexual intercourse or its practical, physical aspects.

What is the best form of sex education program for mentally retarded individuals? McCabe (1993) emphasized that generally the mentally retarded have a real need for information about human sexuality, probably due to the negative thoughts and feelings that parents and caretakers have about this. This writer emphasizes that often the sexuality of the mentally retarded is entirely neglected or not seen as an issue deserving much attention. In her assessment of this issue, McCabe found that existing sex education programs for the mentally retarded do not address a wide enough range of topics, nor do they give much attention to any particular person's unique information needs.

hood. Bhui and Puffett (1994) note that many mentally retarded adults do not have a realistic understanding of their personal rights, cannot tell the difference between expressions of affection and exploitation, and do not understand the importance of avoiding risky situations in which they can be manipulated into doing things they do not understand, want, or like (p. 462).

Specialists in developmental disabilities have created programs to help mentally retarded individuals develop their skills in heterosexual interactions and practice dating behaviors. Valenti-Hein, Yarnold, and Mueser (1994) developed a 12-session Dating Skills Program that they offered to mildly or moderately retarded adults between the ages of 18 and 50, none of whom had perceptual or communication problems. They evaluated these adults' social skills, sexual knowledge, and social anxiety before the program began, again after the subjects finished all 12 sessions, and once more 8 weeks later. Compared with subjects in the control group who did not participate in the program, these subjects had improved social skills and knowledge of sexual issues; however, their social anxiety did not change as a result of having participated in this program. Those who completed the program increased the frequency with which they had interactions with

Reproductive and Contraceptive Considerations

American courts have ruled that individuals with any one of various different psychological problems should be treated in the "least restrictive" environment in keeping with their condition, level of development, and the seriousness of their symptoms. Often this means finding ways to shelter and maintain these individuals within the communities in which they live. For this reason, several sexual issues are basic to their safe and productive functioning in these settings. Elkins, Kope, Ghaziuddin, Sorg, and Quint (1997) developed a program at the University of Michigan Medical Center for mentally retarded individuals. Their aim was to prepare their patients for safe, independent living in noninstitutional settings. Over 100 patients were seen between 1986 and 1989 ranging between 10 and 45 years of age. Of these patients, 52 were women and 51 were men. These patients were typically referred to the center because of sexually inappropriate behavior in their homes, schools, or communities. Females were given complete gynecologic examinations, and all subjects were given a psychosocial evaluation, psychiatric assessment, and group and/or individual counseling when needed. Many sexual issues were introduced in this program, including sexual abuse, requests from clients or their parents and caregivers for sterilization, sexual information, social development, questions about getting married, making decisions about pregnancy, family problems, and abortion counseling. These researchers reported that most of their subjects benefitted from their experience in the program, and only a single unanticipated pregnancy occurred in the 4 years since the end of the program. Apparently, programs like this one are highly beneficial when run by professionals who want to work with mentally retarded people and who are trained thoroughly regarding the sexual concerns of this population.

Because of intellectual deficits, communication difficulties, and the potential for exploitation, mentally retarded females, especially adolescents, must be evaluated for the need for contraception and a choice made from suitable alternatives (Table 16-1). Chamberlain, Rauh, Passer, McGrath, and Burket (1984) evaluated 69 patients between the ages of 11 and 23 years, representing all degrees of mental retardation except for profound deficits. Of the 41 subjects with mild retardation, half had had intercourse. Among those moderately retarded, 32% had had intercourse, and 9% of the severely retarded group reported having intercourse. One-third of the mildly retarded subjects reported that they had been raped or sexually abused, and one-fourth of the moderately retarded subjects reported similar occurrences. Slightly less than half of the subjects reported using barrier methods of contraception at some time in their lives, preferring IUDs or Depo-Provera injections. Many of the subjects who didn't use contraception became pregnant. For this vulnerable population contraceptive counseling is extremely important. At the time this study was published, Norplant was not yet available, but it now offers doctors and patients another effective birth control alternative.

TABLE 16-1

Contraceptive Considerations for Women With Mental Disabilities

Barrier methods:	Condoms, diaphragms, cervical caps, female condoms used with or without spermicidal agents
Requirements:	Manual dexterity, high degree of personal motivation, understanding of mechanism of action
Recommendation:	Not widely recommended for women with mental disabilities
Intrauterine devices:	IUDs
Requirements:	Sufficient dexterity to check placement, must be able to promptly report abdominal discomfort
Recommendation:	Not widely recommended for women with mental disabilities
Oral contraceptives:	Birth control pills
Requirements:	Patient's ability to take regularly, dexterity in handling packaging
Recommendation:	Commonly prescribed in this population

After Sulpizi, 1996.

Legal Issues and Sexuality

The mentally ill have certain legal rights and protections with respect to sexual expression, freedom from abuse and exploitation, and independence in making personal reproductive and contraceptive decisions. One of the more thorough, balanced discussions of these considerations is that of Abramson, Parker, and Weinberg (1988). These authors addressed the issues of the meaning of legal consent and mental competency with respect to mentally retarded people. They emphasize, as noted above, that mentally retarded persons are not often given systematic sex education presented in a way they can understand. They further address the significance of mental "competency" with respect to sexuality. Simply stated, to be mentally competent means that one is capable of coherently and meaningfully expressing themselves. Legal "consent" to sexual activity assumes an intellectual level sufficient to appreciate the act of sexual intercourse, its nature, and some of its likely outcomes (Abramson, Parker, & Weinberg, 1988, p. 328).

All of these issues involve the psychosocial environment in which the mentally retarded individual functions. For example, it has been shown that when these individuals are living in the community their sexual behavior is virtually identical to that seen in their peers, and that when these people live in unusual environments, such as institutions, their sexual behavior is similarly unusual (Gebhard, 1973). Abramson, Parker, and Weinberg write of the beneficial effects of sexual activity on the quality of life of the mentally retarded: "sexual expression is significant to mentally retarded people (Edgerton, 1973; Hall, 1974, 1975; Hall & Morris, 1976). It is related to their personal happiness and enhances the stability of their intimate affiliations" (p. 331).

Abramson, Parker, and Weinberg note that mentally retarded persons as a group tend not to be effectively able to use birth control measures that require foresightful planning and good manual dexterity for their use, such as a diaphragm. Contraception is especially critical in this population because when they become pregnant or are implicated in a pregnancy, the chances of having a mentally retarded child can be very high. Reed and Reed (1965) estimated that when both parents are mentally retarded, there is a 40% chance of the child being born mentally retarded. When one parent is afflicted, the chances are 15%, compared to 1% in mentally "normal" parents. But the role of heredity is not always easy to establish. In mild retardation, other family members are also often mentally retarded, but this is typically seen among individuals who live in substandard housing, do not enjoy adequate nutrition, do not receive important social and environmental stimulation, receive poor or little medical attention, and often receive little emotional nurturance as well. Therefore, in many instances where mental retardation seems to run in families, an impoverished environment early in life may also be an important factor (Hunt, 1995; Zigler, 1995).

Abramson, Parker, and Weinberg suggest that mentally retarded persons be offered the same advantages as other disabled persons, in this case, sex education targeted to their level of understanding. They, and we, believe that whenever legal or policy matters are designed to restrict sexual expression among the mentally retarded, personal freedoms in their most basic sense are compromised.

Ames and Samowitz (1995) constructed standards that can be used to determine if a mentally retarded person is capable of giving sexual consent. These authors believe that there are two separate categories for determining informed consent:

Category A: Determining the ability to give informed consent by examining knowledge, intelligence, and the ability to make a voluntary decision through verbal expression (p. 265).

This implies that the person knows what kind of sexual act is anticipated or being considered and can make a personal, informed decision as to whether or not they want to engage in that behavior. It also implies that the person understands that some sexual behaviors are illegal and could result in harsh, punishing outcomes. Category A also implies that the person understands the means by which conception can be prevented and that diseases can be transmitted through sexual contact. This individual also demonstrates that they understand that "time and place" are very important issues for engaging in sexual behaviors. Finally, the person reveals their understanding that some sexual situations can be exploitative and that they can act foresightfully to remove themselves from such situations. As noted above, verbal expression is basic to the issues included in Category A.

Category B: Determining the ability to give informed consent by communicating through responsible interpersonal behavior.

Category B involves somewhat different criteria. Both parties must be acting voluntarily and be protected from being harmed. Both parties should be free from any coercion and abuse. Both parties have the freedom and ability to discontinue participation in sexual acts. And both parties should demonstrate that they can choose socially appropriate times and places for sexual behavior. Some mentally retarded individuals are not capable of communicating with enough clarity to meet all the requirements in Category A. Because of this, Category B offers families and professionals guidance for evaluating interactions in which clear communication is in some way lacking.

Contraceptive issues affecting mentally retarded individuals have been strongly influenced by the development of Norplant. IUDs also offer effective birth control for those who may be unable to remember to take oral contraceptives regularly or who lack the necessary foresight to obtain and correctly use barrier methods, such as condoms and the diaphragm. In the past, directive legal interventions were more commonly taken. For example, a 17-year-old English woman was the object of a complex legal case in which the young woman's mother and local judicial authorities wanted to have her sterilized (Brahams, 1987). This young woman had the ability to dress and care for herself, as well as to "attend to herself during menstruation." However, she could not leave her home alone because she didn't understand automobile traffic and had no comprehension of money. It was thought at the time that she could be educated to the level of a 5- or 6-year-old child. As she approached her late teens she became more aware of sexual feelings, and so her family, her physician, and legal authorities considered effective contraceptive alternatives. Two means of limiting her fertility were seriously considered: daily oral contraceptives and bilateral tubal ligation. The girl's mother petitioned the judge to have the girl sterilized, and the government's representative appealed this decision, but the appeal was denied. Ultimately, the House of Lords heard this case and approved the decision to have the girl sterilized in 1989 (Brahams, 1989).

SEXUAL EXPRESSION AMONG THE VISUALLY AND HEARING IMPAIRED

The earlier discussion of mental "competency" focused on the individual's ability to communicate and express themselves. Competency involves a person's awareness of their immediate environment and their ability to plan and act in ways that reveal their knowledge of who and what is happening around them. As competency is often affected by mental retardation, so too people who are visually and/or hearing impaired also have a potentially diminished capacity to be aware of what is happening in their immediate surroundings and to express themselves and behave accordingly. The mentally retarded and visually and hearing impaired are *not* challenged in the same ways or to the same degree in their ability to attend to their surroundings or express themselves. Despite the fact that sexual expression is such a basic aspect of our humanity, little research has been done concerning visual and hearing impairments and sexuality. Even though a person may not be able to see or hear, they obviously still have rights to free association and freedom from exploitation. Effective sexual communication can most certainly take place in the absence of visual and/or auditory cues.

Gillman and Gordon (1973) noted that sexual learning and feeling often involve looking at others and being looked at in return. Visual cues are basic to most people's thoughts and feelings about sex. What might then be the impact of blindness on the development of gender identity and later on how one learns and uses sexual information? Some people, blind from birth, are *congenitally blind,* while others lose their vision after varying amounts of time. These people are referred to as *adventitiously blind.* Interestingly, and importantly, children who are blind from birth develop gender roles in the same way as sighted children. The same kind of sex-role typing in play activities, choice of toys, and imaginary heroes occurs among both congenitally blind and sighted children.

As sexuality emerges during adolescence, the more intelligent visually impaired teenager shows virtually no signs of unusual sexual behavior and is quite capable of grasping basic information about sexual anatomy and physiology. Still, many act in a shy, uncertain way as they begin to explore intimate contact during these years. Those who lose their vision later in life often have psychological reactions to this enormous loss and the lifestyle adjustments it demands. Depression is common in these circumstances and often plays a role in sexual repression and in some cases impotence. Those who have successfully adapted to their disability seem able to enjoy an entirely normal sexual repertoire and normal physical responsiveness. Remember that our sense of touch might be the most important sense for fully enjoying sexual activity.

As the visually impaired are challenged by a diminished ability to gain information from their environment, the hearing impaired are too. Relatively little has been written about the impact of deafness on sexuality. One interesting research report emphasizes the disadvantages faced by this population and the need for sex education targeted to this group of people. Joseph, Sawyer, and Desmond (1995) presented questionnaires to 134 deaf and hard of hearing college students that were designed to assess the person's understanding of susceptibility to STDs and risks of unanticipated pregnancy, sexual activities, methods of birth control, personal reproductive health behaviors, sexual health information, and other personal characteristics. Most of the respondents were women (72%). About three-fourths of the subjects were Caucasian. The results of the survey were somewhat disturbing. Generally these subjects were not well informed about their sexual health or sexual issues. Only one-third reported using a condom in their most recent sexual experience. The most commonly reported method of contraception was withdrawal, with only 17% of the subjects using oral contraceptives. About one-third of the women in this sample said that they had experienced forced sex. Overall, these subjects did not have a good knowledge base about a wide variety of sexual issues, particularly those concerning fertility, HIV/AIDS, safe sex, and contraceptive issues. Whether these responses reflected a lack of sex education in general or a lack of the type of sex education readily understood by deaf people is not clear in this study. What did emerge from this study, however, was the fact that like their sighted and hearing counterparts, these subjects relied primarily on their peers for information about sex. Research has yet to demonstrate what kind of sex education would be most appropriate for these groups of individuals.

"IN SICKNESS AND IN HEALTH"

We all get older, more frequently become ill, and eventually die. Yet we are sexual beings from birth to death, as well as "in sickness and in health." A person's sexual value system is based on many diverse issues and influences that have an erotic meaning for that person, and a person's sexual value system doesn't necessarily change because they get sick or develop a chronic or degenerative disease. Continued enjoyment in shared sexual intimacy is the rule, not the exception, for those with chronic illnesses and disabilities. This chapter has sought to *validate and legitimate* the importance of sexual expression among people who are sick. Most of us will experience old age, and part of getting older involves increased vulnerability to disease and diminished physical health.

A person's inner strength, honesty, spontaneity, and authenticity may be of primary importance for sexual attractiveness among those who are ill and/or disabled. Relationships that are characterized by trust, sharing, and good communication typically involve a pattern of lifelong sexual activity, even when one or both partners becomes ill or disabled. All the discussion of good communication in earlier chapters is directly relevant to continued sexual behavior among people who are not in very good health or who may not have long to live.

CONCLUSION

Illness and disabilities may or may not be related to how we live and our lifestyle choices. Certainly, many of our day-to-day decisions concerning diet, exercise, and stress affect our predisposition to disease and disability. However, most of the health problems addressed in this chapter *occur through no fault of the person afflicted.* Many people have done nothing to become sick, infirm, paralyzed, or retarded.

The next chapter will discuss sexually transmitted diseases and AIDS, and a person's lifestyle and daily decisions do play an enormous part in that individual's vulnerability to these disorders. This chapter emphasizes how people *react* to different health problems, but the emphasis of the next chapter is more *proactive,* focusing on lifestyle decisions that can minimize a person's chances of contracting an STD or AIDS. Knowing a lot about STDs is one of the best ways to avoid getting one.

Learning Activities

1. List and discuss common stereotypes about the ill and disabled and their continued expression of sexual feelings. What common social and cultural biases perpetuate these prejudiced beliefs?
2. Speculate as to how a chronically ill or disabled individual might interpret the common belief by the general public that they no longer have any sexual feelings, inclinations, or desires. How can physicians and other health care professionals validate the normality of these desires?
3. In your opinion, should physicians initiate discussions regarding the impact of illness and treatment on sexual expression and functioning, or should the doctor wait until the patient asks specific questions about this subject? Why?
4. If a patient stops taking a prescribed medication, how might a physician tactfully determine whether the person stopped because of diminished sexual functioning as a side effect?
5. When institutional care makes little or no allowance for the sexual needs of residents or patients, how might spouses or grown children do something to create privacy and opportunity for sexual sharing?
6. When one member of a couple is ill or disabled and their desire for intimacy is affected, is this something they should be able to work out on their own, or do you think some type of counseling might be helpful?
7. Contraceptive education should be taught at a level appropriate to an individual's intellectual abilities. In the case of mental retardation among young adults and adults, how do you feel about each of the following statements?
   a. Taking oral contraceptives should be a part of the female's daily hygiene routine if this choice is thought best for her by her parents or guardians.
   b. Norplant should be administered to mentally retarded females at the request of their parents in consultation with a physician. Alternatively, Depo-Provera injections can be used.
   c. Males should be offered explicit information and guidance in the use of condoms, as well as be taught how and where to obtain them.
8. Many women are so anxious about developing breast cancer that they avoid measures that might lead to early detection, such as mammograms. What type of appeal would be effective to motivate these women to be more conscientious about having these examinations and tests done? Is this situation the same for men getting examinations and tests for prostate cancer?
9. Contact your local chapter of the American Cancer Society and the local office of the Ostomy Association to collect educational leaflets. How explicitly do these address the issue of continued sexual expression, and what recommendations are made?
10. What goes through your mind when you hear that a "perfectly healthy" individual has fallen in love with and married a quadriplegic?

Key Concepts

- When people become ill or disabled, we often think of them in terms of the sick role, with attributions of passivity, lack of interest, slow movement, and an inability to take any enjoyment in life.
- Anticipatory guidance involves helping a sick or disabled person to learn about their condition and what is likely to happen to them in the future.
- How we view and evaluate our physical selves is called our body image. Illness and disability have a powerful negative impact on our body image.
- Not all illnesses are treated promptly and aggressively. Watchful waiting involves monitoring the disease closely until the most effective intervention is appropriate.
- Everyone has a personal erotic map based on their own unique sexual experiences. Knowing a person's erotic map helps professionals assist them to continue sexual activity when they are sick or disabled.
- Positive illusions are strategies people employ to see the world as safer than it really is. In a very real sense we "lie" to ourselves about our vulnerabilities and inadequacies and the risks we run daily.
- Common illnesses and disabilities affect a person's sexual functioning and their inclination to enjoy physical intimacy with their partner. Still, for ill and disabled individuals, sexual expression often remains an important personal priority. Some of these ailments and disabilities include:

  Cerebrovascular accidents or "strokes"
  Hemiparesis
  Cancer
  Kidney disease and dialysis treatments
  Osteoarthritis and rheumatoid arthritis
  Ostomy surgery
  Spinal cord injuries involving paraplegia or tetraplegia
  Cerebral palsy
  Multiple sclerosis
  Dementia, including Alzheimer's disease
  Mental retardation

- A person's sexual self-schema is their thoughts about various aspects of their sexuality and the variables (e.g., physical attractiveness) that contribute to it.

■ A person is mentally competent when they can coherently and meaningfully express themselves. Someone who is not mentally competent is entitled to a variety of legal protections from abuse and/or exploitation.

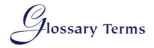

Glossary Terms

cancer	hemiparesis	paraplegia
cerebral palsy	medical model	rheumatoid
cerebrovascular	mental	arthritis
accident	retardation	stoma
dementia	multiple sclerosis	tetraplegia
dialysis	osteoarthritis	

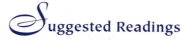

Suggested Readings

Blackburn, M. (1999). Sex and disability. Woburn, MA: Butterworth-Heinemann.

Carlton, L. (1997). In sickness and in health: Sex, love, and chronic illness. New York: Dell Books.

Fegan, L., & Rauch, A. (1993). Sexuality and people with intellectual disability. Baltimore: Paul H. Brookes Publishing Company.

Sandowski, C. L. (1990). Sexual concerns when illness or disability strikes. Springfield, IL: Charles C. Thomas Publishers, Ltd.

Schover, L. R., & Jensen, S. B. (1988). Sex and chronic illness: A comprehensive approach. New York: Guilford Press.

Shakespeare, T., Gillespie-Sells, K., & Davies, D. (1996). The sexual politics of disability: Untold desires. London: Cassell Academic.

17

Sexually Transmitted Diseases and AIDS

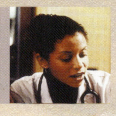

OBJECTIVES

When you finish reading and reviewing this chapter, you should be able to:

1. Recognize that STDs are epidemic in this country as well as other countries throughout the world and that the best way to reduce the prevalence of these is through effective preventive measures.

2. Discuss why many people who have STDs are asymptomatic and explain why delay in treatment is generally more harmful for women than men.

3. Describe how a person can minimize or eliminate their chances of contracting STDs.

4. Discuss how HIV is diagnosed through blood tests and the appearance of clinical signs. Define "seropositive."

5. Explain why HIV has a disproportionately adverse effect on women, children, and minorities.

6. Describe the transmission and clinical manifestations of each of the following STDs:
   - genital herpes
   - human papilloma virus
   - hepatitis
   - chlamydia
   - gonorrhea
   - syphilis
   - chancroid
   - cytomegalovirus
   - molluscum contagiosum

7. Explain the challenges of developing treatments for viral and bacterial STDs, and describe why some of these become resistant over time to the drugs used to treat them.

8. Explain what you should do if you think you have an STD.

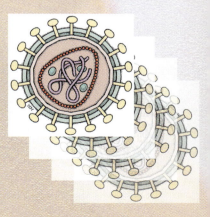

From Dr. Ruth

When I began my radio program in 1980, AIDS was not an issue. I spoke often of avoiding sexually transmitted diseases, but the consequences of those diseases then were not as deadly, at least not if treated in a timely fashion. Obviously the urgency of this message has increased greatly since those days.

That said, I also know that scare tactics don't work, even now with the growing prevalence of AIDS. During World War II, soldiers were told to stay away from prostitutes, and to enforce this message, they were shown films full of horrible images of the symptoms of STDs. Did those films work? Perhaps some men were scared away, but a great many took advantage of any opportunity for sex without worrying about the consequences. These men perhaps had the excuse of being in the heat of battle, but I know that in the heat of passion, two people are also likely to put aside their fears and have unprotected sex rather than listen to reason. That's why the most important time to protect yourself from STDs is before you are in the arms of your partner. Make sure a condom is available, or communicate your wishes not to have sex until the relationship has further developed and you both know more about each other, perhaps including the results of specific tests.

You won't catch me using the phrase "safe sex." I only say "safer sex," because there are always some risks. But just because there are no 100% guarantees in life doesn't mean that you shouldn't do whatever you can to limit the risks.

The five most dangerous words concerning STDs are "It can't happen to me." While I want everyone to get as much enjoyment from sex as possible, you must have a healthy respect for the dangers out there. Even a relatively mild STD, one you don't even know you have, can lead to infertility. Of course, AIDS has fatal consequences. The numbers of people infected with STDs are in the millions in the United States. The fact is that unless you are careful, not only can it happen to you, but it *will* happen. The up side is that if you take precautions so you can have sex without that little voice in the back of your mind constantly asking, "Am I safe?" I promise you that you'll enjoy sex a lot more.

This chapter examines common negative consequences of shared physical intimacy: sexually transmitted diseases, or STDs, often now also referred to as STIs, or sexually transmitted infections. The older term "venereal diseases" is seldom used any more. We will also discuss AIDS in this chapter. Although AIDS can be transmitted also by nonsexual means (such as intravenous drug use), most often this STD is transmitted by sexual means. The viruses and bacteria that cause STDs are amazingly resilient and have been able to survive despite the best efforts of medicine and public health campaigns. Many STDs seem to have become increasingly resistant to the drugs used to treat them. Charles Darwin taught us that a "successful" organism can successfully adapt to changing environments and live long enough to reproduce. This is no less true of the viruses and bacteria that cause STDs than of human beings.

Although this chapter discusses many different STDs and their unpleasant symptoms and consequences, the main focus is *prevention*. Everyone must be individually motivated to take personal responsibility for their own intimate behaviors and to engage in intelligent sexual decision making. We want readers to be informed about these diseases and to feel confident when facing less-than-safe sexual opportunities. If ever the expression, "knowledge is power" was true, this is certainly so with the material in this chapter.

The last chapter closed with the reminder that many illnesses and disabilities occur for no apparent reason and that no one is at "fault." In contrast, STDs do involve a significant element of ignorance, carelessness, magical thinking about one's invulnerability, and negligence. *Our thinking and behavior are directly responsible for our getting or avoiding STDs.* By definition, a sexually transmitted disease is any disease transmitted from one person to another through sexual contact, which also includes oral-genital contact, anal intercourse, and oral-anal contact, and other unusual sexual behaviors. Not all STDs will be discussed in this chapter, as more than 30 have been identified, but the most common ones will be: AIDS, genital herpes, human papilloma virus, hepatitis, chlamydia, gonorrhea, syphilis, nongonococcal urethritis, some skin parasites, chancroid, cytomegalovirus, and molluscum contagiosum. These are the ones you and those you know are most likely to be exposed to. Many different kinds of organisms cause STDs: viruses, bacteria, single-celled animals, parasitic crustaceans, and even fungi. Chapter 5 discussed a number of infections that affect the sexual and reproductive anatomy of both women and men, and some of these also can be transmitted through sexual contact as well. This chapter discusses only those diseases that are transmitted exclusively or primarily through sexual contact.

STDs are very prevalent; in fact, they are among the most prevalent communicable diseases. The term *epidemic* refers to a very high number of cases of a disease in a specific population at any particular point in time, and many STDs are epidemic in many countries, if not continents, throughout the world. In the United States, the Centers for Disease Control and Prevention and the National Institutes of Health have made every effort to inform the American people about STDs of all types. While estimates of prevalence vary somewhat, everyone agrees this is a *huge* problem. By the end of 1997, almost 31 million people throughout the world were HIV-positive or had AIDS. In 1995, an estimated 333 million people had other STDs excluding AIDS, 14 million of whom lived in North America. In 1995 alone, some 478,000 new cases of chlamydia were reported in the United States, along with 393,000 new cases of gonorrhea and 69,000 cases of syphilis–and these are only *three* of the many kinds of STDs. When there are almost a million new cases of three STDs in our country in one year, this is plainly an important public health problem.

In 1996, the World Health Organization estimated that among people between the ages of 15 and 49, there were 12.2 million cases of syphilis, 62.2 million cases of gonorrhea, and 89.1 million cases of chlamydia worldwide. The greatest number of new cases of non-AIDS STDs was found in south and southeast Asia (45.6% increase), sub-Saharan Africa (19.7% increase), and Latin America and the Caribbean (10.9% increase) (Gerbase, Rowley, & Mertens, 1998). Gerbase, Rowley, and Mertens (1998) noted that globally, the prevalence of STDs is higher in cities than in rural areas, higher among the unmarried, and higher among adolescents and young adults. They also noted that STDs generally occur at a younger age among females than males. World health experts note that the increase in STDs in any population depends on a number of variables, including the average number of partners infected, the efficiency with which the virus or bacteria is transmitted from one person to another, the frequency with which infected individuals change sexual partners, and the length of time a person is infectious before they are treated.

One of the most powerful factors contributing to the prevalence of STDs is a lack of adequate sex education and health information (Gerbase, Rowley, & Mertens, 1998). Current data support the fact that adolescents and young adults who receive serious, systematic sex education are far more likely to have positive attitudes about obtaining and using condoms (O'Donnell, San Doval, Duran, & O'Donnell, 1995), although the subjects in this study only reported their attitudes about using condoms, not their actual condom-using behav-

ior. Additionally, middle and high school students who watched video programs about HIV and other STDs demonstrated that they understood that sex takes place as a result of personal, wilful decisions and doesn't "just happen" and that even one sexual experience can involve the transmission of HIV or another STD, and they had clear intentions to obtain and use condoms properly (Noell, Ary, & Duncan, 1997). As with much research in the social and behavioral sciences, follow-up studies are necessary to find out how enduring these behavioral and attitudinal changes are.

Other issues also have an impact on the incidence of any particular STD in a society. For example, because of the social stigma associated with seeking treatment for STDs, many people delay and continue to spread the disease before they receive adequate medical care. Additionally, in many parts of the world medical care is not easily available, a factor people in the United States often have difficulty understanding. In addition, the fact that some STDs have become resistant to certain antibiotics means that some people who are treated are not being cured but continue to harbor the infection, perhaps without knowing it.

THE PROBLEM OF STDS

Basic Facts About STDs

STDs are some of the most common communicable diseases in America. The National Institutes of Health has estimated that the cost of diagnosis, treatment, lost occupational productivity, and lost wages amounts to about $10 billion each year. Following are some facts about STDs compiled by the National Institutes of Health (June 1998 Fact Sheet).

- People of all educational, socioeconomic, religious, political, ethnic, and racial groups contract STDs; no one is immune. Approximately two-thirds of all new cases of STDs are found in individuals under the age of 25.
- The number of new cases of STDs increases each year. One of the reasons for this is that people are more likely today to have multiple sex partners because they begin having sex earlier in their teens and marry later, and therefore are more likely to date (and have sex with) more individuals before they settle down. Additionally, more people are getting divorced, which means that more people are dating other people again and having sex with some of them.
- Many people who have contracted an STD have no symptoms and therefore may continue to have sex with others (sometimes several others) and unknowingly transmit the disease to them.
- The health consequences of STDs are generally worse for women than men. Complications of STDs that are not treated or that are treated long after they have been contracted often involve the uterus and fallopian tubes. This can result in infertility and increased chances of an ectopic pregnancy. Additionally, some STDs are associated with an increased risk of cervical cancer or other genital cancers. Finally, STDs can pass

from an infected woman to her embryo or fetus while she is pregnant.

- Delay in treating chlamydia and gonorrhea in men can also lead to infertility.
- When STDs are diagnosed and treated promptly, effective medical care can reduce the risk of complications and in many cases completely eliminate the bacteria that caused it. Viral STDs are far more difficult to treat, and in most cases the individual will carry the virus as long as they live. While viral STDs might not be curable, most are manageable, and their symptoms can be minimized in most cases. Yet having STDs other than AIDS can increase a person's chances of contracting HIV.

With STDs so common and their effects so negative, why do people neglect to engage in safer sex practices and increase their chances of catching an STD? How can a person be so careless that they engage in behaviors that are likely to lead to their contracting an STD? As frightening, embarrassing, uncomfortable, and potentially lethal as STDs can be, why are people still powerfully motivated to minimize their thinking about the consequences in order to enjoy the pleasures of sexual activity? To some this just seems "human nature," but social, behavioral, and medical scientists are often at a loss to explain the kinds of thinking that lie behind this kind of sexual risk taking. Can behaviors that result in procreation be so powerfully motivated that human beings are "programmed" to override our awareness of the hazards of some sexual activity? We have no good answers to these questions.

History of STDs

For over 3500 years it has been known that diseases can be transmitted sexually, although the apparent relationship between sexual relations and the symptoms of STDs has not always been clear. Michael Waugh's comprehensive history of sexually transmitted diseases (1990) provides the following information.

As early as 1550 B.C. ancient Egyptian papyrus scrolls described symptoms of what today are recognized as vaginitis and infections affecting the vulva. These same documents also note the presence of abnormal narrowing of the genitalia, presumably the urethra, of both women and men, presumed to result from sexual activity. The ancient Egyptians provide a clinical picture of pubic lice, but there are no clear records of syphilis in this ancient civilization. The Biblical Book of Leviticus, Chapter 15, makes specific reference to urethral discharges that were thought to result from sexually transmitted infections. Although these verses certainly describe what we today call urethritis, there is no way of knowing whether this symptom was caused by gonorrhea or some other agent. Greek and Roman writers described a condition that was most assuredly gonorrhea, as well as genital herpes and two other lesser known STDs, chancroid and lymphogranuloma venereum. Anal warts, today called human papilloma virus, were described as a consequence of anal intercourse. We cannot be certain about historical descriptions of sexually related diseases because symptoms

alone are not enough to differentiate different diseases, which today require specific laboratory tests for a definite diagnosis.

Perhaps more so than other STDs, syphilis has been the subject of extensive historical research and debate. Waugh notes that skeletal signs of the disease have been found in remains that predate Columbus's visit to the New World. Because these indications have not been discovered in skeletal remains in Europe before 1493, some scientists speculate that some of Columbus's sailors contracted the disease in the Caribbean and spread it upon their return to Europe. In fact, there was a serious epidemic of syphilis in Europe during that century. The term "pandemic" describes the extremely high prevalence of this disease throughout Europe at this time. A pandemic is more serious than an epidemic because it covers a very large area, such as a country, continent, or even the world. At first, the relationship between sexual activity and the early symptoms were not recognized, perhaps because these symptoms don't appear for about three weeks, which might have

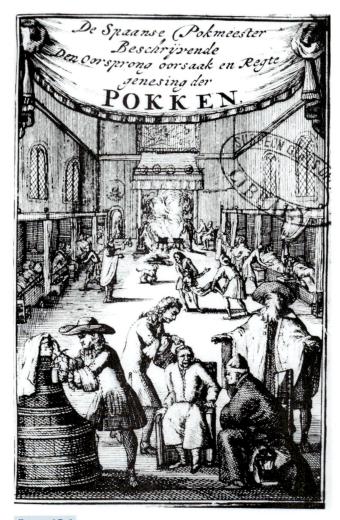

FIGURE 17-1 Many historical documents report the wide prevalence of syphilis, as well as various approaches to the care and treatment of this disease.

made it difficult to appreciate the connection between intercourse and the appearance of the hard, round, red lesions that usually signal syphilis in its earliest stage. As well, syphilis is usually painless at this stage, so there may have been little discomfort to notice. Jacques de Berthencourt first used the term "venereal disease" in 1527, and that term was used until only a few decades ago when "STD" replaced it. The word syphilis did not appear in the English language until 1686 (Fig. 17-1).

During the Middle Ages, and well into the nineteenth century, syphilis and gonorrhea were not recognized as different diseases. In the 1500s, most writers on the subject viewed gonorrhea as an early symptom of syphilis; without microscopes they could not discover that they were caused by two different microorganisms. As early as 1564, the Italian anatomist, Gabriel Fallopius (after whom the fallopian tubes

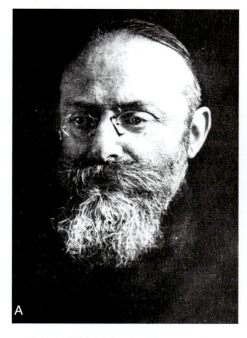

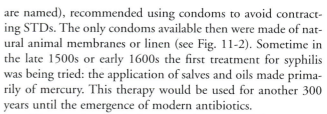

are named), recommended using condoms to avoid contracting STDs. The only condoms available then were made of natural animal membranes or linen (see Fig. 11-2). Sometime in the late 1500s or early 1600s the first treatment for syphilis was being tried: the application of salves and oils made primarily of mercury. This therapy would be used for another 300 years until the emergence of modern antibiotics.

The question of whether gonorrhea and syphilis were two different diseases or different manifestations of the same disease was debated in medical circles for many years to come. In one of the most unusual medical experiments in history, the British physician John Hunter attempted to prove that gonorrhea and syphilis were the same disease. In 1767 he extracted the urethral discharge from one of his patients who was suffering from gonorrhea and inoculated his own foreskin and glans with the infectious pus. Unbeknownst to Hunter, the patient also had syphilis! Medical historians believe that Hunter contracted syphilis as a result of his little experiment.

By the mid 1700s, most large cities in Europe had special hospitals for the diagnosis and treatment of STDs, the most famous of which was the London Lock Hospital, founded by the surgeon William Bromfield. Another important figure in the history of the study of STDs was Philippe Ricord (1800-1889), who was the first person to demonstrate conclusively, based on almost 700 cases, that gonorrhea and syphilis were two different diseases. He was also the first person to recognize that syphilis progresses in three stages. By the mid-1800s, mercury was gradually being replaced as the treatment of choice for syphilis by potassium iodide, which was effective in curing syphilis, particularly during its later stages. Toward the end of the 19th century it became certain that untreated syphilis can affect many of the body's major organ systems, especially the cardiovascular and nervous systems.

With the emergence of bacteriology, investigators could examine the bacteria that cause gonorrhea and syphilis under the microscope and recognize that there are different microorganisms giving rise to different diseases. Albert Neisser (1854-1916) (Fig. 17-2A) first described the bacteria that cause gonorrhea in 1879. Soon afterwards, these bacteria were found in the membranes surrounding the eyes of newborn babies whose mothers had active gonorrhea at the time of birth. This gave rise to the practice of placing silver nitrate eye drops into the eyes of newborn babies to kill any of these bacteria that might be present. A number of investigations between 1875 and 1913 finally isolated the specific bacterium that causes syphilis, called *treponema pallidum*.

The early 20th century saw additional discoveries in the diagnosis and treatment of STDs. In 1907, the German bacteriologist Paul Ehrlich (Fig. 17-2B) discovered a compound de-

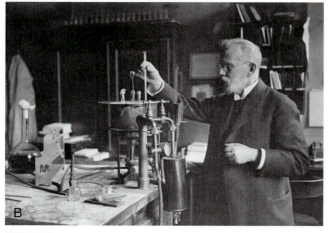

FIGURE 17-2   A. Albert Neisser. B. Paul Ehrlich. C. Julius W. von Jauregg. These men are three early pioneers in the diagnosis and treatment of sexually transmitted diseases.

rived from arsenic, a poison sometimes used as a weed-killer, that he called "Salvarsan." This agent proved to be far more effective than potassium iodide in the treatment of syphilis and became a primary therapeutic weapon against this disease until penicillin became widely available. Another ingenious approach to the treatment of syphilis was invented by Julius W. von Jauregg (1857-1940) (Fig. 17-2C), who discovered that mild malaria could actually cure patients of advanced cases of this STD. Apparently he accidentally introduced a few drops of blood from people with malaria into open skin lesions of syphilis patients and found that the protozoa that cause malaria could actually cure people with syphilis. His results were published in 1921, and this method remained a treatment of choice in dealing with advanced syphilis among the mentally incapacitated until penicillin became available in the 1940s. von Jauregg received the Nobel Prize in Medicine in 1928 for his discovery. The first reported success in using penicillin to treat syphilis was published in 1943, and since that time it has been a primary treatment of choice.

The history of STDs in the United States has also been interesting. The Continental Congress decreed in 1778 that officers would be fined $10 and enlisted men $4 if they went to a hospital seeking treatment for a venereal disease (Moore, 1947). In 1874, it was estimated that 5% of the American population was infected with syphilis and that a woman would live only about 5 years if she became a prostitute. At the onset of World War I, virtually all of the combatant nations took steps to control STDs among their troops. Waugh (1990) noted that at times up to 25% of British and French soldiers were incapacitated by STDs and could not fight. When America entered the war in 1917 there were some 250 "venereal disease control officers," who helped lower the STD rates below those found in the military in peace time. When World War II began, penicillin was not yet available, but a treatment of Koch's Salvarsan given intravenously over the course of 5 to 10 days had high rates of success curing syphilis. When penicillin did become available, however, there was a common misconception that it could cure all STDs. By the early 1970s, gonorrhea and syphilis were again epidemic in the United States. Sexual permissiveness had become more common, and oral contraceptives contributed to fewer condoms being used correctly and consistently. The microorganisms that cause STDs had also become progressively resistant to traditional antibiotic therapies, leading to the development of newer and more powerful drugs.

EFFECTIVENESS OF PROGRAMS TO LOWER STD AND HIV RATES

We have already mentioned the importance of educational programs, community intervention programs, and improved delivery of public health services for lowering STD and HIV infection rates. Aral and Peterman (1998) assessed whether such behavioral interventions actually work. These researchers emphasize some research issues require further study before we can be sure that these prevention efforts actually work. For example:

- There are often differences between what people report they do to minimize the chances of acquiring an STD and what they actually do. This means that it is difficult to establish the validity of measures of behavioral change.
- Whether intervention programs are implemented is often unrelated to any compelling data about their potential effectiveness.
- Collecting data about STD and HIV prevalence in a geographically defined community is extremely difficult to do accurately for any appreciable length of time. What we learn from these trials might be useful, but it is also too late to do anything about prevention failures.
- The relationship between a community's needs and the development of an intervention program may not be clearly outlined, with the result that prevention programs may have little to do with the specific needs of a particular community.

Aral and Peterman emphasize that behavioral intervention programs have been definitively shown to increase people's knowledge of STDs and HIV as well as affect their attitudes about these major health challenges. These programs work to help people feel more effective in making decisions that can enhance their health. Further, data indicate that these educational efforts give people interpersonal communication skills to negotiate safer sex behaviors and use condoms correctly and consistently. Therefore there is reason to be optimistic about their effectiveness.

THE SCOPE OF STDs AND THE NEED FOR PREVENTION

On March 9, 1998, an article on the front page of the *New York Times* proclaimed, "U. S. Awakens to Epidemic of Sexual Diseases," (Stolberg, 1998). To many people, headlines like this seem a little strange as recently as 1998, but in fact, even into the mid-1990s, there was no effective national system for STD prevention. In 1996, the Institute of Medicine's *The Hidden Epidemic* reported that the federal government spent approximately $230 million in 1995 to advertise the availability of diagnostic and treatment services for STDs, not including the costs of similar services for AIDS. The actual cost of treating STDs was approximately $7.5 *billion* in that year alone. The figures are staggering: the number of non-AIDS STD cases reported to the Centers for Disease Control and Prevention is about 80 times the number of new cases of TB, HIV, and AIDS combined. Additionally, a person with chlamydia, gonorrhea, syphilis, or genital herpes is *two to five times* more susceptible to contracting HIV. In light of these data, President Clinton successfully encouraged Congress to appropriate an

Research Highlight

UNETHICAL RESEARCH WITH HORRIBLE LONG-TERM OUTCOMES

Research Highlight sections throughout this book describe various investigations into aspects of human sexuality. Until now all of these have been interesting or important research studies carried out with the approval of Institutional Review Boards (IRBs) that assess research projects to protect the participants. Unfortunately, such safeguards have not always been used in our country. In the study described here there was a virtual absence of attention to ethical principles, resulting in terrible consequences for the participants.

The Tuskegee Syphilis Study was the longest *nontherapeutic* medical study in history. This study has likely contributed to the skepticism of many African Americans regarding the role of the Public Health Service in diagnosing and treating AIDS in African Americans today.

In 1928, the Julius Rosenwald Fund, a philanthropic organization in Chicago, approached the United States Public Health Service with the intention of improving the health of blacks living in the rural South. Significant monies were donated, and thousands of individuals throughout the South were examined and treated for a variety of ailments. Testing for syphilis was a routine aspect of this screening. The prevalence of syphilis was discovered to be extremely high in several areas, especially Macon County Alabama, where 30-40% of African American men tested positive for this disease. At about this time, the Great Depression eliminated the Rosenwald support for this project, and hundreds of African American men with diagnosed syphilis could not begin the treatment phase of the project.

At this time, there were speculations that syphilis affected different races differentially, but no experimental study of this issue had been undertaken. Taliaferro Clark, MD, of the Public Health Service decided in 1932 that these black men diagnosed with syphilis should not be treated in order to monitor the progress and impact of the disease over a significant period of time; some of the impact was planned to be assessed at autopsy. Thus the "Public Health Study of Untreated Syphilis in the Male Negro" began. Here are some important facts about this project:

- Three hundred ninety-nine men with syphilis and 201 control subjects were studied from 1932 to 1972.
- No treatment was administered to the men with syphilis. The role of sexual intercourse in the transmission of the disease was not explained to these men, nor was the threat of the disease to women, pregnant women, and the fetuses they carried.
- The investigators hoped that their data would eventually pressure Southern legislatures to improve health care services for rural blacks.
- The infected men were excluded from military service during World War II without an explanation.
- When penicillin became widely available to the general public in 1951, it was withheld from the infected men.

Particularly noteworthy are the ways subjects were recruited for participation in this horrible enterprise. Black physicians, nurses, schoolteachers, and ministers all encouraged cooperation with the Public Health Service in addition to the farm owners who employed the infected men. Essentially, the disease was allowed to run its course; the men were promised free burial expenses if they agreed to an autopsy.

The terrible ethical and moral failures of this study have had a lasting impact on how African Americans since have viewed the motives and methods of the Public Health Service. Just as doctors, nurses, teachers, and ministers encouraged these unfortunate men to cooperate with the government years ago, these same authority figures now encourage African Americans today to participate in community programs for the prevention, diagnosis, and treatment of AIDS (Thomas & Quinn, 1991). When the story of the Tuskegee Syphilis Study became public on July 25, 1972, black leaders across the country suggested that this investigation was a systematic attempt to carry out genocide in the United States.

additional $10 million for diagnostic and prevention services for STDs in 1999.

The Hidden Epidemic (1996) is a 448-page report that emphasized that there was virtually no federally organized system for the diagnosis and treatment of STDs, even though these disorders account for 5 of the 10 most common diseases reported to the CDC. The report noted that the government spends only $1 on prevention for every $43 spent on treatment (though it is unclear how much cost-effective prevention expenditures are). The report emphasized three areas of focus for enhancing prevention of STDs.

- Integrate STD prevention and treatment into the mainstream of primary care medicine. Very few health care plans invest significant funds in these areas, nor do they typically pay for better training for health care professionals in the area of STDs.
- Focus on teenagers. Changing adolescents' awareness of STDs and their vulnerability to these disorders is a key educational priority. The report recommends that every school district in the country offer students age-appropriate sex education (typically beginning in elementary school), access to latex condoms, and access to medical services for the prevention, diagnosis, and treatment of STDs. The report also emphasizes the fact that no data support the contention that making condoms available to teenagers increases the amount of sexual activity.
- Start a public information campaign in which figures from the entertainment, sports, and political areas of American life promote public discourse and awareness of safer sexual behavior. Because many adolescents are receptive to messages from authoritative figures in the media, this initiative is especially important for this highly susceptible age group.

In all, this document is a realistic appraisal of contemporary health hazards and includes many feasible measures that are likely to effectively diminish the impact of STDs and AIDS on our society and enhance the quality of life of our citizens.

The Critical Role of Prevention

Some might think that a combination of good medication, good public awareness programs, and fear might be enough to prevent STDs, but unfortunately, it's not that simple. The challenge of preventing STDs is important because these diseases can have catastrophic, if not fatal, long-term consequences. According to the Centers for Disease Control (CDC), 20-40% of women infected with chlamydia and 10-40% of women infected with gonorrhea will develop pelvic inflammatory disease (PID). About 20% of women with PID will develop scarring in their fallopian tubes, which often results in infertility. Additionally 9% of these women will have ectopic pregnancies, and almost 20% will experience long-term pelvic discomfort. When these STDs are treated promptly and appropriately, the risks of ectopic pregnancy can be reduced by as much as one-half.

Additionally, the CDC notes that human papilloma virus (HPV) is the single biggest risk factor for the development of cervical cancer. HPV also causes genital warts. While genital warts can be treated in different ways, the virus cannot be completely eliminated from the body. This government agency has estimated that genital herpes is the most common STD in the United States, with as many as 30 million people carrying the virus. Again, there is no cure for genital herpes, but a number of effective drugs help manage it and limit or eliminate the recurrences of symptoms that usually occur without treatment.

As seen earlier, much of the history of STDs involves syphilis, one of the most complex of all sexually transmitted infections. Among pregnant women who have syphilis, approximately 40% will give birth to dead babies or babies who will die shortly after birth. Infants who live may be blind, malformed, paralyzed, or mentally retarded. People who have syphilis are also at an increased risk of contracting HIV if they have sex with an infected partner, because the open sores that characterize syphilis make it easier for HIV to enter the body.

As of this writing, approximately 60% of people who have contracted AIDS have died. While researchers are continually developing better drugs to treat the health problems associated with HIV, prevention remains the most effective means of saving lives and minimizing the impact of this epidemic. Other factors too make prevention especially critical. First, STDs have a disproportionately large effect on women, newborn babies, and members of minority groups, although men are certainly affected, especially in their increased risk of infertility when there is significant delay in the treatment of chlamydia and gonorrhea. As discussed above, STDs affect the development of cancers of the genito-urinary system in women as well as cause increased rates of involuntary infertility and ectopic pregnancy. Second, untreated gonorrhea and syphilis have terrible effects on fetuses and newborn babies, as described above. Finally, the CDC has reported that the prevalence of gonorrhea and syphilis among African Americans is nearly 40 and 60 times that among Caucasians. Syphilis is 4 times more prevalent in Hispanics as in Caucasians. African Americans are 2-3 times more likely than whites to contract genital herpes. We are *not* saying that race involves any special vulnerabilities to STDs, but rather that factors such as access to medical services, low income, illegal drug use, and residence in areas of high STD prevalence plainly increases the risks of infection.

Taking Personal Responsibility for Preventing STDs

We have not yet described what individuals can do to prevent contracting STDs, but this is the most important aspect of sexually transmitted diseases from the perspective of people who might be at risk of getting one. For all the STDs discussed in this chapter, a person can take several simple, effective measures to protect themselves.

- Get the facts. As unpleasant as STDs may seem, a basic part of growing up and taking responsibility for one's actions involves learning the names and symptoms of sexually transmitted diseases and the high-risk sexual behaviors associated with them.

- Seriously consider sexual abstinence. If you are uninformed, unready, or unprepared for sex, don't have sex, and don't engage in behaviors that are likely to lead to sexual behaviors in which STDs can be transmitted. If you think you might be persuaded by the "everybody's doing it" argument, maybe you'll be dissuaded by the "everybody's getting STDs" argument.
- If you make a foresightful decision to have sex, have mutually monogamous sex with someone who does not have any STDs. It is a good idea to be checked for STDs if you have had sex with others.
- Know your partner well and talk about sex before having sex. If you're not comfortable enough to talk with someone about having sex, maybe you shouldn't have sex with them.
- Before having sex (even when using a condom) wash your genitals with soap and warm water, and dry thoroughly. Ideally, use an antibacterial soap. Strong disinfectants are not necessary and are likely to be highly irritating.

- Urinate before having sex. This creates a normal acidity that is inhospitable to many microorganisms that cause STDs affecting the urinary tract.
- Use a new latex condom and apply it properly (or help your partner apply it properly) before making any sexual contact. Latex condoms lubricated with nonoxynol-9 offer additional protection against STDs. Latex is less permeable to bacteria and viruses than natural membrane condoms. Remember, birth control pills offer no protection against STDs. The same is true of IUDs, Norplant, Depo-Provera, and some other contraceptive methods. Using nonoxynol-9 foams and jellies alone is not as effective as using them with condoms.
- Men should grasp the condom where it meets their body before withdrawing their penis from their partner so it won't slip off and allow brief contact with exposed mucous membranes.
- Urinate as soon as possible after having sex. This re-acidifies the urethra and makes it hostile to bacteria and viruses that live and grow in alkaline environments. "Start-stop" Kegel-style urination repeatedly flushes the urethra.

Dear Dr. Ruth

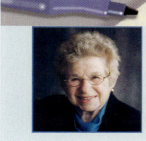

Question:

I am a college student in my early 20s and I recently read that one of the best ways to avoid getting a sexually transmitted disease is to know your partner well and to have open and honest communication about sexual issues. But the problem is, I just don't know how to introduce this subject with a girl; it makes me very uncomfortable to talk about it. I have never had an STD (I believe in always using a condom). Can you give me some advice on how to discuss this complicated subject?

Answer:

First of all, let me congratulate you on using a condom all the time. Talking about sex is difficult for most people. Luckily for our species, people can let each other know when they're willing to have sex without having to express it in words, otherwise we might not have been able to reproduce in sufficient quantities to survive! But when it comes to communicating about STDs, couples have to fall back on words.

Everybody has to use their own approach, but if I were in your situation, I'd find the right time to say something like, "Did you hear that there's a new HIV infection every 13 minutes? I'm sure glad I've never caught any STDs" or "I'm glad all I ever got was a case of the crabs." That gives an opening to the other person to reveal something about their past, which hopefully they'll grab. If they don't, then you might have to assume that they have something to hide and vow to yourself not to go any further in the relationship until you find out what it is.

■ Again wash your genitals with warm water and soap. Because bacteria and viruses cannot survive even small changes in temperature, rinse your genitals with cool water. Dry thoroughly.

If you have had unprotected sex, do *not* douche after intercourse because it will remove bacteria in the vagina that have a protective effect against some STDs. In fact, douching can actually *increase* your risk of contracting an STD. (This is also true of anal douching if you have had anal intercourse.) The suggestions above apply to intercourse. For other sexual behaviors there are other preventive considerations. Because some STDs can be transmitted through oral-genital sex, fellatio with a condom or cunnilingus with a dental dam is recommended. Anal penetration should be accompanied by the use of a condom. Anal penetration is also facilitated and made more comfortable by using sterile, non-petroleum-based surgical lubricant with bacteriostatic qualities. Similarly, since STDs may be transmitted by anilingus (oral stimulation of the anus), the use of a dental dam is recommended in this case as well.

The overall message behind all these suggestions for preventing transmission of STDs is: "You can't be too careful."

Other Prevention Issues

The situation would be simpler if everyone who contracted an STD soon developed symptoms that motivated them to get treated right away. But in fact, many people acquire STDs without knowing it, and this fact has a far-reaching impact on efforts to diagnose and promptly treat these ailments. Many carriers of STDs are asymptomatic, meaning that they do not have any obvious signs of being infected at all. Even visually examining one's partner's genitalia does not always indicate whether a person is harboring an STD. For example, the early sores that characterize syphilis or genital herpes may be inside a woman's vagina or on her cervix, where they cannot easily be seen. With diseases like chlamydia and gonorrhea, most infected women (about 7 out of 10) do not have any obvious symptoms at all. Men who are infected with chlamydia and/or gonorrhea do not always have painful urination and a urethral discharge, the two most common symptoms of these two diseases. Therefore, anyone who is sexually active, particularly with multiple partners, should have regular STD check-ups, perhaps every few months, at a health care facility where they feel comfortable. No one will criticize you as a "hypochondriac" for having a checkup when you aren't having symptoms, and health care professionals will esteem your prudent good sense. These screenings are especially important if you have had unprotected genital or oral sexual contact (sex without using a condom) or have used condoms inconsistently.

People hold a variety of attitudes about STDs, some of which are simply unrealistic or wrong. For example, many have an unwarranted feeling of safety and protection. They believe that bad things, STDs for example, only happen to other people, poor people, uneducated people, or people who live in another part of town. A previous chapter referred to these "delusions of invincibility" and noted that they contribute to risk

taking. In fact, virtually all of us are *equally at risk* of contracting STDs if we have unprotected sex with an infected partner. None of us enjoys a special immunity to the hazards of STDs because we are wealthy, well-educated, or live in a beautiful home.

Even though latex condoms are extremely effective if used properly for preventing the spread of STDs, many people don't want to be reminded of this. Local television stations are often reluctant to air commercials for condoms, although in 1998 the makers of "LifeStyles" condoms ran ads in New York and Los Angeles on a few late-night television programs (Wilke, 1998). LifeStyles condoms were also advertised in *Glamour* magazine in 1998 and in thousands of college newspapers (Fig. 17-3). Still, at the close of the century there remained much nervousness in the media about condom ads. Apparently, society is sending our youth a perplexing double message about disease prevention: "If you plan to behave responsibly about disease prevention, you are planning to be an evil person . . ."

Organizational Approach to STDs

The following sections discuss a number of common, and not so common, STDs. We will explore a number of common issues about each STD. We first describe the microorganism involved and the means by which it is transmitted from one per-

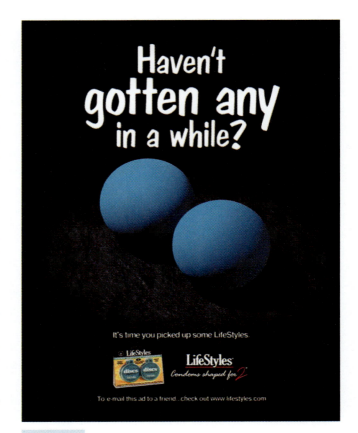

FIGURE 17-3   Advertisements for condoms often contain subtle but significant messages. Here, one ad presents a visual pun on the notion of "blue balls," which is likely to appeal to a broad audience of young adults. Messages such as these seem quite effective in encouraging the use of condoms.

son to another and its incubation period—the amount of time it takes a person to develop symptoms. We will describe the progress of the disease if it is not treated. Effective treatments and disease management strategies are then described, along with a discussion of how the doctor knows when the microorganism is no longer in the body. We'll also see why people don't build immunity to STDs as with other infectious diseases.

STDS CAUSED BY VIRUSES

Viruses are *extremely* small and can be seen only with very powerful electron microscopes. They have an outer coat of protein and have RNA or DNA inside. Unlike bacteria, they do not have a surrounding membrane. Viruses can grow and divide only in living cells, which makes it very difficult to study them in the laboratory. Viruses cause many different kinds of disease, some of which are sexually transmitted. When viruses enter healthy cells, they affect the cell's normal functioning. The virus first attaches itself to a healthy cell and then penetrates it. Only cells with a specific receptor molecule on their surface to which a virus can attach itself can be infected. A viral infection occurs when a virus destroys the cells to which it is attached and then releases copies of itself into surrounding fluids and cells, or the virus may enter the cell, make copies of itself, and live there for some time, sometimes years or decades, without causing any symptoms. Scientists are still studying how some viruses live inside cells for long periods of time without causing problems, as well as the factors that then make them active and cause infections.

Acquired Immunodeficiency Syndrome (AIDS)

In the mid-1970s doctors at Bellevue Hospital in New York City noticed something perplexing and frightening. Many very thin gay men were getting pneumonia and dying, and they were unresponsive to all available antibiotic therapies. The specific

type of pneumonia they had was extremely rare. How could so many cases of this very rare pneumonia appear so suddenly and have such fatal outcomes? As this mystery unfolded, medical scientists throughout the world began noticing this phenomenon, and no one could determine why these people were dying, much less the nature of the disease they had or the infectious agent that caused it. The prospect of a deadly infectious disease with no clear cause and no known cure was very frightening, although many were confident that sooner or later scientists would discover the nature of the problem and develop an effective therapy. The emergence of AIDS generated very little public attention, at least at first. Although some scientists suspected that this disease was viral in nature and possibly sexually transmitted, these facts were not proven conclusively for several years, and not until the early 1980s was the virus that causes AIDS identified by teams working independently in France and the United States. AIDS was first recognized in 1981, although the virus that causes it, **human immunodeficiency virus (HIV)**, certainly had been around for several years by that time. Scientists now know that this virus may be transmitted sexually as well as through needle sharing by intravenous drug users and several other more rare forms of transmission. AIDS is a worldwide epidemic today. There still is no cure, but progressively more effective treatments are being developed to manage the disease and slow or stop its damage to the immune system.

AIDS destroys or impairs the function of various cells of the immune system, specifically the CD4 T cells (Fig. 17-4). Left untreated, HIV gradually destroys the body's capacity to combat certain infections and plays a role in the development of certain cancers. These infections are called opportunistic infections because the microorganisms that cause them take advantage of the opportunity to infect the body when the immune system is not working well. One of the most common opportunistic infections is caused by *Pneumocystis carinii,* the organism causing the type of pneumonia that killed the first

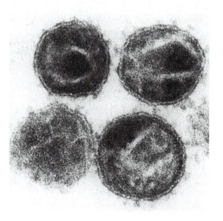

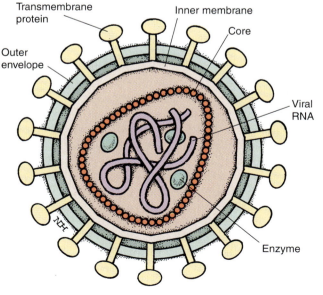

FIGURE 17-4   At left, electron micrograph of HIV. At right, schematic illustration of HIV showing its interior and exterior structures.

(Figure labels: Transmembrane protein, Inner membrane, Core, Outer envelope, Viral RNA, Enzyme)

AIDS victims. HIV can be in a person's body for long periods of time (in some cases up to 15 years) without causing AIDS. Scientists are still attempting to determine what triggers the development of AIDS in someone who has harbored the HIV for long periods of time without symptoms. The duration of the incubation period for AIDS is not well understood.

Although the connection between HIV and AIDS was not to be demonstrated conclusively until 1981, scientists examined frozen blood samples that went back as far as 1978 and established deaths due to AIDS as early as that year. Questions still remained as to how the virus was transmitted. Very early in the study of AIDS, key avenues of transmission emerged: men having sex with men, heterosexual intercourse, drug use involving needle sharing, blood transfusions with blood contaminated with the virus, and giving hemophiliacs blood products manufactured from blood contaminated with HIV. Extremely strict standards for testing blood were then developed, and today there are extremely few cases of accidental transmission of the virus in medical settings. It was also determined that HIV *cannot* be transmitted through mosquito bites or casual contact like shaking hands.

As has happened in the past with highly infectious diseases without cures, AIDS spread with alarming speed throughout the world. The National Institute of Allergy and Infectious Disease estimated that by the end of 1997 there were almost 31 million people infected with HIV worldwide, with about 16,000 new infections occurring every day. By the beginning of 1998, almost 12 million people had already died of AIDS. Since 1981, increasing numbers of AIDS cases have involved women and unborn children. If a pregnant woman is HIV positive or contracts the virus during pregnancy, there is about a 1 in 4 chance that her newborn will also carry the virus. Although much early attention in the United States focused on its prevalence among homosexuals, today about 75% of all HIV infections worldwide are transmitted heterosexually. In the United States alone, there were almost 650,000 cases of AIDS by the beginning of 1998.

How HIV Causes AIDS

HIV is one of a number of viruses called **retroviruses.** Once the virus has entered a cell it uses an enzyme to turn its RNA into DNA and can now actually become a part of the cell's genes. HIV is also characterized as a slow virus, meaning that there can be a long period of time between the moment the virus enters the body's cells and when the person eventually develops symptoms. Once inside a cell, the virus stimulates the production of messenger RNA, which enters the cell's nucleus, and the core of a new virus is made. Messenger RNA creates a sequence of amino acids that become the cell's DNA. These immature virus cores then accumulate in the cell's cytoplasm and are pushed out of the cell's surrounding membrane. These virus particles also have some of the cell's protein molecules and enzymes. The enzyme protease then "clips" these proteins and enzymes into smaller pieces (Fig. 17-5). When this happens, the viral particles become infectious. This step involving protease enzymes is especially important for current HIV and AIDS therapies.

These virus particles eventually make their way through the body into blood, semen, and vaginal and cervical fluids. The virus has also been found in the milk of infected nursing mothers. When one of these body fluids containing these virus particles comes into contact with another person's mucosal membranes in the vagina, vulva, penis, rectum, or, some think, the mouth, the virus may then enter the other person's bloodstream. If this person has any other STDs at this time, especially one involving open lesions as in syphilis or genital herpes, HIV more easily passes through mucous membranes. As soon as HIV enters the body, large numbers of CD4 cells are infected, and the total number of these cells in the body decreases by 20 to 40%. Two weeks to a month after infection, about 7 in 10 infected individuals will manifest the symptoms of a bad case of the flu. As the immune system fights back, HIV levels are significantly reduced, but the virus is never completely eliminated from the body during this early stage of infection.

The average person begins to manifest the symptoms of AIDS about 10 to 12 years after the initial infection. Yet this figure is highly variable, and 10% will develop AIDS in as little as 2 to 3 years, and about 5% will have not developed AIDS after 12 years. Generally, the higher the level of HIV in the individual's bloodstream, the greater the chances that they will develop symptoms associated with AIDS. These HIV levels are also referred to as the "viral load." Additionally, when high levels of HIV are found soon after initial infection, this usually predicts a rapid rate of the progression of the disease. Doctors believe that these patients should be treated as aggressively as possible as early as possible.

While those infected with HIV may show no symptoms of AIDS for many years, data indicate that during this time the virus continues to replicate in the lymphatic system. Cells in lymphatic tissue eventually trap large numbers of the virus until the immune system can begin its protective response. Eventually, however, the lymphatic tissues can no longer contain the ever-increasing number of viral particles, and these then spill out into the bloodstream. When this happens, the person becomes especially vulnerable to a number of different opportunistic infections. Many billions of new viral particles are produced every day, and because of mutation not all copies of the virus are identical. This means that therapies designed specifically to fight one type of virus are ineffective in killing the variants that occur during this period of rapid replication. Therefore, a vaccine developed to protect against one type of virus would not be very effective against other forms of the virus. This is one of the reasons that the development of an effective vaccine against HIV has been such an elusive goal for medical researchers. Ironically, the immune system's initial response to the presence of HIV stimulates a large number of cells that are supposed to combat the virus, which leaves the immune system vulnerable to a number of other illnesses.

Diagnosing HIV

While the effects of HIV on the immune system are dramatic and easy to detect, diagnosing HIV requires definitive proof of

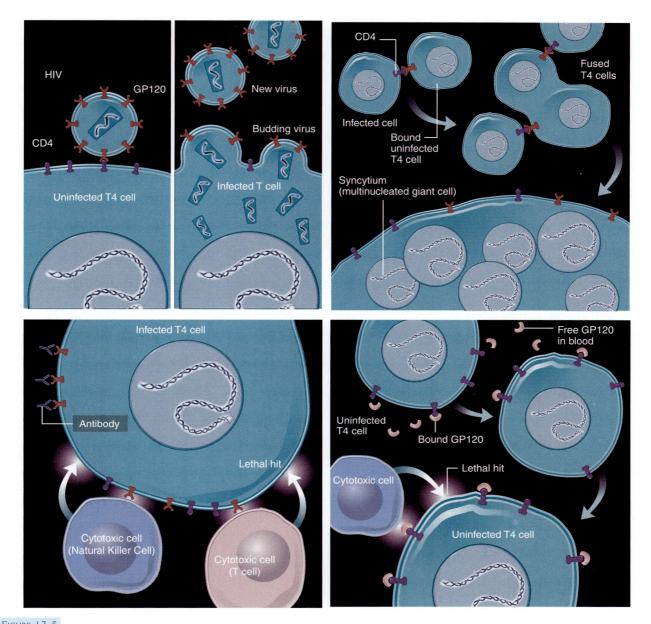

FIGURE 17-5 How HIV destroys T4 cells. **Two upper left panels:** Viral protein GP120 on HIV surface binds with CD4 receptors on surface of healthy T4 cells. This allows HIV to infect the T4 cell. **Upper right:** The infected T4 cells become a multinucleated giant cell called a syncytium. HIV destroys all of these interior cells. **Lower left:** Cytotoxic cells (natural killer cells and T cells) can destroy an infected T4 cell that has HIV proteins on its surface membrane. This can occur with or without the action of antibodies. **Lower right:** Unbound GP120 can travel throughout the blood stream of people who are HIV positive, and bind to the CD4 receptors on uninfected cells. This stimulates an immune response on the part cytotoxic cells, thereby destroying the uninfected T4 cell.

the virus in the bloodstream. In 1993, the Centers for Disease Control changed its clinical definition of AIDS to consist of all those infected with HIV who have fewer than 200 CD4 T cells per cubic centimeter of blood; normal T cell counts vary around 1000 per cubic centimeter of blood. However, definitive diagnosis involves finding antibodies to the virus in the infected person's blood. But the presence of HIV is not the same as having AIDS. These antibodies take at least 1 to 3 months to reach detectable levels in the bloodstream, and in some cases, as much as 6 months. A person who thinks that they

have been exposed to HIV should be tested as soon as possible, for two primary reasons:

1. Doctors can begin prompt, aggressive treatment that will limit the number of viruses and limit the possible development of opportunistic infections.
2. The sooner a person finds out that they are HIV-positive, the sooner they can share this information with their sexual partner and the sooner they can begin taking precautions and preparations to have safer sex.

HIV testing can be done in the doctor's office, local health department, and other local health care facilities such as a neighborhood urgent-care office, as well as confidentially by mail. Ideally, testing is supplemented by counseling. Test results and related information is held in strictest confidentiality. Two tests are used to detect the presence of antibodies to HIV. The ELISA test, which stands for the enzyme-linked immunosorbent assay, reveals the presence of antibodies in the bloodstream. In this case the person is said to be *seropositive* to the virus. A more sensitive and expensive test, the Western blot test, may be used to confirm a positive result. Both tests are very unlikely to indicate that the virus is present when it is not. These tests take only a few days. While these tests detect HIV antibodies, they do not detect the presence of the virus itself, which can be confirmed by other, highly sophisticated medical procedures.

As noted earlier, about 1 in 4 babies whose mothers are HIV positive during pregnancy will be born with the virus, although when the pregnant woman is treated with the drug AZT, the rate of transmission is 1 to 8%. However, a baby can be born with its mother's HIV antibodies and not contract the virus prenatally. Doctors cannot be sure that the baby has the virus itself until about 15 months of age, by which time it will have begun to produce its own antibodies if it has the virus. While we are writing this, new tests are being developed to detect the presence of HIV in infants as early as 3 months of age, perhaps even earlier. This is important in order to give early aggressive treatment when the person is HIV positive.

TREATMENTS FOR HIV AND AIDS

Although there is no cure, treatments have been developed for HIV infection and the opportunistic infections and cancers that often accompany AIDS. A number of drugs have been approved for the treatment of HIV by the Food and Drug Administration. One category of these agents, called reverse transcriptase (RT) inhibitors, stop early viral replication. These include AZT (zidovudine), ddC (zalcitabine), ddl (dideoxyinosine), d4T (stavudine), and 3TC (lamivudine). By limiting viral replication, these act to decrease the viral load and perhaps defer opportunistic infections. The National Institute of Allergy and Infectious Diseases emphasizes that taking these drugs does *not* stop a person from transmitting HIV.

A more recent advance in the treatment of HIV involves a category of drugs called protease inhibitors. These stop viral replication by stopping the last step in the production of infectious viruses. This occurs by blocking the action of the enzyme protease. These agents include such drugs as ritonavir (Norvir), saquinavir (Invirase), indinavir (Crixivan), and nelfinavir (Viracept). Since HIV can become resistant to both of these families of drugs, they are typically used in combination. These drugs do not eliminate HIV from a person's body, however, or cure AIDS if it has developed.

The drugs that are commonly used to treat HIV often cause serious side effects, including nausea, diarrhea, and other gastrointestinal problems. People being treated for HIV often take dozens of pills throughout the day. Patients being treated for HIV may also require treatment to prevent or cure any opportunistic infections that occur, including some cancers. As newer and more powerful drugs are developed for the treatment of HIV, doctors hope that perhaps HIV can be viewed as a chronic disease that can be medically managed over many years.

DETECTING AND TREATING HIV
AFTER EARLY DETECTION OF OTHER STDS

As noted earlier, when someone contracts a curable STD such as syphilis or chlamydia, their chances of contracting HIV increase. In 1997 the Advisory Committee for HIV and STD Prevention (ACHSP) found this strong connection and determined that the earlier other STDs are detected and treated, the better are the chances that the number of new HIV infections might be reduced. ACHSP recommended that:

> *Early detection and treatment of curable STDs should become a major, explicit component of comprehensive HIV prevention programs at national, state, and local levels. In areas where STDs that facilitate HIV transmission are prevalent, screening and treatment programs should be expanded. HIV and STD prevention programs in the United States, together with private and public sector partners, should take joint responsibility for implementing this strategy.*

> —*MORBIDITY AND MORTALITY WEEKLY REPORT,* July 31, 1998

The link between curable STDs and HIV is no longer a matter of speculation (Cohen, 1998). Data indicate that aggressive preventive measures, diagnosis, and treatment of curable STDs is a highly cost-effective way to reduce the prevalence of HIV. Evidence is now accumulating that gonorrhea and bacterial vaginosis may significantly increase the risks of acquiring HIV (Cohen, Hoffman, Royce, et al., 1997; Sewankambo, Gray, Wawer, et al., 1997). Ideally, preventive measures focus on people who are sexually active but who have no obvious symptoms of STDs. Measures such as these would seem essential in both developed and undeveloped nations throughout the world.

THE IMPACT OF HIV ON WOMEN,
CHILDREN, AND MINORITIES

The effects of HIV differ among various groups of people in the population. The impact of HIV is especially severe on women, children, and certain minorities. Between 1985 and 1996, the percentage of reported cases of AIDS among women in the United States increased from 7% to 20%. The National Institute of Allergy and Infectious Diseases estimates that among women between the ages of 25 and 44, AIDS is the second most common cause of death, as it is for men in this age group. As of April 1997, the National Cancer Institute estimated that 107,000 to 150,000 women in the United States were HIV positive (Fig. 17-6). Minority women seem at especially high risk. By the end of 1996, 56% of the cases of AIDS in women were in African Americans, and 20% were in Hispanics. Women who are HIV positive are likely to have problems obtaining good health care, especially if they are single and lack health care benefits. These women are also often re-

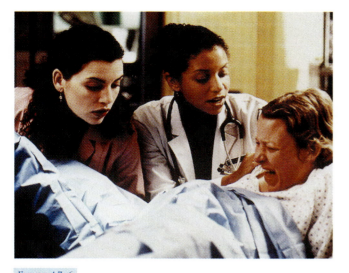

FIGURE 17-6 Actress Gloria Reuben (center) plays nurse Jeanie Boulet on the television show *ER*. Reuben's character reveals the challenges of being an HIV-positive, divorced woman, mother, and health care professional.

sponsible for the care of a child or children, who may also be HIV positive. Therefore, not only are women disproportionately affected by HIV, but they also often must bear the responsibility for taking care of infected children.

In 1996, 40% of AIDS cases in women were attributable to heterosexual intercourse, and 34% could be traced to intravenous drug use. For the remaining 26% of AIDS cases, "no known exposure" was listed although further investigation determined that most of these were in fact due to heterosexual intercourse. On a worldwide basis the World Health Organization estimated that 3 of every 4 cases of AIDS among women are from the heterosexual route of transmission. It seems that women are more easily infected with HIV than are men during unprotected intercourse, for a number of reasons. Women are more likely to have intercourse with partners who have sex with multiple partners, who are intravenous drug users, and who have sex with both women and men. Intercourse is also an efficient means of transmitting the virus to women. However, the data available at this time demonstrates conclusively that correct, consistent condom use dramatically reduces the risk of HIV infection, by some estimates up to 69% (Weller, 1993). Although this isn't perfect protection, it's significantly better than no protection at all. This is also true for couples in committed relationships when one of them is HIV positive and the other is not. A number of gynecologic problems occur in HIV positive women with greater frequency than among women who are not HIV positive:

- vaginal yeast infections
- bacterial vaginosis
- chlamydia
- gonorrhea
- trichomoniasis
- genital herpes
- genital ulcers of unknown origin

- human papillomavirus infections
- pelvic inflammatory disease
- menstrual irregularities

In addition to the health problems experienced by HIV positive women, as noted earlier, when a woman is infected with HIV, the chances of her giving birth to an infected infant are about 1 in 4, although the chances are much lower if the woman is using AZT during her pregnancy. Transmission of the virus to the fetus is thought to occur late during pregnancy or in the process of giving birth. This is not a small health problem. Between 1989 and 1994, the number of women of childbearing age in the United States who were HIV positive remained relatively stable at 1.5 to 1.7 per 1000, with some minor regional differences throughout the country (Davis, Rosen, Steinberg, Wortley, Karon, & Gwinn, 1998). This statistic has remained relatively unchanged even though many women have grown out of this age group, others have experienced progression in their HIV infection to AIDS, and still others have died.

Another unique aspect of HIV infection among women has recently emerged (Grady, 1998). HIV positive women are more likely to develop AIDS than men with the same viral load. This means that a woman may have fewer viral particles in her body but that her immune system is already more damaged than in a man with more viral particles in his body. Women with 5,000 viruses per cubic centimeter of blood have the same risk of developing AIDS as men with 10,000 viruses per cubic centimeter of blood. The reasons for this difference and the importance for changing the way HIV is treated in women are uncertain at this time.

The impact of AIDS on children is especially distressing, since it seems unjust for children to have to "pay" for their parents' actions. By the end of 1996, the World Health Organization estimated that about 2.6 million children were infected with the AIDS virus. This agency also projects that by the year 2000, 5 to 10 million will be infected and another 5 to 10 million left orphans by the worldwide spread of AIDS. With only a few exceptions, children who are HIV positive have acquired the virus from their mothers during pregnancy. While there is some uncertainty about the way the virus is transferred from the mother to her baby, most researchers think that it occurs when the newborn comes into contact with the mother's mucous membranes during birth. Generally, the more advanced the mother's HIV infection and the greater the damage to her immune system, the greater are the chances that the infant will be infected. Nursing mothers can also transmit the virus to their newborns through their milk. By 1994 researchers had learned that when HIV positive pregnant women are given the drug AZT, the risk of the infant contracting the virus drops from a 25% probability to an 8% risk.

As mentioned above, it is not always easy to determine whether a newborn is carrying the AIDS virus. A mother who is HIV positive may pass along antibodies to the virus without actually transmitting the virus itself. Scientists now have sensitive laboratory tests that can detect low levels of the virus in newborns as young as 3 months of age with a high degree of accuracy. Early detection is especially important because it is crucial that treatments begin as soon as possible. The National Institute of Allergy and Infectious Disease has reported that HIV infections in children progress in two different ways. About 1 in 5 infected children will develop AIDS by their first birthday, and most will die by the time they are 4. The other 4 of 5 infected children will manifest a slower progression of AIDS and will not experience their most grave symptoms until they begin school, or in some cases, well into adolescence. Children with AIDS do not grow like their uninfected counterparts, and many develop serious neurologic abnormalities such as mental retardation and seizures. In 1996, 84% of children with AIDS were either African American or Hispanic. Most of these youngsters live in densely populated urban areas where poverty, drug abuse, and inadequate medical care are common.

Generally, minorities are more likely to contract HIV, and this has been true since the epidemic officially began in 1981. The factors noted in the previous paragraph are primarily responsible for this disproportionate victimization of these Americans. By 1996, there were 89.7 cases of AIDS (not those who were HIV positive, but those who had progressed to AIDS) reported per 100,000 African Americans. This figure is more than 6 times that found among Caucasian Americans (13.5) and more than double the prevalence among Hispanics (41.3). It is distressing to note that AIDS is the most common cause of death among African Americans between the ages of 25 and 44, and that despite the fact that Hispanics are less than 10% of the American population, they comprised about 19% of AIDS cases in 1996.

Another American minority is the aging and elderly. Because so many young adults contract HIV, we do not usually think of AIDS as a disease affecting people well into middle age and later life. According to the Centers for Disease Control and Prevention, however, Americans over the age of 50 accounted for about 10% of the cases of AIDS diagnosed in 1995, and 14% of these individuals were over the age of 65 (Lavick, 1998). Older adults may actually be at a higher risk of contracting HIV than their younger counterparts. Lavick (1998) reported that the aging and elderly are less likely to use condoms correctly and consistently than younger adults. Additionally, they are less likely to request HIV testing. Less attention is paid to this population because society generally views them as sexually inactive and nonusers of intravenous drugs. This is a dangerous consequence of ageism, discussed in Chapter 15. Because as women age, there is a gradual thinning of their vaginal membranes, this can increase the chances of an older woman contracting HIV through heterosexual intercourse. As people get older, the immune system does not work as well, and this fact explains the devastating impact of the virus on older individuals. In general, the HIV infected aging and elderly are unlikely to be diagnosed early and unlikely to be treated promptly. A recent case study (Ankrom & Greenough, 1997) described a 78-year-old man who was admitted to the hospital with a number of telling symptoms: significant weight loss, mental confusion, incontinence, and trouble walking. The Western Blot test confirmed that he was HIV positive and his CD4 T cell count was only 103. Tests confirmed that he had no other STDs at the time he was admitted. His medical history revealed that his wife died 10 years ago and he had visited prostitutes, sometimes weekly, and had unprotected sex. He had been treated for syphilis about 10 years ago. While cases like this are unusual, they can make us more aware that the aging and elderly are also vulnerable to HIV infection.

CANCERS RELATED TO AIDS

A number of different kinds of cancer are more common in people with AIDS. Also, some cancers grow faster in these patients. The most common examples include certain types of cancer of the lymphatic system (usually called lymphomas), **Kaposi's sarcoma** (KS), and cancers of the anus and genitalia. The lymphatic system is one of the main components of the immune system. It is made up of vessels that carry a fluid called lymph, which transports the white blood cells that fight infections. The lymphatic system also includes lymph nodes, which are located in the neck, groin, and underarms. Non-Hodgkins lymphoma is the type of lymphoma most commonly associated with HIV infections. In this disease, cells in the lymphatic system grow uncontrollably and form tumors. Therefore, in addition to the person's immune system being already weakened by HIV, it is still further weakened because of the lymphoma.

Kaposi's sarcoma (KS) (Fig. 17-7) involves the growth of malignant cells under the skin and in the mucous membranes of the mouth, nose, or eyes. It can spread to the digestive system, lungs, and liver and may also affect the lymphatic system. The skin has raised, painless discolorations, which may also be found in the mouth. In some cases, this disease does not progress rapidly and can be treated by freezing or surgically removing these lesions. However, in some people KS progresses throughout the body, and in this case chemotherapy is usually recommended.

Because HIV suppresses the immune system, people who have contracted another STD, human papillomavirus, or HPV, are at an increased risk of developing cancers of the cervix or anus. These cancers can be detected by regular vaginal pap smears and visual examination of the anus. Surgical and radiation therapies may be employed to treat these cancers, although they do not affect the progression of AIDS.

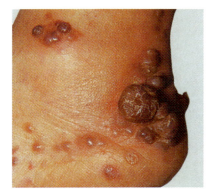

FIGURE 17-7   Skin lesions associated with Kaposi's sarcoma.

PERSONAL RESPONSIBILITY AND AIDS

Of all the STDs discussed in this chapter, AIDS has the most pessimistic prognosis as of this writing. Preventive measures that protect a person against AIDS will also protect them against other STDs. Some simple, inexpensive strategies help minimize or eliminate the chances of contracting any sexually transmitted disease. But *you have to think ahead, take the initiative, and take responsibility for yourself.*

Genital Herpes

Genital herpes is an extremely prevalent STD; some medical specialists believe that it is among the most common STDs in the United States. It results in extremely painful genital sores. The genital herpes virus is related to a large family of viruses that are collectively referred to as herpes. Cold sores around a person's mouth are caused by one variety of the herpes virus called HSV-1 (HSV means herpes simplex virus). Chicken pox is also caused by a virus in the herpes family. Genital herpes is caused by the HSV-2 virus. It is often suggested that HSV-1 is the "above-the waist" version and HSV-2 the "below-the waist" version, although both viruses have been found in both body locations. When a person with a cold sore on or near their mouth orally stimulates the genitals of their partner, the HSV-1 virus can be transmitted this way too. Tayal and Pattman (1994) found that in urban areas in Europe and North America more than half of the newly reported cases of genital herpes were caused by the HSV-1 version of the virus. Therefore the "above-or-below-the-waist" distinction may not always be accurate. Genital herpes is highly contagious, painful, and incurable, although drugs are effective in managing the symptoms on a long-term basis. The Centers for Disease Control and Prevention estimates that about 1 in 4 women and 1 in 5 men in America will become infected with this virus at some point in their lives.

The prevalence of genital herpes in the United States has increased significantly since the 1970s (Fleming, McQuillan, Johnson, et al., 1997). A study done by the Centers for Disease Control and Prevention in cooperation with the Emory University School of Medicine in Atlanta found a 30% increase in the number of people infected since 1976. The disease is more common in women than men over the age of 12 and is also more common in African-Americans (45.9%) than whites (17.6%). Roughly 500,000 new cases of genital herpes are reported every year in this country. Because the genital ulcers characteristic of genital herpes are open sores, this STD increases the chances of contracting HIV as well. Both HSV-1 and HSV-2 can cause lesions on a woman's vagina and a man's penis. Sores are also frequently found on the anus, the thighs, and the buttocks. Once the herpes virus enters a person's body it never leaves, and from time to time a person infected with the virus has recurrent outbreaks of the infection. For this reason, herpes infections are referred to as reactivation infections.

About 2 to 10 days after sexual contact with a person infected with the herpes virus, a person experiences itching, tingling, or burning at the point where the virus entered their body. These early symptoms, sometimes referred to as the pro-dromal period, indicate that soon, clusters of white, translucent blisters will form in that location. In women, these may occur inside the vagina where they cannot readily be noticed or inside the urethra. Shortly after these blisters form, they break open and the fluid inside spreads to adjacent tissue and forms the small, painful sores that characterize this STD (Fig. 17-8). These last from 5 to 10 days and eventually dry out and heal. In some cases, the initial outbreak may last as long as 3 weeks (Corey, Adams, Brown, & Holmes, 1983). These small lesions do not generally leave any scars. A number of other symptoms usually accompany this outbreak, including fever, muscle pains, headaches, painful urination, enlarged lymph nodes in the groin, and in women, a vaginal discharge. These symptoms go away in a few days, although the virus remains in that person's body for the rest of their life. The virus lives in an inactive or dormant state in the dorsal ganglia of the spinal cord. These are clusters of sensory nerve fibers and cell bodies that lie in pairs along each side the dorsal spinal cord. The virus makes its way from the skin, following the nerves that supply the genital area, all the way to these dorsal ganglia and live there without causing much trouble until the individual has another outbreak.

When a person has a recurrence, the viruses travel back to the site of the original outbreak and cause new blisters and lesions to form, preceded by prodromal burning, tingling, and itching. In most cases, recurrences are not as severe, nor do they last as long as the initial outbreak. The future course of genital herpes can be highly unpredictable. While some people have frequent, even monthly recurrences, others have only a few, or even none in the rest of their lives. At this writing, doctors still do not know exactly what triggers recurrences. Some think that prolonged exposure to the sun may play a role, while others think that stress, another illness, or even menstruation can precipitate an outbreak.

In most cases, genital herpes is diagnosed by visual inspection, although laboratory tests may be required to be sure that the genital lesions are caused by the herpes virus and not some other infection. Blood tests can detect antibodies to the virus that have formed or to discriminate between different forms or strains of the herpes virus. It is important to remember that it is possible to spread the virus through sexual contact even when one is not having an active recurrence of genital lesions. Correct, consistent condom usage is an effective way of

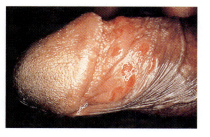

FIGURE 17-8 In genital herpes, small, translucent blisters break open and the fluid within them causes significant local irritation and discomfort.

managing the spread of this STD. Laboratory studies have shown that the virus that causes genital herpes cannot penetrate the membrane of latex condoms, even when left in contact with the condom for up to 8 hours (Conant, Spicer, & Smith, 1984). However, because lesions may also be on the base of the penis, this area not covered by the condom may be involved in transmitting or receiving viral particles. Additionally, incorrect or inconsistent condom use can also contribute to the transmission of this STD. When sex is vigorous or prolonged, the chances of tiny skin abrasions increases, and the virus can easily enter the body through these tiny cracks in the skin. Most cases of genital herpes are transmitted when people are not having any symptoms. In fact, most genital herpes is transmitted by people who are unaware that they have the virus (Mindel, 1998). Genital herpes is transmitted only through direct contact, not through indirect contact with a toilet seat or in a hot tub or bath tub.

Although there is no treatment that can eliminate the virus from an infected person's body, several treatments can help one manage the outbreaks and decrease the frequency with which they occur. Anything that promotes healing of the lesions reduces the length of a recurrence. The National Institute of Allergy and Infectious Diseases recommends that the infected area be kept as clean and dry as possible to reduce the spread of the inflammation. The person should avoid touching the lesions and wash one's hands thoroughly and promptly if this happens. Finally, it is essential to avoid sexual contact after the earliest prodromal symptoms appear until the lesions have healed completely and have been covered with new skin. A number of medications can speed the healing of the sores caused by genital herpes and can also substantially decrease, if not eliminate altogether, recurrences. Drugs such as Zovirax, Famvir, and Valtrex have been approved by the Food and Drug Administration. At this time, doctors cannot reassure their patients that they will not shed contagious viral particles while being treated with these drugs, but patients who have infrequent recurrences of outbreaks are less likely to shed viral particles when not having any symptoms (Patel, Cowan, & Barton, 1997). These drugs are not cures but act to interfere with the replication of the virus.

Dear Dr. Ruth

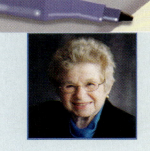

Question:

I have genital herpes. My girlfriend gave it to me. We didn't use a condom and I know that's partly my fault. But I am having a lot of trouble handling my anger. She never told me that she had this disease and she certainly didn't tell me that she was having symptoms when we had sex. I don't know whether to be angrier with her or myself, and we have now broken up. I am really depressed and afraid that nobody will ever want to have sex with me again. If you could tell me how to try to cope with this predicament it would help me a lot.

Answer:

If it's any consolation, you should know that more than 20 million people have genital herpes, and most of them are coping. Linking up with some of these people, either for support or to find a potential partner, is an important part of adapting to this disease. What you mustn't do is crawl into a shell and act like your life is over, because it isn't. Herpes may close some doors, as some people may not want to date someone with herpes; however, since someone else with herpes won't find your condition a problem, and there are many others willing to take the lowered risks of sex using a condom, there's no good reason to spend the rest of your life as a pariah. So rather than trying to hide the fact that you have herpes, be open about it.

I strongly recommend that you do some research about herpes on the Internet. Not only will you find current information about various treatments, but you'll be able to locate support groups, both the on-line variety and local groups, either of which I believe you'll find very useful.

Research Highlight

Developing a Vaccine for the Treatment of Genital Herpes

Vaccines have been developed to immunize humans against many viral diseases, such as polio and hepatitis. Researchers have been working for many years to create a vaccine to protect humans from the HSV-2 virus, which causes genital herpes. As of this writing, these efforts have proven ineffective and frustrating. In 1997, researchers working at the National Institute of Allergy and Infectious Diseases finished their testing of a genetically engineered vaccine against HSV-2. A number of puzzling findings emerged from these early clinical trials. For example, the experimental vaccine was safe and didn't cause any outbreaks of herpes infections, and it caused a specific defensive response in the immune systems of the volunteers who had been inoculated with it. However, the vaccine did not protect individuals who did not have the virus from getting it from their infected partners. Researchers simply don't yet know why this vaccine failed to work. During the 12-year development phase of this vaccine, it was proven effective in preventing the transmission of the herpes virus in several different species of laboratory animals. Yet these data did not predict the vaccine's effectiveness in preventing herpes transmission in humans. Finally, this experimental vaccine reduced the number of outbreaks in humans by about 30%, the same rate of effectiveness found with the use of the antiviral drugs noted above. We are optimistic that eventually a vaccine against genital herpes will be developed, although this research problem seems to particularly complicated.

However, antiviral therapy is very expensive and may not be affordable to all those who need it.

Several factors seem to be associated with a lower probability of giving or getting herpes: knowing prodromal symptoms, using antiviral agents, and avoiding all sexual contact during the prodromal period and especially during the presence of genital (or oral) lesions.

In some cases, genital herpes causes troubling complications. If a pregnant women has genital herpes and the baby is born through an infected birth canal, consequences for the newborn can be extremely serious or fatal. The most significant risks to the newborn occur if the mother contracts genital herpes during her pregnancy. About half of these infants will die of encephalitis, a serious brain infection, or develop other serious neurological problems. If the mother is having her first outbreak around the time of giving birth, the chances are roughly 1 in 3 that the baby will be infected by the virus. However, if the mother is having a recurrence, the chances are much lower. Whenever there is any danger of delivering a baby while a woman is having an outbreak of genital herpes, the obstetrician typically recommends delivering the baby by Cesarean birth, which virtually eliminates the chances of infection. Still, thousands of women with genital herpes give birth vaginally every day to normal, healthy infants with no ill effects to the newborn. Because many women with genital herpes have no symptoms of a recurrence during delivery, they should be seen regularly by their doctors throughout pregnancy for tests to be carried out to determine whether the virus is present inside of the vagina.

Human Papilloma Virus (HPV)

Some STD experts believe that **human papilloma virus (HPV)** is the most common sexually transmitted disease in the world. The Centers for Disease Control and Prevention has estimated that approximately 20 million Americans harbor this virus, and the number of new cases is increasing rapidly every year. Many different varieties of this virus have been isolated, and at this point more than 60 have been identified. Of this number, about one-third may be transmitted sexually and the virus will live only on the genitalia, causing genital warts. Some types of HPV have been implicated in the development of cervical cancer, penile cancer, and anal cancer as well as other genitourinary cancers. According to government estimates, over 95% of cervical cancer cases are attributable to this virus. Many individuals who have contracted HPV do not have, nor have they ever had, any obvious symptoms.

The most common manifestation of HPV is genital warts, historically called "venereal warts." The scientific name for these skin growths is *condylomata acuminata*. They are highly contagious, and roughly 2 of every 3 individuals who have sexual contact with an infected person when the warts are present will eventually develop genital warts. Although the exact incubation period for HPV is not known, warts usually appear within 90 days of contact with an infected partner. The National Institute of Allergy and Infectious Diseases estimates that 1 million new cases of genital warts are diagnosed every year. In women, genital warts may appear on the vulva or within the vagina as well as the anus (Fig. 17-9A). They may also appear on the cervix. Genital warts are often less obvious in men, sometimes occurring on the glans of the penis or the shaft (Fig. 17-9B). Sometimes they appear on a man's anus or scrotum. These growths may be extremely small, or in some instances cover larger areas of genital tissue. Occasionally they appear in small clusters. Although genital warts often go away permanently by themselves, someone who thinks they have them should seek medical attention.

The doctor can usually diagnose genital warts simply by looking at them. Or the doctor may put a few drops of vinegar on suspicious growths, since genital warts become white when vinegar is applied to them. This is especially useful when the growths are inside of the vagina and cannot be seen easily. A pap smear may also reveal indications of genital warts on the cervix.

There are a variety of treatments for genital warts, depending upon how large they are and where they are located. Treatments can eliminate the warts, but the virus never leaves the individual's body. Several chemical agents are effective for removing genital warts. An older agent that is still effective is *podophyllin,* a plant resin with caustic properties. Prescription drugs containing this agent are also available in solution form. Pregnant women should not use podophyllin or drugs containing this substance because it readily enters the bloodstream and can cause birth defects. Other agents such as trichloroacetic acid are also highly effective. In recent years the

United States Food and Drug Administration has approved the use of imiquimod cream and 5-fluorouracil cream. The development of drugs for the treatment of genital warts has become an active area of drug research, and newer and more effective treatments are being developed. Genital warts can also be removed by freezing them (cryosurgery) or burning them off with electrocautery or a laser. If all of these therapeutic approaches fail, surgery may be necessary to remove the growths.

As noted above, some varieties of HPV have been implicated in an increased risk for cancers of the cervix, vulva, anus, and penis. However, HPV infections do not inevitably lead to cancer. A woman with genital warts should have regular pap tests so that any early growth of abnormal cells can be detected and promptly treated. In certain rare cases, untreated genital warts may cause complications of labor and delivery or cause the growth of warts in the newborn's respiratory passageways. At this time, there are no effective vaccines against HPV. Latex condoms, when used correctly, offer some protection against the transmission of the virus.

Hepatitis

Hepatitis is an infectious viral disease that causes inflammation of the liver. The liver is the body's "central processor" for all metabolic reactions. There are several different types of hepatitis, which are transmitted from one person to another by both sexual and non-sexual means. Several different viruses cause the various forms of this disease. For the sake of simplicity, these are usually referred to as hepatitis A, hepatitis B, hepatitis C (which used to be called "non-A, non-B hepatitis"), and hepatitis D, and more recent research has identified hepatitis varieties E, F, and G as well. Because this chapter focuses on sexual routes of transmission, we will not discuss forms of hepatitis caused by exposure to toxic substances or alcohol. The primary means by which hepatitis is transmitted is through contact with various bodily fluids, specifically, feces, blood, semen, vaginal fluids, saliva, and breast milk. Hepatitis is also transmitted by sharing needles used for injecting drugs intravenously, as in the case of HIV. Sexual routes of hepatitis transmission include giving or receiving oral stimulation, penis-in-the-vagina intercourse, anal intercourse, and anilingus. Although the virus is found in saliva, kissing is not a very efficient way of transmitting the virus. Those who work in the health care industry and those receiving kidney dialysis are also at an increased risk of contracting the virus that causes hepatitis. Unborn babies can be infected if their mothers harbor the virus during pregnancy. The incubation period for hepatitis is highly variable, ranging from 3 to 20 weeks.

The symptoms of hepatitis range from uncomfortable to disabling. Many people who contract the virus have no symptoms at all in the early stage of the disease. In those who do have initial symptoms, nausea and vomiting are common. Weakness, persistent headache, and abdominal pain are frequently reported. Chronic fatigue and loss of appetite are common. Because many different disorders can cause these same symptoms, it is essential to have a blood test to determine the exact cause of these problems. As the disease progresses, the in-

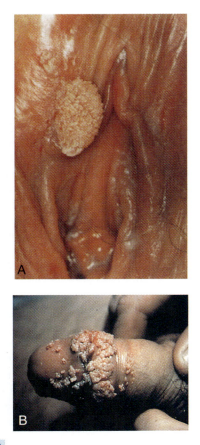

FIGURE 17-9   A, B. Genital warts are a highly contagious manifestation of the human papilloma virus.

dividual experiences swollen lymph nodes throughout the body, and during this time the liver is being damaged. Abdominal pain occurs on the right side, and the person's skin takes on a yellowish tinge, called jaundice. This is another sign that the liver is not functioning properly. According to the Centers for Disease Control and Prevention, there may be up to 320,000 new cases of hepatitis B and 230,000 cases of hepatitis C each year in the United States.

Many who contract hepatitis will develop long-term infections; an estimated 5000 to 10,000 people die each year in the United States as a result of the chronic liver disease caused by hepatitis. Using condoms is an effective way to minimize the risk of giving or getting hepatitis, and individuals with the virus frequently receive counseling about ways to further minimize the transmission of the virus. They are further encouraged not to share toothbrushes, razors, and other personal hygiene items. Since 1982 a vaccine has been available against hepatitis B, and several drugs effectively treat the consequences of this viral infection. At this writing, there are not yet any vaccines available to immunize people against hepatitis A or C. Currently, there are no effective treatment strategies for acute viral hepatitis; the patient is encouraged to rest, eat properly, and avoid drinking alcohol. Since 1993, there has been an increase in the prevalence of hepatitis among heterosexuals with multiple partners, homosexual men, and those who use intravenous drugs.

Cytomegalovirus as a Sexually Transmitted Disease

Cytomegalovirus (CMV) is a very common and usually harmless virus that is carried by about half of all young adults in the United States, according to the National Institute of Allergy and Infectious Diseases. This virus is a member of a large family of viruses that include the herpes family. The virus may be present in saliva, urine, semen, and vaginal fluids. It has been known for about 20 years that CMV may be responsible for chronic inflammation of the cervix and can be spread by sexual intercourse, although it can also be transmitted by kissing. In most cases, no symptoms are associated with the virus, although some people have swollen lymph nodes, fever, and extreme fatigue–symptoms that are often confused with the symptoms of mononucleosis. Because the virus is efficiently transmitted through anal intercourse, homosexual men have a higher prevalence of the virus than heterosexual women or men.

The same general type of blood test used to detect HIV antibodies can also detect CMV antibodies. According to the National Institute of Allergy and Infectious Diseases, there are a number of complex, expensive tests that can reliably and definitively diagnose the presence of CMV in the bloodstream. Even though there are no consistent, obvious symptoms associated with CMV, infected women can transmit the virus to their newborns. Although all affected infants do not have symptoms, some do develop serious, potentially fatal complications that may lead to epilepsy, blindness, deafness, or mental retardation. At this writing, the National Institute of Allergy and Infectious Diseases is developing antiviral agents that may be effective in the treatment of CMV. As with other STDs, people who have CMV are at increased risk of contracting HIV. Currently, there is no known way to prevent CMV, although latex condoms are thought to be very effective.

Molluscum Contagiosum

Molluscum contagiosum is a viral STD that causes tiny bumps on the skin that eventually grow to 3 to 5 mm in diameter. It is not transmitted solely through sexual contact. Small children, for example, may transmit the virus through saliva. The incubation period is roughly 2 to 3 months, although symptoms can appear in as little as 1 week or as long as 6 months (Douglas, 1990). In rare instances skin growths may be as large as 10 to 15 mm in diameter. They are usually gray, yellowish, white, or flesh-colored. They are more commonly found on the buttocks, thighs, and lower abdomen and less often on the genitalia. Most people with molluscum contagiosum have 10 to 20 of these little bumps on their skin. If they are not treated they usually disappear in roughly 2 years, but sometimes they will recur. Because of the unique, pearl-colored appearance of these bumps, molluscum contagiosum is relatively easy to diagnose accurately and quickly. These skin lesions are usually removed by surgery, electrocautery, or local freezing. Occasionally, caustic acidic solutions are used to destroy them.

Personal Responsibility for Viral STDs

One of the most distressing things about viral STDs is the fact that once the virus enters a person's body, it is extremely difficult if not impossible to completely eliminate it. Bouts of infection recur or are reactivated, often by unknown causes. In the case of AIDS, better treatments are being developed, however, but still no cure is in sight. Just as there has been significant improvement in the development of antibiotics for the treatment of bacterial STDs, there has similarly been development of vaccines and topical and systemic antiviral agents for the treatment of viral STDs. Two conclusions clearly emerge from this discussion of these diseases. First, prevention is crucial, especially through the use of latex condoms. Second, one should not become discouraged or fatalistic and thereby avoid or delay seeking treatment. Remember: *you can make important personal decisions to reduce or eliminate your risk of contracting these STDs! YOU are in control.*

STDS CAUSED BY BACTERIA

Bacteria are microscopic single-celled organisms and can be seen under a light microscope. In comparison with viruses, bacteria are enormous. Bacteria have a wide variety of shapes. Some look like little rods, others are round, and still others have a corkscrew-like appearance. They are usually found in groups or clusters called colonies, and some have a little tail that allows them to swim through bodily fluids. Bacteria replicate asexually, which means that two bacteria don't have to join in order to form a third. One bacterium simply divides into two. An important difference between bacteria and viruses is that bacteria can, given the right conditions and necessary nutrients, grow and divide on their own. In contrast, a virus can't replicate itself unless it gets inside a living cell, as we described in the case of HIV. For bacteria to divide, conditions have to be perfect, and this does not always happen when bacteria are in a person's body. All bacteria do not cause diseases. In fact, most don't.

A group of drugs called antibiotics are used to treat bacterial infections. Antibiotics work by interrupting the processes by which bacteria replicate, gradually decreasing the number of bacteria in the body and giving the cells of the immune system the opportunity to find, engulf, and destroy any remaining bacteria. Different kinds of bacteria are affected by different antibiotic drugs. Penicillin was one of the first antibiotics to be developed, but penicillin is not effective in killing all types of bacteria, and the same is true with other drugs. For example, the antibiotic that is effective in treating chlamydia doesn't work at all in the treatment of gonorrhea. In addition, sometimes antibiotics that have been effective in treating a particular STD grow progressively less effective and eventually become totally worthless. The reason for this is that bacteria mutate as they adapt to ever-changing antibiotic environments and thereby become more resistant to antibiotics and eventually do not respond at all. This form of adaptation is what Charles Darwin suggested all "successful" species have to do to survive: adapt flexibly to constantly changing surroundings. For example, one particular strain of gonorrhea not only became resistant to penicillin but actually began to use the drug as a nutrient and grew actively in its presence. There is one more important introductory point to note: no one has any natural immunity to sexually transmitted diseases.

Chlamydia

The most common bacterial STD in the United States is **chlamydia**, and has been for many years. It is a sexually transmitted infection of the genitourinary tract in men and the reproductive tract in women, although in some cases, a woman's urethra too may become infected. The Centers for Disease Control and Prevention estimates that approximately 4 million new cases of chlamydia are reported each year. It is most commonly diagnosed in adolescents between the ages of 15 and 19, although all age groups may potentially be affected. The bacterium that causes chlamydia is *Chlamydia trachomatis,* which can be transmitted by vaginal intercourse, oral stimulation, and anal penetration. For this reason, checking individuals for chlamydia frequently involves culturing fluids from the penis, vagina, throat, and/or rectum just to be sure that all potential sites of infection are studied.

Frequently, chlamydia is a "silent" STD, meaning that a person has acquired the bacteria but has no immediately obvious symptoms. Men may have a urethral discharge (pus coming out of the urethra) and painful urination; inflammation of the lining of the urethra is called urethritis. In some cases, swelling of the scrotum may develop due to a bacterial infection of the epididymis, a condition called epididymitis. Some men may develop prostatitis if their prostate gland becomes infected or proctitis if the lining of the rectum is infected.

Chlamydia produces no specific, consistent symptoms in women, and many women become asymptomatic carriers of the disease without knowing it. It has been estimated that about 15% of women who have chlamydia will have an unusual vaginal discharge and may also feel burning during urination. In those cases where there are symptoms, they usually appear between 1 and 3 weeks after sexual contact. It has been estimated by the National Institute of Allergy and Infectious Diseases that about 1 woman in 3 who has contracted this STD will eventually develop pelvic inflammatory disease (PID). Once these bacteria have entered a woman's fallopian tubes, they may cause significant scarring, thereby eventually causing blockages due to the build-up of scar tissue. Lack of prompt treatment for chlamydia is one of the most common causes of infertility in young women.

An estimated 1 million cases of pelvic inflammatory disease occur each year in the United States, and about 100,000 of these women will become infertile as a result. A woman can have PID for quite some time, sustaining damage to her fallopian tubes, before she begins to experience any symptoms. These symptoms usually include lower abdominal pain. When scarring has occurred in the lining of the fallopian tubes, a fertilized egg can get stuck and begin to develop, causing an ectopic pregnancy. Pelvic inflammatory disease is the most common cause of death during pregnancy among American adolescents. As the prevalence of chlamydia has increased in recent years, so too has the number of ectopic pregnancies among young women.

Diagnosing chlamydia can be difficult. Because its symptoms are somewhat similar to those of gonorrhea, laboratory tests must be carried out to be certain which STD is present. A person may also have both chlamydia and gonorrhea at the same time. Samples of a man's urethral discharge or a woman's vaginal secretions are needed for these tests, which are relatively inexpensive and take little time. The U. S. Food and Drug Administration has approved a urine test for chlamydia that has become widely available; this test can be very convenient in those instances where a regular pelvic examination is not practical. Results from this urine test are available in one day. Accurate laboratory diagnosis is essential because the antibiotics that are effective in the treatment of chlamydia are not effective in the treatment of gonorrhea, and vice versa.

Several antibiotics are effective in the treatment of chlamydia. These include azithromycin (which is taken for one day) and doxycycline (taken for one week). Other antibiotics such as erythromycin and ofloxacin are also effective. Penicillin is ineffective in the treatment of chlamydia. If a woman has or contracts chlamydia during pregnancy, azithromycin, erythromycin, or amoxicillin are effective and will not cause any problems for the developing embryo or fetus. When being treated for chlamydia or any other STD, *it is essential to take the prescribed medication exactly as prescribed until all pills have been taken, even if symptoms disappear before the medication is consumed.* One should refrain from sexual activity until they have been checked by their doctor and it is established that the bacteria are no longer in their body and they are no longer contagious. If symptoms do not disappear within a week or two of finishing the medicine, one should promptly discuss this with their doctor. Of course, it is also necessary to inform one's sex partner(s) when one is diagnosed with an STD and receiving treatment. A person should *never* share medication with their partner(s); she or he may be highly allergic to the drug, and neither individual will get all the medication they need to be cured of the infection.

If a woman gives birth by vaginal delivery while she has chlamydia, her baby may develop an infection of the membranes surrounding the eye, or the baby may be born with pneumonia. Both infections can be treated successfully with antibiotics, but because of the risks, many doctors routinely test pregnant women for chlamydia just to be sure they are not harboring the bacteria without any obvious symptoms.

Latex condoms and diaphragms effectively reduce the risk of transmitting the bacteria that cause chlamydia. Cervical caps are also effective in preventing the bacteria from entering a woman's cervix, a common first site of infection. Inflammation of the cervical canal is called cervicitis. Having unprotected sex with multiple partners dramatically increases a person's risk of contracting virtually all STDs, and many physicians recommend screening for chlamydia for everyone under the age of 25 who has had sex with more than one person. This is important even in the absence of any symptoms. Recent data (Mertz, Levine, Mosure, Berman, & Dorian, 1997) reveal that routinely screening young women who are at a high risk for contracting chlamydia is not particularly effective in reducing rates of infection on a community-wide basis. In fact, a recent study of routine screenings of over 3200 sexually active inner-city adolescent females between the ages of 12 and 19 (Burstein, Gaydos, Diener-West, Howell, Zenilman, & Quinn, 1998) indicated that 24.1% of these young women had active chlamydia during their first visit to family planning centers and school-based clinics. Finally, as noted elsewhere, oral contraceptives, like many other contraceptive methods, do not prevent the transmission of STDs. However, one recent report (Mardh & Hogg, 1998) demonstrates that they may actually mask the symptoms of chlamydia and therefore further delay diagnosis and treatment.

Gonorrhea

After chlamydia, **gonorrhea** is the second most common bacterial STD in the United States. In "street language" gonorrhea is often called the "clap." A recent analysis of demographic and geographic trends in the prevalence of gonorrhea in the United States between 1981 and 1996 (Fox, Whittington, Levine, Moran, Zaidi, & Nakashima, 1998) revealed that since 1981 the incidence of reported cases of gonorrhea has decreased in this country from 431.5 cases per 100,000 people to 124.0 cases per 100,000 people. These scientists found that the prevalence of gonorrhea was 35 times higher in African Americans than in Caucasians in 1996. Among women of all racial groups, those between the ages of 15 and 19 had the highest incidence (716.6 per 100,000), and among men of all racial groups, those between the ages of 20 and 24 had the

highest incidence (512.9 per 100,000). Although the overall prevalence has fallen, this STD continues to present a significant health risk in this country.

The bacterium that causes gonorrhea is *Neisseria gonorrhoeae.* It quickly replicates in warm, moist areas of the body that are slightly alkaline, including the reproductive tract, the mouth and throat, and the rectum. In women, the earliest site of a gonococcal infection is usually the cervical canal. When gonorrhea is not diagnosed and treated promptly, it can quickly spread throughout a woman's fallopian tubes, causing pelvic inflammatory disease. The uterus is another common site of infection. In men, the infection may spread to the epididymis, causing epididymitis, and this can lead to scarring in this structure. Just as pelvic inflammatory disease can lead to scarring of a woman's fallopian tubes with an increased risk of infertility and ectopic pregnancy, epididymitis can also cause infertility because scarring can make it impossible for sperm to enter the vas deferens, and therefore they cannot leave the body during ejaculation. Gonorrhea is most commonly spread through vaginal, rectal, or oral sexual contact. If a woman has a gonococcal vaginal discharge, the fluids may also spread to her anus, thereby causing rectal involvement of the infection. Like chlamydia, gonorrhea can be transmitted from a pregnant woman to her newborn infant as it passes through an infected birth canal.

An estimated 7 of 10 women who have contracted gonorrhea do not have any symptoms in the early, uncomplicated stages of the disease. Because the infection affects a woman's reproductive system and does not usually affect her urinary system, she will have no urethral discharge or pain during urination. The situation is quite different in men, however. Because the urethra in men is part of both the urinary and reproductive systems, most men experience urethral discharge and painful urination between 2 and 14 days after they have been infected (Fig. 17-10). Some men and women have no symptoms whatsoever for many weeks after they have contracted gonorrhea. This is still another reason why individuals who are sexually active, especially with multiple partners, should have

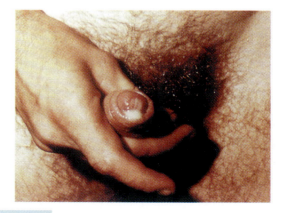

FIGURE 17-10   Urethral discharge associated with gonorrhea. This discharge may vary in color and copiousness and is accompanied by burning during urination.

regular check-ups (perhaps every few months) to find out if they have contracted gonorrhea or any other STDs. When there is a significant delay in diagnosing and treating gonorrhea, women may have a malodorous, yellow, green, white, or gray discharge, occasional vaginal bleeding unrelated to menstruation, and abdominal pain that can be so severe that it causes nausea and vomiting. When gonorrhea has been contracted orally, the infection usually involves a serious sore throat, and when contracted rectally it may be accompanied by rectal itch and very uncomfortable bowel movements.

Sometimes gonorrhea leads to complications distant from the reproductive tract, especially if the infection has been treated with an antibiotic to which it has developed some resistance, as occurs in at least 5% of cases of gonorrhea treated with penicillin. For example, the bacteria may settle in a person's joints and cause a local inflammation. This is called gonococcal arthritis (Wise, 1995). A more rare and worrisome complication involves the spread of the bacteria to a person's heart, a condition called gonococcal endocarditis. In this case, the bacteria can attack and damage the valves in the heart (Cartwright, Petty, Reyes, & Illuminati, 1996). Although these are uncommon, they are serious complications of gonococcal infections.

Diagnosing gonorrhea is not always a straightforward matter. A sample of discharge is taken from a man's penis or a woman's vagina or, when indicated, from the throat or anus. This discharge is mixed with a special dye and examined under a laboratory microscope. Although this test can often reveal the presence of the bacteria that cause gonorrhea, it is generally far more accurate in men than women. Men with gonorrhea almost always have a positive test result using this technique, but only half of women infected with gonorrhea have a positive result. For this reason, a woman may also have a smear taken of the fluids surrounding her cervix and sometimes from her urine as well. Newer tests can detect the genes of the bacteria that cause gonorrhea and are therefore more accurate, although they take longer and are more costly. In still other cases, the discharge is cultured in a laboratory culture dish to see if any bacteria grow. This last test is especially accurate in diagnosing gonorrhea in women. Generally, the results of culture tests and the doctor's clinical judgement may be as valuable for making an accurate diagnosis as the more sensitive DNA tests that discriminate between gonorrhea and chlamydia.

In the past, doctors prescribed penicillin for the treatment of gonorrhea. However, as already noted, gonorrhea has become progressively more resistant to this particular antibiotic. Almost 70% of the cases of gonorrhea in China are highly resistant to some common antibiotics; the comparable figure is almost 60% in Hong Kong and 40% in Korea (Ison, Dillon, & Tapsall, 1998). Fortunately, a number of other drugs are very effective in curing this STD when the bacteria prove resistant to traditional antibiotics or when patients are allergic to them. One especially effective drug is ceftriaxone, which can be injected in the buttocks in a single treatment. Other drugs that can be taken orally are also very effective, including ofloxacin, ciprofloxacin, and cefixime. A single oral dose of ciprofloxacin is almost 100% effective in treating gonorrhea

(Echols, Heyd, O'Keeffe, & Schacht, 1994) at a very low cost (less than $5.00 per dose). The drug selected usually depends on the extent to which the doctor feels the patient will take their medication exactly as prescribed. When a doctor is concerned that the patient may not be compliant in taking all of their pills as directed until all of them are gone, or if the doctor is not sure that the patient will show up for their follow-up check, then a one-dose injectable treatment or one-dose oral treatment may be appropriate. As noted above, some patients have both chlamydia and gonorrhea, and then a combination of antibiotics can be used.

As is the case with chlamydia, delay in treating gonorrhea may lead to pelvic inflammatory disease in women. Similarly, an infant born through a birth canal infected with gonorrhea may cause serious, vision-threatening eye infections. Finally, having gonorrhea increases a person's risk of acquiring HIV, and therefore prompt, effective treatment is extremely important.

Latex condoms lubricated with nonoxynol-9 are very effective in preventing the spread of gonorrhea; female condoms, diaphragms, and cervical caps are also helpful because they block the spread of the bacteria into a woman's cervix. Some research also indicates that nonoxynol-9 vaginal suppositories may be somewhat effective in preventing gonorrhea when condoms are not used (Weir, Feldblum, Zekeng, & Roddy, 1994). Still, barrier methods seem more effective and should be used correctly and consistently if there is any possibility that one's partner may have an STD.

So far this discussion of bacterial STDs has focused primarily on the heterosexual transmission of infections, but of course homosexual transmission is both possible and common and, unfortunately, growing at an alarmingly rapid rate. A thorough study of gonorrhea in gay men between 1993 and 1996 (*Morbidity and Mortality Weekly Report,* September 26, 1997) reveals significant increases in the prevalence of gonorrhea in this population studied in 26 STD clinics across the United States. Importantly, significant increases in the number of reported cases of rectal gonorrhea indicate that large numbers of gay men are engaging in unprotected anal intercourse, which is an efficient means of transmitting HIV as well. In clinics in which data were available about both gonorrhea and HIV, approximately 25% of men having sex with men and contracting gonorrhea were also HIV positive, showing an important relationship between the spread of a viral STD and a bacterial STD.

Pelvic Inflammatory Disease

Although **pelvic inflammatory disease** may occur if prompt, effective treatment is lacking for chlamydia and gonorrhea, PID can also be caused by bacteria that are not sexually transmitted. PID is a very common cause of infertility and ectopic pregnancy in young women. In one study of 58 women with PID (Pavletic, Wolner-Hanssen, Paavonen, Hawes, & Eschenback, 1999), 19 (40%) became infertile as a result of this disease. Note that pelvic inflammatory disease is not, in and of itself, considered a sexually transmitted disease. However, the National Institute of Allergy and Infectious Diseases emphasizes

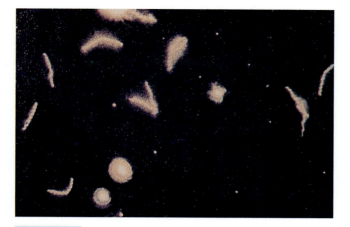

FIGURE 17-11 Syphilis is caused by the corkscrew-shaped microorganism *Treponema pallidum,* shown in this micrograph.

that PID is the second most common complication of STDs, AIDS being the first. PID can affect not only the fallopian tubes but also the uterus, ovaries, and urinary tract. Roughly 1 million American women suffer from an episode of PID each year, most being teenagers. Of these, about 100,000 will become infertile as a result, and another 70,000 will have ectopic pregnancies. These are enormous psychosocial and medical consequences of STDs. Over 90% of women with blocked fallopian tubes had either chlamydia or gonorrhea at some time in the past (World Health Organization Task Force on the Prevention and Management of Infertility, 1995). Women at highest risk for PID are those who have an STD and sexually active adolescents with multiple sex partners.

Diagnosing PID is not always simple. While lower abdominal pain is a common symptom, a pelvic examination is necessary to determine the reason for the discomfort and its location. Tests for chlamydia and gonorrhea are usually carried out, and the patient is evaluated for signs of a fever or any unusual vaginal discharge or inflammation of the cervix. To rule out other problems, the doctor may also carry out an ultrasound examination of the woman's pelvic area, perform a biopsy of her endometrium, or even perform a laparoscopy to view her internal organs. Prompt, aggressive medical attention is very important. With early antibiotic treatment the prognosis for cure and normal future fertility is excellent.

Syphilis

No other sexually transmitted disease has evoked more fear, misinformation, and superstition throughout recorded human history than **syphilis.** In its early stages, syphilis is a highly infectious STD, affecting virtually all of the body's major organ systems. If it is not treated, progressive degenerative changes frequently occur that are often fatal. Between 1986 and 1990, an epidemic of syphilis occurred throughout this country, after which time the incidence began to decline. In the late 1990s, approximately 6,000 cases of primary and secondary syphilis were reported annually to the Centers for Disease Control and

Prevention, representing an 88% decline from the earlier period of the epidemic (*Morbidity and Mortality Weekly Report,* June 26, 1998). Syphilis is more prevalent among African Americans than other racial and ethnic groups in the United States. As with other STDs, having syphilis increases a person's chances of contracting HIV.

Syphilis is caused by the bacterium *Treponema pallidum* (Fig. 17-11), which looks like a little corkscrew under a darkfield microscope. This STD goes through a number of different stages, each with its own symptoms and physical manifestations. Fortunately, syphilis can be treated effectively with a single injection of penicillin. Other antibiotics are also effective for people allergic to penicillin. Because the bacteria that cause syphilis cannot be cultured in the laboratory, a variety of other diagnostic tests are required to accurately confirm a diagnosis of syphilis. These bacteria are extremely sensitive to drying, even slight temperature changes, and mild antiseptics (including soap and water), and therefore the preventive measures outlined at the beginning of this chapter are very effective in preventing syphilis. Each bacterium divides into two bacteria every 30 hours, so the course of the disease can be rapid, especially since thousands are transmitted during sexual contact with an infected partner.

The first, or primary, stage of syphilis is characterized by a small ulcer at the point where bacteria first penetrated the skin or mucous membrane (Fig. 17-12). This ulcer is called a chancre ("chan-ker"), and its appearance can be highly variable. In most cases, it appears between 2 and 6 weeks after exposure to the bacterium. The chancre usually causes no dis-

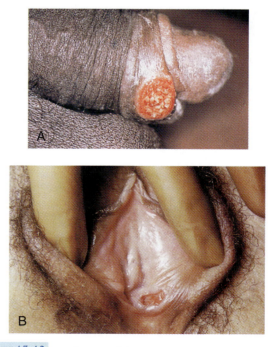

FIGURE 17-12 **A.** Chancre of the penis associated with primary syphilis. **B.** A chancre located on the interior surface of the labia minora.

comfort. In women it may appear on the cervix or inside of the vagina, places where it cannot normally be noticed. The same is true of syphilis transmitted through anal intercourse, when the chancre is located inside the rectum. It is often a hard, red, round, shiny ulcer. Even if syphilis is not diagnosed and treated, the chancre will disappear by itself in a few weeks. If the bacteria were transmitted through oral sex, a chancre may appear on the lips or inside their mouth or throat. If someone with oral syphilis bites their partner, for example, on the shoulder, a chancre will form in that location too.

In its secondary stage, syphilis is characterized by small, round copper-colored skin sores (Fig. 17-13). These appear 3 to 6 weeks after the symptoms of primary syphilis appear. Fatigue, headache, swollen lymph nodes, and sore throat may also occur at this time. The fluid inside these sores has thousands of bacteria in it, so any contact with these sores may transmit syphilis. Like the chancre of primary syphilis, these skin sores will disappear even if the person is not treated. Without treatment, the symptoms of secondary syphilis may reappear a number of times over the next year or two.

If the disease is still not diagnosed and treated, it enters its latent stage, during which there are no longer any symptoms and the person is no longer contagious. But the bacteria are still in the body. Many people with latent syphilis never experience any additional adverse consequences, but 1 in 3 will develop tertiary syphilis, in which the bacteria cause damage to various internal organs, in particular, the heart and brain, as well as bones, joints, and the eyes. When heart muscle cells or brain nerve cells are damaged, they do not regenerate or repair themselves, and this can sometimes lead to heart attacks, damaged blood vessels, blindness, stroke, dementia, and even death. Tertiary syphilis can last for many years.

In some cases, bacteria enter the central nervous system during the earliest stages of infection, and in 3 to 7% of those who are untreated, neurosyphilis will develop. Although some of these people will never have any obvious manifestations of nervous system damage, others will develop serious and often life-threatening neurological problems. In some cases, decades elapse before these health problems become obvious. In general, then, diagnosing syphilis

requires capable medical care because its symptoms can vary so much depending upon the stage the disease has reached. Therefore the best advice remains: if you ever notice *anything* unusual about your genitalia, seek your doctor's opinion immediately and don't have sex with anyone until you do. Syphilis is still epidemic in many parts of the United States and is still a target of aggressive military indoctrination/education programs.

The National Institute of Allergy and Infectious Diseases describes three ways to make a positive diagnosis of syphilis. The first involves a physician's recognition of the physical signs and symptoms of the disease. Because the appearance of a chancre can be highly variable, there is often some doubt based on visual examination alone. The doctor may then want to look at the bacteria inside a chancre or skin sore under the microscope. The doctor presses on the lesion until the fluid inside it oozes out, which is placed on a slide and examined under a microscope to visualize the characteristic corkscrew-shaped bacteria. This offers a more definitive diagnosis than simply examining a skin sore or genital ulcer. Finally, blood tests may be used to detect the presence of the bacteria, although often blood tests for syphilis are negative for several months after initial infection. Two blood tests are frequently used to diagnose syphilis: the Venereal Disease Research Laboratory (VDRL) test and the Rapid Plasma Reagin (RPR) test. These tests detect specific immune system responses to the presence of *Treponema pallidum*, although they may also give positive results when a person has other diseases, such as viral infections. Still other blood tests may be used to diagnose syphilis when the results of these are not clear or do not correspond to obvious physical symptoms of the disease. When neurosyphilis is suspected, cerebrospinal fluid may be removed from the central canal of the spinal cord with a spinal tap to make a definitive diagnosis.

In most cases, penicillin administered by injection is effective in promptly curing syphilis. Some cases may be somewhat resistant to this antibiotic, requiring long-term follow-up blood tests to be certain that the bacteria have been completely eliminated from the patient. Roughly 10% of the population is allergic to penicillin, but doxycycline and tetracycline are also highly effective for those allergic to penicillin. When neurosyphilis has been diagnosed and treated, the patient may require follow-up blood tests for two years. Although syphilis can be effectively treated during any of its stages, the damage it has caused cannot, in most cases, be undone.

As with some other STDs, a pregnant woman who has syphilis can transmit it to her unborn fetus. When syphilis is diagnosed and treated early in pregnancy, there may be no ill effects on the newborn. However, when the disease goes untreated, about 1 in 4 infants will be stillborn or will die shortly after birth. The National Institute of Allergy and Infectious Diseases estimates that 40 to 70% of babies born to mothers with syphilis will themselves be infected with the disease.

Because syphilis is highly infectious in its primary and secondary stages, it is essential to avoid contact with the infected ulcers and skin lesions characteristic of these periods.

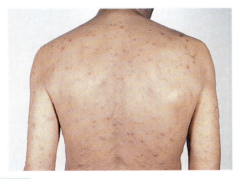

FIGURE 17-13   Skin lesions associated with secondary syphilis.

Latex condoms are very effective in avoiding the transmission of syphilis. Epidemiologists have recently asked whether the eradication of syphilis in the United States is a reasonable goal (Hook, 1998). Despite the availability of effective antibiotics and accurate diagnostic tests, these resources are not generally available to the segments of the population most in need of them. If these people are to be reached, community-wide intervention programs will be necessary. If unequal access to health care resources can be eliminated, we can be more hopeful about eliminating this disease in the United States.

Nongonococcal Urethritis

Inflammation of the urethra may also result from STDs other than gonorrhea. In fact, a number of different bacteria can cause **nongonococcal urethritis (NGU)** and in some cases nonspecific urethritis. Although chlamydia is one cause of nongonococcal urethritis, it may also be caused by a bacteria called *Ureaplasma Urealycticum* as well as a number of other infectious agents. Some women with nongonococcal urethritis may have painful urination, but most women have no symptoms at all. In men with this disease, painful urination is common, as is a thin, watery urethral discharge that is quite different from the thick, yellow discharge characteristic of gonorrhea. Sexual contact is the most common avenue of transmission of nongonococcal urethritis. This STD is effectively treated by tetracycline, doxycycline, or erythromycin. Because a variety of bacteria may cause urethritis, it is important to be diagnosed by a doctor to be sure that the symptoms are treated with an antibiotic that is most likely to be effective.

Chancroid

Chancroid is a significant STD quite common in Africa but less prevalent in the United States, even though there have been periodic outbreaks, particularly in southern and eastern states. The last major epidemic occurred in the late 1980s. Chancroid is a bacterial STD caused by the microorganism *Haemophilus ducreyi*. It causes the appearance of small ulcers, usually on the genitals, and may also be accompanied by swollen lymph nodes in the groin that are tender to the touch. As with syphilis, this ulcer is referred to as a chancre. The chancre may be inside a woman's vagina or on her cervix, a site that makes detection difficult. The incubation period is short, typically between 4 and 7 days (Ronald & Albritton, 1990). Unlike the chancres of syphilis, however, these chancres are quite painful. Chancroid does not spread to the body's major organ systems, nor is it passed to newborns when pregnant women have an active infection. Chancroid is diagnosed by culturing the fluid from the ulcers. Because simply examining this fluid under a microscope may not yield an unambiguous diagnosis of chancroid, culturing the bacteria is important.

Chancroid can be treated effectively with a number of different antibiotics: penicillin, tetracycline, streptomycin, and sulfa drugs such as Bactrim (sulfamethoxazole and trimethoprim). However, like other STDs, *Haemophilus ducreyi* has become somewhat resistant to several commonly used antibiotics. Newer antibiotics such as cephalosporin and ceftriaxone can cure chancroid in a single injection. In a very small percentage of cases a second treatment may be necessary to completely eliminate these bacteria from the body.

Because chancroid causes open genital ulcers, it has been implicated in spreading HIV in Africa. Data reveal that an individual who is HIV positive may not respond to treatment for chancroid. It has been suggested, in fact, that the high prevalence of chancroid in Africa may in part be responsible for the rapid spread of HIV in that part of the world.

STDS CAUSED BY PARASITES ON OR IN THE SKIN

In addition to infections transmitted sexually, sexually transmitted **infestations** involve the spreading or swarming of tiny organisms on or in the skin. **Pubic lice** and **scabies** are ectoparasites, which live on the outer surface of the body. They are not viruses or bacteria but tiny crustaceans. Both can be transmitted readily from one person to another during sexual intercourse or other non-intercourse avenues of intimate pleasuring. While these almost always cause significant itching and discomfort, the infested individual frequently delays seeking medical treatment for fear of embarrassment and may try a number of home remedies, most of which are ineffective for eradicating these tiny organisms.

Pubic lice, often called "crabs" (Fig. 17-14), are related to the same kind of lice that commonly infest the heads of school-

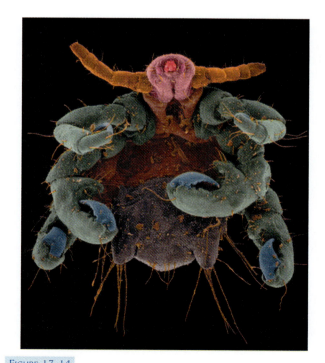

FIGURE 17-14 Scanning electron micrograph of a pubic louse. Note the characteristic crustacean "claws" of the organism.

children. However, these lice are found primarily in pubic hair although they may spread to other areas of the body, such as the arm pits, eyelashes, or facial hair. Pubic lice feed on human blood from tiny capillaries in the skin. A microscope is not needed to see them, although they are quite small. In addition to sexual activity, a person can also get them from infested bedding or the clothing or towels of someone who has them. Because they are transferred so readily from one person to another, it has been estimated that there is about a 95% likelihood of getting pubic lice after only a single contact with someone who has them. They can even be transmitted by furniture and toilet seats. Many young people get crabs in a variety of types of college housing, and people have been known to get them even in hospitals.

Pubic lice lay their eggs at the base of pubic hairs, seen as little discolorations at the base of each affected hair. The crabs themselves can often be seen, and these signs together with the itching make it easy to diagnose pubic lice. The over-the-counter medication Kwell is highly effective in treating pubic lice, although shampooing alone won't completely and permanently get rid of pubic lice. This shampoo usually kills adult lice within a day or so, but the eggs they laid will still hatch in about 6 days. A person has to wash all their clothing and bedding and if necessary treat furniture fabrics as well. Ideally, these items should be dried in a professional clothes dryer at higher temperatures than most home clothes dryers. Infected garments should be placed in sealed plastic bags for one full week after washing (Francoeur, 1991). Anything boiled or dry cleaned can be used immediately. A hot iron should be used on furniture and mattresses. All these precautions show how difficult it is to eliminate these pests.

Scabies is caused by a mite (Fig. 17-15) that is so small it can be seen only with a microscope. This mite is *Sarcoptes scabiei*. It is very effective in burrowing its way into the skin where it deposits its eggs. It causes severe itching, which can be especially painful when a person begins a hot shower. Sometimes little bumps form on the skin's surface, and dark blue or red spots may appear as well. Some people have a more obvious rash, and some may notice tiny flecks of blood on their clothing. While these signs often appear in a person's genital area, the mites can

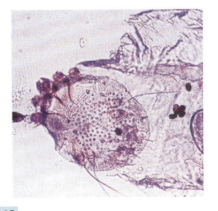

FIGURE 17-15 Micrograph of the mite that causes scabies (*Sarcoptes scabiei*).

infest virtually any area of the body. Scabies is effectively treated by prescription ointments. The person must coat the entire surface of their body with these medications, and often several treatments are required to kill all the mites and their eggs.

Pubic lice and scabies can cause discomfort, annoyance, and embarrassment, but prompt, appropriate treatment is usually effective in very little time.

RECENT ADVANCES IN THE TREATMENT OF STDS

Because STDs affect so many people worldwide and because many have become resistant to traditional antibiotic therapies, the search for better and more effective treatments is a public health research goal. Over the last 15 years there have been both encouraging and discouraging changes in the prevalence of various STDs (Carne, 1998). For example, the number of new cases of gonorrhea had been falling steadily until 1995 when the prevalence again began to rise. New strains of gonorrhea developed that were resistant to both penicillin and tetracycline. A new family of antibiotics called fluoroquinolones was developed, but then new strains of gonorrhea proved resistant to them. Tetracycline family drugs have been the treatment of choice for chlamydia, and a combination of these called Deteclo is proving especially effective. Azithromycin is also very effective in treating chlamydia.

Two relatively new antiviral agents are proving successful for treating genital herpes: Famvir and Valtrex. Until only a few years ago, Zovirax was the only highly effective agent for the treatment of genital herpes. It remains to be seen how well these new drugs will work to stop recurrences of genital lesions and diminish the duration of outbreaks. Of course, none of these treatments entirely eliminates the virus from the body.

Since 1996, protease inhibitors have been used in the treatment of HIV, and their role in the medical management of this virus is now well established. More than a dozen antiretroviral drugs are in use today. Although at this writing there are still no promising signs of a vaccine against HIV, drug combinations have become progressively better in profoundly lowering viral load and increasing life expectancy. Importantly, recent research (Quinn et al., 2000) has demonstrated in a large African population in Uganda that when the viral load is significantly reduced (to fewer than 1500 viral particles per cubic centimeter of blood) through the use of protease inhibitors, heterosexual transmission of HIV becomes highly unlikely.

IF YOU THINK YOU HAVE A SEXUALLY TRANSMITTED DISEASE

Because many of us, especially adolescents and young adults, often feel that bad things happen only to other people, we therefore may actively deny the possibility of getting an STD and resist acknowledging that possibility unless we are plainly

Other Countries, Cultures, and Customs

ADVANCES IN THE TREATMENT OF STDs IN DEVELOPING COUNTRIES

Until AIDS began to take an enormous toll in lives and human misery in the world's less economically developed countries, most of these nations did not have a national agenda for the early diagnosis and treatment of STDs. AIDS was a wake-up call in these impoverished parts of the globe concerning the importance of STDs for the overall health and well-being of their people. Not only are the effects of STDs now being studied far more carefully, but their effects on a person's future reproductive potential as well as the health of yet unborn babies are now major public health priorities in even the world's poorest nations (Mayaud, Hawkes, & Mabey, 1998). It has recently been reported that STDs account for as much as 17% of all significant disease among women of reproductive age in sub-Saharan Africa (Over & Piot, 1993). Additionally, the fact that people with STDs have a markedly increased risk of acquiring HIV infection has forced public health officials around the world to think of procedures and programs for controlling STDs of all types.

For example, it has been shown that public programs promoting the use of condoms can be extremely successful, and that these successes almost always translate into lower STD and HIV infection rates. Condom sales in Ethiopia increased in a 5-year period during the late 1980s and early 1990s from less than 500,000 to almost 20,000,000 (Lamptey & Goodridge, 1996). Increased condom availability and health information programs were primarily responsible for this increase. These figures refer to the number of condoms being *purchased* in a poor country. When condoms are *given* away, comparable or even better progress can be expected in limiting the prevalence of STDs and HIV infections. In other developing countries such as Thailand, condom use has been promoted among prostitutes, brothel owners, and customers, and this has led to a remarkable decrease in the number of STD and HIV cases in that nation.

An especially important example of a community-wide program for the early diagnosis and treatment of STDs is the Mwanza region of Tanzania in Africa (Grosskurth, Mosha, Todd, et al., 1995). Under the guidance of the World Health Organization there was a 40% decrease in the incidence of new HIV infections in a 2-year period. This program had five elements, each of which was essential to the overall success of the entire enterprise:

1. Local STD clinics were set up to train health care workers and to study the various factors that lead to increased rates of STD and HIV infection. These individuals also studied the degree to which the locally prevalent strains of gonorrhea were resistant to antibiotics.
2. Health care workers were trained to manage the course of treatment of various STDs and to learn how to dispense condoms without seeming to be judgmental. Additionally, they were taught how to present basic STD prevention information in simple terms.
3. Large supplies of antibiotics were made available to ensure no interruption or shortage in the availability of these drugs.
4. STD clinics were regularly inspected and care was taken to be sure that staff were well-trained and that supplies of antibiotics were adequate. Patient records were checked to be sure that appropriate care was given and that patients had made their follow-up visits.
5. Public information programs were begun in every village, and residents were taught to recognize early symptoms of STDs and to seek medical treatment promptly.

This program demonstrated dramatically and conclusively that an integrated, thorough approach is indeed effective in significantly lowering the rate of new STD and HIV infections in a specific region. However, one problem encountered in implementing this program concerned the large number of individuals who had active STD infections but showed no symptoms; these people had no idea that they needed to seek the services of these clinics.

In 1994 the International Conference on Population and Development was held in Cairo, Egypt. One of the key recommendations from this meeting was that developing countries make the diagnosis and treatment of STDs and other reproductive health issues a high priority, and that women who attend pre-natal health clinics and family planning centers receive systematic education regarding these infections and prompt treatment and thorough case management when a positive diagnosis is made. A second recommendation was that men should also be approached about these issues. It has been shown that STD clinics located near the workplace are particularly successful in lowering the prevalence of STDs and HIV infections.

A final challenge facing developing countries as they try to lower the rate of STDs and HIV infections is the issue of partner notification. It is necessary to inform one's sexual contacts when one has contracted an STD so that partners can benefit from prompt medical evaluation. But locating and treating the source contact is more essential, and this focus has become a high priority in many developing countries. The source contact is the person from whom an individual's partner acquired HIV, and ideally the person from whom *they* acquired it. This backtracking is basic to effective HIV treatment programs, and public health officials around the world are keenly interested in isolating and treating these source contacts as an essential first step for decreasing the prevalence of STDs and HIV infections.

in physical discomfort. But all STDs do not cause discomfort or obvious, troubling symptoms. Additionally, the early signs of some STDs may not be detectable if they are inside a person's rectum or inside a woman's vagina or on her cervix. Denial is especially likely in people who have an STD but do not have any symptoms, who are referred to as *asymptomatic carriers*. Additionally, because the incubation of some STDs can be quite long, extending over weeks, months, or, in the case of HIV, years, a person can have an STD and give it to others long before they are aware of any signs or symptoms.

Communicating with one's partner or partners about STDs requires maturity, good communication skills, a sense of personal responsibility, and a genuine sense of concern for that other person or persons. If one felt close and trusting enough to have sex with someone in the first place, hopefully one feels close and trusting enough to work through the unhappy consequences that sometimes result. Ideally a couple discusses preventing STDs *before* they have sex, but of course, that doesn't always happen. Working through this together is a good example of adult behavior in which a person assumes responsibility for their own actions and the consequences. Not only is it essential that one talk with their partner if they believe they have given or received an STD, but *promptness* is of the utmost importance for seeking medical assistance. It is absolutely essential that a person refrains from all sexual activity as soon as they suspect that they might have an STD.

Telling Your Partner or Partners

Telling one's partner or partners as soon as one suspects they might have an STD is imperative. This is something one has to do in one's own way, being as genuine and honest as one

possibly can. *Do not do this on the telephone!* These are important, personal issues, and face-to-face communication is imperative. Because both people played a role in transmitting the infection or infestation, both should be willing to share the responsibility and the expense of being treated. This is definitely a private discussion and should take place when two individuals are certain that they will not be interrupted. It is important to make a specific plan and to plan to talk again soon so that both individuals are sure that they are receiving medical attention. Going to the same doctor or health care facility together might be a good idea.

This is not yet the time for the couple to explore the impact of an STD on their relationship, if there is one, and every reasonable effort must be made to engage in productive, mutual problem solving with a minimum of blame and recrimination. These two people can talk about their relationship later; getting treated now is the first priority. It is important to talk about only those issues both individuals *are sure about*. Until they have been to the doctor, they cannot be certain about which, if any, STDs are involved. At this point, the only thing that is really important is getting medical attention as soon as possible.

DO NOT ATTEMPT SELF-MEDICATION

Many people have some leftover antibiotics in their medicine cabinet at home, but it is very important not to start taking any medication without first being diagnosed. First, the medication may be totally ineffective against the STD contracted. Second, even if a person starts taking an antibiotic that is effective, they will probably not have enough of it for a complete course of treatment. That means that the symptoms might go away for a little while, not actually curing the disease but masking the continued progress of the infection. Third, one might be allergic to the medication and have a terrible, life-threatening reaction to it. Finally, the antibiotics a person might have may no longer be effective if they are old. While home remedies might be appropriate for some other types of health problems, they are definitely *not* appropriate for STDs.

WHERE TO GO FOR HELP

Again, ideally one has a close, confidential relationship with their doctor. But everyone doesn't have a personal or family doctor, and many feel embarrassed or humiliated going to their doctor with an STD. Yet part of the professionalism of medical training involves a non-judgmental attitude toward the people one treats and their problems. In most instances, a doctor will not think less of an individual because they have contracted an STD. In fact, the doctor is likely to respect the person's maturity and courage in asking for treatment promptly. All communication with a doctor is confidential, including the diagnosis and any course of treatment prescribed. Pharmacists too are similarly bound by the same professional code and cannot discuss with anyone the medicines a customer is taking or the reason they are taking them.

Still, for many people, a personal or family doctor is not a reasonable option. The local health department can often offer appropriate medical care, however, often for a markedly reduced fee; they also are happy to provide condoms free of charge or at very low cost. The local Planned Parenthood also can generally offer prompt, suitable medical treatment for a reasonable fee. Finally, local urgent care facilities also offer excellent medical care, although they usually cost more than the other two alternatives.

Sometimes people think that they have contracted an STD, seek medical testing, and find out that they have not. Even though this is generally good news, a negative diagnosis involves interesting issues. People who find out that they have not acquired an STD may develop a false sense of security and fail to practice safer sex. This is one reason why people who have had a negative AIDS test are required by law in some states to be counseled about their sexual activity and any high-risk behaviors in which they might be involved.

TAKE MEDICATION AS PRESCRIBED

While in some cases STDs are treated with injectable drugs, often the individual needs to take pills each day for a specified number of days. Needless to say, it is extremely important to take all medications exactly as prescribed and to refrain from all sexual contact until the course of treatment is over and they have been medically checked to ensure that they no longer harbor a sexual infection. In most cases, the doctor will ask the patient to return to the office for tests to confirm that they have been cured, in those cases where a cure is possible. Follow-up check-ups are important because various strains of different STDs have become resistant to some of the antibiotics commonly used to treat them. Sometimes they are somewhat resistant, and in other cases they may be totally resistant. An an-

tibiotic also may be less effective than hoped, and traces of the infection may remain after all the pills have been taken. Another reason follow-up is so important is that it gives the doctor the opportunity to counsel the patient and teach them how to avoid getting another sexually transmitted infection. Often people feel immensely relieved to be treated for an STD and tell themselves that they will never again get into a situation where they could become infected. However, the guidance and expertise of a doctor is especially important in encouraging an individual to practice safer sex in the future.

MEDICAL PROFESSIONALISM

You don't need to read this book to understand that many people are quite judgmental about sexual behavior and its unpleasant outcomes. Unfortunately, some people working in the helping professions also find it difficult to separate their personal beliefs from their professional responsibilities. Everyone has a right to competent, courteous, nonjudgmental interactions with health care professionals when seeking diagnosis and treatment for an STD. Anyone who goes to their doctor, local health department, Planned Parenthood, or student health center should never be made to feel ashamed or "dirty" because they have contracted a communicable disease. Anyone who is treated in this way should seek treatment elsewhere *and make a complaint to the appropriate responsible authorities* such as the local or regional medical society. Everyone has rights as a patient and is always entitled to respect and the highest standards of medical and interpersonal attention.

COUNSELING

Contracting an STD can make a person fearful, anxious, and depressed, feelings which we would call normal under the circumstances. When it comes to diagnosis and treatment for STDs, we believe in the importance of treating the whole person, which might involve some counseling along with medical treatment. The most important thing to do first is get treated for the STD. A good counselor rarely tells a client what to do or think, but often they can help a person understand why they took sexual risks. If one feels that one is not attractive or lovable unless one has sex with someone, then a counselor can help one better understand the faulty assumptions and perhaps gain a better understanding of oneself and one's motives and fears. We are not saying that everyone who has an STD needs counseling, but that in some cases it can be very helpful.

THE FUTURE AFTER AN STD

Contracting and being cured of an STD can teach one some important lessons that might make them a better person. The mistakes a person makes are much less important than what the person *does about their mistakes*. If one learns something about oneself and one's relationships because of an STD, there is an opportunity to adjust one's life and behavior accordingly. With those STDs for which there is no known cure, there are many effective medical interventions to treat recurring symptoms, and new treatment approaches are being developed.

THE PSYCHOSOCIAL CONTEXT OF SEXUALLY TRANSMITTED DISEASES

So far, we have discussed STDs primarily from the point of view of diagnosis and treatment. But of course, it is in a wider psychosocial environment that people engage in health-enhancing behaviors or high-risk behaviors. The relationship between biology and society is close with respect to the prevalence of STDs. The social and psychological aspects of these infections involve a number of questions. For example, how do people approach opportunities for sex in a hazardous social setting? Which populations are at the highest risk for acquiring STDs? Social and psychological factors often have deterministic effects regarding STD and HIV transmission.

Adolescents and Young Adults

Although teenagers seem to be experiencing decreased rates of unanticipated pregnancies and a lower prevalence of STDs, young adults, especially those in their early 20s, are showing an *increase* in both. In this section we will examine the relationship between these adolescent and young adult lifestyles and the high rate of sexually transmitted infections among these individuals. While we are not referring to all individuals and all STDs in these age groups, we are most certainly describing many. Public health organizations have targeted these populations and worked hard to educate them about the prevalence, risks, and consequences of STDs.

To motivate people to avoid getting pregnant or contracting an STD, two basic approaches have been taken: programs that teach safer-sex communication and behavior and programs that encourage sexual abstinence (Fig. 17-16). For many years, social and behavioral scientists have studied the effectiveness of these. Current data related to HIV in African-American youth (Jemmott, Jemmott, & Fong, 1998) indicate that abstinence-only programs are not as effective in delaying sexual intercourse among adolescents as programs that teach safer-sex skills and behaviors. Both sides in this argument agree that STDs and HIV infection are a serious threat to the health of American teenagers. The United States Congress allocated $250 million for the advocacy of abstinence-only programs between 1998 and 2002. Despite the fact that almost $90 million is being used for abstinence-only programs, very few data support the effectiveness of this approach compared with safer-sex programs (DiClemente, 1998).

In research by Jemmott, Jemmott, and Fong (1998), African American adolescents who were sexually active at the beginning of this study were compared with an abstinence-only group. The sexually active youngsters received systematic safer-sex instruction. Three months after the beginning of the study, those receiving abstinence education were less likely to report that they had had sexual intercourse. However, this difference was no longer obvious six months later. Those who were sexually active at the outset were less likely to remain abstinent. Additionally, among those subjects who were sexually active and who received safer-sex instruction, consistent condom use was reported 6 and 12 months after the beginning of

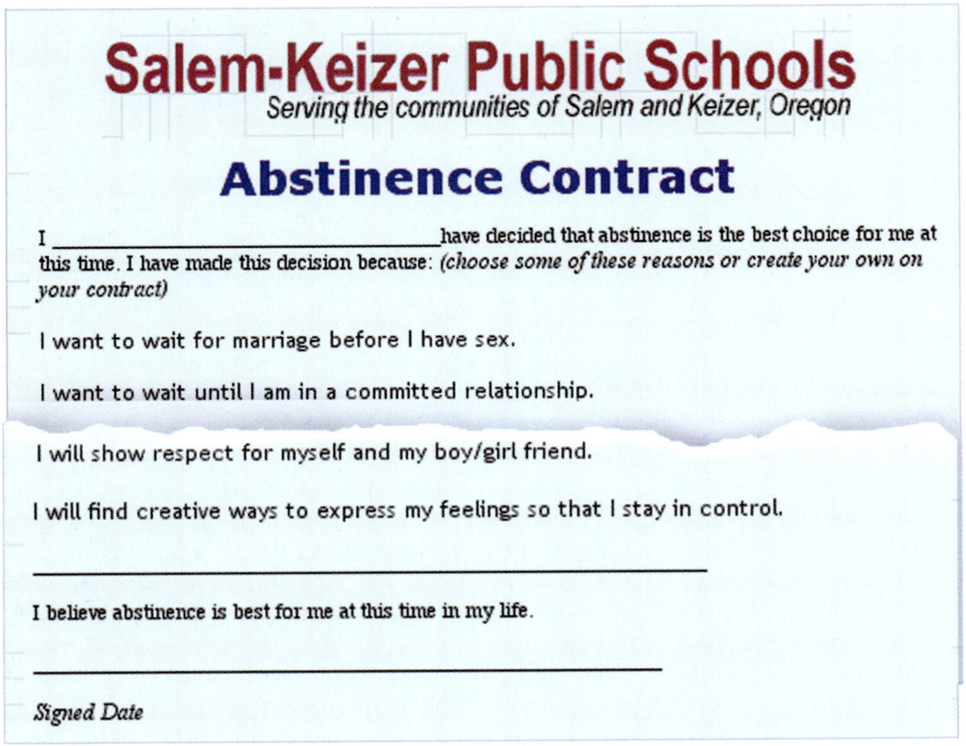

Salem-Keizer Public Schools
Serving the communities of Salem and Keizer, Oregon

Abstinence Contract

I _____ have decided that abstinence is the best choice for me at this time. I have made this decision because: *(choose some of these reasons or create your own on your contract)*

I want to wait for marriage before I have sex.

I want to wait until I am in a committed relationship.

I will show respect for myself and my boy/girl friend.

I will find creative ways to express my feelings so that I stay in control.

_____

I believe abstinence is best for me at this time in my life.

_____

Signed Date

Figure 17-16 Abstinence contracts encourage youngsters to define their personal values and clarify their thinking about becoming involved in sexually intimate relationships.

the investigation. Generally, at this writing, there are few persuasive data to support the effectiveness of programs that encourage abstinence only. A recent editorial in the *Journal of the American Medical Association* (DiClemente, 1998) emphasized that it is difficult to justify the allocation of substantial funds for the implementation of abstinence-only programs. Still, this issue requires continued serious, systematic study with larger sample sizes and more heterogeneous groups of adolescents.

Ideally, adolescents have already received complete, accurate information about sex from their parents, and therefore these programs outside the home might be thought of as supplementary. In fact, this does not always happen. All parents are not well informed themselves about sex, nor are they easily approachable with questions. Raffaelli, Bogenschneider, and Flood (1998) explored the characteristics of communication about sex between parents and teens. They studied 510 pairs of fathers and teens and 666 pairs of mothers and teens. Generally adolescents found it easier to talk with their mothers about sex than with their fathers, and daughters more commonly reported communication about sexual issues with their mothers than did sons. This is not to imply that adolescents *never* talk with their fathers about sex, because in fact they do so frequently. This study focused on three specific topics: the appropriateness or "normality" of adolescent sexual behavior, the risks and consequences of STDs and HIV infection, and various methods of contraception. These authors speculate that one of the reasons communication about sexual topics seems better among girls than boys is that parents are plainly aware that the consequences of sexual activity can be more serious for girls than boys, especially in terms of unanticipated pregnancy. Rosenthal, Cohen, Biro, and DeVellis (1996) found that when female teenagers come from families in which their parents are involved in their lives, attentive to their social activities, and concerned about their academic achievement, they usually feel that their parents would respond supportively if they were to contract an STD. More importantly, when there is good family support and communication on sexual topics, teenagers are far less likely to engage in sexual risk-taking behaviors and more likely to practice safer-sex routinely.

Other researchers have also explored the psychosocial characteristics of teenagers who are most at risk of acquiring an STD (Rosenthal, Biro, Succop, Bernstein, & Stanberry, 1997). In one study 44 males and 88 females were contacted through their primary care physicians. The average age of these subjects was about 17 years, and most had begun having intercourse at around age 14. In this group of subjects, those most likely to report having contracted an STD were somewhat older and female. They were also likely to report having had more sexual partners in their lifetimes, generally thought that STDs were quite common among teenagers, and felt less negative about having had an STD. These data describe some of the psychosocial factors characteristic of teenagers who are most likely to get STDs. This study used a fairly small sample that was not representative of the American population (86% of respondents were African American and 14% were Caucasian). Furby, Ochs, and Thomas (1997) interviewed 48 teenagers using an open-ended

questionnaire. These researchers were particularly interested in learning about teenagers' measures to reduce the risk of acquiring an STD. Interestingly, they found that preventive actions had both positive and negative effects. For example, many respondents reported that taking action to prevent STDs (like using condoms) also were very effective in reducing the chances of pregnancy. However, some subjects reported that if they suggested taking precautionary measures, their partner would interpret it as a gesture of mistrust and it therefore might hurt the quality of the relationship. While many subjects reported that contracting an STD would be viewed in a highly negative way by their peer group, others emphasized that preventive measures such as condoms would diminish the "naturalness" of the sexual experience. In general, taking action to prevent transmission of STDs can have both positive and negative implications for these adolescents, and teenagers frequently consider these pros and cons when they think about having unsafe sex.

While teenagers might not know all they need to know about STDs, recent data indicate that the same might be true about college students. In a study in Australia, Minichiello, Paxton, Cowling, Cross, Savage, Sculthorpe, and Cairns (1996) surveyed over 600 college students regarding the completeness and accuracy of their knowledge about STDs. These students demonstrated a wide degree of variability in their knowledge of the names and nature of diseases that are transmitted sexually. Almost 100% of this sample understood that HIV and AIDS are sexually transmitted, and more than two-thirds understood that genital herpes, HPV, pubic lice, syphilis, hepatitis B, and gonorrhea are also passed from one person to another during physical intimacy. Yet fewer understood the sexual nature of chlamydial infections, scabies, and non-gonococcal urethritis. Although these subjects had a good grasp of the names of STDs, their understanding of symptoms and other medical information about these diseases was not as good, depending on the STD. These respondents had difficulty identifying the means by which genital herpes, chlamydia, hepatitis B, syphilis, and pubic lice are transmitted. The researchers demonstrated that the level of knowledge these students had about STDs did not predict the prevalence of any specific STD in the Australian population, however. While data like these are descriptive, they show the level of information about STDs likely in college students, although these findings cannot necessarily be extended to the entire Australian population. The population of Australia is also likely to differ from the U.S. population in significant ways. Today in the United States there are more than 12 million students in community colleges, colleges and universities, and postgraduate institutions of higher learning—a very large number of individuals who might be less than adequately informed about an extremely significant aspect of their psychosocial environment.

An earlier chapter discussed the fact that some people maintain "positive illusions" of their own competence or safety to avoid confronting real and threatening aspects of modern life. This is certainly true in respect to the risks some people take in relation to STDs. Some of us think that only *other* people need to be vigilant about getting to know their sexual partner or partners and to consistently practice safer-sex behaviors, *but not us.*

Such "illusional beliefs" have been studied through the use of self-report questionnaires in a group of 72 undergraduate college students taking a course in introductory psychology (Wiebe & Black, 1997). This study helps us see what might be going on in someone's mind when they evaluate the risks of engaging in unsafe sexual behaviors. In this sample, Wiebe and Black isolated 16 students whose reports of sexual behavior could be classified as "high risk" but whose reported feelings of actual risk could be classified as "low risk." Clearly, these individuals had illusional beliefs. Subjects were asked how they felt about their chances of getting an STD, becoming pregnant, or getting their partner pregnant; then they read a pamphlet about the behaviors likely to lead to these outcomes. Finally, these students reported their emotions and thoughts regarding their perceived vulnerability to acquiring an STD, becoming pregnant, or impregnating their partner. Subjects who held unreasonable positive illusions about their own safety regarding STDs or unintended pregnancy did not want to learn about the real risks they were facing. Additionally, they claimed that such information was not very pertinent to them, and they did not report any negative emotions when offered information about contraception. These researchers emphasized the fact that these false beliefs tend to protect a person's ego or self-concept. This study offered empirical support to the old adage that people only "hear what they want to hear." These findings are interesting but not new. As long ago as 1987, Bauman and Siegel reported that in a sample of gay men, 83% reported engaging in unsafe sexual practices but thought that these behaviors presented no risks to them personally. Educational programs are generally more effective in changing behavior than are scare tactics, which as noted earlier weren't very effective at all among American soldiers during World War II.

SEXUALLY TRANSMITTED DISEASES AND RISK-TAKING BEHAVIORS

Obviously we do not always do what is good for us, and in fact, we sometimes do stupid, dangerous things. Unfortunately, this aspect of human nature is also related to the risks some of us run in relation to STDs. Social and behavioral scientists have studied the way people think about these risks and how they behave as a consequence. There are some key differences in how women and men take risks.

Sexual Risk-Taking Among Adolescent and Young Adult Women

To fully appreciate the possible risks of acquiring an STD, a person must be able to *think ahead and anticipate the consequences of one's actions*. While these cognitive skills have usually developed by adolescence, there is much variability regarding the age at which these thought processes are operating. Baker and Rosenthal (1998) reviewed the literature concerning the psychological aspects of sexual risk-taking among teenage girls, and their analysis makes clear that in fact, adolescent and young adult females do not always engage in foresightful

thinking about sexual activity. Unless a young woman enjoys the faithful exclusivity of a single sexual partner, there are always risks to consider. It is also important to take into account whether she had any partner or partners before a current, sexually exclusive relationship. When these young women are able to discuss the possibility of STDs with their potential partners, they are not as likely to participate in high-risk sexual behaviors (Sieving, Resnick, Bearinger, et al., 1997). Some young women need to think about many other factors first, such as their need for acceptance from males in general and perhaps one young man in particular, their thoughts about how their girl friends are behaving sexually, and their own mental and emotional maturity and development. Generally, when adolescent and young women feel that they are full partners in a relationship and can make their feelings, fears, and preferences known to their partners, they are more likely to make sexual decisions that are both self-protective and foresightful.

Someone who has never had an STD might think that getting one is about the most terrible thing that can happen, and with HIV infections this might indeed be true. But many people do have sexually transmitted infections and/or infestations, and for them, another STD might not carry with it the shame, fear, and anxiety it would for someone contracting such an infection or infestation for the first time. Someone who starts to think that STDs are a common or "normal" part of life are far less likely to take preventive measures to be sure that they don't get one. Another factor closely related to the care people take in avoiding an STD involves whether they are having any symptoms. If people do not understand that they might be transmitting an STD to their partner even when they are not having any symptoms, then they will be far less likely to take any preventive measures.

Television, movies, and romance novels bombard our society with depictions and promises of exciting sex. However, these media almost never show characters who have acquired an STD or the protective measures they take to be sure they don't. The AIDS epidemic has changed this situation somewhat, but with the exception of HIV infections, women or men are seldom seen talking about having safer sex, buying and using condoms, or candidly discussing their personal sexual histories. The media therefore give the wrong impression that STDs are rare and happen only to other people.

Alcohol and other drugs complicate the situation further. These agents generally contribute to sexual risk-taking because they lower inhibitions and contribute to a person behaving in less than cautious ways. Baker and Rosenthal (1998) note that substance use or abuse play a role in early first intercourse, a lack of condom usage, and the higher risk that one will be "used" sexually. Another problem is negotiating the use of latex condoms. Many men tell their prospective sex partners that they "can't feel anything" if they use a condom and "they really don't work anyway." We recommend that if a man tells a woman that he can't feel as much when he uses a condom, she should tell him that if he doesn't use a condom he won't feel *anything at all*. Someone who truly cares about a woman and respects himself would not fail to use latex condoms.

Sexual Risk-Taking Among Adolescent and Young Adult Men

As with women, there are a number of reasons adolescent and young adult men engage in sexual risk-taking behaviors that are likely to lead to acquiring or transmitting STDs. Hoffman and Bolton (1997) distributed questionnaires to almost 150 self-identified heterosexual men who had visited STD clinics in California. These researchers selected about a dozen sexual behaviors that involved low, moderate, and high risks for acquiring STDs and HIV and asked their respondents whether they engaged in these "always, regularly, sometimes, used to, or do not." On average, these men were about 31 years old, 44% were African American, 36% were Caucasian, and 20% represented other races; 77% were single. Most had some college education, and almost 1 in 5 was a college graduate. At the time of this study, 72% had been diagnosed with an STD and 67% had a history of some type of sexually transmitted infection. From the reports of these subjects, five different reasons for their high-risk sexual behavior could be isolated. These included feelings of being in love, complying with their partner's wishes, the enjoyment of erotic pleasure, sexual behavior while in an altered state of consciousness, and the desire to express dominance and power in a relationship. The "pleasure factor" seemed to be most frequently associated with high-risk sexual behaviors likely to lead to STDs and HIV infection: fellatio without the use of a condom, their partner swallowing their semen, coitus interruptus, vaginal sex without a condom, and anal sex without a condom. This study described heterosexual behaviors that are most likely to lead to the transmission of an STD or HIV and the most common motives behind them.

In a study by Blanton and Gerrard (1997), male undergraduate college students who viewed pictures of women rated as either high or low in "sex appeal" reported that the more attractive women were less likely to have STDs or HIV and therefore would be potentially safer sex partners. These subjects believed that physical attractiveness was in some way related to desirable personality attributes and concluded that they therefore presented a lower risk of having STDs or HIV. Apparently, there is a subtle social stereotype that less attractive individuals are more likely to have more sexual partners or to engage in unsafe sexual practices more often than attractive individuals.

A study in England addressed issues involved in the decision to be tested for HIV. People seeking testing usually have a good reason for doing so. Perhaps they were careless and had frequently engaged in unsafe sexual behaviors, or maybe one of their partners tested positive for HIV. Making a decision to get tested usually carries with it some awareness that one has not been as careful as one should have been. One might therefore hypothesize that those who receive a negative report would begin to be more careful, but an investigation by George, Green, and Murphy (1998) showed this is not necessarily true. In a sample of 114 subjects who tested HIV positive and another 114 subjects who tested HIV negative, 5.3% of those who tested negative acquired an STD in the year after their test, while among those who tested positive, 2.6% acquired an STD during the same period of time. Apparently, the anxiety surrounding HIV testing, even when it yielded a negative result, was not as effective in dissuading unsafe sexual practices as a positive test would have predicted. A negative test result may give a person a false sense of security and unrealistic ideas about the very real risks they are taking. Results like these demonstrate the importance of counseling for individuals who have tested negative for HIV as well as those who have tested positive.

Finally, another study explored the risk of acquiring an STD based on whether a person was engaging in unsafe sexual practices with their monogamous partner or with multiple partners. A study in France explored this issue in a sample of over 1600 subjects who acknowledged having at least two sexual partners over the previous twelve months (Messiah, Pelletier, et al., 1996). These respondents reported engaging in a wide variety of sexual behaviors. Manual stimulation, penis-in-the-vagina intercourse, mutual masturbation, and oral-genital contact were very common in this sample of subjects. Anal sex was uncommon. In most sexual encounters a condom was not used. Condoms were more likely to be used when a person's partner was an "occasional" partner. Similarly, sexual behaviors not involving penetration, including oral stimulation, were more common among occasional partners. Importantly, the women reported that they did not commonly initiate condom usage with their occasional partners; the men, however, were more likely to have done so. By implication, this study emphasizes the importance of condom usage and nonpenetrative sex when considering sex with a partner not known well.

IRREGULAR USE OF CONDOMS

When it comes to preventing STDs, condoms are available, inexpensive, and very effective (Fig. 17-17). So why don't people use them regularly? We have already noted some of the psy-

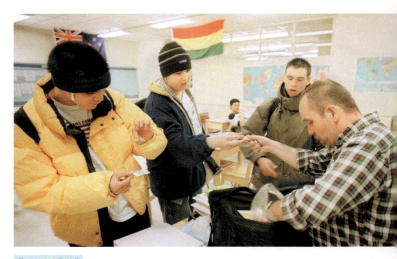

FIGURE 17-17 A community health education counselor (right) hands out condoms in a high school sex education class in Iqaluit, Canada. While condom distribution is controversial, many communities support this simple, effective measure to reduce the number of nonmarital pregnancies and the transmission of STDs.

Dear Dr. Ruth

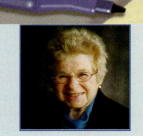

Question:

Is it really true that latex condoms offer enough protection against HIV? They're so cheap and easy, I just can't believe that something so simple works so well. Is there some kind of catch? I am a college student and I see advertisements for condoms all over campus, and I have a hard time understanding why someone wouldn't use them if they work so well. Why would people take such terrible risks?

Answer:

If you were walking down the street and saw a man up ahead waving a gun around, you'd turn around and head in the other direction. The problem with STDs is that they're invisible, and as the old saying goes, "out of sight, out of mind"—particularly if the opportunity for sex is there and both parties are in a high state of arousal. That's why it's important to be prepared with a condom before things go too far.

As to why people actively refuse to use a condom, I can only say that they feel invulnerable or are careless, or both. They think that they can't become a statistic. Now I recognize that in this life one must take some risks to get ahead, but when you weigh the risks of catching an STD against using a condom, the scales tip greatly in favor of using a condom. Luckily many more people are using condoms, and the spread of HIV is slowing, but still far too many people are not practicing safer sex, and sadly, many will regret it.

As to the protection offered by a latex condom, yes, they are effective at preventing both disease and pregnancy. According to the 17th Revised Edition of *Contraceptive Technology*, however, 27,000 condoms slip or break on an average night in the U.S. I don't know how they determine such statistics, but we know enough about the reliability of the condom to say that there is no such thing as safe sex, only safer sex.

---

chosocial factors related to consistent, correct condom usage. Personal attitudes are also important in relation to use or nonuse of condoms. Earlier, we noted the double message of society to teenagers: "If you obtain condoms to take personal responsibility for your sexual behavior, you are planning to behave in an evil, immoral way." It's no wonder that there is a lot of confusion about obtaining and using condoms. Research has shed some light on this issue, however.

Condom Use Among College Students

Beckman, Harvey, and Tiersky (1996) asked almost 200 college students to fill out a questionnaire about their attitudes regarding condom use and oral contraceptives. Approximately 70% of this sample was female. A significant percentage of these subjects emphasized the disease prevention aspects of condoms as basic to their decision to use them. They also found them available and convenient to use. Many students reported that the condom interfered little with sexual spontaneity, a commonly reported reason that many people don't like

using them. However, only 60% of the students in this study reported using condoms during the previous 6 months. Another noteworthy finding was the fact that African American respondents believed more strongly than their Caucasian counterparts that condom use was an important way of preventing pregnancy and sexual infections. While this research dealt exclusively with the male condom, more research is now being published about the female condom, especially its ability to prevent STDs.

Female Condoms and Women at Risk for HIV Infection

Most of what we have written so far about condoms has been about male condoms, but female condoms, while still new, are being used more frequently. Recent research has explored the use of the female condom among women who are at a particularly high risk for acquiring HIV infection (Surratt, Wechsberg, Cottler, Leukefeld, Klein, & Desmond, 1998). These researchers note that few educational programs about

Research Highlight

CONDOM USE IN NEVADA'S LEGAL BROTHELS

Commercial sex workers are certainly at a high risk for STDs if they do not use condoms (Fig. 17-18). In 1988 the Nevada legislature passed a law mandating condom use in legal brothels. Posters reminding prospective customers of this law are placed in conspicuous locations in these establishments. Still, many men who come to these brothels try to negotiate penetrative sex acts without the use of a condom. This issue is the focus of an interesting research study by Albert, Warner, and Hatcher (1998).

These researchers found that most commercial sex workers use condoms regularly and correctly with their customers. The fact that these women are shown free of HIV and other STDs in regular tests supports their consistent use of condoms. Forty licensed commercial sex workers working in two legal brothels in Nevada participated in this study. All were at least 18 years old and had worked in their current establishment for at least 1 month. Of these, 26 women indicated that they had encountered a prospective customer who said that they did not want to use a condom in the previous month. Thirteen women reported that they had been approached by more than one prospective customer who resisted condom use. These women had sex with a total of 3290 customers during the previous month, of whom 90 at first refused to use a condom.

Of the 90 customers who at first refused to use a condom, 65 decided to comply when they were told that the women working there would not have vaginal intercourse or engage in fellatio with them unless they did so. Four of these men had a condom applied to their penises without their knowing it; the woman held a condom in her cheek and applied it to the client's penis during oral stimulation. Condoms lubricated with nonoxynol-9 further protected the woman from risk of oral infection. Of the almost 3300 clients who had visited the brothel during the time of the study, only 14 left without having purchased any sexual services.

When questioned about their personal lives, 38 of these women acknowledged that they had a lover sometime in the previous year, and 14 indicated that they had more than one. In all but three cases, these lovers were men. Virtually all of these women used condoms with all of their clients during penetrative sexual acts, but only 7 of them used condoms consistently with their lovers. Of the 14 women who had more than one lover, 10 reported that they did not use condoms consistently in their private lives. These data suggest that commercial sex workers in this sample may have been at a higher risk of acquiring an STD or HIV infection from a lover in their personal life than from a client with whom they had sex for money.

Social and behavioral scientists have long known that substance abuse and/or alcoholism is common among women and men who engage in sex for money. While the money obtained through prostitution is frequently used to support a drug habit, the implications of this vicious cycle of behavior have only recently been analyzed in terms of the prevalence of STDs in commercial sex workers who smoke crack cocaine, a particularly addictive opiate. Jones, Irwin, Inciardi, Bowser, Schilling, Word, Evans, Faruque, McCoy, and Edlin (1998) studied over 400 prostitutes in 1991 who were addicted to crack cocaine. This population is at an especially high risk for becoming infected with HIV, and these researchers were interested in their high-risk sexual practices. These subjects were approached in urban areas, interviewed, and tested for HIV. In this sample of over 400 female and male prostitutes, a significant number said that they had knowingly had sex with intravenous drug users (30% to 41%) and persons they knew to be HIV positive (8% to 19%). A significant number reported that they had contracted an STD in the past (73% to 93%) but still used condoms irregularly (more than 50% for all types of sex acts reported). Those commercial sex workers working in crack houses were frequently paid with crack and reported engaging in high-risk sexual behaviors. Among these, more than one-fourth were HIV positive, 37.5% had syphilis, and 66.8% had genital herpes.

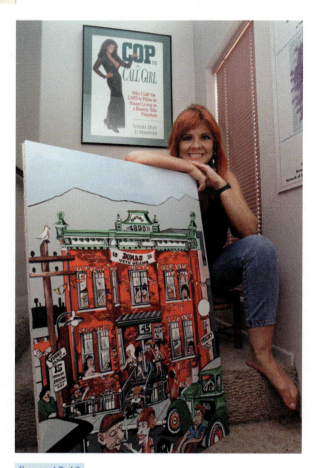

FIGURE 17-18   Norma Jean Almodovar heads a group called the International Sex Worker Foundation for Art, Culture, and Education. She is holding a painting of a brothel in Butte, Montana and is hoping to turn the building into a museum that describes the lives of prostitutes.

HIV are targeted to women. This research focused on women who were receiving treatment for the recent use of injectable drugs and/or crack cocaine, who were also likely to include unsafe sexual behaviors in their drug-related lifestyles. Over 300 women in San Antonio, Texas, St. Louis, Missouri, and Rio de Janeiro, Brazil participated in the study. The average age of these subjects ranged from 28 in Rio de Janeiro to 36 in St. Louis. Most of these women had a history of trading money or drugs for sex, and one-third of the total number of women had multiple sex partners over the course of the last 30 days. About two-thirds of the women from Brazil had used the female condom, while about 20% of those in San Antonio and St. Louis had tried it. Those women who had a history of trading sex for drugs were far more likely to use the female condom. This finding was especially pronounced in the South American women, as was the fact that the women who decided to use the female condom were also 8 times more likely to have been using male condoms. Most of the women in this study reported that they were generally satisfied with the female condom, and in Rio de Janeiro and St. Louis about 75% continued to use them 3 months after the study began. Approximately 40% of

those in San Antonio continued to use them. It is still too early to tell if the female condom will become widely used by women who want a more independent role in pregnancy and STD prevention, but these early data certainly look promising.

Condom Use Among Separated and Divorced Women

When people separate or get divorced, they often begin to date and explore sexual relations with other people. For both women and men, this transitional period can be a time when they have intercourse and share other intimate behaviors with several other people. It is a time when safer-sex practices such as condom use are especially important. Women most often bear the negative consequences of contraceptive negligence or the failure to use condoms correctly and consistently. Marion and Cox (1996) studied condom use in a sample of over 250 separated and divorced women, dividing their sample into women who could still conceive and those who could not. These women were between the ages of 20 and 49, with more than 75% having had some college experience. More than half the subjects had been separated for 3 years or less. All of these women reported having sexual intercourse with someone who was not their spouse in the previous years. The results of this study are troubling: 41% of the subjects reported that they had never used condoms since they became separated or divorced, while "38% reported some-time to half-time condom use, and 21% reported regular condom use. Almost 60% of the respondents never used condoms with regular partners. With last intercourse, 77.7% of the respondents did not use condoms" (p. 114). These women are at a high risk of acquiring an STD or HIV infection. The women who were fertile were far more likely to be careful about using condoms than those who could not conceive. Ideally, separated and divorced women who are sexually active should ensure that condoms are available if sexual intimacy is in any way likely and should communicate their desire to use them to their partners.

SPECIFIC POPULATIONS AND STD RISKS

The incidence and prevalence of STDs vary significantly among different population groups.

Prisoners

It has been estimated that at any point in time in this country, there are approximately 567,000 individuals in local and county jails (*MMWR*, June 5, 1998). People incarcerated in these facilities typically are on short sentences or are waiting for their trial to begin. In a study of women in these facilities, 35% tested positive for syphilis, 27% for chlamydia, and 8% for gonorrhea. With even greater numbers of prisoners in state and federal facilities, this population presents public health officials with special challenges. Since women with STDs do not always have any obvious symptoms, the prevalence of STDs and HIV infection in correctional facilities is generally based on just those who are having symptoms. The Centers for Disease Control and Prevention in 1997 found that most city and county jails test for STDs only when an inmate is having symptoms or specifically requests testing. Voluntary testing to locate inmates who have STDs but are asymptomatic is generally not done, regardless of the consequences of the lack of prompt treatment for sexually transmitted infections. Because conjugal visits are common and because same-sex activity is a part of jail and prison life, these issues seem to warrant serious, systematic, quantitative study.

Military Personnel

Eitzen and Sawyer (1997) studied the questionnaire responses of almost 600 unmarried female army recruits to questions about the consistency with which they used condoms, the number of men they had had sex with in their lives, the variety of sexual behaviors in which they had participated, alcohol use as an accompaniment to sexual activity, their previous reproductive health care history, pregnancy, and personal history of STDs. Ninety percent of these women reported having sexual intercourse at least once, with most women having had three lifetime partners. Of the women in this sample, 26% had at least one pregnancy, and 14% reported having had at least one STD in the past.

The authors of this study described these women's condom use as "erratic," noting that as few as 14% of the women in this sample had used condoms while having sex with a "casual" partner. Alcohol use was commonly incorporated into

Other Countries, Cultures, and Customs

CONDOM USE AMONG COMMERCIAL SEX WORKERS IN THAILAND

There is a new phenomenon in the vacation industry: sex vacations. It has become common for foreign visitors to fly to several countries in Southeast Asia to spend several days as "guests" in brothels. As this industry has grown, so too has the prevalence of HIV infections, placing customers at a high risk of acquiring the virus unless they use condoms conscientiously and consistently. The managers of these brothels took action to support their sex workers and clients with condom use. Because of differences in sex roles and women's rights in other countries, all commercial sex workers may not be able to successfully negotiate condom-only sex with prospective clients, and therefore the support of their brothel manager is an essential first step in creating such a policy. Sakondhavat, Werawatanakul, Bennett, Kuchaisit, and Suntharapa (1997) studied this issue.

These researchers addressed the public health challenge to the commercial sex workers in Khon Kaen City. At the beginning of the study in 1990, only 2 brothels had a condom-only policy enforced by brothel managers. The managers of the city's 24 brothels were encouraged to comply with a condom-only policy. The brothel managers were given a slide presentation about AIDS and they also received additional information about HIV infection and the importance of condom usage in reducing the number of new cases of HIV. They were given condoms to distribute to their sex workers, and their supplies were replenished each month. They received encouragement and reinforcement for their efforts to begin a condom-only policy in their brothels. Commercial sex workers were given free blood tests for HIV and syphilis and then checked again 6 months later. Between 200 and 300 commercial sex workers were working in these 24 brothels at any time.

After 3 months, 74% of all the brothels in Khon Kaen City had a condom-only policy, and clients who refused to use a condom were refused sexual services. When the supply of condoms was uninterrupted, high rates of condom compliance continued. However, when there were inconsistencies in the delivery and availability of condoms, the number of unprotected sex acts increased. When condoms were available without interruption, about 90% of all sexual interactions involved the use of a condom. These researchers believe that the support and encouragement of the brothel managers is critical to the success of their program. Because there is an extremely high rate of turnover among commercial sex workers in Thailand every year, these measures may hopefully play a major role in lowering the rate at which STDs and HIV infections are transmitted.

sexual activity, contributing to lessened inhibitions and less care about taking safer-sex precautions. Alcohol use was generally predictive of a greater number of lifetime sexual partners and fewer screening tests for STDs. Of the women in this sample, those with steady partners and those with casual partners were just as likely to seek testing for STDs. Because there are more than 350,000 women in the military today, these data reveal real and pressing public health issues affecting almost 14% of the total American military establishment. Clearly, health education programs should be developed and implemented for STD prevention and treatment for women in the military. This is especially important because STDs are 5 times more common in the American military population than in the general civilian population in times of peace and 30 times more common in times of war (Eitzen & Sawyer, 1997, p. 686). Between 1985 and 1994, almost 2400 soldiers, sailors, and air personnel tested HIV positive. Although those statistics primarily involve men, the purpose of this study of military women was to highlight the importance of studying more carefully a sample of military personnel at greater risk from unsafe sexual practices and inadequate STD screening. Data like these should encourage greater emphasis on STD education, testing, reporting, and treatment in the armed forces.

Heterosexual Activity Among Self-Identified Homosexual and Bisexual Men

Chapter 9 notes that sexual orientation is a continuum, not a dichotomy. It is rare for a person to have either exclusively heterosexual thoughts, feelings, and fantasies or exclusively homosexual thoughts, feelings, and fantasies. Chapter 9 also noted the difficulties in clearly defining the term "bisexual" unambiguously. When studying the transmission of STDs and HIV, it is important also to explore heterosexual behavior by men who identify themselves as primarily homosexual. Evans, Bond, and MacRae (1998) studied these issues among a sample of 1490 men who had presented themselves at an STD clinic in London. Of them, 1212 were self-identified heterosexuals, 234 homosexuals, and 44 bisexuals. Of the homosexuals in this sample, 8.5% reported having heterosexual sex at least once during the last year, 45.2% said that they had had heterosexual intercourse but not during the past year, and 46.2% reported never having heterosexual intercourse. Among the respondents who identified themselves as bisexual, 34.3% had sex with at least one woman during the previous year, 28.6% had sex with 2 women during this time span, and 11.5% had 3 or more partners. In this sample, 25.7% had not had sex with a woman during the past year. An important finding was a large difference in the frequency with which heterosexuals used condoms consistently (16.9% of the sample) compared with homosexuals and bisexuals (40.9% of the sample). While in the past HIV was more likely to be transmitted during homosexual anal intercourse, today there is a rise in HIV transmission among heterosexuals having vaginal intercourse. Again, these are public health issues of real importance.

CONCLUSION

STDs such as HIV are serious health problems that can happen to good, and sometimes careless people. Despite the unfortunate consequences of STDs, people are still powerfully impelled to engage in sexual behavior when they know the risk, and it is still not completely clear why this so commonly happens. The emphasis here is the importance of taking personal responsibility for one's sexual behavior, making intelligent and cautious sexual decisions, taking appropriate and effective preventive measures, and avoiding sexual risks as a lifestyle issue. Also important are early, accurate diagnosis and effective treatment. Everyone needs to feel responsible for their own health and behaviors.

Learning Activities

1. Discuss social and cultural factors that have prevented or discouraged public awareness of the prevalence and incidence of sexually transmitted diseases.

2. What might be a good way to encourage sexually active women to have periodic STD check-ups, especially since so many of them are asymptomatic carriers of these disorders?

3. Speculate on reasons a person would delay seeking medical treatment for an STD with obvious symptoms.

4. Describe the behavioral changes required by having genital herpes. Comment on sexual, hygiene, and medication issues.

5. When people donate blood, they receive a free test for HIV and hepatitis. Despite this, many who are sexually active, have multiple partners, or are gay do not request to learn the outcomes of these tests. Why do you think this is so?

6. Blood tests for HIV are now available over the counter in many pharmacies with test results assigned a code number. Test results are available over the phone with this code number. Suggest why a person might or might not use such a kit if she or he suspects that they might be carrying the virus.

7. Summarize the psychological, social, and cultural obstacles to the conscientious use of condoms. Why should or shouldn't condom advertising appear on television?

8. The use of drugs and alcohol is commonly linked to unsafe sexual practices that might involve STDs. These agents often lower a person's inhibitions and may lead to risky behaviors.
   a. Describe what population seems most likely to use drugs and/or alcohol concurrently with sexual interaction.
   b. In view of the age and development of this group of people, what medium should be used for cautionary appeals about this combination of behaviors? Would television, radio, or printed matter be most suitable?

c. How might drug and/or alcohol use in conjunction with risky sexual practices be dealt with by public health officials working with prostitutes?

9. Because AIDS is always eventually fatal, the insurance industry has grown justifiably concerned about the impact of this disease and lifestyles that foster its transmission. Yet privacy rights are involved when an insurance company asks questions about a person's family life, relationships, and gender preference and the answers to those questions affect whether the person obtains health or life insurance.

a. What criteria do you think insurers should use to decide who they will insure and who they will not? What criteria do you think they do use?

b. How can an insurer ask a potential customer their health care history without inquiring whether the individual has had HIV testing and/or counseling?

c. Speculate on the impact of the AIDS epidemic on the cost of life insurance.

d. Do you think more parents will purchase life insurance for their very young children?

e. If you are a health worker and are named as a sexual partner of someone who is HIV positive, should your employer have the legal right to require you to be tested for HIV? If so, should the results of this test become part of your permanent personnel file and possibly become available to health insurance companies?

10. Give examples of some good sexual communication skills between two individuals that might help them prevent the transmission of STDs. Be specific.

*K*ey Concepts

■ Prevention of STDs requires an individual to take personal responsibility for their intimate behaviors and to engage in intelligent decision-making so that they will be less likely to participate in high-risk behaviors.

■ Asymptomatic carriers of an STD do not have any obvious signs of being infected. Women infected with chlamydia or gonorrhea, for example, may have no symptoms. When signs of an STD occur inside a woman's vagina or on her cervix, she may be unaware of these.

■ Sexual risk-taking occurs when people do not think ahead and anticipate the possible consequences of their sexual behaviors. It is a basic psychological factor in the transmission of STDs.

■ If you think you have a sexually transmitted disease it is imperative to talk, in person, with your sexual partner or part-

ners and fully, clearly, and honestly tell them your symptoms, your diagnosis (if you have already gone to a doctor), and encourage them strongly to seek prompt, competent medical care, perhaps seeking assistance together.

■ In seeking care for STDs, you are fully entitled to competent, courteous, nonjudgmental medical professionalism without concerns about feeling shameful. Counseling is sometimes beneficial for helping individuals cope with STDs, their treatment, and their long-term effects, if any.

■ Adolescents and young adults often feel that they are immune to the risks inherent in unprotected sex and frequently do not feel vulnerable to STDs. Personal growth and development often involves recognizing these potential problems and acting proactively to avoid them.

■ Irregular and/or inconsistent condom use is not unusual among sexually active adolescents and young adults. Educational, cultural, and religious considerations affect a person's adherence to cautious, prudent condom usage on a regular basis.

■ The risks of transmitting and receiving STDs are no less serious among homosexual and bisexual individuals.

*G*lossary Terms

bacteria
chancroid
chlamydia
cytomegalovirus (CMV)
genital herpes
gonorrhea
hepatitis

human immunodeficiency virus (HIV)
human papilloma virus (HPV)
infestation
Kaposi's sarcoma
molluscum contagiosum

nongonococcal urethritis (NGU)
pelvic inflammatory disease (PID)
pubic lice
retrovirus
scabies
syphilis
virus

*S*uggested Readings

Ebel, C. (1998). *Managing herpes: How to live and love with a chronic STD.* Research Triangle Park, NC: American Social Health Association.

Institute of Medicine. (1997). T. R. Eng & W. T. Butler (Eds.). *The hidden epidemic: Confronting sexually transmitted diseases.* Washington, D. C.: National Academy Press.

Lipman, J. (1998). *Soap, water, and sex: A lively guide to the benefits of sexual hygiene and to coping with sexually transmitted diseases.* Amherst, NY: Prometheus Books.

Marr, L. (1999). *Sexually transmitted diseases: A physician tells you what you need to know.* Baltimore, MD: Johns Hopkins University Press.

Reitano, M. V. (1999). *Sexual health: Questions you have...answers you need.* Allentown, PA: Peoples Medical Society.

18

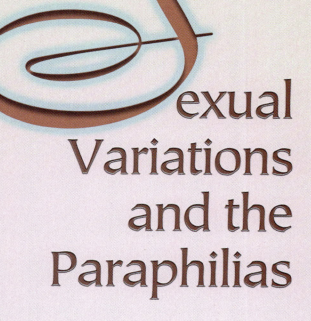

Sexual Variations and the Paraphilias

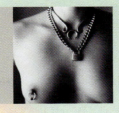

OBJECTIVES

When you finish reading and reviewing this chapter, you should be able to:

1. Briefly describe historical figures and writings relevant to the study of unusual or deviant sexual practices.

2. Discriminate among the meanings of these terms: "atypical," "variation," "deviation," "perversion," and "paraphilia."

3. Discuss why it is difficult to accurately determine the prevalence of paraphilias in the general population.

4. Discuss four theories about the origins of sexual variations and deviations.

5. Explain the diagnostic features of paraphilias that are common to all forms.

6. Describe common and uncommon paraphilias, noting the distinguishing characteristics of each. Discuss the degree to which each may or may not involve legal offenses and the extent to which each victimizes others.

7. Explain the "operating rules" of the sadomasochistic subculture and the "understanding" that governs interactions between sexual sadists and sexual masochists.

8. Review some of the manifestations of paraphilias in everyday life and human relationships. Explain the degree to which these are tolerated or condemned by society as a whole.

9. Discuss the characteristics of sexual addiction. Speculate whether sexual addiction is a true paraphilia.

10. Summarize the approaches to treating paraphilias. Explain the distinguishing features of each and comment on their relative effectiveness.

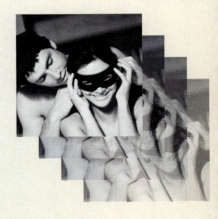

From Dr. Ruth

Many of the questions people ask me about have to do with what is "normal." Many people are very concerned about whether their particular behavior is normal or not. What I think is *much more* important is whether someone is getting hurt by such behavior. If that's the case, it should be avoided, no matter how many other people are doing it.

Certainly, there are particular sexual behaviors that most people do not indulge in. But if somebody gets sexual satisfaction from one of them, and it doesn't cause them any harm or harm anyone else, then I see no reason why they should refrain from this behavior. But it's important that these behaviors are mutually consensual and occur in private.

Many of the behaviors described in this chapter do have negative consequences, however. In those cases, individuals who cannot stop themselves from such behavior need help.

Previous chapters in this book have discussed the more common or "normal" aspects of human sexuality. Some of these sexual topics might be unappealing to some people, but they are generally acknowledged as an ordinary part of the world in which we live. However, some sexual inclinations and behaviors are indeed very unusual, and sometimes frankly against the law. The variations and deviations of human sexual desire know no boundaries, either geographically or in terms of race, religion, educational attainment, or socioeconomic status. Some people are astonished or even disgusted by the sometimes bizarre manifestations of human sexual inclinations (Fig. 18-1). In previous chapters sexual issues have been discussed that are not matters of "right" or "wrong," but this chapter and the next will focus on some aspects of human sexuality that are illegal and exploitative.

COMPLEX LANGUAGE ISSUES

Many different words are used to refer to unusual sexual inclinations and behaviors, and we need to make sense out of these terms and their diverse and sometimes overlapping meanings. Different authors, scientists, experts, psychologists, and psychiatrists often use these terms in idiosyncratic ways, and the suggested meanings here are by no means definitive, only useful in the scope of this chapter. Finally, these terms are *social constructions,* not scientific terms referring to observable, measurable aspects of behavior. Rather they are determined by historical influences, current laws and traditions, and varying social conditions, and may change as new information is acquired.

- *Atypical.* This term is used in a generic sense to refer to anything not characteristic of most people most of the time. It means "unusual" but is value free. Atypical sexual behaviors are not common avenues of intimate expression, but this word does not imply they are bizarre, illegal, or highly peculiar. In a statistical sense, "atypical" means rare when compared with the norm.

- *Variation.* Sexual variations are sexual behaviors engaged in by a minority of individuals in any particular society, but of which there is generally not wide disapproval.

- *Deviation.* Society plainly disapproves of sexual deviations. Still, there may be significant differences between the opinions of society as a whole and psychiatrists or psychologists.

- *Perversion.* This word is not as common today among sexologists as it used to be in the writings of Krafft-Ebing, Freud, and Ellis. It generally refers to deviant sexual behaviors the person *prefers to heterosexual sexual intercourse.* Like the term "deviant," perversion clearly has unpleasant connotations. Sex experts rarely use this term anymore, and when people use the word, it carries a clear value judgment.

- *Paraphilia.* Of these different terms, "paraphilia" has the most contemporary usage and is preferred by sex experts and specialists in the treatment of psychological disorders. It implies persistent, strong atypical sexual urges associated with highly distracting sexual fantasies. Paraphilias may involve erotic feelings for nonhuman objects, age-inappropriate individuals, unwilling or nonconsenting adults, or the allure of punishment or humiliation and degradation as aspects of sexual activity. There are a variety of paraphilias, which will be discussed in this chapter. Paraphilias are included in the *Diagnostic and Statistical Manual of Mental Disorders.* A person with one paraphilia may

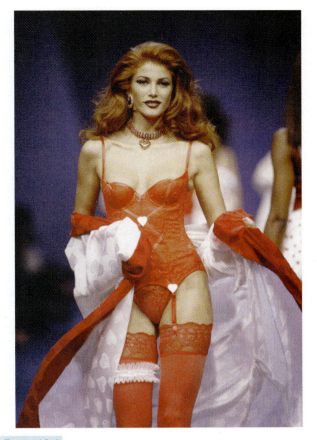

FIGURE 18-1 The public may sometimes react to flamboyant displays of sexual tastes and preferences with undistracted, focused interest. This reveals nothing about the "normality" of the viewer or the viewed.

have others as well. Paraphilias are officially recognized as mental disorders and are thus thought treatable by psychiatrists and psychologists.

HISTORICAL BACKGROUND

For many centuries, uncommon sexual practices have been described, but the serious, systematic exploration of unusual sexual practices began with Krafft-Ebing and Freud in the 19th century. Earlier, descriptions of atypical sexual behavior existed in the context of nonscientific disciplines such as religion, mythology, literature, and the law. This study was generally taken over by more empirical areas of scholarly inquiry, such as anthropology, medicine, psychiatry, psychoanalysis, and sexology (Travin & Protter, 1993). In his famous *Psychopathia Sexualis,* Richard von Krafft-Ebing (1939) originally wrote in Latin about unusual sexual practices in an attempt to diminish what he anticipated would be a huge public outcry over these "indecencies." In this important scholarly treatise, Krafft-Ebing describes a large number of case studies dealing with a large variety of uncommon sexual practices: sadism, masochism, fetishes, exhibitionism, frotteurism, zoophilia, pe-

dophilia, and sadomasochistic behaviors. His clinical examples were drawn from the published psychiatric literature of many different countries in Europe, Russia, and Asia. Part of the tremendous importance of Krafft-Ebing's book is that it was among the first to present an exhaustive, systematic compilation of unusual sexual inclinations and behaviors.

Chapter 2 explored many of the historical antecedents to our culture's current attitudes about human sexuality. Recall that the ancient Greeks were somewhat permissive about many sexual behaviors including sadomasochism, transvestism, zoophilia (sex with animals), and pedophilia (sex with children, although strictly speaking the Greeks used the term *pederasty* to refer to adult men having sexual relations with adolescent boys). According to St. Augustine, however, the only appropriate reason for having sexual intercourse was procreation, and nonprocreative (recreational) sex was considered deviant in this early Christian perspective; Chapter 2 also points out that many fundamentalist Christians today still feel this way. In Victorian England there was an enormous amount of anxiety about the supposedly dangerous effects of masturbation and frequent sexual intercourse, which were considered "deviant" in that historical context.

Two other important historical figures forever changed our culture's view of the diversity of sexual behaviors. The Marquis de Sade (Fig. 18-2), born in 1740, wrote a number of books while a resident in various asylums for the criminally insane. The best known of these include *One Hundred and Twenty Days of Sodom,* and *The Adversities of Virtue.* These books include lucid descriptions of a wide variety of behaviors in which the inflicting of pain is associated with sexual excitement. Various tortures, floggings, and physical mutilations of women are described in minute detail. These books aroused so much public hostility that Napoleon believed that de Sade should be kept under lock and key for his own as well as society's protection (Travin & Protter, 1993). The other person of historical importance in relation to sexual deviations was Leopold von Sacher-Masoch, who was born in 1836. In his book *Venus in Furs,* Sacher-Masoch described in keen detail how a male character was the object of humiliation and degradation by a dominating female character who tormented him with a whip while dressed in high boots and furs. When Krafft-Ebing read these books, he coined the terms "sadism" and "masochism" to refer to how some people become sexually aroused by inflicting pain on others or by being the object of such abuse.

According to Travin and Protter, modern perspectives on sexual deviation began with the publication of Krafft-Ebing's book in 1886. This book had an enormous impact on the psychiatric community of his day. His fame and reputation as a member of the medical faculty at the University of Vienna added weight to his pronouncements, even if they were not entirely correct. Yet there was a serious problem in the general tone and approach of this book. Krafft-Ebing believed that anyone who participated in the unusual sexual behaviors he described was a "degenerate" and could not likely be cured by the therapeutic methodologies of his day. Another very impor-

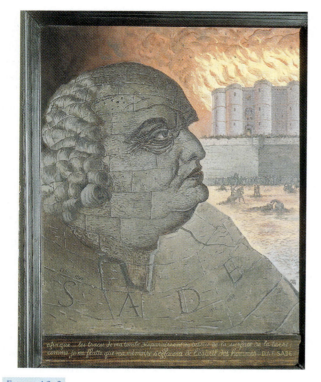

FIGURE 18-2   The Marquis de Sade (1740–1814) explored and wrote about the erotic aspects of administering pain and suffering, as well as restraint and humiliation.

tant figure in the early scientific study of sexual variation and deviation was Magnus Hirschfeld, also introduced in Chapter 2. He founded the Institute of Sexual Science in 1918 in Berlin, where his clinical work involved the study of homosexuality, exhibitionism, sadomasochistic behaviors, and fetishism. Hirschfeld invented the term "transvestism" to refer to what is often called "cross dressing."

Havelock Ellis' important book *Studies in the Psychology of Sex* was of profound significance for the modern approach to sexuality in general and sexual variations and deviations in particular. This book was first published in English in 1897. He was among the first to suggest that homosexuality and masturbation are not sexual perversions but rather variations of normal sexual inclinations and behaviors. Ellis sensitized the professional and lay elements of society to view and interpret sexual behaviors within the framework of the relative social norms of the particular culture, not in an absolute, rigid diagnostic framework. He encouraged serious students of human sexuality to appreciate the psychosocial and interpersonal context in which any sexual activity takes place; his approach was nonjudgmental, foresightful, and professional.

The work of Krafft-Ebing and Ellis had a powerful effect on the thinking of Sigmund Freud, who, in 1905 published one of his most important books: *Three Essays on the Theory of Sexuality.* Freud's psychosexual theory of development (discussed in Chapter 12) was first presented here, and for the first time psychiatrists began to speculate that sexual variations and deviations in adulthood might have their earliest roots in the

experiences of children and young adolescents. Freud argued that if early in life a baby's erogenous zones are incompletely and inconsistently stimulated, the child may grow up to symbolically make up for this early infantile deprivation. Similarly, the overindulgences of childhood may become manifest later in life. Freud believed that here could be found the roots of deviant sexual urges and actions in adulthood.

Another important figure in the brief history of the study of sexual variations and deviations is Alfred Kinsey. Largely through his exhaustive clinical interviews with thousands of people, the public became better informed about the enormous variety of sexual desires and behaviors found in apparently "normal" individuals. For example, Kinsey reported that a sizeable percentage of males with rural origins or residence patterns had had at least one sexual encounter with an animal, but this did not mean that these individuals continued to prefer animals to women or that they were forever "perverted" by this experience.

Contemporary thinking about sexual variations and deviations seems powerfully influenced by policy statements of important professional groups such as the American Psychiatric Association as well as state and federal laws intended to minimize or eliminate sexual victimization and exploitation. The *Diagnostic and Statistical Manual of Mental Disorders* (DSM-IV) includes descriptions and diagnostic criteria of a number of sexual deviations, collectively called paraphilias.

THE *DIAGNOSTIC AND STATISTICAL MANUAL OF MENTAL DISORDERS*

We described the *Diagnostic and Statistical Manual of Mental Disorders* in Chapter 14 in the context of sexual dysfunctions. It represents the final word regarding the criteria and symptoms used to diagnose mental disorders, and virtually all professionals in psychiatry use it consistently to make diagnoses based on a client's signs and symptoms. This book can be extremely helpful in making a distinction between normal sexual interest and behavior and what is abnormal and deviant. Although the DSM-IV is published by the American Psychiatric Association, it is used by sex therapists, clinical psychologists, nurses, mental health technicians, and licensed clinical social workers as well and even has a powerful bearing on legal deliberations concerning deviant sexual behavior.

Diagnostic Features of the Paraphilias

According to the DSM-IV, paraphilias involve "recurrent, intense sexually arousing fantasies, sexual urges, or behaviors generally involving 1) nonhuman objects, 2) the suffering or humiliation of oneself or one's partner, or 3) children or other nonconsenting persons, that occur over a period of at least 6 months" (*Diagnostic and Statistical Manual of Mental Disorders,* 4th edition, 1994, pp. 522–523). These fantasies, urges, and activities are necessarily accompanied by significant subjective inner turmoil and problems interacting with others socially at work or in other arenas of the person's life. These fantasies, urges, and activities might be necessary for the person to experience sexual excitement, while in other cases they may be expressed occasionally, such as during periods of significant personal stress.

In addition to these characteristics, the DSM-IV goes on to note that, "The behavior, sexual urges, or fantasies cause clinically significant distress or impairment in social, occupational, or other important areas of functioning" (*Diagnostic and Statistical Manual of Mental Disorders*, 4th edition, 1994, p. 523). Although all of us become somewhat preoccupied by sexual fantasies and feelings from time to time, these differ in their persistence and potential to cause mental distraction in those with paraphilias. As well, there is a difference between having a fetish and enjoying lingerie or other stimuli that enhance sexual excitement. For example, Chapter 15 describes how many women find using a vibrator very stimulating. In fact, many women do not consistently have orgasms unless they use a vibrator. This situation, however, does not indicate a sexual deviation because these women are rarely distressed about using vibrators—they are generally quite comfortable with them. In most instances, people with a paraphilia do not have a very diversified sex life but are rigidly dependent on a specific constellation of sexual cues and stimuli to feel any erotic excitement or responsiveness at all. This raises another question: Can someone with a paraphilia have "normal" sexual relations? Probably so, but such an experience would not likely be that individual's *preferred* avenue of sexual expression, and in all likelihood they would be fantasizing about the object of their sexual attraction during such sexual relations.

WHAT CAUSES PARAPHILIAS?

The cause of paraphilias is by no means simple, clear, or straightforward. No one really knows if paraphilias may be caused or contributed to by a single, unusual sexual experience. Like all complex human behaviors they are learned, sometimes over a long period of time and sometimes very subtly. Indeed, many factors seem to contribute to the development of the paraphilias. As discussed in a later section, there are a number of different theories about the etiology of the paraphilias.

Brockman and Bluglass (1996) described factors inside an individual and in the wider psychosocial environment that may play a role in the development of paraphilias. They believe that childhood experiences certainly have the potential to affect the way an individual begins to associate a number of social and physical cues with the pleasure derived from erogenous zone stimulation. Second, the individual's physical make-up may also play a role. Feelings of unattractiveness, congenital abnormalities, and atypical urogenital anatomy and physiology might all foster the belief that one is somehow not "acceptable" or "worthy" for normal sexual activities. Third, cognitive factors may certainly contribute to feel-

ings of being "different" and the expectation that one's sexual advances will be rejected. These thought patterns may originate in the interpersonal dynamics of a person's family of origin as well. Fourth, a person's moods and emotions may involve a predisposition to depression, anxiety, anger, or low stress tolerance. Some individuals are noted to engage in paraphilic behaviors only when they are feeling especially stressed, fatigued, or anxious. While these four factors deal mostly with "internal" issues, paraphilic behaviors do not take place in a psychosocial vacuum, and a number of environmental cues or triggers are usually necessary to activate these behavior patterns.

Researchers seldom try to say which factors are likely to lead to the appearance of a specific paraphilia (e.g., fetishism, exhibitionism, etc.). They can only make a number of suggestions about the variables that, working together with and influenced by the psychosocial environment, often lead to strange sexual urges and preferences.

MEASUREMENT PROBLEMS

Social, behavioral, and medical scientists believe it is essential to be able to measure the phenomena one is studying. Laws and O'Donohue (1997) emphasize that it is extremely difficult to measure the nature and manifestations of paraphilias because it is difficult to estimate the frequency of private behaviors and try to reconcile those data with other data from the law enforcement system or the mental health professions. But the scientific methods of the laboratory differ from the scientific methods of the clinic, and both approaches are usually valid and reliable in their respective contexts. Another measurement problem is an ethical one. People have a right to keep their intimate desires and activities to themselves, and it may not be easy to probe these highly sensitive areas of their lives. Just as people are not eager to discuss even apparently normal aspects of their sexuality, people are even less willing to report unusual behaviors.

At this writing, there are virtually no standardized, valid paper-and-pencil questionnaires that have been shown to be reliable in large, representative, randomly selected pools of subjects studied in terms of the prevalence of the paraphilias.

A newer way to get some feeling for how common sexual deviations are in our society involves analyzing how many "hits" various Internet websites get in a set period of time (Fig. 18-3). However, the fact that someone decides to go to one of these websites does *not* mean that they necessarily desire to participate in the types of sexual activity being depicted or even finds such depictions arousing. The same may be said about the apparent growth in the pornography industry. As First Amendment rights have been clarified over the last four decades, many publications have appeared that intend to appeal to individuals with highly unusual and sometimes frankly bizarre sexual behaviors. These types of information can tell us something about the general interest in certain paraphilias but cannot tell us about their prevalence in the population as a whole.

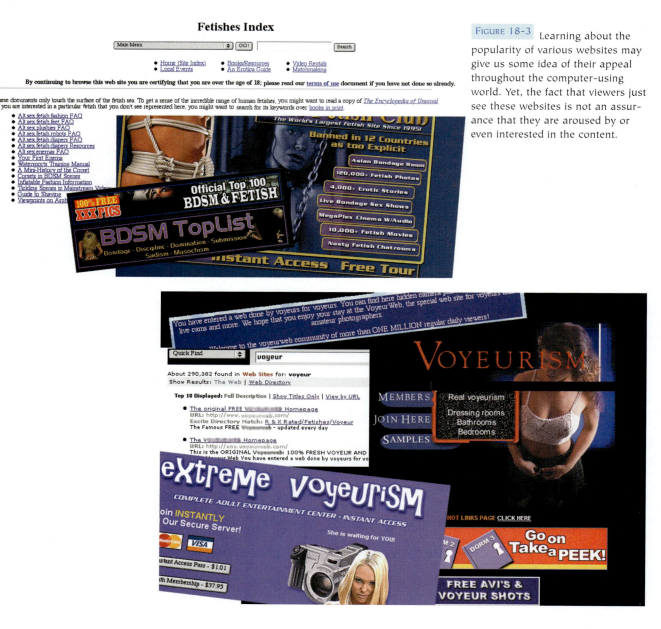

FIGURE 18-3 Learning about the popularity of various websites may give us some idea of their appeal throughout the computer-using world. Yet, the fact that viewers just see these websites is not an assurance that they are aroused by or even interested in the content.

A SOCIOLOGICAL PERSPECTIVE ON SEXUAL DEVIATION

Simon (1994) emphasized that sexuality has grown to have a larger place in most people's lives in the last generation. People can talk about it more easily and enjoy it more unselfconsciously. While not everyone has been influenced equally by this gradual but important social change, it is hard to escape its overt public representations or more covert psychic symbolism that have affected how we think, feel, and act sexually. In a word, our world is colored by symbols of eroticism.

In many contexts this book has emphasized that sexual expression is often divorced from the historically "appropriate" object of its focus; today, sex for recreation is as common as sex for procreation. As societies change over time, so too do their norms about what is acceptable and unacceptable sexual behavior, and, by implication, so too do their perspectives on sexual deviation. Just as masturbation and homosexuality were once considered sexual deviations and perversions, the contemporary social climate has softened that perspective on these behaviors. Similarly, sadomasochism is not viewed as harshly as it once was, mostly because the public generally enjoys a better understanding that it involves consenting adults in private, with no victimization.

PARAPHILIAS AND PERSONALITY DISORDERS

Personality disorders involve persistent, maladaptive ways of interacting with other people that generally result in relationship difficulties and personal unhappiness. People with personality disorders often lack insight into their own behaviors, making it even harder for them to understand why they keep having problems with other people at home, at work, and in other contexts. Recently, the question whether the paraphilias might in fact be a personality disorder has received insightful, serious attention (MacHovec, 1993). In fact, there are some compelling similarities between the paraphilias and personality disorders. Both have their origins in the individual's childhood or adolescence. Both may develop through an individual's interactions with adults with paraphilias or personality disorders. Unrealistic interpersonal expectations and distorted thinking are also common to both clinical categories. Therefore MacHovec builds a case for considering paraphilias a special type of personality disorder.

Like personality disorders, paraphilias very often have their roots in an individual's personal history of inappropriate sexual behavior, usually accompanied by the desire to keep unusual sexual behaviors secret. Paraphilias are clinical manifestations of deviant behaviors widely thought by mental health professionals to be unethical, illegal, highly ritualistic, and socially inappropriate. When these behavior patterns involve unwilling victims, the individual is usually called a sex offender (discussed more in the next chapter). Just as people with personality disorders do not see themselves realistically, individuals with paraphilias may have highly irrational, illogical beliefs about sexuality and what constitutes a meaningful, rewarding sexual relationship. Very often, those with paraphilias have poor impulse control and do not manage the expression of their emotions very well; this too is very common among people with personality disorders. Further, just as those with personality disorders are not very sensitive to the feelings of others, this too is especially true of many people with paraphilias.

People with personality disorders commonly have persistent problems with the basic socialization tasks involved in growing up: impulse control, frustration tolerance, the ability to delay immediate gratification, and the ability and inclination to live with a little uncertainty in one's future. These same problems are almost always seen in individuals with a paraphilia. Further, just as those with personality disorders have a poor self-concept, the same is usually true of those with paraphilias. In fact, their focus on impersonal avenues of sexual gratification reveals a very deep sense of personal inadequacy. Although the DSM-IV has no personality disorder called a "paraphilic personality disorder," MacHovec has encouraged us to think of paraphilias in a different way that might be helpful to social and behavioral scientists as well as clinicians.

THEORIES ABOUT THE ORIGINS OF SEXUAL VARIATIONS AND DEVIATIONS

Productive scientific investigations are generally stimulated by a broad theoretical perspective, a general way of looking at phenomena with which that science deals. The same is true with sexual variations and deviations. The following sections describe different theories about the why and how people develop different sexual tastes and preferences, some of which are deviant. Each theory is useful in its own way, and one should always try to keep an open mind about different explanatory approaches. Remember that theories guide not only research into the causes of variations and deviations but also treatment approaches. Just as no one theory seems best, no one therapeutic strategy is either.

Psychodynamic Approaches

The terms "psychodynamic" and "psychoanalytic" are generally used to refer to the theoretical and clinical contributions of Sigmund Freud. Freud and some of his contemporaries had much to say about the various reasons some people develop unusual sexual tastes, preferences, and behaviors. Chapter 12 introduced Freud's psychosexual theory of development and the basic assumptions underlying it. As infants develop and become young children, they go through a number of stages, each is characterized by a part of the body that when stimulated consistently yields "sexual" pleasure. Remember that Freud used the term "sexual" as the term "sensual" is used today. These body parts are called erogenous zones, and the primary erogenous zones are the mouth, anus, and genitalia. The secondary erogenous zones include parts of our bodies that through personal experiences gradually come to be associated with sexual arousal and response. Freud used the term "perversion" to refer to sexual inclinations that are very powerful but are not anxiety states called neuroses. A perversion according to Freud is a "raw," primitive sexual drive that does not conform to society's expectations of appropriate sexual behavior but that is not apparent as a disturbed mood state that includes anxiety. Perversions have a powerful, compulsive quality that cannot be disguised as other feelings (Travin & Protter, 1993).

In psychodynamic theory, the unresolved Oedipal complex (Fig. 18-4) and its associated castration anxiety are at the heart of the development of sexual deviations. Recall that the Oedipal complex involves a young boy's unconscious sexual feelings for his mother. He does not consciously realize that he is his father's rival for his mother's attention and affection or consciously think that if he were to act on these feelings his father would castrate him. Yet this deep, unconscious fear of castration lies behind the development of sexual deviations according to this approach. Adult sexual deviations, according to Freud, are symbolic attempts to deal with this terrible threat, and as a result men divert their sexual feelings away from women and sexual relations with them because they are a reminder of the castration threat. As explained in Chapter 12, one does not have to believe this speculative theorizing to recognize that these ideas have been of great importance in the development of psychiatric and psychological approaches to sexual variations and deviations. Because men unconsciously feel threatened by reminders of their castration anxiety, they transfer their sexual urges to inanimate or non-human objects, in the case of a fetish. Paraphilias having to do with non-human objects are better explained by another theoretical alternative, however, as we will see soon.

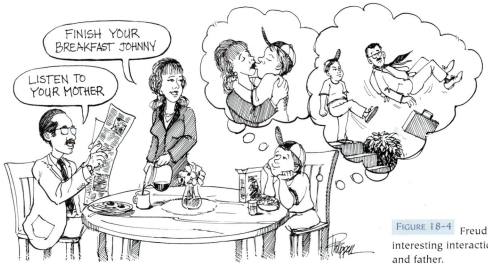

FIGURE 18-4 Freud's Oedipal Complex predicts some interesting interactions between a child and his mother and father.

Because, in Freud's theory, females do not have to negotiate an Oedipal complex and the castration anxiety that goes along with it, sexual deviations are by far less common among women. Other theoretical approaches do not always explain this difference.

Behavioral and Cognitive Perspectives

Another influential theoretical perspective on the development of sexual variations and deviations deals less with supposedly innate biological tendencies to pursue pleasure and more with simple learning and cognitive issues involving pleasure. We learn not only facts but also preferences and emotional habits, because our thoughts, feelings, and actions become associated

with pleasurable consequences. Learning does not only refer to apparent improvements in human behavior; people also learn unusual and sometimes harmful habits if they become connected to highly enjoyable reinforcing feelings. Behavioral theorists suggest that sexual variations and deviations develop as a person grows up because in subtle or obvious ways an erotic focus on objects becomes more pleasurable than an erotic focus on other people. A basic behavioral premise is that when stimuli and pleasurable responses are connected to each other close together in time, the foundations of learned responses have been laid down. This is called the principle of contiguity. When the consequences of a person's actions increase the probability that those actions will be repeated, this is called positive reinforcement. When feelings of unpleasure are stopped by a person's actions, this is called negative reinforcement. If sexual excitement comes to be associated with an article of woman's clothing because a young boy associates that clothing with his mother's warm, loving nurturance, this is an example of positive reinforcement. Similarly, if sexual excitement is associated with such an article of clothing because it is associated with the cessation of feelings of loneliness and isolation, this is an example of negative reinforcement. As these associations are repeated in the course of growing up, a fetish may develop. *Any* behavior consistently associated with either pleasure or the removal of unpleasant feelings has the potential to become a very enduring aspect of an individual's personality (Fig. 18-5).

These are the elementary principles of classical and operant conditioning. But of course, these kinds of associations take place in a diversified social environment too, and we should not minimize the role of imitation and vicarious experience in the early development of sexual variations and deviations. Behavioral and cognitive approaches assume a gradual etiology of variations and deviations because the necessary connections between stimuli and responses generally do not take place in an efficient, consistent way. These associations are often accidental at first and only later become habitual. Finally,

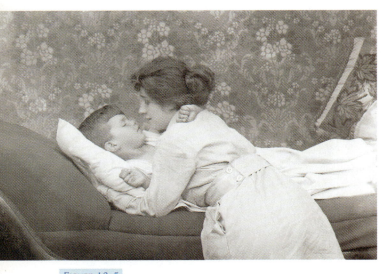

FIGURE 18-5 Lifelong memories of loving, nurtuant interactions with our mothers can, according to Freud, affect later feelings, thoughts, and actions with respect to love and affection for others.

not only do some unusual stimuli come to be associated with sexual fantasies and arousal, but even stimuli associated with the original stimuli. For example, someone with a shoe fetish might gradually begin to develop a fetish for nylon stockings if they are commonly worn with the type of shoe the individual finds exciting. This is called stimulus generalization.

Social Learning Perspectives

Is it possible for some social environments to subtly encourage viewing women (or men) as "sex objects" thereby minimizing the more human, interpersonal nature of intimate relationships? The phrase "sex object" implies that an individual is being "used" for sexual pleasure, independent of their qualities as a thinking, feeling person. This term has generally negative meanings. Implicit is exploitation along with a basic disregard for one's unique personhood and dignity. Some men are socialized to look at women in an exclusively sexual way, and some women too have gradually come to see men in this way.

When images, fantasies, and inanimate objects become the focus of erotic preoccupations, sexual variations and deviations occur. To the degree that commercialized depictions of sexual stimuli sometimes stimulate obsessive interests, the social environment may play a role in the causes of sexual variations and deviations. Additionally, some groups within a culture might discourage widely accepted social norms. For example, if adolescents and young adults are shown that impulse control, frustration tolerance, and delay of gratification are not important, it might be difficult for them to engage in fulfilling, intimate interpersonal sexual relationships involving real sharing and reciprocity. Gratuitous sexual exploitation in the media offers an example.

Biological Perspectives

For decades biological factors have become increasingly important in scientific explanations of psychological functioning and social behavior. For example, descriptions of the biological bases of learning, memory, and emotion have become prominent in the social and behavioral sciences. A number of biological hypotheses have been offered to describe why people develop paraphilias. These explanations usually focus on the way certain neurotransmitter molecules affect the functioning of nerve cells in specific brain areas. Neurotransmitters are chemicals that carry messages from one nerve cell to another by allowing nerve impulses to "jump" across synapses, the tiny gap found between nerve cells. It is too simplistic to say that each specific part of the brain does one thing and one thing only, and therefore there is no single place in the brain for "memory" or "learning." Similarly, there is no single place in the brain where paraphilic behaviors are generated. The brain works on the basis of billions of interconnections among nerve cells. Some of these "circuits" are primarily involved in sexual behaviors. Because certain drugs diminish the frequency of deviant sexual thoughts, feelings, fantasies, and behaviors, and because it is known that these drugs affect how neurotransmitters work, intriguing hypotheses have been developed about the neurological foundations of paraphilic behavior.

In recent years, tantalizing data from the behavioral neurosciences have supported the study of the biological foundations of sexual deviations. These findings bring together what is known about neurotransmitters and sexual behavior, the effects of drugs on sexual appetite, the action of specific neurotransmitters that seem implicated in compulsive sexual behaviors, and the effects of drugs that alter the activity of these neurotransmitters (Kafka, 1997a). This evidence involves both human and animal experiments, of course, and it is still too early to reach definite conclusions.

Neuroscientists have known for more than ten years that a group of chemicals in the brain called monoamines are intimately involved in male sex drive and sexual behavior in laboratory animals. Monoamines include norepinephrine, dopamine, and serotonin. These agents seem to be related to a variety of mood states in humans. Further, studies done on humans show that a variety of prescription drugs can have powerful effects on human sexual behavior, including the desire to engage in sexual activity. Drugs with this effect include some of the antidepressants, stimulants, and drugs used to minimize anxiety. Interestingly, these drugs often act by changing the way monoamines function as neurotransmitters. These drugs do not have this effect on all people all of the time, however. Additional data from human studies reveal that monoamines have an effect on a variety of behaviors associated with impulsive behavior, depression, anxiety, and compulsive behaviors, as well as a variety of "antisocial" behaviors, all of which are frequently involved in the paraphilias. But again, a direct cause-and-effect relationship has not emerged. Perhaps the most important observation is the fact that those drugs that are effective in increasing monoamine activity in certain brain synapses are effective in the treatment of the sexual arousal that accompanies paraphilic behaviors. Sometimes, correcting a biochemical problem in the brain can be effective in the treatment of behavioral and mood disorders.

PARAPHILIAS AND "MENTAL DISORDERS"

Sexual deviations have a compulsive quality: the individual's thoughts, feelings, and fantasies are highly distracting and frequent. These individuals frequently think about their next opportunity to engage in their preferred, unusual sexual practice. Paraphilias do not emerge quickly but result from a long developmental process. As well, paraphilias are difficult to create experimentally in the laboratory, even for brief periods of time. These behaviors vary in both degree and kind, an important characteristic. The following examples illustrate this distinction; they are discussed at greater length later.

One of the more common paraphilias is voyeurism, which involves sexual excitement and gratification while watching a naked person who doesn't know they are being observed. Voyeurs also watch unsuspecting individuals in the act of getting undressed or having sexual intercourse. Women and men who go to clubs with nude dancing are not voyeurs, since the people taking their clothes off certainly know they are being observed (Fig. 18-6). Similarly, women and men who work in these establishments are not exhibitionists simply because they are taking their clothing off and perhaps exposing their genitals to strangers. These dancers generally do not substitute their professional activities for genuine sexual intimacy in their private lives. Most say that "It's just a job."

Similarly, one who enjoys purchasing, wearing, or removing lingerie or sexy underwear does not necessarily have a fetish and is not substituting these clothing-related behaviors for interpersonal sexual activities. For most individuals, these garments are the "frosting on the cake;" they are not the cake itself. If one feels sexually attracted to a younger man or woman, this does not indicate pedophilia, a paraphilia that involves sexual attraction to children; it only means that one finds younger adults sexually interesting. These examples are all matters of degree with respect to sexual stimuli that would not be termed deviant because they do not meet the criteria of deviancy noted earlier. The best description of "true" paraphilias is the *Diagnostic and Statistical Manual of Mental Disorders,* as discussed earlier.

SEXUAL VARIATIONS AND DEVIATIONS

As societies gradually become more liberal and tolerant of a variety of types of sexual expression, behaviors that were once thought unusual are today thought of as less unusual or deviant. Historical context is therefore important in our understanding of many sexual behaviors. For example, transsexuality, discussed in depth in Chapter 3, was once viewed as deviant, but social, behavioral, and medical scientists generally no longer feel that way about it. In a similar vein, "sexual oralism" was once considered an unusual avenue of sexual expression. Today, of course, oral sex is a common aspect of sexual intimacy among most heterosexuals and homosexuals. Similarly, "sexual analism" was once thought of as a deviant, even

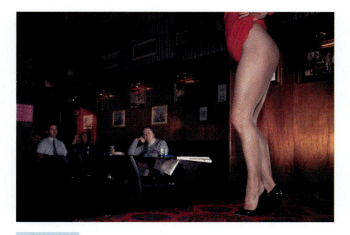

Figure 18-6 Customers of strip-clubs are not voyeurs, nor are those who work there exhibitionists. Observations are not made clandestinely and disrobing takes place in an obviously public environment.

perverted sexual act. Today, of course, anal intercourse is a common avenue of sexual experimentation among heterosexuals and a common aspect of physical intimacy among gay men. Of course, homosexuality itself was once viewed as a mental disorder and was not deleted from the DSM until the early 1970s when the American Psychiatric Association voted to remove it from its catalogue of mental disorders. Although some still may not personally find homosexuality acceptable, most behavioral, social, and medical professionals no longer think of it as aberrant or deviant and certainly not as a paraphilia.

The psychosocial environment often plays a determining role in public conceptualizations of sexual variance and deviance. Interestingly, the sanction or support of professionals usually follows wider public acceptance of sexual tastes and behaviors rather than playing a legitimizing role.

Exhibitionism

Exhibitionism, or "flashing" as it is sometimes called, involves a person (almost always a heterosexual man) exposing his genitals to someone who is unsuspecting and unwilling. These episodes occur in many contexts. For example, a man driving a car pulls over and asks someone for directions while his penis is sticking out of his fly. Or someone opens their raincoat and exposes their penis just as the door of an elevator opens. Exhibitionists generally want to shock, surprise, or provoke embarrassment in their victims, and exposing one's genitals to others clearly victimizes them. Because the desire to engage in these behaviors becomes so compelling and distracting, exhibitionists are usually very preoccupied with their fantasies and urges to expose themselves. Although exhibitionists want to be seen, they do not want to get caught. According to Abel and Rouleau (1990), about half the exhibitionists they interviewed in a sample of over 140 individuals reported that they began exposing themselves to others before they turned 18. Generally, men over the age of 40 are less likely to be exhibitionists than younger men.

Usually the targets of exhibitionists are children and women, but it is not clearly understood whether exposing one's genitals to children is a type of pedophilia or true exhibitionism (Murphy in Laws & O'Donohue, 1997). More than half the exhibitionists who have been studied were married, but little is known about the prevalence of this paraphilia in the general population. Murphy (1997) emphasizes that frequently a variety of psychological disorders are associated with exhibitionism, but none specifically and consistently. Similarly, it is not known if there is a relationship between exhibitionism and other criminal activities; one should not assume, however, that these men, with exception of their paraphilia, are in all other ways "normal." It is not yet possible to point to any specific developmental or family factors isolated as consistent causes of exhibitionistic behavior in adolescence or later. In fact, as of this writing there are too few consistent data to create a profile of exhibitionists. The scientific literature does not support the notion that they are shy, introverted people (Murphy, 1997).

According to Hollender (1997), what we have been describing so far is generally referred to as compulsive exhibi-

CASE STUDY: AN EXHIBITIONIST

*W*hen first seen, the patient was 36 years old, married, the father of six girls. He had recently been fired from his factory job because of his [exhibitionistic] behavior. His exhibitionism began, as he recalled it, when he was 11 or 12 years old when he exposed himself to his teacher, a 30-year-old woman. Shortly thereafter, he had begun exposing himself quite frequently in his own home to his sister's girl friend. This pattern went on for about a year, but during this time he also began exhibiting to a 32-year-old married woman across the street through his window. He exhibited to this woman over a period of about 2 years.

He estimates that he subsequently exposed himself on average of 4 or 5 times a month over the next 22–23 years. The general pattern was constant. No preference was noted regarding the places he chose for exhibiting—beaches, pools, streets, trains, cars, work, home neighborhood. With regard to choice of object, he admitted a preference for "young, pretty girls." He typically exposed in an erect state until he caught the girl's attention, at which time he would fondle and manipulate himself. Never did he manipulate to the point of orgasm while being observed, and rarely, if ever, afterward. On numerous occasions there were sequential repetitive acts of exhibition to the same woman over a period of a half a day. Often he exhibited when depressed "to get me out of the depression."

Despite all this activity, he was "turned in" very infrequently—only three times. Once he was detained overnight and fined. He claims that he rarely, if ever, thought about the consequences, but simply did it because "the pressure built up." Afterwards, he would "feel bad" but not before.

—Reitz & Keil, 1991

tionism, and these actions must be distinguished from other situations in which women and men display their genitals in public places. For example, secondary exhibitionism may occur because an individual is suffering from a psychiatric or neurological disorder, in which their exhibitionism is just another symptom of behavior that does not conform to the expectations of society. Hollender notes a phenomenon called socially sanctioned exhibitionism in which nudity is at least implicitly approved, such as nude sun bathing or the phenomenon known as "streaking," which was quite popular on college campuses in the United States in the 1970s. Nude dancers engage in socially sanctioned exhibitionism when their behavior does not violate local statues regarding standards of public decency. Hollender also notes a variety of exhibitionism called attention seeking, involving displays of nudity usually by women, but this lacks the compulsive quality of true exhibitionism. In other words, the same behavior can have a variety of different motives, which must be understood in order to classify the behavior.

The type of exhibitionism most likely to cause public distress is what Hollender calls compulsive exhibitionism, which is generally referred to as indecent exposure (Fig. 18-7). A comprehensive review of indecent exposure by Gayford in 1981 was based on data collected in England, and the data likely apply to other Western, industrialized countries. These

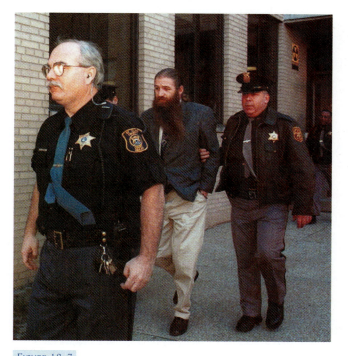

FIGURE 18-7   Gerald Ackerman, former major of Port Huron, Michigan, is led to jail in 1999 after being found guilty of nine counts of indecent exposure involving minors. Mr. Ackerman was sentenced to 1 year in jail.

Research Highlight

THE WORKING ENVIRONMENT OF FEMALE TOPLESS DANCERS

Craig J. Forsyth and Tina H. Deshotels published an in-depth study of the working conditions of female topless dancers. This investigation reveals some very interesting things about women who work in these establishments, their working environments, and their audiences. This environment has some plainly manipulative, often illegal, and unappealing characteristics. It has been estimated that there are nearly 70,000 women in this occupation in the United States. Nude dancing involves much more than just disrobing to music; it may involve highly suggestive body movements, varying degrees of nudity, and allowing patrons to place money on the dancer's body in some way.

Forsyth and Deshotels observed women dancing and also collected data by interviewing them in dance clubs. Their sample included 57 women in a number of American cities: Houston, Texas; New Orleans, Morgan City, and Lafayette, Louisiana; and Newport News, Virginia. Interviews took anywhere from 15 minutes to 4 hours. In addition to interviewing the dancers themselves, Forsyth and Deshotels also interviewed managers, bartenders, and waitresses who worked in these clubs.

Of course, all clubs are not alike, and one of the things that Forsyth and Deshotels found was that most of the women they interviewed expressed the desire to work in a "gentleman's club," the most prestigious type of establishment in which nude dancing takes place. These clubs are often tastefully furnished and often include gyms, tanning facilities, and hair stylists; in separate, darker parts of the club the patrons can enjoy nude dancing and alcoholic beverages. Dancers are separated from patrons by a 3-foot area in which there are no tables. They are expected to dance in a specific sequence, dancing to 1 to 3 songs before another dancer takes over. A customer in a gentleman's club can request a private dance, which usually takes place on a table or in a segregated room with a small stage. The managers of these gentlemen's clubs claimed that there is a rule prohibiting customers from touching dancers and that it is strictly enforced. Yet the dancers themselves reported that this rule is generally ignored. The dancers in gentleman's clubs must follow two rules: they cannot refuse their turn to dance and they cannot refuse a request for a private dance.

In virtually all cases, there is no training to become a nude dancer. Women are usually hired who are attractive and have some dancing ability. A dancer's income generally depends on how many alcoholic beverages she can encourage her customers to buy, and she may receive a flat fee per drink. While many dancers do not interact physically with their customers, others do. Depending on how much money changes hands, customers often fondle the dancers' buttocks and breasts. One of the dancers reported that she sometimes masturbated a customer with her hand or leg and that on at least one occasion she saw another dancer performing fellatio on a client (p. 136).

Finally, Forsyth and Deshotels found that in one way or another, virtually all of the women they interviewed took measures to enhance their attractiveness. Many used body make-up and skin creams, and some used tape to make their nipples erect. Some had plastic surgery to augment the size of their breasts or enhance the shape of their buttocks.

Clearly there is a difference between exhibitionism as a paraphilia and nude dancing, which is an example of what is called pseudoexhibitionism.

data reveal that only somewhat more exhibitionists are married than single and that exhibitionistic behaviors are more likely to occur during daylight hours and on weekdays. Most genital displays last only a few seconds and involve a penis that is not erect, but when the exhibitionist has an erection he is more likely to engage in public masturbatory behaviors. Most genital displays take place outdoors and in warmer weather. The public generally perceives male exhibitionism as a highly aggressive act, while the few instances of female exhibitionism reported in the literature are generally seen as a seductive act.

Gayford emphasizes that most victims of exhibitionists are women or children and that some exhibitionists selectively seek out a particular kind of victim, such as young girls entering puberty, apparently because of their ambivalent responses of curiosity, surprise, and distress.

Fetishism

In **fetishism**, a person has an erotic focus on some nonliving object and enjoys sexual gratification through contact with this item. In a true fetish, this object is the sole, compelling focus of sexual interest and is preferred to sexual intercourse or other interpersonal intimate sharing. Being sexually aroused by a partner dressed in provocative undergarments is not, however, fetishism. As of this writing, the prevalence of fetishism in the general population is not known. The fetishist is obsessed with thoughts, fantasies, and urges about the object of their fetish, is distressed by this preoccupation, and likely experiences problems in a variety of areas of social and interpersonal functioning. Although fetishism is far more common among men than women, the specific reasons for this discrepancy are not clear (Mason in Laws & O'Donohue, 1997). The objects of a fetish are highly diverse and may include various items of clothing, shoes, soft fabrics, leather, and rubber (Fig. 18-8) (Chalkley & Powell, 1983). A fetishist may use these objects during masturbatory rituals or may fondle, suck, steal, burn, slash, or gaze at them (Mason, 1997). While the *DSM-IV* emphasizes visual involvement with the object of a fetish, its tactile or olfactory qualities may be similarly compelling stimuli.

Because a fetish can develop through the repeated association of an object with sexual arousal, fetishes occur also in animals. Pavlov explained more than a century ago that the contiguous pairing of stimuli leads to a situation in which responses to one come to elicit the responses to the other. Epstein (1969) reported an interesting instance of this in a chimpanzee who had lived in captivity for over 17 years. This animal apparently developed a fetish for a rubber boot in its cage. It would approach the boot, stare at it, and touch it. While the animal was doing this, it would become erect and then touch the boot to his penis. Eventually, it engaged in masturbatory movements and then ejaculated. Epstein hypothesized that the shiny boot may have had some similarity to a female chimpanzee's genital display, but if the male had never seen a sexually receptive female, the origins of the fetish would be more obscure; this author believes that fetishes may arise through the contiguity of pleasurable feelings associated with particular stimuli. There may be an innate tendency among higher primates (including both chimpanzees and humans) to learn such stimulus-response connections.

Psychoanalysts have different theories about the etiology of fetishes. Greenacre (1996) suggested that during the child's progression through Freud's psychosexual stages of development (discussed in Chapter 12), he sooner or later recognizes that his mother does not have a penis. This awareness, Freud believed, further fuels the young boy's fears of castration that accompany his progression through the phallic stage. According to this theoretical perspective, the young boy then uncon-sciously focuses his sexual interests (libido) on a part of his mother's clothing associated with his troubling observation. He then comes to associate this inanimate object (clothing, shoes, undergarments, etc.) with his mother's genitalia.

The fact that most paraphilias are seen primarily in men has provoked much scholarly thinking. Gamman and Makinen (1994) explored sexual fetishes in women and found that while rare, women with fetishes may indeed make up a sizeable minority of fetishists. Because only little boys are traumatized by seeing female genitals, Freud believed that girls would not develop the substitute objects of erotic interest that boys do. Gamman and Makinen report that examples of female fetishism are found in about one-third of the psychoanalytic literature they reviewed. They note that Havelock Ellis reported female fetishists, though primarily among lesbians. Gamman and Makinen's review revealed some rather interesting female fetishes, such as a kleptomaniac who after stealing something would caress her genitals with a piece of silk and other women who had compulsive erotic interests in dolls, raincoats, string, books, and rubber. These investigators noted something interesting about female fetishes: while men often fantasize about a woman while masturbating or fondling the object of their fetish, women apparently focus solely on the object itself.

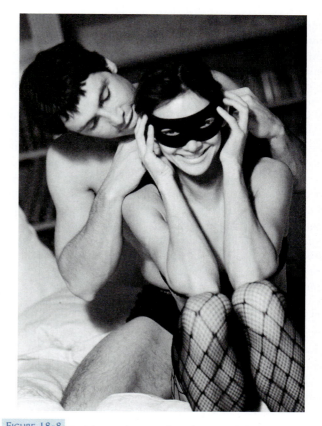

FIGURE 18-8 Fetishism often involves the use of clothing, shoes, soft fabrics, leather, or rubber in both solitary and shared sexual intimacy. The visual, olfactory, and tactile properties of these objects may all be arousing to the fetishist.

Recent research (Freund, Seto, & Kuban, 1996) has distinguished between two types of fetishism. Transvestic fetishism involves what in the past was called "cross dressing," a heterosexual male experiencing sexually arousing fantasies and urges associated with dressing as a woman. The *DSM-IV* lists transvestic fetishism as a separate paraphilia. But are transvestites fetishists when it comes to their clothing, or is the *experience of cross dressing* basic to this paraphilia? Freund, Seto, and Kuban addressed this question. They interviewed 30 fetishists and 78 transvestites and asked a variety of questions about their paraphilic behaviors, childhood development, characteristics of their parents, and feelings of emotional affiliation with their parents. They used an electrical recording device to measure any signs of an erection when presented with photographs of female and male genitalia and other objects that might be stimulating to fetishists. These included nylon stockings, male and female shoes, male and female undergarments, and male and female feet. These two groups did not differ with respect to their childhood development or family relationships, nor were there any differences regarding their response to the photographs they observed. The implications of these data for future revisions of the *DSM* remain to be seen, but these data may be of some help to clinicians when they are diagnosing and treating these paraphilias.

Transvestic Fetishism

As noted above, transvestic fetishism or **transvestism** involves compelling sexual fantasies and urges among heterosexual men that take the form of dressing in women's clothing. Because this is classified as a paraphilia in the *DSM-IV*, these thoughts and behaviors are disturbing to the individual and have the potential to cause problems in interpersonal relationships at home and work. Transvestites buy and keep a variety of women's clothes, and when they are "dressed up" they generally masturbate. However, the nature of their fantasies while masturbating is quite interesting. They imagine themselves as *both* a man having sex with a woman *and* as that woman. We know of no reports in the literature describing transvestic fetishism in women. The manifestations of transvestism vary significantly in their degree and nature. More so than the other paraphilias discussed so far, transvestites may immerse themselves in a subculture that reinforces these fantasies and behaviors. Some of these men choose to dress as women as frequently as possible, wearing make-up, and in some cases having surgery to give their bodies a more feminine form. These individuals especially enjoy being in public and find it exciting to know that they are fooling other men into thinking that they are women (Fig. 18-9). Others, on the other hand, only sometimes dress as women and only when alone. While some transvestites enjoy wearing a complete outfit of female outer and undergarments, others may wear just a pair of women's panties under his male clothing. A transvestite may incorporate cross-dressing into his lifestyle on a regular basis, but some men engage in these behaviors only at times of serious personal stress or anxiety. Transvestites usually identify themselves as primarily heterosexual.

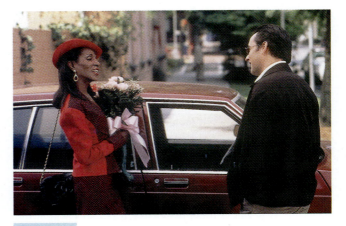

FIGURE 18-9   Cross-dresser Lady Chablis (left) is shown here with John Cusack in *Midnight in the Garden of Good and Evil*.

There is nothing unusual about transvestites when they are "out of uniform," and the *DSM-IV* notes that these men have not had many sexual partners and may have experimented with homosexual behaviors. Although it can be quite shocking to find out that someone you know is a transvestite, this paraphilia does not involve the degree of victimization that others do, if any at all.

A transvestite known to one of us became aware of his interest in cross-dressing while participating in theatrical productions in college. Later, his job often took him to other cities, where he would check in at a motel at which the Rotary Club or Lions Club held their breakfast meetings. The next morning he would dress as a woman and go to the lobby where he would initiate a discussion with one or two club members, telling them that "her" dear departed husband was a member of the Rotary or Lions club and that the fellowship of the organization had meant a very great deal to him. Invariably "she" would be invited to join the members for breakfast, taking an immense delight in knowing that she had successfully deceived the entire room full of men. This particular individual did not report engaging in any masturbatory behaviors while dressed as a female but seemed to derive a keen erotic excitement from the deception itself.

There is an important distinction we wish to emphasize among men who are transvestites, men who are transsexuals, and those who are "transgendered." The discussion of these issues in Chapter 3 introduced these categories, although the specific causes of each remain obscure. Much of the variability seen among transvestites can perhaps be explained through a better understanding of these three terms. According to Brown, Wise, Costa, Herbst, Fagan, and Schmidt (1996), it is difficult to describe typical cross-dressing men because so much of what we know about them comes from subjects who are in significant emotional distress and have received treatment in psychiatric clinics. Only recently has a fuller understanding developed of cross-dressers who are not patients in these facilities. These researchers studied and characterized a sample of 83 transvestites, 44 transsexuals, and 61 transgenderists. The transvestites in this sample never desired a sex change operation, never used female hormones, and had never seriously desired to become a woman. In contrast, the transsexuals reported that they indeed had thought almost daily of changing their sex and becoming a woman, had used female hormones at some time in the past in an effort to change their bodies, and clearly wanted a sex change operation. Finally, the transgenderists engaged in cross-dressing very often, some even daily, and were more likely to think of themselves as having a feminine identity than were transvestites. Clearly, diagnosing and treating transvestism is not a simple, straightforward matter, and the overt act of cross-dressing may be motivated differently in different types of individuals.

Another survey (Docter & Prince, 1997) reported the results of anonymous surveys collected from 1032 cross-dressers, and these data were compared with a similar investigation carried out in 1972 (Prince & Butler) in which similar data were

CASE STUDY: TRANSVESTIC FETISHISM

*M*r. M., 22, is a college senior who complained of a transvestite fantasy that dominated his sex life . . . Early recollections date back to a pre-school memory of fighting with his sister, while taking a bath with her, about who should wear a plastic raincoat in the tub. In kindergarten he remembers being especially attracted to a little girl friend who wore a plastic raincoat. In elementary school he loved to wear a raincoat, especially of the plastic kind, but because he was afraid his friends might call him a sissy, he often desisted [stopped]. By the time he entered junior high school, M.'s affinity for raincoats had extended to girls' boots. In the eighth grade he bought a pair of girls' boots and walked outdoors in deep snow, which hid the boots. To the question: "How do you feel when you put on these boots," he answered: "Nothing special, I just liked the idea of wearing the raincoat and the boots."

One day, at age 14, while rummaging in the basement, he discovered a woman's dress. He slipped it on and inspected himself in a large mirror. After disrobing, he masturbated. The sexual arousal during the early years of his problem was elicited by wearing women's garments. For example, he would put on boots or a raincoat and then proceed to masturbate. For the last 5 years, however, imagining himself in any kind of women's apparel has been a sufficiently exciting stimulus to be followed by masturbation. He enjoyed the act for itself, without associating with it any other thought, feeling, or imagery.

M. made several trips to the basement in his early high school years for the purpose of dressing in women's clothes. One day, after draping himself in an old dress, raincoat and boots, he heard his sister's footsteps on the cellar stairs. He quickly hid, terribly frightened. After she left, he masturbated and removed the clothes. During the next year he had several experiences involving wearing a maid's uniform and his mother's underwear, boots, raincoat and scarf. He would venture outdoors only in the dark, not willing to risk recognition.

Starting with his sophomore year in high school, he dated girls from 1 to 3 times weekly. There was no petting, but after each date, he masturbated. As a junior in high school, he stopped dressing in girl's clothing. The fantasy of imagining himself in girls' attire was sufficient to elicit masturbation. A few years later in college, he participated heavily in sports, and masturbation decreased to approximately twice weekly.

The previous summer he had met a girl, Jessica, at a seashore resort whom he liked very much and with whom he had his first sexual intercourse. This had evoked in him depressed feelings about his sexual potentiality. The intercourse was disappointing: he described it as "Scary—it was just like masturbating." Before and during the sex act, he could not get rid of the image of himself in girl's clothing "It's as if my girl isn't there. The fantasy takes over and sticks with me." This generated the thought that he was perverted. Subsequent sex experiences with Jessica always has the same sequel.

—Gershman, 1991

collected from 504 respondents. The same survey and similar samples were used in both studies. These data tell us something about the lifestyles of transvestites today and also reveal ways in which the self-reports of this group of individuals have changed over the last twenty years (data collection for the latter study was completed in 1992). Some very interesting findings emerged. In 1972, 87% of the subjects identified themselves as heterosexuals compared with 89% in 1992. In the more recent study, 60% of subjects were married at the time of the survey compared with 64% in the early study. Fewer men in the recent research had fathered children compared with the older work (69% and 74% respectively), but the authors point out that this may be due to the increased availability and effectiveness of contraceptives. A sizeable percentage of respondents in both investigations were raised in two-parent homes (76% in 1992 and 82% in 1972), and a large proportion of subjects in both studies reported that their fathers had provided them with a "good masculine image" (76% in 1992 and 72% in 1972). However, in the more recent study a much greater percentage of subjects reported that they had sought counseling for problems related to their transvestism (45%) compared with the earlier study (24%). Those receiving counseling more recently were more likely to report that they had been helped (67%) than in the older sample of subjects (47%). Additionally, subjects in the more recent study reported that they enjoyed their masculine and feminine selves about equally. Empirical findings like these are an important reminder that the psychosocial context in which the transvestite lives may change over time, and it would be unwise to discount this influence in the way we think about these individuals.

Most of the research on transvestites shows that they are primarily heterosexual. Recent research (Bullough &

Bullough, 1997) assessed questionnaire responses submitted by over 370 volunteers, and found that only 2% identified themselves as primarily homosexual, about 10% said that they were primarily bisexual, and almost 20% revealed that sexual activities were no longer a part of their lives. However, Bullough and Bullough emphasize that in addition to one's self-identified sexual orientation, a person's sexual fantasies may also be very important when it comes to determining a person's primary sexual orientation. These researchers asked their subjects about the fantasies they had while they were dressed as women. Their data revealed that about 30% of the bisexual and homosexual respondents reported that they focused on a fantasy man while they were dressed as a woman. Bullough and Bullough note that the clinical description of transvestism in the *DSM-IV* notes that these individuals are heterosexual, but their data suggest that this may not always be the case and that perhaps in the future this description should be reexamined.

Because of the social stigma frequently associated with the paraphilias, many people with sexual deviations go to extraordinary lengths to conceal their circumstances. Travin and Protter (1993) summarized an interesting case study involving a 30-year-old, single lawyer. The young man in this case had consulted a psychotherapist because of anxiety he was experiencing with respect to his upcoming marriage to an achievement-oriented woman who was also an attorney. He was especially troubled by the prospect of making a bad decision and finding himself with a domineering, demanding woman like his mother and seeing himself subjugated by her authoritarian ways just as he had seen this happen to his father. As the wedding date approached, his apprehension became much worse. After he had been receiving therapy for 4 months, the client,

Other Countries, Cultures, and Customs

TRANSVESTISM IN OTHER COUNTRIES

Very few investigators have studied paraphilias in other countries and published their work in the United States. However, Whitham and Mathy (1986) wrote about transvestism in other countries as a part of their broader interest in male homosexuality in Brazil, Guatemala, the Philippines, and the United States. These writers have found that cross dressers in Thailand, Peru, Guatemala, Brazil, and the Philippines are frequently self-identified homosexuals, a somewhat different situation than what has been described in the United States. In summarizing this research, Bullough and Bullough (1997) noted that many of these individuals actually think of themselves as transsexuals who have not yet had surgery. Additionally, the transvestites in these countries are frequently engaged in occupations that are typically chosen by homosexuals in those societies. These include hair styling, prostitution, and a variety of entertainment jobs such as dancing and acting (Bullough & Bullough, 1997, p. 10). The research of Whitam and Mathy shows that outside of North America and Western Europe, transvestites are active members of their gay communities and are frequently primarily homosexual. These data should discourage us from making generalizations about the sexual orientation of transvestites without taking account of the cultures in which they live.

whom Travin and Protter call Mr. E, suddenly announced that he had not been fully disclosing his most troubling concerns. At this point he began to talk in great detail about compelling sexual preoccupations and behaviors with which he had been dealing for a number of years. He told his therapist that recently he had been experiencing powerful compulsions to masturbate while holding women's panties or stockings and that he had then begun to masturbate while holding and then wearing his fiancee's panties. On two occasions he wore her panties and masturbated. For a number of years he had been having similar preoccupations, but the stress of his upcoming marriage was definitely making things a lot worse.

Mr. E's therapist believed that these fantasies, urges, and behaviors all stemmed from a fear of dependency on his new bride-to-be and the diminished masculinity he witnessed in his father under similar circumstances. In the course of therapy Mr. E disclosed that as an adolescent he would masturbate while wearing his [dominant] mother's panties and stockings. These activities continued throughout his adolescence, but by the time he got to college his erotic tastes and interests became more conventionally heterosexual. By helping Mr. E to understand the similarity between his upcoming marriage and the household he had grown up in and by helping him to recognize or monitor the triggering stimuli that led to his transvestic fetishism, his sexual adjustment was eventually improved, helping him make a good adjustment to his marriage (Travin & Protter, 1993, pp. 182-184).

Above we noted that transvestic fetishism rarely if ever is seen among women. Interestingly, historical evidence recently revealed that there may indeed have been a tradition of female cross-dressing in early modern Western Europe. *The Tradition of Female Transvestism in Early Modern Europe,* by Rudolf Dekker and Lotte van de Pol (1989) gives us a fascinating glimpse into female cross-dressing in the Netherlands between 1550 and 1839. Their treatment deals with cross-dressing *per se,* more so than the compulsive erotic preoccupations associated with transvestism in men. These writers carried out a careful analysis of almost 200 women who dressed as men for various reasons and for varying amounts of time. While some were revealed as women within days, others presumably were not discovered until their deaths. Interestingly, much of the motivation for female cross-dressing in Europe at that time involved the economic inequalities between women and men. Being unable to participate fully in commerce, education, or military service, women had few if any opportunities for personal advancement and quality of life within conventional society.

Voyeurism

As noted earlier, **voyeurism** involves looking at another person who is getting undressed, naked, or having sexual relations without their knowledge or consent. For voyeurs, looking is more exciting than doing. Voyeurs do not generally want any sexual contact with the people they observe, although they often masturbate while watching them or later when alone. Voyeurs are frequently called "peeping Toms" (although we will more carefully discriminate between the two shortly), and

while these individuals may fantasize about having sexual relations with those they watch, in fact this is rarely if ever even attempted, much less consummated. As with other paraphilias, voyeurs are very much preoccupied and distracted by their desire to observe others and are often distressed by the disturbing and persistent nature of these thoughts. Their interpersonal relationships or even job performance may suffer. Voyeurs engage in these behaviors as a substitute for interpersonal sexual relations, not because observing stimulates them and makes them more inclined to initiate interpersonal sexual relations. Often people who watch female or male nude dancers become sexually stimulated by the experience, but this is not the same as voyeurism. Part of the arousal of voyeurism lies in the fact that the people who are being watched don't know it and wouldn't consent to it if they did.

For some voyeurs, observing (frequently followed by masturbation) is their only form of sexual behavior, while for others these activities are used to enhance sexual arousal for heterosexual intercourse. For some the desire to observe becomes strongest during periods of stress, tension, and anxiety. Voyeurism becomes a true paraphilia when an individual engages in observing over a prolonged period of time, usually more than 6 months. In most cases, voyeurs begin engaging in these behaviors before they are 15 years old (Abel & Rouleau, 1990). It is difficult if not impossible to estimate the prevalence of voyeurism in the general population. Those known about come to the attention of law enforcement officials because they have been caught looking into someone's home, but there is no way to estimate what percentage of voyeurs are apprehended (Fig. 18-10). Like most of the paraphilias, voyeurism is thought to be extremely rare among women.

Voyeurism represents a fundamental violation of cultural norms that preserve privacy, and Bryant (1982) believes that an interest in seeing others naked may be a basic aspect of our culture as well as many others. In Bali, women often wear no clothing above their waists, and to some extent this has reduced but not eliminated investing breasts with sexual meaning. Yet even in this society, if one were to walk past a stream in which nude women were bathing, it would be considered bad manners to stare at them, and therefore men turn their eyes away as a reflection of their respect for the women's privacy (Bryant, 1982, p. 72). Even in societies in which some public nudity is acceptable there are certain subtle prohibitions against observing entirely nude women.

Appeals to voyeuristic interests has become something of an industry. Bryant refers to this as "commercialized voyeurism" (p. 91). He notes that some houses of prostitution have arranged for some customers to secretively observe other customers engaging in sexual activities with the women who work there, using peep-holes and two-way mirrors. These voyeuristic activities take away much of the risk of getting caught by the law and still allow for the observation of non-consenting adults in the act of having intercourse or engaging in other sexual activities. While the popularity of X-rated videos has led to the closing of movie theaters devoted to showing sexually explicit films, the Internet has become a central focus for the depiction of pornographic

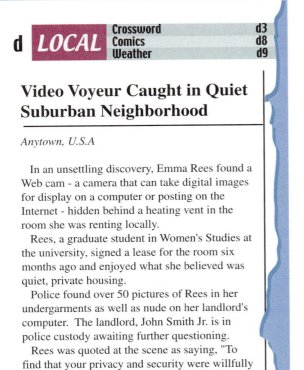

d LOCAL	Crossword	d3
	Comics	d8
	Weather	d9

Video Voyeur Caught in Quiet Suburban Neighborhood

Anytown, U.S.A

In an unsettling discovery, Emma Rees found a Web cam - a camera that can take digital images for display on a computer or posting on the Internet - hidden behind a heating vent in the room she was renting locally.

Rees, a graduate student in Women's Studies at the university, signed a lease for the room six months ago and enjoyed what she believed was quiet, private housing.

Police found over 50 pictures of Rees in her undergarments as well as nude on her landlord's computer. The landlord, John Smith Jr. is in police custody awaiting further questioning.

Rees was quoted at the scene as saying, "To find that your privacy and security were willfully violated is a horrifying experience which will affect me for years."

FIGURE 18-10 This story is based on an actual incident. Technological devices are making it easier to violate a person's right to privacy, even in their own home.

materials in pictorial, prose, and movie formats. Much controversy surrounds this issue and concerns about children having access to such illustrations. When Bryant published his book, *Sexual Deviancy and Social Proscription* in 1982, he couldn't have had any idea of what the Internet would bring.

VOYEURISM "CLUBS"

Voyeurism can also be evaluated from a sociological perspective, according to Forsyth (1996), because:

. . . (a) It [voyeurism] is widespread; (b) it is little different from viewing sex on a screen; (c) a network of mutual voyeurs exists that will continue to recruit new members; (d) the need for lower risk sex has begun to legitimize this form of sexual expression/outlet; and (e) some researchers have used the term 'normal voyeurism' which includes such behaviors as sheet-lifting orderlies or peeping construction workers on high-rise buildings.

—FORSYTH, 1996, 284

In fact, group voyeurism involves structured social interactions, success in making observations on a consistent basis, and a sense of history and understanding that create the group in the first place and contribute to its maintenance over time. Forsyth studied one group of people (all men) who engaged somewhat compulsively in voyeurism together, although some members came and went over the course of 20 years. This group had 9 members who all worked in the downtown area of a large city. They were custodial staff, maintenance workers, and equipment operators in tall buildings. These members had telescopes and arranged by telephone to meet at one of the buildings in which they worked, set up their equipment, and look into hotel rooms and office buildings. They ranged in age from their 30s to their 60s, and after a few hours of watching they would all go to a neighborhood bar, have a few beers, and talk about what (if anything) they had seen that night. They would set up their telescope and begin watching around 9 p.m. and sometimes stop as late as 3 a.m. Interestingly, group members chose to share and take turns looking through a single telescope, even though they all owned their own. In fact, there was an unwritten rule against a member bringing his own telescope and observing on his own. The members of this group bragged to the investigator that they had members who worked in virtually all of the tallest buildings in the city.

We describe this report to emphasize that voyeurism does not involve a simple, consistent pattern of behavior but can even become the object of a well-integrated, organized group's activities. It is unclear in this study whether these observation events for this group stimulated any desire to have intercourse or engage in other sexual activities by those doing the watching.

VIDEOTAPING VOYEURISTIC ACTIVITIES

Portable video cameras have had an enormous impact on the behavior of voyeurs. Simon (1997) published an interesting psychological and legal analysis of this phenomenon. Simon, a psychiatrist, notes that, "In the author's experience, video voyeurs are males, usually under age 40, who operate alone and are acquaintances, friends, coworkers, or neighbors of their victims" (Simon, 1997, p. 884). In most cases, video equipment is set up in dressing rooms, restrooms, and people's bedrooms. This author notes that even though video voyeurs are becoming more common, some voyeurs still prefer direct, "live" viewing of their victims.

When people (almost always women) discover that they have been videotaped, they are "horrified, humiliated, mortified, and extremely fearful" (p. 884). In fact their perceptions of privacy, trust, and safety in their environments are totally violated. While some victims react with justified anger and emotional distress, some are profoundly affected. The situation is worse still when the victim discovers that copies of the tapes have been made and distributed. Simon notes that psychological reactions are more pronounced when the victim has been videotaped engaging in private urination or defecation and sexual activity than when they are just in some state of undress and alone. Young girls, who are often extremely sensitive about

CASE STUDY: A YOUNG MALE VOYEUR

The subject was a 20-year-old unmarried male who referred himself to a mental health clinic because of anxiety, irritability, and depression. His anamnesis [loss of memory] revealed a somewhat directionless life. He left school after Grade VIII and has held down sundry menial jobs, although he is reported to be above average potential.

During the third interview after much reluctance and balking, he admitted peeping in windows for the last 5 years without being caught. His voyeurism occurred about 5 times a week with his preferred object being a young nude female. Sporadically after the session of peeping he would masturbate, thus positively reinforcing the voyeurism on an intermittent schedule.

This behavior was interpreted to him in learning principles, and he manifested great relief and hope when told that this behavior could be extinguished. A survey of potentially exciting stimuli revealed that pornographic pictures had the maximum arousing properties after voyeurism. After that came pictures of nude females such as found in the centerfold of *Playboy*.

It was then suggested that the next time he felt the urge to peep, he would masturbate in the privacy of his bedroom to the most exciting pornographic picture he had in his collection. He was told to focus on the picture at the time of orgasm. This was done for the next 2 weeks, by the end of which he reported no desire to look in windows. The next step involved pairing his orgasm with a nude picture. If he found it necessary he could maintain an erection through imagining a pornographic picture but had to concentrate on the *Playboy* picture at the point of ejaculation. From this juncture, further progress was rapid, and he reported no urges to peep and actually experienced two satisfactory heterosexual relations. Treatment was terminated after 8 sessions. Nine months later, he stated that his desire for voyeurism had dissipated and his sexual energies were directed along more socially acceptable lines.

—Jackson, 1991

their bodies and pubertal development, are often profoundly distressed upon discovering that they have been videotaped. In his assessment of various federal and state laws, Simon notes that video voyeurism can be prosecuted in a civil suit and that compensatory damages (a financial award) may result from such litigation. These behaviors are clear violations of privacy and one's rights to privacy under the 4th Amendment to the United States Constitution.

TROILISM AS A VARIATION OF VOYEURISM

Troilism refers to three people sharing sexual activities. Two might engage in intercourse while a third watches, or all three may share physical intimacies at the same time. This term is sometimes used to describe two couples having sexual intercourse in the visual presence of each other. This issue is similar to voyeurism because there is clearly a powerful visual component to these activities. Troilism often involves a practice (some call it a lifestyle) called "swinging" (Fig. 18-11). Swinging, also sometimes called "comarital sex," involves usually married couples who swap partners for sexual intercourse. Unmarried couples also participate in swinging, but most of what is known about this phenomenon is derived from reports from married couples. Swinging is apparently not very common, and Jencks estimates that only about 2% of married couples in the United States have ever participated.

People become involved in swinging for a variety of reasons, but the most commonly reported ones include the desire

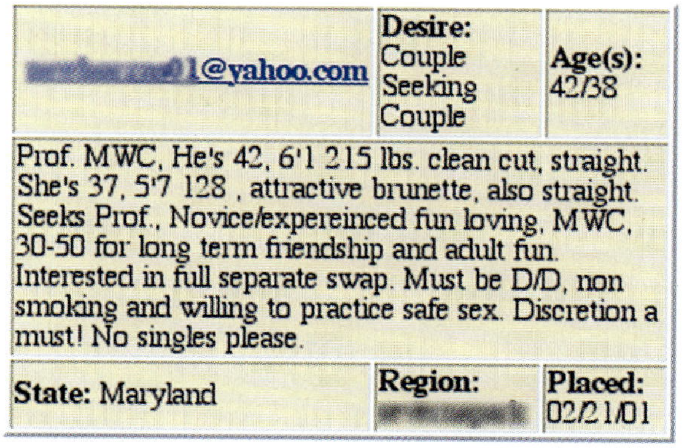

▓▓▓▓▓▓1@yahoo.com	Desire: Couple Seeking Couple	Age(s): 42/38
Prof. MWC, He's 42, 6'1 215 lbs. clean cut, straight. She's 37, 5'7 128 , attractive brunette, also straight. Seeks Prof., Novice/expereinced fun loving, MWC, 30-50 for long term friendship and adult fun. Interested in full separate swap. Must be D/D, non smoking and willing to practice safe sex. Discretion a must! No singles please.		
State: Maryland	Region: ▓▓▓▓▓▓	Placed: 02/21/01

FIGURE 18-11   Internet advertisements for swapping married partners in sexual encounters are common. Troilism and swapping are commonly part of the "swinging" lifestyle.

for sexual variety, pleasure, and excitement (Jenks, 1998). Voyeurism has been reported as one common reason for swinging. Subjects sometimes report that watching another couple have intercourse teaches them new sexual activities and techniques that they can then enjoy with their spouse. Additionally, swingers report that watching others have sex helps them to eliminate some of their own sexual inhibitions.

Frotteurism

Paraphilias vary a great deal in the degree to which they represent depersonalized expressions of sexual urges as well as the extent to which there is a nonconsenting victim. **Frotteurism** involves a fully clothed man rubbing his penis against another person in public, crowded places. This behavior is plainly deviant from normal expressions of sexual intimacy, and the victim in these cases is typically offended, angry, and upset. Related to frotteurism is another paraphilia called "toucherism" in which a man assertively grabs a female stranger's crotch or breasts, usually from behind (Freund, Seto, & Kuban in Laws & O'Donohue, 1997). Encountering either of these individuals in a subway or crowded sporting event is disconcerting and often humiliating for a woman. In both of these deviations the woman is plainly a "sex object" independent of her unique, personal attributes. Fewer than two dozen research articles

have been published on frotteurism in the last quarter century, and there has never been a report of a female frotteur.

Sexual Sadism and Sexual Masochism

The words "sadistic" and "masochistic" have different meanings when they are used in a sexual context and when they are not. A sadist is someone who enjoys inflicting or observing cruelty, either physical or psychological. Similarly, a masochist is someone who enjoys cruelty and pain, again, either physical or psychological. Yet **sexual sadism** and **sexual masochism** are different, as are the interpersonal dynamics between the person creating the pain and the one receiving it. This section discusses sexual sadism and sexual masochism as examples of reciprocal, consensual behaviors with very clear, although implicit, understandings about the boundaries of behaviors involved in creating pain and humiliation.

Sexual sadism involves enjoyable, sexually exciting feelings that derive from hurting or humiliating and degrading another person. Historically, writers point out that it isn't the pain and degradation these individuals enjoy inflicting so much as the sense of total domination and control over another person, thus turning them into an object instead of a person (Hucker in Laws & O'Donohue, 1997). The preva-

---

CASE STUDY: FROTTEURISM

*C*harles was 45 years old when he was referred for psychiatric consultation by his parole officer following his second arrest for rubbing up against a woman in the subway. According to Charles, he had a "good" sexual relationship with his wife of 15 years when he began, 10 years ago, to touch women in the subway. A typical episode would begin with his decision to go into the subway to rub against a woman, usually in her 20s. He would select the woman as he walked into the subway station, move in behind her, and wait for the train to arrive at the station. He would be wearing plastic wrap around his penis so as not to stain his pants after ejaculating while rubbing up against his victim. As riders moved on to the train, he would follow the woman he had selected. When the doors closed, he would begin to push his penis up against her buttocks, fantasizing that they were having intercourse in a normal, noncoercive manner. In about half of the episodes, he would ejaculate and then go on to work. If he failed to ejaculate, he would either give up for that day, or change trains and select another victim. According to Charles, he felt guilty immediately after each episode, but would soon find himself ruminating about and anticipating the next encounter. He estimated that he had done this about twice a week for the last 10 years, and thus had probably rubbed up against approximately a thousand women.

During the interview, Charles expressed extreme guilt about his behavior and often cried when talking about fears that his wife or employer would find out about his second arrest. However, he had apparently never thought about how his victims felt about what he did to them.

His personal history did not indicate any obvious mental problems other than being rather inept and unassertive socially, especially with women.

—DSM-IV Casebook, 1994, 164–165

lence of sexual sadism in the general population is thought to be low, although there is no way of being sure of the exact figures. There may also be a large discrepancy between reported frequency of people engaging in sexually sadistic activities and the frequency with which they merely fantasize about doing so. Similarly, it is difficult to determine whether respondents engage in these behaviors consistently and report that they are their central erotic preference or whether they only experiment with these activities occasionally. We are discussing consensual sexual activities, not extreme cases such as those in which someone tortures and sexually assaults their victims before killing them.

There is a clearly understood "contract" between sexual sadists and sexual masochists (Fig. 18-12). Various terms have been used to describe this arrangement: "bondage and discipline," "dominance and submission," and "sadomasochism" (Hucker, 1997). Those who inflict the discomfort or humiliation do so in a variety of ways. They may whip their partner, who may or may not be restrained at the time. Another common act of sexual sadism is called "fisting," which involves an individual inserting their fist into the vagina or rectum of their partner. Blindfolds and gags are sometimes used in these rituals, as are behaviors which emphasize submission to authority, such as wearing a diaper or licking the boots of one's partner.

Sexual masochism presents sex experts and clinicians with something of a paradox. While pain, discomfort, or humiliation in connection with sexual behavior is perceived as pleasurable, some writers believe that sexual masochism is on the borderline between a normal variation and preference and a pathology (Baumeister and Butler in Laws & O'Donohue, 1997). Baumeister and Butler (1997) emphasize that normal variations are an intrapsychic phenomenon, pretty much all in the individual's mind, while sexual masochism always involves a relationship of some sort (p. 236). These two phenomena therefore are unrelated. Baumeister (1989) estimated that 5% to 10% of the population has engaged in mild forms of sexual masochism involving spanking and blindfolding, but he believes that fewer than 1% of the population participate in sexual masochism on a consistent, regular basis. Again, it seems that males are represented more frequently than females. Interestingly, however, Baumeister and Butler note a relationship between socioeconomic status and the reports of sexual masochism; apparently individuals of higher socioeconomic status are more likely to participate than those who are poor (p. 229). Finally, sexual masochism seems more common than sexual sadism.

Baumeister and Butler have categorized three aspects of sexual masochism: experiencing pain, losing control, and feelings of shame and humiliation. In most cases, pain is inflicted by being spanked by one's partner's hand, although occasionally sexual masochists report being whipped, caned, or paddled (p. 230). Much rarer are reports of pinching the skin with clothespins or the piercing or burning of flesh. This pain is perceived as uncomfortable but not unbearable. Importantly, limits about the amount of pain experienced and its duration

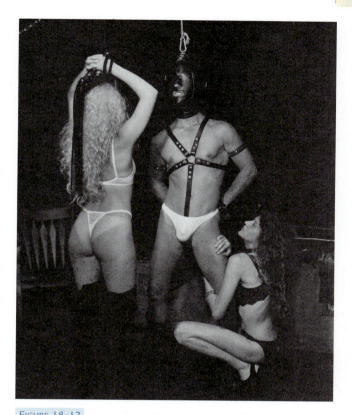

FIGURE 18-12   Despite the obvious bondage, dominance, and submission of sadomasochism, there are clear understandings between the participants about how much discomfort and/or humiliation will occur.

are clearly understood. Sexual masochists report that they enjoy this discomfort only during shared sexual activities. The loss of control noted above is typically created through bondage, being tied up in some way by one's partner. Sexual masochists report varying degrees of bondage as enjoyable. While some prefer moderate restraint, others demand severe and uncomfortable restriction. Being ordered around and told to do certain tasks involves the surrender of control. Baumeister and Butler have concluded that, "The appearance of helplessness and being under another person's power is central to masochism and represents what the masochist often most earnestly seeks" (p. 231). In less common cases, sexual masochists are asked to masturbate in the presence of others, engage in homosexual activities, or observe the infidelity of their spouse.

THE SADOMASOCHISTIC SUBCULTURE

The sociological analysis of sexual sadism and sexual masochism reveals that these two types of people find each other in a variety of ways and imbue their activities with rules, rituals, and implicit understandings of limits. Litman (1997) noted that from the early 1980s, sadomasochistic activities began to gain a popularity and legitimacy on the West Coast of the United States and that many adult bookstores began to cater to this interest with selections of pornographic literature, films, and magazines appealing specifically to these individuals. Certain objects appeared consistently in these shops, including whips, leather collars and costumes, handcuffs, gags, blindfolds, ropes, and other instruments for the administration of pain and torture (Fig. 18-13) (Litman, 1997, p. 256). This investigator discovered when talking with the owners of these establishments that the people who buy this material are "ordinary looking, well-dressed men of all ages" (p. 256), or as one proprietor noted, "People who look just like you, Doc."

In most large cities, underground newspapers appeal directly to people with sadomasochistic inclinations and make it easier for them to get together. Common personal ads involve heterosexuals who "seek S-M services," although the preponderance of males put interested females at a premium. Litman contacted 9 men and 3 women and interviewed them in depth, creating a case study for each, and formulated several generalizations based on this small sample of subjects; all were volunteers, and therefore there may be bias in their reports. Of these subjects, only men reported engaging in behaviors that were potentially dangerous; these formed the nucleus of this study. These were all Caucasian, middle-class subjects, and many reported a history of depression. No history of sexual abuse, cruel family interactions, or unique, traumatic events could be consistently associated with these respondents. Most reported their preferred sexual orientation as homosexual, although many reported having frequent heterosexual encounters. Many joined clubs for sadists and masochists, while others contacted escort services with women trained to cater to a masochistic clientele. Interestingly, some female prostitutes willingly engage in masochistic interactions with their clients for an extremely high fee and an agreement to pay for any medical and/or dental expenses that may be necessary. Prostitutes refer to these interac-

tions as "dumpings" (Bryant, 1982, p. 350). While some of the subjects in this small sample sought painful experiences, others were interested primarily in being humiliated. For these men to have orgasms, they were highly dependent on a sadomasochistic ritual and often also dependent on the objects described earlier. The 3 female subjects in this sample all emphasized that they had participated in masochistic activities entirely to please the sadistic tendencies of their male partners.

When is sadomasochism a sexual variation and when is it a sexual deviation? Storr (1970) has an interesting hypothesis about this question based on the psychodynamic approach. He believes that some individuals are fascinated by the possibility of reaching levels of sexual excitement that they don't usually enjoy during intercourse, and that manageable amounts of pain may, for these people, release an immense passion not normally experienced. For these individuals, sexual intercourse alone is just not exciting enough, and the untamed, reckless feelings that accompany mild pain enhance their sexual excitement and responsiveness. The sexual masochist truly believes that other men routinely and regularly reach these keen levels of passion but he cannot do so without the added pain or the fantasy that the pain may still escalate further. For Storr, these thoughts and feelings are a variation on normal sexual responsiveness. However, when the perception of pain is excessive and intense and has little to do with having intercourse, then he believes it becomes a deviation for that person and their partner. For Storr there is another intriguing aspect of sadomasochism. Common stereotypes often hold that there is an innate, subtle tendency toward sadism in men's relationships with women, but this psychiatrist points out that men often have an explicit desire to experience pain as an adjunct to sexual gratification and that overgeneralizations about male sadism are therefore incomplete and inaccurate. Finally, Storr comments on another aspect of sexual sadism: whether the person inflicting the pain wants his partner to experience pain or pleasure. In his view as a psychiatrist, the sadist truly wants his partner to enjoy the discomfort and/or humiliation he is creating.

THE SADOMASOCHISTIC PACT

A clearly understood set of agreements and understandings govern these complementary sexual variations. Sexual sadists do not, in fact, want to do serious bodily harm, and sexual masochists do not want to be seriously hurt. How does the couple come to some sense of a contract of who will do what to whom, for how long, and how vigorously? According to Gosselin (1987), there are many predictable and negotiable aspects of a sadomasochistic interaction. Indeed, if heterosexuals enjoying foreplay and sexual intercourse had a similar understanding of one another's preferences and limits, their level of erotic enjoyment would often be enhanced by their excellent communication.

While some form of discomfort is basic to sadomasochistic rituals, both the severity and duration of these "beatings" are highly variable. Gosselin notes that this ritual may last a long time and involve perhaps as many as 200 slaps on the but-

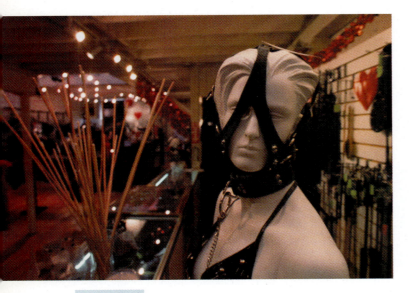

FIGURE 18-13   Shops with diverse merchandise appealing to the sadomasochistic subculture are common and carry a wide diversity of videos, magazines, whips, leather collars and masks, handcuffs, and blindfolds.

tocks using the partner's hand or a paddle. He notes that despite common portrayals of these rituals, whips are seldom used. Between spankings there may be pauses during which the individual playing the dominant role insults or taunts the "victim" and lightly circles the area to be hit to "prime" the recipient for the next stroke. While this is all happening there may be explanations as to why this punishment is necessary and deserved. In most cases these spankings start slowly and escalate in seriousness as the submissive partner becomes progressively more aroused. Gosselin notes that subjects generally respond to these spankings not as if they are experiencing pain but rather with a significant degree of exhilarated excitement. A second routine aspect of sadomasochistic rituals involves bondage, which frequently entails complete immobilization, and once restricted the submissive partner is then "beaten" or otherwise forced to sustain pain and other forms of erotic stimulation upon which they cannot act. In many instances, the dominant partner also deprives them temporarily of sight, sound, smell, taste, and the capacity to speak. In sadomasochistic jargon, this is called "occlusion" (Gosselin, 1987, p. 234). Finally, humiliation is a fundamental feature of sadomasochistic rituals and involves the submissive partner sustaining verbal insults as well as being "forced" to engage in various demeaning behaviors. Once these elements are all in place, the couple then frequently proceeds to some form of sexual interaction. This too is "scripted," with one partner giving explicit directions and the other following passively and unquestioningly. This mutual interaction is sexually exciting to couples enjoying sadomasochistic rituals, not the solitary fantasies of each individual. Ultimately, Gosselin maintains, there is a clear understanding about who will do what to whom, when, and for how long.

CASE STUDY: SEXUAL SADISM

The client was a 21-year-old unmarried white male college senior majoring in history. The university counseling center had received an anxious letter from his parents, requesting help for their son in treating his introversion, procrastination, and "masochism." After working with the student for a few weeks on his tendency to wait until the last minute in his academic work, the psychologist at the center referred him to the author for help with his sexual difficulties.

Mr. M's statement of the problem was: "I'm a sadist." There followed a rather troubled account of a complete absence of "normal" sexual fantasies and activities since age 11. Masturbating about 5 times a week, the client's fantasies had been exclusively sadistic ones, specifically, inflicting tortures on women. He declared emphatically that he had never been sexually aroused by any other kind of image. Although generally uninterested in dating girls, he felt no aversion to them; on the contrary, he sometimes felt a "warm glow" when near them, but did not describe this at all in sexual terms. Because of his extreme concern over the content of his fantasies, however, he had dated very little and expressed no interest in the coeds at the college. He recalled having kissed only two girls in his life, with no sexual arousal accompanying these fleeting episodes. He had never engaged in any homosexual activities or fantasies. Although expressing no guilt about his problem, he was very much worried about it inasmuch as he felt it impossible to ever contemplate marriage. This concern had recently been markedly increased upon reading an account of a Freudian interpretation of "sado-masochism." He was especially perturbed about the poor prognosis for this "illness."

Because his concern over the gravity and implications of his problem seemed at least as disruptive as the problem itself, the therapist spent most of the first session raising arguments against a disease interpretation of unusual behavior. Psychoanalytic notions were critically reviewed, and attention was directed especially to the untestability of many Freudian concepts . . . Instances in the therapist's own clinical work were cited to illustrate the liberating effects observed in many people when they interpret their maladaptive behavior as determined by "normal" psychological processes rather than by insidious disease processes . . . Mr. M. frequently expressed relief at these ideas, and the therapist, indeed, took full advantage of his prestigious position to reinforce these notions.

—Davison, 1991

CHARACTERISTICS OF SEXUAL SADISTS AND SEXUAL MASOCHISTS

John Munder Ross (1997), a training analyst at the Cornell Medical College in New York City, described attributes of sexual sadists and sexual masochists, based on his personal clinical experience and research. Although his ideas have not yet been accepted as definitive, they are a comprehensive, reasonable perspective:

- Sexual sadists and sexual masochists have experienced "lowgrade or mild childhood abuse." This may be in the form of sexual, physical, or emotional abuse, but it typically does not include incest or outright physical assault.
- Because of this, Ross feels that these individuals have "unconscious sadomasochistic and specifically sexual fantasies" which they later try to act out with another person.
- These individuals often experience a sense of "irrational guilt" because they like being hurt and frequently feel anger.
- Ross believes that sexual masochists, contrary to their overt submissive preferences and behaviors, actually have a great reservoir of "unconscious rage and the desire for revenge." Psychologically, they attribute this anger to their sadistic partner who in turn creates physical pain for them.
- According to Ross, sexual sadists have "poor self esteem," which is manifest in their thinking that they don't deserve to be treated better.
- Similarly, Ross believes that sexual masochists have a "fragile sense of identity," which in turn leads to indistinct personal boundaries between themselves and others. These are reflected in the frequently fluid roles played by sexual sadists and sexual masochists.
- Because of these blurred perceptions of themselves and their roles, they in turn "lack self-awareness" and make it seem that they are frequently experiencing unpleasant things.

—After Ross, 1997, 90–91.

Whether these observations will eventually be validated in widespread clinical practice remains to be seen. From a psychodynamic perspective they have a certain compelling logic about them.

Pedophilia

While the "contract" between sexual sadists and sexual masochists entails clearly consensual behaviors and neither individual considers themselves a "victim," the case is very different with **pedophilia,** which involves adults taking advantage of children in a sexual way, usually without their consent and understanding. The term "child molester" is typically used to describe the pedophile. As with other paraphilias, the *DSM-IV* defines pedophilia in terms of frequent, intense urges and vivid fantasies involving sexual behavior with a child. Yet at the same time, there is no diagnostic requirement that the individual actually act on these urges and fantasies, which has been a source of disagreement among clinicians who diagnose pedophilia. A large percentage of people who actually molest children, according to Marshall (1997), are *not* preoccupied by the urges and fantasies described in the *DSM.* For these reasons, many clinicians today make the diagnosis of a child molester regardless of whether they report experiencing any recurring, intrusive sexual fantasies or urges with respect to having sex with children. Marshall also believes that the term "pedophile" is not appropriate because its literal meaning suggests a "child lover," and it is certainly *not* the case that child molesters love the children they assault. Child molesters harass both same- and other-sex children (most are heterosexual), and as in other paraphilias, the great majority are male.

Marshall notes that another issue too makes the diagnosis somewhat ambiguous. The *DSM-IV* asserts that individuals with paraphilias are distressed by their own thoughts, urges, and fantasies and that their interpersonal or occupational relationships are often impaired. In fact, this is often not the case with child molesters. Although child molesters may be attracted exclusively to prepubescent children, many are also engaged in seemingly normal, long-term heterosexual relationships with adult women. While some therapists claim that child molesters are primarily attracted to children under the age of 8, others raise the criterion to 13. In fact, the age of the victim is somewhat arbitrary if she or he has not yet reached adolescence. Ames and Houston (1990) emphasize the importance of the victim's body configuration in legal, social, and biological approaches to pedophilia. They maintain that if an adult has a primary psychological and physiological arousal response to prepubescent body forms, that individual is in all likelihood a pedophile. While the age of the victim has been a factor in diagnosing child molesters, so too has been the age of the perpetrator. Marshall (1997) notes that a diagnosis of pedophilia is not generally made if the offender himself has not yet reached late adolescence. Overall, diagnosing pedophilia involves a number of ambiguous issues. But what isn't ambiguous is the fact that a child is violated sexually, usually against her or his consent and without a full understanding of the exploitation that is taking place. Child molestation is a clear example of an enormous discrepancy in the power of the perpetrator and the ability of the victim to resist being exploited.

The prevalence of child molestation cannot be determined with any accuracy because of the large number of cases that go unreported. Some child molestation involves seemingly "willing" victims, some involves incest, and some is reported instead as homicide. Because of the power differential between adults and children, however, the term "willing victim" may not be accurate. Additionally, cases of kidnapping frequently involve sexual exploitation, and the outcomes of these cases are frequently and tragically unresolved. A conservative estimate of the prevalence of child molestation in the United States is over 300,000 cases each year (Marshall, 1997).

The causes of pedophilia are incompletely understood. Child molesters do not have very much empathy for their victims, although ironically, they report empathy for the victims

Research Highlight

THE LONG-TERM EFFECTS ON MALES OF EARLY SEXUAL ACTIVITY WITH ADULTS

Bauserman and Rind (1997) studied the long-term effects of early sexual activity with adults in a large "non-clinical" sample of males. The term "nonclinical" is used to note that these respondents were not receiving medical, psychiatric, or psychological treatment relevant to this issue at the time of the study and were drawn primarily from college classes and community and national samples. These subjects reported reactions to these early sexual experiences that ranged from very negative to very positive and included emotional outcomes that ranged from severe and negative to none at all. This study revealed that such experiences were not invariably harmful but were assessed by these subjects in many instances as "neutral" or "positive." These researchers were *not* saying that these experiences are harmless, but only that the broad view of a large sample indicated that the commonplace notions on this issue may not be entirely valid.

Bauserman and Rind (1997) also note that there are a number of factors that impact powerfully on the way in which these sexual experiences are evaluated in later life. For example, when these subjects felt that they were being forced into sexual activities against their will, they held a decidedly negative perception of them and all surrounding circumstances. Whether the subjects remember consenting to the sexual interactions and their relationship with the older adult were also important variables that affected their retrospective feelings about the experiences, although again, because of the power differential between adults and children, the term "consent" should be interpreted cautiously. When the subject consented to the sexual activity, long-term outcomes were generally more positive, and when the adult was a family member, the long-term outcomes were plainly more negative. Bauserman and Rind noted that in the various samples they assessed, the older adult was a woman between 40% and 75% of the time—a surprisingly high estimate, given the rarity of women with paraphilias. In research exploring the impact of early sexual experiences on women, the adult is male between 90% and 100% of the time. They note that when contacts with male children and adolescents involved touching and some type of penetration, the respondents reported far more negative perceptions than when contacts involved oral stimulation.

This study also summarized the literature on this issue affecting women, and noted that in the long run, women are far more likely to evaluate their childhood and adolescent sexual experiences with adults far more negatively than males. In most cases, women were involved in heterosexual activities, while males were engaged in about equal amounts of heterosexual and homosexual interactions. Bauserman and Rind were careful to emphasize that their data look very different from studies on similar subjects involving clinical samples, that is, individuals who later in life sought and received some type of psychological or psychiatric assistance for their earlier experiences.

---

of *other* child molesters as well as all other children (Marshall, Fernandez, Lightbody, & O'Sullivan, 1994). Child molesters generally deny and minimize the deviant, exploitative nature of their actions (Pithers, Beal, Armstrong, & Petty, 1989). These researchers also discovered that the early childhood experiences of molesters often reveal highly disturbed and unsettled parent-child relationships, and that it was not uncommon for molesters to have themselves been the victims of childhood sexual abuse, although whether there is a cause-and-effect relationship here remains to be demonstrated.

CHILD VICTIMS OF SEXUAL EXPLOITATION

For a variety of reasons, many still poorly understood, there has been a steady increase in the number of cases of sexual abuse of children over the past few decades. The differential victimization of girls and boys is unclear, although sexual exploitation of female children seems to be far more common.

One can assume that reported cases of child sexual molestation are not single, isolated events but rather reflect a long-standing and consistent pattern of exploitation. Many episodes of molestation are apparently not reported. Bryant (1982)

Research Highlight

YOUNG WOMEN WHO SEXUALLY MOLEST CHILDREN

Pedophilia does not always involve older men and young children, although little is known about females in sexually exploitative activities with children. One research study sheds some light on this interesting issue. Fromuth and Conn (1997) used questionnaires to explore this question in a sample of 546 female students at a large southeastern university in the United States. These researchers defined sexual abuse as involving "(e.g., . . . kissing and hugging in a sexual way, fondling, intercourse, oral-genital contact) and noncontact experiences (e.g., invitation or request to do something sexual, child showing his or her genitals to offender, offender exposing genitals to child)" (p. 459). To meet the criteria for this study, when children were under 13 years old, the offender needed to be at least 5 years older, and when victims were between the ages of 13 and 16, the offender needed to be at least 10 years older.

Of the 546 subjects who completed their questionnaires, 22 acknowledged being involved in at least one episode of sexual abuse as defined. These respondents reported having sexual experiences with a total of 24 different children. The average age of the perpetrator was approximately 12 years, with most of them between the ages of 10 and 14 when these activities took place. The average age of the victim was approximately 6 years, with most being between 5 and 7. In almost 70% of these cases, the victim was a family member of the perpetrator, and 70% of the victims were male. Almost 90% of the perpetrators admitted to having initiated the sexual contact, and a similar percentage reported that they had never disclosed to anyone that they had been involved in such activities. Half of these reports of child molestation involved touching the youngster's genitals and oral-genital stimulation, and sexual intercourse was reported by 25% of these subjects. In retrospect, these experiences had varying effects on these women. For example, 58% of the subjects reported that in general, the long-term effect of initiating molestation had a neutral effect, with 38% noting a clearly negative effect, and only 4% reported a positive effect. When asked explicitly whether they had ever been abused sexually, only 3 of the 22 women indicated that they had. When the psychological status and background of the perpetrators were compared with those of non-perpetrators, no obvious and consistent significant differences were found. There was, however, a slightly higher probability that the women who reported sexually molesting children had themselves been molested in childhood. We have included a summary of this research report because very little is known about women who have engaged in sexual molestation of children. Clearly, more studies are needed before we can make any meaningful generalizations.

points out that it is extremely common for the perpetrator and victim to know one another. They are frequently members of the same nuclear or extended family or may live in the same neighborhood or participate in similar youth-oriented activities together. Additionally, friends of the family and teachers have also been implicated. It is also possible that there is even a close, caring rapport between the perpetrator and the victim, and gentle persuasion might be more commonly used than overt force.

Still, it would be incorrect to assume that these children are informed, consenting partners in these activities, and it would also be wrong to believe that they sustain no or only minor discomfort or injury. In fact, rape is not at all uncommon. These children are also frequently seriously injured physically, suffering cuts, bruises, bites, broken bones, and dramatic damage to their genitalia and anuses. Another issue of genuine importance is the fact that sexually victimized children often acquire sexually transmitted diseases and extremely serious psychological trauma.

Even in those instances in which the child seems to be consenting to the sexual activities, it is important to assess the degree to which she or he fully appreciates the nature and consequences of them. In fact, youngsters may sometimes provoke, solicit, or facilitate such activities in a highly seductive fashion (Bryant, 1982). In these cases, it is not unusual for the victims to initiate some form of genital touching. When children do not have the family background or social skills to learn appropriate ways of receiving the approval and attention of adults, these sexually assertive behaviors are often effective in seducing inclined perpetrators to take "indecent liberties."

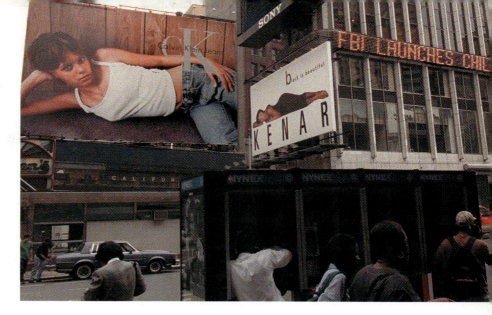

FIGURE 18-14 Many provocative advertisements depict children in more or less explicit, sexually suggestive poses. There is much debate over whether these are authentic examples of child pornography.

Because of the ambiguities involved in accurately defining pedophilia, there is much debate about whether looking at child pornography without ever approaching a child sexually constitutes pedophilia. Bryant (1982) refers to this as "vicarious pedophilia," and the huge market in child pornography shows this is a widespread phenomenon (Fig.18-14). Magazines, films, videotapes, and other periodicals cater to adults with these interests.

CHILD PORNOGRAPHY AND THE INTERNET

Does pornography stimulate or provoke child sexual abuse? Howitt (1995) assessed case study data on the relationship between exposure to pornography and later child molesting activities. Howitt evaluated the case histories of 11 male pedophiles undergoing psychological treatment in a private sex offenders clinic in England. His subjects were all volunteers and agreed to be interviewed at length and in depth about their pedophilic behaviors and the role of pornography in possibly stimulating these illegal sexual activities. Interestingly, most of these subjects reported that they had been exposed to pornography before their first experience with sexual abuse. In none of these subjects did there seem to be any clear cause-and-effect relationship between early experience with pornography and a later pattern of pedophilic behavior. Although many of these men did report that they found pictures of children sexually arousing, this was not a primary source of sexual stimulation in their lives; indeed, they found child pornography highly distasteful. These subjects reported erotic arousal instead from reading the newspaper, watching television, viewing non-pornographic movies, and looking at clothing catalogs in which children were depicted wearing undergarments.

Until recently, gaining access to pornography was a difficult, quiet, and potentially embarrassing enterprise (Fig. 18-15). With the expansion of First Amendment rights and the gradual liberalization of our society over the last 50

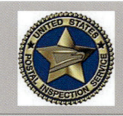

United States
Postal Inspection Service

Mailing of Child Pornography

FIGURE 18-15 The United States Postal Service has created strict policies and sanctions with respect to the production and distribution of child pornography and works together with law enforcement officials to apprehend those who break the law.

It is illegal to send child pornography through the U.S. Mails. Child pornography includes the visual depiction of sexual activities or overtly sexual poses involving children, legally defined as persons under age 18.

The Postal Inspection Service is interested in combating the production and distribution of child pornography and the sexual exploitation of children. Therefore, the mailing of child pornography receives priority attention as a part of the effort to eliminate this form of child abuse. If acts of physical child abuse are discovered incident to a Postal Inspection Service investigation, immediate referral is made to local law enforcement authorities for additional attention to protect the children.

If you have information the U.S. Mails were used to send child pornography, please contact the Postal Inspection Service immediately. Postal Inspectors may be listed in the white pages years, this situation has changed markedly. Nowhere has this revolution been more pronounced and controversial than on the Internet. Durkin (1997) explored some of the implications of this issue for law enforcement and probation officials.

In a nonempirical analysis Durkin highlights a number of issues important to the law enforcement community. He believes that the availability of pornography to pedophiles on the Internet is cause for significant social concern, and because much more research is needed, it may be premature to minimize the potential threat in the availability of pornography on the Internet. Specifically, he highlights various ways in which pedophiles are abusing the freedoms inherent on the Internet.

- It is a fact that pedophiles sometimes engage in the trafficking of child pornography on the Internet.
- It is a fact that pedophiles have contacted children on the Internet for the purpose of engaging in sexual activities with them.
- It is a fact that pedophiles have used "chat rooms" to communicate with children about sexual subjects and the potential for meeting them.
- It is a fact that pedophiles communicate with other pedophiles on the Internet and sometimes plan illegal activities while doing so.

—Durkin, 1997, 17

In fact, Durkin believes that the Internet is a socially facilitating influence on pedophiles for the exploitation of children (Fig. 18-16). This writer emphasizes that most law enforcement agencies today are unprepared to deal with these potential threats to children and their well-being and that it is extremely difficult to detect the identity of these potential perpetrators, much less discourage or stop their actions.

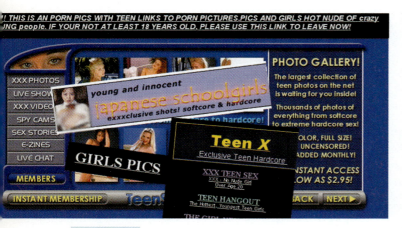

FIGURE 18-16 Many social and behavioral scientists believe that the Internet has the potential to stimulate pedophiles to find and exploit children.

LABORATORY PROCEDURES FOR THE DIAGNOSIS OF PEDOPHILIC INTEREST

So far, the data described here on sexual interactions with children were derived primarily from questionnaire, clinical, and case study investigations. Other research has sought to determine whether pedophiles are preferentially responsive to depictions of children, clothed or unclothed, in a physiological way. Abel, Huffman, Warberg, and Holland (1998) used two different laboratory techniques while working with a group of 56 men who had been accused of sexually inappropriate behaviors involving children. The first involved measuring changes in the diameter of the subject's penis while observing slides of males and females 4, 8, 12, 16, and 22 years of age. Each slide depicted a frontal view of individuals in these age levels. The second technique involved presenting subjects with slides of females and males in three age groups: 8–10 years of age, 14–17, years of age, and over 22 years of age, all of whom were clothed and depicted as the victims of exhibitionistic behavior, voyeurism, frotteurism, a suffering female, a suffering male, two males hugging, two females hugging, a male and a female hugging, and unrelated photographs of landscapes (p. 86). Subjects were asked to rate the desirability or sexually arousing qualities of these pictures on a scale from 1 to 7, and the amount of time they took to make these judgements was recorded.

Both of these techniques effectively showed an empirical relationship between accusations of pedophilic interest and enhanced physiological responsiveness to pictures of undressed children and adolescents as well as faster reaction times and ratings of greater sexual arousal to pictures of clothed children and adolescents while being victimized by paraphilic behavior. Although it might be risky to use such techniques to make a definitive diagnosis of pedophilic interests, they do lend some support to the notion that this particular paraphilia can be meaningfully studied by laboratory methods as well as data from the clinic or questionnaires.

THE PEDOPHILE'S THOUGHTS AND FEELINGS

In a recent case study investigation, Ivey and Simpson (1998) recorded lengthy, open-ended discussions with 6 men who had been legally identified as child molesters. These men were asked to talk about their feelings about being sexually attracted to children and interacting with them intimately. These researchers did not ask direct questions but let the interviewee determine the agenda and details they chose to disclose. The tapes of these interviews were analyzed for any significant commonalities among the subjects and any consistent themes.

These respondents all spoke about how their own childhood needs for love and validation were never met. They felt inadequate in their families and rejected by their parents. In many cases their parents were wilfully abusive and neglectful; these abusive experiences may have been sexual and/or physical in nature. Because of these childhood experiences, the subjects gradually came to perceive the intimacy of adult sexual sharing as risky and fraught with the ever-present threat of renewed rejection. The child molester gradually came to see the immaturity and vulnerability of children as a substitute for the love and intimacy they were afraid to pursue with other adults. These authors came to the conclusion that the gender of the child is not as important as the belief that they offer the kind of validation and love the molester never received in childhood. Finally, the subjects in this study reported that they take every precaution against hurting their victims physically, but they seemed to have very little awareness that they may be doing profound emotional harm. Whether the insights from these interviews can be generalized to large numbers of child molesters requires further scientific investigation.

Uncommon Paraphilias

The paraphilias described so far are not unusual in the general population. Other paraphilias are much rarer in the general population. Almost all of these other paraphilias involve a nonconsenting victim or in some cases no other human at all.

Telephone Scatologia. **Telephone scatologia** refers to the experience of sexual arousal, and sometimes orgasm, while making obscene telephone calls. These usually involve highly suggestive sexual statements and propositions. Most obscene callers are men who generally have a poor self-image and often feelings of anger towards women (Matek, 1988). This sexual deviation has practically become an industry with the proliferation of "phone sex" services. Inherent in telephone scatologia is a highly depersonalized approach to sexual feelings; the telephone is used instead of interpersonal communication and interaction. Some people become "addicted" to phone sex and spend thousands of dollars each year making these calls, almost always without the knowledge or consent of their partner.

Gerontophilia. In **gerontophilia**, an individual, typically a young man, has a compulsive, compelling interest in having sexual relations with an elderly woman. There are extremely few reports of gerontophilia in the medical, psychological, or psychiatric literature. An interesting case study published by Ball (1998) described a 24-year-old man who came from a large family and had been physically assaulted by his father, who was an alcoholic. During his late teenage years he began a behavior pattern of seeking secluded outdoor areas, waiting for an "older" woman to walk by, and then exposing himself. At this time in his life, most of his victims were in their 30s and 40s. After exposing his erect penis he would then masturbate. The offense for which he was eventually put in jail began with exposing himself to a 58-year-old woman accompanied by her 2-year-old grandson. He forcibly inserted his penis into the victim's mouth before raping her. There was significant evidence to demonstrate that he had followed this particular woman for a long time. Although there are not many reports of gerontophilic behavior in the scholarly literature, there is a particularly thorough one in the true story called *The Boston Strangler*, by Gerold Frank (Fig. 18-17).

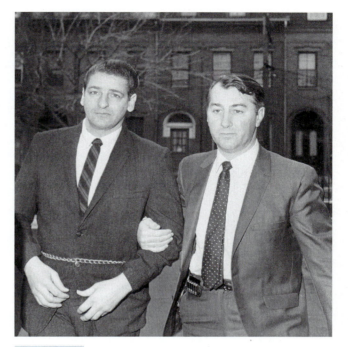

FIGURE 18-17   Albert DeSalvo (left), also known as the Boston Strangler, is here being led to jail after a trial had proven that he raped and murdered 13 women in Boston, many of whom were aging and elderly.

Partialism. If an individual has a sole and exclusive sexual focus on just one part of a person's body to the total disinterest and neglect of others, this deviation is referred to as "partialism." This is not the same as a man being attracted to a woman's legs or breasts when these are not the sole focus of sexual attraction. Partialism is sometimes thought of as a variation on fetishism, but fetishes, by definition, involve inanimate objects.

Necrophilia. Some individuals feel compelled to have sex with corpses (Fig. 18-18). Suspects have been caught after a break-in at a funeral home, leading to reports of "defiling a corpse." Serial killers have also been known to kill victims to obtain their corpses for sexual purposes (Fig. 18-19). **Necrophilia** may involve vaginal penetration, anal penetration, fondling, fellatio, and cunnilingus with a corpse (Milner in Laws & O'Donohue, 1997). Very few data are available regarding the prevalence of necrophilia, but Rosman and Resnick (1989) studied 122 reported cases of this deviation and found that 92% were male and 8% female; the average age of this clinical sample was 34. Approximately 70% of these subjects reported that they were heterosexual, 15% bisexual, and 15% homosexual. Interestingly, 57% of these individuals had occupations in which they normally came into contact with corpses, such as hospital workers, cemetery workers, and funeral home workers.

Zoophilia. Sometimes called "bestiality," **zoophilia** involves having penetrating sex with a nonhuman animal. Zoophilic behaviors may also involve masturbating an animal,

Des Moines Regist

Ban on necrophilia sent to Branstad
Feb. 29, 1996

By The Associated Press

DES MOINES -- A bill to outlaw sexual abuse of a human corpse, or necrophilia, has cleared the Legislature.

The bill was drafted after a 1995 incident in which a man was found fondling a woman's corpse in a Des Moines funeral home. Authorities determined there was no law against such actions on the books in Iowa.

The House approved the bill Wednesday on a 90-0 vote after being told of its serious nature.

"I don't believe any of us would believe it was a joke if it involved a family member or friend of ours," the bill's manager, Rep. Jeffrey Lamberti, R-Ankeny, told the House.

Rep. Ed Fallon, D-Des Moines, said he knows the family of the woman whose corpse was fondled.

"It was a traumatic experience for them," Fallon said.

The bill makes such actions a felony punishable by up to five years in prison and a $7,500 fine. It was earlier approved by the Senate and now goes to Gov. Terry Branstad, who is expected to sign it into law.

ge 3

 FIGURE 18-18   While stories about necrophilia are not common in the media, occasionally stories like this one about a funeral home break-in inform the public that these acts may not be too unusual.

performing fellatio or cunnilingus on the animal, or penetrating the animal anally. Very often, the animal the individual selects is one with which he lived in close proximity earlier in childhood. Little is known about the prevalence of this paraphilia in the general population, but Kinsey's study of male sexuality reported that 40% to 50% of males with rural origins and residence patterns reported having had some sexual interaction with a nonhuman animal. Zoophilia is far less common among females, like most of the paraphilias.

Klismaphilia. An enema involves introducing liquids through the anus into the rectum, often in the treatment of constipation. But because the anus is such a sensitive area, and one endowed with significant libido according to Freud, ene-

mas for some are powerfully associated with sexual pleasure. Both women and men report **klismaphilic** interests. According to Agnew (1982), a tube is inserted through the anus into the rectum, the rectum filled with some liquid substance, and the contents of the rectum expelled. Warm water is commonly used, as well as a variety of other substances including alcoholic beverages such as beer, wine, or whisky or cocaine mixed into a solution. These agents are readily absorbed through the membranes of the rectum and enter the bloodstream very quickly, creating feelings of euphoria in many instances. While some klismaphiliacs administer enemas to themselves privately, others engage in these behaviors with another person who is also self-administering an enema. Agnew's research has suggested that filling the rectum with fluids presses on a man's prostate gland, as well as seminal vesicles and similarly exerts pressure on the posterior side of a woman's vagina, and these perceptions are similar to feelings experienced during both masturbation and sexual intercourse.

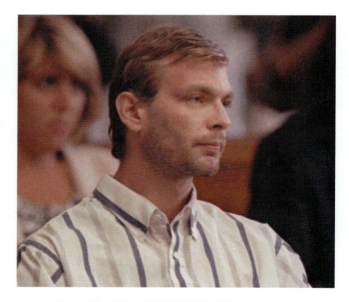

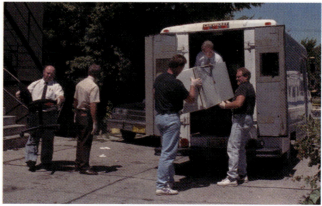

FIGURE 18-19   Top: Jeffrey Dahmer shown in 1991. Dahmer tortured and killed his 17 victims, had sex with their corpses, mutilated them, and stored their remains in his apartment. Below: police remove evidence from Dahmer's apartment on July 24, 1991.

Coprophilia. One of the most unusual of the rare paraphilias is **coprophilia,** the desire to incorporate human feces into sexual activity. This may take the form of defecating on one's partner or in manually manipulating feces during sexual interactions.

Urophilia. Others feel impelled to include urine in their sexual activities. **Urophilia** refers to sexual activities concentrating on urination or urine itself. The street terms for urophilia are "water sports" or "golden showers." In some cases, people drink urine as a part of a sexual ritual. Because there are often aggressive connotations to the act of urination, Milner and Dopke (in Laws & O'Donohue, 1997) suggest that urophilia may be a variety of sexual sadism or sexual masochism, depending on whether one urinates on someone else or desires to be urinated on.

Stigmatophilia. When a person feels a strong sexual attraction to someone who has tatoos or scars, this is called **stigmatophilia.** It may also involve sexual interest in someone who has had part or parts of their body pierced with ornamentation attached. People have had almost every corner of their bodies pierced, including their tongues, penises, and labia (Fig. 18-20).

Asphyxiophilia. The paraphilias described so far range from the unusual to the bizarre, but none is frankly dangerous or potentially fatal. This is not the case with **asphyxiophilia,** or hypoxyphilia. It sometimes involves applying pressure to the carotid arteries in one's neck, reducing blood flow to the brain, which in turn leads to an increase in carbon dioxide in the bloodstream. In other instances a person puts a plastic bag over their head or wears a tight mask. This lack of oxygen reaching the brain, called asphyxia, is for these people associated with profoundly enhanced feelings of sexual arousal and similar increases in the pleasure accompanying orgasm. Unfortunately, in some cases the individual is unable to loosen the pressure applied, or there is a delay in

restoring breathing, and death may result. Accidental hangings have been reported. It is difficult to judge the prevalence of asphyxiophilia in the general population, but some have suggested that suicide by hanging should be evaluated carefully by medical examiners for the possibility that death occurred as a result of this paraphilia (Kirkley, Holt-Ashley, Williamson, & Garza, 1995).

PARAPHILIAS IN PSYCHOSOCIAL CONTEXT

So far this discussion of paraphilias has focused mostly on the nature of the thoughts, feelings, and behaviors involved in deviant sexual activities and some of the legal aspects of these activities. Now we will look at the impact of sexual variations and deviations on a person's functioning in the broader psychosocial environment. Because of the taboo nature of these activities, people who engage in them do not often disclose this information. A good source of information regarding this issue is *The Kinsey Institute New Report on Sex* (Reinisch, 1990), from which we quote the following case studies to illuminate the psychosocial context of some paraphilias.

The first of these involves a question from a young woman engaged to be married to a transvestite:

> *I'm engaged to marry a man who I'm completely in love with, but he has just told me something I can't understand. He says he loves me too (and acts like he does, if you know what I mean) and wants to get married and have kids, but he wears ladies' panties!*
>
> *I don't know what to think. He acts just like other men I've gotten serious with. Does this mean he's secretly a homosexual? He doesn't seem like anything but a real man. What should I do?*
>
> —REINISCH, 1990, 155–156

Many transvestites are successfully secretive about their cross-dressing and may never be discovered in a woman's clothing. Most transvestites are heterosexuals and are aroused and responsive with women in intimate situations. In this case we do not know a crucial factor: the degree to which women's undergarments are *necessary* for this particular man to become sexually aroused and responsive.

The following anecdote is an example of sexual sadism. The individual writing seems to be very open and honest about his inclinations but, as is commonly the case with paraphilias, has little insight into the deeper motivations for his urges and behaviors:

> *I enjoy spanking women! I feel that most women not only need, but in their deep subconscious mind WANT a man to spank them. The problem is that far too many females have been brainwashed by the feminists into thinking that if they meet a man's needs then something is wrong with them.*

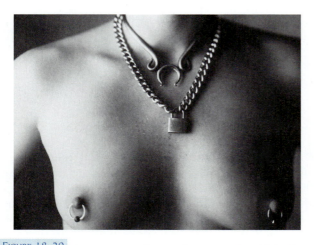

FIGURE 18-20   A strong sexual attraction to people with body piercings, tattoos, and scars is called "stigmatophilia."

> *How can I help a woman understand that a little game playing can be a healthy expression of human emotion? The male drive is to dominate and the female drive is to be the object of attention. To spank the bottom of a woman, and then caress her is such an exciting thing that I fail to see why the women I know are afraid to really let themselves go and find release of passion. I'd like any advice you can give me on dealing with women who want to be spanked but who do not want to admit they want and/or need a good spanking.*
>
> —REINISCH, 1990,162

While this individual is unlikely to be able to convince a woman to participate in his preferred sexual activities, some troubling issues are raised in this passage. First, this man seems very comfortable in making sweeping generalizations about what "all" men and women "really" want sexually. It is an enormous leap of logic to presume that all women secretly desire to be spanked. Second, his perceptions of the influence of feminism on female sexuality are utter nonsense. Finally, his pronouncements about male and female sex drives are highly personal and idiosyncratic and are offered here only as a justification for his own erotic preferences. While the sadomasochistic contract *may* bear some similarity to his speculations, these generalizations are by no means true of most people most of the time.

Following is another example of a person's perplexity and curiosity about the public manifestation of exhibitionism. Presumably, the person who wrote this is a woman. It conveys some of the anxiety that the lay public often experience when confronted by a "flasher."

> *Yesterday a man exhibited himself to me on the bus. I was terrified and couldn't sleep because I was convinced he had followed me home and would break into my apartment. When I asked the landlady if anyone had been hanging around and told her why, she laughed about it and said I didn't have to worry about men who did that. I can't believe that a man who did what he did isn't dangerous.*
>
> —REINISCH, 1990, 163

As discussed earlier, it is extremely unusual for an exhibitionist to engage in the behaviors this woman worries about. Most exhibitionists want to surprise their victim and derive their primary sexual gratification from doing so, not attempting to have sexual relations with them. But it is not unusual for the public to be uninformed or misinformed about exhibitionists, resulting in anxiety. Although the man who did this may not be dangerous, he is nonetheless behaving in an offensive way that should not be minimized. This is one reason for laws against indecent exposure.

The lay public also has little understanding of what motivates a person to make obscene telephone calls. Here is an example of a common strategy employed by those who use the telephone as a vehicle for their paraphilia:

> *I had a phone call from a man who said he was a doctor doing research for The Kinsey Institute. He asked me very intimate questions and I told him things I have never even told my husband. I told a friend about the interview and she said I'd better check with you because he might be some kind of weirdo. Now I'm scared. Does this man work for you?*
>
> —REINISCH, 1990, 164

Dr. Reinisch emphatically noted that the Kinsey Institute does not collect information on the telephone. In fact, we are aware of no reputable sex researcher who does so. Yet men with this paraphilia have persistent and distracting thoughts about making telephone calls that focus on sexual activities and are powerfully aroused when doing so. Like exhibitionists, men who do this almost never make a second call, and it is even more rare for them to even attempt any personal contact. If you ever receive such a telephone call, hang up as soon as you realize something inappropriate is going on. Because of "caller ID" devices that reveal the identity and telephone number of callers, obscene telephone calls have diminished significantly.

The earlier discussion of fetishism focused primarily on men who find women's undergarments and clothing erotically exciting and fondle them, stare at them, or incorporate them into their masturbatory behaviors. But almost anything associated with a woman has the potential to become the object of a fetish. Here is a rather interesting example, also from The Kinsey Institute:

> *I am a male of 34 years. This will be a strange one for you. Ever since I was 6 or older, a woman's hair has given me fascination and sexual arousements. I took hair styling for a few months. But quit because when the girls young or old came in and wanted their long hair cut short, it gave me an erection. I wanted to cut it, then didn't want to cut it, at different times, so I quit.*
>
> *Just the thought of a girl sitting in the chair after I have the cape on, I pile the hair up and clip it, then let it down. It's beautiful hair, then she says cut it off short. It gives me an erection. What's going on here? Am I crazy or queer?*
>
> —REINISCH, 1990, 166

When someone doesn't understand about paraphilias, urges and thoughts like those just described are indeed puzzling. Of course, what we don't know, in this brief passage, is whether this is the only way in which this individual can become erect, serving as a substitute for normal sexual intercourse. Still, this man is clearly preoccupied by his attraction to cutting women's hair. The last question he raises is an interesting one. Just as the general population may not know much about paraphilias, they are often similarly uninformed about homosexuality.

The last example here of the impact of a paraphilia on interpersonal behavior concerns a very rare deviation, *acrotomophilia*, which involves powerful feelings of erotic arousal for sexual partners who have lost a limb. This example suggests that there are an enormous variety of ways in which sexual feelings can become associated with highly unusual objects and circumstances.

> *I lost my leg in an auto accident at age 16 and, until recently, had assumed that no man would ever find me attractive. I am now happily married, but uncertain about my husband's behavior. I know about other types of fetishes and wonder if that's what's going on.*
>
> *My husband seems fascinated by my stump, as though it is sexually a plus. (In my eyes, my stump looks grotesque.) My husband cannot explain what is behind this, but a friend who is also an amputee told me her husband is that way too.*
>
> *We've been calling it our "fringe benefit" for losing legs, and it's a small consolation that helps make life a little more bearable. Still, we are very curious as to what is behind this attraction.*
>
> —REINISCH, 1990, 168

Little is known about people with this paraphilia, but there is some suggestion that they first become aware of this attraction during adolescence; we are not sure if there are common etiological factors in the development of this sexual preference. This anecdote raises an interesting question. Do these men become attracted to others who have had amputations *because* of their disability, or does interest in the stump follow upon an already established, "solid" relationship? We are not certain of the answer but strongly suspect the former.

Although little cases do not exemplify all the paraphilias we have discussed, they show something about the impact of a sexual deviation on a person's lifestyle and relationships. People with paraphilias are rarely entirely isolated from normal human bonds and interactions. A subtle issue in these examples is that these individuals typically have to establish a great deal of trust with another before revealing their paraphilia and how it affects them.

Contact Among People With the Same Paraphilia

Until recent years, contact among people with the same paraphilia was far more difficult and dangerous than it is today. With increasing liberalization and freedom of the press, a variety of magazines, newspapers, and newsletters that focus on the interests of individuals with a specific paraphilia have become numerous and popular. With the exception of laws against the manufacture, distribution, and possession of child pornography, there are few legal restrictions on materials related to most paraphilias. One prominent feature of these publications is personal ads that may facilitate people getting together to explore their paraphilias, although many paraphilias involve highly solitary, private activities. Additionally, an increasing number of websites and chat rooms make it much easier for people with similar sexual tastes to quickly find one another and get together if they desire. There are always inherent dangers in meeting people this way, as discussed in an earlier chapter. Bars in urban areas cater to those with some paraphilic interests, such as sexual sadism and sexual masochism. There is an implicit understanding about who is welcome in these places, and curious outsiders are sometimes politely but plainly informed that they are not welcome. There seems to be a delicate etiquette for meeting others and exploring the possibility of intimate contact. For example, in some bars there is an understanding that men who wear a large key ring on their left hip are interested in sexual sadism, while those who wear their keys on their right hip are interested in sexual masochism. State and local statutes may be more or less tolerant of these establishments, as long as overt public expressions of sexuality, violence, and excessive alcohol consumption or the use of other illicit drugs are not involved, and patrons are typically left alone.

Through these various avenues of communication these individuals also reinforce one another and perhaps reassure themselves that they are still productive citizens despite their private sexual preferences. Any stigmatized minority often gain safety and consolation by sharing their feelings and fears with other similar individuals.

"SEXUAL ADDICTION"

The word "addiction" usually is used to describe psychological and/or physiological or metabolic dependency on a drug, such as alcohol or cocaine. Another aspect of an addiction is increasing tolerance, in which progressively larger amounts of the substance have to be used to attain the same (usually pleasurable) feelings. The term "sexual addiction" is surrounded by much controversy, and there is by no means uniform agreement among social, behavioral, and medical scientists that sexual addiction is a legitimate "addiction." While many people may be frequently preoccupied with sexual thoughts and fantasies, this is not the same as sexual addiction. Abundant reports in the scholarly literature point to the possibility that pursuing sexual partners and consummating a sexual interaction can become a compulsive and sometimes uncontrollable behavior pattern, similar to what occurs with drug addictions. There is also discussion whether such a sexual addiction may be a paraphilia.

Although people who are apparently addicted to sex typically engage in heterosexual intercourse with consenting adults in private places, it is the persistent, compulsive, and some would say uncontrollable nature of their sexual appetites that prove most troubling. As is commonly the case with the paraphilias, the sought object of these sexual urges becomes an object independent of whatever personal attributes (usually she) might possess. She may be only the target of the addict's sexual compulsion. Sexual addictions can hurt or destroy marriages, relationships, friendships, job performance, and job permanence. Sexual addiction is similar to paraphilias because of the objectified nature of the sexual partner as well as the subjective inner turmoil that frequently accompanies the compulsive nature of these behaviors and the ultimately unsatisfying nature of feelings following these sexual activities.

The important element in this behavior pattern is the apparent lack of control over one's sexual urges and behaviors. We earlier defined an obsession as uncontrollably recurrent thoughts, and compulsions as uncontrollably recurrent behaviors. It can be argued that sexual addiction has both of these attributes. Sexual addicts are *always* looking for an opportunity to make a new conquest, and when they discover a receptive, willing individual they never hesitate to engage in sexual activities with them. The uncontrollable nature of these urges and behaviors often overrides any potentially negative consequences of the sexual activity. For example, sex addicts are typically not dissuaded by the possibility of being discovered by their partner's spouse, the chances of being found out by their own spouse or partner, the possibility of an unanticipated pregnancy, the likelihood of acquiring HIV or another sexually transmitted disease, or the chances of losing their job.

Patrick Carnes' book *Out of the Shadows* (1992) offers an excellent, concise summary of the issues surrounding sexual addiction. Carnes suggests that there is an "addiction cycle" that describes a person's experiences as they become progressively more entrenched in an addictive lifestyle, and these feelings get stronger the longer she or he is engaged in these activities:

1. *Preoccupation*—the trance or mood wherein the addicts' minds are completely engrossed with thoughts of sex. This mental state creates an obsessive search for sexual stimulation.
2. *Ritualization*—the addicts' own special routines which lead up to the sexual behavior. The ritual intensifies the preoccupation, adding arousal and excitement.
3. *Compulsive sexual behavior*—the actual sex act, which is the end goal of the preoccupation and ritualization. Sexual addicts are unable to control or stop this behavior.
4. *Despair*—the feeling of utter hopelessness addicts have about their behavior and their powerlessness.
   —Carnes, 1992, 9

These four stages raise an interesting issue. Do similar stages occur with other paraphilias? We know of no systematic clinical or empirical examination of this question.

Carnes suggested that there are varying degrees of immersion in this behavior pattern and that a number of different behaviors may be associated with each one. For example, he asserts that addictive preoccupations and behaviors concern not only heterosexual intercourse but may ultimately involve the compulsive use of pornography, frequent masturbation, homosexual experimentation, visiting prostitutes, and other paraphilias such as exhibitionism, voyeurism, making obscene telephone calls, and child molestation. In other words, the sex addict's drive seems to be an *uncontrollable, diffuse expression of eroticism*. However, most instances of sexual addictions are primarily concerned with heterosexual erotic behaviors and intercourse. Carnes suggested that the mental life of the sex addict is characterized by four core beliefs:

1. Self-image: I am basically a bad, unworthy person.
2. Relationships: No one would love me as I am.
3. Needs: My needs are never going to be met if I have to depend on others.
4. Sexuality: Sex is my most important need.
   —Carnes, 1992, 120

Addictions, whether physiological or behavioral, are difficult to break. One of the more successful strategies may be the philosophy and methods of the Twelve Steps of Alcoholics Anonymous, which Carnes adapted for sex addicts. While some are uncomfortable with the spiritual element of 12-step programs, many people find this ingredient genuinely helpful and supportive. As of this writing, we are not unaware of any systematic data that demonstrate the effectiveness of a 12-step program for sex addicts.

Because of the gradual liberalization of the media with respect to sexuality, other writers have suggested other versions of the clinical manifestations of sexual addiction. Levin (1998) adapted the *DSM-IV* criteria for an addiction for sexual addictions. The *DSM-IV* includes no diagnostic category dealing solely with sexual addiction, but Levin applied the criteria for addictions in general to sexual addictions. According to Levin, there are 11 criteria for a diagnosis of sexual addiction:

1. Repeated sexual activity resulting in a failure to fulfill major role obligations at work, school, or home.
2. Sexual activity in potentially dangerous situations.
3. Repeated sex-related legal problems.
4. Continued sexual activity despite persistent or recurrent social or interpersonal problems.
5. Tolerance.
6. Withdrawal.
7. Larger amounts of sexual activity over longer periods of time than originally intended.
8. An enduring desire to control sexual activity and simultaneous failed attempts to do so.
9. Increased time spent in activities necessary to obtain sexual activity and/or to recover from its effects.

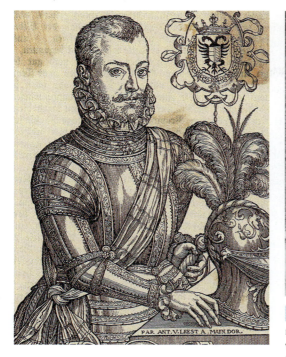
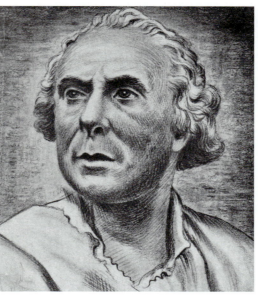

FIGURE 18-21   Left: Don Juan. Right: Casanova. These two historical figures are renown for their many sexual exploits and the women they seduced. Don Juan was a fictional character and a symbol of libertinism who was introduced in a Spanish drama in 1630. Casanova was an Italian adventurer who lived from 1725 to 1798.

10. Decreased social, occupational, or recreational activities directly related to sexual activity.

11. Continued sexual activity despite knowledge of persistent or recurrent physical or psychological problems that are caused or exacerbated by the activity.

—Levin, 1998, 27–28

In the thinking of both Carnes and Levin, sexual addicts often have serious problems in their relationships and jobs, frequently experience significant personal distress, and still may have little insight into the nature of their addiction, its causes, or its consequences.

Historically, other terms have been used to refer to sexual addiction or compulsive sexual activity. Among the most common are "nymphomania" (referring to woman) and Don Juanism (referring to men) (Fig. 18-21). These syndromes are usually considered similar. According to the American Psychiatric Association Glossary (cited in Shainess, 1997), nymphomania involves "abnormal and excessive needs or desire for sexual intercourse in the female . . . most nymphomaniacs, if not all, fail to achieve orgasm in the sexual act." Similarly, Don Juanism is a "compulsive or anxiety-ridden sexual overactivity in males." The term "satyriasis" is also used, and this implies "pathologic or exaggerated sexual desire or excitement in the male - analogous to nymphomania" (Shainess, 1997, p. 57). Shainess makes a subtle but very important distinction among these terms. She emphasizes that both nymphomania and Don Juanism are focused primarily on the activities related to sexual seduction, while satyriasis

has as its central defining feature frequent sexual intercourse. Another subtle issue is the "double standard" we have discussed elsewhere in this book. Since males may be socialized to believe that it is normal and healthy to desire and have many sexual partners, this seems to make Don Juanism a less serious problem than nymphomania, because women are often socialized to be far more sexually discriminating and to desire few or only one sexual partner.

When considering whether sexual addictions are genuine psychological problems falling into a group of disorders that include the paraphilias, investigators have sought to define a unitary clinical syndrome in which those afflicted are very similar with respect to their common "problem." However, people who report that they struggle with compulsive sexual urges may in fact be a highly diversified group of individuals. For example, Black, Kehrberg, Flumerfelt, and Schlosser (1997) carried out an in-depth study of 36 individuals who openly acknowledged that they had a problem, and sometimes a longstanding problem, with compulsive sexual behavior. This sample included 28 men and 8 women. After these volunteers completed several paper-and-pencil psychological tests, each was interviewed in depth. What was most interesting about these subjects was the fact that *several other psychological problems often accompanied their compulsive sexual urges.* Fourteen of these subjects reported a history of depression, 15 said that they have suffered from phobias, and 23 revealed that they had engaged in substance abuse in the past. Additionally, personality disorders were commonly found in these subjects. In some cases, the compulsive sexual behavior was manifest in cross-dressing, and other subjects reported a compelling desire to masturbate frequently. The basic conclusion of this study is that it is too simplistic to try to characterize the "typical" sexual addict because so many other psychological problems may be involved. One might assume that other paraphilias also may be accompanied by similar personality disorders.

TREATING PARAPHILIAS

The following sections examine the potential benefits and pitfalls of three broad approaches to the treatment of the paraphilias: the psychodynamic approach, cognitive-behavioral approaches, and biological-medical treatments.

Psychodynamic Approaches to Therapy for the Paraphilias

Recall that psychodynamic theories deal with the development of emotions and their impact on adult behavior. The British psychiatrist Anthony Storr (1970) offered a psychodynamic perspective on the development of paraphilias. He believes that individuals with paraphilias have strong feelings of sexual guilt and sexual inferiority and that a better understanding of the factors that give rise to these emotions can be helpful in therapy. Storr points out that few adults reared in Western civilizations can entirely escape sexual guilt, and he believes that the normal family is the source of much of this guilt. Very few people grow up in a home where caretakers openly praise expressions of sexuality or say anything positive about it (Storr, 1970, p. 21). His own experience as a therapist has taught Storr that most adults who seek help for a paraphilia were extremely impressionable as children and tend to be both withdrawn and unsociable as adults. As a result, they often fabricate a vivid fantasy world that serves as a substitute for any genuine intimacy with another adult. Most of us gradually get rid of this guilt as we become adults and establish relationships with others, but those who develop sexual deviations do not, and their sexual value system is focused primarily on their inner fantasies rather than their adult relationships. A fantasy can't refuse or rebuke you; it is available at will and you can determine its contents in the most minute detail. Storr believes that this profound inability to initiate and maintain a genuine, adult sexual relationship is a result of leftover childhood sexual guilt.

For Storr, the psychological consequence of sexual guilt is a sense of sexual inferiority—the feeling that somehow one is deficient, flawed, or inadequate. Storr notes that adults with paraphilias have not really learned to adopt contemporary versions of male and female roles. In psychodynamic terms, this is a failure in "identification," the subconscious desire to become like someone whom we love, admire, or respect. Storr notes that in his clinical practice, adults with paraphilias do not feel that they have had an adult sexual role model of their own gender. When therapists explore the paraphiliac's inner sexual fantasies, they usually find unresolved childhood emo-

tional issues coupled with ambiguous thoughts and dreams about the future.

Travin and Protter (1993) summarized the assumptions and methods involved in psychodynamic approaches to the treatment of paraphilias. They emphasize that some of Freud's initial speculations about sexual deviations have required revision throughout the 20th century. For example, Freud believed that while neurotic patients repress their unconscious conflicts and wait for the therapist to uncover and discuss them, the paraphiliac instead represses nothing but acts on his or her subconscious motives. The client, from this perspective, stands to gain very little by surrendering behaviors that have come to have highly rewarding qualities. More recent advances in psychodynamic thinking have sought to come to a better understanding of the meaning of the patient's deviant behavior and its place in that person's whole personality. Travin and Protter emphasized that the psychotherapist offers the client a "corrective emotional experience" (p. 139) and can refashion many of the individual's older, distorted thoughts, fantasies, and urges. In this therapeutic process the therapist comes to represent an adult with a well-integrated personality and a capacity for impulse control, frustration tolerance, and the ability to delay gratifications. Such a role model is thought to be of great importance in facilitating change in the client. Remember, in this model of therapy the client's enhanced self-awareness is thought to have powerful curative value.

Modern psychodynamic therapists often utilize a group therapy approach, one never explored by Freud himself, and it is now thought that this avenue of assistance may have some very special and powerful benefits for the client. Members of a therapeutic group can directly confront the client and not allow him or her to use denial or rationalization to avoid taking responsibility for their actions. Group members can also emphasize the exploitative, dangerous, and sometimes frankly illegal nature of their actions. Very often, the paraphiliac's open revelations are a good source of information, which can then become the focus of further therapy sessions. Finally, Travin and Protter noted that contrary to traditional Freudian methods, psychodynamic therapists today are becoming more directive in an attempt to change behaviors more quickly. This is especially important when the client's behaviors have involved sexual offenses that have come to the attention of law enforcement authorities.

As of this writing, we are unaware of research using large, randomly selected samples of individuals with paraphilias that reveal the relative effectiveness of psychodynamic therapies in comparison with other therapeutic approaches. But we are reminded of Freud's own belief that while psychoanalysis may not necessarily cure you or make you feel any better, it will help you to better understand your problematic behaviors and why they frequently involve genuine human misery. Some insight is better than none and may perhaps serve as the foundation for gradual behavioral change and improved psychological well-being.

Cognitive-Behavioral Approaches to Therapy for the Paraphilias

Recall that one of the basic premises behind behavioral approaches to human nature is the fact that human beings have the capacity to learn from the consequences of their actions and to make necessary adjustments in their behavior accordingly. While this is a bit simplistic, it is generally true. Travin and Protter (1993, pp. 141-147) also summarized the nature of cognitive-behavioral approaches to the treatment of the paraphilias, described in the following sections.

SELF-CONTROL TECHNIQUES

For a long time behavioral scientists had very little understanding of how people acquired will-power and self-control. We now know that these apparently important skills can be *learned*. People can acquire will-power and self-control when they are reinforced for doing so. Techniques called "thought-shifting" and "thought-stopping" can be very effective in an individual's attempts to distract him- or herself when engaged in deviant thoughts, fantasies, and urges. These are wilful strategies in which an individual practices deliberately changing the focus of their thoughts or stopping them altogether. Sometimes the client may be asked to keep a personal journal that describes the circumstances under which they begin to have deviant thoughts and the ways in which they were able to interrupt them. One of the most important things about these self-control techniques is the fact that the client no longer feels at the mercy of their urges but can instead play an active role in completely re-focusing their thoughts. They gradually come to better understand their cravings and the stimuli that seem to elicit them.

STRESS MANAGEMENT

As noted earlier, stresses can trigger deviant thoughts, fantasies, and urges. Therefore, some cognitive-behavioral therapists have reasoned that if the person can be taught techniques to control, minimize, and eliminate such stressors, ultimately they will be successful in refraining from becoming obsessed with deviant thoughts. These techniques can be used to help people assess the reality of ideas and threats that in fact may be entirely irrational. In some cases, the client is taught relaxation techniques that allow them to remain calm and focused when they feel besieged by provocative environmental stimuli. Ultimately, for stress management techniques to be successful, they must be both *emotion focused* and *problem focused*. That is, the client needs to recognize the distinction between eliminating problems that cause stress and managing the feelings evoked by stress. When both of these are done, stress management techniques are likely to be highly effective.

COGNITIVE RESTRUCTURING

Counselors and therapists now know with certainty that they can help their clients recognize irrational thought patterns and distorted thinking and eliminate these counterproductive mental habits. Such distortions allow the para-philiac to be less than honest with themselves about the nature and repercussions of their actions and to deny its deviant nature and the fact that it may exploit others. Clients commonly diminish the significance of their behaviors in their own minds, and the therapist can disabuse them of their self-deception. Sometimes paraphiliacs genuinely believe that they have been provoked into a demonstration of deviant behavior by the very individual who is victimized by it. When the therapist can strip the client of these illusions and deceptions, they have made an important first step in altering the thinking processes that compulsively govern deviant behaviors.

SOCIAL REHABILITATIVE TECHNIQUES

The word "rehabilitate" means to "restore," and these techniques have as their objective the restoration of normal forms of social and sexual interaction. For example, clients may receive systematic instruction in learning to better assess the impact of their emotions and actions on others as well as explore their basic assumptions about what constitutes normal human relationships. Travin and Protter emphasize that paraphiliacs need to learn better skills concerning sexual communication and various socially acceptable ways of initiating and maintaining intimate relationships with an appropriate partner. The client may be asked to model or role-play different scenarios that have in the past precipitated erotic thoughts and fantasies. Special attention is given to maladaptive and exploitative ways of behaving and to changing these to actions with a more respectful, reciprocal nature. This may take many therapeutic sessions.

SEX EDUCATION

Finally, Travin and Protter point out that in many cases, paraphiliacs have very little basic knowledge about human sexuality, especially human sexual arousal and response. Often a paraphiliac has a sexual dysfunction that they do not understand and that may contribute to feelings of sexual guilt and sexual inferiority. As Storr (1970) noted, these often play a major contributing role in the development and expression of the deviant sexual behavior.

As classical and operant learning paradigms are fundamental to behavioral approaches to learning and behavior change, they too are used in therapies for paraphilias. One type of learning experiment attempts to eliminate certain behaviors from an animal's repertoire by pairing those behaviors (and presumably the thoughts and feelings that accompany them) with aversive (painful) stimuli. Although aversive conditioning experiments have been used to try to change a wide variety of human behaviors, such as for smoking cessation and in attempts to "change" a person's sexual orientation from homosexual to heterosexual, these are no longer felt to be either effective or humane and in some cases may even be unethical. One such investigation attempted to treat sexual deviations through the use of electrical shock paired with pictures depicting paraphilic behaviors

(Callahan & Leitenberg, 1973). In a limited investigation of 6 subjects in a clinical setting, an attempt was made to diminish or eliminate sexual arousal when these individuals were presented with 5 erotic slides that depicted deviant sexual practices and 2 erotic slides illustrating common heterosexual practices. Of the 6 subjects in this study, 2 were exhibitionists, 1 a transvestic-fetishist, 2 homosexuals, and 1 a pedophilic homosexual. This study was published in 1973, a time when homosexuality was believed to be a sexual deviation and behavioral therapy was administered to individuals with diverse paraphilias.

Each subject had a penile plethysmograph affixed to his penis to measure changes in the circumference (and by inference, erection) in response to the erotic visual stimuli, each of which was presented for a little over 2 minutes. Electrodes attached to the subject's right hand delivered brief, tolerable shocks when penile responses reached 15% of full erectile dimensions. The shocks lasted from 0.1 to 0.5 seconds and were evaluated by these volunteers as ranging between "pain" and "tolerance." The results of this study revealed that this aversive conditioning procedure involving shock paired with sexual arousal was relatively ineffective in diminishing sexual arousal. A single therapeutic procedure is not likely to be equally effective in treating all subjects, many of whom demonstrated highly variable patterns of deviant sexual behavior, and the impact of multiple procedures remains uncertain. Also, the sample size was far too small to allow for valid, predictive generalizations. Although behavioral techniques can be highly effective in altering many types of human behavior, it remains unclear as to whether they are clinically effective in the treatment of paraphilias.

Biological/Medical Approaches to the Treatment of Paraphilias

Our society has grown used to the idea of taking a pill to feel better, cure disease, or alter how we react to people and events in our environments. The same is true with the treatment of paraphilic behaviors. To the degree that paraphilias are accompanied by obsessions and compulsive behaviors, there is a medical rationale for treating them with medications effective for these psychological problems. Some researchers believe that paraphilias are best understood as behaviors on an obsessive-compulsive continuum. Kruesi, Fine, Valladares, Phillips, and Rapoport (1992) studied a small sample of paraphiliacs who volunteered to be in a study on the effects of antidepressant agents on the intrusive nature of paraphilic thoughts, fantasies, and urges. Their subjects were exhibitionists, fetishists, transvestites, and obscene telephone callers. Two engaged in compulsive masturbation. Of the 15 subjects in this study, 10 reported engaging in two or more paraphilic behaviors during the previous 6 months. Subjects received daily doses of two common antidepressant agents that have been effective in the treatment of obsessive-compulsive disorder, clomipramine and desipramine. Both drugs seemed to diminish the severity of paraphilic preoccupations when compared with the subjects' pre-treatment reports. This was a double-blind study in which neither the subject nor the person administering the drugs knew which drug the patient was receiving or whether a placebo was being dispensed. It would be unwise to recommend pharmacological treatment for paraphilias based on this very small study, but the rationale for using these drugs is legitimate, and further research is needed in this area. These data are suggestive but require replication.

Kafka (1997c) suggested that brain neurotransmitters called monoamines may be involved in the compulsive behaviors frequently occurring in paraphiliacs and that altering monoamine brain chemistry may have beneficial therapeutic effects in treating sexual deviations. Common monoamines include norepinephrine, dopamine, and serotonin. Kafka points out that these agents seem to play a powerful role in impulsive sexual behaviors, anxiety, depression, compulsive behaviors, and antisocial sexual activities, and that altering monoamine concentrations in the brain may lessen or eliminate these difficulties in humans. Still, it is not yet clear whether drugs that alter monoamines in the brain are ultimately effective in treating individuals with paraphilias. One research team investigated the effects in paraphiliacs of three antidepressants (Luvox, Prozac, and Zoloft) that alter serotonin activity in the brain (Greenberg, Bradford, Curry, & O'Rourke, 1996). In a sample of 58 subjects, most volunteers reported a marked reduction in the number of sexual fantasies they experienced as well as in their persistence and distractability. Any effects of these drugs in fostering more "normal" sexual functioning were not addressed in this study. No significant differences were found among these drugs in therapeutic effectiveness. These drugs have been used in the treatment of other compulsive habits such as gambling with marked success. Clearly, drug therapies may indeed be of some genuine benefit in the treatment of paraphilias, although such therapy would ideally be supplemented by counseling or psychotherapy.

Recall from our earlier discussion of gender that various hormones can have powerful effects on sex drive and that their absence can have similarly dramatic effects diminishing sexual interest and behavior. This has been used as a therapeutic approach in the treatment of paraphilias. Rosler and Witztum (1998) explored the impact of a long-acting chemical version of gonadotropin-releasing hormone on paraphilic behaviors in men. This particular chemical agent decreases the pituitary gland's stimulation of a man's testes, thus diminishing the output of testosterone, a hormone intimately involved in a man's sex drive. These researchers suggested that diminished sex drive in men with paraphilias might decrease their propensity to engage in deviant behaviors. In an investigation involving 30 men with a serious, longstanding history of paraphilia, primarily pedophilia, monthly injections of this hormone blocker were administered in conjunction with regular therapy sessions for up to 42 consecutive months. These hormone-blocker injections caused a profound decrease in blood levels of testosterone. All subjects in this study reported a marked decrease in the number of fantasies and urges they experienced; indeed, the combination of the hormone blocker and therapy virtually eliminated all such fantasies and urges. This treatment entirely eliminated all paraphilic behaviors for the duration of the combined drug and psychotherapy regimen. These therapeutic gains were obvious between 3 and 10 months of treatment and continued for the 1-year duration of the study. These authors did not report whether these subjects began to engage in more "normal" types of sexual thoughts, feelings, and behaviors.

All social and medical scientists do not, however, support or sanction the use of hormones to alter sexual thoughts, fantasies, and urges. Tsang (1995) cautioned investigators that using such drugs as Depo-Provera to alter the expression of paraphilic behaviors may represent an example of "social control" that may violate ethical scientific principles. This writer emphasized the importance of gaining the subject's informed consent, and described some of the side effects of the drug. This author cautions against chemically altering the sexual experience and expression of "sexual minorities." While we believe that these concerns are important, our analysis of the primary literature failed to reveal any substantive abuses of this treatment strategy, and worries about the activities of "mad scientists" do not seem justified at this time. Ultimately, the therapeutic effects of such agents must, of course, be weighed against any unpleasant side effects. Yet in the treatment of paraphilias, the benefits to society of a particular therapeutic approach are as important as these ethical and medical considerations. As with behavioral therapies, the effectiveness of medical treatments requires much further research.

Sociological Approaches to Therapy for the Paraphilias

Although the psychological and medical approaches to treatment of paraphilias involve specific methods, sociological perspectives are more general. As of this writing, there is no coherent social-environmental approach to the treatment of sexual deviations, except for imprisonment to prevent repeated sex offenses. We are unaware of any sociologically based theories dealing with treatments for paraphiliacs who are not sex offenders. Such a theory would likely require broad permanent changes in the entire culture, and this is unfeasible.

WOMEN AND PARAPHILIAS

Almost all the sexual paraphilias we have discussed involve males. While a few pedophiles are women, the great majority are men. In those few cases in which paraphilias have been noted in women, it has typically been within the context of sex offenders. Extremely little is known about women who might have a paraphilia not involving sex offenses.

In a review of sexual deviation among women, Hunter and Mathews (1997) noted that in recent years researchers have become more aware of female child molestation and that these behaviors frequently begin in adolescence and involve family members and friends but almost never strangers. The adult manifestations of female child molestation are less likely to involve force or coercion than male child molestation. There is also some suggestion that adult women who engage in these activities frequently do so together with a male co-offender. Among adolescent females who have been involved in these activities, a small percentage (about 15%) have also engaged in exhibitionistic activities, and a very small number (about 3%) have made obscene telephone calls. Generally very little is known about women with paraphilias that do not involve child molestation.

CONCLUSION

This chapter discusses a wide variety of highly unusual sexual tastes and behaviors. Most involve solitary activities or consenting adults in private places. However, the darker side of aberrant sexual tastes and practices involves coercion, exploitation, and abuse. The next chapter explores many of these issues. Sexual abuse is discussed in more detail, along with other unsavory ways in which people are "used" sexually or use others. This discussion includes rape, pornography, and prostitution as well. While these aspects of human sexuality involve issues remote from love, intimacy, and nurturance, they are a prominent part of the sexual scene in every culture.

*L*earning Activities

1. Often we emphasize the importance of privacy and the inappropriateness of coercion in sexual behavior. Describe how these criteria bear on how society decides what is normal and what is atypical sexually.

2. "Caller ID" devices display the telephone number of the calling party. When people receive obscene telephone calls, do you think they usually explore legal means of identifying and prosecuting the caller. If so, why? If not, why not?

3. Explain how the advertising and film industries may foster voyeuristic tendencies in individuals who would otherwise deny any such inclinations.

4. Many transvestites claim that a particularly arousing aspect of their cross-dressing rituals involves the feeling that they are fooling men into thinking they actually are women. How would you respond to the discovery that you had been deceived?

5. When individuals participate in rare, bizarre, or highly unconventional paraphilias, do you think they have any guilt, shame, or self-depreciation about their actions? Or are the reinforcing aspects of their behavior so powerful that these feelings would not occur?

6. Explain the relationship between a "bad habit" and an addiction in light of the recent cultural emphasis on the great variety of addictions (e.g., drugs, alcohol, gam-

bling, compulsive overeating, compulsive sexual behavior) to which we are supposedly vulnerable.

7. Speculate on some of the biological, psychological, or social influences that might predispose more males than females to develop atypical sexual preferences and behaviors.

8. What factors might encourage a person to seek therapy for a paraphilia on his own, without the direction or intervention of the judicial system?

9. Give some examples of unusual sexual behaviors that many people engage in from time to time but that would not be considered "deviant."

10. Has a partner ever suggested or strongly encouraged a type of sexual behavior with which you felt more or less "forced" to comply? Did you indicate any hesitancy or misgivings? If so, how were these received by your partner?

11. In early August of 1991, Milwaukee police entered Apartment 213 in the Oxford Apartments on the city's west side. Within, they found a freezer covered with photographs of mutilated human corpses. Inside the freezer were two severed heads, with another in the refrigerator. Closets and filing cabinets contained skulls and a large metal kettle with the remains of human hands and a penis. A variety of acids and chemical preservatives were present. This was the residence of Jeffrey L. Dahmer, who had just lost his job at a chocolate factory. The more police learned, the more terrible the tale became. Eleven murders were confirmed and another six suspected. There was ample evidence that Mr. Dahmer had sexual relations with his victims after he killed them.

- Speculate on formative life experiences that might have played a role in the development of this particular paraphilia.
- Is someone with a sexual fascination with corpses necessarily suffering from a psychological disorder?
- Do you think that psychotherapy might have been effective in helping Mr. Dahmer regain some semblance of normality and stop his sexual obsession with corpses? (Mr. Dahmer was later murdered in prison.)

*K*ey Concepts

- Atypical sexual behaviors do not conform to common avenues of intimate expression, but this term does not imply anything bizarre, illegal, or highly peculiar.
- Sexual variations are sexual behaviors sometimes enjoyed by "normal" people as a part of a diverse sexual repertoire.

- Because of discrepancies between the actual prevalence of sexual deviations and the reported prevalence, it is difficult to accurately determine how widespread these behaviors are in a society as a whole.
- Sexual deviations are not considered normal by society and may include behaviors that are frankly illegal, that involve coercion, that involve victimization, or that involve sexual expression in public places.
- The term "perversion" generally refers to deviant sexual behaviors that are preferred to normal sexual intercourse. Experts in human sexuality rarely use this term any more.
- A paraphilia involves persistent, strong sexual urges as well as highly distracting sexual fantasies. Paraphilias may involve erotic feelings for nonhuman objects, age-inappropriate sexual partners, unwilling or unconsenting adults, or the allure of punishment or humiliation and degradation as aspects of sexual activity.
- There are some interesting similarities between paraphilias and personality disorders. Both have their origins in the individual's childhood or adolescence. Both may develop through an individual's interactions with adults with paraphilias and personality disorders. Unrealistic interpersonal expectations and distorted thinking are also common to both.
- Various learning principles may be involved in the development of paraphilias. The principle of contiguity emphasizes that when two stimuli are consistently experienced together, one comes to be associated with the other. Reinforcements increase the probability of behaviors that precede them.
- The term sexual addiction refers to the fact that pursuing sexual partners and consummating sexual interactions can become a truly compulsive and sometimes uncontrollable behavior pattern.
- Psychodynamic, cognitive-behavioral, and biological/medical approaches are used in the treatment of paraphilias. It is difficult to determine the relative effectiveness of these three approaches to therapy.

*G*lossary Terms

asphyxiophilia	necrophilia	transvestism
coprophilia	pedophilia	troilism
exhibitionism	sexual	urophilia
fetishism	masochism	voyeurism
frotteurism	sexual sadism	zoophilia
("frottage")	stigmatophilia	(bestiality)
gerontophilia	telephone	
klismaphilia	scatologia	

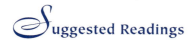
Suggested Readings

Bakos, S. C. (1995). Kink. New York: St. Martins Press.

Dailey, D. M. (Ed.). (1989). The sexually unusual: A guide to understanding and helping. Binghamton, NY: Haworth Press.

Goldberg, A. (1995). The problem of perversion: The view from self psychology. New Haven, CT: Yale University Press.

Henkin, W., & Holiday, S. (1996). Consensual sadomasochism. How to talk about it & how to do it safely. San Francisco, CA: Daedalus Publishing.

Money, J. (1989). Lovemaps. Clinical concepts of sexual-erotic health & pathology, paraphilia & gender transposition in childhood, adolescence, & maturity. New York: Irvington Publishers.

Skeen, D. (1991). Different sexual worlds. Contemporary case studies of sexuality. Lanham, MD: Lexington Books.

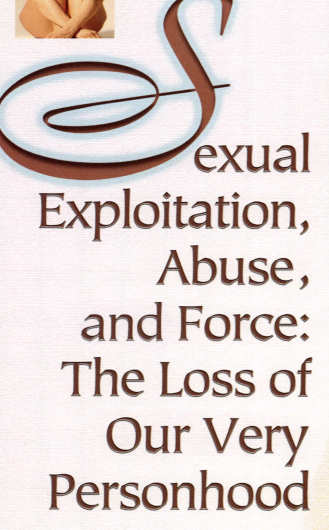

19

Sexual Exploitation, Abuse, and Force: The Loss of Our Very Personhood

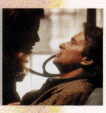

OBJECTIVES

When you finish reading and reviewing this chapter, you should be able to:

1. Discuss various meanings of the term "sexual consent," and summarize key perspectives on the origins of sexual abuse, exploitation, and coercion.

2. Describe the different settings in which prostitutes work.

3. Describe motives men have for visiting prostitutes and the types of sexual interactions they pay for.

4. Characterize common aspects of different types of pornographic materials, and discuss problems inherent in defining the term "obscenity."

5. Describe similarities and differences in how women and men react to pornography.

6. Define "sexual harassment" according to the United States Equal Employment Opportunity Commission (EEOC).

7. Describe the behaviors usually involved in the sexual abuse of children and the ways in which children react to these events.

8. Discuss the consequences of sexual abuse of both females and males.

9. Define "incest," describe its most common manifestations, and note its long-term impact on an individual.

10. Discuss various legal options for dealing with sex offenders, and comment on their ability to dissuade further sexually abusive behaviors.

11. Define "rape" and describe the frequency with which it occurs in American society.

12. Discuss motives men have for raping women, and note how these are expressed differently in the act of rape.

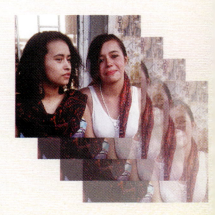

From Dr. Ruth

For most people, sex is an exciting and fulfilling way to share their lives with another person. The feelings of closeness and intimacy that go along with good sex are hard to find in other parts of our lives. Sex involves closeness and mutual respect that are aspects of a good relationship as well as acceptance in a loving way by another person.

But as you know, sex for some people involves abuse, exploitation, and harm — and it is now to these less happy aspects of human sexuality that we turn. No human sexuality textbook would be complete without examining ways people use and victimize others sexually, and this chapter might be one of the most important in terms of how you take care of yourself and maintain your sexual self-respect. Isn't it paradoxical that sex can be such a rewarding part of most people's lives while being something terrible, painful, and humiliating for others? Here you will read about pornography, prostitution, sexual harassment, sexual abuse, and rape.

If there is a key message in this chapter, it is that we all must learn to define our sexual value system and live comfortably with it. In this way we can do our best to avoid the kinds of manipulation, rudeness, and assault described in this chapter.

The last chapter explored some very unusual sexual inclinations and behaviors, many of which are classified as abnormal from a psychological or social perspective. This chapter focuses on behaviors our society has deemed illegal because they obviously infringe on the rights and well-being of others.

Some feel that some of the topics discussed in this chapter should not be against the law. For example, some have argued that prostitution is a "victimless crime" in which prostitutes and their clients mutually consent to engage in a variety of sexual activities for a fee. So why should this be illegal in most places? People who become prostitutes are often coerced to do so and continue to sell sex for money because they are drug dependent and cannot easily break out of a highly self-injurious life style. Similarly, while *consumers* of prostitution might be behaving in accordance with their own free will, the women, men, and, unhappily, children who are exploited are being victimized. This thread will run through the topics discussed in this chapter: in one way or another, they all involve some degree of coercion, exploitation, and victimization, even though this may not be immediately apparent. Because legal traditions throughout the world have their roots in the role of society for protecting people and their property, the subject matter of this chapter involves clear legal implications.

ISSUES OF CONSENT

Whenever sexual coercion, victimization, or exploitation occurs, there is usually a problem with consent. When it comes to sex, consent is more complicated than just voluntary agreement or permission. Sex educators have emphasized the central role of communication in sexual consent (Haffner, 1995). For sexual consent to occur, two people have to talk clearly about their expectations, responsibilities, and wishes. However, the Sexuality and Education Council of the United States has emphasized that this kind of communication might not mean much when the media constantly presents the message that the most exciting and fulfilling sexual experiences happen spontaneously, when we "lose our heads" and are carried away with the romantic or lustful feelings of the moment. Sex educators therefore generally believe that true consent implies genuine verbal communication of a highly specific and personal nature.

Throughout the legal history of our country, experts have had various ideas about how old a person has to be in order to give consent to engage in sexual activities, and there is still some degree of variability from state to state in this country today and some debate regarding inflexible definitions of sexual consent. Elshtain (1998) has noted that, "Consent carries with it the presupposition that an individual is capable of making up his or her own mind and of being responsible for his or her behavior" (p. 8). As straightforward as this definition might seem, many so-called adults still have a very poor understanding of the consequences of their behavior. Still, children are almost universally believed to be incapable of offering informed consent to sexual relations, and even when those who are supposed to be legally competent to make such a decision at the age of about 16, we must remember that what is legal is not always a good idea, nor does it reflect an ability to fully consider the consequences of one's behaviors. Elshtain emphasizes that the term "consent" has a narrow legal meaning, and although a person may knowingly enter into sexual relations with another, this does not mean that consent is based on "wisdom, decency, discretion, fairness, maturity, and judgment" (p. 9). What may legally justify an action may not fully explain its morality.

William N. Eskridge (1995) offered a thorough discussion of sexual consent from a legal point of view. While the standard of his argument happens to be the laws of the State of Virginia, each of these points is relevant in most other states and similar statutes may be found throughout the United States. His analysis is relevant to much of the content of this chapter. In general, consent is dependent upon "the identities of the parties, their relationship, and precisely what form of intercourse takes place" (p. 49).

Eskridge notes that "Consent [is] negated by serious physical injury, physical coercion, or economic inducement" (pp. 49-50). He further notes that consent does not have anything to do with the nature of sexual activity which takes place

(e.g., oral sex, anal sex, or oral-anal stimulation), and is negated if one of the parties is under a specific age (usually 16), is a non-human animal, or was persuaded to have intercourse because of a mental disability. In simple terms, just saying "yes" to sexual activity may not be consensual under certain well-defined circumstances in a state's legal code.

In a sense, sexual exploitation and victimization may be defined indirectly in terms of the lack of consent involved. Is it possible to be too careful about how sexual consent is defined? In the early 1990s, Antioch College in Ohio (see display) instituted a policy that required men or women to ask for, and the other person to consent to or decline to consent, progressively more intimate behaviors in their interactions with one another (Grenier, 1993). In fact, the college held workshops so that all students had a clear understanding of what was considered consensual sexually.

Issues surrounding consent present an interesting question: "Do women who are the victims of sexual exploitation give off subtle cues that they are vulnerable to coercion?"

ANTIOCH COLLEGE'S POLICY ON CONSENSUAL SEXUALITY

The following was taken from J. Giles and S. Holmes, "There's a time for talk, and a time for action," in the March 7, 1994, issue of *Newsweek*.

THE OFFICIAL RULES OF THE GAME
Antioch Dean Marian Jensen [apparently no longer there] says students are abiding by the college's nine-page sexual-conduct code "to the extent that they feel comfortable." A few excerpts:

Fair Play and Foreplay
If sexual contact and/or conduct is not mutually and simultaneously initiated, then the person who initiates sexual contact/conduct is responsible for getting the verbal consent of the other individual(s) involved.

Are We Having Fun Yet?
Obtaining consent is an on-going process in any sexual interaction. Verbal consent should be obtained with each new level of physical and/or sexual contact/conduct in any given interaction, regardless of who initiates it. Asking "Do you want to have sex with me?" is not enough. The request for consent must be specific to each act.

Sex and Drugs
To knowingly take advantage of someone who is under the influence of alcohol, drugs, and/or prescribed medication is not acceptable behavior in the Antioch community.

Putting on the Brakes
If someone has initially consented but then stops consenting during a sexual interaction, she/he should communicate withdrawal verbally and/or through physical resistance. The other individual(s) must stop immediately.

Richards, Rollerson, and Philips (1991) showed college men videotapes of women being interviewed about a number of nonsexual subjects. During the interviews the women were challenged about the correctness of their views by the interviewer. Based on the way these subjects dealt with this challenge, they were categorized as either "submissive" or "dominant." This study revealed that men observing the taped interviews were easily able to differentiate submissive from dominant subjects, that their assessments were based primarily on gestural, nonverbal cues, that submissive and dominant subjects exhibited very different nonverbal cues, and that the male subjects believed that they could more easily persuade a submissive subject to do something she might not ordinarily want to do. Perhaps those who are inclined to sexually exploit or victimize another can perceive subtle cues that may imply vulnerability. Maybe some people who sexually abuse or exploit others have grown adept at recognizing these subtle cues and coercing a victim into nonconsensual sexual activities.

Stalking: A Special Case of Abuse

Social and behavioral scientists use the term **obsessive relational intrusion** to refer to stalking behaviors, defined as the "repeated and unwanted pursuit and invasion of one's sense of physical or symbolic privacy by another person, either stranger or acquaintance, who desires and/or presumes an intimate relationship" (Cupach & Spitzberg, 1998, pp. 234-235) (Fig. 19-1). In a sense, stalking is a *threat of victimization,* and is therefore a special case of sexual abuse. One question involved is whether stalking is likely to result in some form of sexual coercion. Until recently, there have not been any empirical data to support or disclaim this hypothesis. We do know, however, that most stalkers are male and that in about half of the cases, he is either an estranged husband (38%) or cohabiting partner (10%) (Tjaden & Thoennes, 1997). In other cases, women were stalked by a man they had dated (14%), a relative (4%), an acquaintance (19%), or a stranger (23%). Spitzberg and Rhea (1999) have shown, however, that stalking and sexual coercive episodes are correlated and that the chances of a woman being sexually victimized are far higher if she is being stalked than if she is not. According to Spitzberg and Rhea (1999), "jealousy, possessiveness, and insecure attachment styles can work as predictors of both perpetration and victimization, because they all indicate a tendency to cling to a partner, even if the relationship is destructive."

THEORETICAL APPROACHES

Although there are no simple explanations for sexual abuse or exploitation, a number of theories describe why people behave in these ways, how victims sustain the insult or assault, whether perpetrators can be helped, and how those afflicted recover, if ever.

Social Learning Theory

This approach emphasizes the roles of observation and vicarious experience in learning. According to social learning theory, our psychosocial environment may include various activities our own experiences may have predisposed us to engage in and to allow us to gauge the possible consequences of our behaviors without engaging in those behaviors. Observation alone is often sufficient to teach, but the reinforcements and punishments that come from the environment are often basic to the behaviors we choose to imitate or model. When a person models actions on the basis of what they see others doing and presumably enjoying, they too expect to experience positive consequences from the experience. For example, a young man at a big party where a lot of drinking is going on will probably see other boys "putting the moves" on women. He will probably see other boys acting decidedly aggressive in a sexual way. If he observes these women yielding or acting ambivalently about these sexual overtures, he may learn that one way to get sex is to act in a similarly aggressive, forward fashion. Events like these may be instrumental in condoning date rape or perhaps even marital rape. When observations such as these do not seem to entail any immediate negative consequences for the perpetrator, they further imply that abusive or exploitative behaviors will not be punished.

In addition to the fact that observers may witness others engaging in supposedly enjoyable sexual activities, the observer may attend selectively to the imposition of power of one person over another, and forceful activities may in fact be perceived as more exciting than the sexual aspects of those behaviors. The "eye of the beholder" determines what is stimulating or potentially punishing about what is observed, and this depends in large part on a person's sexual value system.

The main distinction between behavioral theories and social learning theories is that in the latter observation alone is sufficient for learning to occur, while in the former the indi-

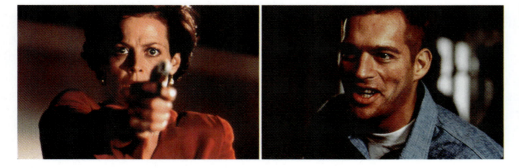

FIGURE 19-1 The movie *Copy Cat*, starring Sigourney Weaver (left) and Harry Connick, Jr. (right), depicts the persistent, menacing, and threatening nature of a stalker who is obsessed with a number of women, most of whom he kills.

vidual her- or himself behaves in a way that leads to either rewards or punishments.

Sociological Theory

While psychological theories focus on the behavior of individuals in certain circumstances, sociological theories instead deal primarily with the ways in which groups of individuals (for example, men) behave in similar circumstances. Some might argue that sexual abuse, exploitation, and coercion are more a manifestation of a "sick society" than sick individuals. For example, sociologists often claim that these behaviors result from the different amounts of power women and men have in a culture. The desire of men to feel powerful may be provoked by feminism, women's rights, gender equity, and the hiring and advancement of women in educational, business, or domestic settings; they may retaliate with the aggressive imposition of their own masculinity through abuse, exploitation, or coercion (such as rape). Although these are the behaviors of particular men, general social pathology related to these issues may be very prevalent and reflected in explicit ways in society as a whole. Differential power relations between the sexes may therefore be involved in sexual victimization, and a sociological perspective is one useful way of looking at these phenomena. Yet sociological theory does not explain why relatively few men become rapists or engage in sexual abuse.

PROSTITUTION

Prostitution is included in this chapter even though it has often been referred to as a "victimless crime." In other words, people who are prostitutes and the clients they cater to are said to enter into "sexual contracts" in a mutually consenting fashion. Yet very often someone is indeed being victimized in sex-for-money transactions. Most prostitutes are women, although many boys, girls, and men are also prostitutes.

Community standards have a role in condoning, condemning, or being indifferent to sex for sale. With a few exceptions, prostitution is illegal everywhere in the United States. But other countries and cultures have different customs, and in some places governments play an active role in monitoring legalized prostitution and ensuring that those engaged in these jobs remain disease free.

Types of Prostitutes and Occupational Settings

Location is generally a key factor in prostitution. When prostitutes can locate potential clients they can negotiate a sexual transaction and have sex with them. But they have to locate them first, and many communities have a number of well-traveled places (bars, hotels, motels, clubs, etc.) where prostitutes approach men. Different places have very different types of clients, or "johns" as they are called in the trade.

CALL GIRLS

Call girls usually work alone, arranging dates with clients by themselves or sometimes through pimps. Some entertain their clients in their own homes and apartments, while others go to the client's residence or a hotel. Encounters are prearranged by telephone or e-mail. Most call girls are comparatively young, and many charge steep fees because they are often very attractive physically (Fig. 19-2). These women are clear about when and where they can be contacted and are very careful about keeping their personal and occupational lives separate. Some call girls identify themselves as lesbians but cater only to men, without revealing their gender orientation. Others are receptive to female clients or couples. Call girls may offer bondage or sadomasochistic activities or emphasize "sensual straight sex." Some call girls work through escort services, and sometimes even advertise "exotic entertainments." Many of these women model lingerie for their clients, allow themselves to be photographed nude, and even provide their customers with expensive, rare cigars. These women tend to seek men who want to be pampered and enjoy a woman who behaves in a passive, subservient way.

Call girls often put on shows for individual clients or groups of men. These invariably involve stripping and often lap dancing. Call girls may have oral, vaginal, or anal sex with the men who watch her perform. These women usually make themselves available for an entire evening (unlike other types of prostitutes who engage in brief sexual activities), and some

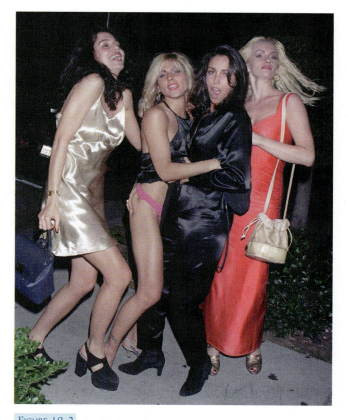

FIGURE 19-2   Heidi Fleiss (second from right in black) with some of her friends in September 1995. Ms. Fleiss was found guilty of arranging "dates" for a number of female acquaintances who worked for her as prostitutes.

Research Highlight

HOW DOES SOMEONE BECOME A CALL GIRL?

The ways in which women become call girls has been studied, such as the informative analysis by James H. Bryan in 1965. His analysis probes the emotional and interpersonal aspects of how young women become prostitutes and the subculture they join.

Bryan's study is based on interviews with 33 women who were or had been call girls in Los Angeles and who ranged in age between 18 and 32. Most of his subjects were in their mid-20s; none participated in this study because they had been apprehended by legal or mental health officials. All voluntarily agreed to be interviewed and fully understood the scope and objectives of the investigation. The study focused on the ways in which women are recruited into this career and their apprenticeship experiences. When a women expresses an interest in becoming a call girl, she is "assigned" to someone working in the trade to learn the values and procedures of the business. During this period a pimp establishes his "ownership" of the woman even though the information and guidance are provided by a prostitute who was already a call girl. Then the apprenticeship proper begins.

At this point the young woman usually moves into the apartment of the trainer or commutes there daily. This lasts for about 2 to 3 months. During this time, the trainer teaches the recruit the "do's" and "don'ts" of the trade, focusing on how to stay out of dangerous situations or those likely to lead to an arrest by the police. The values of the profession are shared. For example, call girls often perceive men as corrupt and dishonest, and see themselves as more open and honest about what they do than the customer, who is hiding his sexual activities in a clandestine encounter with a prostitute. Bryan believes that many call girls share this belief and that this contributes to a sense of cohesiveness among them. Part of a call girl's indoctrination also involves learning acceptable ways of using alcohol and/or drugs to minimize their impact on her earning potential. She is also given specific instructions about negotiating fees and collecting cash, as well as making small talk with her johns. Training may also include information about avoiding sexually transmitted diseases. Bryan notes that trainees don't very much like making telephone contacts with prospective customers. He believes that one reason for this is that many females are socialized to believe that it is inappropriate for them to initiate conversations with men.

Interestingly a call girl's training does not generally include much information about sexual techniques, although Bryan notes that usually techniques of performing fellatio are discussed. At the end of a call girl's training, her trainer may eavesdrop on her first interactions with clients to offer constructive criticism. The final issue in a call girl's training concerns her income and her enhanced value in the trade because of her newness. In most cases, the apprenticeship ends abruptly. As the new call girl begins to develop her own clientele, she creates a "book" of customers. This item is enormously important in the trade, and sometimes a call girl may steal another's to increase her earning potential.

are willing to travel with their clients, especially men who like to "wear an expensive looking woman," like they would wear an expensive suit or drive an expensive car. Some call girls specialize in having sex with men in their places of business. Because call girls sometimes have no manager or pimp to find them clients and protect them from the threat of abuse or violence, they must constantly be attentive to their own safety and security; some carry guns.

STREETWALKERS

From the standpoint of personal safety, streetwalkers have the most dangerous job as prostitutes. These women make their availability to clients known by walking along well-traveled streets, "cruising" in cars, or frequenting restaurants and bars. Interestingly, prostitutes in crowded Italian cities have begun wearing running shoes to better pursue vehicles and strike a deal on the run. Streetwalkers are frequently called "hookers," a term coming from the large number of prostitutes who followed the troops of Joseph Hooker, a Union army officer in the American Civil War. These women charge less money than call girls, and their clients are usually less well off as well. Their sexual encounters are typically brief and usually take place in inexpensive hotels and motels, although sometimes cars, elevators, and alleys are also used. Streetwalkers must be far more assertive in displaying and marketing their "wares" and on that account frequently get into trouble with the police. They choose attire to display their best "assets" and appeal to customers with particular physical preferences in women. They must be sufficiently sexually suggestive but not seem coarse or impatient.

A streetwalker has to manage some fairly complex social logistics. After finding a willing client she must take him to a place where the sexual activity can take place, get paid first, take appropriate measures to avoid contracting a sexually transmitted disease or become pregnant, perform the desired/negotiated sex act, keep an eye on the client so that he doesn't assault her and rob her, and avoid getting caught by the police. For streetwalkers more so than call girls, "time is money," and streetwalkers generally try to turn as many "tricks" as they can in a day while still trying to be friendly and responsive with her customers. Streetwalkers generally work for pimps who arrange "dates," offer protection, manage finances (and take a

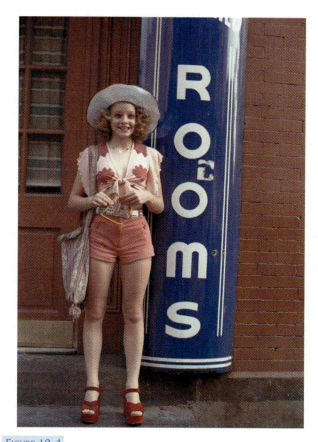

FIGURE 19-4 Actress Jodie Foster in the movie *Taxi Driver.* Ms. Foster plays a 12-year-old streetwalker in this 1976 film.

large cut for themselves), and often supply them with drugs (Fig. 19-3). Because most pimps are men, the pimp-prostitute relationship is often viewed as a form of sexual exploitation and gender inequality. Pimps manage many streetwalkers at a time and sometimes have sex with them too. According to various estimates, the pimp takes between 40% and 60% of the prostitute's earnings. Because the pimp is being supported by the prostitute, he often obtains whatever drugs she might need to tolerate the often depressing and dangerous aspects of her work. Streetwalkers are often assaulted by their clients (Fig. 19-4).

BROTHEL WORKERS

From the days of the old Wild West through the era of prominent organized crime in the United States, "whorehouses" have been common. These institutions were frequently associated with a hotel and bar, and a number of girls were available, often at all hours. The terms "brothel" and "bordello" refer to the same thing. Historically, these establishments were quite ornate and opulent, and the women who worked in them made every effort to appear clean, poised, and stylish. But things have changed, and with the exception of a few places in Nevada, brothels today are decidedly unsavory places. When a client enters a brothel he is introduced to a number of women

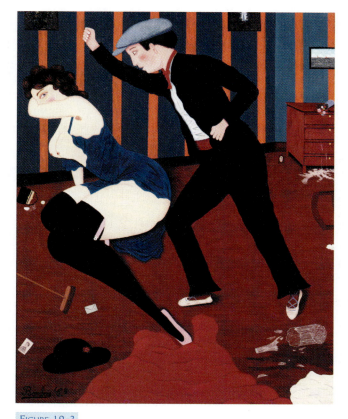

FIGURE 19-3 Pimps arrange sexual contacts for prostitutes and take a share of their earnings. Many pimps coerce their prostitutes with violence, and give them drugs and alcohol to keep them dependent on them.

and he chooses the one whom he finds most appealing. They then proceed to a room where cash changes hands and sexual activities take place. Women who work in brothels are sometimes called "house prostitutes." Unlike streetwalkers, they are managed by a "madam" who handles the money, pays the rent, provides protection, and occasionally bribes the police to look the other way. In many cases, the madam is a former prostitute. At the turn of the twentieth century, every large American city had a "red light district" with a number of brothels. The appearance of a red light on the building was the cue that sexual services could be purchased within.

In 1971, the state legislature of Nevada passed a law allowing each county to decide if it would legalize prostitution and license its sex workers. Many of these facilities consist of a number of mobile homes. Security is tight and guards are always on the premises. Alcoholic beverages are often sold. Women who work in these brothels are examined and tested regularly by health officials approved by the state to ensure that they have not contracted any sexually transmitted diseases. All sexual activities involving penetration of any kind require the use of a condom. Most of the girls who work on these "ranches" decline to kiss their clients as well. Violence is almost unheard of in these establishments (Fig. 19-5).

MASSAGE PARLORS

Another arena in which prostitutes work is the so-called massage parlor, where men go ostensibly to get the kinks rubbed out of their neck and back. Often women who work in these businesses also provide sexual services. Clients negotiate sex for money, and these acts may include masturbation, sexual intercourse, oral sex, or other forms of erotic stimulation. These transactions are typically extremely brief, lasting only a few

minutes in some cases. Like prostitutes who work in other settings, women who work in massage parlors (sometimes called a "masseuse") often require their clients to wear condoms during all forms of physical contact.

BAR GIRLS

The previous chapter discussed nude dancing in connection with pseudoexhibitionism and voyeurism and noted that in some venues the dancers also engage in sexual services with clients for a fee. Technically, this is prostitution too when some type of sex is being exchanged for money, even though a topless bar might seem different from a brothel. Although most women who work in topless bars do not meet their clients away from the workplace, some do so occasionally.

■ ■ ■

In all, the job descriptions and work environments of prostitutes vary enormously. There are big differences in the incomes of different types of prostitutes, their reliance on pimps, and the risks they put themselves at by soliciting sex with strangers. Some work in modern, expensive hotels while others perform sex acts in seedy back rooms and cars. But as long as there is any element of human exploitation, danger of injury or assault, or probability of contracting a sexually transmitted disease, prostitution is *not* a victimless crime.

What Types of Sex Do Clients Buy From Prostitutes?

Reinisch (1990) summarized the literature on this question and emphasized that the most common reason men go to prostitutes is to purchase sex acts that their "regular" partner finds objectionable. In the years before World War II, most men went to prostitutes to have sexual intercourse. But things have changed since, and today the most commonly purchased sexual activity is fellatio. Men today are more likely to request fellatio and anal penetration prior to vaginal sex. Reinisch notes that research conducted by the Kinsey Institute shows not only that oral sex is requested more frequently than vaginal intercourse, but also that prostitutes themselves seem to prefer this avenue of sexual intimacy "because it is faster (it doesn't involve taking off clothes), less tiring, and doesn't necessarily involve the expense of renting a room" (p. 151). According to Kinsey Institute research, about 1 in 3 American men have had some type of sexual interaction with a prostitute during their lives.

Men have a variety of motives for visiting prostitutes. In addition to desiring some type of sexual activity their partner doesn't like, others visit prostitutes because they are away from home for extended periods of time, do not want to become "involved" with a woman, or desire an uninhibited sexual experience that will not threaten their marriage. Reinisch points out that some men go to prostitutes because of physical or mental disabilities that they feel make them somewhat undesirable partners for other women.

Another important and interesting question is whether clients, knowing that prostitutes have sex with many men, rec-

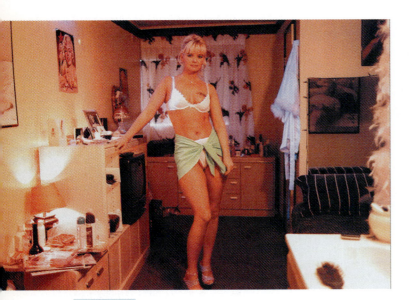

FIGURE 19-5 Nevada legal prostitute "Princess Rio" at the Moonlight Bunnyranch Bordello.

ognize that they run a substantially increased risk of contracting HIV or other sexually transmitted diseases. This is especially important because many men who solicit a prostitute's services adamantly refuse to wear a condom. Plumridge, Chetwynd, Reed, and Gifford (1996) interviewed 20 men between the ages of 23 and 78. These subjects were approached through a massage parlor, newspaper advertisements, and prostitutes. Most of these subjects reported that in visiting prostitutes they believed that they were not running any more "unusual" risks than any person might encounter in daily life.

How and Why Individuals Become Prostitutes

A website devoted to serious social science research concerning prostitution (www.prostitutionresearch.com) includes an ironic "Help Wanted" job description for a prostitute. It describes the nature of this occupation and notes the following:

- No experience required. No high school diploma needed.
- No minimum age requirement. On-the-job training provided.
- Special opportunities for poor women—single women—women of color.

Women and girls applying for this position will provide the following services:

- Being penetrated orally, anally, and vaginally with penises, fingers, fists, and objects, including but not limited to, bottles, brushes, dildos, guns and/or animals.
- Being bound and gagged, tied with ropes and/or chains, burned with cigarettes, or hung from beams or trees.
- Being photographed or filmed performing these acts.

Workplace: Job-related activities will be performed in the following locations: in an apartment, a hotel, a "massage parlor," car, doorway, hallway, street, executive suite, fraternity house, convention, bar, public toilet, public park, alleyway, military base, on a stage, in a glass booth.

Of course, anyone reading this would wonder who would want to do this and why. In many cases, past experiences with sexual abuse and/or incest may play a role in the development of the "prostitution persona" (Russell, 1998a). Such experiences may profoundly affect a woman's feelings of self-worth and her sense of adequacy in a later relationship with a husband, lovers, and other members of her family. Cause-and-effect statements cannot be made, however, between early sexual victimization and later likelihood of becoming a prostitute. Unger et al. (1998) studied the living habits of almost 250 youngsters between the ages of 12 and 15 who were living on the streets of Los Angeles. About 40% of these youths reported being involved in prostitution as well as selling drugs, muggings, and theft. These researchers emphasized that when youth this young become involved in these activities, there is a very strong possibility that they are creating a foundation for a

later lifestyle. Nadon, Koverola, and Schludermann (1998) explored the factors that predispose young women to become prostitutes and note that when an adolescent runs away from an abusive, intolerable home environment, she is at an especially high risk of becoming a prostitute, although again, there is no clear cause-and-effect relationship.

Other research has addressed this question, especially the impact of sexual abuse and drug use on becoming a prostitute. Potterat, Rothenberg, Muth, Darrow, and Phillips-Plummber (1998) recruited 237 women from a sexually transmitted disease (STD) clinic and an HIV counseling and testing center in Colorado Springs over a 2-year period in the early 1990s. Subjects presented themselves at these facilities either voluntarily or because they had been arrested for prostitution. Women who were prostitutes were compared with other women who were not prostitutes visiting these facilities in terms of the roles of sexual abuse and drug use during their adolescent years. They found several trends in their data. For example, 86% of the women who became prostitutes reported drug use, while only 23% of the subjects in the control group acknowledged a similar behavior pattern. Additionally, 32% of the prostitutes revealed that they had been victimized by nonconsensual sex before adolescence, compared with only 13% of the control group. The subjects who became prostitutes reported that they had experimented with drugs before they became involved in prostitution, and had used intravenous drugs before they began to engage in sex for money. These findings indicate that sexual abuse and drug use are common, important milestones in becoming a prostitute, but that they do not necessarily and inevitably lead to this lifestyle.

A Prostitute's Lifestyle

The childhood and adolescence of many women who become prostitutes is generally not a positive experience, nor is their current lifestyle. Many powerful stressors are associated with this way of making a living, even for "high-class" call girls. Not only can the job itself be unpleasant and dangerous, but even when these women have any "time off" they don't necessarily enjoy freedom from anxiety and fear. El-Bassel and colleagues studied almost 350 women in New York City who exchanged sex for money, drugs, or both. These subjects were between the ages of 18 and 29, were poor, and lived in a depressed inner-city environment. These researchers were particularly interested in the degree to which this lifestyle affected a prostitute's inclination to adopt safer sex practices with her clients. Slightly over half of this sample were African American, and Hispanics accounted for almost 41%. The remaining women were Caucasian. Most reported that welfare payments were their primary source of income. Many were homeless and reported that they had been raped during the previous year. Questionnaire and interview data revealed that these prostitutes were extremely likely to experience severe psychological distress daily. Anxiety, hostility, depression, phobias, and paranoia were everpresent. Needless to say, these women were seriously stressed and distressed as a result of their trading sex for money or illegal drugs. These respondents reported having sex with a large number of partners but used condoms inconsistently, putting them at an extremely high risk for becoming infected with HIV and other STDs.

The Sexual Exploitation Education Project (SEEP)

With prostitution, who is "most" guilty, the vendor or the customer? Through an arrangement with the district court in Portland, Oregon, the Sexual Exploitation Education Project (SEEP) seeks to make men more accountable for prostitution in that city (Monto, 1998). Men who have been convicted of soliciting sex from prostitutes are required to take part in an intensive, 17-hour weekend workshop experience. The purpose of these workshops is to make these men more aware of the nature of prostitution and to help them recognize its basically exploitative nature. A major message in this program is that sex between a prostitute and a client may in fact not be consensual or victimless, since many prostitutes are forced by their pimps to perform sex acts for money, much against their genuine intentions and preferences. Because law enforcement efforts to remove prostitutes from the streets have been less than effective, the people at SEEP feel that focusing on the customer may be a better approach, especially when he is sensitized to the fact that he is participating in what amounts to a conspiracy of oppression of women. One of SEEP's most important goals involves "Stressing the choice and responsibility that men have to create egalitarian relationships without coercion or violence."

The good work of SEEP and other similar organizations is one example of the role of sociological and feminist theory applied to prostitutes and their clients. Monto (1998) notes that when men go to prostitutes and pay them for sex acts, they are really silencing them about reporting what in the context of another relationship might be called "abuse." A major focus of the SEEP training program for men is encouraging men to willingly acknowledge what they are doing and to take responsibility for their behavior. The SEEP program has several specific objectives that aim both to protect women who are prostitutes and to discourage men from buying their services. Monto enumerates these:

1. While discouraging men from purchasing sex from prostitutes is a central, important objective of this organization, an even more significant goal is to help women find a way out of the violent and dangerous lifestyle inherent in prostitution.

2. SEEP seeks to encourage the development of a pro-feminist attitude in men. Workshops involve facilitators who are both female and male so that those attending will have the opportunity to see what productive, equal interactions between women and men can be like.

3. If a community wants an organization like SEEP, it will have to organize both financial and political support for it. A major objective of SEEP involves the coordination of resources of a variety of women's

groups and the recognition of those women who have the potential to become leaders and coordinators of these organizations.

4. The development of a coherent curriculum with specific behavioral objectives is central to the mission of this organization. Seminar topics, role-play exercises, and consciousness-raising activities are all basic to this goal.

Male Prostitution

The discussion of prostitution thus far has focused on women only because there are far more female than male prostitutes. But male prostitution is not rare or different from the victimization explicit in female prostitution. Australia Browne and Minichiello (1996a) carried out an in-depth qualitative study of the psychosocial context of male prostitutes between the ages of 19 and 34. These men worked in settings similar to women who are call girls, streetwalkers, and massage parlor workers. The amount of time these men had been prostitutes ranged from 6 months to 12 years. These men did not adopt passive or feminine roles in their interactions with their clients, unless explicitly requested to do so to cater to a particular client's preferences. Interestingly, all of these subjects emphasized that it is a decidedly masculine privilege to get sex any time they want it, and this is one need they see themselves serving for their clients. These respondents emphasized that by using condoms they were putting an explicit barrier between themselves and a business "contact." These subjects reported that condom use was nonnegotiable with a client.

While the qualitative data of Browne and Minichiello depict male prostitutes who seem in control of their lives, this is by no means the case for all or even most male prostitutes. Like young female runaways who become prostitutes to survive on the streets, young men often find themselves in dangerous circumstances and turn to prostitution to "make it" on the streets. The men interviewed by Browne and Minichiello seemed to feel they had a choice about who they would have sex with, when, and what the nature of the sexual interaction would be. But young male "hustlers" often have no such alternatives and often have risky, dangerous, and abusive interactions with their clients (Fig. 19-6).

In a more general review of male prostitution Browne and Minichiello (1996b) emphasized that in the past the study of male prostitution generally considered it an example of social deviance. Today the study of male prostitution is a rich area of inquiry within the contexts of the social and behavioral sciences and urban economics. While older research commonly labeled the male prostitute a social outcast, current data reveal that this person is not less well educated than other males or any more likely to come from dysfunctional homes (Earls & David, 1989). Their data reveal that male prostitutes seem to enjoy good mental health relative to the dangerous and exploitative nature of their work. Still, some plainly unsavory lifestyle issues are frequently involved in being a male prostitute. The number of male prostitutes who are HIV-positive is thought to be at least 10% in Western industrialized countries

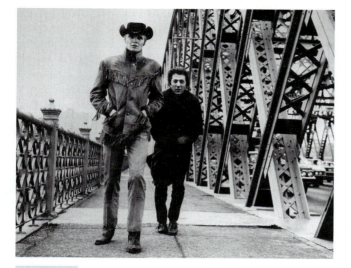

FIGURE 19-6   Jon Voight and Dustin Hoffman in the movie *Midnight Cowboy* (1969). While destitute and homeless in New York City, Voight's character turns to male prostitution to support the pair.

and may even be as high as 50% (Bloor, Barnard, Finlay, & McKeganey, 1993).

Those who have sex with male prostitutes are an extremely diverse group. They are rarely female. Clients are married and unmarried, widowed, divorced, bisexual, heterosexual, and homosexual men, usually from the upper middle class. Many want to have sex without condoms, but how male prostitutes and their clients negotiate safer sex practices is still being studied, and as yet no generalizations can be made.

The Personality of Prostitutes

The term "personality" is not easy to define, but generally it refers to what is predictable about a person to other people. Many social and behavioral scientists have wondered whether there is a common thread in the personalities of prostitutes. While little is known about how being a prostitute might adversely affect someone's personality, surprisingly little research has tried to characterize the personality of the "typical" prostitute. In a study by O'Sullivan, Zuckerman, and Kraft (1996), 32 self-identified prostitutes were interviewed and took a

Other Countries, Cultures, and Customs

CHILD PROSTITUTION IN ASIA

An especially distressing example of the sexual exploitation of children is the enormous child prostitution business in southeast Asia. In this case, consent to have sexual relations is explicitly lacking for two reasons. First, the prostitute is a child or young adolescent, and second, there is significant pressure to engage in sexual relations with adults for money because of the crushing poverty of the region. In September of 1996, the first World Congress Against the Commercial Sexual Exploitation of Children met in Stockholm, Sweden to consider the enormous sexual exploitation and victimization of children around the world. The United Nations Children's Fund has estimated that one million children under the age of 18 are working as prostitutes in Asia (Chidey, 1996). Thailand alone supposedly has more than 800,000 children working as prostitutes, and it is believed that in the United States there are approximately 300,000 children involved in this trade. This organization estimates that in addition, another million youngsters become prostitutes each year throughout the world. Clearly this is a huge, distressing problem.

Chidey (1996) notes that in recent years there has been an attempt to try to curb the sex tourism industry in Asia. An organization called End Child Prostitution in Asian Tourism has been instrumental in publicizing the enormity of the industry and the terrible victimization of children in the Philippines, Taiwan, Thailand, and Sri Lanka. Virtually all child prostitutes live in terrible conditions, are frequently physically abused, and are virtually certain to contract a variety of STDs, including HIV. Because of the appalling poverty in these countries, families commonly sell a daughter into the sex trade to gain income from her activities. In nations with an explicit sexist attitude toward women, female children are somehow seen as worth very little. Many men apparently believe that having sex with a virgin will make them live longer. Yet the social conditions that subtly sanction this exploitation of children do not fully account for the demand among adults for these sexual services. Clearly, culturally sanctioned sex with juveniles in conditions of suffocating poverty makes the notion of sexual consent almost irrelevant (Fig. 19-7).

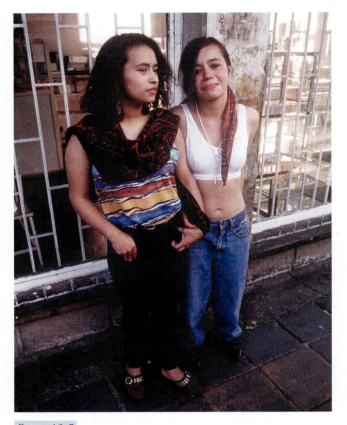

FIGURE 19-7   Child prostitutes often live in appalling squalor and confront dangerous clients, the risk of unanticipated pregnancy, and STDs and AIDS. A number of organizations have attempted to end the sexual exploitation of minors.

paper-and-pencil personality test and were compared with a control group of similar women who were not prostitutes. The prostitutes scored especially high on a personality dimension called "impulsive sensation seeking," and the subjects who used cocaine scored higher on this dimension than women who used other drugs and higher than women who used no drugs at all. These investigators believe that this personality trait is also frequently associated with "antisocial" personality traits.

People with an **antisocial personality disorder** often have a number of characteristics in common. They often disregard the rights of other people and frequently fail to obey the law. Lying is common in their interactions with others, and they act impulsively and demonstrate a reckless disregard for the safety and welfare of others. They often manifest irritability and aggressive behaviors and rarely feel sorry for any harm they have caused (DSM-IV, 1994). It would be unwise to suggest that *all* prostitutes have an antisocial personality disorder, however, as this is not true.

Prostitution and Posttraumatic Stress Disorder

Just as a prostitute frequently runs the risk of physical injury, her personality can be "injured" as well. Recently, evidence has begun to accumulate that indicates that because of the stresses

and dangers of their jobs, prostitutes sometimes develop *posttraumatic stress disorder* (PTSD). Much has been written about this psychological disorder in the military as a result of terrible experiences in combat. It is a complex cluster of persistent and distressing symptoms. According to the *Diagnostic and Statistical Manual of Psychological Disorders* (4th edition, 1994), PTSD involves a person experiencing a traumatic event in which:

(1) the person experienced, witnessed, or was confronted with an event or events that involved actual or threatened death or serious injury, or a threat to the physical integrity of self or others
(2) the person's response involved intense fear, helplessness, or horror.

Additionally, the stressful event or events are experienced repeatedly in reality, fantasy, or memory. The individual comes to carefully avoid any cues associated with the stressful event or events and frequently experiences "difficulty falling or staying asleep, irritability or outbursts of anger, difficulty concentrating, hypervigilance, [or an] exaggerated startle response." Studying a group of 130 prostitutes, Farley and Barkan (1998) discovered that a significant number of their subjects reported symptoms of posttraumatic stress disorder and that the likelihood of this happening was related to the number of violent events they had experienced as prostitutes. For example, 82% of these respondents had been physically assaulted, 83% reported being threatened with a weapon, 68% were raped while working as prostitutes, and 84% had experienced a period of homelessness as adults. Of all the subjects interviewed in this investigation, 68% met the criteria for posttraumatic stress disorder.

Leaving Prostitution

Although some research on prostitution includes interviews with women in their 40s, 50s, and even their 60s, we have not found a single report indicating that the female and male prostitutes studied are satisfied with their work and plan to continue it as long as possible. Much research frankly acknowledges that prostitutes frequently think about ways to quit their work and reclaim their lives–to live free of sexual exploitation, victimization, and frequently alcohol and drug dependency as well (Fig. 19-8). More organizations are emerging in large American cities to help women get off the streets and out of the trade and assist them in rebuilding their health and self-esteem and live more normal, satisfying lives.

Genesis House is located on the north side of Chicago. In a sense, it's a "safe house" for prostitutes, a place where they can bathe, have a decent meal, and share their fears and worries with paid staff workers and volunteers, many of whom have been prostitutes themselves. There is no pressure to change or abruptly give up their work on the streets. But they are given the opportunity to decide for themselves if they would like to move in and begin a complete transformation of their lives while living there (Cole, 1998). Unfortunately, federal support for such projects is not always forthcoming.

Other Countries, Cultures, and Customs

POSTTRAUMATIC STRESS AMONG PROSTITUTES IN OTHER COUNTRIES

Some argue that prostitutes, female and male, around the world, probably encounter similar, severe stressors on almost a daily basis. Therefore it is reasonable to wonder whether commercial sex workers in other countries also suffer from posttraumatic stress disorder. This question has been addressed by Farley, Baral, Kiremire, and Sezgin (1998). These researchers undertook this investigation to further assess whether prostitution is a "job" or a "violation of human rights." The sociological theoretical approach has led to much fruitful research into sexual exploitation and victimization, and this study is another example of that perspective. At the very outset of their report, these authors assert that prostitution is "an act of violence against women" that is "intrinsically traumatizing to the person being prostituted" (p. 405). In all, 475 prostitutes were interviewed in South Africa, Thailand, Turkey, the United States, and Zambia. Subjects participated in a short interview and filled out a 23-item questionnaire that explored such issues as physical and sexual assault during encounters with clients, the individual's lifelong experience with physical and sexual assault, and whether the individual had participated in the making of pornographic materials. Finally, the researchers sought to determine whether their subjects displayed the symptoms of posttraumatic stress disorder described in the DSM-IV. Subjects were contacted in San Francisco, California; Lusaka, Zambia; Istanbul, Turkey; Capetown, South Africa; and two undesignated cities in Thailand. In two of these countries, the United States and South Africa, the subjects represented a number of different races.

In most cases, pimps, boyfriends, brothel owners, and madams tried to interfere with the collection of these data. When data from these five countries were pooled together, it was discovered that 81% of these subjects reported that they had been threatened physically in some manner while working as prostitutes, and 73% had been physically assaulted (p. 412-413). Since becoming prostitutes, 62% of the subjects reported that they had been raped by their customers, with almost half of this number having been raped more than five times. Of all the subjects in this study, almost half reported that they had participated in the making of pornography while working as prostitutes. Further, 72% of the respondents reported that they were currently homeless or had been homeless at some time in the recent past. About half reported that they were addicted to alcohol, and 45% said that they had a problem with drug addiction. When evaluated for posttraumatic stress disorder, the averaged data from these five countries revealed a prevalence of PTSD slightly higher than that reported for American Vietnam veterans. Among these prostitutes, 67% met the diagnostic criteria for this psychological disorder. Even though there were significant cultural differences in these five countries, the prevalence of PTSD did not differ appreciably among these prostitutes.

These researchers found that streetwalkers were physically assaulted more frequently than those working as call girls or in brothels, but there were no differences in the prevalence of PTSD in prostitutes working in these different venues. The authors conclude that this is due to the fact that "psychological trauma is intrinsic to the act of prostitution" (p. 419). Among the American prostitutes who participated in this study, 3 reported that they had worked in legal brothels, presumably in Nevada. Reports of their experiences in these facilities reveal a highly exploitative, abusive environment. Specifically, these respondents noted that during their tenure in a legal brothel they had virtually no autonomy and were entirely under the control of the owner. They could not refuse to have sex with any particular customer and generally were not allowed to leave the facility for 8 days at a time.

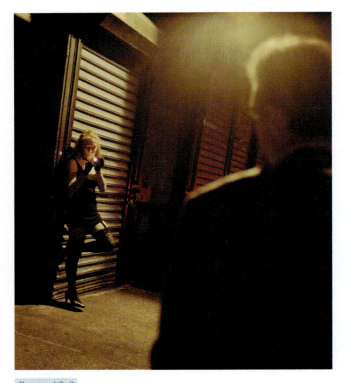

FIGURE 19-8 Leaving prostitution and reclaiming one's life can be a daunting task for many women who have grown economically dependent on their pimps and have substance abuse problems as well.

Workers at Genesis House have approached local judges in an attempt to persuade them to send prostitutes to their facility instead of jail. They have a very strong case to make: 70% of the women who begin their rehabilitation complete the program, of those who do so, 4 out of 5 stay off the streets. Workers at Genesis House help many women regain custody of their children as well. Sociological/feminist theories might contend that programs such as these achieve nothing less than a psychosocial transformation in a woman that allows her to again enjoy her roles as a productive member of society and perhaps as a parent too. Prostitutes can indeed regain their self-respect and live more normal lives.

PORNOGRAPHY

Pornography in one form or another has been present from the beginning of human civilization and is revealed in a wide variety of art forms. This cross-cultural reality suggests there may be some deep human interest in visual depictions of human bodies participating in acts that are usually highly pleasurable. What many people call pornographic has appeared independently in virtually all of the world's cultures at one time or another.

The word "pornography" derives from an old Greek word that means to write about harlots or prostitutes. The term is most commonly associated with depictions of sexual activity in which women are obviously exploited, degraded, or victimized. Rather than being full and willing partici-

pants in these sexual activities, they are shown in a submissive, subservient light. They are pleasing their partners with little focus on their own pleasures. Traditions of male supremacy are explicit in pornography, as is a woman's role as sex object. In contrast, "erotica" refers to representations of sexual activity in which women and men are coequally enjoying explicitly their sexual sharing. "Sensuality" is more obvious in erotica than pornography (Fig. 19-9). Pornography and erotica can involve pictures, films, or prose accounts of sexual activity, as well as listening to sexually stimulating talk, like the type found on telephone sex services. Both prose and pictorial depictions of sexual activity have existed for thousands of years.

How is a distinction made between historical erotic art and literature and modern "smut" as it is sometimes called? Several times in this book we have referred to cultural universals, which are aspects of societies that seem to be found in most societies. It is interesting that virtually every society, both historical and contemporary, has had producers and consumers of pornography. People everywhere seem to have some propensity to view/read/ listen to various forms of sexually arousing information as well as create them. A case could also be made for the fact that historically, less "civilized" societies felt fewer restraints or inhibitions in creating images portraying powerfully pleasurable feelings and that maybe what today is called pornography is a societal concept that has evolved over time. We are *not* suggesting, of course, that all cultures have wilfully created depictions of nudity and sexual activity with the intent of victimizing or humiliating women, as is true of much pornography today.

Pornography involves emotional issues in the United States, although this is not always true in other countries. Many other cultures often have decidedly liberal attitudes about pornography. Perhaps this issue is so contentious here because of the lack of a clear distinction among pornography, erotica, and obscenity. We will discriminate among these terms, although there is no unambiguous way to do so.

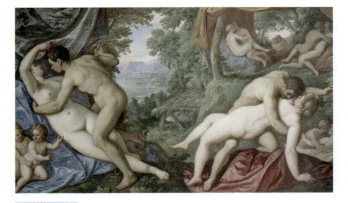

FIGURE 19-9 Unlike pornography, erotica tastefully depicts sexual acts in which women and men are full, sharing partners in enjoying physical intimacy together.

"Obscenity" and "indecency" are difficult to define concretely (Fig. 19-10). In 1957, the United States Supreme Court in *Roth v. United States* ruled that expression that is "utterly without redeeming social importance" does *not* deserve constitutional protection as freedom of expression. As vague as this criterion might be, it is fundamental to the obscenity laws with which we are living today. In *Miller v. California* (1973), the Supreme Court formulated a three-part test that can be used to determine if an expression is obscene. All three criteria must be met if a legal attribution of obscenity is to be upheld:

1. the average person, applying contemporary community standards, would find that the work, taken as a whole, appeals to the prurient [involving indulgence in lewd, sexual ideas] interest; and
2. the work depicts or describes, in a patently offensive way, sexual conduct [activity] specifically defined by the applicable state law [as illegal]; and
3. the work, taken as a whole, lacks serious literary, artistic, political or social value.

For many years, this definition seemed to work in most controversies involving a definition of obscenity. Yet recently, interpretations of one word in this decision have muddied the waters: "community." When people kept abreast of one another's doings by word of mouth, the telephone, or a local newspaper, this term was relatively straightforward. But now that we live in a "global village" and stay in touch with one another almost instantaneously by electronic media and the Internet, the whole notion of a "community" has become rather ambiguous. Do community standards refer to the location of the group presenting materials on the Internet, or is it the community of the individual downloading that material? An historical case sheds some light on this question. In *United States v. Thomas*, a United States postal inspector living in Tennessee bought pornography through a company located in California. The proprietors of this company were arrested for using the United States postal system to send obscene materials. The courts ruled that the relevant community standards were those of the place in which the person receiving the materials lived. Yet this question is far from decided and will likely be a focus of legal debate for many years. Another complication surrounds another word often associated with pornography: "indecency." Legally, the meanings of obscenity and indecency seem to overlap. In 1978, the Federal Communications Commission defined indecency as "that which is offensive to community standards for broadcasting." One Supreme Court Justice has been quoted as saying that although he had trouble defining pornography with any specificity, he knew it when he saw it.

Another matter of definition about which there is much discussion and debate and still little resolution is the distinction between "soft core" and "hard core" pornography. While much has been written about this, little clarity seems to have emerged concerning legal understandings of terms like "obscenity" or "indecency." We will try to make a tentative discrimination between soft core and hard core pornography. In contemporary cultural standards of publishing for the general

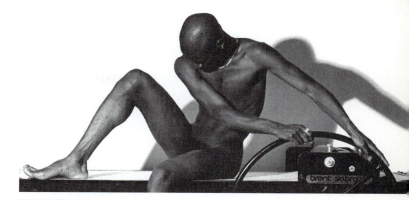

FIGURE 19-10   The photographs of Robert Mappelthorpe have provoked much discussion and, in some cases, even legal suppression with respect to the nature of obscenity and decency in art.

population, soft core pornography typically involves the depiction of women and/or men who are undressed and in sexually provocative poses. Their genitalia may or may not be visible, and they are not touching each other's genitalia. In contrast, hard core pornography usually involves the depiction of nude women and/or men in which manual stimulation of the other individual, penis in the vagina penetration, anal penetration, or oral-genital contact is obvious. Further, male or female ejaculation may be explicit. Group sexual activities and the use of inanimate objects may also be explicit.

The definitions of these two terms need qualifying, however. Sadomasochistic behaviors can be depicted in ways representative of both soft core and hard core pornography, for example. Bestiality would certainly be an example of hard core pornography, as would child pornography. To judge the differences between soft core and hard core pornography it is also necessary to assess the degree of degradation, exploitation, and victimization depicted.

The federal government has studied the impact of pornography in its attempts to protect citizens from flagrantly offensive depictions of sexual behavior. Presumably, "outlawing" pornography would be considered an example of such protective efforts.

The first study was carried out over 30 years ago. Two years in the making, the White House Commission systematically explored the hypothesized effects of pornography on American citizens. This early government study suggested that neither hard-core nor soft-core pornography has a clear cause-and-effect relationship with antisocial behaviors, and therefore recommended that with the exception of those statutes that prohibit minors from viewing pornography, obscenity laws should be eliminated. Many members on the commission felt that pornography may actually provide a safe release of pent-up sexual urges and may therefore be instrumental in reducing sexual offenses. President Nixon declined to accept the report, and the United States Senate rejected its findings by an overwhelming vote of 60 to 5.

Two government studies published in 1986 also failed to provide a clear verdict on the societal effects of pornography, although both have continued to frame the legal arguments surrounding pornography as an example of free speech protected by the First Amendment. President Reagan asked Edwin Meese, Attorney General of the United States, to head a committee to examine the relationship between pornography, violent pornography in particular, and rapes and sexual assaults. With very little time to carry out the President's mandate (and very little funding as well), the Meese Commission did more of a literature review than an independent research study like the one carried out earlier. This committee determined that based on the published scientific literature, there was indeed a cause-and-effect relationship between viewing violent pornography and committing acts of rape and sexual assault. (More current data do not come to this conclusion.) The legal implications of the Meese Commission report were important, for they recommended strict legal penalties for the producers and purchasers of obscene materials. The methods used in the Meese Commission report are flawed in several ways, however. The figures who testified before the committee did not represent a cross-section of the American public; most were decidedly conservative and unscientific in their stated allegiances. Also, this commission systematically excluded the social policy and legal opinions of a number of scholars in the academic community.

A more cautious, well-reasoned approach to the scientific evidence about pornography also appeared in 1986. The Surgeon General of the United States, Dr. C. Everett Koop, published a report on pornography in which he wrote that we are still unsure about the behavioral, emotional, or intellectual consequences of observing pornography. This report noted the problems in generalizing information obtained in the laboratory to the real world and urged caution about making any inferences that may not be supported by the data.

Pornography on the Internet

Because of the incredible technological advances that have taken place since earlier Supreme Court rulings about definitions of pornography, potentially "questionable" images and materials are reaching the public through new sources. Magazines continue to cater to customers with highly diverse sexual tastes and preferences. Videos depict explicit images of sexual intercourse and other sexual activities. Many family video stores have an "Adult" section. Cable and closed-circuit television systems show pornography and erotica. CD-ROMs with plainly sexual content have become very popular. The movies continue to be a focus of controversy regarding standards of obscenity and decency. And of course, the Internet has an enormous number of websites that appeal to individuals interested in viewing sexually frank pictures (Fig. 19-11). In fact, the Internet is the area of greatest growth in the production of pornography for the American consumer. Pornography was close to a billion dollar a year industry in 1998 after having generated about 40% in annual growth over the few previous years. This is a large share of the total amount of revenue from the Internet of $4.8 billion in 1998. In the second quarter of 1998, 43% of all Internet traffic found its way to sexually related websites (Tedesco, 1998). Pornography is clearly big business.

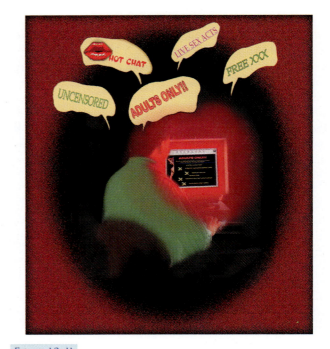

FIGURE 19-11   On the Internet, one can visit websites that appeal to virtually every sexual interest, taste, and preference. Issues surrounding free speech have been introduced into the public discussion of these websites.

One of the most controversial issues involving the availability of sexually explicit material on the Internet is the access minors may have to these materials. Although most agree there is a problem with children and teens viewing pornography on their home or school computers, policing Internet access involves a number of legal issues such as those of free speech. However, blocking and filtering software is effective in stopping the transmission of images from pornographic websites. Late in 1998, when the Child Online Protection Act (COPA) was to become law, the American Civil Liberties Union (ACLU) along with the Electronic Privacy Information Center and the Electronic Frontier Foundation sought in federal district court in Philadelphia to delay the application of the law. These groups are not pro-pornography but are pro-free speech. If this law goes into effect, commercial websites would be required to solicit identification numbers or credit card numbers before allowing access to hard core pornography. Those who are convicted of violating the law will have to pay a fine of $50,000 and/or serve a 6-month jail term (Albiniak, 1998).

An interesting legal analysis of this issue (Cate, 1996) notes that the amount of sexually related material on the Internet accounts for a relatively small percentage of its current content (estimates range from 1% to 10%), especially in light of the amount of attention given to this issue by the media and the government. Cate emphasizes that generally this attention is not sensitive to important legal considerations involved.

In a particularly lengthy and careful assessment of the feasibility of censorship on the Internet, Simon (1998) notes that the government does indeed have the legal authority and precedent of creating laws that selectively protect minors, but at the same time, the government does not have "unlimited" powers to do so. Additionally, many pornographic websites are located outside of the United States. Further, there is precedent in Supreme Court decisions to examine the potential for regulation, review, and censorship in different communications media rather than applying a single blanket standard to television, print media, radio, the Internet, etc. For the protection of free speech under the first amendment to operate, the *content* of the message may *not* be censored, but the viewpoint of the presenter *may* be censored. For a strategy of censorship to have legal authority, it must be feasible, and as of this writing, there is no technological or practical means by which the true identity (and age) of someone requesting information on the Internet can be established authoritatively. Therefore, Simon asserts that as of this writing, the Internet will remain fundamentally free of censorship or arbitrary restrictions.

The Effects of Pornography on the Observer

Just as people have somewhat different sexual tastes and preferences and thoughts about sexual behavior, so too are we likely to have different tastes, preferences, and thoughts about *observing* sexual behavior. For example, some people enjoy watching sexual behaviors among consenting adults, especially behaviors of reciprocal enjoyment. There may be an important element of vicarious experience in viewing pornography. However, others have come to enjoy sexual activities involving force and aggression. In 1970, the findings of the Presidential Commission on Obscenity and Pornography caused quite a stir because at that time the data indicated that there were no harmful effects associated with viewing pornographic materials (Donnerstein & Malamuth, 1997). The current state of knowledge about the different effects of aggressive and nonaggressive pornography is far from clear, however. Donnerstein and Malamuth (1997) summarized this literature and noted the following findings. Among men who are normally somewhat aggressive individuals, exposure to nonaggressive pornography may increase their aggressive behavior, as if exposure to this material somehow lowered their behavioral threshold to act in a way to which they may have already been predisposed. However other data reveal just the opposite: exposing these men to nonaggressive pornography may in fact diminish later aggressive behaviors. These writers suggest that as pornography becomes progressively more aggressive, it also becomes more arousing to some viewers. Nonaggressive pornography may in fact distract or even relax people, while aggressive pornography may make some individuals more aroused and likely to act out their anger and hostilities. From a behavioral perspective, when aggressive feelings are consistently paired with sexual feelings, sexual arousal may ultimately come to precipitate aggression.

Another issue is how the recipients of sexual aggression and violence react in the pornography. If the viewer is led to believe that women being treated aggressively and roughly during sex actually enjoy the violence as an aspect of their sexual arousal, then he may begin to think that such an assault is in fact justified and acceptable. An individual with highly aggressive tendencies may in fact be somewhat provoked by images portraying aggressive sex.

The selective impact of pornography on males of various ages has long been an active area of research. In an excellent review of this topic, Stock (1997) emphasizes that a young boy's first exposure to sexuality and sexual imagery is often through pornography, and this medium therefore has a powerful potential to shape his developing sexuality as well as his perceptions of females. Most pornography illustrates what is called **nonrelational sex.** Levant and Brooks (1997) define nonrelational sex as, "the tendency to experience sex primarily as lust without any requirements for relational intimacy or emotional attachment" (p. 1). When strong pleasurable feelings associated with orgasm take place while a person is viewing depictions of nonrelational sex, a powerful association is created, one which may be difficult or impossible to "unlearn." Stock also suggests that when males view pornography, they often use these experiences to create a personal belief system about male roles in sexual relationships. Exposure to pornography can contribute to some problems in the way males view themselves, their bodies, and their partner's bodies. Stock (1997) reported that 60% of males in her study compared themselves unfavorably to actors they see in pornographic films and videos. Of these subjects, 22% felt that they were not tall enough, 48% thought that they were not sufficiently muscular, and 29% believed that their penises were too small. These males also made comparisons between their partners and the bodies of actresses portrayed in films and videos, and 51% reported feelings of disappointment with their partners, 27% felt that their partner's breasts were too small, 35% reported that their partner's buttocks were unattractive in such a comparison, 27% felt that their partner's legs were unappealing, and 23% reported that their partners weighed too much. Data like these indicate that pornography may contribute to the way men view women as sex objects rather than as individuals in an intimate relationship.

In an attempt to find out whether different kinds of pornography affect men's attitudes and thoughts about women, Bauserman (1998) presented slides of mutually enjoyable sex, exploitative sex, and aggressive sex to 115 male undergraduates. All depicted female-male sexual interactions. While this researcher was unable to demonstrate any attitudinal shift among these subjects based on the type of pornography they viewed, subjects did, however, report that they had the most positive thoughts and feelings after viewing scenes in which a couple enjoyed mutual, egalitarian sexual interactions. It is heartening to note that in this sample of young men, many reported an aversion to viewing scenes of exploitative and aggressive sexual behavior by men. As noted in earlier chapters, attitudes are relatively stable and enduring personality traits, and it is unlikely that these men's attitudes would change noticeably as a result of exposure to stimulus materials such as pornography.

Remember that social learning theory asserts that when we observe the behavior of others we often experience vicariously what we imagine they are experiencing, and that through these observations we learn ways of acting without actually practicing those behaviors. Therefore social and behavioral scientists have had some very serious concerns about the impact of watching sexually aggressive pornography, although the relationship between viewing these images and later sexually aggressive acts is by no means clear. Bauserman (1996) reviewed the research exploring the correlation between viewing aggressive pornography and later sexual offenses. A correlation only describes the magnitude of the relationship between two things, of course, and does not reveal a cause-and-effect relationship. When he examined the research on this issue, Bauserman found no apparent relationship between exposure to pornography during childhood or adolescence and committing sexual offenses later in life. Importantly, this researcher also reports that there is no apparent relationship between the regular use of pornography and acts of rape. Other research has focused on the relationship between exposure to pornography and men's attitudes about feminism and rape. Davies (1997) collected data from 194 men who rented pornographic films from a video rental business in a large metropolitan area in the late 1980s. Subjects were asked their opinions about the Equal Rights Amendment, a statute against marital rape, and penalties for date and marital rape. No correlation was found between the number of X-rated videos a man rented and his attitudes about these feminist and rape issues. Data like these suggest that there may not be a clear relationship between men's viewing of pornographic videos and their thoughts and feelings about women. To say that rapists regularly view pornographic materials (and not all do) is *not* to say that these experiences provoke sexual assaults in many or most men. While viewing pornography may be physically arousing, it is premature to suggest that this arousal is readily channeled into sexually offensive attitudes and behaviors.

Still other writers, however, notably Russell (1998b), do not accept the validity of findings like these but have constructed a powerful case linking men's viewing of pornography and their predisposition to rape women. In her book, *Dangerous Relationships,* Diana E. H. Russell presents a theoretical analysis that suggests that pornography may predispose *some* men to want to rape women and that viewing pornography may diminish a man's internal inhibitions against restraining their desire to rape. Further, she suggests that pornography, particularly degrading and violent pornography, may also lessen social inhibitions against their desire to rape.

We noted at the beginning of this discussion of pornography that this is a very emotional issue that has generated a great deal of research, and some contradictory conclusions have been reached. Since no one has yet settled this controversy once and for all, it is important to see both sides of the issue.

Women's Responses to Pornography

So far this discussion has focused primarily on how men respond to various kinds of pornography. A recent study has explored the impact of male-oriented and female-oriented pornography on women. Male-oriented pornography tends to focus on visual depictions of a variety of penetrative sexual behaviors in which the male is more or less in charge of the sexual interaction. This may or may not imply coercion or aggression. Additionally, male-oriented pornography is likely to focus on depictions of a woman's anatomy and usually includes "close-up" film views of penetration and sometimes ejaculation, which usually takes place outside of the woman's vagina. While female-oriented pornography may include many of the elements just described, it typically focuses on co-equal sexual sharing and the depiction of intimate behaviors in which there isn't a "leader" or "director." There is much more kissing and hugging as well as nurturant verbalization. Presumably, female-oriented pornography is manufactured because it appeals to erotic preferences of women not addressed by male-oriented pornography. In 1997, Pearson and Pollack published a study in which women's reports of sexual arousal were associated with their viewing male- or female-oriented pornography. The subjects in this research, between the ages of 18 and 26, filled out questionnaires that explored their sexual experiences, degree of sexual guilt, and demographic and personal characteristics. While they were watching these videos, the subjects rated their degree of sexual arousal. The results were clear: subjects who observed the female-oriented videos reported significantly higher levels of sexual arousal than subjects in the group who observed the male-oriented video. In analyzing their data further, Pearson and Pollack found that subjects with previous experience with pornographic films, novels, and magazines reported higher levels of sexual arousal after viewing female-oriented pornography. However, sexual arousal was not related to the subject's age or previous sexual experience.

In a different study Laan, Everaerd, van Bellen, and Hanewald (1994) studied the physiological responses of women presented with female- and male-oriented pornography. Photoplethysmographic responses were measured in a group of 47 subjects who observed short segments of female- and male-oriented erotic films. Interestingly, there were no differences in the amplitude of the physiological responses while viewing these two types of films. However, as in the research cited above, *subjective* sexual arousal among these women was reported to be significantly greater while viewing the female-oriented films.

The Special Case of Sadomasochistic Pornography

The somewhat unique nature of sadomasochistic pornography has received a good bit of serious, scholarly attention (Shortes, 1998). Sadomasochistic pornography is clearly different from "traditional" pornography in which nudity and/or the depiction of heterosexual or homosexual sexual acts is the centerpiece. S/M pornography, instead, focuses on the complex roles of fantasy and power as aspects of sexual expression and very often does not reveal genitalia, genital, or oral-genital contact (Fig. 19-12). Shortes (1998) notes that it wasn't until the mid-1980s that S/M pornography could be recognized as clearly

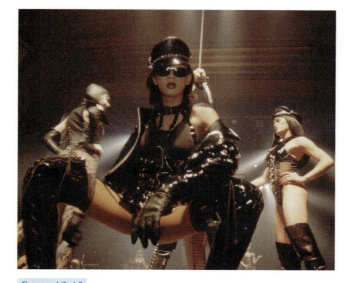

FIGURE 19-12 Unlike other kinds of pornography, sadomasochistic pornography focuses on complex roles of dominance and power and may not reveal much nudity at all.

different from what she calls "mainstream pornography." Before this time, any depictions of S/M activities were often "pretend" representations of common sadomasochistic activities and focused on our culture's recognition of the powerful and violent aspects of many sexual desires and interactions. Andrea Dworkin, a well-known feminist, believes that *all* pornography is basically sadomasochistic because it reveals an exploitative difference in power between women and men. However, Shortes' analysis is more discriminating in the way she describes and discusses S/M pornography. Interestingly, S/M pornography involves a loophole in laws describing obscene and/or indecent materials. Such legal definitions usually emphasize the fact that most people would find traditional pornography offensive and stimulating. Yet most people have little understanding of or attraction to S/M sexual activities and therefore find them more odd than erotic. In a trial in which a jury is shown films that local prosecutors deem obscene, the more unusual or astonishing the images, the greater the chances that these materials would be judged obscene. In summary, Shortes makes a strong case for a clear distinction between S/M and mainstream pornography.

SEXUAL HARASSMENT

The 1990s will be remembered as the beginning of an era in which women who were sexually embarrassed, harassed, and exploited in the work place said "Enough!" Along with this demand for respect came a puzzling diversity of definitions of the term "sexual harassment." There have been complaints of sexual harassment in virtually every sphere of American life: workplaces, schools, colleges, corporate boardrooms, the courts, and health care settings, to name just a few. More people are talking about it, acknowledging its presence, making complaints about it, and bringing legal action over it. One of the more unfortu-

nate aspects of gender inequality in human relations has been the prevalence of sexual harassment. Although women have made tremendous strides in this country over the past 40 years, addressing this issue has been long overdue.

One very public, very important event brought sexual harassment into clear focus for the entire nation (Borger, 1991). On October 6, 1991, a law professor at the University of Oklahoma, Ms. Anita Hill, claimed that while working for Judge Clarence Thomas, a nominee to the United States Supreme Court, she had been exposed to behaviors on the part of Judge Thomas that were both "unwelcome and unwanted" and of an explicitly sexual nature (Fig. 19-13). Clarence Thomas, an African American, politically conservative judge was being accused of appalling behaviors. His accuser, Ms. Hill, also an African American, had pulled herself up from a background of poverty to become a highly respected attorney and law school professor. To make the case even more pressing in the eyes of the public was the fact that the United States Senate, at that time 98% male, had to vote on Judge Thomas' confirmation. A vote to confirm would seem to deny the truthfulness of Ms. Hill's statements as well as the mental anguish she had experienced as a direct result of Judge Thomas's alleged behavior. Ms.

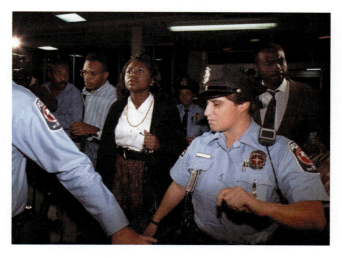

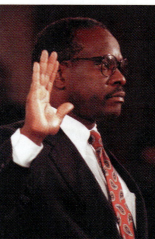

FIGURE 19-13 Top: Professor Anita Hill, who accused U.S. Supreme Court nominee Judge Clarence Thomas of sexual harassment, leaves Washington's National Airport amid heavy police protection on October 10, 1991. Below: Judge Clarence Thomas is sworn in before testifying before the Senate Judiciary Committee on October 11, 1991. Judge Thomas categorically denied all of Hill's allegations.

Hill's testimony was especially graphic, lurid, and detailed. Ms. Hill testified that Judge Thomas told her that his penis was much larger than normal and that he was adept at giving women sexual pleasure during oral sex. He was also accused of talking in the workplace about pornography he had seen. In his powerful and consistent denials, Judge Thomas made it clear that he believed he was being persecuted and that his accuser had fabricated her accusation. It became a very public case of "her word against his," which in fact is often the case with sexual harassment. Still, Ms. Hill impressed many in Congress and throughout the country as a credible individual of the highest personal integrity. Ms. Hill said that the stress created by these encounters led to her being hospitalized. Many important questions were unanswered during these proceedings. For example, there was no clear explanation why Ms. Hill declined to bring charges against Judge Thomas until 10 years after the events had allegedly occurred. Another unanswered question centered on the well-documented fact that Ms. Hill changed jobs in 1982 to continue working with Judge Thomas when he transferred from the United States Department of Education to the Equal Employment Opportunity Commission (EEOC). A number of telephone logs demonstrated that Hill had stayed in touch with Thomas frequently during the time after she left Washington. In the end, of course, Judge Thomas was confirmed by the Senate and took his place on the highest court of the land.

The Clarence Thomas - Anita Hill confrontation demonstrates many of the elements of accusations of sexual harassment. Women do not often promptly report sexual harassment. A longstanding tradition of male dominance in legal and judiciary circles may discourage women from promptly and assertively filing a complaint of sexual harassment, and some even feel that women provoke harassment. Sexual banter in the workplace, while common, is not always interpreted in the same way it is offered. This section will explore the nature of sexual harassment, the behaviors commonly involved, and personal, legal, and institutional measures that have been taken to minimize and eliminate sexual harassment from the workplace and other settings in American life.

One of the issues that has received keen attention since 1991 is liability. Who is legally accountable for sexual harassment—the person supposedly committing the offensive behavior or the organization or agency they work for? If a company, college or university, agency, or other organization has created a policy that addresses, discourages, and punishes sexual harassment, then it is appropriate to assume that everyone who works there knows the policy and follows it. In the event that an employee engages in behaviors interpreted as sexually harassing by another or others, she or he must personally answer to any charges and is personally liable for their behavior. However, if the corporate entity does not have a public, well-articulated policy against sexual harassment and one of its employees engages in these behaviors, the organization is then liable for the employee's behaviors.

This issue caught the attention of corporate America, educational establishments, and a large number of workplaces with relative suddenness. After 30 years of social progress in creating gender equality in American life, the time was clearly ripe for this particular issue to take center stage. In the 1990s there was much strident anger and activism about this issue that has since abated, replaced by a more well-reasoned climate of discourse.

The United States Equal Opportunity Commission and the Office of Civil Rights have published guidelines about what exactly constitutes sexual harassment. Sexual harassment is a form of discrimination which violates Title VII of the Civil Rights Act of 1964. The EEOC defines sexual harassment, in part, as follows:

> *Unwelcomed sexual advances, requests for sexual favors, and other verbal or physical conduct of a sexual nature constitutes sexual harassment when submission to or rejection of this conduct explicitly or implicitly affects an individual's employment, unreasonably interferes with an individual's work performance or creates an intimidating, hostile or offensive work environment. (EEOC, 1980)*

The EEOC makes clear the fact that both women and men can be sexually harassed and the person doing the harassing does not necessarily have to be a member of the opposite sex. The harasser can be a boss, supervisor, someone working on behalf of the employer, a co-worker, someone working elsewhere in the organization, or even someone on the premises of an organization who is not an employee of that organization. The victim of sexual harassment does not necessarily have to be the person who is being harassed. For example, if someone in an organization is being given preferential treatment of some type because she or he is succumbing to sexual harassment, others in that organization who are not receiving similar preferential treatment are legally also victims of the harasser. The EEOC notes that a person does not have to suffer any economic hardship because of the harassment, nor do they have to be fired for not complying with requests for sexual favors in order to be sexually harassed under the law. Finally, the conduct of the harasser must be unwelcomed in order for sexual harassment to exist. Victims of sexual harassment should use whatever mechanism an employer or organization has put in place to make a formal complaint.

The Office of Civil Rights published a pamphlet about sexual harassment in the academic world that was updated in May 1997. Entitled "Sexual Harassment: It's Not Academic," it is available without charge from the United States Government Printing Office. Anyone can call their representative in Congress and request a copy. This pamphlet gives specific examples of illegal sexual conduct, including "sexual advances, touching of a sexual nature, graffiti of a sexual nature, displaying or distributing sexually explicit drawings, pictures and written materials, sexual gestures, sexual or 'dirty' jokes, pressure for sexual favors, touching oneself sexually or talking about one's sexual activity in front of others, and spreading rumors about or rating other students as to sexual activity or performance." This is not an exhaustive list but includes some of the more common manifestations of what the government deems sexual harassment.

Two issues of special importance are what is called "quid pro quo" harassment and the creation of a "hostile environment." In **quid pro quo sexual harassment**, there is a clearly implied "deal" or "bargain" that involves the exchange of sexual favors in return for some special consideration or evaluation. When a teacher tells a student that he will give her an "A" for the course if she has sex with him, this is a clear example of quid pro quo sexual harassment. It is also quid pro quo sexual harassment if the student tells the teacher that she will have sex with him if he gives her an "A." The same is true of educators who include students on athletic teams, promise to write strong letters of recommendation, or work to secure financial aid in exchange for sexual favors. Regardless of whether the student complies with the "offer," illegal sexual harassment has occurred.

Although it is usually relatively easy to determine quid pro quo sexual harassment, the hostile environment issue may not always be so clear. In academic settings, college administrators are not usually attorneys and may make decisions about the issue of a hostile environment in the absence of valid legal evidence or corroboration.

When is Sexual Harassment Likely to Occur?

O'Hare and O'Donohue (1998) have identified a number of perspectives on the causes of sexual harassment. Each of these may provide a potential explanation for the prevalence and implications of this widespread personal and occupational problem.

THE NATURAL/BIOLOGICAL MODEL
According to this perspective sexual harassment is a "common" manifestation of the "natural" sexual attraction between women and men. This approach holds that because men supposedly have a stronger sex drive than women, they are more inclined to behave in a sexually assertive manner and sexual harassment is but one form of this. While some of the sexual harassment men inflict on women might be unwanted and unwelcomed, this is just a routine aspect of a man's sex drive according to this perspective.

THE ORGANIZATIONAL MODEL
Tangri, Burt, and Johnson (1982) believe that the power hierarchy of the workplace creates a situation in which those with more power and authority are likely to abuse their roles to satisfy their sexual needs by harassing those who work for them. This model holds that sexual harassment is a means by which those in authority may threaten and exploit their employees. The number of women in the organization, their rank and job tasks, and the existence of procedures for filing grievances are all variables that affect the prevalence of sexual harassment according to this view.

THE SOCIOCULTURAL MODEL
This approach views sexual harassment as an occupational form of male dominance that serves to keep men in positions of leadership and intimidates women into leaving the work environment. According to this view, women and men experience different socialization experiences. Men are often brought up to be active and assertive while women are frequently raised to be passive and submissive. The sociocultural model maintains that sexual harassment is one way men try to maintain their assertive roles while subjugating women to less powerful positions in society.

THE SEX-ROLE SPILLOVER MODEL
This perspective views sexual harassment in the workplace as a "spillover" from expectations about women that have nothing to do with work. According to this view, sexual harassment is most likely to occur when there are either a lot more men than women or a lot more women than men in the workplace. In both instances, traditional sex roles become extremely obvious. When the workplace is dominated by men, women are viewed as somewhat unique, and therefore their sex is more obvious than their occupational tasks. In contrast, when the workplace has far more women than men, a woman's occupational productivity and traditional conceptions of feminine passivity become somewhat blurred, and again, according to Gutek and Morasch (1982), a woman's sexuality may be more conspicuous than her professional role, perhaps leading to sexual advances. O'Hare and O'Donohue believe that this model includes elements of both the organizational and sociocultural approaches and is a more powerful predictor of sexual harassment.

O'Hare and O'Donohue recognized potential causes of sexual harassment at the individual, organizational, and social level and explored the usefulness of a model characterizing variables that are likely to lead to sexual harassment in the workplace. Using a theory about the origins of child sexual abuse (Finkelhor, 1984), O'Hare and O'Donohue applied the same suspected causes to the study of sexual harassment. This led to the development of what they called the four-factor model. Each of the following factors is explicitly related to these theoretical approaches to the study of sexual harassment in the workplace.

1. Motives for sexual harassment. These often focus on a man's need for power and dominance, his need for control, and his sensitivity to a woman's physical attractiveness. Sexual advances are an expression of these needs for power.
2. Overcoming internal inhibitions against sexual harassment. These factors are related to a man's understanding of the illegalities involved in harassment, the immoral and unethical nature of harassment behaviors, and the ability to imagine what a woman might be experiencing when she is being sexually harassed.
3. Overcoming external inhibitions against sexual harassment. These factors involve the existence of a clear grievance policy and procedure and an understanding of the outcomes of one's actions and the negative personal and professional consequences of harassing activities.

4. Overcoming victim resistance. These factors focus on a man's awareness of a woman's recognition of harassing behaviors and her capacity to thwart those behaviors.

—O'Hare and O'Donohue, 1998

Their study of 266 female university professors, staff members, and students found that these four factors are highly accurate in predicting the occurrence of sexual harassment in academic settings. These subjects filled out two questionnaires reporting their experiences with sexual harassment. It remains to be seen whether these factors will also predict sexual harassment in other workplaces and interpersonal settings.

Sexual Harassment in the Workplace

Because of the legal issues surrounding sexual harassment and the possibility that a relationship gone sour can be thoroughly disruptive in a work climate, companies of all sizes have hired consultants to stop or prevent sexual harassment. Sexual harassment has become something of a legal industry in its own right. Attorneys, consultants, private investigators, labor mediators, psychotherapists, and counselors have all gotten into the act (*U. S. News & World Report,* December 14, 1998). For when a company is faced with the choice of possibly paying out hundreds of thousands (or millions) of dollars in a sexual harassment lawsuit, spending a few thousand dollars for a day-long workshop about sexual harassment in the workplace makes good sense. Training seminars are widely believed to be the most effective preventive measure against sexual harassment in the workplace. According to the EEOC, more than 15,000 sexual harassment suits are filed each year. And the payouts can be enormous. In 1998, the Mitsubishi Motor Corporation settled out of court for *$34 million* to end long-standing sexual harassment practices at its factory in Normal, Illinois. Employees now are far more careful about what they say and do for fear that their superiors and subordinates might get the wrong idea.

Different companies take somewhat different approaches to sexual harassment issues. Some have a rigid "no dating" rule. Others have adopted a policy in which co-workers who are romantically involved agree to be very open about it and inform supervisors and fellow employees promptly to ensure that what is happening is mutually agreeable to both parties. Of course, the most controversial relationships are those between supervisors and employees who work directly for them. Fear of accusations of sexual harassment has changed some business practices too. For example, when on business travel together female and male employees may book rooms on different floors of a hotel and hold all business meetings in conference rooms instead of regular hotel rooms with beds (*U. S. News & World Report,* December 14, 1998).

Sexual harassment has led to so many expensive lawsuits that many companies now purchase "employee practice liability insurance" to protect them in case they must pay attorneys to defend them in sexual harassment suits (Solomon, 1998). About half of America's Fortune 500 companies have such policies. In 1997 the amount paid in a sexual harassment case stood at $10 million, compared with $1.3 million only the year before. Solomon (1998), however, points out an important fact about this liability insurance: if people know that a company has it, they may be more likely to sue in an attempt to recover money. Other investigators (Pierce & Aguinis, 1997) suggested that it is practically impossible to eliminate sexual harassment from the workplace, especially through the use of legalistic, rigid administrative mandates. Perhaps the best one can hope for are clear organizational policies about a human relations issues in conjunction with regular training seminars that focus on all forms of sexual harassment.

Measuring Sexual Harassment

Although the hallmark of scientific investigation is quantitative measurement, the study of sexual harassment has focused on the description and documentation of isolated, unquantified instances of offensive behavior. Murdoch and McGovern (1998) emphasize the importance of recognizing sexual harassment as quickly as possible because of the many adverse physical and psychological consequences associated with it. Specifically, anxiety, depression, posttraumatic stress disorder, alcohol abuse, and such ailments as ulcers, migraine headaches, and high blood pressure have all been documented in individuals who reported being sexually harassed.

Using EEOC guidelines, Murdoch and McGovern developed a paper-and-pencil questionnaire to assess both "quid pro quo" and "hostile environment" types of sexual harassment. They first tested their instrument with women on active duty in the military as well as other employees of the federal government. Following is their test. Although it was developed for military and government personnel, there is no reason it cannot be adapted to other occupational groups. Items 1 through 20 are answered yes or no, and the last item allows the respondent to offer more personal, qualitative data.

The Sexual Harassment Inventory (Military Version)

1. People with whom I worked made sexual jokes that made me feel uncomfortable.
2. I was touched by a co-worker or supervisor in ways that made me feel uncomfortable.
3. A coworker frequently asked me out for dates, even though I had asked him/her to stop.
4. A supervisor or superior officer asked me out for dates, even though I had asked him/her to stop.
5. A supervisor or superior officer threatened to block my promotion unless I agreed to have sex with him/her.
6. A supervisor or superior officer threatened to block a favorable transfer unless I agreed to have sex with him/her.
7. Coworkers made sexual comments about my body.
8. My supervisor or superior officer made sexual comments about my body.
9. My coworkers or superior officer exposed themselves to me in a sexual way.

10. I was offered favorable assignments in exchange for sex with my supervisor or commanding officer.

11. I was offered promotions in exchange for having sex with my supervisor or commanding officer.

12. A coworker or coworkers attempted to have sex with me without my consent.

13. My coworkers made demeaning comments to me because I was a woman/man.

14. I was given the most unpleasant, difficult assignments because I was a woman/man.

15. The people I work with put up posters of women/men in provocative poses.

16. My supervisor or superior officer attempted to have sex with me without my consent.

17. Some of the people I worked with leered at me in a sexual way.

18. Some of the people I worked with made catcalls or sexual remarks when I walked by.

19. I was forced by a coworker or supervisor to have sex without my consent.

20. Were you ever prevented from getting a promotion, favorable assignment, or transfer because you refused to have sex with someone?

21. Were there other things of a sexual nature that happened to you while you were in the military? (Please list)

Murdoch and McGovern sought to determine which of these questions provided clues to the most and least severe interpretations of sexual harassment. Question 19, which asks if an individual had been forced to have sex with a coworker or supervisor against their consent, was judged to be the most severe manifestation of sexual harassment, while Question 1, sexual jokes, was judged least severe. Research like this can provide counselors and human resource personnel with specific information about the various forms of sexual harassment in the workplace as well as the differential seriousness of various offenses.

Policies to Eliminate Sexual Harassment

Measures can be taken to create more civil, egalitarian workplace and educational environments. Although lawsuits sometimes resolve sexual harassment complaints, it would be better if institutional procedures were in place to reduce their frequency or eliminate them altogether. In the *Employee Responsibilities and Rights Journal,* Peirce, Rosen, and Hiller (1997) analyzed reasons women are frequently harassed sexually but infrequently report these abuses and explored the requirements for creating "user-friendly" sexual harassment reporting procedures. These researchers surveyed a sample of 1500 working women to find out what kind of sexual harassment policies would help women feel more comfortable reporting their complaints. These authors isolated three broad factors important in such policies, as follows:

Strong Management Support. When senior administrative and supervisory officials take a clear public stand against sexual harassment and create a "no tolerance" policy, employees feel supported and are more likely to report incidents of sexual harassment and to believe that management will take them seriously and investigate their complaints.

Offer Employees Privacy and Anonymity. Almost 4 of 5 respondents reported that access to confidential counseling would help them feel more comfortable reporting sexual harassment. Importantly, 84.4% of these subjects believed that some authority outside the organization would make them feel even more comfortable registering their complaints. Because sexual harassment often occurs between supervisors and subordinates, the latter often believe that they will suffer reprisal for making a complaint and are therefore hesitant to do so unless they are offered privacy and anonymity. Almost 9 of 10 of these subjects believed that sexual harassment complaints should be kept separate from their permanent personnel files and that they should have to give their consent to anyone who wanted to investigate these documents.

Investigating Complaints. Virtually all respondents in this study believed that there should be no adverse consequences for women who make sexual harassment complaints that have been supported through investigation. Respondents overwhelmingly supported the importance of a neutral negotiator to serve as a liaison between the person making the complaint and the organization.

In addition to these three primary preconditions for a "user-friendly" sexual harassment policy, most respondents also felt that it was important for employees to see real consequences for these workplace abuses and for such penalties to be promptly imposed.

Historically there has been much sexual harassment in settings of higher education. For a variety of reasons, professors and their students have had sexual relationships since colleges and universities were first founded. These relationships have not always been consensual, and even when they are consensual there is some well-founded concern about the unequal power status of professor and student. Of course, it would be virtually impossible to have policies against student-professor relationships because of the guaranteed right to "freedom of association" under the United States Constitution. Both quid pro quo and hostile environment types of sexual harassment are common in collegiate settings. In recent years there has been more serious discussion about these potentially explosive relationships and their impact on the educational setting and the people involved intimately. Because female students have been sexually harassed more frequently than male students, most of the literature on sexual harassment in higher education has focused on male professors and female students.

The controversy surrounding the Clarence Thomas - Anita Hill confrontation played a major role in sensitizing women, especially in universities, to the nature of sexual harassment and its potentially adverse consequences for all parties involved. The publicity of these hearings motivated women at a large, public New England university to form an organization called Women Against Sexual Harassment (WASH). This organization sought to educate students and faculty about the importance of avoiding sexist behaviors, preserving privacy, legitimizing feminist viewpoints, and refraining from all activities that might be interpreted as quid pro quo sexual harassment or the creation of a hostile environment for women on campus (Lott & Roccio, 1998). WASH publicized its agenda at the department, individual, university, and community levels. While there was some resistance to the strident feminist philosophy behind this group, most people on campus believed that this group had opened an important dialogue and sought to end doubt and confusion about a potentially very contentious issue. Clearly, WASH played a pivotal role in "consciousness raising" concerning this very troubling subject. Students felt less vulnerable and better informed. Professors and teaching assistants gained a clearer sense of institutional opinion with respect to potential sexual exploitation. We are especially impressed with WASH in part because it is an effective program that developed from the bottom up. The people who stood to gain the most by opening discussion and organizing interested parties were instrumental in starting this organization.

Responses to Sexual Harassment

While colleges, universities, and other organizations and workplaces may develop procedures for reporting, investigating, and resolving sexual harassment complaints, the personality of the person being harassed probably determines whether these resources are ultimately used. Perry, Kulik, and Schmidtke (1997) studied the factors that determine women's responses to sexual harassment. Their work examines whether a woman's feelings of personal power, the power of her position in an organization, and the organization's record of resolving incidents of sexual harassment can predict how a woman will behave if she is sexually harassed. Over 400 women responded to a hypothetical example of sexual harassment involving "Lisa," a 26-year-old, college-educated, single employee; this describes the type of individual most likely to be sexually harassed. In general, the factors noted above were shown relevant to the way these subjects responded to Lisa's situation. But feelings of personal power did not predict who would be likely to report sexual harassment. In fact, the more power a woman had, the *less likely* she was to report a real instance of sexual harassment. Also, the respondent's level of education was not significantly related to the likelihood that she would report sexual harassment. In another investigation, Adams-Roy and Barling (1998) found that measures of a woman's personal assertiveness predict who will report harassment. These writers also found that clear organizational procedures for reporting, investigating, and punishing harassment are powerful predictors of who is likely to register a formal complaint.

Feminism and Sexual Harassment

Feminist ideology is a central focus in the American psychosocial landscape. Since the early 1960s the rights of women have been an extremely important issue in efforts to achieve equal rights in all avenues of American life. While major social changes take place very slowly, there have been important advances in women's rights over the last two generations. We are not saying that full equality among women and men has been achieved in all spheres, but progress has certainly been made. In 1978, Catharine A. MacKinnon wrote *Sexual Harassment of the Working Woman: A Case of Sex Discrimination.* Largely because of the impact of this work, the United States Supreme Court decided in 1986 that sexual harassment in the workplace was indeed a violation of the law. Yet women and men today still experience conflicted working relations and remain somewhat mistrustful of one another with respect to the "letter of the law" defining sexual harassment (Shalit, 1998). Shalit notes that it is possible for a sexual interaction between two people to be much desired and entirely consensual and still be problematic in the workplace.

This is a good example of how the laws of the land have created a standard of behavior that in fact may be unattainable because of long-held, stubborn misperceptions about the autonomy and integrity of women in commercial, professional, and educational settings (Fig. 19-14).

Shalit emphasizes that sexual harassment is an example of a very pervasive cultural lack of civility toward women. Television talk shows today reveal unbelievably rude and offensive utterances and behaviors toward women. Common profanities on the street and the many men who abandon their partners are further examples of this distressing social trend.

Unfortunately, sexual harassment has focused the public's attention on only *one* aspect of feminism, neglecting an enormous and rich body of scholarship about women. This is only one forum in which women have asked for respect and equality; it is certainly not the only one. Benedict (1998) raised an interesting parallel between the central focus of feminism in the 1990s (sexual harassment) and the central focus of feminism in

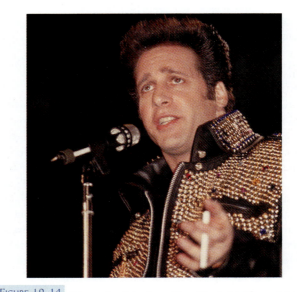

FIGURE 19-14   "Comedian" Andrew Dice Clay's highly sexist act is routinely perceived by woman as insulting, offensive, and crude. When shared in the workplace, jokes like his may be construed as sexual harassment.

the 1970s (rape). She notes that the interests of women are often reflected in the way the media treats issues. In the 1970s, the media seemed obsessed with the idea that rape is a conspiracy among men to subjugate all women and that women who firmly resist rape are denying men's techniques of sexual persuasion. Benedict also notes that in the 1970s, feminists were invited to comment on the distinction between rape and consensual sex, just as they are today being asked to clarify the difference between consensual sex and sexual harassment.

Sexual Harassment of Specific Groups of Women

In most discussions of sexual harassment, one easily imagines an office worker or college student. Yet sexual harassment occurs in virtually all arenas in which women work. Women in all professions and occupations are harassed sexually, as shown by the examples in the following sections.

THE CASE OF THE HARVARD BUSINESS SCHOOL

In April 1998, six graduate students at the Harvard Business School were disciplined for sexually harassing a number of their female classmates (*Inc.,* 1998). The numbers of women graduating from this program had fallen steadily since the middle of the 1980s, and it has nothing to do with ability, talent, or persistence. It has been widely acknowledged that this institution has some very serious problems with sexual harassment. No matter how prestigious the institution or organization, no matter how smart the students or employees, no matter how egalitarian the policies on paper, sexual harassment can still occur. Some of the male students in the business school at Harvard had sent their female classmates "lewd and sexually explicit notes." The administration at the business school conducted an investigation, and six individuals who had engaged in these harassing behaviors were required to apologize to the entire Harvard Business School, both students and faculty, as a condition of their graduation.

If the professional work environments of tomorrow are to be free of sexual harassment, the institutions in which these people are being trained need to be more sensitive about the seriousness of these behaviors and more aggressive in investigating and resolving serious complaints. There is something subtle but important about the case at Harvard. No one came forward and openly took responsibility for their actions; all those accused tried to weasel out of the accusations without admitting any personal role in these embarrassing and painful events.

FEMALE LAWYERS

Laband and Lentz (1998) studied the impact of sexual harassment on women in law school and later during their employment in a law firm. Astonishingly, two-thirds of these women acknowledged that they had been sexually harassed themselves or had observed acts of sexual harassment by coworkers, supervisors, or even clients during the two-year period preceding the survey. In 1990, the American Bar Association carried out a survey of "Career Satisfaction/Dissatisfaction." This questionnaire attempted to learn about the prevalence of sexual ha-

rassment in the legal profession. Women were asked whether they had been subjected to remarks of a sexually suggestive nature, including off-color humor, pornographic pinups, leering, unwanted physical touching, or perceived coercion to engage in sexual activities. About 1 in 4 male attorneys in private practice reported having observed sexual harassment of female attorneys, while about 2 out of 3 women made similar observations about their female peers. Sexual harassment of male attorneys was extremely rare.

Not surprisingly, women who had been sexually harassed by coworkers or clients reported significantly less job satisfaction than those who had not. However, there was no evidence in this sample that women who were sexually harassed experienced an adverse impact on their income. Additionally, women who had been sexually harassed were far more likely to report that they were interested in leaving their current job more than women who had not been sexually harassed. Laband and Lentz conclude with an important message: women are subjected to sexual harassment in ways so subtle that they cannot bring a legal complaint against the responsible individual(s). This study did not address the frequency or seriousness of sexual harassment in the workplace, only its impact on job satisfaction, income, and the desire to leave the organization.

WOMEN IN THE MILITARY DURING WAR

Wolfe, Sharkansky, Read, Dawson, Martin, and Ouimette (1998) studied a group of 160 women who had been sexually harassed verbally, sexually harassed physically (unwanted touching or fondling), and sexually assaulted physically (forced sex or attempts at forced sex) during the Persian Gulf war. In all instances, the sexual approaches were unwanted. These researchers were interested in the effects of these forms of sexual harassment as well as the stresses of combat on the development of posttraumatic stress disorder. It is widely known that sexual harassment takes place in the military in times of peace, but the combination of harassment and combat on the development of posttraumatic stress disorder had not been thoroughly studied previously. In this sample of women, 33.1% were sexually harassed physically, 7.3% were sexually assaulted, and 66.2% were subjected to verbal sexual harassment while serving in the Gulf region.

Being sexually assaulted was more powerfully predictive of posttraumatic stress disorder than exposure to combat, and the more often a woman was assaulted, the greater were the chances that she would later suffer from posttraumatic stress disorder. Those women who were sexually assaulted *and* sexually harassed physically *and* exposed to combat conditions were the most likely to experience long-term psychological problems as a result of these combined stressors.

FEMALE DOCTORS

In addition to students, office workers, business leaders, attorneys, and military personnel female physicians also report being sexually harassed, by both their professional peers and their patients. Schneider and Phillips (1997) carried out a qualitative analysis of sexual harassment of female physicians by their patients. These writers note that in addition to common examples of sexual harassment, doctors have professional interactions with their patients that offer the opportunity for unusual sexual harassment practices. Over 400 female physicians returned questionnaires, indicating that they had experienced both common forms of sexual harassment such as unwanted touching, leering, and being asked out for dates repeatedly, as well as forms of sexual harassment involving patient interactions and care. For example, many of these doctors reported that some of their male patients had complaints of genital discomfort, only to find that these patients became erect during their examination and were plainly experiencing no discomfort at all. One doctor noted that two male patients returned to her office on three separate occasions with this ploy. In another case a doctor reported her interactions with a patient who came to her with many explicit questions about masturbation, sexual intercourse, and proper genital hygiene. After three visits, this doctor asked her nurse to be present during these question-and-answer sessions, and soon the patient stopped returning.

Some patients have exploited the closeness of a physical examination to engage in inappropriate touching with their female doctor. Even more flagrant examples of sexual harassment were sometimes noted:

> A patient came into the office with nonspecific complaints then complained of some pain in the genitals. I left the room and asked him to remove the lower half of his clothes and gave him a sheet to cover himself. When I reentered the room the patient was smiling, hands behind his head with an erection. I spoke with him in a professional manner and asked him to cover himself until it was time for the examination. I then asked the RN to accompany me in the room. After the exam the RN left the room . . . the patient asked me for a date (p. 673).

FEMALE PSYCHOLOGISTS

Like other professional women who work closely with coworkers and clients, female psychologists are likely to be sexually harassed, and understanding sexual harassment doesn't mean that one is less likely to be victimized. deMayo (1997) collected data from over 350 female psychologists to learn more about the prevalence of sexual harassment of female psychologists. Of this number, slightly over half reported at least one instance in which they were sexually harassed. In 85% of these cases, the harassing party was male. Most of these psychologists said that the most blatant examples of sexual harassment occurred in outpatient settings (their private offices), while 20% noted that these approaches took place in inpatient settings (hospitals and psychiatric facilities). The age range of the harassers was 18 to 73. deMayo calculated the chances of a female psychologist being sexually harassed by a patient as approximately 1 offense in every 5,553.9 hours of psychotherapy. While sexual harassment is almost always very unsettling, these preliminary data indicate that it is not very common among female psychologists. Most instances of harassment involved

"inappropriate remarks," but a few sexual assaults were reported by these subjects. Almost half of these subjects reported instances of patients making highly sexualized statements that included or implied attraction to the therapist.

While these data are preliminary and are based on a relatively small sample of female psychologists, they affirm our earlier statement that sexual harassment takes place in virtually every occupational setting, regardless of the professional status of the victim or the nature of the relationship between the victim and the harasser.

Sexual Harassment of Men

So far, this discussion of sexual harassment has focused primarily on women for the simple reason that women are harassed sexually far more frequently than men in virtually all educational and occupational arenas. Yet this does not mean that sexual harassment of men is rare or that men are any less distressed by harassment than women (Fig. 19-15). Sometimes men are harassed by women and sometimes by other men. Waldo, Berdahl, and Fitzgerald (1998) analyzed a number of legal cases involving the sexual harassment of men. Since the movie version of Michael Crichton's book *Disclosure* starring Demi Moore and Michael Douglas was released in the early 1990s, the public has become more aware of some of the circumstances in which men might be harassed sexually.

Researchers have considered whether circumstances that women describe as harassment are perceived similarly by men. While quid pro quo sexual harassment is apparently very rare among men, hostile environment harassment does indeed occur. Yet even when sexual statements, jokes, or leering involve males as victims, some men actually welcome these behaviors. Generally speaking, men report much less anxiety about sexual harassment in the workplace than women. Berdahl, Magley, and Waldo (1996) discovered a form of sexual harassment that

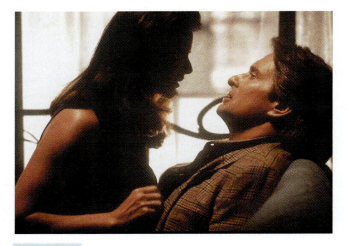

FIGURE 19-15   The movie *Disclosure,* starring Demi Moore and Michael Douglas, is about a woman (Moore) who is a supervisor and an ex-girlfriend of Douglas' character. Explicit sexual harassment and coercion reveal the flip-side of the common scenario seen in business, industry, and education.

Other Countries, Cultures, and Customs

SEXUAL HARASSMENT FROM A CROSS-CULTURAL PERSPECTIVE

In 1997, Pryor, DeSouza, Fitness, Hutz, Kumpf, Lubbert, Pesonen, and Erber published a comprehensive analysis of gender differences in the judgments people make about sexual harassment in Australia, Brazil, Germany, and the United States. Subjects included 402 male and 425 female college students ranging in age from 17 to 47. Their focus was a number of hypothetical interactions between students and professors in higher education settings. Subjects were asked whether a specific scenario was or was not an example of sexual harassment and were asked to provide their personal definition of sexual harassment. While most research on perceptions of sexual harassment are based on data collected in the United States, these researchers explored this issue in a cross-cultural perspective. Many studies of sexual harassment have found that women are much better at recognizing it than men. Pryor and colleagues sought to explore both gender differences and cross-cultural differences in recognizing sexual harassment.

Questionnaires were initially written in English and translated into Portuguese (for the Brazilian sample) and German. Volunteers read the following scenario and were then asked about the degree to which the interaction represented an example of sexual harassment.

> *Professor J. W. teaches a senior seminar class at a large state university. Sandra is one of the students currently in that seminar. Early one evening, Professor J. W. encounters Sandra walking across campus. After talking about a research paper she wrote in his class for a short while, Professor J. W. asks Sandra to join him for dinner in the coming weekend. (Pryor et al., 1997, p. 515)*

Subjects were asked to rate the degree to which they felt this did or did not represent sexual harassment, using a 7-point scale in which point values ranged from "definitely not sexual harassment" with a point value of 1 to "definitely sexual harassment" with a point value of 7.

Among students in the American sample, women were more likely than men to evaluate this scenario as an example of sexual harassment. Interestingly, these researchers found the opposite effect among students in the Brazilian sample, in which men were more likely to see this scenario as an example of sexual harassment. When providing their personal definitions of sexual harassment, both female and male Brazilian students were much more likely to see the invitation to dinner as "relatively harmless sexual behavior" than their American counterparts and to focus less on the power differential between professor and student or the discriminatory aspects of the request. The German and Australian subjects both viewed this scenario negatively and saw it as a clear example of sexual harassment, but there were no differences between the female and male subjects in these two groups. In general, there were no major gender differences in the way women and men evaluated sexual harassment in the Brazilian, German, or Australian samples.

While the American subjects in this study were aware of both EEOC and university standards regarding sexual harassment, undergraduates in Brazil, Germany, and Australia were more influenced by the policies of their universities than any government regulations. Perhaps because the Thomas-Hill case dramatically affected the way Americans think about harassment, we are more likely to be aware of governmental laws and standards about these behaviors. These writers introduced the "reasonable woman" standard by which behaviors potentially indicating sexual harassment might be judged: would a "reasonable woman" react to specific behaviors as harassment? Apparently, a reasonable woman in the United States might not judge behavior by the same standards as her peers in other countries.

Barak (1997) examined the literature on sexual harassment in many different countries. This cross-cultural analysis included data from Australia, Austria, Belgium, Canada, former Czechoslovakia, Denmark, Egypt, Finland, France, Germany, India, Israel, Italy, Japan, Luxembourg, Mexico, Netherlands, New Zealand, Northern Ireland, Norway, Pakistan, Portugal, Russia and the Former USSR, Spain, Sweden, South Africa, Switzerland, the United Kingdom, and the United States. Because research on sexual harassment carried out in these countries has involved highly diverse methods, samples of subjects, methods of interviewing or questioning subjects, terminology, guarantees of confidentiality, and statistical analyses, it is virtually impossible to compare the prevalence or manifestations of sexual harassment with these cross-cultural data. Further, the manifestations and variety of behaviors that might be called sexual harassment are also extremely diverse. Barak concludes this analysis by noting that virtually all important information about sexual harassment comes from economically developed, industrialized nations.

troubles men that has no counterpart among women, concerning behaviors and statements by both female and male coworkers that demand that a man act like a "real man." As Waldo, Berdahl, and Fitzgerald note, "This form of behavior includes ridiculing men for acting too 'feminine' and pressuring them to engage in stereotypical forms of 'masculine' behavior" (p. 61). Sexual harassment of men includes not only the same kinds of exploitative and derogatory comments women often hear but also taunting comments that quietly challenge their "genuine" masculinity.

Much of the sexual harassment men experience in the workplace comes from male harassers. Waldo and his colleagues report that between one-fourth and one-third of men who are harassed sexually are harassed by other men. This may involve homosexual solicitations as well as the type of ridicule described above. Just as numerous court cases have clarified the behaviors that constitute sexual harassment of women, several court cases have dealt with sexual harassment of men. In the case of *Polly v. Houston Lighting and Power Company*, a man was persistently harassed by his male co-workers because his appearance and demeanor were effeminate and those who worked with him thought he was gay. Waldo, Berdahl, and Fitzgerald (1998) cite the court record, which, in part reads:

> The plaintiff had been "kissed by one or more of the [male] defendants, that the other defendants exposed their genitalia to him, that his genitals were grabbed and squeezed, that the defendants would pinch his buttocks and chest, and that on one occasion, [a defendant] forced a broom handle against [his] rectum." (p. 62)

When men sexually harass other men in this way, this is an example of what is legally known as "unwanted sexual pursuit" and has been interpreted as an example of the misuse of organizational power precipitated by the sex of the person who is harassed. Waldo, Berdahl, and Fitzgerald note that in cases involving the sexual harassment of men, the sexual orientations of the plaintiff and defendant(s) are generally not revealed. Because many gay men do not want their coworkers to know they are homosexual, cases of gay men sexually harassing "straight" men are extremely rare.

Waldo, Berdahl, and Fitzgerald (1998) collected data from three samples of male employees to learn more about sexual harassment of men. The first sample was 378 men at a large utility company in the Northwest, the second sample was 209 men who were faculty and staff members at a large university in the Midwest, and the final sample was 420 men who worked in a large food processing factory. The subjects ranged in age from 35 to 44 years of age. Subjects filled out questionnaires that sought to determine the frequency of male sexual harassment and the sex of the harasser. They were also asked how distressed they were as a result of being sexually harassed. Collectively, about half of the men in these three samples reported that they had felt sexually harassed on at least one occasion. Only 2% reported that they had been the victims of sexual coercion, and between 11.5% and 29% reported that they had experienced "unwanted sexual attention"

in one form or another. Lewd, offensive comments and negative remarks about men were the most common types of sexual harassment, conforming closely to the notion of a "hostile environment" discussed earlier in connection with female sexual harassment.

In all three samples, men reported that the person who harassed them was in most cases another man. This was the case in 52.7% of the men in sample 1, 50.2% of the men in sample 2, and 39.8% of the men in sample 3. Female-to-male sexual harassment was clearly less common with 30.1% of the men in sample 1, 31.7% of the men in sample 2, and 31.9% of the men in sample 3. In sample 1, 17.2% of the men identified both female and male harassers, while the comparable figures in samples 2 and 3 were 19.1% and 28.3% respectively. An analysis of the degree to which subjects were distressed by sexual harassment was carried out with the men in sample 2. Lewd comments and negative comments about men proved to be the most "upsetting" forms of sexual harassment in this group of subjects, with unwanted sexual attention ranking third.

One of the most important findings to emerge from this study are the facts that male-to-male sexual harassment may be far more common that most people think and that this form of sexual harassment is rarely reported in the media. As well, although quid pro quo sexual harassment is common among females, it is relatively unknown among men. Men in these samples evaluated harassment taunting them to behave in more masculine ways as particularly distressing. While quid pro quo and hostile environment sexual harassment have been punished by the courts, demands for conformity to masculine roles have not, and it is doubtful whether they are amenable to legal penalties. Interestingly, another study that explored male sexual harassment (DuBois, Knapp, Faley, & Kustis, 1998) interpreted many instances of male-to-male harassment as examples of "hazing," a form of bullying.

Current State Laws Concerning Sexual Harassment

Legal opinions on sexual harassment seem to be debated daily and will likely be a focus for the courts for many years to come. Three decisions handed down by the United States Supreme Court in the summer of 1998 are of particular importance. Lavelle (1998) writes that these are likely to foster a number of changes in educational and workplace environments. For example, in the past, the person being harassed had to demonstrate that she resisted the harassment and because she did so her income, job duties, and advancement were adversely affected. But in 1998 the court ruled that sexual harassment has occurred even if the person being harassed has been treated well and suffered no apparent professional adverse consequences as a result of resisting the harassment. Secondly, in the past, managers who were unaware that one of their employees was harassing another employee were generally not responsible for the actions of the perpetrator. However, current law now holds that the manager can indeed be responsible for an employee's sexual harassment unless the company has a clear, strong sexual harassment policy. Finally, the Supreme Court ruled that if a person feels that they have been sexually harassed, it is not sufficient to tell just anyone about it in order to make it a matter of record. The person being harassed must inform a responsible individual within the organization who is in a position to do something about the complaint.

SEXUAL ABUSE

Sexual abuse involves criminal behavior, as was introduced in the previous chapter's discussion of pedophilia. Because Chapter 18 discusses sexual abuse as a paraphilia, this chapter will examine other aspects of sexual abuse. There are no simple explanations why some people sexually abuse others, and there is much debate about why the victims of sexual abuse don't always report being victimized. The connection between coercion and abuse on one hand and our most intimate sexual selves on the other is both perplexing and provocative. Women and men of all ages are vulnerable to sexual abuse.

Short-Term Consequences of Child Sexual Abuse

Although some children report that sexual contact with adults has neutral or even beneficial effects, generally these behaviors can have adverse short- and long-term consequences for the child. Even though sexual abuse does not always have prompt, detrimental outcomes for the child, subtle problems are often apparent. McLeer, Dixon, Henry, Ruggerio, Escovitz, Niedda, and Scholle (1998) studied a sample of 80 subjects between 6 and 16 years of age who were referred to the investigators by the Philadelphia Department of Human Services. None of these youngsters actually seemed to need clinical assistance as a result of the abuse experiences. All acknowledged that they had been sexually abused, and the abuse had been revealed and stopped in the previous 30 to 60 days. These researchers found that posttraumatic stress disorder was diagnosed in 36.3% of the youngsters who had been sexually abused; these children were preoccupied with vivid, unpleasant, recurrent memories of their abuse experiences. These subjects also experienced as much clinically apparent anxiety and depression as those subjects with more obvious psychological problems resulting from their abusive experiences.

Hall, Matthews, and Pearce (1998) studied sexual behavior problems children developed presumably as a result of being sexually abused. Chapter 12 discussed many aspects of normal sexual development in children, and it is reasonable to consider whether being sexually abused might disturb this regular pattern of sexual development. Hall and her colleagues explored this question. These researchers collected data from 100 sexually abused boys and girls between the ages of 3 and 7 years. These subjects were grouped into three categories: those who were apparently developing normally with respect to sexuality, those whose behavior revealed problems in sexual interest and expressiveness, and those who were engaging in inappropriate contact and touching with others. The children in

the third group had more interpersonal sexual problems. Hall and her colleagues found that four factors seemed to predict whether a sexually abused child would later have problems with sexual development. In general, those children who were most likely to experience difficulties in sexual development as a result of their sexual abuse had the following characteristics:

1. They become sexually aroused during abusive experiences. This is not uncommon. Many perpetrators take special pains to create trust and feelings of safety with their victims, who become excited or aroused during episodes of abuse.
2. Children who are treated sadistically during abusive experiences are likely to have long-term problems with their sexual development. In this case, the abuser not only creates fear and anxiety in the victim, but also *relieves* that fear and anxiety by "freeing" the child from the abusive situation. These feelings of fear and relief have been called a "trauma bond" and are an example of negative reinforcement. If children become excited or aroused during abusive experiences they may also experience a sense of shame. Interestingly, when children are molested rarely and the episodes are painful, they find it much easier to put the experience behind them.

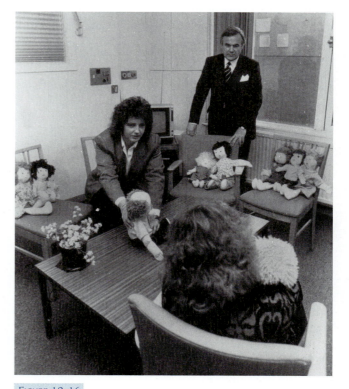

FIGURE 19-16 One informative way to determine the accuracy of a child's memories surrounding alledged child sexual abuse involves the use of dolls. Children are asked to point to parts of the dolls body and indicate the nature of possibly abusive actions related to those areas of the body.

3. When a child has experienced harsh physical punishments in their family of origin, this more or less sanctions the use of force in attempts to control the child's behavior, even much later when the child has become an adult. Yet this abuse can be emotional as well as physical, and its long-term effects are very much the same.

A subtle but important finding implicit in this research is that sometimes children who experience sexual abuse and adolescents who report these experiences are in a father-absent home. This may make a child at risk of abuse from other males in the household or be associated with a number of emotional vulnerabilities in the child. The research of Hall and her colleagues directs attention to children who are most likely to suffer the long-term effects of child sexual abuse. Knowing that a child has been sexually abused can help a counselor or therapist later on if that individual has any psychological or sexual problems (Fig. 19-16).

Sometimes the consequences of child sexual abuse are immediate and obvious. In many instances, children who are sexually abused by adults contract STDs as a result. The diagnosis of an STD may be the first sign that sexual molestation has occurred (Hammerschlag, 1998). In a few cases, STDs may result from infections acquired congenitally, and these may go undiagnosed for a long period of time, in some cases up to 3 years. This is especially true in the case of chlamydia. Recent research has demonstrated that screening tests for chlamydia have not been widely used in children. Further, bacterial vaginosis has been diagnosed in children who have and have not been sexually abused (Hammerschlag, 1998), and the techniques used to diagnosis this disorder in adults have generally not been used in children. At this writing, researchers are still uncertain about how frequently HIV is transmitted to children by sexual abuse, nor are they certain about which children should be tested for the virus. Diagnosing an STD in children involves several unanswered medical and legal questions (Fig. 19-17).

Sexual Abuse of Boys

Holmes and Slap (1998) reviewed the literature on sexual abuse of boys between 1985 and 1997. They focused on studies that analyzed the abuse experiences of at least 20 boys and that used sound research designs. They reviewed 166 different investigations that summarized data from 149 samples of sexually abused boys. These investigators characterized the boy at highest risk of sexual abuse as being under the age of 13, non-Caucasian, of low socioeconomic status, and not living with his biological father. Most abuse was perpetrated by older males known to but unrelated to the child. Most often, the abusive episodes took place outside of the child's home. In most cases, oral or anal penetration took place, and perpetrators repeatedly abused their victims. Commonly these boys later became involved in substance abuse. As Hall's data revealed, these boys often exhibited problems in sexual development. This literature review emphasizes that sexual abuse of

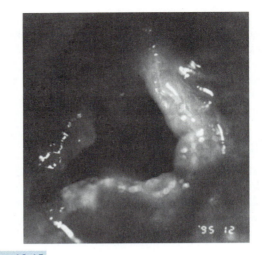

FIGURE 19-17 Enlarged photograph of a lacerated hymen of a toddler. Sexual abuse of children is often a violent crime with serious injuries.

boys is "common, underreported, underrecognized, and undertreated" (Holmes & Slap, 1998, p. 1855).

Long-Term Consequences of Child Sexual Abuse

Just as few people would feel comfortable acknowledging their submissiveness in the face of aggressive intimate gestures, so too many would be troubled about revealing that they have been sexually coerced, exploited, or victimized or that they had engaged in nonconsensual sex. It is remarkable when someone who has been a victim reveals the fact publicly. In 1984, Florida Senator Paula Hawkins was to deliver the welcoming address at the National Conference on Sexual Victimization of Children, but as the attendees took their seats she said something of far more personal importance. Senator Hawkins said, "When I was five years old, I was abused by a neighbor, a man around the corner" (*Time,* May 7, 1984) (Fig. 19-18). The 1,300 listeners fell silent and were astonished by her courage in making this statement. The Senator went on, "I told my mother. Fortunately, she believed me. . . . We went to court, and I was one of the witnesses. But the man was let go. The judge decided that children had to be lying" (p. 27). At the time she revealed this episode, Senator Hawkins was 57 years old and had never told anyone about the incident, not even her husband. She hoped that her revelation would make it easier for parents to believe their children about such incidents when they report them. Since commonly the victim of sexual exploitation or coercion feels that they somehow provoked the behavior that victimized them, courageous statements like those of Senator Hawkins are important to the thousands of individuals who may feel responsible in some way for their circumstances.

Memories of child sexual abuse are usually extremely unpleasant and may last throughout a person's life. This fact raises an interesting question: when the victim is asked to remember and recount the particulars of an abuse experience, might this stir up old, terrible recollections that could make it even more difficult to understand the event and put it in its proper perspective? This issue was studied by Walker, Newman, Koss, and Bernstein in 1997. These investigators were interested in the long-term impact of sexual abuse and administered a questionnaire to 500 randomly selected women in a health maintenance organization. Among other questions, these subjects were asked to respond to inquiries concerning any previous history of sexual, physical, and emotional abuse or neglect. They were also asked to report how they felt about answering these questions. Importantly, most of these respondents noted that they were not especially distressed about being asked these questions, implying that these types of research tools are accepted well by respondents rather than interpreted as provoking powerful, terrible memories. This is a good example of a research problem involving ethical discussion about the appropriateness of certain questions and how they might be perceived by subjects.

Much literature has described the highly diverse consequences of sexually abusive experiences. Sheldon and Bannister (1998) pointed out problems faced by survivors of child sexual abuse. These include the denial that the event(s) ever occurred, fear of reporting the abuse, the inability to stop thinking about the abuser as a powerful, controlling person, and continued feelings of female inferiority when the abuse involved girls. Often these thoughts and feelings become manifest in posttraumatic stress disorder, described earlier. In working with adults who were sexually abused as children, many counselors consider "breaking the silence" a critical step in the victim's recovery. As the issues of power and control are often an important part of an abusive experience, they are also issues of extreme importance in the counseling relationship. For this

reason, therapists often face the same interpersonal communication challenges that were involved in the original abusive experience. Those who treat adults who were sexually abused as children must make every effort to reassure the client that she or he is a full, active partner in the therapeutic process and that the counselor will not be playing a powerful or controlling role in counseling. Many people who seek counseling because they have been sexually abused don't know very much about sexual abuse in general even though they know a lot about their own personal experiences. Therefore therapists must often teach their abused clients basic facts about sexual abuse, similar to what is described in this chapter. The issue of the therapist's sex has also been debated. While some researchers believe that a male therapist should not work with women who have been sexually abused by men, others claim that it doesn't matter very much.

In recent years group therapy has proved especially effective for helping adults come to terms with child sexual abuse experiences (Sheldon & Bannister, 1998). A group of individuals with common experiences is often very helpful in getting members to explore the reasons they have kept their experiences a secret, their current mistrustfulness towards certain individuals, their feelings of isolation, their low self-esteem, and their feelings of humiliation and personal responsibility for the abusive experiences. Often group meetings center on issues that seem problematic for most group members. These include trust, power, control, anger, sexuality, and the loss of one's innocent childhood (Sheldon & Bannister, 1998).

This book has repeatedly emphasized the importance of self-esteem and body image as an aspect of one's sexual value system (SVS). The impact of child sexual abuse on the adult's later perceptions of their bodies has been studied by Wenninger and Heiman (1998). In an analysis of 57 adult females who were sexually abused as children, these researchers found that these individuals assessed their general health far more negatively than a control group of similar women who had not been sexually abused in childhood. Survivors of sexual abuse had extremely negative "body self-esteem" and similarly saw themselves as far less attractive sexually than the subjects in the control group. These differences between abused women and non-abused women were significant even after controlling for the influence of body weight.

To analyze the literature on child sexual abuse and its effects on individuals later in life, Rind, Tromovitch, and Bauserman (1998) carefully evaluated almost 60 different studies that explored the impact of child sexual abuse on women in college. The data overall revealed that although women who had been sexually abused as children were, on average, somewhat less well adjusted psychologically than those who weren't, the individual's family environment was a far more powerful predictor of these adjustment problems than were sexually abusive experiences. Women's self-reports about sexual abuse revealed that a negative impact did not occur in all abused women, nor were the effects of these experiences particularly strong. Additionally, men who had been abused experienced less negative emotional consequences than

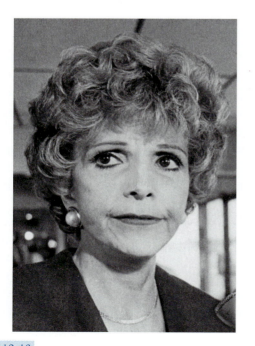

FIGURE 19-18 Former U.S. Senator Paula Hawkins of Florida.

Research Highlight

Are Memories of Child Sexual Abuse Accurate?

One of the most active and controversial areas of research in child sexual abuse involves the accuracy of memories of abusive episodes and the possibility that therapists may actually "implant" memories of abusive experience when none in fact occurred. Importantly, when children say that they have been sexually molested, no one should doubt the accuracy of their statement but should proceed on the assumption that such behaviors did occur unless demonstrated conclusively that they did not. On the other hand, is it possible to have been sexually abused and to have forgotten the experience? Of special interest is the question whether memories of child sexual abuse might lie dormant for many years and then suddenly become conscious in the recollections of the abused individual. Although many want every perpetrator punished to the fullest extent of the law, others worry about accusing, convicting, and punishing someone who may in fact be innocent. Lawsuits have cropped up everywhere, and some therapists have been sued and found guilty of influencing their clients to fabricate recollections of sexual abuse when none occurred. While much media attention is given to accusations of sexual abuse, far less is presented later when a supposed perpetrator is found innocent. Lives, careers, and reputations can be ruined by allegations that are not supported in court.

Loftus (1993) summarized the primary literature and concluded that the creation of false memories is not at all unusual or difficult to achieve under laboratory circumstances; in fact it is quite common (Fig. 19-19). Nonetheless, genuine memories of child sexual abuse can also fall below an individual's level of awareness. Studies on this issue do not yield consistent data. For example, Briere and Conte (1993) found in a large sample of 450 subjects receiving therapy for childhood sexual abuse that 59% said that there had been times before age 18 when they could not remember the abusive experience(s). In a similar study published in 1998, Epstein and Bottoms reported the results of survey data from over 1,700 female young adults. These subjects were asked about childhood sexual abuse, the persistence of their memories of these events, and whether they had been influenced by others who tried to persuade them to acknowledge a history of child sexual abuse. Very few of the subjects in this study reported that they had forgotten their abuse, even temporarily.

Why might therapists persistently try to uncover "forgotten" memories of child sexual abuse, even when, perhaps, none occurred? Part of the answer to this question may lie in the powerful influence of Freud's theory on the way we think about many different sexual issues today. Recall that according to Freud, any experience that creates much anxiety will cause the mind to find some way of defending itself against the highly unpleasant recollections. One such defense mechanisms is **repression**, and there is reason to believe that some people who have been sexually abused as children stifle any memories of it simply because it would cause too much anxiety to remember it. When a therapist believes that her or his client may be repressing some important memory, some memory that might help clarify the client's current psychological complaints and problems, they are likely to try their best to find out what that memory is. In the process of doing this, they may plant the seeds of events that never took place. It is not known exactly why this happens, but apparently it happens often enough to cause heartache for many adults who are completely innocent of child sexual abuse.

People may confuse memories of events they have heard about with memories of events in which they were personally involved. Memory experts call this **confabulation**, and it is quite common in everyone. Accurate memories are highly detailed and distinctive, however, and these attributes of authentic memories do not change over time. In contrast, false memories often lack the detail and distinctiveness of real memories, and their content often changes with continued clinical probing. Still, people often have difficulty separating an embellished, detailed fantasy about which they have perhaps often thought from the unembellished truth.

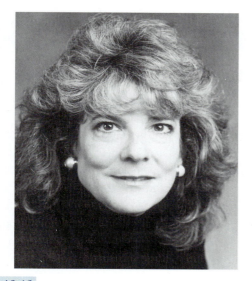

FIGURE 19-19   Dr. Elizabeth Loftus, one of the world's best known researchers in the field of eyewitness recollections and victim's memories, frequently testifies in court cases.

women. This analysis further emphasizes the differences between the public's perceptions of the effects of child sexual abuse and research findings.

An additional issue deserves some discussion. Sexually abused children live in a family, of course, and the family is generally the focus of the relationship between the individual and the wider psychosocial environment. Here we are referring only to abuse perpetrated by individuals outside the child's nuclear family. Ray and Jackson (1997) investigated whether a close, supportive family might lessen the impact of sexually abusive experiences, and whether nonsupportive, noncohesive families might magnify the negative outcomes of child sexual abuse. No clear-cut relationship emerged between the nature of family organization and support and the long-term outcomes of child sexual abuse. Yet these researchers found that victims of child sexual abuse may have coped better with their experience or experiences because they lived in a close, structured, supportive family and that children who don't live in this kind of a family might have more trouble adapting to their abuse. Perhaps this helps explain some big differences in the way adults cope with their abusive experiences.

Incest

We have already noted that the victim of child sexual abuse is frequently acquainted with the perpetrator and sometimes related to that individual. Although the physical acts entailed in incest do not differ from other child sexual abuse, the close family ties and constant domestic proximity between the victim and the perpetrator make incest a special case of child sexual abuse (Fig. 19-20). Johnson (1983) estimated that at least one million cases of incest occur each year in the United States, but only approximately 10% of these are reported to law enforcement authorities. Forward and Buck (1989) define incest as "any overtly sexual contact between closely related persons

or between persons who believe themselves to be related." By this definition, in-laws who may assume responsibility for a child also are said to engage in incest even though they are not biologically related to the child. Taboos against incest have developed in virtually every world culture that has been studied. Because of the close living arrangements in which incest often occurs, the victims of incest often have feelings of helplessness about a situation in which they typically feel "trapped." Father-daughter, mother-son, and sibling incest are the most common varieties. In the case of parent-child incest, these behaviors are plainly illegal because the child cannot be said to consent to the sexual acts because of the older age of the parent, the powerful caretaker role of the parent, and the parent's capacity to use deception and trickery to coerce the youngster to participate in sexual acts (Finkelhor, 1994). Despite possible cross-cultural differences, a study of incest carried out in Brazil isolated a number of predisposing risk factors that may play a role in the intra-familial sexual victimization of children:

1. Problems of family structure
2. Extreme poverty
3. Mother's incapacitating illness
4. Mental illness in the aggressor
5. Extreme violence in the family environment
6. Social interaction difficulties
7. Multiple victims
8. Incest recurrence in the family
9. Mental retardation in the victim

—Flores & Mattos, 1998

Although the presence of one or more of these factors does not indicate a high probability of incest occurring, these factors can sensitize social and behavioral scientists, mental health workers, and law enforcement authorities of an elevated risk of child sexual victimization in some families. In those rare cases in which a child is born as the result of an incestuous union,

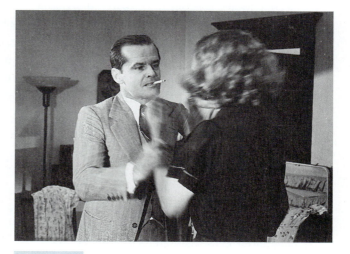

FIGURE 19-20   The movie *Chinatown*, starring Jack Nicholson (left) and Faye Dunaway (right), is one of the few films that explores the complex nature of an incestuous father-daughter relationship. An aging John Huston plays Ms. Dunaway's character's father.

Other Countries, Cultures, and Customs

SEXUAL TRAUMA AMONG CHINESE CHILDREN AND ADOLESCENTS IN TAIWAN

We have repeatedly emphasized that the manifestations and meanings of sexual behaviors can vary much depending on the culture in which they occur, and this is true as well about sexual abuse of children. In China powerful patriarchal traditions exist as well as the belief that female chastity is especially important, and within this context Tsun-Yin (1998) analyzed the impact of child and adolescent sexual abuse. An estimated 4,200 cases of child sexual abuse take place each year in Taiwan, or 42% of the total number of sexual abuse and/or assault incidents. Even more than in the West, child sexual abuse has been a "taboo and silenced issue for centuries in Chinese society" (Tsun-Yin, 1998, p. 1014). In this society men have traditionally and without question exercised almost total control over female sexual expression and have created a psychosocial environment in which there is enormous condemnation for the premature loss of a woman's virginity. This investigation included detailed, lengthy interviews with 19 young women who had been sexually abused as children, some only once and one repeatedly for a period of 10 years. In 5 cases, the perpetrator was a stranger, but in all the rest the victim knew the abuser.

With virtually all these subjects, feelings of betrayal and disempowerment were obvious in their judgments about the impact of the abusive experiences, and in this sense these Chinese women do not differ from their counterparts in the United States. However, feelings of stigmatization were especially powerful and prominent in the Chinese subjects. They all reported profound feelings of guilt and shame over the loss of their virginity by sexual victimization. These Chinese women had uniformly low self-esteem and felt very different from other young women, so different in fact that they felt like outcasts in their culture. They commonly isolated themselves, and many reported serious problems in their interpersonal relationships. The path to recovery from child sexual abuse therefore seems more complex and tortuous in Taiwan than in North America, although it is never easy. Survivors of child sexual abuse in Taiwan seemed to manifest a "polarized sexuality," that is, they were either highly fearful or even phobic about sexual feelings and intimacy or they were frequently preoccupied with their sexual feelings and often behaved in openly promiscuous ways. All of these women expressed deep feelings of anger, mistrust, and betrayal toward other people, especially men.

While it is not uncommon in the United States for survivors of child sexual abuse to later become involved in drug abuse, have serious marital problems, or even become child sexual abusers themselves, no data in this sample of Taiwanese subjects suggested these outcomes. Tsun-Yin believes that the obsessive concern with the loss of their virginity and terrible anxiety about their attractiveness as potential marital partners are unique cultural features of child sexual abuse among women in Taiwan. This study shows that the long-term impact of child sexual abuse in any culture depends in part on traditional male and female roles and power structures.

there is an increased risk of mental and physical abnormalities thought to result from the influence of recessive genes. Retardation, physical malformations, and problems in motor coordination are common.

Sibling incest is the most common form of incest, followed in frequency by father-daughter and mother-son sexual contact, respectively (Waterman & Lusk, 1986). Sibling incest is typically instigated by the brother, or older male in cases of same sex contact. Often, siblings do not see their behavior as

unnatural. Father-daughter incest often begins with "casual" affectionate touching and then proceeds to more explicit breast and genital touching and then vaginal and/or anal penetration. Alcohol is sometimes but not always involved. Some men approach their daughters sexually if they feel rebuffed sexually by their wives.

Because mother-son incest is the rarest form of incest, less is known about it. One study examined 13 men who had been sexually abused by women, 7 by their mothers (Etherington,

1997). Although 7 case studies are not a very large sample, mother-son incest is so rare that this study can give us at least a glimpse into the dynamics and consequences of this type of incest. None of these subjects were studied because they approached mental health professionals with psychological complaints; all responded to newspaper advertisements for adult survivors of child sexual abuse (a common, ethical way to create a pool of subjects). All 7 reported difficulties in the process of male socialization, and all had developed psychological defense mechanisms that protected them from anxiety-provoking interactions with women. As with other forms of incest, the long-term effects of mother-son incest can be very troubling in later life.

In a study of the long-term effects of incest on women, Newman and Peterson (1996) found very high levels of anger in a sample of 68 subjects. When their fathers were the perpetrators of the abuse, these subjects expressed very high levels of anger toward *both* their mothers and fathers. They were angry with their fathers for obvious reasons, but they were also especially upset that their mothers seemed to have condoned the abuse or at least refused to acknowledge that it was happening. The anger these subjects experienced also had many diffuse, nonspecific characteristics; these subjects were generally angry about many things, and when compared with a control group of women who were not incest survivors, these differences were consistent and significant. Another interesting finding by Newman and Peterson was that female survivors of incest who were sympathetic to feminist ideals and those who had received psychotherapy were apparently more angry than those who had not. Apparently, holding feminist beliefs and having explored their incest with a therapist seemed to facilitate the expression of their hostility and made them more comfortable about revealing their outrage.

People often have difficulty believing that the spouse of a perpetrator of incest did not know about the abuse or failed to act to stop it. This is an extremely complex subject. Crawford, Hueppelsheuser, and George (1996) studied 132 perpetrators of incest, 155 spouses of incest perpetrators, and a control group of 100 women in an attempt to discover the characteristics of women who were married to men who sexually abused their children. These researchers found that the spouses of incest perpetrators had a number of maladaptive compulsive behaviors of their own that suggested that the abuser was controlling or influencing his spouse to refrain from stopping him. Further, spouses of incest perpetrators in this study seemed to support the perpetration of the incest through either active or passive acquiescence. Finally, this research demonstrated that in this sample of subjects both the incest perpetrators and their wives were highly likely themselves to have suffered physical, emotional, and sexual abuse when they were children.

As in other cases of child sexual abuse, there is frequently a public outcry about the exploitation and injury inherent in incest, and this is often reflected in the ways in which professionals react to perpetrators. Trute, Adkins, and MacDonald (1996) presented clinical case studies to community mental health professionals, police officers, and child welfare workers

in an attempt to find out if these groups favored treatment or punishment of incest perpetrators. In a sense, this study sought to determine if these groups viewed incest perpetrators as mentally ill or as criminals. Community mental health workers and child welfare workers were more likely to see the perpetrator as mentally ill, while the police plainly saw him as a criminal who should be punished. However, all groups supported the clinical assessment and treatment legally required by the court system.

Sexual Abuse by Therapists

Sexual abuse occurs in domestic settings, in preschools and elementary schools, and other settings as well. Studies have explored the nature and prevalence of sexual abuse in settings in which psychiatric care is administered. Sloan, Edmond, Rubin, and Doughty (1998) surveyed licensed clinical social workers in Texas. In their sample of 450 subjects who replied to a mailed questionnaire, 17% of respondents had provided therapy to at least one client who had been involved in sexual activities with a psychotherapist at some time during the past 12 months; 5% had provided therapy to more than one client who had been involved with their therapist. Social workers at all levels and working in a variety of therapeutic settings worked with victims of professional sexual exploitation at some time in the previous 12 months. With more than 12,000 social workers in Texas alone, these data indicate that approximately 1 in 6 social workers is likely to work with victims of professional sexual exploitation by a psychotherapist in any given year. As a deterrent to this type of unprofessional behavior, the Texas legislature passed a law defining this type of activity as nonconsensual sexual assault and a second degree felony. Additionally, these offenses must be reported to civil authorities for prosecution.

Borruso (1991) assessing these issues from a legal perspective, raises some interesting questions, and makes an important recommendation. This writer emphasizes that despite the fact that all professional organizations have a code of ethics that prohibits sexual contact between therapists and their clients, the boards responsible for licensing therapists do not have sufficient legal authority to discourage or prevent this behavior. There is no requirement in many states that a person become licensed to practice therapy, and therefore licensing boards have no authority to censure or punish unlicensed therapists who engage in sexual activities with their patients (Fig. 19-21).

Borruso believes, however, that all states should adopt a uniform statute applying to both licensed and unlicensed therapists that makes it a criminal offense to have sex within the therapist-client relationship. Further, the client's participation in sexual activities with (usually) her therapist should not be interpreted legally as if she consented.

What Should Be Done With Sex Offenders?

Sexual abuse of children and teenagers is a terrible thing, and sometimes the consequences last a long time. But as there are issues related to the victim, so too are there issues related to the

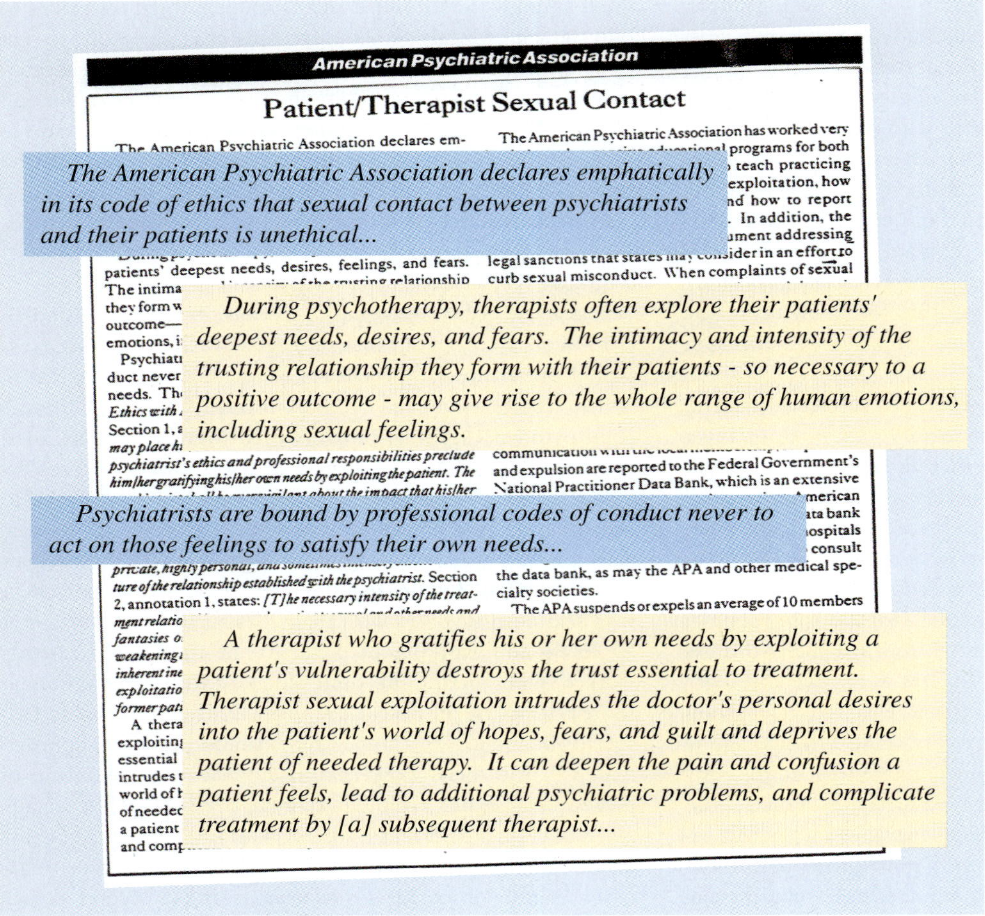

American Psychiatric Association

Patient/Therapist Sexual Contact

The American Psychiatric Association declares emphatically in its code of ethics that sexual contact between psychiatrists and their patients is unethical...

During psychotherapy, therapists often explore their patients' deepest needs, desires, and fears. The intimacy and intensity of the trusting relationship they form with their patients - so necessary to a positive outcome - may give rise to the whole range of human emotions, including sexual feelings.

Psychiatrists are bound by professional codes of conduct never to act on those feelings to satisfy their own needs...

A therapist who gratifies his or her own needs by exploiting a patient's vulnerability destroys the trust essential to treatment. Therapist sexual exploitation intrudes the doctor's personal desires into the patient's world of hopes, fears, and guilt and deprives the patient of needed therapy. It can deepen the pain and confusion a patient feels, lead to additional psychiatric problems, and complicate treatment by [a] subsequent therapist...

FIGURE 19-21 The American Psychiatric Association has published an explicit "fact sheet" that outlines the organization's position on patient/therapist sexual contact.

perpetrator. Why do adults sexually abuse children? Were sexual abusers themselves abused as children? Can a child molester ever be "cured" of a compulsion to victimize young people? If child molesters receive psychotherapy, how frequently will they again victimize youngsters? Are there any effective treatments for child molesters? While there are no clear, unequivocal answers to these important questions, they are important areas for basic and applied research.

Dhawan and Marshall (1996) studied the backgrounds of men in jail who had been convicted of various sex crimes. This group included 45 men: 29 rapists, 9 child molesters unrelated to their victims, and 7 men found guilty of father-daughter incest. The purpose of this study was to try to find out if sexual abusers were sexually abused as children. These subjects had either completed a course of psychiatric treatment or were currently receiving therapy. Questionnaires and interviews were used to explore their backgrounds. While the results of this study point to frequent sexual abuse in the childhoods of these perpetrators, there was clearly no direct cause-and-effect relationship. Of the 29 rapists in this sample, 18 were sexually abused as children, and 8 of the 17 child molesters and incest perpetrators had been similarly abused. In a control group of 20 nonsexual offenders, only 4 of the subjects had been abused as children. Overall, a statistical analysis of these data revealed that having been sexually abused as a child put a man at a significantly increased risk of becoming a perpetrator himself. But again, this is not a clear cause-and-effect relationship, only a statement of a statistical association. In almost 80% of these subjects, the perpetrator of their child sexual abuse was a man. More than 4 of 5 abusers reported that they had been sexually molested repeatedly, and 69% reported that they had been victimized by more than one perpetrator. Genital fondling was the most frequently reported abusive behavior. The abused perpetrators generally reported that their childhood experiences were unpleasant and had a powerful long-term impact on them. Finally, adults who were sexually abused as children came from families with weaker organization, poor relationships, verbal abuse, physical abuse, and parental neglect. Data like these should remind us that it is often hard to disentangle the effects of child sexual abuse from the impact of disruptive family functioning.

In recent years, much attention has been given to the "recidivism rate" of sexual offenders, which refers to the chances someone will again abuse or victimize others sexually after receiving a course of psychotherapy as part of his (and sometimes her) punishment for sexual crimes. As you might be able to tell, low recidivism rates generally point to more effective treatment strategies or perhaps offenders who have committed less serious offenses or engaged in abusive behaviors infrequently. Or perhaps offenders have learned how to better conceal their actions. Because it is hard to compare the effectiveness of different types of psychotherapy, it is similarly hard to be sure about how to predict recidivism rates for these types of offenses. In a literature review of 61 published research reports concerning the factors that are most likely to lead to repeat sexual offenses, Hanson and Bussiere (1998) found that in an analysis of over 23,000 cases of sexual abuse reported in research articles between 1943 and 1995, recidivism rates were relatively low: 13.4% of these cases involved repeat offenses in the 4 or 5 years these individuals were followed. Yet these researchers believe this recidivism figure may be low due to the fact that many cases of child sexual abuse or violent sexual crime are not reported to the authorities. We are not saying that this is an "acceptable" level of repeat offense because we very much want sex offenders to completely stop their victimization of others. But these authors point out that recidivism rates for nonviolent sexual offenses are similar to those found for crimes of a nonsexual nature. However, these researchers found that recidivism rates were highest with more deviant sexual offenses and when the individual had a prior arrest record for sex crimes. Additionally, when the focus of the offender's abuse was highly inappropriate, such as young children, recidivism rates were also high. Importantly, when sex offenders failed to complete a course of treatment, the chances of their continuing to sexually assault and/or abuse others was much higher than if they finished treatment. These data do not support the popular belief that "once an offender, always an offender."

There is another important issue we wish to raise in connection with recidivism figures. Even low recidivism rates *are totally independent of some of the terrible long-term consequences of child sexual abuse or violent sexual crimes.* Simply stated, first offenses are terrible, even when the question of repeat offenses might lead to encouraging data. The review of Hanson and Bussiere also points to another aspect of sex crime recidivism. When sex offenders become distressed, anxious, depressed, hostile, or suffer from other bad feelings they are at an increased risk of reoffending. In other words, they seem to manifest poor impulse control when they are experiencing subjective inner turmoil. One of the most important conclusions of this literature review is that when sex offenders cooperate with their therapists in treatment programs they are much less likely to repeat their crimes.

Hanson and Bussiere's review of the recidivism literature included several studies carried out in other countries. One particularly interesting approach to the treatment of paraphilic sex offenders has been developed in the Czech Republic and has involved the treatment of 953 individuals since its inception in 1976 (Weiss, 1997). This therapeutic approach involves three interrelated steps.

1. A group of sex offenders is formed and members are encouraged to share information about themselves

and the history of their offending behaviors. They are instructed to describe the sometimes compulsive, uncontrollable nature of their urges and to explore one another's motives for engaging in these behaviors.

2. The second stage of treatment promotes self-analysis and the social, personal, and familial factors which may have been instrumental in the development of the client's abusive behavior pattern. In this stage, the focus is on the individual recognizing their independence and their responsibility for their actions.

3. Finally, in stage three, the client is offered sex therapy, often involving their partner. Clients and couples engage in role-playing exercises and become more focused on self-rewarding thoughts which emphasize personal accountability and self-esteem. The nature of the client's re-entry to society is discussed along with some of the inevitable temptations he will face.

Weiss reports that over the course of the last two decades and the treatment of over 900 individuals, the recidivism rate of sexual offending among those who have completed this program is 17.1%, not very different from the data reported by Hanson and Bussiere.

Other data concerning recidivism are not so encouraging, and this discrepancy may be due to different criteria being used to assess whether or not child molesters and violent sex offenders reoffend. In a study of 136 rapists and 115 child molesters who were discharged from treatment and/or incarceration over a 25-year period, Prentky, Lee, Knight, and Cerce (1997) found that both types of perpetrators did indeed remain at a risk to commit similar crimes, in some cases, even 15 or 20 years after treatment. These researchers also found that there was good reason to believe that the reported percentages of perpetrators who had reoffended was probably a significantly lower than realistic estimate.

Therapy for Sex Offenders

There is often much confusion and disagreement regarding the diagnosis of sexual offenders, treatment plans to rehabilitate them, and the best way to determine whether they may sexually victimize others in the future. Physicians and social and behavioral scientists would benefit from standardization in diagnosis and treatment of sex offenders. MacHovec (1994) developed a "Sex Offender Treatment Needs Assessment And Progress Summary" for evaluating and treating perpetrators in diverse psychosocial settings. With this paper-and-pencil instrument, MacHovec believes that a number of issues can be isolated and explored and appropriate treatment strategies formulated. It also monitors therapeutic progress and points out future directions for clinical assistance. MacHovec isolated 10 different treatment factors that the counselor or therapist rates on a scale using the following rating categories: 0 (none), 1 (poor), 2 (low average), 3 (average), 4 (good), and 5 (very good):

1. *Responsibility/readiness,* without denial, minimization or blaming; amenable to therapy

2. *Cognitive distortion,* overcomes denial, fantasy, and avoidance

3. *Deviant fantasy,* knows and able to modify to socially appropriate level

4. *Processes own victimization,* loss, rejection, abandonment, or family dysfunction

5. *Offense cycle* understood, how to interrupt/control it; sexual arousal pattern, how and when to get help

6. *Impulse control:* anger, power need, frustration, helplessness; improved coping skills; meeting affective needs appropriately; role of substance abuse

7. *Remorse/empathy* for victim, the victim's family, offender's family, friends, society; restitution (victim, community)

8. *Resocialization:* Appropriate life, social, and interpersonal skills, verbal and nonverbal, public and private; building trust; family issues

9. *Normalization:* Understands what appropriate sexual outlets, what is and is NOT considered normal, lawful behavior; consequences

10. *Self concept,* sex role, identity, and preference; appropriate arousal and outlet; stability and spirituality

—MacHovec, 1994, 99–100

MacHovec's classification for the diagnosis and treatment of sex offenders seems a useful way of creating some uniformity for examining the effectiveness of various treatments. Without a consistent way of monitoring the progress of treatment and its effectiveness, there will continue to be significant confusion regarding highly variable recidivism rates (Fig. 19-22).

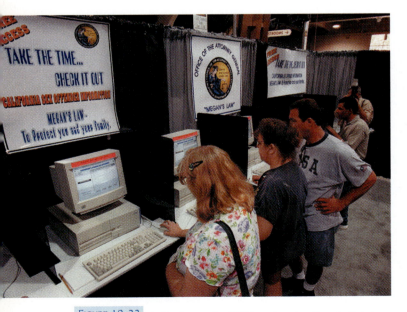

FIGURE 19-22 A display at the 75th Los Angeles County Fair in 1997 allowed California residents to search a sex offender registry with over 64,000 names listed in that state.

Medical Therapy for Sex Offenders

Over the last decade, researchers have evaluated the effectiveness of drugs that may inhibit sexual drive and interest in individuals who have been convicted of sexual offenses. The best known of these is medroxyprogesterone acetate, or **Depo-Provera.** In clinical trials, some involving very small samples, results do not clearly support the sexually suppressive effects of this agent (Cooper, Sandhu, Losztyn, & Cernovsky, 1992; Meyer, Cole, & Emory, 1992). Although diminished sexual interest, lowered testosterone levels, fewer sexual fantasies, and lowered frequency and enjoyment of masturbation have all been reported with this drug, larger samples and more consistent results are needed before Depo Provera is used more frequently in the treatment of sex offenders.

RAPE

Rape is the forcible sexual assault of an unwilling victim, someone who definitely does not want to participate in the sexual interaction with the assailant. Rape is a sexual crime motivated by a need for power, dominance, and intimidation. In most definitions of rape, the rapist uses some type of physical intimidation or force, or a weapon of some type or the threat of force. The *victim's perception* of the reality or imminence of that force is central to legal aspects of rape. Both women and men can be raped. Spouses can be raped. Dates can be raped. Children can be raped. Sometimes the victim knows the rapist, and sometimes he is a stranger.

The prevalence of rape in the United States is frightening. An organization called Rape, Abuse & Incest National Network (RAINN), a clearinghouse of information and support about these crimes, has collected statistics about rape, which are truly troubling. According to the U. S. Department of Justice an American woman is raped *every 2 minutes.* In 1996 alone, 307,000 women were raped, and in 1995 and 1996 over 670,000 women were the victims of rape, attempted rape, or other forms of sexual assault (such as sodomy). Of all serious violent crime in the United States, rape is the most likely to be unreported to law enforcement authorities. Some women feel deeply shameful, perhaps thinking that they may in some way have provoked the attack. They are also extremely fearful that the assailant will be found innocent and then find them and rape them again or commit other violence. According to the Bureau of Justice Statistics, about 31% of rapes and sexual assaults were reported in 1996, and approximately two-thirds of rape victims knew the person who assaulted them. In 1994 the Bureau of Justice Statistics data revealed that 28% of rape victims were raped by their husbands or boyfriends, 35% by acquaintances, and 5% by other relatives.

A 1994 report, *Violence Against Women,* published by the Bureau of Justice Statistics, U. S. Department of Justice, revealed the following data about rape in the United States:

- One of every four rapes takes place in a public area or in a parking garage.

- 29% of female victims reported that the offender was a stranger.
- 68% of rapes occur between the hours of 6 p.m. and 6 a.m.
- At least 45% of rapists were under the influence of alcohol or drugs.
- In 29% of rapes, the offender used a weapon.
- In 47% of rapes, the victim sustained injuries other than rape injuries.
- 75% of female rape victims required medical care after the attack.

—RAINN statistics, www.rainn.org, 1999

As with many aspects of human sexuality, there is much discussion and debate about the causes, manifestations, and consequences of rape. But there is no argument that this is a very big problem that affects the quality and security of a woman's psychosocial environment. This is a terribly violent crime, involving the unwanted and unwelcomed imposition of power of one person over another. Most social and behavioral scientists agree that interpersonal subjugation is more central to rape than sexual gratification for the rapist.

Data reveal that both incarcerated rapists and nonincarcerated sexually aggressive college men have important motivational characteristics in common (Lisak & Roth, 1988). Both overcompensate for feelings of weakness by expressing aggression against women. Both feel a disproportionate degree of anger against women who they perceive have hurt, rejected or slighted them. Lisak and Roth note that sexual frustration is generally not an important motivational factor in the groups they studied and emphasize that many rapists and sexually aggressive college men have regular legal sexual outlets, often within the context of a marriage. Finally, rapists and nonincarcerated sexually aggressive men have poor impulse control with respect to their sexual urges. This may be because of a high sensitivity to sexual cues in the environment or a character problem in monitoring and controlling their sexual feelings. Still, it is extremely difficult to point with certainty to cause-and-effect relationships between personality characteristics and the tendency to engage in sexually aggressive acts.

Is Rape a Sexual Deviation?

In addition to rape being a sexual offense, some have suggested that it may also be a sexual deviation (Groth & Burgess, 1977). This is not a common perspective but one worth examining briefly. A number of years ago this question received careful analysis, and current thinking about rapists' motivations and actions have been powerfully influenced by this early work (Groth & Burgess, 1977). For a long time rape had been viewed as the result more of certain high-risk situations and circumstances than of the personality of the perpetrator. Now that certain personal attributes are basic to the understanding of rapists, however, it seems that such characteristics might comprise a sexual deviation. Groth and

Burgess as well as many others believe that sexual deviations involve sexual activities that are part of nonsexual personal needs. In the case of rape, this involves the need to express anger and hostility rather than genital sexual intimacy. They believe that when force and intimidation become a part of sexual expression, a number of nonsexual needs are involved. These investigators carried out in-depth interviews and made numerous clinical observations of 133 sex offenders, a sizeable sample for a qualitative study. This study has educated the public about a number of common misperceptions about men who rape.

There had been a common belief that men who rape could not otherwise find sexual partners. This study showed that one-third of this sample were married at the time of their arrest and were having regular sexual relations with their spouses. Among the rapists who were not married, most were currently involved with at least one woman (and many with more than one) with whom they had regular sexual relations. These findings disconfirmed the hypothesis that rapists are typically starved for sexual outlets. The act of rape itself did not, among the men in this study, involve any effort to seduce or persuade their victims. Virtually all effort was given to trying to penetrate their victims. Verbal threats, weapons, physical overpowering, and physical violence were used to subdue the victim so that an attempt at penetration could take place. Over half of the victims of these sexual assaults sustained serious physical injuries, with 40% suffering from genital trauma. Over half of the 133 sex offenders studied had been convicted previously of rape, and perhaps most troubling, the majority used even more violence and force in second and subsequent sexual assaults. *None* of the subjects became less assertive or aggressive in second or subsequent rapes or rape attempts.

A significant number of rapists have trouble attaining and maintaining erections when attempting penetration. Others experience retarded ejaculation once they penetrate their victims, and still others ejaculate immediately. In their sample, Groth and Burgess found that 3 of 4 of their subjects experienced some type of sexual dysfunction during the sexual assault and attempted penetration. In their study of 92 victims of rape, Groth and Burgess reported that 45 women had no sperm in their vaginas after the assault. Findings like these also go against the idea of rape as an act of uncontrollable sexual desire.

This research also concerned the various motives of rapists. Based on their clinical experience, Groth and Burgess discriminated between men who raped because they were angry and those who raped because of a need for power and domination of their victim in particular and perhaps women in general. "Anger rape" usually involved vicious physical violence and much more force than was necessary to subdue the victim. During the attack, the rapist would commonly use profanity and other abusive language and would sometimes demand that the victim submit to degrading and humiliating acts. Anger rapes were usually not planned beforehand. Groth and Burgess learned that anger rapists attributed to their victims a hatred for the rejection they had suffered in interactions with other women in their lives. The "power rapist," in contrast, usually planned his assault carefully over a long period of time, often stalking his victim long before he attacked her. The power rapist wants to experience feelings of domination and control over his victim. This individual wants to experience the feeling that his victim cannot reject him and must submit to his sexual demands without question. Both types of rapists obviously still have much in common.

Groth and Burgess found that in their sample of 133 rapists, 40% had personality disorders, and many others suffered from anxiety disorders. Some were even plainly psychotic and may not have entirely been in touch with reality. Yet giving a diagnostic label to a psychological disorder does not explain how a person developed the problem. These researchers believe, based on their clinical interviews, that something very wrong occurs in the development of men who become rapists, often during their adolescence. Specifically, these men often experience "a failure to achieve an adequate sense of self-identity and self-worth." They point to the frustrations such a young man might experience as he tries to formulate a basic masculine picture of himself and the feelings of failure and inadequacy that sometimes result.

Groth and Burgess believe that because many of the psychological dynamics of rapists are a result of problems in development, and because their troubling personality characteristics are stable and enduring, there may be clinical justification for thinking of rape as a sexual deviation more than as the result of certain circumstances or provocations. It is noteworthy that men who rape almost never come to the attention of counselors or therapists until *after* they have committed a crime. Instead of asking for help, apparently the rapist acts out his old, frustrating emotional difficulties (Groth & Burgess, 1977, p. 405-406). Yet these writers also make the important point that if we begin to see rape as the result of the perpetrator's pathology, we may be less likely to attribute blame to the victim.

Brownmiller's Perspective on Rape

In 1975, Susan Brownmiller published a book that focused public attention and debate on the nature of male-female rape. *Against Our Will* opened a cultural dialogue on rape that revealed long-held misconceptions about this crime as well as its perpetrators and victims. Although we do not agree with all of Brownmiller's claims, her book has been important in stimulating fruitful social discussion and analysis about rape.

Brownmiller wants the reader to understand clearly that rape victims are not always young, attractive women, but that rape victimizes children, the elderly, and women not generally thought of as "pretty." Second, it is absolutely false that rape can be justified or defended by claims that the victim "really wanted it." Third, and most controversially, Brownmiller believes that rape has evolved over the course of human evolution

as an instrument of male power and intimidation, a terrible expression of "male dominance." Brownmiller states:

> *Man's discovery that his genitals could serve as a weapon to generate fear must rank as one of the most important discoveries of prehistoric times, along with the use of fire and the first crude stone axe. From prehistoric times to the present, I believe, rape has played a critical function. It is nothing more or less than a conscious process of intimidation by which all men keep all women in a state of fear.*
>
> —BROWNMILLER, 1975, 5

Brownmiller addresses an important question in human history: Why, in times of war, social unrest, revolution, genocide, or abuses of law enforcement has rape *always* been a basic instrument of interpersonal coercion and punishment? Why have "dominant" races and religions turned a blind eye to the rape of women who are members of minority races and religions? Why is the victim often "on trial" herself? Brownmiller's thinking on male-female rape does not characterize all feminist perspectives about rape, but it is a powerful perspective worthy of our attention.

Incorrect Perceptions of Rape

Because the general public is often uninformed about rape, a number of myths have developed about this crime. Johnson, Kuck, and Schander (1997) studied three categories of myths about rape: (1), when women are raped, it is their own fault, (2), there are good reasons that men should be exonerated for raping women, and (3), there are justifications for rape when women and men know each other. Surprisingly, some people still believe some of these. A sample of 149 female and male American undergraduates completed surveys assessing their beliefs about these three categories of myths about rape. Subjects were between 17 and 43 years of age. Almost all respondents answered all of the questions in this 30-item questionnaire. Johnson, Kuck, and Schander were particularly interested in the social and demographic characteristics of subjects who subscribed to these myths about rape. Below is a sampling of the results of this study. The percentage of respondents agreeing with each statement is presented. These authors combined data from female and male subjects, so we cannot determine how each sex responded to each item.

Rape Myth Category I: Blaming the Woman

Women provoke rapes	17.4
Women secretly want to be raped	6.6
A woman's reputation should be an issue	26.3
Women can't be raped without a weapon	1.9
Healthy women can resist rape	15.6

Rape Myth Category II: Excusing the Man

Most men are capable of rape	43.9
Men have sexual urges they can't control	32.2
Men who rape hate women	32.0

Rape Myth Category III: Justifications for Acquaintance Rape

Rapists are almost always strangers	20.1
A man had the right to assume a woman wants to have sexual intercourse with him if:	
she allows him to touch her in a sexual way	22.9
she touches him in a sexual way	30.3
she has an oral sexual encounter with him	42.4
If a woman has had previous sex with a man, she cannot claim that she was raped if the same man has sex with her again	7.9
If a man pays for everything on a date, a woman is obligated to have sex with him	0 .7

Many of the subjects in this sample believe a number of common myths about rape. While students of human sexuality have long known about myths about rape, empirical data were lacking on this subject. Further, note that a greater proportion of these subjects believed myths that exonerate the perpetrator rather than blame the victim of the assault. It is surprising that fully 43.9% of these respondents believed that most men are capable of raping a woman. Generally speaking, far more men agreed with the statement about males having uncontrollable sexual urges (41.9%) than women (25.3%).

CONFUSING LAWS CONCERNING RAPE

While rape might legally seem relatively straightforward, legal arguments about "force," "consent," and "sexual autonomy" reveal that much confusion exists—in the psychosocial environment as well as the courts—about exactly what these and other concepts actually mean in terms of the interactions between women and men. In a provocative analysis of these legal issues, Schulhofer (1998) emphasizes that while laws exist to protect our property, right to work, privacy, and a number of other freedoms and possessions, there is a tremendous and troubling amount of ambiguity concerning shared sexual intimacy. For example, this author emphasizes the fact that legal standards about what constitutes force on a man's part and what constitutes consent on a woman's part are frustratingly ambiguous. In the past, laws that dealt with rape required that if a woman was assaulted sexually, she was required to combat the assailant "to the utmost." Yet today, Schulhofer notes, "reasonable" resistance is apparently an adequate requirement for resisting sexual assault. Still, this writer notes that in virtually all states, forms of intimidation that do not involve overt physical threats are viewed by the courts as "persuasion" (Schulhofer, 1998, p. 56). In fact, pushing a woman to the ground or picking her up to throw her onto a bed to have sex with her are often legally insufficient examples of physical force.

Ambiguous also is the issue of consent. Alcohol and drugs present a common and controversial case for the courts. For example, if a woman is profoundly impaired and/or incoherent because of the effects of alcohol and/or drugs, how can she be certain that she has *not* given her implied or real consent to have sex (Fig. 19-23). Apparently, courts have found rapists innocent because it could not be proven that the defendant did not in some way consent to sexual intercourse or other sexual acts.

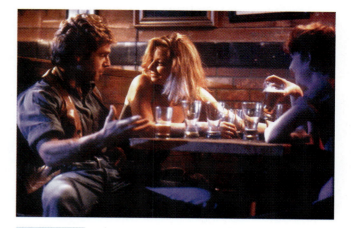

FIGURE 19-23 Jodie Foster (center) plays the victim of a gang rape in the movie, *The Accused*. Ms. Foster's character refuses to be intimidated by a legal system that assumes she has provoked the crime.

While there is a compelling simplicity in the statement that "no means no," even such a direct way of considering resistance to sexual coercion involves some confusion. In fact, whether "no *really* means no" has been surrounded by significant legal controversy. For example, Schulhofer asks whether "no" is always final and unarguable. If a man is told "no," can he attempt to persuade a woman to have sex with him at a later time? This too has not been decided with any clarity in the legal arena.

Schulhofer emphasizes that the right to sexual autonomy has two aspects. One involves *active personal decisions* about what a woman will and will not do sexually. Second is also a passive component in which a person has a right to decide who they will *not* have sexual relations with. Protest is assuredly an important way to preserve sexual autonomy, but when women are being sexually assaulted, they do not always have the opportunity to make their protest or resistance clear and unambiguous. Importantly, some states have tried to clarify the notion of sexual consent. Schulhofer notes that in New Jersey, Wisconsin, and Washington, consent involves "actual words or conduct indicating freely given agreement to have sexual intercourse" (Schulhofer, 1998, p. 66). And many social and behavioral scientists as well as feminist writers believe that a clear and unambiguous verbal "yes" is an absolute requirement for consensual sex.

RAPE FANTASIES

When women are surveyed about their sexual fantasies, one of the more common fantasies reported involves being taken sexually in a powerful, assertive way. Does this mean that women who report having this fantasy subconsciously want to be raped? In fact, having this fantasy most definitely does *not* mean that a woman wants to be raped. Reinisch (1990) points to a body of literature that suggests that women who have these fantasies might experience some ambivalence about initiating sex. Some girls are raised to believe that only men initiate sex and that it is somehow "unladylike" for a woman to make the first move, even if she feels especially interested in sharing sexual intimacy. Fantasies of being "taken" therefore remove guilt and reservations about having sex because the imaginary figure removes all choice in the matter as well as any need for potentially embarrassing behaviors with which a woman signals her sexual receptivity. These fantasies may also reveal a woman's underlying guilt about enjoying sexual excitement and pleasure. Men too have fantasies of being forced to have sex by beautiful, assertive, dominant women. Finally, while some men fantasize about raping women, these individuals consistently report that they would never even think of doing so in real life. Therefore, when women report having fantasies about being raped it does not in any way mean that they really want to be raped.

A recent study investigating sexual fantasies in women (Strassberg & Lockerd, 1998) evaluated reports of sexual fantasies in 137 college students and found that more than half of the subjects in this investigation reported having fantasies of being forced to have sex against their will. However, the women who reported these fantasies also had *less* guilt about sex than women who did not have them and scored higher in erotophilia than subjects not having these fantasies. Another important finding in this study is the fact that women who had forced sex fantasies had no consistent history of experiences involving sexual force. These researchers conclude that instead of forced sex fantasies being indications of sexual guilt, they are a sign that a woman has a diversified, lively, and open perspective on her own sexual expression. However, the fact that these women volunteered to report their sexual fantasies in the first place may suggest that this sample of subjects was relatively open about their sexuality and therefore less likely to report guilt feelings in connection with their sexual thoughts, feelings, and behaviors.

Different Kinds of Rapists

Since Groth and Burgess first characterized the differences between "anger rapists" and "power rapists," other researchers further examined the different predispositions behind different kinds of rapes and expanded this categorization. Knight, Warren, Reboussin, and Soley (1998) summarized this research and demonstrated that in some cases, a careful analysis of the crime-scene can tell law enforcement officials what kind of rapist probably committed the crime. These researchers suggested that there may be four basic motives involved in most rapes, related consistently to four different patterns of rapist behavior:

The Opportunity Rapist. These rapes are highly impulsive, unplanned attacks and are more the result of particular circumstances than the rapist's fantasies or general feelings about women. For example, Knight, Warren, Reboussin, and Soley suggest that if a woman is present when another, nonsexual crime is being committed she may be assaulted as a peripheral, unintended aspect of the initial crime. The same may be true if a man meets a woman at a bar or party and finds her attractive and interesting and fails to exercise proper impulse control.

The Pervasive Anger Rapist. These rapists are angry at everything, not just women. A compelling and unfocused anger permeates every aspect of this person's life, and very commonly these individuals have a record of other antisocial behaviors. This individual is also likely to assault men, and his attacks almost always result in significant physical injury.

The Sexual Gratification Rapist. These offenders are highly and obsessively preoccupied with sexual matters. They often experience deep needs for dominance but have profound feelings of personal inadequacy. These individuals often engage in sexual fetishes; they also often have the sexual dysfunctions noted above. This type of rapist seeks some sign that his victim is "enjoying" having sex with him and engages in sex acts in a highly ritualistic way.

The Vindictive Rapist. Vindictive rapists hate women, who are the key and central object of their enormous anger. These men want to hurt their victims as well as offend, degrade, humiliate, and insult them. They too sometimes experience sexual dysfunctions while assaulting their victims.

Crime scene analysis and victim interviews often show some consistency within each of these types of rape, although there is a great deal of variability within each category. Information like this can help identify and find the rapist. Note that scientists are often uncomfortable with classification schemes because they sometimes give the impression that every individual case fits neatly into one and only one category, and this is not the case with the different motives of rapists.

Not all men who rape women fit neatly into one of the above categories. Many men who have raped women or who may be inclined to do so score high on such personality traits as aggressiveness, manipulativeness, and impulsivity on a personality test called the "Schedule for Nonadaptive and Adaptive Personality" (SNAP). These traits frequently characterize a psychopathic personality, also sometimes called an antisocial personality. These individuals frequently find themselves in conflict with society's expectations of law-abiding behavior and do not feel any guilt for their transgressions. Nor do they learn from the consequences of their actions. Hersh and Gray-Little (1998) administered this test and others to a large group of men taking an Introductory Psychology course at a large, Southern public university. They presumed that this sample of subjects would most probably engage in sexually aggressive acts with their acquaintances rather than strangers, if they were to do so at all. The testing procedures used in this study did not allow the researchers to determine the identity of any of the 191 men in this study or whether any had ever been accused or convicted of rape. Importantly, subjects who reported engaging in aggressive sexual behaviors scored far higher on the SNAP aggressiveness scale than subjects who had reported that they had engaged only in consensual sex. The same was true of their ratings on the manipulativeness scale. These subjects were also asked whether they believed in the truthfulness of common rape myths. Those subjects who reported having engaged in sexually aggressive acts were more likely to support these erroneous myths than subjects who scored lower in the aggression, manipulativeness, and impulsivity scales. Very few of the subjects in this investigation had severe antisocial tendencies, however. Data like these tend to support the general connection between what people think and feel and how they act, although this is by no means always the case. A key question remains unanswered, however: can data based on responses to personality tests *predict* who is and is not likely to sexually assault a woman? At this time no one can answer with any certainty.

Resisting Rape

It has been debated whether a woman should vigorously resist a rapist's attempts, defend herself, and fight back or do as little as possible to further incite and anger the attacker. Ullman (1998) studied whether offender violence escalates when the victim resists and fights back. This study analyzed over 2,000 rapes and attempted rapes reported to the Chicago police department between 1979 and 1981. Police files were examined to learn more about the violent sexual assaults and how the behaviors of the rapists and victims affected the prevalence and seriousness of injuries incurred during the rape. The data revealed that when women forcefully resisted an attacker, either verbally or physically, this resistance did not lead to increased violence by the rapist, and that in general, resistance activities were associated with the diminished likelihood of being raped. The various motives of the apprehended rapists were not reported in this study. This author notes that it is rare for rape to result in serious injuries or death and that active avoidance and resistance strategies are more frequently associated with escaping the attacker and resisting penetration than with worse physical injuries.

When physical injuries are the result of a sexual assault, they are often genital injuries. Biggs, Stermac, and Divinsky (1998) studied the prevalence and nature of genital injuries following sexual assaults in women who had had prior sexual intercourse and those who had not. A total of 132 subjects were examined in this study. These researchers noted that "nonperforating soft-tissue injuries, lacerations, or current bleeding" often occurred up to 10 days after the attack, especially in women without prior sexual intercourse experience (65.2% of those injured). Among women without prior sexual experience, only about 9% had any tearing of their hymen, a finding consistent with comments above about the prevalence of sexual dysfunctions in many rapists. Some women do not have visible genital injuries after a sexual assault.

Rape in War and Political Conflict

It is extremely common in times of war for members of the military to rape women in the territory of the enemy. This is an example of Brownmiller's idea that rape is an instrument of masculine aggression against women. These sexual assaults are often premeditated and reveal a deliberate decision to demoralize and humiliate the victims of such attacks. Many military leaders have in the past openly encouraged their men to rape the wives, mothers, and daughters of soldiers on the other side to demonstrate their control of geographical areas and the broader sociopolitical environment. Ancient Greek and Roman history reveals that rape and pillage are often considered

the "right" of the victor over the vanquished. Rape in war is a powerful weapon that profoundly discourages and subdues the citizens and military of opposition forces. Far from being a rare action undertaken by "uncivilized" or "barbaric" armies, rape in war has unfortunately been noted in virtually all of the world's military forces at some time (Fig. 19-24).

Recent conflicts in eastern Europe involved mass rapes of women in Bosnia-Herzegovina (Stiglmayer, 1994). The earliest reports of planned, systematic rapes first arrived in the West in 1991. It is not easy to identify women who have been raped in this political and military conflict, but estimates of the number of women raped ranged from 20,000 to 60,000. Many women who were raped hid that fact out of shame or perhaps because they feared retribution and ostracism from their spouses and family members. When asked about rape by relief workers, about 1 woman in 5 declined to respond at all. Apparently the rapes in eastern Europe were condoned by commanding officers in the field. Rapes and sexual assaults on men have also been reported in this military conflict. Many prisoners in detention camps were raped or suffered genital mutilation while incarcerated.

In 1998 reports of mass, systematic rapes by members of the Burmese military gained attention in the West, although as early as 1988 the new military ruling party encouraged a "strategy of mixing blood" that condoned if not openly encouraged these attacks (Bernstein & Kean, 1998). These attacks were against not members of an adversarial nation but Burmese women themselves. In one case, two young women were abducted from their rural village and "raped continually for six nights by two or three men each night, including the soldiers'

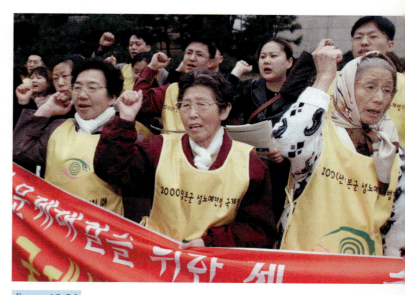

FIGURE 19-24   During World War II, Japanese soldiers made sex slaves of nearly 200,000 women of various races and nationalities. A number of these "military comfort women" sued the Japanese government in 1991. Here, survivors of this sexual exploitation demonstrate their outrage.

Research Highlight

RAPE IN THE MILITARY

In the late 1990s an enormous controversy erupted in the Canadian popular press when a notable Canadian newsmagazine, *Maclean's*, ran a cover story on rape in the military. Immediately, defenders of the military status quo and many women and men who had been raped, assaulted, or sexually harassed in the past came forward to support or criticize the military's climate of opinion in regard to sexual assault. Many felt that women were fully enfranchised in the military and enjoyed more esteem and admiration than ever before. Others believed that it was time to reveal a longstanding pattern of avoiding prosecuting and punishing men who sexually victimized others. Military officials rejected claims that Canadian armed services are a highly permissive environment with regard to sexual assault and harassment. Yet one senior woman who had resigned from the military in 1994 and who was the first female to fly the CF-18 fighter acknowledged that in her 21-year career she had been raped, sexually harassed, and sexually assaulted. One wonders if there are any fundamental differences between the Canadian military and the United States military, or between the military and other large organizations.

The documentation showing problems in the Canadian military is enormous and compelling. Following are a few important cases that surfaced during this highly publicized discussion:

1. Apparently, senior military authorities squelched a story about the violent gang rape of a mentally handicapped woman by a number of soldiers in 1988.
2. At a military base north of Toronto, military police investigated 27 separate sexual assault charges in the summer of 1994. In one case, a local 13-year-old girl was one of the victims of these attacks.
3. A military base in Alberta was believed to be so dangerous for female soldiers that they had to be in their quarters by a stated curfew, and then the building was locked and surrounded by guards.
4. A military physician was suspected of sexually assaulting at least 12 female patients in the mid-1980s. His superiors filed no charges against him.
5. A former member of the reserve military police who worked at military facilities in Saskatchewan and British Columbia between 1991 and 1994 became aware of over two dozen cases of rape, sexual molestation, and sexual assault. He was quoted as saying, "We were told to shut our mouths, that these things would be handled by the chain of command" (O'Hara, 1998, p. 16). Apparently they were not; he quit.

By most estimates, events like these reveal serious problems. Yet many female and male members of the military felt that these cases do not offer a fair and accurate portrait of the general climate regarding women in the Canadian military. Still, as the investigation unfolded, it was found that military superiors commonly suppressed or obstructed inquiries of these complaints. Authorities felt that if such cases were reported in civilian courts instead of military courts, far more publicity would surround them. By the end of 1998, however, many women in the military believed that the situation was improving, at least somewhat.

An analysis of reactions to rape of women in the military was published in the journal *Military Medicine* by Ritchie in 1998. This investigator analyzed about 100 cases in which rape was alleged to have occurred in the military. In most cases, the author evaluated the victim, and other data were drawn from military records. Based on this sample of United States Army personnel, Ritchie characterized the most common military rape scenario. As with civilians, military rape commonly involves two people who know each other, and often they have both been drinking and are intoxicated. While physical force is commonly reported, the use of weapons is very rare. Ritchie's analysis also revealed that there is frequently a delay in reporting the rape. Victims report that when the assailant is of superior rank, they feel strongly coerced to comply with the sexual demand, and when and if legal proceedings result from complaints of sexual assault, it almost always becomes a case of one person's word against another's, a situation that reveals humiliating information with little satisfactory legal resolution to show for it. Ritchie noted the following common reactions among women in the military who have been raped:

1. she delays reporting for days to months;
2. she washes or douches her genitals;
3. she refuses a medical examination;
4. she continues to have contact with the assailant;
5. she only divulges the information after others report being sexually assaulted by the assailant;
6. she has sexual relations shortly after being assaulted; or
7. her behavior seems otherwise "inconsistent" for someone who has been raped.

—Ritchie, 1998, 506

Whether these findings are pertinent to sexual assaults in the military forces of other countries remains to be determined. Yet if we assume that a country's military personnel represent a microcosm of the entire society, we should anticipate the same types of antisocial behaviors in the military as seen in the general population.

Yet the rape of women seems far more prevalent in the military than in the population as a whole. Martin, Rosen, Durand, Stretch, and Knudson (1998) distributed questionnaires to 555 male and 573 female soldiers serving in combat missions or in combat support units. A surprising 22.6% of the women in this sample reported a completed rape, and 6.7% of the men reported being sexually assaulted by another man, but the overwhelming majority of these cases occurred *before* these individuals entered the military. These data imply that a disproportionately large percentage of women entering the military have been victimized by sexual assaults and abuse, although the precise causes or implications of these statistics remain unclear.

commander" (Bernstein & Kean, 1998, p. 5). Most attacks like this one involve soldiers who have been given permission by their officers to engage in such behavior and sustain no punishment. Another report from Burma published in 1997 refers to an incident in which "120 troops led by Capt. Htun Mya found forty-two women and fifty-seven men hiding in the forest last September. The troops gang-raped all the women for two days and two nights, and then killed all ninety-nine villagers" (Bernstein & Kean, 1998, p. 5).

Rape as an instrument of terror does not occur only in times of war. Other forms of political unrest as well as economic turmoil may also precipitate such attacks on women. In late 1998 evidence surfaced that up to 170 Chinese women may have been raped in Indonesia. Because the Indonesian economy was in a state of near collapse, riots broke out in a number of cities and Chinese residents were the focus of the rioters' rage. News stories reported that gangs of men, many apparently members of the military, ransacked businesses, threatened residents, and raped and murdered women. One 17-year-old girl who counseled victims of these sexual assaults was murdered in an especially violent way, almost decapitated. Another report described how a 12-year-old girl and her mother were raped beside each other. When the woman's husband tried to stop the attack he was hanged. Events like these reveal old, long-held animosities that sometimes boil over in

time of economic turmoil. Unfortunately, many women were the scapegoats of this anger.

Statutory Rape

In the past, the term "statutory rape" was used to describe sexual intercourse between an adult and a minor, even if the minor consented. The reason this is illegal is simple: minors are not thought to be cognitively or emotionally capable of making a decision to consent to sexual intercourse. This is a complex legal issue. In some states, adults who have intercourse with consenting minors are charged with sexual assault, and if physical force or coercion is used, the adult may be charged with aggravated sexual assault. Generally the penalties for adults are more severe when they hold positions of authority and trust. In reference to the crime of statutory rape, the term "jail bait" has been used to describe flirtatious minors who appear willing to have sexual relations with an adult. Often, local and regional customs influence how this crime is defined, prosecuted, and punished. Prosecuting statutory rape has become both politically popular and socially complex.

In an interesting analysis of the rise in prosecutions for statutory rape, Elton (1997) explored ways in which statistics have been oversimplified and case-by-case considerations neglected. For example, Elton points out that statistics released in 1996-97 revealed that "two-thirds of teen pregnancies involve adult fathers" (p. 12). Yet when these individual cases are explored in depth, cases of exploitative "older men" and innocent, passive teenage girls are the exception rather than the rule. Elton reviews a Wisconsin case in which a 19-year-old man was prosecuted for sexual assault for getting his 15-year-old girlfriend pregnant, even though the two were planning to marry and raise their child together. Further, the names of young men like this would be entered into a national registry for sex offenders. Many social critics feel this punishment absurd and unfair. It seems that many states have decided to fight high teen pregnancy rates with more severe punishments for statutory rape; California, Delaware, Florida, and Georgia have already done so. Elton quotes then-Governor Pete Wilson of California as saying, "It's not macho to get a teenager pregnant, but if you lack the decency to understand this yourself we'll give you a year to think about it in county jail" (cited in Elton, 1998, p. 12). A more careful analysis of this issue by the Urban Institute found that about 8% of teenage pregnancies among unmarried women between the ages of 15 and 17 involved fathers who were at least five years older, and that 13% of these girls became pregnant by men who were at least four years older.

Many of these young girls do not feel that they have been sexually victimized, and because of this many prosecutors are hesitant to take on these cases. In one case, social workers in California suggested that a 13-year-old girl marry her 20-year-old boyfriend because they were certain that such a marriage would create order and predictability in this girl's life, which had involved habitual truancy and drug abuse. Elton points out another important consideration in cases like this: pregnant teenage girls may hesitate to seek prenatal counseling or care for fear that it will lead to the arrest of their boyfriends.

Legal opinions also vary on whether female minors should be held accountable for precipitating sexual intercourse with an adult male while knowing it is against the law. Guerrina (1998) has written persuasively that assigning legal penalties to females in these cases as a way of reducing the punishment for the adult male further punishes the young woman and may limit consideration of unique, extenuating circumstances such as those described in the previous paragraph.

Researchers in Kansas surveyed the district attorneys in that state using a questionnaire and some in-depth follow-up telephone interviews (Miller, Miller, Kenney, & Clark, 1998). Of the 105 district attorneys in that state, 92 returned their surveys. The results reveal the legal and psychosocial climate of opinion about enforcement of statutory rape in that state. While 74% of those returning their surveys favored the aggressive prosecution of cases of statutory rape, only 37% felt that they would have broad public support for doing so and only 24% believed that such prosecutions would have any measurable impact on reducing teen pregnancy in Kansas; 57% supported the current legal age of consent (16 years) at the time of the study. Importantly, 17% of district attorneys felt that prosecuting cases of statutory rape would inhibit young women from seeking adequate prenatal medical care. These data point to an important area of potential collaboration among the legal, medical, and social work professions and a wider understanding of the place of statutory rape in the psychosocial setting.

Date Rape

As already noted, most rapes involve people who know each other. Date rape recently gained the public's attention and remains an especially problematic issue on college campuses. The fact that the assailant and victim know each other in no way diminishes the seriousness of the crime or mitigates prosecution and sentencing for rape. Much attention has been given to this subject in the context of family life education courses in high school and other forums in higher education settings. Date rape is usually defined as nonconsensual sex between two people who are in an affectionate and/or romantic relationship of varying duration and intensity. A literature review on this subject was carried out by Rickert and Wiemann (1998) who compared various research studies regarding the prevalence of date rape among women in different age groups as well as factors that might predispose men toward this type of sexual assault. There is a large range in the reported prevalence of date rape in the primary literature. Estimates range from 13% to 27% of women in college and from 20% to 68% of adolescent females. The subject samples in which date rape has been studied are highly diverse, and it is difficult to estimate the prevalence of date rape in the general population.

These researchers found that a number of factors are correlated with an increased risk of a woman being raped on a date, although many of these are not directly related to dating behaviors or interpersonal skills. These characteristics include women who are younger at the time of their first date and women who become sexually active earlier in adolescence. Further, females with an earlier age of menarche (and presumably other early signs of puberty) are also more likely to be raped on a date. Females who have been sexually abused as children or otherwise victimized sexually are also at an increased risk of date rape. Females who believe common rape myths, such as those outlined earlier, and who are more tolerant of violence against females are also more likely to be raped by a date. Additionally, Shapiro and Schwarz (1997) reported that an important potential risk factor for date rape was a larger lifetime number of sexual partners and more frequent sexual intercourse. None of these points to a cause-and-effect relationship with date rape, but all reflect the conspicuousness of sexual issues in a young woman's self-esteem and perhaps her interpersonal relationships.

The use of alcohol and illegal drugs further increases the likelihood of date rape because of the impact of these drugs on a person's ability to accurately interpret the behaviors, gestures, and mannerisms of others. Rickert and Wiemann believe that alcohol and drugs increase the chances that a male might misjudge a female's friendly behaviors as a sexual "come-on" when in fact they are not. Finally, other subtle factors related to date rape are the degree to which males are socialized to fully understand that "no means no" and whether their peer group encourages restraint and respect for women who set clear limits and boundaries.

Refusing a sexual advance depends on various factors too. Yescavage (1999) has reported that in questioning a group of 46 college men, the timing of a woman's refusal predicts how the subjects will respond to a description of a date-rape scenario. She found that when a female engages in some sexual activity with a male and then refuses similar activity on a later occasion, most of the males in this sample report that her responsibility for date rape "increases dramatically" (p. 806). Indeed, many respondents reported that women are accountable for forced sex for permitting the earlier sexual activity to occur in the first place; male responsibility in this scenario was decreased drastically in their estimations. Similarly, if the couple in the scenario has been together for a long period of time and has been sexually active, again the male is seen as less culpable. McCaw and Senn (1998) asked women and men to write short essays about a date rape scenario and found that the men in their study were very cognizant of specific behaviors women were likely to perceive as sexually coercive and that it was most unusual for a man to engage in sexually coercive behaviors without knowing what he was doing.

Another study examined negative dating experiences of both younger and older women, including rape. Kalra, Wood, Desmarais, Verberg, and Senn (1998) compared unpleasant dating experiences in a sample of 115 women between 18 and 85 years of age and found much similarity in these experiences among both younger and older women. The older subjects, however, were more likely to believe myths about rape and to blame negative dating experiences on themselves rather than their male partners. Data like these are important because many women and men begin dating later in life as a result of marital separation, divorce, or the death of their spouses. These individuals might benefit from reexamining their assumptions about dating and their short- and long-term expectations of their companions. Of the women over 40 in this study, almost 70% reported that they had experienced unwanted physical contact on a date.

One of the factors that has increased the prevalence of date rape, especially among younger individuals, is the drug flunitrazepam, called **Rohypnol**, a powerful sedative that as of this writing is not approved for distribution in the United States. This agent has been available by prescription in Europe since the mid-1990s as well as Mexico and some South American countries. Pills can be obtained on the black market for $1 to $5 per tablet. Rohypnol has no odor, taste, or color and promptly dissolves in any beverage. In addition to being a powerful sedative, it often eliminates the subject's memory for up to 6 or 8 hours after it has been swallowed. It takes only about 20 minutes to take effect, and many date rapes take place while females are under the influence of this agent. On the street Rohypnol is called "roach," "rope," "roofies," or "the forget pill." It is common for women to remember virtually nothing while under the influence of this drug. This drug is about 10 times stronger than the common anti-anxiety agent Valium. When Rohypnol is taken with alcohol its sedative-hypnotic effects are tremendously magnified, although those who have never taken it are usually unaware of this danger. In some cases this drug does not have sedative effects but instead causes unprovoked anger and sometimes hallucinations. If you have any suspicions that you have ingested Rohypnol, call 911 immediately. The "Drug-Induced Rape Prevention and Punishment Act of 1996" made it a felony to give Rohypnol or any similar-acting agent to any person without their knowledge intending to inflict violence, including rape, on that individual.

The consequences of date rape are many and diverse. Shapiro and Schwarz (1997) studied a sample of 41 college women who reported they had been date raped and a control group of 125 college women who had not been date raped. Those who had been assaulted reported significantly more symptoms of psychological trauma, including anxiety and depression as well as many of the characteristics of posttraumatic stress disorder. They also had significantly lower sexual self-esteem than the women in the control group. Importantly, the women who had been date raped revealed these symptoms whether they were in a "committed sexually active relationship" with the rapist, were in an "uncommitted sexually active relationship" with the rapist, or were "sexually inexperienced."

After a Rape

Rape is a demoralizing, dehumanizing crime. Women who have been raped experience powerful emotions ranging from shame and guilt to anger and rage. Confusion, emotional and physical pain, and anxiety and depression are also common. However, some women who have been raped seem calm and composed after the attack. A woman's initial reaction to sexual assault may differ significantly from her long-term psychological reaction, and there is no way of predicting the duration and severity of these outcomes. Following a rape the woman is typically interviewed, examined, and treated, often in the emergency room of a hospital, which in itself carries the implication of injury and disease. In a hospital it may be difficult to focus on the emotional aspects of the assault, but generally this is the best place to have these interactions. The following descriptions of these procedures are summarized from Petter and Whitehill (1998).

Information about the sexual assault. Petter and Whitehill emphasize the importance of using a private, quiet place for discussing the attack. It is recommended that at first the police be excused. A victim's permission should be obtained during every step of the interview and examination. She should give her permission to be questioned and examined as well as for the collection of physical samples and specimens or any photographs that might be important. Petter and Whitehill recommend doctors try to learn the following types of information, which is especially helpful in treating patients who have been sexually assaulted:

1. age and identifying information for both the victim and the assailant (if available);
2. date, time and location of the alleged assault;
3. circumstances of the assault;
4. details of sexual contact, such as penile, digital or object penetration, and route, such as vaginal, oral or anal intercourse, as well as documentation of any ejaculation or urination by the assailant;

5. type of physical restraints used, such as weapons, drugs or alcohol;
6. activities of the victim after the assault, such as change of clothing, bathing, douching, dental hygiene, urination or defecation; and
7. gynecologic history — last menstrual period, contraceptive use, pregnancy history, last voluntary sexual encounter, any recent episode of gynecologic infection and pelvic surgery.

—Adapted from Beebe, 1991

Physical examination. Following rape there are two important reasons for a thorough physical examination: determination of the presence, nature, and extent of any injuries and the collection of evidence that might be used in any legal action against the assailant. The victim needs to understand that evidence collected more than 48 to 72 hours after the assault may not be very helpful in prosecuting a rape suspect. Examining physicians use a "rape kit" to collect evidence (see Fig. 1-16). Following are items or specimens typically collected after a sexual assault, according to Petter and Whitehill:

Patient's clothing

Fingernail scrapings, broken fingernail piece

Hair strands

Oral and throat swabbing

Pubic hair sample

Vaginal swabbing

Vaginal washings

Pap smear

Blood samples

Laboratory tests. A pregnancy test is recommended in most cases of sexual assault, as is a test for most common STDs. Additionally, blood tests for hepatitis B and HIV are commonly performed. HIV tests are ideally repeated 3, 6, and 12 months after the assault.

Treatment. Petter and Whitehill estimate that 1% to 5% of sexual assault victims will become pregnant and that the risk of acquiring an STD is 5% to 10%. In many instances, emergency contraception measures are taken (see Chapter 11). Treating victims of sexual assault generally requires four approaches: treating any physical injuries that may have occurred, after-intercourse pregnancy prevention measures, treatment for any STDs that may have been contracted, and preparing the victim for any psychological and/or social consequences of her attack. Medical, surgical, and drug interventions are sometimes required as well as crisis counseling and long-term psychotherapy follow-up.

Long-Term Consequences of Rape. Women who have been raped often have long-term problems with interpersonal relationships. Thelen, Sherman, and Borst (1998) studied problems in creating emotional attachments and fear of intimacy in a sample of 44 college women who reported being raped. Their questionnaire responses were compared to those of a control group of 57 college women who had not been sexually as-

saulted. It was not possible to determine how much time had elapsed since the women who reported having been raped had been victimized. These investigators found that rape survivors had significantly greater fear of emotional intimacy, were less confident in the dependability of other people, and were more uncomfortable with emotional closeness. Additionally, they had significantly more fear of interpersonal abandonment. Longitudinal studies may illuminate how persistent and enduring these characteristics might be. The psychological consequences of rape can be devastating, sometimes involving posttraumatic stress disorder as the following case study indicates.

Support for Rape Victims

Women who have been raped often have access to services that address the medical, emotional, and financial needs of sexual assault victims (Campbell & Aherns, 1998). Local agencies provide psychosocial support services and attempt to meet victim needs at various times after the assault. In some communities, Sexual Assault Response Teams are available, located in hospital emergency rooms and including physicians, police officers, legal prosecutors, rape crisis counselors, and hospital social workers. Such a single facility is often highly effective in providing diverse support services and efficiently assessing and meeting various victim needs. Drug and Alcohol Programs attempt to explore any relationship between sexual assault and the abuse of drugs and/or alcohol. They are typically staffed by mental health workers and also offer rape crisis counseling. While these facilities do not offer all the support services of sexual assault response teams, they are highly effective in addressing the special problems they deal with. Campbell and Aherns emphasize that many rape survivors never approach medical or law enforcement authorities but instead seek counseling from clergy within a religious institutional setting. While this provides the victim with important emotional assistance, this resource rarely can meet all of the victim's needs after a sexual attack. Another source of support for rape victims are Domestic Violence Shelters for women in a battering relationship; they often act as legal advocates of women in these circumstances. They also provide emergency housing, which can be extremely important in cases of marital and date rape. The last type of community resource studied by Campbell and Aherns are Crime Reparation Assistance Programs. These organizations provide funds to pay for medical and psychological treatment necessitated by sexual assault. Together, these agencies and organizations provide for an integrated, supportive system of resources to rape victims, and usually there is excellent coordination of assistance measures for women who are trying to deal with these terrible stresses.

Treatment for Rapists

Earlier we noted that rapists often feel uncontrollable compulsions to sexually assault women. Research has considered whether these powerful and persistent urges can be treated effectively and the chances of future assaults decreased. This predisposition varies in seriousness, and all men who rape are not

CASE STUDY: JoAnn

JoAnn is a 20-year-old woman who works as a secretary for a small business. She was attacked one evening when she stepped outside to the back of the apartment building where she lived alone to take out the trash. A young man she had never seen before was outside and followed her back into the building. When she opened her door he lunged at her and pushed her inside where he raped and sodomized her at knifepoint. After he left she was in a state of shock, and just sat, staring, the rest of the night. Once, she tried to call a friend who was not home. The next morning her co-workers took her to the rape crisis center.

JoAnn's boyfriend was supportive and wanted to do anything he could for her. He suggested she move in with him but agreed not to try to have sex until she was ready. During the next few weeks she was unable to work and had to quit her job, after which she stayed at home doing nothing, rarely even bothering to dress. She had nightmares, difficulty sleeping and eating, and lost a lot of weight. Her boyfriend did everything for her, comforted her constantly, and was careful not to push her into doing anything she did not feel like, even eating. His kindness was not helpful, however, making her feel dependent and incapable of doing anything for herself. She began to think about suicide all the time.

The one thing JoAnn was able to do was to visit the rape crisis center where she saw a counselor. She began going daily and staying there a lot during the day, talking to the staff or just sitting. She felt she could not communicate with any of her old friends because she spoke constantly about the assault, which seemed to make them uncomfortable. Her counselor allowed her to talk as much as she wanted about the assault. She went over it again and again, focusing on why it happened, and what she could have done to prevent it or defend herself. Whereas her friends tried to keep her from expressing any self-blame, her counselor helped her put it in perspective.

After 3 or 4 months, JoAnn's depression began to lift and the suicidal thoughts decreased. Her nightmares became infrequent and she began to sleep and eat more regularly, regaining some of the weight she lost. She was still dependent on her boyfriend but took a job and was able to function adequately in spite of her anxiety when strange men came into the office. At first her boyfriend took her home from work every day, but she told him that she needed to learn to do more things for herself and become more independent.

Calhoun & Atkeson, 1991

---

equally afflicted; many rapists are not habitually preoccupied with the prospect of raping someone.

A case in Kansas increased the public debate on the punishment of rapists. Donald Gideon was convicted of rape in 1982. He was released from prison and was on parole for less than a year when he murdered a young college student during a rape in 1993. As a consequence, the Kansas state legislature passed a law requiring all sex offenders, upon completion of their prison sentence, to be "involuntarily committed to treatment of indefinite duration if a jury decides he is likely to commit sex crimes again because of 'a mental abnormality or personality disorder'" (Stoil, 1998, p. 6). The Supreme Court of Kansas ruled this law unconstitutional because it required psychological treatment in the absence of proof that the individual was in fact mentally ill (Stoil, 1998). The United States Supreme Court overturned the Kansas decision, allowing the law to stand.

In Kansas, the Sexual Predator Treatment Program began at the Larned Correctional Mental Health Facility with each resident receiving about 30 hours of psychological treatment each week, mostly in group therapy sessions. The men in this program are physiologically monitored for arousal to nonerotic photographs. Stoil notes that the Kansas statute might change the way state hospital systems are managed. Mental health administrators and practitioners do not always agree about whether committing sex offenders to inpatient treatment is an effective way to minimize repeat rape offenses. In fact, the American Psychological Association does not think the Kansas statute will be very effective in the long run. Instead, this organization recommends longer initial prison sentences with in-jail evaluation and treatment programs. The University of Hawaii, for example, runs a program in that state's prisons that includes group therapy sessions and sometimes aversion therapy (in which the patient may receive electrical shocks if he shows signs of sexual arousal while listening to depictions of sexual assault or viewing pictures of a sexual attack). This program continues on an outpatient basis when the prisoner leaves jail on parole and has been shown to lower the recidivism rate for sexual offenses. In Kansas, in contrast, after this statute was enacted there was a 16% *increase* in forcible rape while comparable statistics declined throughout most of the country.

Firestone, Bradford, McCoy, Greenberg, Curry, and Larose (1998) studied the recidivism of rapists in Canada. These investigators analyzed data on 86 men who had been out of jail for up to 12 years, with a mean of almost 8 years. About half of these men had committed some legal offense in the first 5 years they were out of prison, a disheartening statistic. While these researchers reported that the rate of recidivism for sexual offenses was about 16% (a figure comparable to those cited in our earlier section on sexual abuse), this actually is lower than recidivism rates for violent crimes (26%) and all criminal activities considered collectively (53%). Additionally, this research indicates that it is very difficult to predict which men are likely to reoffend and which are not. However, the more frequently a man had been in trouble with the law and the more violent the crimes he committed, the more likely it was that he would be a sexual crime reoffender. Reoffenders were also generally younger than those not prosecuted a second or subsequent time. Reoffenders were also more likely to have a problem with alcohol abuse. Overall, a number of psychosocial variables may help determine whether someone convicted of rape will later victimize others, but there is no sure way to make a completely accurate prediction.

CONCLUSION

As with most aspects of human nature, there are boundaries between what is common, acceptable, and decent and what is not. This last chapter has discussed some of the less attractive aspects of human sexual expression, especially when it seems entirely divorced from erotic intentions, and our legal system has developed explicit guidelines for defining and punishing sexual transgressions. This book begins with an emphasis on two essential criteria that lend dignity to human sexual expression: privacy and the lack of coercion. The topics in this chapter involve problems with both. We have seen that "victimless crimes" really are not "victimless." Exploitation in prostitution and sexual harassment is much in the public's consciousness and will likely continue so for a long time. Difficulties in defining pornography and limiting its availability to minors will trouble legal experts for the foreseeable future. The sexual abuse of children as well as adolescents and adults involves violations of the most basic of human rights. And the assertion of male dominance through rape will occupy the pages of our newspapers and magazines as long as we live.

Yet victims often feel in some way responsible for their victimization. Therefore we would like to emphasize that if you are ever the nonconsenting recipient of anyone's sexual expression, verbalization, innuendo, or hostile assertions or actions, you are, by definition, a victim, not to be blamed yourself.

*L*earning Activities

1. Soft-core pornography is sometimes sold in convenience stores in brown wrappers so that the cover cannot be seen by customers in the store. X-rated videos are rented in a variety of clubs and outlets. Speculate on how community sensitivities approving or disapproving of the sale of these items can be assessed and communicated to local government officials.

2. Speculate as to why the legalization of pornography in Denmark has not been accompanied by an increase in reported sex offenses.

3. Should those who manufacture pornography be responsible for sexual offenses committed by those who buy it?

4. Support or refute the notion that prostitution is a "victimless crime."

5. Speculate on how being physically or sexually abused as a child might play a role in women becoming prostitutes.

6. Should law enforcement officials publish the names of persons who are arrested with prostitutes?

7. Consensual sexual relations are common in many occupational settings. If this is true, why might someone need to use coercion to gain sexual favors from an associate, co-worker, subordinate, or student?

8. Is it legal harassment if someone sexually harasses an individual in the educational or work setting who holds a role of seniority or authority over them? Think about your own experiences before answering this question.

9. Explain why there are often difficulties clearly defining "sexual harassment" and why the same behaviors are often interpreted in very different ways by different people. If someone is unjustly accused of sexual harassment, what legal protections does she or he have and how might these be exercised?

10. In your opinion, can someone who has sexually abused children ever be fully "cured?" Why or why not?

11. Does the incidence of child sexual abuse grow every year, or does the more frequent reporting of these crimes make it seem so?

12. Do you think that the victim of child sexual abuse is best treated with one-on-one counseling or with group therapy? Why?

13. In your opinion, what is the best way to tell children about the dangers of sexual abuse without frightening them?

14. To what extent do you think that rape has historically, adversely, and persistently affected relations between women and men?

15. Describe why it is so difficult to obtain accurate statistics about attempted and completed rapes in the United States.

16. Discuss why the idea of "resistance" has become so important in legal definitions of rape. Is it possible to agree upon what "earnest resistance" might entail?

17. When a person learns that a friend or acquaintance has been raped, a number of thoughts go through the head. Speculate about what these thoughts might be.

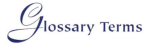

Key Concepts

■ For sexual consent to occur, two people have to talk clearly about their expectations, responsibilities, and wishes. Sexual exploitation and victimization involve the lack of sexual consent.

■ Social learning theory emphasizes the role of observation in learning as well as the importance of vicarious experience. This is one approach to the way individuals might learn to sexually abuse or exploit others.

■ Prostitution involves exchanging sexual behaviors for money. These behaviors may or may not involve sexual intercourse. Male prostitutes work in settings similar to women, including call girls, streetwalkers, and massage parlor workers. Individuals become prostitutes for reasons that may involve dysfunctional families of origin, economic stresses, drug dependency, and psychological problems. Many individuals go to prostitutes because they do not enjoy diverse sexual activities with their current partner.

■ Prostitutes often develop posttraumatic stress disorder after experiencing events that involve actual or threatened death or injury. Their responses involve intense fear, helplessness, or horror (*Diagnostic and Statistical Manual of Psychological Disorders,* 4th edition, 1994).

■ Pornography involves depictions of sexual behavior intended to arouse the viewer, including pictures, films, or prose accounts of sexual activity.

■ The United States Supreme Court has declared that materials are obscene if:

the average person, applying contemporary community standards, would find that the work, taken as a whole, appeals to the prurient interest; and the work depicts or describes, in a patently offensive way, sexual conduct specifically defined by the applicable state law; and the work, taken as a whole, lacks serious literary, artistic, political or social value.

■ According to the United States Equal Employment Opportunity Commission:

Unwelcomed sexual advances, requests for sexual favors, and other verbal or physical conduct of a sexual nature constitutes sexual harassment when submission to or rejection of this conduct explicitly or implicitly affects an individual's employment, unreasonably interferes with an individual's work performance or creates an intimidating, hostile or offensive work environment.

■ According to the American Academy of Pediatrics, child sexual abuse involves

. . . any sexual act with a child that is performed by an adult or an older child. Such acts include fondling the

child's genitals, getting the child to fondle the adult's genitals, mouth to genital contact, rubbing the adult's genitals on the child, or actually penetrating the child's vagina or anus.

■ Incest involves "any overtly sexual contact between closely related persons or between persons who believe themselves to be related" (Forward & Buck, 1989).

■ Rape involves sexual coercion and the forcible sexual assault of an unwilling victim. Rapists are motivated by aggression, anger, vindictiveness, and desire for sexual gratification.

■ Statutory rape is sexual intercourse between an adult and a minor, even if the minor consents to the sexual activity. Much legal confusion surrounds the prosecution of statutory rape today, especially if the two individuals know each other, are planning to marry, and consent to sexual relations.

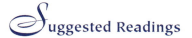

Glossary Terms

antisocial personality disorder	nonrelational sex	*quid pro quo* sexual harassment
confabulation	obsessive relational intrusion	repression
Depo-Provera		Rohypnol

Suggested Readings

Alexander, S., & Karaszewski, L. (1996). The people vs. Larry Flynt. New York: Newmarket Press.

American Academy of Pediatrics Staff (1998). A guide to references and resources in child abuse & neglect. Elk Grove Village, IL: American Academy of Pediatrics.

Baird, R. M., & Rosenbaum, S. E. (Eds.) (1998). Pornography: Private right or public menace. Amherst, NY: Prometheus Books.

Baker, R. A. (1998). Child sexual abuse & false memory syndrome. Amherst, NY: Prometheus Books.

Bergen, R. K. (1998). Issues in intimate violence. Thousand Oaks, CA: Sage Publishing.

Chapkis, W. (1996). Live sex acts: Women performing erotic labor. New York: Routledge.

DeKeseredy, W. S., & Schwartz, M. D. (1997). Women abuse on campus: Results from the Canadian national survey. Thousand Oaks, CA: Sage Publishing.

Fitzwater, T. (1998). Manager's pocket guide to preventing sexual harassment. Amherst, MA: Human Resource Development Press.

Hill, A. (1998). Speaking truth to power. New York: Doubleday.

Juffer, J. (1998). At home with pornography: Women, sexuality, & everyday life. New York: New York University Press.

McKeganey, N., & Barnard, M. U. (1996). Sex work on the streets: Prostitutes & their clients. Bristol, PA: Taylor & Francis.

Parrot, A. (1998). Coping with date rape & acquaintance rape. New York: The Rosen Publishing Group.

Phoenix, J. (1999). Making sense of prostitution. New York: St. Martin's Press.

Stamler, V. L., & Stone, G. L. (1998). Faculty-student sexual involvement: Issues & interventions. Thousand Oaks, CA: Sage Publishing.

West, T. C. (1999). Spirit-wounding violence against black women. New York: New York University Press.

GLOSSARY

A

Abstinence: refraining from sexual intercourse and any and all sexual behavior in which semen might come into proximity to a woman's external or internal genitalia.

Adherence: the inclination or willingness of a person to follow a doctor's advice, recommendations, or treatment directives.

Affection: a term used to mean liking or fondness, but usually without any deep emotional or passionate connotations.

Ageism: a prejudice that stereotypes aging or elderly people as somehow weak, impaired, unwholesome, or asexual.

American Association of Sex Educators, Counselors, and Therapists (AASECT): the primary accreditation body for those who work in sex therapy; provides an important credential that assures potential clients of a high level of training and experience.

Amniocentesis: a procedure in which a needle is inserted into the uterus through the wall of the abdomen. A small amount of amniotic fluid is removed and sent to a laboratory where cells in it are grown and examined for signs of genetic abnormalities.

Anal intercourse: the insertion of a man's penis into the anus of his partner.

Analingus: oral stimulation of the anal area.

Anaphrodisiac: drugs that are thought to inhibit or diminish sexual arousal and that may foster disinterestedness in sexual interaction.

Anatomy: the systematic study of the structure of an organism's body and the names and relationships of its various parts.

Androgen insensitivity syndrome: a chromosomal abnormality in which the body cells of a genetic male are insensitive to androgens, testosterone in particular, and as a consequence the male develops normal-appearing female sexual characteristics. Also called testicular feminization.

Androgens: a family of male sex hormones secreted by the testes in men and the adrenal glands in both women and men.

Androgyny: having the psychological attributes of both females and males.

Andrologist: a medical specialist who evaluates and treats men's fertility problems.

Anorexia athletica: an eating disorder typically seen in female athletes in which food restriction is coupled with prolonged, intense physical exercise.

Anorexia nervosa: an eating disorder typically seen in women involving systematic self-starvation.

Antisocial personality disorder: a psychological disorder in which an individual disregards the rights of other people and frequently fails to behave in accordance with the law.

Aphrodisiac: substances that are supposed to enhance erotic perceptions and sexual performance.

Areola: the area of a woman's breast surrounding the nipple.

Artificial insemination: a procedure in which semen is injected directly into a woman's uterus through her cervix; also called intrauterine insemination.

Asphyxiophilia: a paraphilia that involves the application of pressure to the carotid arteries in one's neck or putting a plastic bag over one's head during masturbation or shared sexual intercourse. When the flow of blood to the brain is diminished, the enjoyment of orgasm is intensified. This is a very dangerous practice with potentially fatal consequences.

Assortative mating: the pairing of individuals based on their similarity in one or more characteristics.

Attribution theory: a psychological theory that attempts to explain why people behave as they do. Some attributions emphasize the importance of environmental expectations while others focus on the individual's own characteristics.

Autonomic nervous system: part of the peripheral nervous system, made up of two separate branches, the sympathetic nervous system and the parasympathetic nervous system. Internal organs, blood vessels, and endocrine glands receive nerve fibers from the autonomic nervous system.

Autosome: a chromosome that is not a sex chromosome.

B

Bacteria: microscopic single-celled organisms. Unlike viruses, they have a membrane surrounding them.

Bartholin's glands: small glands located on each side of the opening to the vagina. Their function is not clearly understood.

Basilar squeeze technique: a technique used in the treatment of premature ejaculation, in which a man grasps the base of his penis and squeezes for 3 or 4 seconds, usually eliminating the desire to ejaculate.

Behavioral theory of development: a theoretical perspective that asserts that rewarding or punishing consequences of our behaviors are critical in shaping our development as we grow older.

Bestiality: see Zoophilila.

Bilateral tubal ligation: a surgical procedure involving the surgical sectioning, clipping, or cauterizing of a woman's fallopian tubes, making it impossible for sperm to penetrate and fertilize eggs. It should be thought of as permanent, although surgical reversal is sometimes possible.

Bimanual pelvic examination: a gynecological examination in which a doctor places a finger from one hand in a woman's vagina while putting the other hand on top of her abdomen. This allows the doctor to feel the cervix, ligaments supporting the uterus, ovaries, and fallopian tubes.

Birth control pills: perhaps the most reliably effective contraceptives, they act by inhibiting the pituitary gland's secretion of FSH and LH and also thicken cervical mucus so that sperm cannot swim into the uterus and then up into the fallopian tubes. Also called oral contraceptives.

C

Cancer: a term that refers to the uncontrolled division of some of the body's cells and the tendency of these cells to spread to other parts of the body. Eventually, affected organs do not function properly because of this process.

Candida albicans: the microorganism causing a type of vaginal infection; usually referred to as a yeast infection.

Carnal love: the sensual aspects of physical intimacy.

Celibacy, complete: abstinence from both masturbation and interpersonal sexual behavior.

Celibacy, partial: abstinence from sexual intercourse, but not necessarily abstinence from masturbation.

Cerebral Palsy: a condition caused by brain injury at or around the time of birth. This disease is incurable; it does not get worse nor does it improve. Movement disorders and/or impaired cognitive functioning in varying degrees characterize cerebral palsy.

Cerebrovascular Accident: also known as a "stroke." An abnormal event involving the circulatory system of the brain. A stroke may involve blood vessels that are blocked by clots or burst. This can lead to the loss of large areas of the brain and impaired behavioral, emotional, and cognitive functioning.

Cervical cap: a thimble-shaped rubber or plastic cup that fits snugly over a woman's cervix, acting as a barrier to sperm. It can be left in place longer than a diaphragm and is also used in conjunction with a spermicide.

Cesarean section: a procedure in which an incision is made through a woman's abdominal wall and uterus so that a baby can be delivered without having to pass through the birth canal; also called C-section.

Chancroid: a bacterial sexually transmitted disease (STD) that is quite common in Africa. It involves the appearance of small ulcers, usually on the genitals, and may also be accompanied by swollen lymph nodes in the groin.

Chlamydia: one of the most common STDs in the United States. It is a bacterial infection of the genitourinary tract in both women and men.

Chorionic villi sampling: a procedure in which a needle is inserted into the uterus through the abdominal wall, and chorionic villi are removed and examined in the same way as the cells removed through amniocentesis.

Chorionic villi: microscopic "fingers" of tissue that attach a zygote to the lining of the uterus.

Circumcision: surgical removal of the foreskin of the penis covering the glans.

Climacteric: a "turning point" in a person's life at middle age, generally between their mid 40s and early 60s, when some of their youthful energy has begun to decline.

Clinical perspective: a research method that usually combines a combination of observation and in-depth interview.

Clitoris: a female homologue of the penis that carries information from erotic stimuli into the central nervous system. Its tip is the glans.

Codependency: a term that describes a relationship in which a clearly unhealthy interdependence exists. A codependent person is secure in their sense of being only when someone else defines their desires and autonomy for them.

Cognitive developmental theory: a theory concerning the way children learn traditional sex roles. This theory emphasizes the importance of the feedback children receive from their peers for acting like females or males and how this information guides their social interactions in the future.

Cohabitation: a situation in which a couple sharing an intimate relationship lives together without being married.

Coital alignment technique: an intercourse position in which a woman is lying on her back and her partner enters her in the traditional man-on-top position, but in which he now moves his entire body forward so that each time his penis enters her vagina it also directly stimulates her clitoris.

Coitus interruptus: a highly ineffective attempt at avoiding conception, also called "withdrawal." A man attempts to withdraw his uncovered penis from his partner before he ejaculates but usually still leaves significant numbers of sperm in the vagina.

Coitus: a man inserting his penis into a woman's vagina; also often called sexual intercourse.

Concordance rate: the percentage of twins who both manifest a particular characteristic under study.

Condom: latex or natural membrane sheath that fits over the erect penis. It is a highly effective contraceptive that offers significant protection against acquiring sexually transmitted diseases (STDs).

Confabulation: an error in memory in which a person confuses a recollection of events of which they are aware with personal involvement in those events.

Congenital virilizing adrenal hyperplasia: a condition in which a female human embryo is exposed to androgens and develops male-like genitalia as a result.

Conization: a procedure in which a cone-shaped area of the cervix is cut out with a scalpel or laser for examining the cells under a microscope.

Contraceptive negligence: the behavior of individuals who, for one of a variety of reasons, either are ambivalent about becoming pregnant or may actually want to become pregnant to remove themselves from troubling life circumstances, such as a hostile, abusive home environment.

Contraceptive: any device or behavioral strategy that is intended to minimize or eliminate the chances of conception following sexual intercourse.

Contragestational agents: agents that technically do not stop conception from occurring, but instead inhibit the implantation of a fertilized egg in the lining of the uterus and thus stop pregnancy from progressing.

Coprophilia: a paraphilia in which a person desires to incorporate feces (human excrement) into sexual activity.

Coronal ridge: the crease separating the glans from the shaft of the penis.

Coronal squeeze technique: a technique used in the treatment of premature ejaculation in which a man's partner grasps the penis with the thumb on the frenum and two fingers on either side of the coronal ridge and squeezes once, firmly, for 3 or 4 seconds, usually eliminating the desire to ejaculate.

Corpora cavernosa: two expandable spongy cylindrical bodies composing the interior of the penis. These become engorged with blood during erection.

Corpus luteum: a collection of cells in the ovary that contain an ovum before it is released during ovulation.

Corpus spongiosum: an expandable spongy cylindrical body inside the penis that surrounds the urethra.

Cowper's glands: located on the underside of the prostate, these glands secrete a substance into the urethra during sexual arousal and are thought to lubricate the inside of the urethra.

Crabs: see Pubic lice.

Cross-dressing: see Transvestism.

Crura: spongy bodies that attach the clitoris to the pubic bone.

Cryotherapy: a procedure in which a well-localized lesion on the surface of the cervix is frozen.

C-section: see Cesarean section.

Cunnilingus: oral stimulation of a woman's vulva.

Cytomegalovirus (CMV): a common and usually harmless virus that is carried by about half of all young adults in the United States. It can be spread during sexual intercourse and may lead to swollen lymph nodes, fever, and extreme fatigue.

D

Delusions of invincibility: false beliefs that bad things happen to other people but never to oneself.

Dementia: diminished intellectual functioning and behavioral deficits associated with degenerative diseases of the brain. The most common kind of dementia is Alzheimer's disease.

Depo-Provera: trade name for medroxyprogesterone acetate, a contraception injection taken in the buttocks once every 3 months. It is highly effective and also works to block ovulation and thicken cervical mucus. Depo-Provera is also sometimes used for the chemical suppression of sex drive in men.

Determinism: the belief that adult thoughts, feelings, and behaviors are the result of events that happened in infancy and childhood.

Detumescence: a shortening and softening of an erect penis. Ejaculation may or may not precede detumescence.

DHT deficiency syndrome: an unusual abnormality in prenatal sexual differentiation in which testosterone is not metabolized to dyhydrotestosterone (DHT) and as a result the testes do not descend into the scrotum and the genitalia have a feminine appearance.

Diagnostic hysteroscopy: a procedure in which a very thin fiberoptic telescope is inserted through the cervix into the uterus so that selected areas may be isolated for biopsy and later evaluation.

Dialysis: a medical procedure in which wastes in the blood are filtered by a machine rather than our kidneys.

Diaphragm: a plastic or rubber dome-shaped cup that fits over a woman's cervix. Diaphragms are used together with spermicidal foams, creams, or jellies. This combination is an effective contraceptive, although spermicides alone do not work nearly as well as when they are used with condoms or a diaphragm.

Double-blind study: a research investigation in which neither the researcher nor the subject knows what treatment (if any) is being administered to the subject.

Double standard: the assumption that males are somehow "entitled" to things that their female partners are not, as if there were one set of standards and expectations for men and another for women.

Douche: to introduce various types of fluids into the vagina under low pressure, usually with a hand-held squeeze bottle.

Dyspareunia: discomfort associated with vaginal penetration, apparent during penetration or after intercourse. It can result from organic and/or psychosocial factors.

Dysplasia: the abnormal growth and development of cells; typically used to describe cells examined in a Pap smear.

E

Ectopic pregnancy: a pregnancy in which a fertilized egg is implanted someplace other than in the lining of the uterus (e.g., the pelvic cavity, on an ovary, or in a fallopian tube).

Ego-dystonic homosexuality: a psychological disorder in which a homosexual person is adamant and persistent about not wanting to be gay. It involves a person's extreme and pervasive distress about being a homosexual.

Ejaculatory ducts: a passageway formed at the junction of the vas deferens and the seminal vesicle. Sperm pass through this duct as they proceed through the prostate gland and then into the urethra.

Ejaculatory inevitability: the feeling that a man has when he is certain that he can no longer delay ejaculation.

Embryology: the scientific study of the growth and development of animals before birth.

Embryoscopy: a procedure in which a slender fiber optic telescope is inserted through the cervix and into the uterus where the developing embryo or fetus may be visualized and examined; also called fetoscopy.

Emergency contraception: any of various strategies intended to reduce the risk of pregnancy after having intercourse. Various regimens of oral contraceptives can be used in this way, as can the insertion of an IUD.

Endocrine glands: glands that secrete hormones directly into the bloodstream. Endocrine glands are discrete bundles of tissue closely linked to the circulatory system.

Endocrine system: the body's ductless glands that secrete hormones directly into the bloodstream.

Endometrium: inner layer of the uterus, made up of glandular tissue and a network of blood vessels.

Epicureanism: an ancient Roman philosophy in which the highest human pleasures are thought to be associated with intellectual understanding and mastery of the use of information, often mistakenly associated with an un-controlled pursuit of physical, sensual pleasures.

Epididymis: a comma-shaped structure located along the posterior surface of each testis. Sperm are temporarily stored here.

Episiotomy: an incision made between the back of a woman's vagina and her anus to facilitate the passage of the baby's head through her birth canal.

Erikson's psychosocial theory of development: a theory that suggests that all humans go through eight successive stages of development from in-fancy through old age. Each stage is associated with a specific develop-mental challenge. Problems in development at one time during the life span do not necessarily predict problems later. Similarly, positive develop-mental experiences at one stage do not necessarily predict positive ones later.

Erogenous zones: according to Freud, parts on the surface of the body that when stimulated yield keen sensual pleasures; thought to include the mouth, anus, and genitals; see also Primary erogenous zones and Sec-ondary erogenous zones.

Erotic: associated with sensual and/or sexual pleasures.

Estrogens: a family of eight different female hormones that are responsible for a woman's secondary sexual characteristics, menstrual cycle, and fertility.

Ethnocentrism: the belief that the standards, norms, and customs of one's own culture are right and superior to those of other cultures.

Exhibitionism: the perceived urge to expose one's genitals to strangers. It may or may not involve masturbation. Often there is a motive to shock or startle the victim.

F

Fallopian tubes: tubes connecting the uterus with the area around each of a woman's ovaries. They open directly into the abdominal cavity.

Fecundity: a person's maximum biological potential to procreate.

Fellatio: oral stimulation of the penis and/or scrotum.

Female condom: a long polyurethane sleeve with one closed end that fits in-side a woman's vagina. This is an effective contraceptive and also protects women from sexually transmitted diseases (STDs).

Female orgasmic disorder: the inability of a woman to have orgasms regu-larly, reliably, and consistently. This condition is also known as anorgas-mia; there are several types of this sexual dysfunction.

Female sexual arousal disorder: reduced or absent vaginal lubrication and swelling of the tissues surrounding the opening to the vagina making pen-etration awkward and/or uncomfortable. This may be due to organic and/or psychosocial factors.

Femininity: thoughts, feelings, and behaviors often associated with female roles.

Fertility: a person's reproductive performance, or the number of live births they have had.

Fertilization: the union of a sperm and an egg. A fertilized egg is also called a zygote.

Fetal alcohol syndrome: a condition in which women who drink alcohol during pregnancy give birth to babies with physical abnormalities and sometimes psychological and behavioral problems as well.

Fetal viability: that point in time when a fetus can survive independently of its mother.

Fetishism: a paraphilia in which nonliving objects are the focus of sexual urges and arousal.

Fetoscopy: see Embryology.

Fibroadenoma: a type of breast lump made up of glandular and connective tissue.

Fibrocystic disease: generalized, multiple, benign breast lumps that are de-scribed as "knotty," "ropy," or of a "granular" texture.

Fisting: a sexual practice in which a woman puts her closed fist into the vulva, and sometimes the vagina, of her partner. Among gay men, fisting involves one partner putting his closed fist into the rectum of his partner.

Follicle-stimulating hormone (FSH): a pituitary hormone responsible for the early growth of primary follicles in the ovaries during each menstrual cycle. The same hormone regulates sperm production in men.

Foreplay: any one of a number of behaviors in which two people touch each other or stimulate one another orally, usually as a prelude to intercourse.

Frenulum: the part of the penis connecting the ventral portion of the glans with the underside of the shaft. One of the most sensitive parts of the penis.

Frottage: see Frotteurism.

Frotteurism: A paraphilia in which a person engages in rubbing or pressing up against another person, usually in very crowded places (that the "frot-teur" seeks out); also called frottage.

G

G spot: named after Dr. Ernest Grafenberg, a supposedly highly sensitive area located along the anterior wall of the vagina. Stimulation of this area manually or during intercourse has been associated with strong orgasmic response and, in some cases, ejaculation.

Gamete intrafallopian transfer (GIFT): a procedure in which a woman's eggs are removed from her ovaries and combined with sperm in the labo-ratory. The eggs and sperm are then implanted directly into her fallopian tube through a small incision using laparoscopy.

Gamete: a sex cell. Sperm and ova are gametes.

Gender identity: one's self-perceptions as either a female or male person ac-cording to the customs and traditions of a particular culture.

Gender role: the beliefs and behaviors a person acts out in accordance with their thoughts about being a male or female person.

Gender role conflict: the feeling or belief that one's gender identity does not conform to the expectations of one's culture.

Gender schema theory: a theory of gender role development in which chil-dren think and act upon a culture's notions of how females and males should behave. The feedback they get from their peers and/or adults may confirm or disconfirm the degree to which their behavior conforms to these norms.

Genital herpes: an extremely prevalent sexually transmitted disease (STD), causing the appearance of painful genital sores and sometimes affecting in-ternal structures of the genitourinary system.

Gerontophilia: a paraphilia in which an individual, usually a young man, has a compulsive sexual interest in having sexual relations with an old or elderly woman.

Glans: the name for the tip of a man's penis or the tip of a woman's clitoris.

Gonads: sex glands. A woman's gonads are her ovaries; a man's gonads are his testes.

Gonorrhea: the second most common bacterial sexually transmitted disease (STD) in the United States, an infection of the genitourinary tract in both women and men.

Gynecology: the medical specialty concerned with the health of a woman's sexual and reproductive organs as well as the diagnosis and treatment of maladies affecting them.

H

Habituation: a very simple form of learning in which repeated presentations of a stimulus lead to progressively diminished behavioral responses.

Hemiparesis: paralysis of half of a person's body due to the effects of a stroke.

Hepatitis: an infectious viral disease that causes inflammation of the liver. It can be transmitted from one person to another by both sexual and non-sexual means.

Hormonal sex: an individual's sexual characteristics resulting from the predom-inant secretion of testosterone from the testes or estrogens from the ovaries.

Hormone: a chemical substance secreted by an endocrine gland into the bloodstream that travels to some distant target organ in the body and changes its activity.

Human chorionic gonadotropin: a hormone produced when an embryo becomes firmly implanted in the lining of the uterus. The presence of this hormone in a woman's urine is detected with pregnancy tests.

Human immunodeficiency virus (HIV): a virus that may be transmitted sexually and usually leads to AIDS.

Human papilloma virus (HPV): perhaps the most common sexually trans-mitted disease (STD) in the world. Its most common manifestation in-volves the appearance of genital warts.

Hymen: thin layer of tissue that often covers the opening to the vagina be-fore first intercourse.

Hypoactive sexual desire disorder: a very notable absence of any desire to have sexual intercourse, engage in any other form of sexual activity, and the absence of sexual fantasies.

Hypogonadism: diminished secretion of testosterone from a man's testes. In some cases, this condition can impair sexual arousal and response.

Hypothalamus: an area at the base of the brain involved in a number of im-portant motivational and procreational behaviors.

I

Ideal self: people's image of themselves when they have developed into the individual they would like to become.

Identification: the subconscious desire to become like someone we love, admire, or respect.

Impotence: see Male erectile disorder.

In vitro fertilization: a procedure in which an ovum is fertilized by sperm in a laboratory dish, allowing early cellular division to begin. The zygote is then implanted in the lining of a woman's uterus with the hope that pregnancy results.

Infestation: the spreading or swarming of tiny organisms on or in the skin. Pubic lice and scabies are examples of infestations.

Interdependence: how one feels and reveals an authentic concern for the happiness and welfare of one's partner while remaining aware of one's own needs and autonomy.

Interfemoral intercourse: a type of sexual behavior in which a man puts his penis between his partner's thighs and engages in pelvic thrusting, commonly ejaculating.

Intermarriage: marriage between two people of different cultural, racial, religious, or ethnic groups.

Interstitial cell stimulating hormone: see Luteinizing hormone (LH).

Intrauterine device (IUD): any foreign object in the uterus that is intended to act as a contraceptive. Modern IUDs typically include small amounts of copper; copper is highly toxic to sperm and slightly irritates the lining of a woman's uterus.

Intrauterine insemination: see Artificial insemination.

Introitus: area immediately adjacent to the opening of the vagina.

J

Jealousy: an emotion related to fears and anxieties surrounding betrayal and deception involving intimate attachments outside a relationship.

K

Kaposi's sarcoma: a type of cancer commonly associated with AIDS that involves the growth of malignant cells under the skin and throughout the mucous membranes of the mouth, nose, or eyes.

Klismaphilia: a paraphilia in which an individual experiences sexual gratification during an enema. Sometimes the individual administers the enema while alone, and sometimes two people administer enemas to themselves while together. A variety of different fluids, including beer, whisky, or drugs in solution may be used.

L

Labia majora: prominent skin folds lateral to the vestibule.

Labia minora: delicate, soft skin folds immediately surrounding the opening to the vagina.

Lamaze technique: a method of prepared parenthood in which a woman uses focused concentration, abdominal massage, and breathing exercises to give birth without local or general anesthesia. Her partner is usually involved as a "coach."

Laparoscopy: a procedure in which a doctor inserts a fiber-optic telescope into a woman's abdomen through a small incision in her umbilicus (belly button) or elsewhere in the abdomen, allowing the doctor to see her fallopian tubes, ovaries, and pelvic cavity.

Libido: a primitive, motivational force in the personality, usually associated with powerful aggressive and sexual inclinations.

Limbic system: a circuit of subcortical brain structures that play an important role in the experience and expression of emotions.

Loop electrocautery excision procedure (LEEP): a procedure in which abnormal cervical tissue is cut out with a sharp wire loop and the area is then cauterized.

Love: an emotion that is often thought of as unselfish and loyal and often involves a feeling of sexual attraction.

Luteinizing hormone (LH): a pituitary hormone responsible for the release of a mature ovum from an ovary during each menstrual cycle. Also called interstitial cell stimulating hormone (ICSH), which stimulates cells in a man's testes to produce testosterone.

M

Male erectile disorder: the inability or diminished ability of a man to attain and maintain an erection of sufficient hardness for a long enough time to enjoy sexual intercourse. It is frequently referred to as impotence.

Masculinity: thoughts, feelings, and behaviors often associated with male roles.

Masochism: a sexual inclination in which a person derives erotic gratification from experiencing physical or psychological pain or humiliation.

Masturbation: genital self-stimulation with some anticipation of rewarding erotic feelings. Some women masturbate by touching their breasts as well.

Mature minor doctrine: a common-law rule that permits mature teenagers to give their own consent for medical care even if they have not yet reached the age of majority.

Mechanistic perspective: the belief that the human body (and mind) are "machines" and can best be understood by comprehending the nature and interrelationships of their parts.

Medical Model: a perspective that views illness and abnormality as amenable to diagnosis and treatment from the standpoint of a physician and the many interventions at her or his disposal: medication, surgery, physical therapy, psychotherapy, and so forth.

Menstrual synchrony: a phenomenon in which women (not using oral contraceptives) living together and interacting frequently gradually develop similar menstrual cycles.

Menstruation: the relatively regular sloughing off of the endometrium and the vaginal bleeding that accompanies it.

Mental Retardation: below average intellectual functioning and problems in functioning adaptively to one's environment.

Miscarriage: see Spontaneous abortion.

Mittelschmerz: lower abdominal discomfort, usually on one side of the body, that accompanies the release of an ovum from an ovary.

Molluscum contagiosum: a viral sexually transmitted disease (STD) that causes bumps on the skin than eventually grow to 3-5 mm in diameter. It is not transmitted solely through sexual contact.

Mons veneris: a small compact cushion of fat located on top of a woman's pubic bone.

Multiple Sclerosis: a progressive, degenerative, incurable disease of the nervous system. Symptoms often include muscular weakness, spasticity, problems in keeping one's balance while walking, tremors, visual difficulties, bladder and/or bowel problems, depression, pain, and poor temperature sensitivity.

Myometrium: outer, muscular layer of the uterus.

N

Naturalistic observation: a research method in which consenting subjects agree to being observed behaving in their own settings in a comfortable, unselfconscious way.

Necrophilia: a paraphilia in which individuals feel impelled to have sex with human corpses. It is one of the most bizarre and disturbed paraphilias and fortunately is extremely rare.

Nocturnal emission: penile erection and ejaculation during sleep, usually accompanied by erotic dreams.

Nocturnal penile tumescence: penile erections during sleep.

Nongonococcal urethritis (NGU): an inflammation of the urethra resulting from STDs other than gonorrhea.

Nonrelational sex: "the tendency to experience sex primarily as lust without any requirements for relational intimacy or emotional attachment" (Levant & Brooks, 1997).

Norplant: a contraceptive technique involving the insertion of 6 thin capsules beneath the skin on the underside of a woman's upper arm. These contain a hormone, levonorgestrel, that acts in much the same way as oral contraceptives.

Nucleus: a well-defined, discrete collection of nerve cells inside the central nervous system.

O

Obsessive relational intrusion: a technical term used to describe "repeated and unwanted pursuit and invasion of one's sense of physical or symbolic privacy by another person, either stranger or acquaintance, who desires and/or presumes an intimate relationship" (Cupach & Spitzberg, 1998).

Oral contraceptives: see Birth control pills.

Osteoarthritis: the gradual erosion and sometimes eventual destruction of the cartilage in our joints.

Outercourse: the mutual enjoyment of a variety of sexual behaviors with the exception of vaginal or anal penetration.

Ovaries: a woman's gonads, or sex cell producing glands.

Ovulation: the physiological and hormonal process by which a woman's body produces a mature ovum.

Ovum: an egg cell.

P

Pap smear: an accurate diagnostic test for cervical cancer involving scraping the cervix with a wooden spatula and placing the cells on a glass slide for microscopic examination.

Paraplegia: a spinal cord injury in which someone loses the use of the legs, but still has normal feeling and movement in the arms.

Parasympathetic branch of the autonomic nervous system: regulates heart rate, respiratory rate, and metabolic and digestive activity under normal physiological conditions.

Parental notification laws: laws that require a minor to obtain the consent of at least one parent to have an abortion. In some cases, a judge's consent is also sufficient.

Passive-aggressive behavior: an expression of anger in which a person behaves in a stubborn, obstructionistic, or deliberately ineffective way.

Pederasty: physical sexual expression between an adult male and male child or adolescent.

Pedophilia: a paraphilia in which sexual urges are directed toward children. The focus of erotic attention has generally not yet reached puberty.

Pelvic inflammatory disease (PID): a bacterial infection involving the lining of the fallopian tubes that often results in female infertility. PID is a possible consequence of a lack of prompt, effective treatment for chlamydia or gonorrhea.

Penile implants: semi-rigid or expandable plastic cylinders that can be surgically implanted inside a man's penis. These are often helpful in treating erectile dysfunction that does not respond to drug therapies.

Penile strain gauge: a narrow metallic or rubber noose that fits around the base of the penis and sends electrical messages to devices that record increases in the circumference of the penis during erection.

Penis: the male organ for sexual intercourse; also an excretory structure facilitating urination.

Perceived self: people's current, honest, undistorted perception of themselves.

Perineum: small patch of very smooth skin extending from the vaginal opening to the anus.

Personal space: the area immediately adjacent to the surface of our bodies, over which we wish to control intrusions.

Personality disorders: longstanding patterns of thinking, feeling, and behaving that are very much at odds with common social expectations. It is not unusual for personality disorders to contribute to incompatibilities that foster sexual dysfunctions.

Pessary: a vaginal suppository that is supposed to act as a form of contraception. Ancient pessaries were made of a variety of substances, including plants, fermented dough, and even crocodile dung.

Pheromone: air-borne hormones that affect complex behaviors in some subhuman species. Some of these agents act as sex attractors. The existence of human pheromones is debated.

Physiology: the systematic study of the functions and interrelationships of the major organ systems of animals and plants.

Pituitary gland: the body's "master endocrine gland," which coordinates the activities of all other endocrine glands.

Pleasure principle: Sigmund Freud's belief that humans are powerfully motivated to pursue pleasures and avoid pain and frustrations.

Premature ejaculation: a condition in which a man ejaculates before his partner has experienced some significant sense of sexual satisfaction. Very often he will ejaculate as soon as he penetrates his partner or only after brief pelvic thrusting.

Primary anorgasmia: a condition in which a woman has never had an orgasm by any means, including masturbation, fantasizing, or oral, anal, or vaginal penetration.

Primary erogenous zones: the mouth, genitalia, and anus; areas of the body that when stimulated yield feelings of intense sensual and/or sexual pleasure; see also Secondary erogenous zones.

Progesterone: a hormone secreted by the corpus luteum that prepares the endometrium for the implantation of a fertilized ovum. Along with estrogen, it coordinates the regulation of the menstrual cycle and the maintenance of pregnancy.

Prostaglandins: naturally occurring hormones in women and men. In women, these play a role in initiating contractions of the muscular layer of the uterus.

Prostate gland: a gland at the base of a man's bladder, surrounding the urethra. It secretes fluids that combined with sperm help neutralize the acidic environment inside the vagina. It is composed of both glandular and muscular tissues.

Prostatic specific antigen (PSA): a substance found in a man's blood stream thought to be strongly associated with prostate cancer.

Psychoanalysis: a method of psychotherapy invented by Sigmund Freud in which the client's subconscious is made conscious, in the anticipation that this knowledge will eliminate anxiety and associated abnormal behaviors, thoughts, and feelings.

Psychoanalytic theory: Sigmund Freud's theory that asserts that adult thoughts, feelings, and actions are powerfully determined by subconscious forces, of which we are often unaware or have only a dim awareness.

Psychobiological approach: a way of analyzing and interpreting behavior that is based on an understanding of the functions of the nervous and endocrine systems.

Psychosocial theory: a theory of human growth and development that asserts that a person's experiences in their wider social environment play a central role in their psychological development over the lifespan.

Psychotherapy: a form of treatment for behavioral, emotional, or cognitive disorders that usually involves counseling, the disclosure of personal information, and an attempt to change maladaptive psychological habits.

Puberty: the appearance of secondary sexual characteristics. These are called "secondary" because they are the result of increasing levels of sex hormones in the bloodstream.

Pubic lice: tiny crustaceans, often referred to as crabs.

Pubococcygeal muscles: muscles that surround the opening to the vagina.

Q

Quid pro quo sexual harassment: a clearly implied "deal" or "bargain" that involves the exchange of sexual favors in return for some special consideration or evaluation.

R

Random anorgasmia: a condition in which orgasms do not occur regularly and dependably even when a woman feels sexual desire and arousal.

Reality principle: a Freudian notion attributed to a part of the personality called the ego that suggests that we try to deal with the realistic aspects of our daily lives while balancing sexual and aggressive impulses against our moral beliefs and conscience.

Reductionism: an approach to explaining things that breaks complex things down into simple components.

Reflex: the simplest stimulus-response connection of which the nervous system is capable.

Refractory period: the post-ejaculatory interval in men during which continued erotic stimulation is ineffective in rearousing the individual.

Repression: a psychological defense mechanism in which a person "forgets" highly unpleasant recollections of an event and the circumstances surrounding it. Repression is involuntary and takes place without a person trying to forget the event.

Retarded ejaculation: a condition in which a man can attain and maintain an erection, penetrate his partner, and engage in prolonged pelvic thrusting but not ejaculate readily or at all.

Retrovirus: a type of virus that upon entering a cell uses an enzyme to turn its RNA into DNA, which incorporates the virus into the cell's genes.

Rheumatoid Arthritis: a form of arthritis characterized by swelling, inflammation, and stiffness in several of the body's joints.

Rohypnol: trade name for flunitrazepam, a drug that is a powerful sedative and sometimes used to incapacitate women for the purposes of rape.

S

Sadism: deriving enjoyment from inflicting emotional or physical pain on another person; see also Sexual sadism.

Scabies: an infestation caused by a microscopic mite that burrows into the skin and lays eggs. This may be in the genital area as well as other parts of the body.

Scrotum: the soft skin sac containing the testes.

Secondary anorgasmia: a condition in which a woman has lost a previously reliable pattern of orgasmic responsiveness.

Secondary erogenous zones: areas on the surface of the body that, through learning, yield feelings of intense sensual or sexual pleasure when stimulated; see also Primary erogenous zones.

Self-concept: people's view of themselves based on the degree to which their perceived self approximates their ideal self.

Seminal vesicles: glands that lie along the posterior portion of the bladder. These produce fluids that combine with sperm in the ejaculatory ducts.

Seminiferous tubules: a long, fine network of tubules in the testes. Spermatogenesis occurs in the walls of these tubules.

Sex chromosomes: the twenty-third pair of human chromosomes, which determine one's genetic sex as either female or male.

Sex preselection: procedures intended to allow a woman and man to choose the sex of their baby.

Sex: an individual's biological designation as either female or male.

Sexual aversion disorder: an extremely strong and pervasive dislike of the prospect of shared sexual activity and the avoidance of any physical contact or verbal interaction that is likely to lead to sexual interaction.

Sexual dysfunctions: physical, psychological, and/or interpersonal problems that might impair sexual desire, arousal, or response.

Sexual intercourse: see Coitus.

Sexual masochism: a paraphilia in which a person derives sexual gratification from being humiliated, physically beaten, tied up, or made to experience pain in some other way.

Sexual objectification: the impersonal focusing of sexual thoughts, feelings, and actions on an individual, disregarding their individual, unique attributes as a woman or a man.

Sexual pain disorder: sexual dysfunction associated with significant discomfort during sexual intercourse.

Sexual response cycle: a sequence of physical changes accompanying sexual arousal, orgasm, and the return to a pre-arousal state of excitement.

Sexual sadism: a paraphilia in which a person derives sexual gratification from humiliating or hurting others during sexual interactions.

Sexual strategies theory: a theoretical perspective describing some of the possible evolutionary influences on how females and males view sexual exclusivity and marital fidelity.

Sexual value system: the sum of all thoughts, feelings, and behaviors that have an erotic meaning for a particular individual.

Sexuality: sensual pleasure that comes from the stimulation of the body, often with the anticipation of an enjoyable, erotic feeling. Sexual behaviors may or may not involve the desire to procreate.

Sissy boy syndrome: a syndrome in which boys in childhood dress as girls on a consistent basis, play with dolls, prefer female playmates, and in many cases state that they wish they had been born girls.

Situational anorgasmia: a condition in which a woman can only have orgasms by means of a limited (and often highly stereotyped) pattern of stimulation.

Social attraction: a feeling of interpersonal closeness based on proximity, familiarity, physical attractiveness, similarity, and self-disclosure.

Social learning theory: a theory that asserts that learning can occur vicariously by observing the behavior of others. Imitation, behavioral modeling, and social skills training are all aspects of social learning theory.

Sociality: interpersonal attraction of a nonsexual nature.

Sociobiology: a discipline that tries to explain the degree to which (and the ways in which) social behavior might be genetically determined and, therefore, influenced by the long, gradual process of evolution.

Somatic cells: body cells, as distinguished from gametes.

Speculum: a metal or plastic instrument that allows a doctor to see inside the vagina, visualizing the cervix as well.

Spermatogenesis: the process of cellular division by which sperm are produced in the testes.

Spinal cord: part of the central nervous system located inside of the vertebral column. Sensory messages ascend to the brain and motor messages descend from the brain through the spinal cord.

Spontaneous abortion: separation of the embryo from the endometrium, thus ending pregnancy; also called miscarriage.

Steroids: a class of chemical compounds sharing the same general molecular structure. Sex hormones are steroids.

Stigmatophilia: a feeling of strong sexual attraction to someone who has tattoos or scars.

Stoicism: a Roman philosophy that suggests that the highest good lies in living in harmony with nature and accepting whatever life offers with a sense of dignity and poise.

Stoma: an opening in the body created by a surgical procedure in which diseased parts of the body are removed. This is often called "ostomy" surgery. Bodily fluids may be collected through this opening in a bag worn by the patient.

Sympathetic branch of the autonomic nervous system: activates physiological responses in "fight-or-flight" conditions.

Syphilis: a highly infectious bacterial sexually transmitted disease (STD) that can affect virtually all of the body's major organ systems. The first, or primary stage of syphilis is characterized by a small ulcer at the point where the bacteria first penetrated skin or mucus membranes. This ulcer is called a chancre.

T

Telephone scatologia: the experience of sexual arousal, and sometimes orgasm, while making obscene telephone calls.

Teratology: the study of birth defects.

Testicular feminization: see Androgen insensitivity syndrome.

Testosterone: male sex hormone. Testosterone is a form of androgen.

Tetraplegia: a spinal cord injury in which someone has lost the use of both their arms and legs. Formerly called "quadriplegia."

Transsexuality: a phenomenon in which a person's physical sexual characteristics are different from their psychological, gender-based characteristics.

Transvestism: a paraphilia in which a heterosexual male derives sexual excitement from dressing as a woman. This is also sometimes called cross dressing.

Tribadism: a type of lesbian sexual behavior in which two women lie abdomen-to-abdomen and engage in mutual pelvic thrusting. In tribadism, the mons veneris of both partners is in contact.

Troilism: three or sometimes four people sharing sexual activities. It may involve two persons having intercourse with the third watching and then the third person engaging in sex with one of the persons she or he was observing. Troilism may also involve two couples having sexual intercourse in the visual presence of each other.

U

Ultrasound imaging: a procedure in which high-frequency sound waves are presented to a pregnant woman's abdomen and penetrate into the expanded uterus. The resulting reflected sound waves reveal the developing embryo or fetus.

Urethra: the short passageway that carries urine from the bladder out of the body.

Urologist: a medical specialist in the diagnosis and treatment of disorders of the excretory system and urinary tract in both women and men.

Urophilia: a paraphilia in which individuals feel impelled to include urine or urination in their sexual activities.

Uterus: a large hollow multilayered muscle in which the fertilized egg implants itself and begins to grow into an embryo and then a fetus; also known as a woman's womb.

V

Vagina: a collapsed sleeve of tissue composed of muscle, connective tissue, and mucous membrane layers. It is a woman's primary organ of sexual intercourse, a passageway for the elimination of menstrual discharge, the arrival point for incoming semen during intercourse, and the birth canal during vaginal birth.

Vaginal plotoplethysmograph: a small device inserted into the vagina that measures the engorgement of blood vessels during sexual arousal.

Vaginal sponge: a circular piece of synthetic soft foam impregnated with a common spermicide, nonoxynol-9. This spermicide is somewhat effective in killing the bacteria and viruses that cause sexually transmitted diseases (STDs) and HIV. The vaginal sponge is no longer readily available to American women.

Vaginismus: a condition in which a woman experiences a spastic contraction of the musculature at the opening to her vagina, as well as the outer one-third of the vagina. It may also occur during only the expectation of vaginal penetration. These muscular contractions cannot be controlled and make penile penetration difficult or impossible.

Vas deferens: the tubule that carries mature sperm from the testes to the ejaculatory ducts.

Vasectomy: a surgical procedure involving the surgical sectioning of the vas deferens, making it impossible for sperm to leave the body during ejaculation. It should be thought of as permanent, although surgical reversal is sometimes possible.

Vasocongestion: the gradual accumulation of blood in blood vessels. Vasocongestion in the genitalia and lower pelvis accompanies sexual arousal in women and men.

Vasodilators: drugs that cause blood vessels to expand. Vasodilators that locally affect the genitalia are used in the treatment of male erectile disorder.

Vestibular bulbs: bodies located alongside the opening to the vagina. These become engorged with blood during sexual arousal.

Vestibule: smooth tissue surrounding a woman's urethral opening.

Vicarious learning: a type of learning in which a person can acquire information, remember it, and use it through the observation of others.

Virus: a very simple microorganism with an outer coat made of protein and RNA or DNA inside.

Voyeurism: a paraphilia that involves watching another person who is naked, undressing, or having sexual intercourse without their knowledge or consent.

Vulva: another term for a woman's external genitalia, everything a woman sees when using a mirror for a genital self-examination.

Vulvovaginitis, or vaginitis: An infection involving irritation, inflammation, and itching at the opening to the vagina.

W

Withdrawal: see Coitus interruptus.

Womb: see Uterus.

Y

Yeast infection: see Candida albicans.

Z

Zoophilia: a paraphilia in which an individual has penetrative sex with a non-human animal; also called bestiality. Zoophilic behaviors may also involve masturbating an animal or performing fellatio or cunnilingus on the animal.

Zygote intrafallopian transfer (ZIFT): a procedure in which a woman's eggs are harvested through the use of laparoscopy and then combined with sperm in the laboratory. After fertilization has taken place, the zygote is implanted inside the fallopian tube, also through the use of laparoscopy.

REFERENCES

A senator recalls a wrong. (1984, May 7). Time, 123, 27.

Abarbanel, A. R. (1978). Diagnosis and treatment of coital discomfort. In J. LoPiccolo & L. LoPiccolo (Eds.), Handbook of sex therapy (pp. 241–259). New York: Plenum Press.

Abbott, D. A., & Walters, J. (1985). Parenthood is a question of free choice, and there should be no societal pressure. In H. Feldman & M. Feldman (Eds.), Current controversies in marriage and family (pp. 183–192). Beverly Hills, CA: Sage Publications.

Abel, E. L. (1981). Behavioral teratology of alcohol. Psychological Bulletin, 90, 564–581.

Abel, E. L. (1981). Marijuana and sex: A critical survey. Drug and Alcohol Dependence, 8, 1–22.

Abel, G. G., & Rouleau, J. L. (1990). The nature and extent of sexual assault. In W. L. Marshall, D. R. Laws, & H. E. Barbaree (Eds.), Handbook of sexual assault: Issues, theories, and treatment of the offender (pp. 9–21). New York: Plenum Press.

Abel, G. G., Huffman, J., Warberg, B., & Holland, C. L. (1998). Visual reaction time and plethysmography as measures of sexual interest in child molesters. Sexual Abuse: A Journal of Research and Treatment, 10, 81–95.

Abou-Saleh, M. T., & Ghubash, R. (1997). The prevalence of early postpartum psychiatric morbidity in Dubai: A transcultural perspective. Acta Psychiatrica Scandinavica, 95, 428–432.

Abplanalp, J. M. (1983). Psychologic components of the premenstrual syndrome. Evaluating research and choosing the treatment. The Journal of Reproductive Medicine, 28, 517–523.

Abrahams, M. F. (1994). Perceiving flirtatious communications: An exploration of the perceptual dimensions underlying judgments of flirtatiousness. The Journal of Sex Research, 31, 283–292.

Abrahamson, D. J., Barlow, D. H., & Abrahamson, L. S. (1989). Differential effects on performance demand and distraction on sexually functional and dysfunctional males. Journal of Abnormal Psychology, 98, 241–247.

Abramowitz, S. I. (1986). Psychosocial outcomes of sex reassignment surgery. Journal of Consulting and Clinical Psychology, 54, 183–189.

ACOG Patient Information. Gynecologic Problems. (1991). Important Facts About Endometriosis. [Brochure]. Washington, DC: Author.

ACOG Patient Information. Gynecologic Problems. (1992). Urinary Tract Infections. [Brochure]. Washington, DC: Author.

ACOG Patient Information. Gynecologic Problems. (1994). Vaginitis: Causes and Treatments. [Brochure]. Washington, DC: Author.

Adams, J., McClellan, J., Douglass, D., McCurry, C., & Storck, M. (1995). Sexually inappropriate behaviors in seriously mentally ill children and adolescents. Child Abuse & Neglect, 19, 555–568.

Adams, Jr., S. G., Dubbert, P. M., Chupurdia, K. M., Jones, Jr., A., Lofland, K. R., & Leermakers, E. (1996). Assessment of sexual beliefs and information in aging couples with sexual dysfunctions. Archives of Sexual Behavior, 25, 249–260.

Adams, R. S. (1997). Preventing verbal harassment and violence toward gay and lesbian students. Journal of School Nursing, 13, 24–28.

Adams-Roy, J., & Barlint, J. (1998). Predicting the decision to confront or report sexual harassment. Journal of Organizational Behavior, 19, 329–336.

Addiego, F., et al. (1981). Female ejaculation: A case study. Journal of Sex Research, 17, 13–21.

Agnew, J. (1982). Klismaphilia: A physiological perspective. American Journal of Psychotherapy, 36, 554–566.

Ainsworth, M. D. S. (1989). Attachments beyond infancy. American Psychologist, 44, 709–716.

Akesode, F. A., & Iyang, U. E. (1981). Some social and sexual problems experienced by Nigerians with limb amputation. Tropical and Geographical Medicine, 33, 71–74.

Alan Guttmacher Institute. (1994). Sex and American teenagers. New York: Author.

Albarran, J. W., & Bridger, S. (1997). Problems with providing education on resuming sexual activity after myocardial infarction: Developing written information for patients. Intensive & Critical Care Nursing, 13, 2–11.

Albert, A. E., Warner, D. L., & Hatcher, R. A. (1998). Facilitating condom use with clients during commercial sex in Nevada's legal brothels. American Journal of Public Health, 88, 643–646.

Albiniak, P. (1998). ACLU files suit against Internet porn act. Broadcasting & Cable, 128, 18.

Alcoe, S. Y., Gilbey, V. J., McDermot, R. S. R., & Wallace, D. G. (1995). The practice of breast self-examination over a six-year period following teaching. Patient Education & Counseling, 25, 183–196.

Alexander, C. J., Sipski, M. L., Findley, T. W. (1993). Sexual activities, desire, and satisfaction in males pre- and post-spinal cord injury. Archives of Sexual Behavior, 22, 217–228.

Alexander, S., & Karaszewski, L. (1996). The people vs. Larry Flynt. New York: Newmarket Press.

Alksnis, C., Desmarais, S., & Wood, E. (1996). Gender differences in scripts for different types of dates. Sex Roles, 34, 321–336.

Allen, Jr., J. L. (1997). Homosexual children a "gift" bishops say. National Catholic Reporter, 33, 9.

Allison, A. (1994). Nightwork: Sexuality, pleasure, and corporate masculinity in a Tokyo hostess club. Chicago: University of Chicago Press.

Allport, G. W. (1961). Pattern and Growth in Personality. New York: Holt, Rinehart and Winston.

Altschul, M. S. (1997). Cultural bias and the urinary tract infection (UTI) circumcision controversy. [on line].

American Academy of Pediatrics Staff (1998). A guide to references and resources in child abuse & neglect. Elk Grove Village, IL: American Academy of Pediatrics.

American Medical Association. Council on Scientific Affairs. (1999, June). Implications of brain development research (Report 15 - A99). Chicago, IL: Author.

American Psychiatric Association. (1994). Diagnostic and statistical manual of mental disorders (4th ed.). Washington, DC: Author.

Americans growing more tolerant of gays. (1996, December 14). Gallup organization. Saad, L.

Ames, M. A., & Houston, D. A. (1990). Legal, social, and biological definitions of pedophilia. Archives of Sexual Behavior, 19, 333–342.

Ames, T-R. H., & Samowitz, P. (1995). Inclusionary standard for determining sexual consent for individuals with developmental disabilities. Mental Retardation, 33, 264–268.

Andersen, S. L., & Pollack, R. H. (1994). The making of an oral sex questionnaire. Journal of Sex Education and Therapy, 20, 123–133.

Anderson, B. L., Woods, X. A., & Copeland, L. J. (1997). Sexual self-schema and sexual morbidity among gynecologic cancer survivors. Journal of Consulting & Clinical Psychology, 65, 221–229.

Anderson, B. L., Woods, X. A., & Cyranowski, M. A. (1994). Sexual self-schema as a possible predictor of sexual problems following cancer treatment. The Canadian Journal of Human Sexuality, 3, 165–170.

Anderson, D. A. (1993–94). Lesbian and gay adolescents: Social and developmental considerations. High School Journal, 77, 13–19.

Anderson, J. E., Brackbill, R., & Mosher, W. D. (1996). Condom use for disease prevention among unmarried U. S. women. Family Planning Perspectives, 28, 25–28.

Angier, N. (1997, July 15). Doctors favor ultrasound use in right hands. The New York Times. [http://www.nytimes.com/].

Angier, N. (1997, July 15). Sonogram dilemma: Tales of joy and grief. The New York Times. [http://www.nytimes.com/].

Ankney, C. D. (1992). Sex differences in relative brain size: The mismeasure of women, too? Intelligence, 16, 329–336.

Ankrom, M., & Greenough, W. B. (1997). Delayed diagnosis: A 78-year-old man with AIDS. Journal of the American Geriatrics Society, 45, 1282–1283.

Annan, N. (1995, June 22). Under the Victorian bed. The New York Review, 48–51.

Annon, J. (1976). The behavioral treatment of sexual problems: Brief therapy. New York: Harper & Row.

Annual mammograms urged at 40. (1997, March 23). The New York Times. [http://www.nytimes.com].

Apt, C., Hurlbert, D. F., Sarmiento, G. R., & Hurlbert, M. K. (1996). The role of fellatio in marital sexuality: An examination of sexual compatibility and sexual desire. Sexual & Marital Therapy, 11, 383–392.

Aral, S. O., & Peterman, T. A. (1998). Do we know the effectiveness of behavioural interventions? Lancet, 351, Supplement 3, 33–36.

Aranow, H., & Wood, W. B. (1942). Staphylococcic infection simulating scarlet fever. Journal of the American Medical Association, 119, 1491–1495.

Araoz, D. L. (1998). The new hypnosis in sex therapy. Northvale, NJ: Jason Aronson Inc.

Arellano Lara, S., Gonzalez Barrera, J. L., Hernandez Ono, A., Moreno Alcazar, O. & Espinosa Perez, J. (1997). No-scalpel vasectomy: Review of the first 1,000 cases in a family medicine unit. Archives of Medical Research, 28, 517–522.

Aristotle. (1976). The ethics of Aristotle. (J. A. K. Thompson, Trans.). Harmondsworth, England: Penguin.

Asali, A., Khamaysi, N., Aburabia, Y., Letzer, S., Halihal, B., Sadovsky, M., Maoz, B., & Belmaker, R. H. (1995). Ritual female genital surgery among Bedouin in Israel. Archives of Sexual Behavior, 24, 571–575.

Assessment of sexually transmitted diseases services in city and county jails - United States, 1997. Morbidity and Mortality Weekly Reports, 47, June 5, 1998, 429–431,

Atkins, E., Solomon, L. J., Worden, J. K., & Foster, R. S. (1991). Relative effectiveness of methods of breast self-examination. Journal of Behavioral Medicine, 14, 357–367.

Atlanta Reproductive Health Centre WWW. (1997). Routine fertility workup. International Council on Infertility Information Dissemination. [http://www.ivf.com/art.html].

Attneave, C. (1982). American Indians and Alaska Native families: Emigrants in their own homeland. In M. McGoldrick, J. Pierce, & J. Giordano (Eds.), Ethnicity and family therapy (pp. 55–83). New York: Guilford.

Aune, K. S., & Comstock, J. (1997). Effect of relationship length on the experience, expression, and perceived appropriateness of jealousy. The Journal of Social Psychology, 137, 23–31.

Bachmann, G. A. (1995). Influence of menopause on sexuality. International Journal of Fertility and Menopausal Studies, 40, Supplement 1, 16–22.

Bachmann, G. A., Leiblum, S. R., & Grill, J. (1989). Brief sexual inquiry in gynecologic practice. Obstetrics and Gynecology, 73, 425–427.

Background and Mission of RESOLVE. (1996). Resolve of Maryland. [http://www.resolve.org/famfrend.htm].

Bailey, J. M., & Pillard, R. C. (1991). A genetic study of male sexual orientation. Archives of General Psychiatry, 48, 1089–1096.

Bailey, J. M., & Pillard, R. C. (1995). Genetics of human sexual orientation. Annual Review of Sex Research, VI, 126–150.

Bailey, J. M., Pillard, R. C., Neale, M. C., & Agyei, Y. (1993). Heritable factors influence sexual orientation in women. Archives of General Psychiatry, 50, 217–223.

Baird, D. D., Weinberg, C. R., Voigt, L. F., & Daling, J. R. (1996). Vaginal douching and reduced fertility. American Journal of Public Health, 86, 844–850.

Baird, R. M., & Rosenbaum, S. E. (Eds.) (1998). Pornography: Private right or public menace. Amherst, NY: Prometheus Books.

Baker, J. G., & Rosenthal, S. L. (1998). Psychological aspects of sexually transmitted infection acquisition in adolescent girls: A developmental perspective. Developmental and Behavioral Pediatrics, 19, 202–208.

Baker, R. A. (1998). Child sexual abuse & false memory syndrome. Amherst, NY: Prometheus Books.

Bakos, S. C. (1995). Kink. New York: St. Martins Press.

Baldwin, D. S. (1996). Depression and sexual function. Journal of Psychopharmacology, 10, Supplement 1, 30–34.

Ball, H. (1998). Offending pattern in a gerontophilic perpetrator. Medicine, Science, and the Law, 38, 261–262.

Ballard, C. G., Solis, M., Gahir, M., Cullen, P., George, S., Oyebode, F., & Wilcock, G. (1997). Sexual relationships in married dementia sufferers. International Journal of Geriatric Psychiatry, 12, 447–451.

Balon, R., Yeragani, V. K., Pohl, R., & Ramesh, C. (1993). Journal of Clinical Psychiatry, 54, 209–212.

Bancroft, J. (1983). Human sexuality and its problems. Churchill Livingstone, New York.

Bancroft, J. (1984). Hormones and human sexual behavior. Journal of Sex and Marital Therapy, 10, 3–21.

Bancroft, J. (1991). Human sexuality and its problems. New York: Churchill Livingstone.

Bancroft, J., Sherwin, B. B., Alexander, G. M., Davidson, D. W., & Walker, A. (1991). Oral contraceptives, androgens, and the sexuality of young women: I. A comparison of sexual experience, sexual attitudes, and gender role in oral contraceptive users and nonusers. Archives of Sexual Behavior, 20, 105–120.

Bancroft, J., Tennent, T. G., Loucas, K., & Cass, J. (1974). Control of deviant sexual behaviour by drugs: Behavioural effects of oestrogens and antiandrogens. British Journal of Psychiatry, 125, 310–319.

Bandura, A. (1965). Influence of a model's reinforcement contingencies on the acquisition of imitative responses. Journal of Personality and Social Psychology, 1, 589–595.

Bandura, A. (1977). Social learning theory. Englewood Cliffs, NJ: Prentice Hall.

Banks, A., & Gartrell, N. K. (1995). Hormones and sexual orientation: A questionable link. Journal of Homosexuality, 28, 247–268.

Barak, A. (1997). Cross-cultural perspectives on sexual harassment. In W. O'Donohue (Ed.), Sexual harassment. Theory, research, and treatment (pp. 263–300). Boston: Allyn and Bacon.

Barak, Y., Achiron, A., Elizur, A., Gabbay, U., Noy, S., & Sarova-Pinhas, I. (1996). Sexual dysfunction in relapsing-remitting multiple sclerosis: Magnetic resonance imaging, clinical, and psychological correlates. Journal of Psychiatry and Neuroscience, 21, 255–258.

Barbach, L. G. (1976). For yourself: The fulfillment of female sexuality. Garden City, NY: Anchor.

Barclay, L. M., McDonald, P., & O'Loughlin, J. A. (1994). Sexuality and pregnancy. An interview study. Australian and New Zealand Journal of Obstetrics and Gynaecology, 34, 1–7.

Bardoni, B., Zanaria, E., Guioli, S., Floridia, G., Worley, K., Tonini, G., Ferrante, E., Chiumello, G., McCabe, E., Fraccaro, M., Zuffardi, O., & Camerino, G. (1994). A dosage sensitive locus at chromosome Xp21 is involved in male to female sex reversal. Nature Genetics, 7, 497–501.

Barling, N. R., & Moore, S. M. (1996). Prediction of cervical cancer screening using the theory of reasoned action. Psychological Reports, 79, 77–78.

Barnhart, K., Furman, I., & Devoto, L. (1995). Attitudes and practice of couples regarding sexual relations during the menses and spotting. Contraception, 51, 93–98.

Barques, G. S., Lapinski, R. H., Dolgin, S. E., Gazella, G, et al. (1993). Prevalence and natural history of cryptorchidism. Pediatrics, 82, 44–49.

Barret, R., & Barzan, R. (1996). Spiritual experiences of gay men and lesbians. Counseling and Values, 41, 4–15.

Bartoi, A. G., & Kinder, B. N. (1998). Effects of child and adult sexual abuse on adult sexuality. Journal of Sex and Marital Therapy, 24, 75–90.

Bassol, S., Hernandez, C., Nava, M. P., Trujillo, A. M., Luz de la Cruz, D. (1995). A comparative study on the return to ovulation following chronic use of once-a-month injectable contraceptives. Contraception, 51, 307–311.

Bauman, L. J., & Siegel, K. (1987). Misperception among gay men of the risk for AIDS associated with their sexual behavior. Journal of Applied Social Psychology, 17, 329–350.

Baumeister, R. F. (1989). Masochism and the self. Hillsdale, NJ: Erlbaum.

Baumeister, R. F., & Butler, J. L. (1997). Sexual masochism. Deviance without pathology. In D. R. Laws & W. O'Donohue (Eds.), Sexual deviance. Theory, assessment, and treatment (pp. 225–239). New York: The Guilford Press.

Bauserman, R. (1996). Sexual aggression and pornography: A review of correlational research. Basic and Applied Social Psychology, 18, 405–427.

Bauserman, R. (1998). Egalitarian, sexist, and aggressive sexual materials: Attitude effects and viewer responses. The Journal of Sex Research, 35, 244–253.

Bauserman, R., & Davis, C. (1996). Perceptions of early sexual experiences and adult sexual adjustment. Journal of Psychology and Human Sexuality, 8, 37–59.

Bauserman, R., & Rind, B. (1997). Psychological correlates of male child and adolescent sexual experiences with adults: A review of the nonclinical literature. Archives of Sexual Behavior, 26, 105–141.

Beach, E. K., Maloney, B. H., Plocica, A. R., Sherry, S. E., Weaver, M., Luthringer, L., & Utz, S. (1992). The spouse: A factor in recovery after acute myocardial infarction. Heart & Lung, 21, 30–38.

Beard, M. K. (1992). Atrophic vaginitis. Postgraduate Medicine, 91, 257–260.

Bechtel, S., & Stains, L. R. (1996). Sex. A man's guide. Emmaus, PA: Rodale Press.

Beck, A. T. (1988). Love is never enough. New York: Harper & Row.

Beck, J. G. (1993). Vaginismus. In W. O'Donohue & J. H. Geer (Eds.), Handbook of sexual dysfunctions. Assessment and treatment (pp. 381–397). Boston: Allyn and Bacon.

Beck, J. G. (1995). Hypoactive sexual desire disorder: An overview. Journal of Consulting and Clinical Psychology, 63, 919–927.

Becker, J. V. (1989). Impact of sexual abuse on sexual functioning. In S. R. Leiblum & R. C. Rosen (Eds.), Principles and practice of sex therapy. Update for the 1990s (2nd ed) (pp. 298–318). New York: The Guilford Press.

Beckman, L. J., & Ackerman, K. T. (1995). Women, alcohol, and sexuality. Recent Developments in Alcoholism, 12, 267–285.

Beckman, L. J., Harvey, S. M., & Tiersky, L. A. (1996). Attitudes about condoms and condom use among college students. Journal of American College Health, 44, 243–250.

Beckmann, C. R. B., Ling, F. W., Herbert, W. N. P., Laube, D. W., Smith, R. P., & Barzansky, B. M. (1998). Obstetrics and gynecology (3rd ed.). Baltimore, MD: Williams & Wilkins.

Beebe, D. K. (1991). Emergency management of the adult female rape victim. American Family Physician, 43, 2041–2046.

Belcher, A. E. (1992). Cancer nursing. St. Louis: Mosby.

Bell, A. P., & Weinberg, M. S. (1978). Homosexualities. New York: Simon and Schuster.

Bell, A. P., Weinberg, M. S., & Hammersmith, S. K. (1981). Sexual preference. Bloomington: Indiana University Press.

Bell, C. S., Johnson, J. E., McGillicuddy-Delisi, A. V., & Sigel, I. E. (1980). Normative stress and young families. Family Relations, 29, 453–458.

Bell, R. R., & Chaskes, J. B. (1970). Premarital sexual experiences among coeds, 1958 and 1968. Journal of Marriage and the Family, 32, 81–84.

Bell, S., Porter, M., Kitchener, H., & Fraser, C., et al. (1995). Psychological response to cervical screening. Preventive Medicine: An International Journal Devoted to Practice & Theory, 24, 610–616.

Bem, D. J. (1996). Exotic becomes erotic: A developmental theory of sexual orientation. Psychological Review, 103, 320–335.

Bem, S. L. (1974). The measurement of psychological androgyny. Journal of Consulting and Clinical Psychology, 42, 155–162.

Bem, S. L. (1975). Sex role adaptability: One consequence of psychological androgyny. Journal of Personality and Social Psychology, 31, 634–643.

Bem, S. L. (1976). Probing the promise of androgyny. In A. G. Kaplan & J. P. Bean (Eds.), Beyond sex-role stereotypes: Readings toward a psychology of androgyny. Boston: Little, Brown & Co.

Ben-Ari, A. T. (1995). Coming out: A dialectic of intimacy and privacy. Families in Society, 76, 306–314.

Benazon, N., Wright, J., & Sabourin, S. (1992). Stress, sexual satisfaction, and marital adjustment in infertile couples. Journal of Sex and Marital Therapy, 18, 273–284.

Benbow, C. P. (1988). Sex differences in mathematical reasoning ability in intellectually talented preadolscents: Their nature, effects, and possible causes. Behavioral and Brain Sciences, 11, 169–232.

Benedict, H. (1998, May 11). Fear of feminism. The Nation, 266, 10.

Benign Prostatic Hypertrophy Guideline Panel. (1994). Benign prostatic hyperplasia: diagnosis and treatment. American Family Physician, 49, 1157–1165.

Bennett, P. (1992, January 3). Bunking down together. Los Angeles Times, M. E1–2.

Berdahl, J. L., Magley, V., & Waldo, C. R. (1996). The sexual harassment of men? Exploring the concept with theory and data. Psychology of Women Quarterly, 20, 527–547.

Berek, J. S., & Hacker, N. F. (Eds.). (1989). Practical gynecologic oncology. Baltimore: Williams & Wilkins.

Berenson, A. B., Wiemann, C. M., Rickerr, V. In., & McCombs, S. L. (1997). Contraceptive outcomes among adolescents prescribed Norplant implants versus oral contraceptives after one year of use. American Journal of Obstetrics and Gynecology, 176, 586–592.

Bergen, R. K. (1998). Issues in intimate violence. Thousand Oaks, CA: Sage Publishing.

Berger, R. M. (1982). Gay and gray. Urbana, IL: University of Illinois Press.

Berkman, A. H., Katz, L. A., & Weissman, R. (1982). Sexuality and the life-style of home dialysis patients. Archives of Physical Medicine and Rehabilitation, 63, 272–275.

Berkman, C. S., & Zinberg, G. (1997). Homophobia and heterosexism in social workers. Social Work, 42, 319–332.

Berman, E. M., Miller, W. R., Vines, N., & Lief, H. I. (1977). The age 30 crisis and the 7-year-itch. Journal of Sex and Marital Therapy, 3, 197–204.

Bernstein, D., & Kean, L. (1998). Burma's military rapists. The Nation, 267, 5–6.

Berry, R. E., & Williams, F. L. (1987). Assessing the relationship between quality of life and marital and income satisfaction: A path analytic approach. Journal of Marriage and the Family, 49, 107–116.

Bess, B. E. (1997). Human sexuality and obesity. International Journal of Mental Health, 26, 61–67.

Betchen, S. J. (1991). Male masturbation as a vehicle for the pursuer/distancer relationship in marriage. Journal of Sex and Marital Therapy, 17, 269–278.

Betzig, L. (1989). Causes of conjugal dissolution: A cross-cultural study. Current Anthropology, 30, 654–676.

Bhui, K., & Puffett, A. (1994). Sexual problems in the psychiatric and mentally handicapped populations. British Journal of Hospital Medicine, 51, 459–464.

Bieber, I., et al. (1962). Homosexuality: A psychoanalytic study of male homosexuals. New York: Basic Books.

Bienenfeld, D. (1990). Physical changes with aging. In D. Bienenfeld (Ed.), Verwoerdt's clinical geropsychiatry (pp. 3–16). Baltimore: Williams & Wilkins.

Biggs, M., Stermac, L. E., & Divinsky, M. (1998). Genital injuries following sexual assault of women with and without prior sexual intercourse experience. CMAJ, 159, 33–37.

Biglan, A., Meltzer, C. W., Wirt, R., Ary, D., Noell, J., Ochs, L., French, C., & Hood, D. (1990). Social and behavioral factors associated with high-risk sexual behavior among adolescents. Journal of Behavioral Medicine, 13, 245–261.

Bills, S. A., & Duncan, D. F. (1991). Drugs and sex: A survey of college students' beliefs. Perceptual and Motor Skills, 72, 1293–1294.

Billy, J. O. G., Tanfer, K., Grady, W. R., & Klepinger, D. H. (1993). The sexual behavior of men in the United States. Family Planning Perspectives, 25, 52–60.

Birch, A. J. (1992). Steroid hormones and the Luftwaffe. A venture into fundamental strategic research and some of its consequences: The Birch reduction becomes a birth reduction. Steroids, 57, 363–377.

Bird, S. R. (1996). Welcome to the men's club. Homosociality and the maintenance of hegemonic masculinity. Gender and Society, 10, 120–132.

Black, D. W., Kehrberg, L. L. D., Flumerfelt, D. L., & Schlosser, S. S. (1997). Characteristics of 36 subjects reporting compulsive sexual behavior. American Journal of Psychiatry, 154, 243–249.

Blackburn, M. (1999). Sex and disability. Woburn, MA: Butterworth-Heinemann. Carlton, L. (1997). In sickness and in health: Sex, love, and chronic illness. New York: Dell Books.

Blakeslee, S. (1993, June 2). New therapies are helping men to overcome impotence. The New York Times, C12.

Blaney, C. (1995). New approaches seek greater safety, appeal. Network, 15, 26–29.

Blanton, H., & Gerrard, M. (1997). Effect of sexual motivation on men's risk perception for sexually transmitted disease: There must be 50 ways to justify a lover. Health Psychology, 16, 374–379.

Blee, K. M., & Tickamyer, A. R. (1995). Racial differences in men's attitudes about women's gender roles. Journal of Marriage and the Family, 57, 21–30.

Bloch, I. (1937). The sexual life of our time. New York: Falstaff Press, Inc.

Bloor, M. J., Barnard, M. A., Finlay, A., & McKeganey, N. P. (1993). HIV-related risk practices among Glasgow male prostitutes: Reframing concepts of risk behavior. Medical Anthropology Quarterly, 7, 152–169.

Blumstein, P., & Schwartz, P. (1983). American couples: Money, work, sex. New York: Morrow.

Bly, R. (1990). Iron John. Reading, MA: Addison-Wesley Publishing Company, Inc.

Blyth, E. (1994). "I wanted to be interesting. I wanted to be able to say 'I've done something interesting with my life'": Interviews with surrogate mothers in Britain. Special issue: Ethics at the beginning of life. Journal of Reproductive & Infant Psychology, 12, 189–198.

Boehm, S., Coleman-Burns, P., Schlenk, E. A., Funnell, M. M., et al. (1995). Prostate cancer in African-American men: Increasing knowledge and self-efficacy. Journal of Community Health Nursing, 12, 161–169.

Bohlen, J. G., Held, J. P., Sanderson, M. O., & Boyer, C. M. (1982). Development of a woman's multiple orgasm pattern: A research case report. Journal of Sex Research, 18, 130–145.

Bohon, J. S. (1997). Teaching on the edge: The psychology of sexual orientation. Teaching of Psychology, 24, 27–32.

Boldrini, P., Basaglia, N., & Calanca, M. C. (1991). Sexual changes in hemiparetic patients. Archives of Physical Medicine and Rehabilitation, 72, 202–207.

Boolell, M., Allen, M. J., Ballard, S. A., et al. (1996). Sildenafil: an orally active type 5 cyclic GMP-specific phosphodiesterase inhibitor for the treatment of penile erection dysfunction. International Journal of Impotence Research, 8, 47–52.

Bordens, K. S., & Abbott, B. B. (1996). Research design and methods. A process approach. Mountain View, CA: Mayfield Publishing Company.

Borelli-Kerner, S., & Bernell, B. (1997). Couple therapy of sexual disorders. In R. S. Charlton (Ed.), Treating sexual disorders (pp. 165–199). San Francisco: Jossey-Bass.

Borger, G. (1991, October 21). Judging Thomas. U. S. News & World Report, 111, 32–36.

Borruso, M. (1991). Sexual abuse by psychotherapists: The call for a uniform criminal statute. American Journal of Law & Medicine, 17, 289–311.

Bortolotti, A., Parazzini, F., Colli, E., & Landoni, M. (1997). The epidemiology of erectile dysfunction with its risk factors. International Journal of Andrology, 20, 323–334.

Bostick, R. M., Sprafka, J. M., Virnig, B. A., & Potter, J. D. (1994). Predictors of cancer prevention attitudes and participation in cancer screening examinations. Preventive Medicine: An International Journal Devoted to Practice & Theory, 23, 816–826.

Boston Women's Health Book Collective. (1992). The new our bodies, ourselves: Updated and expanded for the 90s. New York: Simon & Schuster.

Boswell, J. (1980). Christianity, social tolerance and homosexuality. Chicago: University of Chicago Press.

Boswell, J. (1994). Same-sex unions in premodern Europe.. New York: Villard.

Bowlby, J. (1969). Attachment and Loss. Vol. 1: Attachment. New York: Basic Books.

Boyd, R. L. (1989). Childlessness and social mobility during the baby boom. Sociological Spectrum, 9, 425–438.

Bozett, F. W. (1981). Gay fathers: Evolution of the gay-father identity. American Journal of Orthopsychiatry, 51, 552–559.

Bozman, A. W., & Beck, J. G. (1991). Covariation of sexual desire and sexual arousal: The effects of anger and anxiety. Archives of Sexual Behavior, 20, 47–60.

Brahams, D. (1987). Court of appeal agrees to sterilisation of 17-year-old mentally handicapped girl under wardship jurisdiction. The Lancet, March 28, 1 (8535), 757–758.

Brahams, D. (1989). Sterilisation of mentally handicapped woman approved by House of Lords. Lancet, May 13, 1 (8646), 1089.

Bram, S. (1985). Childlessness revisited: A longitudinal study of voluntarily childless couples, delayed parents, and parents. Lifestyles, 8, 46–66.

Brant, H. (1978). The psychosexual problems of women. Part 2: Female sexual dysfunctions. Community Nurse, 14, 73–76.

Brecher, E. M. (1984). Love, sex, and aging. New York: Little, Brown & Co.

Breedlove, S. M. (1994). Sexual differentiation of the human nervous system. Annual Review of Psychology, 45, 389–418.

Brehm, S. S. (1985). Intimate Relationships. New York: Random House.

Brennan, K. A., & Morris, K. A. (1997). Attachment styles, self-esteem, and patterns of seeking feedback from romantic partners. Personality & Social Psychology Bulletin, 23, 23–31.

Briere, J., & Conte, J. (1993). Self-reported amnesia for abuse in adults molested as children. Journal of Traumatic Stress, 6, 21–31.

Briley, H. D., Walker, M. M., Luzzi, G. A., Bell, R., Taylor-Robinson, D., Byrne, M., & Renton, A. M. (1993). Clinical features and management of recurrent balanitis; association with atopy and genital washing. Genitourinary Medicine, 69, 400–403.

Britain ends ban on gays, begins code for all forces. (2000, January 13). The Daily Press, Newport News, VA, A8.

Brockman, B., & Bluglass, R. (1996). A general psychiatric approach to sexual deviation. In I. Rosen (Ed.), Sexual deviation (3rd ed.) (pp. 1–42). Oxford: Oxford University Press.

Bronstein, P. (1988). Father-child interaction: Implications for gender role socialization. In P. Bronstein & C. P. Cowan (Eds.), Fatherhood today: Men's changing role in the family. New York: Wiley.

Brookey, R. A. (1996). A community like Philadelphia. Western Journal of Communication, 60, 40–56.

Brookoff, D. (1994). Compliance with doxycycline therapy for outpatient treatment of pelvic inflammatory disease. Southern Medical Journal, 87, 1088–1091.

Brothers, J. (1982). What every woman should know about marriage. New York: Simon & Schuster.

Brott, A. A., & Ash, J. (1995). The expectant father. Facts, tips, and advice for the dad-to-be. New York: Abbeville Press.

Brown, G. R., Wise, T. N., Costa, P. T., Herbst, J. H., Fagan, P. J., & Schmidt, C. W. (1996). Personality characteristics and sexual functioning of 188 cross-dressing men. The Journal of Nervous and Mental Disease, 184, 265–273.

Brown, H. (1976). Familiar faces hidden lives. The story of homosexual men in America today. New York: Harcourt Brace Jovanovich.

Brown, L. (1989). Is there sexual freedom for our aging population in long-term care institutions? Journal of Gerontological Social Work, 13, 75–93.

Brown, R. D., Whisnant, J. P., Sicks, J. D., et al. (1996). Stroke incidence, prevalence, and survival: Secular trends in Rochester, Minnesota through 1989. Stroke, 27, 373–380.

Brown, T. J., & Allgeier, E. R. (1995). Managers' perceptions of workplace romances: An interview study. Journal of Business and Psychology, 10, 169–176.

Browne, J., & Minichiello, V. (1996a). The social and work context of commercial sex between men: A research note. Australian and New Zealand Journal of Sociology, 32, 86–92.

Browne, J., & Minichiello, V. (1996b). Research directions in male sex work. Journal of Homosexuality, 31, 29–56.

Brownmiller, S. (1975). Against our will: Men, women and rape. New York: Simon and Schuster.

Bruess, C. J. S., & Pearson, J. C. (1997). Interpersonal rituals in marriage and adult friendship. Communication Monographs, 64, 25–46.

Brustein, R. (1998). Sex, art, and the supreme court. The New Republic, 219, 28–30.

Bryan, J. H. (1965). Apprenticeships in prostitution. Social Problems, 12, 287–297.

Bryant, C. D. (1982). Sexual deviancy and social proscription. New York: Human Sciences Press.

Bullough, B., & Bullough, V. (1997). Are transvestites necessarily heterosexual? Archives of Sexual Behavior, 26, 1–12.

Bullough, V. L. (1994). Science in the bedroom. New York: Basic Books.

Bullough, V. L., & Bullough, B. (1997). The history of the science of sexual orientation 1880–1980: An overview. Journal of Psychology & Human Sexuality, 9, 1–16.

Bumpass, L. L., & Sweet, J. A. (1989). National estimates on cohabitation. Demography, 26, 615–625.

Bumpass, L., Sweet, J., & Martin, T. C. (1990). Changing patterns of remarriage. Journal of Marriage and the Family. 52, 747–756.

Burch, B. (1993). On intimate terms. The psychology of difference in lesbian relationships. Urbana, IL: University of Illinois Press.

Burger, C. W., & Kenemans, P. (1998). Postmenopausal hormone replacement therapy and cancer of the female genital tract and breast. Current Opinion in Obstetrics and Gynecology, 10, 41–45.

Burger, H. G. (1994). Reproductive hormone measurements during the menopausal transition. In G. Berg & M. Hammar (Eds.), The modern management of the menopause (pp. 103–108). New York: The Parthenon Publishing Group.

Burns, A. (1992). Mother-headed families: An international perspective and the case of Australia. Society for Research in Child Development: Social Policy Report, 6, 1–22.

Burns-Cox, N., & Gingell, C. (1997). The andropause: fact or fiction? Postgraduate Medical Journal, 73, 553–556.

Burstein, G. R., Gaydos, C. A., Diener-West, M., Howell, R., Zenilman, J. M., & Quinn, T. C. (1998). Incident Chlamydia trachomatis infections among inner-city adolescent females. Journal of the American Medical Association, 280, 521–526.

Buss, D. M. (1985). Human mate selection. American Scientist, 73, 47–51.

Buss, D. M. (1989). Sex differences in human mate preferences: An evolutionary hypothesis tested in 37 different cultures. Behavioral and Brain Sciences, 12, 1–49.

Buss, D. M. (1994). The evolution of desire: Strategies of human mating. New York: Basic Books.

Buss, D. M., & Schmitt, D. P. (1993). Sexual strategies theory: An evolutionary perspective on human mating. Psychological Review, 100, 204–232.

Butler, R., & Lewis, M. (1973). Aging and mental health. St. Louis: C. V. Mosby.

Buunk, B. P. (1995). Sex, self-esteem, dependency and extradyadic sexual experience as related to jealousy responses. Journal of Social & Personal Relationships, 12, 147–153.

Byrne, D., & Griffitt, W. (1973). Interpersonal attraction. Annual Review of Psychology, 24, 317–336.

Byrne, D., & Murnen, S. (1988). Maintaining loving relationships. In R. Sternberg & M. Barnes (Eds.), The psychology of loving. New Haven, CT: Yale University Press.

Cairns, K. V., Collins, S. D., & Hiebert, B. (1994). Adolescents' self-perceived needs for sexuality education. Canadian Journal of Human Sexuality, 3, 245–251.

Caldwell, J. C., & Caldwell, P. (1996). The African aids epidemic. Scientific American, 274, 62–63, 66–68.

Calhoun, K. S., & Atkeson, B. M. (1991). Treatment of rape victims: Facilitating psychosocial adjustment. New York: Pergamon Press.

Callahan, E. J., & Leitenberg, H. (1973). Aversion therapy for sexual deviation: Contingent shock and covert sensitization. Journal of Abnormal Psychology, 81, 60–73.

Callahan, S. (1993, December 17). Memory can play tricks. Commonweal, 120, 6–7.

Callan, V. J. (1983). The voluntarily childless and their perceptions of parenthood and childlessness. Journal of Comparative Family Studies, 14, 87–96.

Cameron, P., & Cameron, K. (1998). What proportion of newspaper stories about child molestation involves homosexuality. Psychological Reports, 82, 863–871.

Campbell, R., & Aherns, C. E. (1998). Innovative community services for rape victims: An application of multiple case study methodology. American Journal of Community Psychology, 26, 537–571.

Can contraception reduce the underclass? (1990, December 12). The Philadelphia Inquirer, A18.

CancerNet [on line] (1995). Cancer Facts. Benign breast lumps and other benign breast changes.

Candela hopeful that FDA clearance will lead to acceptance of prostate cryoablation. (1996, June). Health Industry Today, 59, 6.

Card, C. (1995). Lesbian choices. New York: Columbia University Press.

Carey, M. P., & Johnson, B. T. (1996). Effectiveness of yohimbine in the treatment of erectile disorder: Four meta-analytic integrations. Archives of Sexual Behavior, 25, 341–360.

Cargan, L. (1982). Singles: Myths and realities. Beverly Hills, CA: Sage Publications.

Carlson, K. J. (1997). Outcomes of hysterectomy. Clinical Obstetrics and Gynecology, 40, 939–946.

Carlson, K. J., Eisenstat, S. A., & Ziporyn, T. (1996). The Harvard guide to women's health. Cambridge, MA: Harvard University Press.

Carlstedt, I., & Sheehan, J. K. (1989). Structure and macromolecular properties of cervical mucus glycoproteins. Symposia of the Society for Experimental Biology, 43, 289–316.

Carne, C. (1998). Sexually transmitted diseases: Recent advances. British Medical Journal, 317, 129–132.

Carnes, P. (1991). Don't call it love: Recovery from sexual addiction. New York: Bantam Books.

Carnes, P. (1992). Out of the shadows (2nd ed.). Center City, MN: Hazelden.

Carney, A., Bancroft, J., & Mathews, A. (1978). Combination of hormonal and psychological treatment for female sexual unresponsiveness: A comparative study. British Journal of Psychiatry, 132, 339–346.

Cartwright, I. D., Petty, M., Reyes, M., & Illuminati, L. (1996). Gonococcal endocarditis. Sexually Transmitted Diseases, 23, 181–183.

Casey, S. (1994). Homosexual parents and Canadian child custody law. Family & Conciliation Courts Review, 32, 379–396.

Caspi, A., & Herbener, E. S. (1990). Continuity and change: Assortative marriage and the consistency of personality in adulthood. Journal of Personality and Social Psychology, 58, 250–258.

Cass, V. C. (1979). Homosexual identity formation: A theoretical model. Journal of Homosexuality, 4, 219–235.

Castaneda, D. M. (1993). The meaning of romantic love among Mexican-American. Journal of Social Behavior and Personality, 8, 257–272.

Cate, F. H. (1996). Cybersex: Regulating sexually explicit expression on the Internet. Behavioral Sciences & the Law, 14, 145–166.

Cederholm, M., & Axelson, O. (1997). A prospective comparative study on transabdominal chorionic villus sampling and amniocentesis performed at 10–13 week's gestation. Prenatal Diagnosis, 17, 311–317.

Chalkley, A., & Powell, G. E. (1983). The clinical description of forty-eight cases of sexual fetishism. British Journal of Psychiatry, 142, 292–295.

Chamberlain, A., Rauh, J., Passer, A., McGrath, M., & Burket, R. (1984). Issues in fertility control for mentally retarded female adolescents. I. Sexual activity, sexual abuse, and contraception. Pediatrics, 73, 445–450

Chan, C. (1987). Asian lesbians: Psychological issues in the "coming out" process. Journal of the Asian American Psychological Association, 12, 16–18.

Chandler, C. K. (1993). "Homosexuality as a compulsion neurosis": Comment. Individual Psychology: Journal of Adlerian Theory, Research & Practice, 49, 223–225.

Chapkis, W. (1996). Live sex acts: Women performing erotic labor. New York: Routledge.

Charlton, R. S. (1997). Treating sexual disorders. San Francisco: Jossey-Bass.

Charlton, R. S., & Brigel, F. W. (1997). Treatment of arousal and orgasmic disorders. In R. S. Charlton (Ed.), Treating sexual disorders (pp. 237–280). San Francisco: Jossey-Bass.

Charlton, R. S., & Yalom, I. D. (Eds.). (1996). Treating sexual disorders. San Francisco: Jossey-Bass.

Chasteen, A. L. (1994). "The world around me": The environment and single women. Sex Roles, 31, 309–328.

Chelala, C. (1998). Algerian abortion controversy highlights rape of war victims. The Lancet, 351, 1413.

Chidey, J. (1996). The fight to save the children: Activists battle the sexual exploitation of kids. Maclean's, 109, 20–23.

Chittister, J. (1995). Low status of Turkish women. National Catholic Reporter, 31, 13.

Chodorow, N. (1978). The reproduction of mothering: Psychoanalysis and the sociology of gender. Berkeley: University of California Press.

Chollar, S. (1994). Mind over cancer? American Health, 13, 74–75, 100.

Chow, W. H., Daling, J. R., Weiss, N. S., Moore, D. E., and Soderstrom, R. (1985). Vaginal douching as a potential risk factor for tubal ectopic pregnancy. American Journal of Obstetrics and Gynecology, 153, 727–729.

Cicerello, A., & Sheehan, E. P. (1995). Personal advertisements: A content analysis. Journal of Social Behavior and Personality, 10, 751–756.

Cicero, M. T. (1971). Laelius: On friendship. London: Penguin Books.

Cimbalo, R. S., & Novell, D. O. (1993). Sex differences in romantic love attitudes among college students. Psychological Reports, 73, 15–18.

Clanton, G., & Kosin, D. J. (1991). Developmental correlates of jealousy. In P. Salovey (Ed.), The Psychology of Jealousy and Envy (pp. 132–177). New York: Guilford.

Clanton, G., & Smith, L. G. (Eds.). (1977). Jealousy. Englewood Cliffs, NJ: Prentice-Hall.

Clark, J. M., & McNeir, B. (1997). An extended case study. (Doing the work of love, part 2). The Journal of Men's Studies, 5, 333–350.

Clement, U., & Schmidt, G. (1983). The outcome of couple therapy for sexual dysfunctions using three different formats. Journal of Sex & Marital Therapy, 9, 67–78.

Coale, A. J., & Banister, J. (1994). Five decades of missing females in China. Demography, 31, 459–479.

Cobb, J. C. (1997). Outercourse as a safe and sensible alternative to contraceptives. American Journal of Public Health, 87, 1380–1381.

Cohen, B. A. (1994). In search of human skin pheromones. Archives of Dermatology, 130, 1048–1051.

Cohen, M. S. (1998). Sexually transmitted diseases enhance HIV transmission: No longer a hypothesis. Lancet, 351, Supplement 3, 5–7.

Cohen, M. S., Hoffman, I. F., Royce, R. A., et al. (1997). Reduction of concentration of HIV-1 in semen after treatment of urethritis: Implications for prevention of sexual transmission of HIV-1. Lancet, 349, 1868–1873.

Cohen, R. S. (1995). Subjective reports on the effects of the MDMA ("ecstasy") experience in humans. Progress in Neuro-Psychopharmacology & Biological Psychiatry, 19, 1137–1145.

Cohen, S. (1976). The 94 day cannabis study. Annals of the New York Academy of Sciences, 282, 211–220.

Colapinto, J. (1997, December 11). The true story of John/Joan. Rolling Stone, 54–97.

Colarusso, C. A. (1995). Traversing young adulthood: The male journey from 20 to 40. Psychoanalytic inquiry, 15, 75–91.

Cold, C. J., Storms, M. R., & Van Howe, R. S. (1997). Carcinoma in situ of the penis in a 76-year-old circumcised man. Journal of Family Practice, 44, 407–410.

Cole, C. M., Emory, L. E., Huang, T., & Meyer, W. J. III. (1994). Treatment of gender dysphoria (transsexualism). Texas Medicine, 90, 68–72.

Cole, W. (1998, November 16). Life off the streets. Time, 152, 8.

Coleman, M., McCowan, L., & Farquhar, C. (1997). The levonorgestrel-releasing intrauterine device: A wider role than contraception. Australian and New Zealand Journal of Obstetrics and Gynaecology, 37, 195–201.

Collins, N. L., & Miller, L. C. (1994). Self-disclosure and liking: A meta-analytic review. Psychological Bulletin, 116, 457–475.

Colton, F. B. (1992). Steroids and "the pill": Early steroid research at Searle. Steroids, 57, 624–630.

Comfort, A. (1972). The joy of sex. New York: Crown.

Conant, M. A., Spicer, D. W., & Smith, C. D. (1984). Herpes simplex virus transmission: Condom studies. Sexually Transmitted Diseases, 11, 94–95.

Conklin, S. C. (1997). Sexuality education in seminaries and theological schools: Perceptions of faculty advocates regarding curriculum and approaches. Journal of Psychology & Human Sexuality, 9, 143–174.

Connell, R. W. (1992). A very straight gay: Masculinity, homosexual experience, and the dynamics of gender. American Sociological Review, 57, 735–751.

Contraceptive practices before and after intervention promoting condom use to prevent HIV infection and other sexually transmitted diseases among women - selected U. S. sites, 1993–1995. (1997, May 2). Morbidity and Mortality Weekly Report, 46, 373–377.

Contreras, R., Hendrick, S. S., & Hendrick, C. (1996). Perspectives on marital love and satisfaction in Mexican American and Anglo-American Couples. Journal of Counseling & Development, 74, 408–415.

Cook, R. R., & Perkins, L. L. (1996). The prevalence of breast implants among women in the United States. Current Topics in Microbiology and Immunology, 210, 419–425.

Cooper, A. J., Sandhu, S., Losztyn, S., & Cernovsky, Z. (1992). A double-blind placebo controlled trial of medroxyprogesterone acetate and cyproterone acetate with seven pedophiles. Canadian Journal of Psychiatry, 37, 687–693.

Corey, L., Adams, H. G., Brown, Z. A., & Holmes, K. K. (1983). Genital herpes simplex virus infections: Clinical manifestations, course, and complications. Annals of Internal Medicine, 98, 958–972.

Cottrell, A. B. (1990). Cross-national marriages: A review of the literature. Journal of Comparative Family Studies, 21, 151–165.

Courtois, F. J., Charvier, K. F., Leriche, A., & Raymond, D. P. (1993). Sexual function in spinal cord injury men. I. Assessing sexual capability. Paraplegia, 31, 771–784.

Cowley, J. J., & Brooksbank, B. W. (1991). Human exposure to putative pheromones and changes in aspects of social behaviour. Journal of Steroid Biochemistry and Molecular Biology, 39, 647–659.

Craib, I. (1987). Masculinity and male dominance. The Sociological Review, 38, 721–743.

Crandall, B. F., & Chua, C. (1997). Risks for fetal abnormalities after very and moderately elevated AF-AFPs. Prenatal Diagnosis, 17, 837–841.

Crawford, P., Hueppelsheuser, M., & George, D. (1996). Spouses of incest offenders: Coaddictive tendencies and dysfunctional etiologies. Sexual Addiction & Compulsivity, 3, 289–312.

Creatsas, G. (1997). Sexually transmitted diseases and oral contraceptive use during adolescence. Annals of the New York Academy of Sciences, 816, 404–410.

Crenshaw, T. L. (1985). The sexual aversion syndrome. Journal of Sex and Marital Therapy, 11, 285–292.

Crenshaw, T. L., & Goldberg, J. P. (1996). Sexual pharmacology: Drugs that affect sexual function. New York: W. W. Norton.

Crepault, C., & Couture, M. (1980). Men's erotic fantasies. Archives of Sexual Behavior, 9, 565–581.

Cromer, B. A., Blair, J. M., Mahan, J. D., Zibners, L., & Naumovski, Z. (1996). A prospective comparison of bone density in adolescent girls receiving depot medroxyprogesterone acetate (Depo-Provera), levonorgestrel (Norplant), or oral contraceptives. Journal of Pediatrics, 129, 671–676.

Cromer, B. A., Frankel, M. E., Hayes, J., & Brown, R. T. (1992). Compliance with breast self-examination instruction in high school students. Clinical Pediatrics, 31, 215–220.

Crowe, L. C., & George, W. H. (1989). Alcohol and human sexuality: Review and integration. Psychological Bulletin, 105, 374–386.

Crowe, M. J., & Ridley, J. (1990). Therapy with couples. London: Blackwell.

Crowe, M., & Ridley, J. (1990). Therapy with couples: A behavioural systems approach to marital and sexual problems. Maldon, MA: Blackwell Science Inc.

Cupach, W. R., & Spitzberg, B. H. (1998). Obsessive relational intrusion and stalking. In B. H. Spitzberg & W. R. Cupach (Eds.), The dark side of close relationships (pp. 233–263). Hillsdale NJ: Lawrence Erlbaum.

Cupid's cubicles. (1998, December 14). U. S. News & World Report, 44–51.

Curbing prostitution on demand side. (1992, April 20). The New York Times, B8.

Current Biography, (1968). Masters, William H(owell), 247–249.

Cushman, L. F., Kalmuss, D., Davidson, A. R., Heartwell, S., & Rulin, M. (1996). Beliefs about Depo-Provera among three groups of contraceptors. Advances in Contraception, 12, 43–52.

Dailey, D. M. (1997). The failure of sexuality education: Meeting the challenge of behavioral change in a sex-positive context. Journal of Psychology & Human Sexuality, 9, 87–97.

Dailey, D. M. (Ed.). (1989). The sexually unusual: A guide to understanding and helping. Binghamton, NY: Haworth Press.

Dallas, J. (1996). In defense of clinical treatment for homosexuality. Journal of Psychology & Christianity, 15, 369–372.

Daniels, P., & Weingarten, K. (1982). Sooner or later. The timing of parenthood in adult lives. New York: W. W. Norton & Company.

Dankoski, M. E., Payer, R., & Steinberg, M. (1996). Broadening the concept of adolescent promiscuity: Male accountability made visible and the implications for family therapists. American Journal of Family Therapy, 24, 367–381.

Darling, C. A., & Davidson, J. K. Sr. (1986). Coitally active university students: Sexual behaviors, concerns, and challenges. Adolescence, 21, 403–419.

Darling, C. A., & Davidson, J. K. Sr. (1987). Guilt: A factor in sexual satisfaction. Sociological Inquiry, 57, 251–271.

Darling, C. A., Davidson, J. K., & Cox, R. P. (1991). Female sexual response and the timing of partner orgasm. Journal of Sex and Marital Therapy, 17, 3–21.

Darling, C. A., Davidson, J. K., & Jennings, D. A. (1991). The female sexual response revisited: Understanding the multiorgasmic experience in women. Archives of Sexual Behavior, 20, 527–540.

Darling, C. A., Davidson, Sr., J. K., & Passarello, L. C. (1992). The mystique of first intercourse among college youth: The role of partners, contraceptive practices, and psychological reactions. Journal of Youth and Adolescence, 21, 97–117.

Davey Smith, G., Frankel, S., & Yarnell, J. (1997). Sex and death: Are they related? Findings from the Caerphilly Cohort Study. British Medical Journal, 315 (7123), 1641–1644.

Davidson, A. R., & Kalmuss, D. (1997). Topics for our times: Norplant coercion - an overstated threat. American Journal of Public Health, 87, 550–551.

Davidson, J. K., & Darling, C. A. (1993). Masturbatory guilt and sexual responsiveness among post-college-age women: Sexual satisfaction revisited. Journal of Sex and Marital Therapy, 19, 289–300.

Davidson, J. K., & Moore, N. B. (1994). Masturbation and premarital sexual intercourse among college women: Making choices for sexual fulfillment. Journal of Sex and Marital Therapy, 20, 178–199.

Davidson, J. K., Darling, C. A., & Conway-Welch, C. (1989). The role of the Grafenberg spot and female ejaculation in the female orgasmic response: An empirical analysis. Journal of Sex & Marital Therapy, 15, 102–120.

Davidson, Sr., J. K., Darling, C. A., & Conway-Welch, C. (1989). The role of the Grafenberg Spot and female ejaculation in the female orgasmic response: An empirical analysis. Journal of Sex & Marital Therapy, 15, 102–120.

Davies, H. D., Zeiss, A., & Tinklenberg, J. R. (1992). 'Til death do us part: Intimacy and sexuality in the marriages of Alzheimer's patients. Journal of Psychosocial Nursing and Mental Health Services, 30, 5–10.

Davies, K. A. (1997). Voluntary exposure to pornography and men's attitudes toward feminism and rape. The Journal of Sex Research, 34, 131–137.

Davis, C. M., Blank, J., Lin, H-Y., & Bonillas, C. (1996). Characteristics of vibrator use among women. Journal of Sex Research, 33, 313–320.

Davis, J. P., Chesny, P. J., Wand, P. J., LaVenture, M., & the Investigation and Laboratory Team. (1980). Toxic-shock syndrome - epidemiologic features, recurrence, risk factors, and prevention. New England Journal of Medicine, 303, 1429–1435.

Davis, L. G., Riedmann, G. L., Sapiro, M., Minogue, J. P., & Kazer, R. R. (1994). Cesarean section rates in low-risk private patients managed by certified nurse-midwives and obstetricians. Journal of Nurse-Midwifery, 39, 91–97.

Davis, S. R., Rosen, D. H., Steinberg, S., Wortley, P. M., Karon, J. M., & Gwinn, M. (1998). Trends in HIV prevalence among childbearing women in the United States, 1989–1994. Journal of Acquired Immunodeficiency Syndromes and Human Retrovirology, 19, 158–164.

Davison, G. C. (1977). Elimination of a sadistic fantasy by a client controlled counterconditioning technique: A case study. In J. Fischer & H. L. Gochros (Eds.), Handbook of behavior therapy with sexual problems (pp. 542–551). New York: Pergamon Press.

Dawkins, R. (1976). The selfish gene. New York: Oxford University Press.

Day, N. (1995). Abortion: Debating the issue. Springfield, NJ: Enslow.

Day, S. M. (1995). American Indians: Reclaiming cultural and sexual identity. SIECUS Report, 23, 6–7.

Dayringer, R., Paiva, R. E., & Davidson, G. W. (1983). Ethical decision making by family physicians. Journal of Family Practice, 17, 267–272.

De Aguilar, M. A., Altamirano, L., Leon, D. A., De Fung, R. C., Grillo, A. E., Gonzalez, J. D., Canales, J. R., Sanchez, J del C., Pozuelos, J. L., Ramirez, L., Rigionni, R., Salgado, J. S., Torres, L., Vallecillos, G., Zambrano, E. J., & Zea, C. (1997). Current status of injectable hormonal contraception, with special reference to the monthly method. Advances in Contraception, 13, 405–417.

De Gaston, J. F., Weed, S., & Jensen, L. (1996). Understanding gender differences in adolescent sexuality. Adolescence, 31, 217–231.

de Lignieres, B. (1993). Transdermal dihydrotestosterone treatment of 'andropause.' Annals of Medicine, 25, 235–241.

de Veciana, M. (1998). Diabetes and female sexuality. Diabetes Reviews, 6, 54–64.

Deacon, S., Minichiello, V., & Plummer, D. (1995). Sexuality and older people: Revisiting the assumptions. Educational Gerontology, 21, 497–513.

DeKeseredy, W. S., & Schwartz, M. D. (1997). Woman abuse on campus: Results from the Canadian national survey. Thousand Oaks, CA: Sage Publishing.

Dekker, R., & van de Pol, L. (1989). The tradition of female transvestism in early modern Europe. New York: St. Martin's Press.

DeKoker, B. (1996). Sex and the spinal cord. Scientific American, 275, 30–32.

DeLameter, J., & MacCorquodale, P. (1979). Premarital sexuality: Attitudes, relationships, behavior. Madison, WI: University of Wisconsin Press.

Delaney, J., Lupton, M. J., & Toth, E. (1976). The curse, a cultural history of menstruation. New York: E. P. Dutton and Co.

deMayo, R. A. (1997). Patient sexual behavior and sexual harassment: A national survey of female psychologists. Professional Psychology: Research and Practice, 28, 58–62.

Denil, J., Ohl, D. A., & Smythe, C. (1996). Vacuum erection device in spinal cord injured men: Patient and partner satisfaction. Archives of Physical Medicine and Rehabilitation, 77, 750–753.

Dennerstein, L. (1994). In pursuit of happiness: Well-being during the menopausal transition. In G. Berg & M. Hammar (Eds.), The modern management of the menopause (pp. 151–159). New York: The Parthenon Publishing Group.

Dennerstein, L. (1995). Mental health, work, and gender. International Journal of Health Services, 25, 503–509.

Denny, N. W., Field, J. K., & Quadagno, D. (1984). Sex differences in sexual needs and desires. Archives of Sexual Behavior, 13, 233–245.

DePuy, C., & Dovitch, D. (1997). The healing choice: Your guide to emotional recovery after an abortion. New York: Simon & Schuster.

Derlega, V. J., Wilson, M., & Chaikin, A. L. (1976). Friendship and disclosure reciprocity. Journal of Personality and Social Psychology, 34, 578–582.

Derouesne, C., Guigot, J., Chermat, V., Winchester, N., & Lacomblez, L. (1996). Sexual behavioral changes in Alzheimer's disease. Alzheimer Disease and Associated Disorders, 10, 86–92.

deVincenzi, I., & Mertens, T. (1994). Male circumcision: A role in HIV prevention? AIDS, 8, 153–160.

Dewaraja, R., & Sasaki, Y. (1991). Semen-loss syndrome: A comparison between Sri Lanka and Japan. American Journal of Psychotherapy, 45, 14–20.

DeWit, M. L., & Rajulton, F. (1992). Education and timing of parenthood among Canadian women: A cohort analysis. Social Biology, 39, 109–122.

Dhawan, S., & Marshall, W. L. (1996). Sexual abuse histories of sexual offenders. Sexual Abuse: A Journal of Research and Treatment, 8, 7–15.

Diaz, A., Jaffe, L. R., Leadbeater, B. J., & Levin, L. (1990). Frequency of use, knowledge, and attitudes toward the contraceptive sponge among inner-city black and Hispanic adolescent females. Journal of Adolescent Health Care, 11, 125–127.

DiBartolo, P. M., & Barlow, D. H. (1996). Perfectionism, marital satisfaction, and contributing factors to sexual dysfunction in men with erectile disorder and their spouses. Archives of Sexual Behavior, 25, 581–588.

DiClemente, R. J. (1998). Preventing sexually transmitted infections among adolescents. A clash of ideology and science. Journal of the American Medical Association, 279, 1574–1575.

Dignan, M., Michielutte, R., Wells, H. B., & Bahnson, J. (1994). The Forsyth county cervical cancer prevention project - I. Cervical cancer screening for black women. Health Education Research, 9, 411–420.

Ditto, P. H., Moore, K. A., Hilton, J.L., & Kalish, J. R. (1995). Beliefs about physicians: Their role in health care. Basic and Applied Social Psychology, 17, 23–48.

Docter, R. F., & Prince, V. (1997). Transvestism: A survey of 1032 cross-dressers. Archives of Sexual Behavior, 26, 589–605.

Donnelly, D. A. (1993). Sexually inactive marriages. Journal of Sex Research, 30, 171–179.

Donnerstein, E., & Malamuth, N. (1997). Pornography: Its consequences on the observer. In L. B. Schlesinger & E. Revitch (Eds.), Sexual dynamics of anti-social behavior (2nd ed.) (pp. 30–49). Springfield, IL: Charles C. Thomas.

Dorfman, R., Walters, K., Burke, P., Hardin, L., Karanik, T., Raphael, J., & Silverstein, E. (1995). Old, sad, and alone: The myth of the aging homosexual. Journal of Gerontological Social Work, 24, 29–44.

d'Oro, L. C., Parazzini, F., Naldi, L., & La Vecchia, C. (1994). Barrier methods of contraception, spermicides, and sexually transmitted diseases: A review. Genitourinary Medicine, 70, 410–417.

Douglas, J. M., Jr. (1990). Molluscum contagiosum. In K. K. Holmes, Mardh, P. A., Sparling, P. F., & Wiesner, P. J. (Eds.), Sexually transmitted diseases (2nd ed.) (pp. 443–447). New York: McGraw-Hill Information Services Company.

Downing, J. (1996). Dreams and nightmares. A book of Gestalt therapy sessions (2nd ed.). Highland, NY: Gestalt Journal Press.

Drife, J. O. (1997). The benefits and risks of oral contraceptives today. New York: Parthenon Publishing Group.

Drory, Y., Fisman, E. Z., Shapira, Y., & Pines, A. (1996). Ventricular arrhythmias during sexual activity in patients with coronary artery disease. Chest, 109, 922–924.

Dubois, C. L. Z., Knapp, D. E., Faley, R. H., & Kustis, G. A. (1998). An empirical examination of same- and other-gender sexual harassment in the workplace. Sex Roles: A Journal of Research, 39, 731–749.

Dunbar-Jacob, J., Begg, L., Yasko, J., & Belle, S. (1991). Breast self-examination compliance among older high risk women. Patient Education & Counseling, 18, 223–230.

Dunlap, D. W. (1995, May 10). Two universities with religious links, with two distinct approaches to dealing with gay groups. The New York Times, B11.

Dunlap, D. W. (1996, January 31). Judge voids an Alabama law against gay campus groups. The New York Times, B6.

Dunn, M. W., & Trost, J. E. (1989). Male multiple orgasms: A descriptive study. Archives of Sexual Behavior, 18, 377–387.

Dupont, S. (1996). Sexual function and ways of coping in patients with multiple sclerosis and their partners. Sexual & Marital Therapy, 11, 359–372.

Duran-Aydintug, C., & Causey, K. A. (1996). Child custody determination: Implications for lesbian mothers. Journal of Divorce & Remarriage, 25, 55–74.

Durkin, K. F. (1997). Misuse of the Internet by pedophiles: Implications for law enforcement and probation practice. Federal Probation, 61, 14–18.

Durodoye, B. A. (1994). Intermarriage and marital satisfaction. TCA Journal, 22, 5–9.

Dykstra, P. A. (1995). Loneliness among the never and formerly married. The importance of supportive friendships and a desire for independence. Journals of Gerontology: Series B: Psychological Sciences & Social Sciences, 50B, S321–S329.

Eagly, A. H. (1995). The science and politics of comparing women and men. American Psychologist, 50, 145–158.

Earl, D. T., & David, D. J. (1994). Depo-Provera: An injectable contraceptive. American Family Physician, 49, 891–894.

Earls, C. M., & David, H. (1989). A psychosocial study of male prostitution. Archives of Sexual Behavior, 18, 401–419.

Ebbesen, E. B., Kjos, G. L., & Konecni, V. J. (1976). Spatial ecology: Its effects on the choice of friends and enemies. Journal of Experimental Social Psychology, 12, 505–518.

Ebel, C. (1998). Managing herpes: How to live and love with a chronic STD. Research Triangle Park, NC: American Social Health Association.

Echols, R. M., Heyd, A., O'Keeffe, B. J., & Schacht, P. (1994). Single-dose ciprofloxacin for the treatment of uncomplicated gonorrhea: A worldwide summary. Sexually Transmitted Diseases, 21, 345–352.

Edge, V., & Miller, M. (1994). Women's health care. St. Louis: Mosby.

Edgerton, R. B. (1973). Some socio-cultural research considerations. In F. F. De La Cruz & G. D. LaVeck (Eds.), Sexuality and the mentally retarded. New York: Brunner-Mazel.

Edwards, S. (1996). Balanitis and balanoposthitis: A review. Genitourinary Medicine, 72, 155–159.

Ehrhardt, A. A. (1996). Our view of adolescent sexuality: A focus on risk behavior without the developmental context. American Journal of Public Health, 86, 1523–1525.

Ehrhardt, A. A., Meyer-Bahlburg, H. F. L., Rosen, L. R., Feldman, J. F., Veridiano, N. P., Zimmerman, I., & McEwen, B. S. (1985). Sexual orientation after prenatal exposure to exogenous estrogen. Archives of Sexual Behavior, 14, 57–78.

Ehrlich, P. (1975). The population bomb. Mattituck, NY: Amereon, Ltd.

Eicher, E. (1994). Sex and trinucleotide repeats. Nature Genetics, 6, 221–223.

Eisenberg, A., Murisoff, H. E., & Hathaway, S. E. (1996). What to expect when you're expecting. New York: Workman Publishing.

Eisler, R. M., & Blalock, J. A. (1991). Masculine gender role stress: Implications for the assessment of men. Clinical Psychology Review, 11, 45–60.

Eitzen, J. P., & Sawyer, R. G. (1997). Sexually transmitted diseases: Risk behaviors of female active duty U. S. army recruits. Military Medicine, 162, 686–689.

Elash, A. (October 2, 1995). The shock effect. Advertisers face a backlash over sexual images. Maclean's, 108, 36–37.

El-Bassel, N., Schilling, R. F., Irwin, K. L., Faruque, S., Gilbert, L. Von Bargen, J., Serrano, Y., & Edlin, B. R. (1997). Sex trading and psychological distress among women recruited from the streets of Harlem. American Journal of Public Health, 87, 66–70.

Elias, M. (1997, April 3). New sexual revolution taking place on Net. USA Today, D1.

Elkins, T. E., Kope, S., Ghaziuddin, M., Sorg, C., & Quint, E. (1997). Integration of a sexuality counseling service into a reproductive health program for persons with mental retardation. Journal of Pediatric and Adolescent Gynecology, 10, 24–27.

Ellis, H. (1933). The psychology of sex (2nd ed.). New York: Harcourt Brace Jovanovich.

Ellis, H. (1936). Studies in the psychology of sex (Vols. 1–2). New York: Random House.

Elshtain, J. B. (1998). Beyond consent. The New Republic, 218, 8–9.

Elton, C. (1997). Jail baiting: Statutory rape's dubious comeback. The New Republic, 217, 12–13.

Eng, T. R., & Butler, W. T. (Eds.) (1997). The hidden epidemic: Confronting sexually transmitted diseases. Washington, D. C.: National Academy Press.

Engel, J. D., & McVary, K. T. (1998). Transurethral alprostadil as therapy for patients who withdrew from or failed prior intracavernous injection therapy. Urology, 51, 687–692.

Entwisle, B., & Kozyreva, P. (1997). New estimates of induced abortion in Russia. Studies in Family Planning, 28, 14–23.

Epel, E. S., Spanakos, A., Kasl-Godley, J., & Brownell, K. D. (1996). Body shape ideals across gender, sexual orientation, socioeconomic status, race, and age in personal advertisements. International Journal of Eating Disorders, 19, 265–273.

Episcopal bishop goes on trial for ordaining gay priest. (1996, February 20). OutNOW. [on-line].

Epstein, A. W. (1969). Fetishism: A comprehensive review. In J. H. Masserman (Ed.), Science and psychoanalysis, Vol. 15 (pp. 81–87). New York: Grune and Stratton.

Equal Employment Opportunities Commission (1980). Guidelines on discrimination because of sex. Federal Register, 45, 74676–74677.

Erickson, P. I., Bastani, R., Maxwell, A. E., Marcus, A. C., Capell, F. J., & Yan, K. X. (1995). Prevalence of anal sex among heterosexuals in California and its relationship to other AIDS risk behaviors. AIDS Education and Prevention, 7, 477–493.

Erikson, E. (1963). Childhood and Society. (2nd ed.). New York: W. W. Norton & Company.

Erikson, E. H. (1962). Young man Luther. New York: W. W. Norton.

Erikson, E. H. (1968). Identity, youth, and crisis. New York: Norton.

Escala, J. M., & Rickwood, A. M. (1989). Balanitis. British Journal of Urology, 63, 196–197.

Eskridge, W. N. (1995). The many faces of sexual consent. William and Mary Law Review, 37, 47–67.

Etherington, K. (1997). Maternal sexual abuse of males. Child Abuse Review, 6, 107–117.

Ethical Standards for Psychologists. (1992). Washington, D. C.: American Psychological Association.

Eurenius, K., Axelsson, O., Gallstedt-Fransson, I., & Sjoden, P. O. (1997). Perception of information, expectations and experiences among women and their partners attending a second-trimester routine ultrasound scan. Ultrasound in Obstetrics and Gynecology, 9, 86–90.

Evans, B. A., Bond, R. A., & MacRae, K. D. (1998). Heterosexual behaviour, risk factors and sexually transmitted infections among self-classified homosexual and bisexual men. International Journal of STD and AIDS, 9, 129–133.

Evans, S. (1994). Counseling: A crucial aspect of care. Washington Post Health, 10, 21.

Everhardt, E., Dony, J. M., Jansen, H., Lemmens, W. A., & Doesburg, W. H. (1990). Improvement of cervical mucus viscoelasticity and sperm penetration with sodium bicarbonate douching. Human Reproduction, 5, 133–137.

Fagot, B. I., & Hagan, R. (1991). Observations of parental reactions to sex-stereotyped behaviors: Age and sex effects. Child Development, 62, 617–628.

Fagot, B. I., Leinbach, M. D., & O'Boyle, C. (1992). Gender labeling, gender stereotyping, and parenting behaviors. Developmental Psychology, 28, 225–230.

Faison, S. (1997, September 2). Tolerance grows for homosexuals in China. The New York Times. [http://www.nytimes.com].

Falcone, T., Goldberg, J. M., & Miller, K. F. (1996). Endometriosis: Medical and surgical intervention. Current Opinion in Obstetrics and Gynecology, 8, 178–183.

Falk, G. T. (1996). Review of "The African aids epidemic," by J. C. Caldwell and Pat Caldwell, Scientific American, March 1996. [on line]. Family Physician, 51, 1531–1542.

Farley, M., & Barkan, H. (1998). Prostitution, violence, and posttraumatic stress disorder. Women & Health, 27, 37–49.

Farley, M., Baral, I., Kiremire, M., & Sezgin, U. (1998). Prostitution in five countries: Violence and post-traumatic stress disorder. Feminism & Psychology, 8, 405–426.

Farr, G., Gabelnick, H., Sturgen, K., & Dorflinger, L. (1994). Contraceptive efficacy and acceptability of the female condom. American Journal of Public Health, 84, 1960–1964.

Faulkner, A. H., & Cranston, K. (1998). Correlates of same-sex sexual behavior in a random sample of Massachusetts high school students. American Journal of Public Health, 88, 262–266.

Fee-Fulkerson, K., Conaway, M. R., Winer, E. P., Fulkerson, C. C., Rimer, B. K., & Georgiade, G. (1996). Factors contributing to patient satisfaction with breast reconstruction using silicone gel implants. Plastic and Reconstructive Surgery, 97, 1420–1426.

Fegan, L., & Rauch, A. (1993). Sexuality and people with intellectual disability. Baltimore: Paul H. Brookes Publishing Company.

Feldman, H., & Feldman, M. (Eds.). (1985). Current controversies in marriage and family. Beverly Hills, CA: Sage Publications.

Fenell, D. L. (1993). Characteristics of long-term first marriages. Journal of Mental Health Counseling, 15, 446–460.

Fennell, T. (1998, November 9). The evidence of rape. Indonesia's Chinese live in fear. Maclean's, 111, 30–31.

Fenster, L., Katz, D. R., Wyrobek, A. J., Pieper, C., Rempel, D. M., Oman, D., & Swan, S. H. (1997). Effects of psychological stress on human semen quality. Journal of Andrology, 18, 194–202.

Ferdinand, P. (1996, June 21). Youthful trek ends in 'Net loss for love. Boston Globe, 1.

Ferrell, M., Tolone, W., & Walsh, R. (1977). Maturational and societal changes in the sexual double-standard: A panel analysis (1967–1971; 1970–1974). Journal of Marriage and the Family, 39, 255–271.

Filer, R. B., & Wu, C. H. (1989). Coitus during menses. Its effects on endometriosis and pelvic inflammatory disease. Journal of Reproductive Medicine, 34, 887–890.

Fine, R. (1987). Psychoanalytic theory. In L. Diamant (Ed.), Male and female homosexuality (pp. 81–95). New York: Hemisphere Publishing Corporation.

Finkelhor, D. (1984). Child sexual abuse: New theory and research. New York: Free Press.

Finkelhor, D. (1994). Current information on the scope and nature of child sexual abuse. Future of Children, 4, 31–53.

Finkelstein, M. A., & Brannick, M. T. (1997). Making decisions about sexual intercourse: Capturing college students' policies. Basic & Applied Social Psychology, 19, 101–120.

Firestone, P., Bradford, J. M., McCoy, M., Greenberg, D. M., Curry, S., & Larose, M. R. (1998). Recidivism in convicted rapists. Journal of the American Academy of Psychiatry and Law, 26, 185–200.

Fishbein, M., & Burgess, E. W. (Eds.). (1947). Successful marriage. Garden City, NY: Doubleday & Company.

Fishbein, M., & Burgess, E. W. (Eds.). (1947). Successful marriage. Garden City, NY: Doubleday & Company.

Fisher, W. A. (1988). Erotophobia-erotophilia as a dimension of personality. Journal of Sex Research, 25, 123–151.

Fisher, W. A., & Byrne, D. (1978). Sex differences in response to erotica. Love versus lust. Journal of Personality and Social Psychology, 36, 117–125.

Fisher, W. A., Byrne, D., White, L. A., & Kelley, K. (1988). Erotophobia-erotophilia as a dimension of personality. Journal of Sex Research, 25, 123–151.

Fitness, J., & Fletcher, G. J. O. (1993). Love, hate, anger, and jealousy in close relationships: A prototype and cognitive appraisal analysis. Journal of Personality and Social Psychology, 65, 942–958.

Fitzwater, T. (1998). Manager's pocket guide to preventing sexual harassment. Amherst, MA: Human Resource Development Press.

Fleming, D. T., McQuillan, G. M., Johnson, R. E., et al. (1997). Herpes simplex virus type 2 in the United States, 1976–1994. New England Journal of Medicine, 337, 1105.

Flieger, K. (1995). Testosterone. Key to masculinity and more. FDA Consumer, May, 27–31.

Flores, R. Z., & Mattos, L. F. C. (1998). Incest: Frequency, predisposing factors, and effects in a Brazilian population. Current Anthropology, 39, 554–558.

Ford, C. S., & Beach, F. A. (1951). Patterns of sexual behavior. New York: Harper and Brothers, Publishers and Paul B. Hoeber, Inc., Medical Books.

Forrest, G. G. (1995). Alcohol and human sexuality. Northvale, NJ: Jason Aronson.

Forsyth, C. J. (1996). The structuring of vicarious sex. Deviant Behavior: An Interdisciplinary Journal, 17, 279–295.

Forsyth, C. J., & Deshotels, T. H. (1997). The occupational milieu of the nude dancer. Deviant Behavior: An Interdisciplinary Journal, 18, 125–142.

Forward, S., & Buck, C. (1989). A traicao da inocencia: O incesto e suas consequencias. Rio de Janeiro: Rocco.

Fox, K. K., Whittington, W. L., Levine, W. C., Moran, J. S., Zaidi, A. A., & Nakashima, A. K. (1998). Gonorrhea in the United States, 1981–1996. Demographic and geographic trends. Sexually Transmitted Diseases, 25, 386–393.

Fox, R. (1993). Male masturbation and female orgasm. Society, 30, 21–25.

Francoeur, R. T. (1991). Becoming a sexual person (2nd ed.). New York: Macmillan Publishing Company.

Franzoi, S. L., & Shields, S. A. (1984). The body esteem scale: Multidimensional structure and sex differences in a college population. Journal of Personality Assessment, 48, 173–178.

Frazee, C. A. (1988). The origins of clerical celibacy in the western church. Church History, 57, supplement, 108–126.

Freud, S. (1905). Three essays on the theory of sexuality. New York: Basic Books.

Freud, S. (1943). A general outline to psychoanalysis. Garden City, NY: Garden City Publishing.

Freud, S. (1965). The interpretation of dreams (J. Strachey, Trans.). New York: Avon Books. (Original work published 1900).

Freund, K., & Blanchard, R. (1986). The concept of courtship disorder. Journal of Sex and Marital Therapy, 12, 79–92.

Freund, K., Seto, M. C., & Kuban, M. (1996). Two types of fetishism. Behavior Research and Therapy, 34, 687–694.

Freund, K., Seto, M. C., & Kuban, M. (1997). Frotteurism. Frotteurism and the theory of courtship disorder. In D. R. Laws & W. O'Donohue (Eds.), Sexual deviance. Theory, assessment, and treatment (pp. 111–130). New York: The Guilford Press.

Friday, N. (1991). Women on top: How real life has changed women's sexual fantasies. New York: Simon & Schuster.

Friedrich, W. N., Fisher, J., Broughton, D., Houston, M., & Shafran, C. R. (1998). Normative sexual behavior in children: A contemporary sample. Pediatrics, 101 [electronic article].

Froelicher, E. S., Kee, L. L., Newton, K. M., Lindskog, B., & Livingston, M. (1994). Return to work, sexual activity, and other activities after acute myocardial infarction. Heart & Lung, 23, 423–435.

Fromm, E. (1962). The art of loving. New York: Harper & Row.

Fromuth, M. E., & Conn, V. E. (1997). Hidden perpetrators: Sexual molestation in a nonclinical sample of college women. Journal of Interpersonal Violence, 12, 456–465.

Frye, C. A., & Weisberg, R. B. (1994). Increasing the incidence of routine pelvic examinations: Behavioral medicine's contribution. Women & Health, 21, 33–55.

Funke, B. L., & Nicholson, M. E. (1993). Factors affecting patient compliance among women with abnormal Pap smears. Patient Education & Counseling, 20, 5–15.

Furby, L., Ochs, L. M., & Thomas, C. W. (1997). Sexually transmitted disease prevention: Adolescents' perceptions of possible side effects. Adolescence, 32, 781–809.

Futterman, E. (1996, February 22). Finding a man: Some cold, hard facts. St. Louis Post-Dispatch, 55.

Gagnon, J. H. (1990). The explicit and implicit use of the scripting perspective in sex research. Annual Review of Sex Research, 1, 1–43.

Gagnon, J. H., & Simon, W. (1987). The sexual scripting of oral genital contacts. Archives of Sexual Behavior, 16, 1–25.

Gamman, L., & Makinen, M. (1994). Female fetishism. New York: New York University Press.

Ganem, J. P., Lucey, D. T., Janosko, E. O., & Carson, C. C. (1998). Unusual complications of the vacuum erection device. Urology, 51, 627–631.

Garcia, L. T., Brennan, K., DeCarlo, M., McGlennon, R., & Tait, S. (1984). Sex differences in sexual arousal to different erotic stories. The Journal of Sex Research, 20, 391–402.

Gaston, M. H., & Moody, L. E. (1995). Improving utilization of breast and cervical cancer screening in your office practice. Journal of the National Medical Association, 87, 700–704.

Gayford, J. J. (1981). Indecent exposure: A review of the literature. Medicine, Science, and the Law, 21, 233–242.

Geasler, M. J., Croteau, J. M., Neineman, C. J., & Edlund, C. J. (1995). A qualitative study of students' expressions of change after attending panel presentations by lesbian, gay, and bisexual speakers. Journal of College Student Development, 36, 483–492.

Gebhard, P. (1973). Sexual behavior of the mentally retarded. In F. F. De La Cruz & G. D. LaVeck (Eds.), Human sexuality and the mentally retarded. New York: Brunner-Mazel.

Gebhard, P. M., & Johnson, A. B. (1979). The Kinsey data: Marginal tabulation of the 1938–1963 interviews conducted by the Institute of Sexual Research. Philadelphia: Saunders.

Genius, S. J., & Genius, S. K. (1996). Orgasm without organisms: Science or propaganda? Clinical Pediatrics, 35, 10–17.

George, N., Green, J., & Murphy, S. (1998). Sexually transmitted disease rates before and after HIV testing. International Journal of STD and AIDS, 9, 291–293.

Gerbase, A. C., Rowley, J. T., & Mertens, T. E. (1998). Global epidemiology of sexually transmitted diseases. Lancet, 351, Supplement 3, 2–4.

Gergen, K. J., & Gergen, M. M. (1986). Social psychology (2nd ed.). New York: Springer Verlag.

Ghizzani, A., Pirtoli, A., Bellezza, A., & Velicogna, F. (1995). The evaluation of some factors influencing the sexual life of women affected by breast cancer. Journal of Sex & Marital Therapy, 21, 57–63.

Ghubash, R., & Abou-Saleh, M. T. (1997). Postpartum psychiatric ilness in Arab culture: Prevalence and psychosocial correlates. British Journal of Psychiatry, 171, 65–68.

Giblin, P. (1994). Premarital preparation: Three approaches. Pastoral Psychology, 42, 147–161.

Gibran, K. (1977). The prophet. New York: Alfred A. Knopf.

Giddens, A. (1992). The transformation of intimacy. Stanford, CA: Stanford University Press.

Gil, V. E. (1990). Sexual fantasy experiences and guilt among conservative Christians: An exploratory study. The Journal of Sex Research, 27, 629–638.

Giles, J. (1994). A theory of love and sexual desire. Journal for the Theory of Social Behaviour, 24, 339–357.

Gillespie, B. L., & Eisler, R. M. (1992). Development of the feminine gender role stress scale. Behavior Modification, 16, 426–438.

Gilligan, C. (1982). In a different voice: Psychological theory and women's development. Cambridge, MA: Harvard University Press.

Gillman, A. E., & Gordon, A. R. (1973). Sexual behavior in the blind. Medical Aspects of Human Sexuality, 7, 49–50, 53, 59–60.

Gladue, B. A. (1987). Psychobiological contributions. In L. Diamant (Ed.), Male and female homosexuality (pp. 129–154). New York: Hemisphere Publishing Corporation.

Gladue, B. A., Green, R., & Hellman, R. E. (1985). Neuroendocrine response to estrogen and sexual orientation. Science, 225, 1496–1499.

Glascock, J., & LaRose, R. (1993). Dial-a-porn recordings: The role of the female participant in male sexual fantasies. Journal of Broadcasting & Electronic Media, 37, 313–324.

Glass, S. P., & Wright, T. L. (1992). Justifications for extramarital relationships: The association between attitudes, behaviors, and gender. Journal of Sex Research, 29, 361–387.

Glenn, N. D., & McLanahan, S. (1982). Children and marital happiness: A further specification of the relationship. Journal of Marriage and the Family, 44, 63–72.

Gloeckner, M. R. (1983). Partner reaction following ostomy surgery. Journal of Sex & Marital Therapy, 9, 182–190.

Goldberg, A. (1995). The problem of perversion: The view from self psychology. New Haven, CT: Yale University Press.

Golden, J. S., Price, S., Heinrich, A. G., & Lobitz, W. C. (1978). Group vs. couple treatment of sexual dysfunctions. Archives of Sexual Behavior, 7, 593–602.

Golding, J., Henriques, J., & Thomas, P. (1986). Unmarried at delivery. II. Perinatal morbidity and mortality. Early Human Development, 14, 217–227.

Goldstein, I., Lue, T. F., Padma-Nathan, H., et al. (1998). Oral sildenafil in the treatment of erectile dysfunctions. Sildenafil study group. New England Journal of Medicine, 338, 1397–1404.

Golis, A. M. (1996). Sexual issues for the person with an ostomy. Journal of Wound, Ostomy, and Continence Nursing, 23, 33–37.

Golombok, S., & Tasker, F. (1996). Do parents influence the sexual orientation of their children? Findings from a longitudinal study of lesbian families. Developmental Psychology, 32, 3–11.

Gonorrhea among men who have sex with men—selected sexually transmitted disease clinic, 1993–1996. Morbidity and Mortality Weekly Report, September 26, 1997, 46, 889–892.

Good, G. E., & Mintz, L. B. (1990). Depression and the male role: Evidence for compounded risk. Journal of Counseling and Development, 69, 17–21.

Goodale, I. L., Domar, A. D., & Benson, H. (1990). Alleviation of premenstrual syndrome symptoms with the relaxation response. Obstetrics and Gynecology, 75, 649–655.

Goodson, P., & Edmundson, E. (1994). The problematic promotion of abstinence: An overview of Sex Respect. Journal of School Health, 64, 205–210.

Gordon, S., & Gilgun, J. F. (1987). Adolescent sexuality. In V. B. Van Hasselt & M. Hersen (Eds.), Handbook of adolescent psychology (pp. 147–167). New York: Pergamon Press.

Gosselin, C. C. (1987). The sadomasochistic contract. In G. D. Wilson (Ed.), Variant sexuality: Research and theory (pp. 229–258). Baltimore: The Johns Hopkins University Press.

Gottman, J. (1994). The seven principles for making marriage work. New York: Simon and Schuster.

Gould, S. J. (1981). The mismeasure of man. New York: Norton.

Govier, F., McClure, R., & Kramer-Levien, D. (1996). Endocrine screening for sexual dysfunction using free testosterone determinations. Journal of Urology, 156, 405–408.

Grady, D. (1998, November 6). Study says H.I.V. tests misstate women's risk. The New York Times, [http://www.nytimes.com].

Graham, C. A., & Sherwin, B. B. (1993). The relationship between mood and sexuality in women using an oral contraceptive as a treatment for premenstrual symptoms. Psychoneuroendocrinology, 18, 273–281.

Gravelle, K., & Gravelle, J. (1996). The period book. Everything you don't want to ask (but need to know). New York: Walker and Company.

Green, D. S., & Green, B. (1965, March). Double sex. Sexology, 561–563.

Green, R. (1974). Sexual identity conflict in children and adults. New York: Basic Books.

Green, R. (1987). The "sissy boy syndrome" and the development of homosexuality. New Haven: Yale University Press.

Greenacre, P. (1996). Fetishism. In I. Rosen (Ed.), Sexual deviation (3rd ed.) (pp. 88–110). Oxford: Oxford University Press.

Greenberg, D. M., Bradford, J. M., Curry, S., & O'Rourke, A. (1996). A comparison of treatment of paraphilias with three serotonin reuptake inhibitors: A retrospective study. Bulletin of the American Academy of Psychiatry and the Law, 24, 525–532.

Greenspoon, J., & Lamal, P. A. (1987). A behavioristic approach. In L. Diamant (Ed.), Male and female homosexuality (pp. 109–128). New York: Hemisphere Publishing Corporation.

Greenwald, J. (November 11, 1996). Barbie boots up. Time, 148, 48–50.

Greider, K. (1995). Medical chaperones. Self, 17, 100–103.

Grenier, G., & Byers, S. (1997). The relationships among ejaculatory control, ejaculatory latency, and attempts to prolong heterosexual intercourse. Archives of Sexual Behavior, 26, 27–47.

Grenier, R. (1993). Some advice on consent: This is going way too far. Insight on the News, 9, 28–29.

Greydanus, D. E., Pratt, H. D., & Dannison, L. L. (1995). Sexuality education programs for youth: Current state of affairs and strategies for the future. Journal of Sex Education & Therapy, 21, 238–254.

Grief, E. B., & Ulman, K. J. (1982). The psychological impact of menarche on early adolescent females: A review of the literature. Child Development, 53, 1413–1430.

Grosskopf, D. (1983). Sex and the married woman. New York: Simon & Schuster.

Grosskurth, H., Mosha, F., Todd, J., et al. (1995). Impact of improved treatment of sexually transmitted diseases on HIV infection in rural Tanzania: Randomised controlled trial. Lancet, 346, 530–536.

Grosskurth, P. (1980). Havelock Ellis. New York: Alfred A. Knopf.

Groth, A. N., & Burgess, A. W. (1977). Rape: A sexual deviation. American Journal of Orthopsychiatry, 47, 400–406.

Gruner, O-P. N., Naas, R., Fretheim, B., & Gjone, E. (1977). Marital status and sexual adjustment after colectomy. Scandinavian Journal of Gastroenterology, 12, 193–197.

Grunseit, A., Kippax, S., Aggleton, P., Baldo, M., & Slutkin, G. (1997). Sexuality education and young people's sexual behavior: A review of studies. Journal of Adolescence Research, 12, 421–453.

Guerrero, L. K., Andersen, P. A., Jorgensen, P. F., Spitzberg, B. H., & Eloy, S. V. (1995). Coping with the green-eyed monster: Conceptualizing and measuring communicative responses to romantic jealousy. Western Journal of Communication, 59, 270–304.

Guerrina, B. (1998). Mitigating punishment for statutory rape. University of Chicago Law Review, 65, 1251–1277.

Guinan, M. E. (1988). Virginity and celibacy as health issues. Journal of the American Medical Women's Association, 43, 60.

Gupta, M. C., Singh, M. M., Gurnani, K. C., & Pandey, D. N. (1990). Psychopathology of delayed resumption of sexual activity after myocardial infarction. Journal of the Association of Physicians of India, 38, 545–548.

Gupton, A., Heaman, M., & Ashcroft, T. (1997). Bed rest from the perspective of the high-risk pregnant woman. Journal of Obstetric, Gynecologic, and Neonatal Nursing, 26, 423–430.

Gutek, B. A., & Morasch, B. (1982). Sex-ratios, sex-role spillover, and sexual harassment of women at work. Journal of Social Issues, 38, 55–74.

Guyton, A. C. (1992). Human physiology and mechanisms of disease (3rd ed.). Philadelphia: W. B. Saunders Company.

Hadfield, R., Mardon, H., Barlow, D., & Kennedy, S. (1996). Human Reproduction, 11, 878–880.

Haffner, D. W. (1995). The essence of "consent" is communication. SIECUS Report, 24, 2–3.

Hage, J. J. (1995). Medical requirements and consequences of sex reassignment surgery. Medicine, Science, and Law, 35, 17–24.

Hailey, B., & Bradford, A. C. (1991). Breast self-examination and mammography among university staff and faculty. Women & Health, 17, 59–77.

Halberstam, D. (1993, May/June). Discovering sex. American Heritage, 39–58.

Hale, V. E., & Strassberg, D. S. (1990). The role of anxiety on sexual arousal. Archives of Sexual Behavior, 19, 569–581.

Hall, D. K., Mathews, F., & Pearce, J. (1998). Factors associated with sexual behavior problems in young sexually abused children. Child Abuse & Neglect, 22, 1045–1063.

Hall, J. (1974). Sexual behavior. In J. Wortis (Ed.), Mental retardation and developmental disabilities: An annual review IV. New York: Brunner-Mazel.

Hall, J. (1975). Sexuality and the mentally retarded. In R. Green (Ed.), Human sexuality: A health practitioner's text (p. 181–195). Baltimore: Williams & Wilkins.

Hall, J. E., & Morris, H. L. (1976). Sexual knowledge and attitudes of institutionalized retarded adolescents. American Journal of Mental Deficiency, 80, 382–387.

Hall, M. (1996). Unsexing the couple. Women & Therapy, 19, 1–11.

Halvorsen, J. G., & Metz, M. E. (1992). Sexual dysfunction, Part I: Classification, etiology, and pathogenesis. Journal of the American Board of Family Practice, 5, 51–61.

Hamer, D. H., Hu, S., Magnuson, V. L., Hu, N., & Pattatucci, A. M. L. (1993). A linkage between DNA markers on the X-chromosome and male sexual orientation. Science, 261, 321–327.

Hamer, D., & Copeland, P. (1994). The science of desire. The search for the gay gene and the biology of behavior. New York: Simon & Schuster.

Hammerschlag, M. R. (1998). Sexually transmitted diseases in sexually abused children: Medical and legal implications. Sexually Transmitted Infections, 74, 167–174.

Handel, N., Jensen, J. A., Black, Q., Waisman, J. R., & Silverstein, M. J. (1995). The fate of breast implants: A critical analysis of complications and outcomes. Plastic and Reconstructive Surgery, 96, 1521–1533.

Hanrahan, S. N. (1994). Historical review of menstrual toxic shock syndrome. Women & Health, 21, 141–165.

Hanson, R. K., & Bussiere, M. T. (1998). Predicting relapse: A meta-analysis of sexual offender recidivism studies. Journal of Consulting and Clinical Psychology, 66, 348–362.

Haqq, C., King, C., Ukiyama, E., Falsafi, S., Haqq, T., Donahoe, P., & Weiss, M. (1994). Molecular basis of mammalian sexual determination: Activation of Mullerian inhibiting substance gene expression by SRY. Science, 266, 1494–1499.

Hardy, J. B., Astone, N. M., Brooks-Gunn, J., Shapiro, S., & Miller, T. L. (1998). Like mother, like child: Intergenerational patterns of age at first birth and associations with childhood and adolescent characteristics and adult outcomes in the second generation. Developmental Psychology, 34, 1220–1232.

Harlow, S. D., & Park, M. (1996). A longitudinal study of risk factors for the occurrence, duration and severity of menstrual cramps in a cohort of college women. British Journal of Obstetrics and Gynaecology, 103, 1134–1142.

Harris, R. H. (1994). It's perfectly normal. Cambridge, MA: Candlewick Press.

Harris, S. M. (1995). Psychosocial development and black male masculinity: Implications for counseling economically disadvantaged African American male adolescents. Journal of Counseling and Development, 73, 279–287.

Hartmann, B. (1995). Reproductive rights and wrongs: The global politics of population control. Boston, MA: South End Press.

Harvey, J. (1995). Odyssey of the heart: The search for closeness, intimacy, and love. New York: Freeman.

Harvey, S. M., Beckman, L. J., & Murray, J. (1989). Factors associated with use of the contraceptive sponge. Family Planning Perspectives, 21, 179–183.

Hassan, E. O., el-Nahal, N., & el-Hussein, M. (1994). Acceptability of the once-a-month injectable contraceptives Cyclofem and Mesigyna in Egypt. Contraception, 49, 469–488.

Hatala, M. N., & Prehodka, J. (1996). Content analysis of gay male and lesbian personal advertisements. Psychological Reports, 78, 371–374.

Hatch, J. P. (1981). Voluntary control of sexual responding in men and women: Implications for the etiology and treatment of sexual dysfunction. Biofeedback and Self-Regulation, 6, 191–205.

Hatfield, E., & Rapson, R. L. (1987). Passionate love: New directions in research. In W. H. Jones & D. Perlman, Advances in personal relationships (pp. 109–139). Greenwich, CT: JAI.

Hatterer, L. J. (1976). Changing homosexuality in the male. New York: Dell.

Haugaard, J. J. (1996). Sexual behaviors between children: Professionals' opinions and undergraduates' recollections. The Journal of Contemporary Human Services, 77, 81–89.

Haugh, S., Hoffman, C., & Cowan, G. (1980). The eye of the very young beholder: Sex typing of infants by young children. Child Development, 51, 598–600.

Hawton, K. (1984). Sexual adjustment of men who have had strokes. Journal of Psychosomatic Research, 28, 243–249.

Hawton, K. (1985). Sex therapy: A practical guide. New York: Oxford University Press.

Hawton, K. (1998). Integration of treatments for male erectile dysfunction. The Lancet, 351, 7–8.

Hawton, K., Gath, D., & Day, A. (1994). Sexual function in a community sample of middle-aged women with partners: Effects of age, marital, socioeconomic, psychiatric, gynecological, and menopausal factors. Archives of Sexual Behavior, 23, 375–395.

Hayes, A. F. (1995). Age preferences for same- and opposite-sex partners. Journal of Social Psychology, 135, 125–133.

Hazan, C., & Shaver, P. R. (1987). Romantic love conceptualized as an attachment process. Journal of Personality and Social Psychology, 52,270–280.

Heath, C. B. (1993). Helping patients choose appropriate contraception. American Family Physician, 48, 1115–1124.

Hedon, B. (1990). The evolution of oral contraceptives. Maximizing efficacy, minimizing risks. Obstetricia y Gynecologica Scandinavica Supplement, 152,7–12.

Heiman, J. R. (1977). A psychophysiological exploration of sexual arousal patterns in females and males. Psychophysiology, 14, 266–274.

Heiman, J. R., Rowland, D. L., Hatch, J. P., & Gladue, B. A. (1991). Psychophysiological and endocrine responses to sexual arousal in women. Archives of Sexual Behavior, 20, 171–186.

Hellberg, D., Zdolsek, B., Nilsson, S., & Mardh, P. A. (1995). Sexual behavior of women with repeated episodes of vulvovaginal candidiasis. European Journal of Epidemiology, 11, 575–579.

Help wanted: Women and girls. Retrieved February 25, 1999 from the World Wide Web: http://www.prostitutionresearch.com/prosAD.html

Henderson, D. J., Boyd, C. J., & Whitmarsh, J. (1995). Women and illicit drugs: Sexuality and crack cocaine. Health Care for Women International, 16, 113–124.

Henderson-King, D. H., & Veroff, J. (1994). Sexual satisfaction and marital well-being in the first years of marriage. Journal of Social and Personal Relationships, 11, 509–534.

Hendrick, C., & Hendrick, S. S. (1993). Romantic love. Newbury Park, CA: Sage Press.

Hendrick, S., & Hendrick, C. (1992). Liking, loving, and relating (2nd ed.). Pacific Grove, CA: Brooks/Cole.

Henkin, W., & Holiday, S. (1996). Consensual sadomasochism. How to talk about it & how to do it safely. San Francisco, CA: Daedalus Publishing.

Henriques, J., Golding, J., & Thomas, P. (1986). Unmarried at delivery. I. The mothers and their care. Early Human Development, 14, 201–216.

Henshaw, S. K. (1987). Characteristics of U. S. women having abortions, 1982–1983. Family Planning Perspectives, 19, 5–9.

Henshaw, S. K. (1992). Research note: Abortion trends in 1987 and 1988—Age and race. Family Planning Perspectives, 24, 85–86.

Henshaw, S. K., & Kost, K. (1996). Abortion patients in 1994–1995: Characteristics and contraceptive use. Family Planning Perspectives, 28, 140–147.

Henton, C. L. (1976). Nocturnal orgasm in college women: It's relation to dreams and anxiety associated with sexual factors. Journal of Genetic Psychology, 129, 245–251.

Herdt, G. (1987). The Sambia: Ritual and gender in New Guinea. New York: Holt, Rinehart and Winston.

Herman, S. H., & Prewett, M. (1974). An experimental analysis of feedback to increase sexual arousal in a case of homosexual and heterosexual impotence: A preliminary report. Journal of Behavior Therapy and Experimental Psychiatry, 5, 271–274.

Herold, E., Corbesi, B., & Collins, J. (1995). Attitudes toward female topless beach behaviour: A study of male Australian university students. The Canadian Journal of Human Sexuality, 4, 177–182.

Hersh, K., & Gray-Little, B. (1998). Psychopathic traits and attitudes associated with self-reported sexual aggression in college men. Journal of Interpersonal Violence, 13, 456–471.

Hessellund, H. (1976). Masturbation and sexual fantasies in married couples. Archives of Sexual Behavior, 5, 133–147.

Hickey, A. R., Boyce, P. M., Ellwood, D., & Morris-Yates, A. D. (1997). Early discharge and risk for postnatal depression. Medical Journal of Australia, 167, 244–247.

Hill, A. (1998). Speaking truth to power. New York: Doubleday.

Hill, D. A., Weiss, N. S., Voigt, L. F., & Beresford, S. A. (1997). Endometrial cancer in relation to intra-uterine device use. International Journal of Cancer, 70, 278–281.

Himelein, M. J., Vogel, R. E., & Wachowiak, D. G. (1994). Nonconsensual sexual experiences in precollege women: Prevalence and risk factors. Journal of Counseling and Development, 72, 411–415.

Hines, M., & Collaer, M. L. (1993). Gonadal hormones and sexual differentiation of human behaviors: Developments from research on endocrine syndromes and studies of brain structure. Annual Review of Sex Research, 4, 1–48.

Hite, S. (1981). The Hite report on male sexuality. New York: Alfred A. Knopf.

HIV prevention through early detection and treatment of other sexually transmitted diseases—United States. Recommendations of the Advisory Committee for HIV and STD prevention. (1998, July 31). MMWR Morbidity and Mortality Weekly Reports, 47 (RR-12), 1–24.

Hobbins, J. (1997). Morphology of fetal growth. Acta Paediatrica Supplement, 423, 165–168.

Hoch, Z. (1986). Vaginal erotic sensitivity by sexological examination. Acta Obstetricia et Gynecologica Scandinavica, 65, 767–773.

Hodge, F. S., Fredericks, L., & Rodriguez, B. (1996). American Indian women's talking circle. A cervical cancer screening and prevention program. Cancer, 78, 1592–1597.

Hoeffer, B. (1981). Children's acquisition of sex-role behavior in lesbian-mother families. American Journal of Orthopsychiatry, 51, 536–544.

Hoffman, V., & Bolton, R. (1997). Reasons for having sex and sexual risk-taking: A study of heterosexual male STD clinic patients. AIDS CARE, 9, 285–296.

Hollender, M. H. (1970). The wish to be held. Archives of General Psychiatry, 22, 445–453.

Hollender, M. H. (1997). Genital exhibitionism in men and women. In L. B. Schlesinger & E. Revitch (Eds.), Sexual dynamics of anti-social behavior (2nd ed.) (pp. 119–131). Springfield, IL: Charles C. Thomas.

Holley, J. L., Schmidt, R. J., Bender, F. H., Dumler, F., & Schiff, M. (1997). Gynecologic and reproductive issues in women on dialysis. American Journal of Kidney Diseases, 29, 685–690.

Holmberg, A. R. (1946). The Siriono. Unpublished doctoral dissertation, Yale University, New Haven, Connecticut.

Holmes, A. S. (1995). The double standard in the English divorce laws, 1857–1923. Law & Social Inquiry: Journal of the American Bar Foundation, 20, 601–620.

Holmes, W. C., & Slap, G. B. (1998). Sexual abuse of boys: Definition, prevalence, correlates, sequelae, and management. Journal of the American Medical Association, 280, 1855–1862.

Homosexuals targeted for abuse. (1997, February 26). The Washington Post, A15.

Hook, E. W. (1998). Is elimination of endemic syphilis transmission a realistic goal for the USA? Lancet, 351, Supplement 3, 19–21.

Hooper, A. (1992). The ultimate sex book. New York: Dorling Kindersley, Inc.

Horner, M. S. (1970). Femininity and successful achievement: A basic inconsistency. In J. Bardwick, E. Douvan, M. S. Horner, & D. Gutmann (Eds.), Feminine personality and conflict. Monterey, CA: Brooks/Cole.

Horner, M. S. (1972). Toward an understanding of achievement related conflicts in women. Journal of Social Issues, 28, 157–176.

Horwood, L. J., & Fergusson, D. M. (1998). Breastfeeding and later cognitive and academic outcomes. Pediatrics, 101, E9.

Hosken, F. P. (1978). The epidemiology of female genital mutilations. Tropical Doctor, 8, 150.

How reliable are condoms? (1995, May). Consumer Reports, 60, 320–325.

Howitt, D. (1995). Pornography and the paedophile: Is it criminogenic? British Journal of Medical Psychology, 68, 15–27.

Hoyt, M. F. (1978). Primal scene experiences as recalled and reported by college students. Psychiatry, 41, 57–71.

Hoyt, M. F. (1979). Primal scene experiences: Quantitative assessment of an interview study. Archives of Sexual Behavior, 8, 225–245.

Hsu, J. H., & Shen, W. W. (1995). Male sexual side effects associated with antidepressants: A descriptive clinical study of 32 patients. The International Journal of Psychiatry in Medicine, 25, 191–201.

Hubinont, C., Kollmann, P., Malvaux, V., Donnez, J., & Bernard, P. (1997). First-trimester diagnosis of conjoined twins. Fetal Diagnosis and Therapy, 12, 185–187.

Hucker, S. J. (1997). Sexual sadism. Psychopathology and theory. In D. R. Laws & W. O'Donohue (Eds.), Sexual deviance. Theory, assessment, and treatment (pp. 194–209). New York: The Guilford Press.

Hunsberger, B. (1996). Religious fundamentalism, right-wing authoritarianism, and hostility toward homosexuals in non-Christian religious groups. International Journal for the Psychology of Religion, 6, 39–49.

Hunt, E. (1995). The role of intelligence in modern society. American Scientist, 83 (July-August), 356–368

Hunt, M. (1974). Sexual behavior in the 1970s. New York: Dell Books.

Hunter, J. (1990). Violence against lesbian and gay male youths. Journal of Interpersonal Violence, 5, 295–300.

Hunter, J. A., & Mathews, R. (1997). Sexual deviance in females. In D. R. Laws & W. O'Donohue (Eds.), Sexual deviance. Theory, assessment, and treatment (pp. 465–480). New York: The Guilford Press.

Hunter, M. S. (1994). The effects of estrogen therapy on mood and well-being. In G. Berg & M. Hammar (Eds.), The modern management of the menopause (pp. 177–184). New York: The Parthenon Publishing Group.

Hurlbert, D. F. (1992). Factors influencing a woman's decision to end an extramarital sexual relationship. Journal of Sex & Marital Therapy, 18, 104–113.

Hurlbert, D. F., & Apt, C. (1995). The coital alignment technique and directed masturbation: A comparative study on female orgasm. Journal of Sex & Marital Therapy, 21, 21–29.

Huston, A. C. (1983). Sex-typing. In P. H. Mussen (Ed.), Handbook of child psychology: Vol. 4. Socialization, personality and social development. New York: Wiley.

Hyde, J. S. (1979). Understanding human sexuality. New York: McGraw-Hill.

Imperato-McGinley, J. (1976). Gender identity and hermaphroditism: An exchange with J. Money. Science, 191, 872.

Ingersoll-Dayton, B., Campbell, R., Kurokawa, Y., & Saito, M. (1996). Separateness and togetherness: Interdependence over the life course in Japanese and American marriages. Journal of Social and Personal Relationships, 13, 385–398.

Inkeles, G. (1992). The new sensual massage. New York: Bantam Books.

Institute of Medicine. (1997). T. R. Eng & W. T. Butler (Eds.). The hidden epidemic: Confronting sexually transmitted diseases. Washington, D. C.: National Academy Press.

Ison, C. A., Dillon, J. R., & Tapsall, J. W. (1998). The epidemiology of global antibiotic resistance among Neisseria gonorrhoeae and Haemophilus ducreyi. Lancet, 351, Supplement 3, 8–11.

Itzhaki, J. (1996). The sperm that fail to get a grip. New Scientist, 150, 16.

Ivey, G., & Simpson, P. (1998). The psychological life of paedophiles: A phenomenological study. South African Journal of Psychology, 28, 15–20.

Jaarsma, T., Dracup, K., Walden, J., & Stevenson, L. W. (1996). Sexual function in patients with advanced heart failure. Heart and Lung, 25, 262–270.

Jackson, B. T. (1977). A case of voyeurism treated by counterconditioning. In J. Fischer & H. L. Gochros (Eds.), Handbook of behavior therapy with sexual problems (pp. 554–555). New York: Pergamon Press.

Jackson, L. A., & McGill, O. D. (1996). Body type preferences and body characteristics associated with attractive and unattractive bodies by African-Americans and Anglo Americans. Sex Roles, 35, 295–307.

Jacobs, C., & Wolf, E. (1995). School sexuality education and adolescent risk-taking behavior. Journal of School Health, 65, 91–95.

Jacobsen, S. J., Girman, C. J., Guess, H. A., Oesterling, J. E., Lieber, M. M. (1995). New diagnostic and treatment guidelines for benign prostatic hyperplasia. Potential impact in the United States. Archives of Internal Medicine, 155, 477–481.

Jacobson, C. K., & Heaton, T. B. (1991). Voluntary childlessness among American men and women in the late 1980s. Social Biology, 38, 79–93.

Jacobson, J. N. (1987). Anorgasmia caused by an MAOI. American Journal of Psychiatry, 144, 527.

Jagstaidt, V., Golay, A., & Pasini, W. (1997). Relationship between sexuality and obesity in male patients. New Trends in Experimental & Clinical Psychiatry, 13, 105–110.

Jamieson, D. J., & Steege, J. F. (1996). The prevalence of dysmenorrhea, dyspareunia, pelvic pain, and irritable bowel syndrome in primary care practices. Obstetrics and Gynecology, 87, 55–58.

Jankowiak, W. R., & Fischer, E. F. (1998). A cross-cultural perspective on romantic love. In J. M. Jenkins & K. Oatley (Eds.), Human emotions: A reader (pp. 55–62). Malden, MA: Blackwell Publications.

Janus. S. S., & Janus, C. L. (1993). The Janus report on sexual behavior. New York: John Wiley & Sons.

Jemmott, J. B., Jemmott, L. S., & Fong, G. T. (1998). Abstinence and safer sex HIV risk-reduction interventions for African American adolescents: A randomized controlled trial. Journal of the American Medical Association, 279, 1529–1536.

Jenkins, M. E., Friedman, H. I., & von Recum, A. F. (1996). Breast implants: Facts, controversy, and speculations for future research. Journal of Investigative Surgery, 9, 1–12.

Jenks, R. J. (1998). Swinging: A review of the literature. Archives of Sexual Behavior, 27, 507–521.

Jensen, L. C., de Gaston, J. F., & Weed, S. E. (1994). Societal and parental influences on adolescent sexual behavior. Psychological Reports, 75, 928–930.

Jimmerson, S. D., & Becker, J. D. (1980). Vaginal ulcers associated with tampon usage. Obstetrics and Gynecology, 56, 97–99.

Johnson, B. E., Kuck, D. L., & Schander, P. R. (1997). Rape myth acceptance and sociodemographic characteristics: A multidimensional analysis. Sex Roles: A Journal of Research, 36, 693–707.

Johnson, D. W. (1987). Human relations and your career. Englewood Cliffs, NJ: Prentice-Hall, Inc.

Johnson, M. S. (1983). Recognizing the incestuous family. Journal of the National Medical Association, 75, 757–761.

Johnston, S. (1994). On the fire brigade: Why liberalism won't stop the anti-gay campaigning of the right. Critical Sociology, 20, 3–19.

Jones, D. L., Irwin, K. L., Inciardi, J., Bowser, B., Schilling, R., et al. (1998). The high-risk sexual practices of crack-smoking sex workers recruited from the streets of three American cities. The Multicenter Crack Cocaine and HIV Infection Study Team. Sexually Transmitted Diseases, 25, 187–193.

Jones, J. C., & Barlow, D. H. (1990). Self-reported frequency of sexual urges, fantasies, and masturbatory fantasies in heterosexual males and females. Archives of Sexual Behavior, 19, 269–279.

Jones, M. M. (1997). Lessons from gay marriages. Psychology Today, 30, 22.

Joseph, J. M., Sawyer, R., & Desmond, S. (1995). Sexual knowledge, behavior and sources of information among deaf and hard-of-hearing college students. American Annals of the Deaf, 140, 338–345.

Joshi, V. N., & Money, J. (1995). Dhat syndrome and dream in transcultural sexology. Journal of Psychology and Human Sexuality, 7, 95–99.

Jossens, M. O., Eskenazi, B., Schacter, J., & Sweet, R. L. (1996). Risk factors for pelvic inflammatory disease. A case control study. Sexually Transmitted Diseases, 23, 239–247.

Jovanovic, L. (1998). Sex and the diabetic woman: Desire versus dysfunction. Diabetes Reviews, 6, 65–72.

Juffer, J. (1998). At home with pornography: Woman, sexuality, & everyday life. New York: New York University Press.

Juhn, G. (1994). Understanding the pill: A consumer's guide to oral contraceptives. Binghamton, NY: Haworth Press.

Kafka, M. P. (1997a). A monoamine hypothesis for the pathophysiology of paraphilic disorders. Archives of Sexual Behavior, 26, 343–358.

Kafka, M. P. (1997b). Hypersexual desire in males: An operational definition and clinical implications for males with paraphilias and paraphilia-related disorders. Archives of Sexual Behavior, 26, 505–526.

Kahn, M. J. (1991). Factors affecting the coming out process for lesbians. Journal of Homosexuality, 21, 47–70.

Kall, K. I. (1992). Effects of amphetamine on sexual behavior of male I.V. drug users in Stockholm—a pilot study. AIDS Education and Prevention, 4, 6–17.

Kalra, M., Wood, E., Desmarais, S., Verberg, N., & Senn, C. Y. (1998). Exploring negative dating experiences and beliefs about rape among younger and older women. Archives of Sexual Behavior, 27, 145–153.

Kantner, J. F., & Zelnik, M. (1973). Contraception and pregnancy: Experience of young unmarried women in the United States. Family Planning Perspectives, 5, 21–35.

Kaplan, H. S. (1974). The new sex therapy: Active treatment of sexual dysfunctions. New York: Brunner/Mazel.

Kaplan, H. S. (1988). Illustrated manual of sex therapy. New York: Brunner/Mazel.

Kaplan, H. S. (1989). How to overcome premature ejaculation. New York: Brunner/Mazel.

Kaplan, H. S. (1990). Sex, intimacy, and the aging process. Journal of the American Academy of Psychoanalysis, 18, 185–205.

Kaplan, H. S. (1994). A neglected issue: The sexual side-effects of current treatments for breast cancer. The Canadian Journal of Human Sexuality, 3, 151–163.

Kaplan, H. S. (1995). The sexual desire disorders: Dysfunctional regulation of sexual motivation. New York: Brunner/Mazel.

Kaplan, H. S., & Klein, D. F. (1987). Sexual aversion, sexual phobias, and panic disorder. New York: Brunner/Mazel.

Kaplan, H. S., & Passalacqua, D. (1988). Illustrated manual of sex therapy. New York: Brunner/Mazel.

Karlen, N. (1996). Jacked like me. GQ, 66, 206–211.

Karney, B. R., & Bradbury, T. N. (1995). The longitudinal course of marital quality and stability: A review of theory, method, and research. Psychological Bulletin, 118, 3–34.

Kash, K. M., Holland, J. C., Halper, M. S., & Miller, D. G. (1992). Psychological distress and surveillance behaviors of women with a family history of breast cancer. Journal of the National Cancer Institute, 84, 24–30.

Katz, P. A. (1987). Variations in family constellation: Effects on gender schemata. In L. S. Liben & M. L. Signorella (Eds.), Children's gender schemata. San Francisco: Jossey-Bass.

Kaufert, P. A. (1994). Menopause and depression: A sociological perspective. In G. Berg & M. Hammar (Eds.), The modern management of the menopause (pp. 161–168). New York: The Parthenon Publishing Group.

Kaunitz, A. M. (1996). Long-acting contraceptive options. International Journal of Fertility and Menopausal Studies, 41, 69–76.

Kazdin, A. E. (1980). Investigating generality of findings from analogue research: A rejoinder. Journal of Consulting and Clinical Psychology, 48, 772–773.

Kehoe, M. (1986). Lesbians over 65: A triply invisible minority. Journal of Homosexuality, 12, 139–152.

Kehoe, M. (1988). Lesbians over 60 speak for themselves. Journal of Homosexuality, 16, 1–111.

Kelaher, M., Ross, M., Rohrsheim, R., Drury, M., & Clarkson, A. (1994). Dominant situational determinants of sexual risk behavior in gay men. AIDS, 8, 101–105.

Keller, J. F., Eakes, E., Hinkle, D., & Hughston, G. A. (1978). Sexual behavior and guilt among women: A cross-generational comparison. Journal of Sex and Marital Therapy, 4, 259–265.

Kellett, J. (1991). Sexuality of the elderly. Sexual and Marital Therapy, 6, 147–155.

Kelly, H. H. (1973). The process of causal attribution. American Psychologist, 28, 107–128.

Kelly, J. (1977). The aging male homosexual. The Gerontologist, 17, 328–332.

Kelly, M. P., Strassberg, D. S., & Kircher, J. R. (1990). Attitudinal and experiential correlates of anorgasmia. Archives of Sexual Behavior, 19, 165–177.

Kennedy, H. (1997). The riddle of "man-manly" love: The pioneering work on male homosexuality (Vols. 1 and 2). By Karl Heinrich Ulrichs. Translated by Michael A. Lombardi-Nash. [Book review]. Archives of Sexual Behavior, 26, 220–224.

Kenrick, D. T., & Keefe, R. C. (1992). Age preferences in mates reflect sex differences in human reproductive strategies. Behavioral and Brain Sciences, 15, 75–133.

Kenrick, D. T., Keefe, R. C., Bryan, A., Barr, A., & Brown, S. (1995). Age preferences and mate choice among homosexuals and heterosexuals: A case for modular psychological mechanisms. Journal of Personality and Social Psychology, 69, 1166–1172.

Key, T. C., & Kreutner, A. K. (1980). Menstrual extraction in the adolescent. Journal of Adolescent Health Care, 1, 127–131.

Khoudary, K. P., DeWolf, W. C., Bruning, C. O. 3rd, & Morgentaler, A. (1997). Immediate sexual rehabilitation by simultaneous placement of penile prosthesis in patients undergoing radical prostatectomy: Initial results in 50 patients. Urology, 50, 395–399.

Kieler, H., Haglund, B., Waldenstrom, U., & Axelsson, O. (1997). Routine ultrasound screening in pregnancy and the children's subsequent growth, vision, and hearing. British Journal of Obstetrics and Gynaecology, 104, 1267–1272.

Kilmann, P. R., Boland, J. P., West, M. O., Jonet, C. J., & Ramsey, R. E. (1993). Sexual arousal of college students in relation to sex experiences. Journal of Sex Education and Therapy, 19, 157–164.

Kim, A., Galanter, M., Castaneda, R., Lifshutz, H., & Franco, H. (1992). Crack cocaine use and sexual behavior among psychiatric inpatients. The American Journal of Drug and Alcohol Abuse, 18, 235–246.

Kimmel, D. C. (1977, November). Patterns of aging among gay men. Christopher Street, 7–26.

Kimmel, M. (1996). Great moments in American masculinity. Psychology Today, 29, 12–15.

King, B. M., & Lorusso, J. (1997). Discussions in the home about sex: Different recollections by parents and children. Journal of Sex & Marital Therapy, 23, 52–60.

Kinsey, A., Pomeroy, W., & Martin, C. (1948). Sexual behavior in the human male. Philadelphia: Saunders.

Kinsey, A., Pomeroy, W., Martin, C., & Gebhard, P. (1953). Sexual behavior in the human female. Philadelphia: Saunders.

Kinzl, J. F., Mangweth, B., Traweger, C., & Biebl, W. (1996). Sexual dysfunction in males: Significance of adverse childhood experiences. Child Abuse & Neglect, 20, 759–766.

Kinzl, J. F., Traweger, C., & Biebl, W. (1995). Sexual dysfunctions: Relationship to childhood sexual abuse and early family experiences in a nonclinical sample. Child Abuse & Neglect, 19, 785–792.

Kirby, D., Korpi, M., Barth, R. P., & Cagampang, H. H. (1997). The impact of the Postponing Sexual Involvement curriculum among youths in California. Family Planning Perspectives, 29, 100–108.

Kirksey, K. M., Holt-Ashley, M., Williamson, K. L., & Garza, R. O. (1995). Autoerotic asphyxia in adolescents. Journal of Emergency Nursing, 21, 81–83.

Kjerulff, K. H., Erickson, B. A., & Langenberg, P. W. (1996). Chronic gynecological conditions reported by US women: Findings from the national health interview study, 1984–1992. American Journal of Public Health, 86, 195–199.

Klassen, A. D., Williams, C. J., & Levitt, E. E. (1989). Sex and morality in the U. S.: An empirical enquiry under the auspices of the Kinsey Institute. Middletown, CT: Wesleyan University Press.

Klassen, A. D., & Wilsnack, S. C. (1986). Sexual experience and drinking among women in a U. S. national survey. Archives of Sexual Behavior, 15, 363–392.

Klebanoff, M. A., Nugent, R. P., & Rhoads, G. G. (1984). Coitus during pregnancy: Is it safe? Lancet, 8408, 914–917.

Kleinberg, S. (1980). Alienated affections: Being gay in America. New York: St. Martin's Press.

Kleinplatz, P. J. (1992). The erotic experience and the intent to arouse. Canadian Journal of Human Sexuality, 1, 133–139.

Knight, R. A., Warren, J. I., Reboussin, R., & Soley, B. J. (1998). Predicting rapist type from crime-scene variables. Criminal Justice and Behavior, 25, 46–80.

Kockott, G., & Fahrner, E. M. (1987). Transsexuals who have not undergone surgery: A follow-up study. Archives of Sexual Behavior, 16, 511–522.

Koenig, R. (1995, November 25). Fifteen hundred, but only one rape. The Spectator, 57–58.

Koetsawang, S. (1994). Once-a-month injectable contraceptives: Efficacy and reasons for discontinuation. Contraception, 49, 387–398.

Koff, E., Rierdan, J., & Sheingold, K. (1982). Memories of menarche: Age, preparation, and prior knowledge as determinants of initial menstrual experience. Journal of Youth and Adolescence, 11, 1–9.

Kolata, G. (1998, January 4). Infertile foreigners see opportunity in the U.S. The New York Times. [http://www.nytimes.com].

Kolb, B., & Whishaw, I. Q. (1996). Fundamentals of human neuropsychology (4th ed.). New York: W. H. Freeman and Company.

Kolodny, R. C. (1974). Depression of plasma testosterone levels after chronic intensive marijuana use. New England Journal of Medicine, 290, 872–874.

Kolodny, R. C. (1981). Evaluating sex therapy: Process and outcome at the Masters & Johnson Institute. Journal of Sex Research, 17, 301–318.

Kolodny, R. C. (1981, February). Effects of Marijuana on Sexual Behavior and Function. Paper presented at the Midwestern Conference on Drug Use, St. Louis, MO. Cited in Masters, W. H., Johnson, V. E., & Kolodny, R. C. (1992). Human sexuality. New York: HarperCollins.

Kolodny, R. C., Masters, W. H., & Johnson, V. E. (1979). Textbook of sexual medicine. Boston: Little, Brown & Co.

Komisaruk, B. R., Gerdes, C. A., & Whipple, B. (1997). 'Complete' spinal cord injury does not block perceptual processes to genital self-stimulation in women. Archives of Neurology, 54, 1513–1520.

Korn, E. (1995, June 16). Sex sherpas of the Victorians. Times Literary Supplement, 16–17.

Korn, J. H., Huelsman, T. J., Reed, C. S., Aiello, M., et al. (1992). Perceived ethicality of guided imagery in rape research. Ethics and Behavior, 2, 1–14.

Koukounas, E., & Over, R. (1993). Habituation and dishabituation of male sexual arousal. Behaviour Research and Therapy, 31, 575–585.

Kraaimaat, F. W., Bakker, A. H., Janssen, E., & Bijlsma, J. W. (1996). Intrusiveness of rheumatoid arthritis on sexuality in male and female patients living with a spouse. Arthritis Care & Research, 9, 120–125.

Krafft-Ebing, R. V. (1939). Psychopathia sexualis. New York: Pioneer Publications.

Kreher, N. E., Hickner, J. M., Ruffin, M. T., & Lin, C. S. (1995). Effect of distance and travel time on rural women's compliance with screening mammography: A UPRNet study. Journal of Family Practice, 40, 143–147.

Kreiss, J. L., & Patterson, D. L. (1997). Psychosocial issues in primary care of lesbian, gay, bisexual, and transgender youth. Journal of Pediatric Health Care, 11, 266–274.

Kreiss, J., Ngugi, E., Holmes, K., Ndinya-Achola, J., Waiyaki, P., Roberts, P. L., Ruminjo, I., Sajabi, R., Kimata, J., Fleming, T. R., et al. (1992). Efficacy of nonoxynol-9 contraceptive sponge use in preventing heterosexual acquisition of HIV in Nairobi prostitutes. Journal of the American Medical Association, 268, 477–482.

Kreuter, M., Sullivan, M., & Siosteen, A. (1994). Sexual adjustment after spinal cord injury (SCI) focusing on partner experiences. Paraplegia, 32, 225–235.

Kruesi, M. J. P., Fine, S., Valladares, L., Phillips, Jr., R. A., & Rapoport, J. L. (1992). Paraphilias: A double-blind crossover comparison of clomipramine versus desipramine. Archives of Sexual Behavior, 21, 587–593.

Kukula, K. C. (1996). Reach out, the surprising benefit of hugs, handshakes and heart-to-hearts. Women's Day, 49, 40–41.

Kumar, P., & Makwana, S. M. (1991). Factors affecting sexual satisfaction in married life. Journal of the Indian Academy of Applied Psychology, 17, 31–34.

Kurgan, A., Nunnelee, J. D., & Zilberman, M. (1994). The importance of the early detection of varicocele in adolescent males. Nurse Practitioner, 19, 36–37.

Kuriansky, J. (1995). Sex simmers, still sells. Advertising Age, 66, p. 49.

Kurki, T., & Ylikorkala, O. (1993). Coitus during pregnancy is not related to bacterial vaginosis or preterm birth. American Journal of Obstetrics and Gynecology, 169, 1130–1134.

Kurtz, M. E., Wyatt, G., & Kurtz, J. C. (1995). Psychological and sexual well-being, philosophical spiritual views, and health habits of long-term cancer survivors. Health Care for Women International, 16, 253–262.

Kushner, M. (1977). The reduction of a long-standing fetish by means of aversive conditioning. In J. Fischer & H. L. Gochros (Eds.), Handbook of behavior therapy with sexual problems (pp. 443–447). New York: Pergamon Press.

Kuwabara, Y. (1989). The current status of oral contraceptive clinical development in Japan. International Journal of Fertility, 34, 18–20.

Kwan, M., Greenleaf, W. J., Mann, J., Crapo, L., and Davidson, J. M. (1983). The nature of androgen action on male sexuality: A combined laboratory self-report study on hypogonadal men. Journal of Clinical Endocrinology and Metabolism, 57, 557–562.

Laan, E., & Everaerd, W. (1995). Habituation of female sexual arousal to slides and film. Archives of Sexual Behavior, 24, 517–541.

Laan, E., Everaerd, W., Van Aanhold, M. T., & Rebel, M. (1993). Performance demand and sexual arousal in women. Behaviour Research and Therapy, 31, 25–35.

Laan, E., Everaerd, W., van Bellen, G., & Hanewald, G. (1994). Women's sexual and emotional responses to male- and female-produced erotica. Archives of Sexual Behavior, 23, 153–169.

Laan, E., Everaerd, W., van der Velde, J., & Geer, J. H. (1995). Determinants of subjective experience of sexual arousal in women: Feedback from genital arousal and erotic stimulus content. Psychophysiology, 32, 444–451.

Laband, D. N., & Lentz, B. F. (1998). The effects of sexual harassment on job satisfaction, earnings, and turnover among female lawyers. Industrial and Labor Relations Review, 51, 594–617.

Labbate, L. A., Grimes, J. B., & Arana, G. W. (1998). Serotonin reuptake antidepressant effects on sexual function in patients with anxiety disorders. Biological Psychiatry, 43, 904–907.

Ladas, A. K., Whipple, B., & Perry, J. D. (1982). The G spot and other recent discoveries about human sexuality. New York: Holt, Rinehart, & Winston.

Laforge, R. G., Green, G. W., & Prochaska, J. O., (1994). Psychosocial factors influencing low fruit and vegetable consumption. Journal of Behavioral Medicine, 17, 361–374.

Lampman, C., & Dowling-Guyer, S. (1995). Attitudes toward voluntary and involuntary childlessness. Basic and Applied Social Psychology, 17, 213–222.

Lamptey, P. R., & Goodridge, G. (1996). Condoms. In G. Dallabetta, M. Laga, & P. Lamptey (Eds.), Control of sexually transmitted diseases. A handbook for the design and management of programs (pp. 73–103). Arlington, VA: AIDSCAP/FHI.

Lane, C. (1995). The liminal iconography of Jodie Foster. Journal of Popular Film and Television, 22, 149–153.

Langeland, W., & Hartgers, C. (1998). Child sexual and physical abuse and alcoholism: A review. Journal of Studies on Alcohol, 59, 336–348.

Langer, L. M., Zimmerman, R. S., & Katz, J. A. (1995). Virgins' expectations and nonvirgins' reports: How adolescents feel about themselves. Journal of Adolescent Research, 10, 291–306.

LaRossa, R. (1986). Becoming a parent. Beverly Hills, CA: Sage Publications.

Larsen, A. S., & Olson, D. H. (1989). Predicting marital satisfaction using PREPARE: A replication study. Journal of Marital and Family Therapy, 15, 311–322.

Larson, J. H. (1992). "You're my one and only": Premarital counseling for unrealistic beliefs about mate selection. American Journal of Family Therapy, 20, 242–253.

Lashmar, P. (March 8, 1996). The men's gloom. New Statesman and Society, 9, 33.

Laumann, E. O., Gagnon, J. H., Michael, R. T., & Michaels, S. (1994). The social organization of sexuality: Sexual practices in the United States. Chicago: University of Chicago Press.

Lavee, Y. (1991). Western and non-western human sexuality: Implications for clinical practice. Journal of Sex & Marital Therapy, 17, 203–213.

Lavelle, M. (1998, July 6). The new rules of sexual harassment. U. S. News & World Report, 125, 30–31.

Lavick, J. (1998, May 25). An overlooked HIV population. Los Angeles Times. [on-line].

Lawrence, D. L. (1988). Menstrual politics: Woman and pigs in rural Portugal. In T. Buckley & A. Gottlieb (Eds.), Blood magic (pp. 117–136). Berkeley, CA: University of California Press.

Laws, D. R., & O'Donohue, W. (1997). Sexual deviance. Theory, assessment, and treatment. New York: The Guilford Press.

Leathers, S. J., Kelley, M. A., & Richman, J. A. (1997). Postpartum depressive symptomatology in new mothers and fathers: Parenting, work, and support. Journal of Nervous and Mental Disease, 185, 129–139.

Leboyer, F. (1975). Birth without violence. New York: Knopf.

Lee, J. A. (1977). A typology of styles of loving. Personality and Social Psychology Bulletin, 3, 173–182.

Lee, P. H., O' Leary, L. A., Songer, N. J., Coughlin, M. T., et al. (1996). Paternity after unilateral cryptorchidism: A controlled study. Pediatrics, Part 1, 98, 676–679.

Leff, J. J., & Israel, M. (1983). The relationship between mode of female masturbation and achievement of orgasm in coitus. Archives of Sexual Behavior, 12, 227–236.

Leigh, B. C., Morrison, D. M., Trocki, K., & Temple, M. (1994). Sexual behavior of American adolescents: Results from a U. S. national survey. Journal of Adolescent Health, 15, 117–125.

Leiker, J. J., Taub, D. E., & Gast, J. (1995). The stigma of AIDS: Persons with AIDS and social distance. Deviant Behavior: An Interdisciplinary Journal, 16, 333–351.

Leitenberg, H., & Henning, K. (1995). Sexual fantasy. Psychological Bulletin, 117, 469–496.

Leitenberg, H., Detzer, M. J., & Srebnik D. (1993). Gender differences in masturbation and the relation of masturbation experience in preadolescence and/or early adolescence to sexual behavior and sexual adjustment in young adulthood. Archives of Sexual Behavior, 22, 87–98.

Lemere, F., & Smith, J. W. (1973). Alcohol-induced sexual impotence. American Journal of Psychiatry, 130, 321–332.

Lemieux, R. (1996). Picnics, flowers, and moonlight strolls: An exploration of routine love behaviors. Psychological Reports, 78, 91–98.

Leong, G. B., Silva, J. A., Garza-Trevino, E. S., Oliva, Jr., D., Ferrari, M. M., Komanduri, R. V., & Caldwell, J. C. B. (1994). The dangerousness of persons with the Othello syndrome. Journal of Forensic Sciences, 39, 1445–1454.

Lerman, C., Daly, M., Sands, C., Balshem, A., Lustbader, E., Heggan, T., Goldstein, L., James, J., & Engstrom, P. (1993). Mammography adherence and psychological distress among women at risk for breast cancer. Journal of the National Cancer Institute, 85, 1074–1080.

Lerner, R. M., Karabenick, S. A., & Stuart, J. L. (1973). Relations among physical attractiveness, body attitudes, and self concept in male and female college students. Journal of Psychology, 85, 119–129.

Levant, R. F., & Brooks, G. R. (1997). Men and the problem of nonrelational sex. In R. F. Levant & G. R. Brooks (Eds.), Men and sex (pp. 1–6). New York: John Wiley & Sons.

Levay, A. N., & Kagle, A. (1977). Ego deficiencies in the areas of pleasure, intimacy, and cooperation: Guidelines in the diagnosis and treatment of sexual dysfunctions. Journal of Sex and Marital Therapy, 3, 10–18.

LeVay, S. (1991). A difference in the hypothalamic structure between heterosexual and homosexual men. Science, 253, 1034–1037.

LeVay, S. (1993). The sexual brain. Cambridge, MA: MIT Press.

Leventhal, E. A., Leventhal, H., Shacham, S., & Easterling, D. V. (1989). Active coping reduces reports of pain from childbirth. Journal of Consulting and Clinical Psychology, 57, 365–371.

Lever, J. (1995). Bringing the fundamentals of gender studies into safer-sex education. Family Planning Perspecitves, 27, 172–174.

Levin, J. D. (1998). The Clinton syndrome. Rocklin, CA: Forum.

Levine, S. B., & Fones, C. S. L. (1998). Psychological aspects at the interface of diabetes and erectile dysfunction. Diabetes Reviews, 6, 41–49.

Levinson, D. (1980). Toward a conception of the adult life course. In N. J. Smelser & E. H. Erikson (Eds.), Themes of work and love in adulthood (pp. 265–290). Cambridge, MA: Harvard University Press.

Levinson, D. (1986). A conception of adult development. American Psychologist, 41, 3–13.

Levinson, D. J. (1978). The seasons of a man's life. New York: Knopf.

Levitt, E. E. (1975). Sexual counseling. What the busy physician can, and cannot do. Postgraduate Medicine, 58, 91–97.

Lewinsohn, R. (1958). A history of sexual customs. Greenwich, Connecticut: Fawcett.

Lewis, R. W. (1995). Long-term results of penile prosthetic implants. Urologic Clinics of North America, 22, 847–856.

Leznoff, M. (1954). The homosexual in urban society. Unpublished master's thesis, McGill University, Montreal, Quebec, Canada. Cited in Murray, S. O., American gay. Chicago: University of Chicago Press, 194.

Li, S. Q., Goldstein, M., Zhu, J., & Huber, D. (1991). The no-scalpel vasectomy. Journal of Urology, 145, 341–344.

Lickona, T. (1996, May). Ten consequences of premature sexual involvement. US Catholic, 32–34.

Lipman, J. (1998). Soap, water, and sex: A lively guide to the benefits of sexual hygiene and to coping with sexually transmitted diseases. Amherst, NY: Prometheus Books.

Lisak, D., & Roth, S. (1988). Motivational factors in nonincarcerated sexually aggressive men. Journal of Personality and Social Psychology, 55, 795–802.

Litman, R. E. (1997). Bondage and sadomasochism. In L. B. Schlesinger & E. Revitch (Eds.), Sexual dynamics of anti-social behavior (2nd ed.) (pp. 252–270). Springfield, IL: Charles C. Thomas.

Litz, B. T., Zeiss, A. M., & Davies, H. D. (1990). Sexual concerns of male spouses of female Alzheimer's disease patients. Gerontologist, 30, 113–116.

Liu, D. L., & Ng, M. L. (1995). Sexual dysfunction in China. Annals of the Academy of Medicine, Singapore, 24, 728–731.

Liu, D. L., Ng, M. L., & Chou, L. P. (1992). Sexual behavior in modern China—A report of the nationwide sex-civilization survey on 20,000 subjects in China [in Chinese, cited in Liu & Ng, (1995)]. Shanghai: Joint Publishing.

Liu, P., & Rose, G. A. (1995). Social aspects of >800 couples coming forward for gender selection of their children. Human Reproduction, 10, 968–971.

Livingston, J. A. (1996). Love and illusion. Psychoanalytic Quarterly, 65, 548–560.

Lobitz, W. C., & Baker, E. L. Jr. (1979). Group treatment of single males with erectile dysfunction. Archives of Sexual Behavior, 8, 127–138.

Loftus, E. (1993). The reality of repressed memories. American Psychologist, 48, 518–537.

Lothstein, L. M., Fogg-Waberski, J., & Reynolds, P. (1997). Risk management and treatment of sexual inhibition in geriatric patients. Connecticut Medicine, 61, 609–618.

Lott, B., & Roccio, L. M. (1998). Standing up, talking back, and taking charge: Strategies and outcomes in collective action against sexual harassment. In L. H. Collins, J. C. Chrisler, & K. Quina (Eds.), Career strategies for women in academe. Arming Athena (pp. 249–273). Thousand Oaks, CA: Sage Publications.

Lovey, H. (1996, April 14). On-line 'love' can lead to date or danger. Detroit News & Free Press, A1.

Lowe, J. C., & Mikulas, W. L. (1975). Use of written material in learning self-control of premature ejaculation. Psychological Reports, 37, 295–298.

Lund, L., & Nielsen, K. T. (1996). Varicocele testis and testicular temperature. British Journal of Urology, 78, 113–115.

Lytton, H., & Romney, D. M. (1991). Parents' differential socialization of boys and girls: A meta-analysis. Psychological Bulletin, 109, 267–296.

Maccoby, E., & Jacklin, C. (1974). The psychology of sex differences. Stanford, CA: Stanford University Press.

MacHovec, F. (1993). Is there a paraphilic personality disorder? Treating Abuse Today, 3, 5–10.

MacHovec, F. (1994). A systematic approach to sex offender therapy: Diagnosis, treatment, and risk assessment. Psychotherapy in Private Practice, 13, 93–108.

MacPhee, D. C., Johnson, S. M., & Van der Veer, M. M. (1995). Low sexual desire in women: The effects of marital therapy. Journal of Sex and Marital Therapy, 21, 159–182.

Maden, C., et al. (1993). History of circumcision, medical conditions, and sexual activity and risk of penile cancer. Journal of the National Cancer Institute, 85, 19–24.

Madey, S. F., Simo, M., Dillworth, D., Kemper, D., et al. (1996). They do get more attractive at closing time, but only when you are not in a relationship. Basic & Applied Social Psychology, 18, 387–393.

Mahler, M. S., Pine, F., & Bergman, A. (1975). The psychological birth of the human infant. New York: Basic Books.

Mahoney, J. M., & Strassberg, D. S. (1991). Voluntary control of male sexual arousal. Archives of Sexual Behavior, 20, 1–16.

Mainiero, L. A. (1989). Office romance: Love, power, and sex in the workplace. New York: Rawson Associates.

Major, B., Cozzarelli, C., Sciacchitano, A. M., Cooper, M. L., Testa, M., & Mueller, P. M. (1990). Perceived social support, self-efficacy, and adjustment to abortion. Journal of Personality and Social Psychology, 59, 452–463.

Malina, R. M., & Bouchard, C. (1991). Growth, maturation, and physical activity. Champaign, IL: Human Kinetics Books.

Malott, R. W. (1996). A behavior-analytic view of sexuality, transsexuality, homosexuality, and heterosexuality. Behavior & Social Issues, 6, 127–140.

Mangam, K. S. (1995, October 6). U. of Texas plans workshops on sexual abstinence. The Chronicle of Higher Education, 42, A44.

Mann, K., Klinger, T., Noe, S., Roschke, J., Muller, S., & Benkert, O. (1996). Effects of yohimbine on sexual experiences and nocturnal penile tumescence and rigidity in erectile dysfunction. Archives of Sexual Behavior, 25, 1–16.

Many women make no link between abortion and politics. (1998, January 22). The New York Times. [http://nytimes.com].

Marano, H. E. (1997). Rescuing marriages before they begin. The New York Times. [http://nytimes.com].

Marano, H. E. (1997, July 1). Puberty may begin at 6, contrary to Freud's view. The New York Times. [http://nytimes.com].

Mardh, P. A., & Hogg, B. (1998). Are oral contraceptives masking symptoms of chlamydial cervicitis and pelvic inflammatory disease. European Journal of Contraception and Reproductive Health Care, 3, 41–43.

Margolin, L. (1990). Gender and the stolen kiss: The social support of male and female to violate a partner's sexual consent in a noncoercive situation. Archives of Sexual Behavior, 19, 281–291.

Marion, L. N., & Cox, C. L. (1996). Condom use and fertility among divorced and separated women. Nursing Research, 45, 110–115.

Markus, H. R., & Kitayama, S. (1994). A collective fear of the collective: Implications for selves and theories of selves. Personality & Social Psychology Bulletin, 20, 568–579.

Marr, L. (1999). Sexually transmitted diseases: A physician tells you what you need to know. Baltimore, MD: Johns Hopkins University Press.

Marshall, D. (1971). Sexual behavior on Mangaia. In D. Marshall & R. Suggs (Eds.), Human sexual behavior: Variations in the ethnographic spectrum. Englewood Cliffs, NJ: Prentice-Hall.

Marshall, J. R., & Neill, J. (1977). The removal of a psychosomatic symptom: Effects on the marriage. Family Process, 16, 273–280.

Marshall, W. L. (1997). Pedophilia. Psychopathology and theory. In D. R. Laws & W. O'Donohue (Eds.), Sexual deviance. Theory, assessment, and treatment (pp. 152–174). New York: The Guilford Press.

Marthin, T., Liedgren, S., & Hammar, M. (1997). Transplacental needle passage and other risk-factors associated with second trimester amniocentesis. Acta Obstetricia et Gynecologica Scandinavica, 76, 728–732.

Martin, A. (1993). The lesbian & gay parenting handbook. New York: HarperTrade.

Martin, L., Rosen, L. N., Duand, D. B., Stretch, R. H., & Knudson, K. H. (1998). Prevalence and timing of sexual assaults in a sample of male and female U. S. Army soldiers. Military Medicine, 163, 213–216.

Martz, D. M., Handley, K. B., & Eisler, R. M. (1995). The relationship between feminine gender role stress, body image, and eating disorders. Psychology of Women Quarterly, 19, 493–508.

Mason, F. L. (1997). Fetishism. Psychopathology and theory. In D. R. Laws & W. O'Donohue (Eds.), Sexual deviance. Theory, assessment, and treatment (pp. 75–91). New York: The Guilford Press.

Mason, M. (1995). The making of Victorian sexuality. Oxford: Oxford University Press.

Masters, W. H., & Johnson, V. E. (1966). Human sexual response. Boston: Little, Brown & Company.

Masters, W. H., & Johnson, V. E. (1970). Human sexual inadequacy. Boston: Little, Brown & Company.

Masters, W. H., Johnson, V. E., & Kolodny, R. C. (1992). Human sexuality (4th ed.). New York: HarperCollins.

Matek, O. (1988). Obscene phone callers. Journal of Social Work and Human Sexuality, 7, 113–130.

Matthews, A., Bancroft, J., Whitehead, A., Hackmann, A., Julier, D., Gath, D., & Shaw, P. (1976). The behavioural treatment of sexual inadequacy: A comparative study. Behaviour Research and Therapy, 14, 427–436.

Mauck, C. K., Allen, S., Baker, J. M., Barr, S. P., Abercrombie, T., & Archer, D. F. (1997). An evaluation of the amount of nonoxynol-9 remaining in the vagina up to 4 h after insertion of a vaginal contraceptive film (VCF) containing 70 mg nonoxynol-9. Contraception, 56, 103–110.

Mauck, C. K., Baker, J. M., Barr, S. P., Abercrombie, T. J., & Archer, D. F. (1997). A phase I comparative study of contraceptive vaginal films containing benzalkonium chloride and onoxynol-9. Postcoital testing and colposcopy. Contraception, 56, 89–96.

May, R. (1968). Love and will. New York: Dell Publishing Company.

Mayaud, P., Hawkes, S., & Mabey, D. (1998). Advances in control of sexually transmitted diseases in developing countries. Lancet, 351, Supplement 3, 29–32.

Mazur, D. J., & Merz, J. F. (1995). Older patients' willingness to trade off urologic adverse outcomes for a better chance at five-year survival in the clinical setting of prostate cancer. Journal of the American Geriatrics Society, 43, 979–984.

McCabe, M. P. (1993). Sex education programs for people with mental retardation. Mental Retardation, 31, 377–387.

McCann, C. R. (1994). Birth control politics in the United States, 1916–1945. Ithaca, NY: Cornell University Press.

McCarthy, B. W. (1987). Developing positive intimacy cognitions in males with non-intimate sexual experiences. Journal of Sex and Marital Therapy, 13, 253–259.

McCarthy, B. W. (1995). Bridges to sexual desire. Journal of Sex Education and Therapy, 21, 132–141.

McCaw, J. M., & Senn, C. Y. (1998). Perceptions of cues in conflictual dating situations. A test of the miscommunication hypothesis. Violence Against Women, 4, 609–624.

McClellan, J. (1997, February 6). Love caught in the Net: Singles are turning to the Internet in their search for the perfect partner. Jim McClellan weighs up the odds of finding your Valentine in cyberspace. Guardian, Online 2.

McConnell, E. A., & Zimmerman, M. F. (1983). Care of patients with urologic problems. Philadelphia: J. B. Lippincott Company.

McCoy, K., & Wibbelsman, C. (1992). The new teenage body book. New York: The Body Press/Perigee Books.

McCoy, N. L. (1994). Survey research on the menopause and women's sexuality. In G. Berg & M. Hammar (Eds.), The modern management of the menopause (pp. 581–587). New York: The Parthenon Publishing Group.

McDonald, G. J. (1982). Individual differences in the coming out process for gay men: Implications for theoretical models. Journal of Homosexuality, 8, 47–60.

McGoldrick, M., & Preto, N. (1984). Ethnic intermarriage. Family Process, 23, 347–364.

McGuire, T. R. (1995). Is homosexuality genetic? A critical review and some suggestions. Journal of Homosexuality, 28, 115–145.

McKay, A. (1993). Research supports broadly-based sex education. Canadian Journal of Human Sexuality, 2, 89–98.

McKay, A. (1996). Rural parents' attitudes toward school-based sexual health education. Canadian Journal of Human Sexuality, 5, 15–23.

McKeganey, N., & Barnard, M. U. (1996). Sex work on the streets: Prostitutes & their clients. Bristol, PA: Taylor & Francis.

McLeer, S. V., Dixon, J. F., Henry, D. Ruggiero, K., Escovitz, K., Niedda, T., & Scholle, R. (1998). Psychopathology in non-clinically referred sexually abused children. Journal of the American Academy of Child and Adolescent Psychiatry, 37, 1326–1333.

McLoughlin, D. (1994). Women and sexuality in nineteenth century Ireland. Irish Journal of Psychology, 15, 266–275.

McMullen, S., & Rosen, R. C. (1979). Self-administration masturbation training in the treatment of primary orgasmic dysfunction. Journal of Consulting and Clinical Psychology, 47, 912–918.

Meisler, A. W., & Carey, M. P. (1991). Depressed affect and male sexual arousal. Archives of Sexual Behavior, 20, 541–554.

Mengel, M. B., & Davis, A. B. (1992). Recurrent bacterial vaginosis: Association with vaginal sponge use. Family Practice Research Journal, 12, 283–288.

Meredith, S. (1985). Understanding the facts of life. London: Usborne Publishing Ltd.

Mertz, K. J., Levine, W. C., Mosure, D. J., Berman, S. M., & Dorian, K. J. (1997). Trends in the prevalence of chlamydial infections: The impact of community-wide testing. Sexually Transmitted Diseases, 24, 169–175.

Messiah, A., Blin, P., & Fiche, V. (1995). Sexual repertoires of heterosexuals: Implications for HIV/sexually transmitted disease risk and prevention. AIDS, 9, 1357–1365.

Messiah, A., Pelletier, A., and the ACSF Group (1996). Partner-specific sexual practices among heterosexual men and women with multiple partners: Results from the French National Survey, ACSF. Archives of Sexual Behavior, 25, 233–247.

Messner, M. (1990). Boyhood, organized sports, and the construction of masculinities. Journal of Contemporary Ethnography, 18, 416–444.

Meston, C. M. (1997). Aging and sexuality. Western Journal of Medicine, 167, 285–290.

Meston, C. M., & Gorzalka, B. B. (1996). The effects of immediate, delayed, and residual sympathetic activation on sexual arousal in women. Behavioural Research and Therapy, 34, 143–148.

Metz, M. E., Pryor, J. L., Nesvacil, L. J., Abuzzahab, Sr., F, & Koznar, J. (1997). Premature ejaculation: A psychophysiological review. Journal of Sex & Marital Therapy, 23, 3–23.

Metzenbaum, H. M. (September 18, 1992). National defense authorization act. Congressional Record, S13982–S14026.

Meuwissen, I., & Over, R. (1990). Habituation and dishabituation of female sexual arousal. Behaviour Research and Therapy, 28, 217–226.

Meuwissen, I., & Over, R. (1992). Sexual arousal across phases of the human menstrual cycle. Archives of Sexual Behavior, 21, 101–119.

Meuwissen, I., & Over, R. (1993). Female sexual arousal and the law of initial value: Assessment at several phases of the menstrual cycle. Archives of Sexual Behavior, 22, 403–413.

Mewhinney, D. M., Herold, E. S., & Maticka-Tyndale, E. (1995). Sexual scripts and risk-taking of Canadian university students on spring break in Daytona Beach, Florida. Canadian Journal of Human Sexuality, 4, 273–288.

Meyer, J. H. Jr. (1983). Early office termination of pregnancy by soft cannula vacuum aspiration. American Journal of Obstetrics and Gynecology, 147, 202–207.

Meyer, W. J. 3d., Cole, C., & Emory, E. (1992). Depo provera treatment for sex offending behavior: An evaluation of outcome. Bulletin of the American Academy of Psychiatry and Law, 20, 249–259.

Michael, R. T., Gagnon, J. H., Laumann, E. O., & Kolata, G. (1994). Sex in America: A definitive survey. Boston: Little, Brown & Company.

Michielutte, R., Dignan, M., Bahnson, J., & Wells, H. B. (1994). The Forsyth county cervical cancer prevention project - II. Compliance with screening follow-up of abnormal cervical smears. Health Education Research, 9, 421–432.

Milde, F. K., Hart, L. K., & Fearing, M. O. (1996). Sexuality and fertility concerns of dialysis patients. ANNA Journal, 23, 307–313.

Miller, H. L., Miller, C. E., Kenney, L., & Clark, J. W. (1998). Issues in statutory rape law enforcement: The views of district attorneys in Kansas. Family Planning Perspectives, 30, 177–181.

Miller, R. S. (1978). The social construction and reconstruction of physiological events: Acquiring the pregnancy identity. Studies in Symbolic Interaction, 1, 181–204.

Miller, W. B. (1976). Sexual and contraceptive behavior in young unmarried women. Primary Care; Clinics in Office Practice, 3, 427–453.

Milner, J. S., & Dopke, C. A. (1997). Paraphilia not otherwise specified. Psychopathology and theory. In D. R. Laws & W. O'Donohue (Eds.), Sexual deviance. Theory, assessment, and treatment (pp. 424–423). New York: The Guilford Press.

Mindel, A. (1998). Genital herpes - how much of a public-health problem. Lancet, 351, Supplement 3, 16–18.

Minichiello, V., Paxton, S., Cowling, V., Cross, G., Savage, J., Sculthorpe, A., & Cairns, B. (1996). University students' knowledge of STDs: Labels, symptoms, and transmission. International Journal of STD & AIDS, 7, 353–358.

Minton, H. L. (1997). Queer theory: Historical roots and implications for psychology. Theory & Psychology, 7, 337–353.

Mishkind, M. E., Rodin, J., Silberstein, L. R., & Striegel-Moore, R. H. (1986). The embodiment of masculinity. American Behavioral Scientist, 29, 545–562.

Miyaji, N. T., & Lock, M. (1994). Monitoring motherhood: Sociocultural and historical aspects of maternal and child health in Japan. Daedalus, 123, 87–112.

Mogilevkina, I., Markote, S., Avakyan, Y., Mrochek, L., Liljestrand, J., & Hellberg, D. (1996). Induced abortions and childbirths: Trends in Estonia, Latvia, Lithuania, Russia, Belarussia and the Ukraine during 1970 to 1994. Acta Obstetricia et Gynecologica Scandinavica, 75, 908–911.

Mondimore, F. M. (1996). A natural history of homosexuality. Baltimore: The Johns Hopkins University Press.

Money, J. (1976). Gender identity and hermaphroditism. Science, 191, 872.

Money, J. (1989). Lovemaps. Clinical concepts of sexual-erotic health & pathology, paraphilia & gender transposition in childhood, adolescence, & maturity. New York: Irvington Publishers.

Money, J. (1991). Semen-conservation theory vs. semen-investment theory, antisexualism, and the return of Freud's seduction theory. Journal of Psychology and Human Sexuality, 4, 31–45.

Money, J., & Tucker, P. (1975). Sexual signatures: On being a man or a woman. Boston: Little, Brown & Company.

Monga, T. N., Lawson, J. S., & Inglis, J. (1986). Sexual dysfunction in stroke patients. Archives of Physical Medicine and Rehabilitation, 67, 19–22.

Monga, T. N., Monga, M., Raina, M. S., & Hardjasudarma, M. (1986). Hypersexuality in stroke. Archives of Physical Medicine and Rehabilitation, 67, 415–417.

Montagne, D. K., Barada, J. H., Belker, A. M., et al. (1996). Clinical guidelines panel on ED: Summary report on the treatment of organic erectile dysfunction. Journal of Urology, 156, 2007–2011.

Montagu, A. (1971). Touching. The significance of the skin. New York: Harper & Row.

Montague, D. K. (1988). Disorders of male sexual function. Chicago: Year Book Medical.

Monto, M. A. (1998). Holding men accountable for prostitution. The unique approach of the Sexual Exploitation Education Project (SEEP). Violence Against Women, 4, 505–517.

Mooney, D. K. (1995). The relationship between sexual insecurity, the alcohol expectation for enhanced sexual experience, and consumption patterns. Addictive Behaviors, 20, 243–250.

Moore, J. E. (1947). The modern treatment of syphilis (2nd ed.). Springfield, IL: C. C. Thomas.

Morley, J. E. (1998). Sex hormones and diabetes. Diabetes Reviews, 6, 6–15.

Morris, D. (1967). The naked ape: A zoologist's study of the human animal. New York: McGraw-Hill.

Morris, J. (1974). Conundrum. New York: Harcourt Brace Jovanovich, Inc.

Morrison, T. L., Goodlin-Jones, B. L., & Urquiza, A. J. (1997). Attachment and the representation of intimate relationships in adulthood. The Journal of Psychology, 131, 57–71.

Mosher, D. L., & MacIan, P. (1994). College men and women respond to X-rated videos intended for male or female audiences: Gender and sexual scripts. Journal of Sex Research, 31, 99–113.

Mosher, D. L., & White, B. B. (1980). Effects of committed or casual erotic imagery on females' subjective sexual arousal and emotional response. The Journal of Sex Research, 16, 273–299.

Mosher, W. D., & McNally, J. W. (1991). Contraceptive use at first premarital intercourse: United States, 1965–1988. Family Planning Perspectives, 23, 108–116.

Mossman, D., Perlin, M. L., & Dorfman, D. A. (1997). Sex on the wards: Conundra for clinicians. Journal of the American Academy of Psychiatry and the Law, 25, 441–460.

Motluk, A. (1996). Men respond to the scent of a woman. New Scientist, 151, 16.

Mueller, P., & Major, B. (1989). Self-blame, self-efficacy, and adjustment to abortion. Journal of Personality and Social Psychology, 57, 1059–1068.

Muir, J. G. (1996). Sexual orientation: Born or bred. Journal of Psychology and Christianity, 15, 313–321.

Munjack, D. J., & Kanno, P. H. (1979). Retarded ejaculation: A review. Archives of Sexual Behavior, 8, 139–150.

Murdoch, M., & McGovern, P. G. (1998). Measuring sexual harassment: Development and validation of the Sexual Harassment Inventory. Violence and Victims, 13, 203–216.

Murphy, W. D. (1997). Exhibitionism. Psychopathology and theory. In D. R. Laws & W. O'Donohue (Eds.), Sexual deviance. Theory, assessment, and treatment (pp. 22–39). New York: The Guilford Press.

Murray, S. L., Holmes, J. G., & Griffin, D. W. (1996). The self-fulfilling nature of positive illusions in romantic relationships: Love is not blind, but prescient. Journal of Personality and Social Psychology, 71, 1155–1180.

Murray, S. O. (1996). American gay. Chicago: The University of Chicago Press.

Murry, V. M., & Ponzetti Jr., J. J. (1997). American Indian female adolescents' sexual behavior: A test of the life-course experience theory. Family and Consumer Sciences Research Journal, 26, 75–95.

Nadon, S. M., Koverola, C., & Schludermann, E. H. (1998). Antecedents to prostitution. Childhood victimization. Journal of Interpersonal Violence, 13, 206–221.

Nagata, C., Matsushita, Y., Inaba, S., Kawakami, N., & Shimizu, H. (1997). Unapproved use of high-dose combined pills in Japan: A community study on prevalence and health characteristics of the users. Preventive Medicine, 26, 565–569.

Nairne, K. D., & Hemsley, D. R. (1983). The use of directed masturbation training in the treatment of primary anorgasmia. British Journal of Clinical Psychology, 22, 283–294.

National Institutes of Health. (1997). Consensus Development Statement. Breast Cancer Screening for Women Ages 40–49. [Draft]

Nave-Herz, R. (1989). Childless marriages. Marriage and Family Review, 14, 239–250.

Negro-Vilar, A. (1993). Stress and other environmental factors affecting fertility in men and women: An overview. Environmental Health Perspectives, 101 Supplement 2, 59–64.

Nemeth, C., & Wachtler, J. (1974). Creating the perceptions of consistency and confidence: A necessary condition of minority influence. Sociometry, 37, 529–540.

Newcomer, S. F., & Udry, J. R. (1985). Oral sex in adolescent population. Archives of Sexual Behavior, 14, 41–46.

Newell, A. G. (1978). A case of ejaculatory incompetence treated with a mechanical aid. In J. LoPiccolo & L. LoPiccolo (Eds.), Handbook of sex therapy (pp. 291–293). New York: Plenum Press.

Newkirk, G. R. (1996). Pelvic inflammatory disease: A contemporary approach. American Family Physician, 53, 1127–1135.

Newman, A. L., & Peterson, C. (1996). Anger of women incest survivors. Sex Roles: A Journal of Research, 34, 463–474.

Nichols, M. (1988). Low sexual desire in lesbian couples. In S. R. Leiblum & R. C. Rosen (Eds.), Sexual desire disorders (pp. 387–412). New York: Guilford Press.

Nilsson, L. (1990). A child is born. New York: Dell Publishing Group, Inc.

Noell, J., Ary, D., & Duncan, T. (1997). Development and evaluation of a sexual decision-making and social skills program: "The choice is yours— preventing HIV/STDs." Health Education and Behavior, 24, 87–101.

Notelovitz, M. (1994). Non-hormonal management of the menopause. In G. Berg & M. Hammar (Eds.), The modern management of the menopause (pp. 513–523). New York: The Parthenon Publishing Group.

Nowell, R. (1997, July 14). 19 bishops ordained gays, says group on eve of debate. The Irish Times on the Web. [on-line].

O' Brien, J. (1994). With a little help from my friends. Your Health, 33, 20–21.

O'Connor, M. (1996, November 27). Man accused of having sex with girl, 13. Chicago Tribune, 2C, 4.

Odlind, V. (1996). Modern intra-uterine devices. Baillieres Clinical Obstetrics and Gynaecology, 10, 55–67.

O'Donnell, L., San Doval, A., Duran, R., & O'Donnell, C. R. (1995). The effectiveness of video-based interventions in promoting condom acquisition among STD clinic patients. Sexually Transmitted Diseases, 22, 97–103.

O'Donohue, W., & Geer, J. (1993). Research issues in the sexual dysfunctions. In W. O'Donohue & J. H. Geer (Eds.), Handbook of sexual dysfunctions. Assessment and treatment (pp. 1–14). Boston: Allyn and Bacon.

O'Farrell, T. J., Choquette, K. A., & Birchler, G. R. (1991). Sexual satisfaction and dissatisfaction in the marital relationships of male alcoholics seeking marital therapy. Journal of Studies on Alcohol, 52, 441–447.

Office of Civil Rights. (1997). Sexual harassment: It's not academic [Brochure].

Office of Educational Research and Improvement. (1990). Child sexual abuse: What it is and how to prevent it: ERIC Digest. Washington, DC: U. S. Government Printing Office.

Ogawa, N., & Retherford, R. D. (1991). Prospects for increased contraceptive pill usage in Japan. Studies in Family Planning, 22, 378–383.

O'Hara, J. (1998, June 1). Rape in the military. Speaking out. Maclean's, 111, 14–20.

O'Hare, E. A., & O'Donohue, W. (1998). Sexual harassment: Identifying risk factors. Archives of Sexual Behavior, 27, 561.

Okami, P. (1995). Childhood exposure to parental nudity, parent-child co-sleeping, and "primal scene": A review of clinical opinion and empirical evidence. The Journal of Sex Research, 32, 51–64.

Okami, P., Olmstead, R., Abramson, P. R., & Pendleton, L. (1998). Early childhood exposure to parental nudity and scenes of parental sexuality ("primal scenes"): An 18-year longitudinal study of outcome. Archives of Sexual Behavior, 27, 361–384.

O'Leary Cobb, J. (1994). Why women choose not to take hormone therapy. In G. Berg & M. Hammar (Eds.), The modern management of the menopause (pp. 525–532). New York: The Parthenon Publishing Group.

Oliver, M. B., & Hyde, J. S. (1993). Gender differences in sexuality: A meta-analysis. Psychological Bulletin, 114, 29–51.

On the road. Inc., 20, 33.

Orbuch, T. L., House, J. S., Mero, R. P., & Webster, P. S. (1996). Marital quality over the life course. Social Psychology Quarterly, 59, 162–171.

Orr, S. P., Lasko, N. B., Metzger, L. J., Berry, N. J., Ahern, C. E., & Pitman, R. K. (1998). Psychophysiological assessment of women with posttraumatic stress disorder resulting from childhood sexual abuse. Journal of Consulting and Clinical Psychology, 66, 906–913.

Osman, A. K. A., & Al-Sawaf, M. H. (1995). Cross-cultural aspects of sexual anxieties and the associated dysfunction. Journal of Sex Education & Therapy, 21, 174–181.

Osterling, R. N. (1993, October 4). A refinement of evil. Time, 142, 75.

O'Sullivan, D. M., Zuckerman, M., & Kraft, M. (1996). The personality of prostitutes. Personality & Individual Differences, 21, 445–448.

Over, M., & Piot, P. (1993). HIV infection and sexually transmitted diseases. In D. T. Jamison, W. H. Mosley, A. R. Measham, & J. L. Bobadilla (Eds.), Disease control priorities in developing countries (pp. 455–527). New York: Oxford University Press.

Over, R., & Phillips, G. (1997). Differences between men and women in age preferences for a same-sex partner. Behavioral & Brain Sciences, 20, 138–140.

Palace, E. M. (1995). A cognitive-physiological process model of sexual arousal and response. Clinical Psychology: Science & Practice, 2, 370–384.

Pan, S., Wu, Z., & Gil, V. E. (1995). Homosexual behaviors in contemporary China. Journal of Psychology & Human Sexuality, 7, 1–17.

Papalia, D. E., & Olds, S. W. (1995). Human development (6th ed.). New York: McGraw-Hill.

Pariser, S. F., Nasrallah, H. A., & Gardner, D. K. (1997). Postpartum mood disorders: Clinical perspectives. Journal of Womens Health, 6, 421–434.

Parker, L. (1998). Ambiguous genitalia: Etiology, treatment, and nursing implications. Journal of Obstetrics, Gynecology, and Neonatal Nursing, 27, 15–22.

Parks, M. R., & Floyd, K. (1996). Meanings for closeness and intimacy in friendship. Journal of Social & Personal Relationships, 13, 85–107.

Parrot, A. (1998). Coping with date rape & acquaintance rape. New York: The Rosen Publishing Group.

Parsonnet, J., Modern, P. A., & Giacobbe, K. D. (1996). Effect of tampon composition on production of toxic shock syndrome toxin-1 by Staphylococcus aureus in vitro. The Journal of Infectious Diseases, 173, 98–103.

Patel, R., Cowan, F. M., & Barton, S. E. (1997). Advising patients with genital herpes: Aciclovir reduces asymptomatic viral shedding, but effect on transmission is unclear. British Medical Journal, 314, 85–86.

Patterson, C. J. (1997). Children of lesbian and gay parents. Advances in Clinical Child Psychology, 19, 235–282.

Patterson, C. J., & Redding, R. E. (1996). Lesbian and gay families with children: Implications of social science research for policy. Journal of Social Issues, 52, 29–50.

Patterson, M. J., Hill, R. P., & Maloy, K. (1995). Abortion in America: A consumer-behavior perspective. Journal of Consumer Research, 21, 677–694.

Patton, D., Kolasa, K., West, S., & Irons, T. G. (1995). Sexual abstinence counseling of adolescents by physicians. Adolescence, 30, 963–969.

Pauly, I. B. (1974). Female transsexualism: Part II. Archives of Sexual Behavior, 3, 509–526.

Pauly, I. B. (1981). Outcome of sex reassignment surgery for transsexuals. Australian and New Zealand Journal of Psychiatry, 15, 45–51.

Pauly, I. B. (1990). Gender identity disorders: Evaluation and treatment. Journal of Sex Education and Therapy, 16, 2–24.

Pavletic, A. J., Wolner-Hanssen, P., Paavonen, J., Hawes, S. E., Eschenbach, D. A. (1999). Infertility following pelvic inflammatory disease. Infectious Diseases in Obstetrics and Gynecology, 7, 145–152.

Pearson, S. E., & Pollack, R. H. (1997). Female responses to sexually explicit films. Journal of Psychology & Human Sexuality, 9, 73–88.

Pederson, D. M., & Shoemaker, M. T. (1993). Dimensions of romantic attitudes. Perceptual & Motor Skills, 77, 623–633.

Pegalis, L. J., Shaffer, D. R., Bazzini, D. G., & Greenier, K. (1994). On the ability to elicit self-disclosure: Are there gender-based and contextual limitations on the opener effect? Personality and Social Psychology Bulletin, 20, 412–420.

Pennebaker, J. (1990). Opening up: The healing power of confiding in others. New York: William Morrow.

Peplau, L. A., & Cochran, S. D. (1981). Value orientations in the intimate relationships of gay men. Journal of Homosexuality, 6, 1–19.

Perry, E. L., Kulik, C. T., & Schmidtke, J. M. (1997). Blowing the whistle: Determinants of responses to sexual harassment. Basic and Applied Social Psychology, 19, 457–482.

Peters, B. (1988). Terrific sex in fearful times. New York: St. Martin's Press.

Peters, M. (1991). Sex differences in human brain size and the general meaning of differences in brain size. Canadian Journal of Psychology, 45, 507–522.

Petrie, T. A., Austin, L. J., Cowley, B. J., Helmcamp, A., et al. (1996). Sociocultural expectations of attractiveness for males. Sex Roles, 35, 581–602.

Petter, L. M., & Whitehill, D. L. (1998). Management of female sexual assault. American Family Physician, 58, 920–928.

Pfeiffer, N. (1995). The prostate-problem solvers. Longevity, 7, 74.

Phoenix, J. (1999). Making sense of prostitution. New York: St. Martin's Press.

Piepert, J. F., & Gutmann, J. (1993). Oral contraceptive risk assessment. Obstetrics and Gynecology, 82, 112–117.

Pierce, C. A., & Aguinis, H. (1997). Bridging the gap between romantic relationships and sexual harassment in organizations. Journal of Organizational Behavior, 18, 197–200.

Pierce, C. A., Byrne, D., & Aguinis, H. (1996). Attraction in organizations: A model of workplace romance. Journal of Organizational Behavior, 17, 5–32.

Pillari, V. (1997). Shadows of pain: Intimacy and sexual problems in family life. Northvale, NJ: Jason Aronson.

Pina, D. L., & Bengston, V. (1993). The division of household labor and wives' happiness: Ideology, employment, and perceptions of support. Journal of Marriage and the Family, 55, 901–912.

Pithers, W. D., Beal, L. S., Armstrong, J., & Petty, J. (1989). Identification of risk factors through clinical interviews and analysis of records. In D. R. Laws (Ed.), Relapse prevention with sex offenders (pp.77–87). New York: Guilford Press.

Pitts, M., Burtney, E., & Dobraszczyc, U. (1996). "There is no shame in it any more": How providers of sexual advice view young people's sexuality. Health Education Research, 11, 1–9.

Plant, R. (1986). The pink triangle. New York: Henry Holt and Company.

Plaut, A., & Kohn-Speyer, A. C. (1947). The carcinogenic action of smegma. Science, 105, 391–392.

Plumridge, E. W., Chetwynd, S. J., Reed, A., & Gifford, S. J. (1996). Patrons of the sex industry: Perceptions of risk. AIDS Care, 8, 405–416.

Pope, M., & Schulz, R. (1990). Sexual attitudes and behavior in midlife and aging homosexual males. Journal of Homosexuality, 20, 169–177.

Popov, A. A., Visser, A. P., & Ketting, E. (1993). Contraceptive knowledge, attitudes, and practice in Russia during the 1980s. Studies in Family Planning, 24, 227–235.

Porst, H. (1997). Transurethral alprostadil with MUSE (medicated urethral system for erection) vs intracavernous alprostadil—a comparative study in 103 patients with erectile dysfunction. International Journal of Impotence Research, 9, 187–192.

Porter, R., & Hall, L. (1995). The facts of life. New Haven: Yale University Press.

Portwood, S. G. (1995). Employment discrimination in the public sector based on sexual orientation: Conflicts between research evidence and the law. Law & Psychology Review, 19, 113–152.

Postrado, L. T., & Nicholson, H. J. (1992). Effectiveness in delaying the initiation of sexual intercourse of girls aged 12–14: Two components of the Girls Incorporated Preventing Adolescent Pregnancy Program. Youth and Society, 23, 356–379.

Potterat, J. J., Rothenberg, R. B., Muth, S. Q., Darrow, W. W., & Phillips-Plummer, L. (1998). Pathways to prostitution: The chronology of sexual and drug abuse milestones. The Journal of Sex Research, 35, 333–340.

Prager, K. J. (1995). The psychology of intimacy. New York: The Guilford Press.

Prentky, R. A., Lee, A. F. S., Knight, R. A., & Cerce, D. (1997). Recidivism rates among child molesters and rapists: A methodological analysis. Law and Human Behavior, 21, 635–659.

Price, J. H., Colvin, T. L., & Smith, D. (1993). Prostate cancer: Perceptions of African-American males. Journal of the National Medical Association, 85, 941–947.

Primary and secondary syphilis - United States, 1997. (1998, June 26). Morbidity and Mortality Weekly Reports, 47, 493–497.

Prince, V., & Bentler, P. M. (1972). Survey of 504 cases of transvestism. Psychological Reports, 31, 903–917.

Prins, K. S., Buunk, B. P., & VanYperen, N. W. (1993). Equity, normative disapproval and extramarital relationships. Journal of Social and Personal Relationships, 10, 39–53.

Procci, W. R., & Martin, D. J. (1985). Effect of maintenance hemodialysis on male sexual performance. Journal of Nervous and Mental Disease, 173, 366–372,

Proctor, F., Wagner, N., & Butler, J. (1974). The differentiation of male and female orgasm: An experimental study. In Wagner, N. (Ed.), Perspectives on human sexuality. New York: Behavioral Publications.

Prostate gland enlargement. (1996, May). Mayo Clinic Health Letter, 14, 1–2.

Pryor, J. B., DeSouza, E. R., Fitness, J., Hutz, C., Kumpf, M., Lubbert, K., Pesonen, O., & Erber, M. W. (1997). Gender differences in the interpretation of social-sexual behavior. A cross-cultural perspective on sexual harassment. Journal of Cross-Cultural Psychology, 28, 509–534.

Psychoyos, A., Creatsas, G., Hassan, E., Georgoulias, V., & Gravanis, A. (1993). Spermicidal and antiviral properties of cholic acid: Contraceptive efficacy of a new vaginal sponge (Protectaid) containing sodium cholate. Human Reproduction, 8, 866–869.

Purnine, D. M., Carey, M. P., & Jorgensen, R. S. (1994). Gender differences regarding preferences for specific heterosexual practices. Journal of Sex & Marital Therapy, 20, 271–287.

Quadagno, D., Sly, D. F., Harrison, D. F., Eberstein, I. W., & Soler, H. R. (1998). Ethnic differences in sexual decisions and sexual behavior. Archives of Sexual Behavior, 27, 57–76.

Quam, J. K., & Whitford, G. S. (1992). Adaptation and age-related expectations of older gay and lesbian adults. The Gerontologist, 32, 367–374.

Quevillon, R. P. (1993). Dyspareunia. In W. O'Donohue & J. H. Geer (Eds.), Handbook of sexual dysfunctions. Assessment and treatment (pp. 367–380). Boston: Allyn and Bacon.

Quinn, T. C. (2000). Viral load and heterosexual transmission of human immunodeficiency virus type I. The New England Journal of Medicine, 342, 921–929.

Quinsey, V. L., Bergersen, S. G., & Steinman, C. M. (1976). Changes in physiological and verbal responses of child molesters during aversion therapy. Canadian Journal of Behavioural Science, 8, 202–212.

Quintero, R. A., Romero, R., Mahoney, M. J., Abuhamad, A., Vecchio, M., Holden, J., & Hobbins, J. C. (1993). Embryoscopic demonstration of hemorrhagic lesions on the human embryo after placental trauma. American Journal of Obstetrics and Gynecology, 168, 756–760.

Radkowsky, M., & Siegel, L. J. (1997). The gay adolescent: Stressors, adaptations, and psychosocial interventions. Clinical Psychology Review, 17, 191–216.

Rafaelli, M., Bogenschneider, K., & Flood, M. F. (1998). Parent-teen communication about sexual topics. Journal of Family Issues, 19, 315–333.

Rand, E. (1995). Barbie's queer accessories. Durham, NC: Duke University Press.

Rane, T. R., & Draper, T. W. (1995). Negative evaluations of men's nurturant touching of young children. Psychological Reports, 76, 811–818.

Rao, K. V., & Demaris, A. (1995). Coital frequency among married and cohabiting couples in the United States. Journal of Biosocial Science, 27, 135–150.

Rawlins, W. K., & Holl, M. (1987). The communicative achievement of friendship during adolescence: Predicaments of trust and violation. Western Journal of Speech Communication, 51, 345–363.

Ray, K. C., & Jackson, J. L. (1997). Family environment and childhood sexual victimization. A test of the buffering hypothesis. Journal of Interpersonal Violence, 12, 3–17.

Read, S., King, M., & Watson, J. (1997). Sexual dysfunction in primary medical care: Prevalence, characteristics and detection by the general practitioner. Journal of Public Health Medicine, 19, 387–391.

Redman, S., Henrikus, D., Clover, K., & Sanson-Fisher, R. (1993). Responses of women and their doctors to the occurrence of a breast symptom: A community study. Health Promotion International, 8, 177–187.

Reece, E. A., Homko, C. J., Koch, S., & Chan, L. (1997). First-trimester needle embryofetoscopy and prenatal diagnosis. Fetal Diagnosis and Therapy, 12, 136–139.

Reece, E. A., Whetham, J., Rotmensch, S., & Wiznitzer, A. (1993). Gaining access to the embryonic-fetal circulation via first-trimester endoscopy: A step into the future. Obstetrics and Gynecology, 82, 876–879.

Reece, R. (1988). Special issues in the etiologies and treatments of sexual problems among gay men. Journal of Homosexuality, 15, 43–57.

Reed, B. D., & Eyler, A. (1993). Vaginal infections: Diagnosis and management. American Family Physician, 47, 1805–1816.

Reed, E. W., & Reed, S. C. (1965). Mental retardation: A family study. Philadelphia: Saunders.

Reed, J. S., & Klebanoff, M. A. (1993). Sexual intercourse during pregnancy and preterm delivery: Effects of vaginal microorganisms. The Vaginal Infections and Prematurity Study Group. American Journal of Obstetrics and Gynecology, 168, 514–519.

Reese, S. (1997). The law and gay-bashing in schools. Education Digest, 62, 46–49.

Regan, P. C. (1996). Sexual outcasts: The perceived impact of body weight and gender on sexuality. Journal of Applied Social Psychology, 26, 1803–1815,

Regan, P. C., & Sprecher, S. (1995). Gender differences in the value of contributions to intimate relationships: Egalitarian relationships are not always perceived to be equitable. Sex Roles, 33, 221–238.

Reifsnider, E. (1997). On the horizon: New options for contraception. Journal of Obstetric, Gynecologic, and Neonatal Nursing, 26, 91–100.

Reinholtz, R. K., & Muehlenard, C. L. (1995). Genital perceptions and sexual activity in a college population. Journal of Sex Research, 32, 155–165.

Reinisch, J. M. (1990). The Kinsey institute new report on sex. New York: St. Martin's Press.

Reinstein, L., Ashley, J., & Miller, K. H. (1978). Sexual adjustment after lower extremity amputation. Archives of Physical Medicine and Rehabilitation, 59, 501–504.

Reisman, J. A. (1986). A content analysis of Playboy, Penthouse, and Hustler magazines with special attention to the portrayal of children, crime and violence: Supplementary testimony given to the United States Attorney General's Commission on Pornography. Arlington, VA: Institute for Media Education.

Reiss, I. (1960). Premarital sexual standards in America. New York: Free Press.

Reitano, M. V. (1999). Sexual health: Questions you have … answers you need. Allentown, PA: Peoples Medical Society.

Reitz, W. E., & Keil, W. E. (1977). Behavioral treatment of an exhibitionist. In J. Fischer & H. L. Gochros (Eds.), Handbook of behavior therapy with sexual problems (pp. 485–488). New York: Pergamon Press.

Remez, L. (1996). Nevada's licensed sex workers achieve minimal condom breakage rates. Family Planning Perspectives, 28, 35.

Renshaw, D. C. (1988). Sexual problems in later life: A case of impotence. Clinical Gerontologist, 8, 73–76.

Renshaw, D. C., & Karstaedt, A. (1988). Is there (sex) life after coronary bypass? Comprehensive Therapy, 14, 61–66.

Renwick, S. B. (1996). Silicone breast implants: Implications for society and surgeons. Medical Journal of Australia, 165, 338–341.

Reubinoff, B. E., & Schenker, J. G. (1996). New advances in sex preselection. Fertility and Sterility, 66, 343–350.

Reynolds, E. L., & Wines, J. V. (1948). Individual differences in physical changes associated with adolescent girls. American Journal of Diseases of Children, 75, 329–350.

Rice, G., Anderson, C., Risch, N., & Ebers, G. (1995, September). Male homosexuality: Absence of linkage to micro satellite markers on the X-chromosome in a Canadian study. Paper presented at the annual meeting of the International Academy of Sex Research, Provincetown, MA.

Rice, T. W., & Coates, D. L. (1995). Gender role attitudes in the southern United States. Gender and Society, 9, 744–756.

Richards, L., Rollerson, B., & Phillips, J. (1991). Perceptions of submissiveness: Implications for victimization. The Journal of Psychology, 125, 407–411.

Rickert, V. I., & Wiemann, C. M. (1998). Date rape among adolescents and young adults. Journal of Pediatric and Adolescent Gynecology, 11, 167–175.

Riddle, J. M. (1997). Eve's herbs: A history of contraception and abortion in the west. Cambridge, MA: Harvard University Press.

Riddle, J. M. (1997). The history of contraception. [http://rtt.colorado.edu/~mcck/Home.html].

Rifkind, L. J., & Harper, L. F. (1994). The Branch Davidians and the politics of power and intimidation. Journal of American Culture, 17, 65–72.

Rind, B., Tromovitch, P., & Bauserman, R. (1998). A meta-analytic examination of assumed properties of child sexual abuse using college samples. Psychological Bulletin, 124, 22–53.

Ritchie, E. C. (1998). Reactions to rape: A military forensic psychiatrist's perspective. Military Medicine, 163, 505–509.

Roberts, E. (Ed.). (1997). Am I the last virgin? Ten African American reflections on sex and love. New York: Aladdin Paperbacks.

Roberts, L. (1991). Does egg beckon sperm when the time is right? Science, 252, 214.

Robinson, J. W., Scott, C. B., & Faris, P. D. (1994). Sexual rehabilitation for women with gynecological cancer: Information is not sufficient. Canadian Journal of Human Sexuality, 3, 131–142.

Rofe, Y., Blittner, M., & Lewin, I. (1993). Emotional experiences during the three trimesters of pregnancy. Journal of Clinical Psychology, 49, 3–12.

Rohde, L. A., Busnello, E., Wolf, A., Zomer, A., Shansis, F., Martins, S., & Tramontina, S. (1997). Maternity blues in Brazilian women. Acta Psychiatrica Scandinavica, 95, 231–235.

Rojansky, N., Reubinoff, B., Tanos, V., Shushan, A., & Weinstein, D. (1997). High risk pregnancy outcome following induction of labour. European Journal of Obstetrics, Gynecology, and Reproductive Biology, 72, 153–158.

Romano, D. (1988). Intercultural marriage: Promises and pitfalls. Yarmouth, ME: Intercultural Press.

Ronald, A. R., & Albritton, W. (1990). Chancroid and Haemophilus ducreyi. In K. K. Holmes, Mardh, P. A., Sparling, P. F., & Wiesner, P. J. (Eds.), Sexually transmitted diseases (2nd ed.) (pp. 263–271). New York: McGraw-Hill Information Services Company.

Rosal, M. C., Downing, J., Littman, A. B., & Ahern, D. K. (1994). Sexual functioning post-myocardial infarction: Effects of beta-blockers, psychological status and safety information. Journal of Psychosomatic Research, 38, 655–667.

Rosen, R. C., & Leiblum, S. R. (1989). Assessment and treatment of desire disorders. In S. R. Leiblum & R. C. Rosen (Eds.), Principles and practice of sex therapy. Update for the 1990s (2nd ed.) (pp. 19–50). New York: The Guilford Press.

Rosen, R. C., & Leiblum, S. R. (1995). Case studies in sex therapy. New York: Guilford Press.

Rosen, R. C., & Leiblum, S. R. (1995). Hypoactive sexual desire. The Psychiatric Clinics of North America, 18, 107–121.

Rosenberg, D. (1992). Trends: Circumcision and circumspection. Technology Review, 95, 17

Rosenberg, M. J., & Phillips, R. S. (1992). Does douching promote ascending infection. Journal of Reproductive Medicine, 37, 930–938.

Rosenberg, M. J., Phillips, R. S., & Holmes, M. D. (1991). Vaginal douching. Who and why? Journal of Reproductive Medicine, 36, 753–758.

Rosenfeld, J. A. (1992). Emotional responses to therapeutic abortion. American Family Physician, 45, 137–140.

Rosenkrantz, P., Vogel, S., Bee, H., Broverman, I., & Broverman, D. (1968). Sex-role stereotypes and self-concepts in college students. Journal of Consulting and Clinical Psychology, 32, 287–295.

Rosenthal, S. L., Cohen, S. S., Biro, F. M., & DeVellis, R. F. (1996). How do family characteristics relate to interpersonal expectations regarding STD acquisition among adolescent girls? Families, Systems & Health, 14, 465–474.

Rosenzweig, J. M., & Dailey, D. M. (1991). Women's sex roles in their public and private lives. Journal of Sex Education and Therapy, 17, 75–85.

Rosler, A., & Witztum, E. (1998). Treatment of men with paraphilia with a long-acting analogue of gonadotropin-releasing hormone. The New England Journal of Medicine, 338, 416–422.

Rosman, J., & Resnick, P. (1989). Sexual attraction to corpses: A psychiatric review of necrophilia. Bulletin of American Academic Psychiatry and Law, 17, 153–163.

Ross, J. M. (1997). The sadomasochism of everyday life. New York: Simon & Schuster.

Rotheram-Borus, M. J., & Fernandez, M. I. (1995). Sexual orientation and developmental challenges experienced by gay and lesbian youths. Suicide and Life-Threatening Behavior, 25, Supplement, 26–34.

Rotherman-Borus, M. J., Rosario, M., Beyer-Bahlburg, H., Koopman, C., Dopkins, S., & Davies, M. (1994). Sexual and substance use acts among gay and bisexual male adolescents in New York City. Journal of Sex Research, 31, 47–57.

Rothschild, A. J. (1995). Selective serotonin reuptake inhibitor-induced sexual dysfunction: Efficacy of a drug holiday. American Journal of Psychiatry, 152, 1514–1516.

Rotmensch, S., Liberati, M., Bronshtein, M., Schoenfeld-Dimaio, M., Shalev, J., Ben-Rafael, Z., & Copel, J. A. (1997). Prenatal sonographic findings in 187 fetuses with Down syndrome. Prenatal Diagnosis, 17, 1001–1009.

Rowland, D. L., Kallan, K., & Slob, A. K. (1997). Yohimbine, erectile capacity, and sexual response in men. Archives of Sexual Behavior, 26, 49–62.

Rubenstein, G. (1995). The decision to remove homosexuality from the DSM: Twenty years later. American Journal of Psychotherapy, 49, 416–427.

Ruminjo, J. K., Steiner, M., Joanis, C., Mwathe, E. G., & Thagana, N. (1996). Preliminary comparison of the polyurethane female condom with the latex male condom in Kenya. East African Medical Journal, 73, 101–106.

Runkel, G. (1998). Sexual morality of Christianity. Journal of Sex & Marital Therapy, 24, 103–122.

Russell, D. E. H. (1998a). The making of a whore. In R. K. Bergen, et al., (Eds), Issues in intimate violence (pp. 65–77). Thousand Oaks, CA: Sage Publications.

Russell, D. E. H. (1998b). Dangerous relationships: Pornography, misogyny, and rape. Thousand Oaks, CA: Sage Publications.

Russell, G. M., & Greenhouse, E. M. (1997). Homophobia in the supervisory relationship: An invisible intruder. Psychoanalytic Review, 84, 27–42.

Rutledge, D. N. (1992). Effect of age on lump detection accuracy. Nursing Research, 41, 306–308.

Ryan, S. A., Millstein, S. G., & Irwin, C. E. (1996). Puberty questions asked by early adolescents: What do they want to know? Journal of Adolescent Health, 19, 145–152.

Rybczynski, W. (1986). Home. A short history of an idea. New York: Viking.

Sagarin, E. (1973). Power to the peephole. Sexual Behavior, 3, 2–7.

Sakondhavat, C., Werawatanakul, Y., Bennett, A., Kuchaisit, C., & Suntharapa, S. (1997). Promoting condom-only brothels through solidarity and support for brothel managers. International Journal of STD and AIDS, 8, 40–43.

Salovey, P. (Ed.). (1991). The psychology of jealousy and envy. New York: Guilford.

Salter, M. J. (1992). Aspects of sexuality for patients with stomas and continent pouches. Journal of ET Nursing, 19, 126–130.

Saltzburg, S. (1996). Family therapy and the disclosure of adolescent homosexuality. Journal of Family Psychotherapy, 7, 1–18.

Sanchez-Guerrero, J., Colditz, G. A., Karlson, E. W., Hunter, D. J., Speizer, F. E., & Liang, M. H. (1995). Silicone breast implants and the risk of connective-tissue diseases and symptoms. New England Journal of Medicine, 332, 1666–1670.

Sandowski, C. L. (1990). Sexual concerns when illness or disability strikes. Springfield, IL: Charles C. Thomas Publishers, Ltd.

Sang, G. W., Shao, Q. X., Ge, R. S., Ge, J. L., Chen, J. K., Song, S., Fang, K. J., He, M. L., Luo, S. Y., Chen, S. F., et al. (1995). A multi-centered phase III comparative clinical trial of Mesigyna, Cyclofem and injectable no. 1 given monthly by intramuscular injection to Chinese women. I. Contraceptive efficacy and side effects. Contraception, 51, 167–183.

Sangi-Haghpeykar, H., Poindexter, A. N. 3rd, & Bateman, L. (1997). Consistency of condom use among users of injectable contraceptives. Family Planning Perspectives, 29, 67–69.

Sapadin, L. (1986). Friendship patterns: A comparison of professional men's and women's cross-sex and same-sex friendships. Dissertation Abstracts International, 47–09B, 4009.

Sapire, K. E. (1995). The female condom (Femidom)—a study of user acceptability. South African Medical Journal, 85, 1081–1084.

Sarrel, L. J. (1984). Sexual turning points: The seven stages of adult sexuality. New York: Macmillan.

Sarrel, P., Dobay, B., & Wiita, B. (1998). Estrogen and estrogen-androgen replacement in postmenopausal women dissatisfied with estrogen-only therapy. Sexual behavior and neuroendocrine responses. Journal of Reproductive Medicine, 43, 847–856.

Satoh, K. (1989). The importance of the worldwide contraceptive experience of Japanese physicians. International Journal of Fertility, 34 Supplement, 8–13.

Sbrocco, T., Weisberg, R. B., & Barlow, D. H. (1995). Sexual dysfunction in the older adult: Assessment of psychosocial factors. Sexuality and Disability, 13, 201.

Schacter, S. (1951). Deviation, rejection and communication. Journal of Abnormal and Social Psychology, 46, 190–207.

Schaefer, L. C., & Wheeler, C. C. (1995). Harry Benjamin's first ten cases (1938–1953): A clinical historical note. Archives of Sexual Behavior, 24, 73–93.

Schechterman, A. L., & Hutchinson, R. L. (1991). Causal attributions, self-monitoring, and gender differences among four virginity status groups. Adolescence, 26, 659–678.

Schiavi, R. C., Stimmel, B. B., Mandeli, J., & White, D. (1995). Chronic alcoholism and male sexual function. American Journal of Psychiatry, 152, 1045–1051.

Schlesinger, B. (1996). The sexless years or sex rediscovered. Journal of Gerontological Social Work, 26, 117–131.

Schmidt, G., Sigusch, V., & Schafer, S. (1973). Responses to reading erotic stories: Male-female differences. Archives of Sexual Behavior, 2, 181–199.

Schneider, M., & O'Neill, B. (1993). Eligibility of lesbians and gay men for spousal benefits: A social policy perspective. The Canadian Journal of Human Sexuality, 2, 23–31.

Schneider, M., & Phillips, S. P. (1997). A qualitative study of sexual harassment of female doctors by patients. Social Science & Medicine, 45, 669–676.

Schover, L. R., & Jensen, S. B. (1988). Sex and chronic illness: A comprehensive approach. New York: Guilford Press.

Schraag, J. A. (1989). Sexual education in schools: Concepts and possibilities. International Journal of Adolescent Medicine & Health, 4, 239–250.

Schuklenk, U., & Ristow, M. (1996). The ethics of research into the cause(s) of homosexuality. Journal of Homosexuality, 31, 5–30.

Schulhofer, S. (1998). Unwanted sex. The Atlantic Monthly, 282, 55–66.

Schuster, M. A., Bell, R. M., & Kanouse, D. E. (1996). The sexual practices of adolescent virgins: Genital sexual activities of high school students who have never had vaginal intercourse. American Journal of Public Health, 86, 1570–1576.

Schuster, M. A., Bell, R. M., Petersen, L. P., & Kanouse, D. E. (1996). Communication between adolescents and physicians about sexual behavior and risk prevention. Archives of Pediatrics and Adolescent Medicine, 150, 906–913.

Schwartz, M. D., Lerman, C., Miller, S. M., Daly, M., & Masny, A. (1995). Coping disposition, perceived risk, and psychological distress among women at increased risk for ovarian cancer. Health Psychology, 14, 232–235.

Sdoro, L. M. (1993). Psychology (2nd ed.). Madison, WI: WCB Brown & Benchmark.

Seagraves, R. T. (1995). Antidepressant-induced orgasm disorder. Journal of Sex and Marital Therapy, 21, 192–201.

Sedney, M. A. (1989). Conceptual and methodological sources of controversies about androgyny. In R. K. Unger (Ed.), Representations: Social constructions of gender. Amityville, NY: Baywood Press.

Segraves, R. T., & Segraves, K. B. (1995). Human sexuality and aging. Journal of Sex Education and Therapy, 21, 88–102.

Seidl, M. M., & Stewart, D. E. (1998). Alternative treatments for menopausal symptoms. Systematic review of scientific and lay literature. Canadian Family Physician, 44, 1299–1308.

Seidman, S. N., & Reider, R. O. (1994). A review of sexual behavior in the United States. American Journal of Psychiatry, 151, 330–341.

Seitz, C. R. (1995). Human sexuality viewed from the Bible's understanding of the human condition. Theology Today, 52, 236–246.

Sellers, T. A., Mink, P. J., Cerhan, J. R., Zheng, W., Anderson, K. E., Kushi, L. H., & Folsom, A. R. (1997). The role of hormone replacement therapy in the risk for breast cancer and total mortality in women with a family history of breast cancer. Annals of Internal Medicine, 127, 973–980.

Sellwood, W., & Tarrier, N. (1994). Demographic factors associated with extreme noncompliance in schizophrenia. Social Psychiatry and Psychiatric Epidemiology, 29, 172–177.

Semans, J. H. (1956). Premature ejaculation: A new approach. Southern Medical Journal, 49, 353–357.

Shaban, S. F. (1996). Male infertility overview. Atlanta Reproductive Health Centre WWW. [on-line].

Shackelford, T. K., & Buss, D. M. (1996). Betrayal in mateships, friendships, and coalitions. Personality & Social Psychology Bulletin, 22, 1151–1164.

Shafer, R. J. (Ed.). (1980). A guide to historical method (3rd ed.). Homewood, Illinois: Dorsey.

Shah, D. (1996). Critical review of group interventions for sexual dysfunction: Advances in the last decade. Sexual & Marital Therapy, 11, 187–195.

Shainess, N. (1997). Nymphomania, sexual alienation, hostile sex, and superego development. In L. B. Schlesinger & E. Revitch (Eds.), Sexual dynamics of anti-social behavior (2nd ed.) (pp. 50–75). Springfield, IL: Charles C. Thomas.

Shakespeare, T., Gillespie-Sells, K., & Davies, D. (1996). The sexual politics of disability: Untold desires. London: Cassell Academic.

Shalit, W. (1998, April 6). Feminism lives! In sexual harassment law, there is a nugget of truth that keeps feminism vital. National Review, 50, 36–38.

Shapiro, B. L., & Schwarz, J. C. (1997). Date rape. Its relationship to trauma symptoms and sexual self-esteem. Journal of Interpersonal Violence, 12, 407–419.

Sharf, B. F., & Freimuth, V. S. (1993). The construction of illness on entertainment television: Coping with cancer on *thirtysomething*. Health and Communication, 5, 141–160.

Sheldon, H., & Bannister, A. (1998). Working with adult female survivors of childhood sexual abuse. In A. Bannister (Ed.), From hearing to healing. Working with the aftermath of child sexual abuse (pp. 96–117). New York: John Wiley & Sons.

Shepperdson, B. (1995). The control of sexuality in young people with Down's syndrome. Child Care, Health, and Development, 21, 333–349.

Shortes, C. (1998). The containment of S/M pornography. Journal of Popular Film and Television, 26, 72–79.

Shults, C. (1995). Sexual harassment as sexual addiction. Sexual Addiction & Compulsivity, 2, 128–141.

Shumate, R. (1995, March 9). Gay marriage issue is a political time bomb. Bay Windows. [on-line].

Siegert, J. R., & Stamp, G. H. (1994). "Our first big fight" as a milestone in the development of close relationships. Communication Monographs, 61, 345–360.

Sieving. R., Resnick, M. D., Bearinger, L., et al. (1997). Cognitive and behavioral predictors of sexually transmitted disease risk behavior among sexually active adolescents. Archives of Pediatrics and Adolescent Medicine, 151, 243–251.

Sigman, G. S., & O'Connor, C. (1991). Exploration for physicians of the mature minor doctrine. Journal of Pediatrics, 119, 520–525.

Silber, T. J. (1982). Ethical considerations concerning adolescents consulting for contraceptive services. Journal of Family Practice, 15, 909–911.

Silverstein, B., Peterson, B., & Perdue, L. (1986). Some correlates of the thin standard of bodily attractiveness for women. International Journal of Eating Disorders, 5, 895–905.

Simerly, T. (1996). Longtime companions: Gay couples in the era of AIDS. Transactional Analysis Journal, 26, 8–14.

Simkin, P. (1989). The birth partner. Everything you need to know to help a woman through childbirth. Boston, MA: Harvard Common Press.

Simon, G. E. (1998). Cyberporn and censorship: Constitutional barriers to preventing access to internet pornography by minors. The Journal of Criminal Law & Criminology, 88, 1015–1048.

Simon, R. I. (1997). Video voyeurs and the covert videotaping of unsuspecting victims: Psychological and legal consequences. Journal of Forensic Sciences, 42, 884–889.

Simon, W. (1994). Deviance as history: The future of perversion. Archives of Sexual Behavior, 23, 1–20.

Simon, W., & Gagnon, J. H. (1986). Sexual scripts: Permanence and change. Archives of Sexual Behavior, 15, 97–120.

Simonds, J. F. (1980). Sexual behaviors in retarded children and adolescents. Journal of Developmental and Behavioral Pediatrics, 1, 173–179.

Singh, K., & Ratnam, S. S. (1997). A comparison of the clinical performance, contraceptive efficacy, reversibility and acceptability of Norplant implants and Ortho Gynae T380 intrauterine copper contraceptive devices. Advances in Contraception, 13, 385–393.

Sipski, M. L. (1991). The impact of spinal cord injury on female sexuality, menstruation and pregnancy: A review of the literature. Journal of the American Paraplegia Society, 14, 122–126.

Sipski, M. L., Alexander, C. J., & Rosen, R. C. (1995a). Physiological parameters associated with psychogenic sexual arousal in women with complete spinal cord injuries. Archives of Physical Medicine and Rehabilitation, 76, 811–818.

Sipski, M. L., Alexander, C. J., & Rosen, R. C. (1995b). Orgasm in women with spinal cord injuries: A laboratory-based assessment. Archives of Physical Medicine and Rehabilitation, 76, 1097–1102.

Sipski, M. L., Alexander, C. J., & Rosen, R. C. (1997). Physiologic parameters associated with sexual arousal in women with incomplete spinal cord injuries. Archives of Physical Medicine and Rehabilitation, 78, 305–313.

Siston, A. K., List, M. A., Schleser, R., & Vokes, E. (1997). Sexual functioning and head and neck cancer. Journal of Psychosocial Oncology, 15, 107–122.

Sjogren, K. (1983). Sexuality after stroke with hemiplegia. II. With special regard to partnership adjustment and to fulfilment. Scandinavian Journal of Rehabilitation Medicine, 15, 63–69.

Sjogren, K., Damber, J. E., & Liliequist, B. (1983). Sexuality after stroke with hemiplegia. I. Aspects of sexual function. Scandinavian Journal of Rehabilitation Medicine, 15, 55–61.

Skeen, D. (1991). Different sexual worlds. Contemporary case studies of sexuality. Lanham, MD: Lexington Books.

Slavis, S. A., Novick, A. C., Steinmuller, D. R., Streem, S. B., Braun, W. E., Straffon, R. A., Mastroianni, B., & Graneto, D. (1990). Outcome of renal transplantation in patients with a functioning graft for 20 years or more. Journal of Urology, 144, 20–22.

Slemenda, C. (1978). Sociocultural factors affecting acceptance of family planning services by Navajo women. Human Organization, 37, 190–194.

Sloan, L., Edmond, T., Rubin, A., & Doughty, M. (1998). Social workers' knowledge of and experience with sexual exploitation by psychotherapists. Social Work, 43, 43–53.

Slob, A. K., Erneste, M., & van der Werff ten Bosch, J. J. (1990). Menstrual cycle phase and sexual arousability in women. Archives of Sexual Behavior, 20, 567–577.

Sloggett, K. J., & Herold, E. S. (1996). Single women with high sexual interest. Canadian Journal of Human Sexuality, 5, 211–219.

Slonim-Nevo, V. (1991). The experiences of women who face abortions. Health Care for Women International, 12, 283–292.

Slovenko, R. (1995). People seeking people. The Journal of Psychiatry & Law, Number 2, 333–343.

Slusher, M. P., Mayer, C. J., & Dunkle, R. E. (1996). Gays and lesbians older and wiser (GLOW): A support group for older gay people. Gerontologist, 36, 118–123.

Sly, D. F., Quadagno, D., Harrison, D. F., Eberstein, I. W., Riehman, K., & Bailey, M. (1997). Factors associated with use of the female condom. Family Planning Perspectives, 29, 181–184.

Small, M. F. (1992). The evolution of female sexuality and mate selection in humans. Human Nature, 3, 133–156.

Smith, D. E., Wesson, D. R., & Apter-Marsh, M. (1984). Cocaine- and alcohol-induced sexual dysfunction in patients with addictive disease. Journal of Psychoactive Drugs, 16, 359–361.

Smith, D., & Over, R. (1990). Enhancement of fantasy-induced sexual arousal in men through training in erotic imagery. Archives of Sexual Behavior, 19, 477–489.

Smith, E. M., & Bodner, D. R. (1993). Sexual dysfunction after spinal cord injury. Urologic Clinics of North America, 20, 535–542.

Smith, P. M., & Schwartz, P. E. (1993). Social work role in an early ovarian cancer detection program. Social Work in Health Care, 19, 67–80.

Smith, T. W. (1991). Adult sexual behavior in 1989: Number of partners, frequency of intercourse, and risk of AIDS. Family Planning Perspectives, 23, 102–107.

Snaith, P., Tarsh, M. J., & Reid. R. (1993). Sex reassignment surgery. A study of 141 Dutch transsexuals. British Journal of Psychiatry, 162, 681–685.

Snyder, E. E., & Spreitzer, E. (1976). Attitudes of the aged toward nontraditional sexual behavior. Archives of Sexual Behavior, 5, 249–254.

Sober orgies only! (1993, October 11). Time, 142, 24.

Solomon, J. (1998, March 16). An insurance policy with sex appeal. Newsweek, 131, 44.

Southern Baptists vote to boycott Disney. (1997, July 2–9). Christian Century, 114, 623–624.

Spector, I. P., & Carey, M. P. (1990). Incidence and prevalence of the sexual dysfunctions: A critical review of the empirical literature. Archives of Sexual Behavior, 19, 389–408.

Spector, I. P., & Fremeth, S. M. (1996). Sexual behaviors and attitudes of geriatric residents in long-term care facilities. Journal of Sex & Marital Therapy, 22, 235–246.

Spence, S. H. (1991). Psychosexual therapy: A cognitive-behavioral approach. New York: Chapman & Hall.

Spica, M. M., & Schwab, M. D. (1996). Sexual expression after total hip replacement. Orthopaedic Nursing, 15, 41–44.

Spitzberg, B. H., & Rhea, J. (1999). Obsessive relational intrusion and sexual coercion victimization. Journal of Interpersonal Violence, 14, 3–20.

Spitzer, R. L., Gibbon, M., Skodol, A. E., Williams, J. B. W., & First, M. D. (1994). DSM-IV casebook. Washington, DC: American Psychiatric Press.

Sprecher, S., & Felmlee, D. (1993). Conflict, love and other relationship dimensions for individuals in dissolving, stable, and growing premarital relationships. Free Inquiry in Creative Sociology, 21, 115–125.

Sprecher, S., Metts, S., Burleson, B., Hatfield, E., & Thompson, A. (1995). Domains of expressive interaction in intimate relationships. Associations with satisfaction and commitment. Family Relations, 44, 203–210.

Spring, W. D. Jr., Willenbring, M. L., & Maddux, T. L. (1992). Sexual dysfunction and psychological distress in methadone maintenance. The International Journal of the Addictions, 27, 1325–1334.

Stack, S., & Gundlach, J. H. (1992). Divorce and sex. Archives of Sexual Behavior, 21, 359–367.

Stamler, V. L., & Stone, G. L. (1998). Faculty-student sexual involvement: Issues & interventions. Thousand Oaks, CA: Sage Publishing.

Stearns, P. (1989). Jealousy: The evolution of an emotion in American history. New York: New York University Press.

Stein, T. J. (1996). Child custody and visitation: The rights of lesbian and gay parents. Social Service Review, 70, 435–450.

Steinhauer, J. (1998, June 23). Viagra's other side effect: Upsets in many a marriage. The New York Times. [http://www.nytimes.com].

Steinke, E. E. (1994). Knowledge and attitudes of older adults about sexuality in aging: A comparison of two studies. Journal of Advanced Nursing, 19, 477–485.

Stenager, E., Stenager, E. N., & Jensen, K. (1996). Sexual function in multiple sclerosis. A 5-year follow-up study. Italian Journal of Neurological Sciences, 17, 67–69.

Stenson, J. (1998, June 4). Sex, nursing homes and Viagra: Drug focuses new attention on ongoing dilemma. Medical Tribune. [on line].

Stepakoff, S. (1998). Effects of sexual victimization on suicidal ideation and behavior in U.S. college women. Suicide and Life-Threatening Behavior, 28, 107–126.

Stern, S. H., Fuchs, M. D., Ganz, S. B., Classi, P., Sculco, T. P., & Salvati, E. A. (1991). Sexual function after total hip arthroplasty. Clinical Orthopaedics and Related Research, 269, 228–235.

Sternberg, R. J. (1988). Triangulating love. In R. J. Sternberg & M. L. Barnes (Eds.), The psychology of love (pp. 24–30). New Haven: Yale University Press.

Sternglanz, S. H., & Serbin, L. A. (1974). Sex-role typing in children's television programming. Developmental Psychology, 10, 710–715.

Stevens, V. M., Hatcher, J. W., & Bruce, B. K. (1994). How compliant is compliant? Evaluating adherence with breast self-exam positions. Journal of Behavioral Medicine, 17, 523–534.

Stewart, D. E. (1992). Reproductive functions in eating disorders. Annals of Medicine, 24, 287–291.

Stewart, D. E., Robinson, E., Goldbloom, D. S., & Wright, C. (1990). Infertility and eating disorders. American Journal of Obstetrics and Gynecology, 163 (4 Part 1), 1196–1199.

Stiglmayer, A. (Ed.). (1994). Mass rape: The war against women in Bosnia-Herzegovina. Lincoln, NE: University of Nebraska Press.

Stock, W. E. (1997). Sex as commodity: Men and the sex industry. In R. F. Levant & G. R. Brooks (Eds.), Men and sex (pp. 100–132). New York: John Wiley & Sons.

Stoil, M. J. (1998). Do rapists belong in mental hospitals? Behavioral Health Management, 18, 6–8.

Stokes, J. P., McKirnan, D. J., Doll, L., & Burzette, R. G. (1996). Female partners of bisexual men. What they don't know might hurt them. Psychology of Women Quarterly, 20, 267–284.

Stolberg, S. G. (1997, December 14). For the infertile, a high-tech treadmill of despair. The New York Times. [http://www.nytimes.com].

Stolberg, S. G. (1998, March 9). U.S. awakens to epidemic of sexual diseases. The New York Times, A1.

Stordahl, V. (1995). Changing roles in Sami families—a case illustration. Arctic Medical Research, 54, 42–46.

Storr, A. (1970). Sexual deviation. Baltimore, MD: Penguin Books.

Strassberg, D. S., & Lockerd, L. K. (1998). Force in women's sexual fantasies. Archives of Sexual Behavior, 27, 403–414.

Strouse, J. S., Buerkel-Rothfuss, N., & Long, E. C. J. (1995). Gender and family as moderators of the relationship between music video exposure and adolescent sexual permissiveness. Adolescence, 30, 505–521.

Struckman-Johnson, C., & Struckman-Johnson, D. (1993). College men's and women's reactions to hypothetical sexual touch varied by initiator gender and coercion level. Sex Roles, 29, 371–385.

Stumpf, P. G., Byers, G., & Lloyd, T. (1986). Effect of vaginal contraceptive sponges on growth of toxic shock syndrome-associated Staphylococcus aureus in vitro. Contraception, 33, 395–399.

Sturgeon, S. R., Brinton, L. A., Berman, M. L., Mortel, R., Twiggs, L. B., Barrett, R. J., Wilbanks, G. D., & Lurain, J. R. (1997). Intrauterine device use and endometrial cancer risk. International Journal of Epidemiology, 26, 496–500.

Sue, D. (1979). Erotic fantasies of college students during coitus. Journal of Sex Research, 15, 299–305.

Suggs, R., & Miracle, A. (Eds.). (1993). Culture and human sexuality. Pacific Grove, CA: Brooks/Cole.

Suppe, F. (1984). Classifying sexual disorders: The diagnostic and statistical manual of the American Psychiatric Association. Journal of Homosexuality, 9, 9–28.

Surratt, H. L., Wechsberg, W. M., Cottler, L. B., Leukefeld, C. G., Klein, H., & Desmond, D. P. (1998). Acceptability of the female condom among women at risk for HIV infection. American Behavioral Scientist, 41, 1157–1170.

Sussman, J. R., & Levitt, B. B. (1989). Before you conceive. The complete pregnancy guide. New York: Bantam Books.

Swaab, D. F., & Hofman, M. A. (1990). An enlarged suprachiasmatic nucleus in homosexual men. Brain Research, 537,141–148.

Swaab, D. F., Gooren, L. J. G., & Hofman, M. A. (1992). The human hypothalamus in relation to gender and sexual orientation. Progress in Brain Research, 93, 205–219.

Swankambo, N., Gray, R. H., Wawer, M. J., et al. (1997). HIV-1 infection associated with abnormal vaginal flora morphology and bacterial vaginosis. Lancet, 350, 546–550.

Sweet, R. L. (1995). Role of bacterial vaginosis in pelvic inflammatory disease. Clinical Infectious Diseases, 20, S271–S275.

Tamaki, R., Murata, M., & Okano, T. (1997). Risk factors for postpartum depression in Japan. Psychiatry and Clinical Neurosciences, 51, 93–98.

Tamkins, T. (1995). New PSA test may reduce biopsy need. Medical Tribune, 36, 1, 4.

Tanfer, K., & Horn, M. C. (1985). Contraceptive use, pregnancy and fertility patterns among young single American women in their 20s. Family Planning Perspectives, 17, 10–19.

Tang, C., Siu, B., Lai, F., & Chung, T. (1996). Heterosexual Chinese women's sexual adjustment after gynecologic cancer. Journal of Sex Research, 33, 189–195.

Tangri, S. S., Burt, M. R., & Johnson, L. B. (1982). Sexual harassment at work: Three explanatory models. Journal of Social Issues, 38, 33–54.

Tannahill, R. (1980). Sex in history. New York: Stein and Day.

Tatchell, P. (1995). Sweet fourteen. New Statesman & Society, 8, 25.

Tayal, S. C., & Pattman, R. S. (1994). High prevalence of herpes simplex virus type 1 in female anogenital herpes simplex in Newcastle upon Tyne. International Journal of STD and AIDS, 5, 359–361.

Taylor, S. E. (1989). Positive illusions: Creative self-deception and the healthy mind. New York: Basic Books.

Taylor, S. E., & Armor, D. A. (1996). Positive illusions and coping with adversity. Journal of Personality, 64, 873–898.

Tedesco, R. (1998). Porn sites making hay. Broadcasting & Cable, 128, 64.

The PDR Family Guide to Woman's Health and Prescription Drugs. (1994). Montvale, NJ: Medical Economics.

Thelen, M. H., Sherman, M. D., & Borst, T. S. (1998). Fear of intimacy and attachment among rape survivors. Behavior Modification, 22, 108–116.

Thiel, G. (1997, February 25). No gay clergy say SA churches. Electronic Mail & Guardian. [online].

Thienhaus, O. J., Conter, E. A., & Bosmann, H. B. (1986). Sexuality and ageing. Ageing and Society, 6, 39–54.

Thoen, L. D., & Creinin, M. D. (1997). Medical treatment of ectopic pregnancy with methotrexate. Fertility and sterility, 68, 727–730.

Thomas, S. B., & Quinn, S. C. (1991). The Tuskegee syphilis study, 1932 to 1972: Implications for HIV education and AIDS risk education programs in the black community. The American Journal of Public Health, 81, 1498–1505.

Thompson, H. A. (1989). Consent requirements for treatment of minors. Texas Medicine, 85, 56–59.

Tidwell, M-C. O., Reis, H. T., & Shaver, P. R. (1996). Attachment, attractiveness, and social interaction: A diary study. Journal of Personality and Social Psychology, 71, 729–745.

Tiefer, L., & Melman, A. (1989). Comprehensive evaluation of erectile dysfunction and medical treatments. In S. R. Leiblum & R. C. Rosen (Eds.), Principles and practice of sex therapy. Update for the 1990s (2nd ed.) (pp. 207–236). New York: The Guilford Press.

Tipton, K. (1998). In the eye of the beholder. The Humanist, 58, 45–47.

Tissot, S. A. D. (1832). A treatise on the diseases produced by onanism. New York: Collins and Hannay.

Tjaden, R., & Thoennes, N. (1997, July). Stalking in America: Findings from the National Violence Against Women Survey (N.I.J. Grant No. 93-1J-CX-0012). Washington, DC: National Institutes of Justice/Centers for Disease Control.

Tokatlidis, O., & Over, R. (1995). Imagery, fantasy, and female sexual arousal. Australian Journal of Psychology, 47, 81–85.

Trachtenberg, P. (1988). The Casanova complex. New York: Poseidon Press.

Traeen, B., & Kvalem, I. L. (1996). Sexual socialization and motives for intercourse among Norwegian adolescents. Archives of Sexual Behavior, 25, 289–302.

Trainer, J. B. (1979). Pre-marital counseling and examination. Journal of Marital and Family Therapy, 5, 61–78.

Travin, S., & Protter, B. (1993). Sexual perversion. New York: Plenum Press.

Trevathan, W. R., Burleson, M. H., & Gregory, W. L. (1993). No evidence for menstrual synchrony in lesbian couples. Psychoneuroendocrinology, 18, 425–435.

Trudel, G., Aubin, S., & Matte, B. (1995). Sexual behaviors and pleasure in couples with hypoactive sexual desire. Journal of Sex Education and Therapy, 21, 210–216.

Trudel, G., Landry, L., & Larose, Y. (1997). Low sexual desire: The role of anxiety, depression and marital adjustment. Sexual and Marital Therapy, 12, 95–99.

Trussell, J., Strickler, J., & Vaughan, B. (1993). Contraceptive efficacy of the diaphragm, the sponge and the cervical cap. Family Planning Perspectives, 25, 100–105.

Trute, B., Adkins, E., & MacDonald, G. (1996). Professional attitudes regarding treatment and punishment of incest: Comparing police, child welfare, and community mental health. Journal of Family Violence, 11, 237–249.

Tsang, D. C. (1995). Policing "perversions": Depo-Provera and John Money's new sexual order. Journal of Homosexuality, 28, 397–426.

Tserotas, K., & Merino, G. (1998). Andropause and the aging male. Archives of Andrology, 40, 87–93.

Tsun-Yin, E. L. (1998). Sexual abuse trauma among Chinese survivors. Child Abuse and Neglect, 22, 1013–1026.

Tucker, L. A. (1982). Effect of a weight-training program on the self-concepts of college males. Perceptual and Motor Skills, 54, 1055–1061.

Tugrul, C., & Kabakci, E. (1997). Vaginismus and its correlates. Sexual and Marital Therapy, 12, 23–34.

Turkington, C. A. (1999). Miscarriage. Gale Encyclopedia of Medicine (p. 1928). Farmington, MI: Gale Publishing Group.

Turner, J. C., Garrison, C. Z., Korpita, E., Waller, J. L., et al. (1994). Promoting responsible sexual behavior through a college freshman seminar. AIDS Education and Prevention, 6, 266–277.

Turner, R. (March/April 1992). Births to women in their middle and late 30s have risen among both blacks and whites since 1980. Family Planning Perspectives, 24, 91–92.

Twohig, F., & Furnham, A. (1998). Lay beliefs about overcoming four sexual paraphilias: Fetishism, paedophilia, sexual sadism, and voyeurism. Personality and Individual Differences, 24, 267–278.

U. S. college women. Suicide and Life-Threatening Behavior, 28, 107–126.

U. S. Department of Health and Human Services (1996). Advance data from vital and health statistics of the National Center for Health Statistics. Washington, D. C.: U. S. Government Printing Office.

Udry, J. R. (1980). Changes in the frequency of marital intercourse from panel data. Archives of Sexual Behavior, 9, 319–325.

Uhlenberg, P., Cooney, T., & Boyd, R. (1990). Divorce for women after midlife. Journal of Gerontology, 45, S3–S311.

Unger, J. B., Simon, T. R., Newman, T. L., Montgomery, S. B., Kipke, M. D., & Albornonz, M. (1998). Early adolescent street youth: An overlooked population with unique problems and service needs. Journal of Early Adolescence, 18, 325–348.

United States Equal Employment Opportunity Commission. (1997). Facts about sexual harassment [Brochure].

Valenti-Hein, D. C., Yarnold, P. R., & Mueser, K. T. (1994). Evaluation of the dating skills program for improving heterosocial interactions in people with mental retardation. Behavior Modification, 18, 32–46.

Van De Walle, E., & Muhsam, H. V. (1995). Fatal secrets and the French fertility transition. Population and Development Review, 21, 261–279.

Van Mechelen, R. (1994). Values & ideologies. [on line].

van Nijnatten, C. H. C. J. (1995). Sexual orientation of parents and Dutch family law. Medicine & Law, 14,359–14,368.

van Turnhout, A. A., Hage, J. J., & van Diest, P. J. (1995). The female corpus spongiosum revisited. Acta Obstetricia et Gynecologica Scandinavica, 74, 767–771.

Van Winter, J. T., Harmon, M. C., Atkinson, E. J., Simmons, P. S., & Ogburn Jr., P. L. (1997). Young Mom's Clinic: A multidisciplinary approach to pregnancy education in teens and young single women. Pediatric and Adolescent Gynecology, 10, 28–33.

Vartiainen, H., Saarikoski, S., Halonen, P., & Rimon, R. (1994). Psychosocial factors, female fertility and pregnancy: A prospective study—Part I: Fertility. Journal of Psychosomatic Obstetrics and Gynaecology, 15, 67–75.

Vartiainen, H., Suonio, S., Halonen, P., & Rimon, R. (1994). Psychosocial factors, female fertility and pregnancy: A prospective study—Part II: Pregnancy. Journal of Psychosomatic Obstetrics and Gynaecology, 15, 77–84.

Vaughan, D. (1986). Uncoupling: Turning points in intimate relationships. New York: Oxford University Press.

Verkauf, B. S., Von Thron, J., & O'Brien, W. F. (1992). Clitoral size in normal women. Obstetrics and Gynecology, 80, 41–44.

Vermeulen, A. (1994). Andropause, fact or fiction? In G. Berg & M. Hammar (Eds.), The modern management of the menopause (pp. 567–577). New York: The Parthenon Publishing Group.

Vermeulen, A., & Kaufman, J. M. (1995). Ageing of the hypothalamo-pituitary-testicular axis in men. Hormone Research, 43, 25–28.

Viinamakil, H., Niskanen, L., Pesonen, P., & Saarikoski, S. (1997). Evolution of postpartum depression. Psychosomatic Obstetrics and Gynaecology, 18, 213–219.

Vinik, A., & Richardson, D. (1998). Erectile dysfunction in diabetes. Diabetes Reviews, 6, 16–33.

Visser, A. P., Bruyniks, N., & Remmenick, L. (1993). Family planning in Russia: Experience and attitudes of gynecologists. Advances in Contraception, 9, 93–104.

Visser, A.P., Pavlenko, I., Remmenick, L., Bruyniks, N., & Lehert, P. (1993). Contraceptive practice and attitudes of former Soviet women. Advances in Contraception, 9, 13–23.

Von Gruenigen, V. E., & Karlen, J. R. (1995). Carcinoma of the endometrium. American Family Physician, 51, 1531-1536, 1541–1542.

Vonk R., & Ashmore, R. D. (1993). The multi-faceted self: Androgyny reassessed by open-ended self-descriptions. Social Psychology Quarterly, 56, 278–287.

Vreeland, C. N., Gallagher, B. J., & McFalls, J. A. (1995). The beliefs of members of the American Psychiatric Association on the etiology of male homosexuality: A national survey. Journal of Psychology, 129, 507–517.

Vyras, P. (1996). Neglected defender of homosexuality: A commemoration. Journal of Sex and Marital Therapy, 22, 121–129.

Wade, G. N., Schneider, J. E., & Li, H. Y. (1996). Control of fertility by metabolic cues. American Journal of Physiology, 270 (1 Part 1), E1–E19.

Wainaina, N. (1997). Kenya: gender equality—the role of men. WIN News, 23, 38.

Waldo, C. R., Berdahl, J. L., & Fitzgerald, L. F. (1998). Are men sexually harassed? If so, by whom? Law and Human Behavior, 22, 59–79.

Walker, E. A., Newman, E., Koss, M., & Bernstein, D. (1997). Does the study of victimization revictimize the victims. General Hospital Psychiatry, 19, 403–410.

Wallen, K. (1995). The evolution of female sexual desire. In P. R. Abramson & S. D. Pinkerton (Eds.), Sexual nature/sexual culture (pp. 57–79). Chicago: The University of Chicago Press.

Wallerstein, E. (1985). Circumcision. The uniquely American enigma. Urologic Clinics of North America, 12, 123–132.

Wallerstein, J. S. (1994). The early psychological tasks of marriage: Part I. American Journal of Orthopsychiatry, 64, 640–650.

Walrath, J., Fayerweather, W. E., & Spreen, K. A. (1992). A survey of the prevalence of epididymitis in an industrial setting. Journal of Occupational Medicine, 34, 170–172.

Ward, A., & Morgan, W. (1984). Adherence patterns of healthy men and women enrolled in an adult exercise program. Journal of Cardiac Rehabilitation, 4, 143–152.

Ward, M. (1995). Talking about sex: Common themes about sexuality in the prime-time television programs children and adolescents view most. Journal of Youth and Adolescence, 24, 595–615.

Ward, R. A. (1993). Marital happiness and household equity in later life. Journal of Marriage and the Family, 55, 427–438.

Wardell, D. (1980). Margaret Sanger: Birth control's successful revolutionary. American Journal of Public Health, 70, 736–742.

Wardle, J., Steptoe, A., Burckhardt, R., Vogele, C., et al. (1994). Testicular self-examination: Attitudes and practices among young men in Europe. Preventive Medicine: An International Journal Devoted to Practice & Theory, 23, 206–210.

Warner, P., & Bancroft, J. (1988). Mood, sexuality, oral contraceptives and the menstrual cycle. Journal of Psychosomatic Research, 32, 417–427.

Waterman, J., & Lusk, R. (1986). Scope of the problem. In K. MacFarlane, et al. (Eds.), Sexual Abuse of Young Children: Evaluation and Treatment (pp. 3–14). New York: Guilford Press.

Wattenberg, B. (1997, December 7). Population boom is going bust. Daily Press, H1, H4.

Waugh, M. A. (1990). History of clinical developments in sexually transmitted diseases. In K. K. Holmes, Mardh, P. A., Sparling, P. F., & Wiesner, P. J. (Eds.), Sexually transmitted diseases (2nd ed.) (pp. 3–18). New York: McGraw-Hill Information Services Company.

Weaver, A. J., Koenig, H. G., & Larson, D. B. (1997). Marriage and family therapists and the clergy: A need for clinical collaboration, training, and research. Journal of Marital and Family Therapy, 23, 13–25.

Weaver, C. H., & Mengel, M. B. (1988). Bacterial vaginosis. Journal of Family Practice, 27, 207–215.

Wein, A. J., & Van Arsdalen, K. N. (1988). Drug-induced male sexual dysfunction. Urologic Clinics of North America, 15, 23–31.

Weir, S. (1992). Crimes passionnels: Gender differences in perceived justification for murder in the face of marital infidelity. Irish Journal of Psychology, 13, 350–360.

Weir, S. S., Feldblum, P. J., Zekeng, L., & Roddy, R. E. (1994). The use of nonoxynol-9 for protection against cervical gonorrhea. The American Journal of Public Health, 84, 910–914.

Weis, D. L. (1985). The experience of pain during women's first sexual intercourse: Cultural mythology about sexual initiation. Archives of Sexual Behavior, 14, 421–437.

Weiss, P. (1997). Psychotherapy of paraphilic sex offenders. Medicine and Law, 16, 753–764.

Weitz, R., & Bryant, K. (1997). The portrayals of homosexuality in abnormal psychology and sociology of deviance textbooks. Deviant Behavior, 18, 27–46.

Weller, L., & Weller, A. (1993). Menstrual synchrony between mothers and daughters and between roommates. Physiology and Behavior, 53, 943–949.

Weller, L., Weller, A., & Avinir, O. (1995). Menstrual synchrony: Only in roommates who are close friends? Physiology and Behavior, 58, 883–889.

Weller, S. (1993). A meta-analysis of condom effectiveness in reducing sexually transmitted HIV. Social Science of Medicine, 36, 1635–1644

Wells, B. L. (1986). Predictors of female nocturnal orgasms. Journal of Sex Research, 22, 421–437.

Wells, J. W. (1990). The sexual vocabularies of heterosexual and homosexual males and females for communicating erotically with a sexual partner. Archives of Sexual Behavior, 19, 139–147.

Wells, W. D., & Siegel, B. (1961). Stereotyped somatotypes. Psychological Reports, 8, 77–78.

Wenninger, K., & Heiman, J. R. (1998). Relating body image to psychological and sexual functioning in child sexual abuse survivors. Journal of Traumatic Stress, 11, 543–562.

Werlinger, K., King, T. K., Clark, M. M., Pera, V., et al. (1997). Perceived changes in sexual functioning and body image following weight loss in an obese female population: A pilot study. Journal of Sex & Marital Therapy, 23, 74–78.

Werner, A. A. (1947). Sex behavior and problems of the climacteric. In M. Fisbein & E. W. Burgess (Eds.), Successful marriage (pp. 470–487). Garden City, NY: Doubleday & Company, Inc.

Werthman, P., & Rajfer, J. (1997). MUSE therapy: Preliminary clinical observations. Urology, 50, 809–811.

West, D. J. (1998). Boys and sexual abuse: An English opinion. Archives of Sexual Behavior, 27, 539–559.

West, T. C. (1999). Spirit-wounding violence against black women. New York: New York University Press.

Westgren, N., Hultling, C., Levi, R., Seiger, A., & Westgren, M. (1997). Sexuality in women with traumatic spinal cord injury. Acta Obstetricia et Gynecologica Scandinavica, 76, 977–983.

Westheimer, R. (1998). Dr. Ruth talks to kids. New York: Aladdin Paperbacks.

Westheimer, R. K. (1988). Dr. Ruth's guide to good sex. New York: Crown Publications Group.

Westheimer, R. K. (1995). Sex for dummies. Boston: International Data Group.

Westin, A. F. (1967). Privacy and freedom. New York: Atheneum.

Westoff, C. F. (1974). Coital frequency and contraception. Family Planning Perspectives, 6, 136–141.

Whipple, B., Josimovich, J. B., & Komisaruk, B. R. (1990). Sensory thresholds during the antepartum, intrapartum and postpartum periods. International Journal of Nursing Studies, 27, 213–221.

Whipple, B., Ogden, G., & Komisaruk, B. R. (1992). Physiological correlates of imagery-induced orgasm in women. Archives of Sexual Behavior, 21, 121–133.

Whitam, F. L., & Mathy, R. M. (1986). Male homosexuality in four societies: Brazil, Guatemala, the Philippines, and the United States. New York: Prager.

White, C. B. (1982). Sexual interest, attitudes, knowledge, and sexual history in relation to sexual behavior in the institutionalized aged. Archives of Sexual Behavior, 11, 11–21.

White, M. J., Rintala, D. H., Hart, K. A., Young, M. E., & Fuhrer, M. J. (1992). Sexual activities, concerns and interests of men with spinal cord injury. American Journal of Physical Medicine and Rehabilitation, 71, 225–231.

Whitehead, B. K. (1996). Lesbianism: Causality and compassion. Journal of Psychology & Christianity, 15, 348–363.

Wiebe, D. J., & Black, D. (1997). Illusional beliefs in the context of risky sexual behaviors. Journal of Applied Social Psychology, 27, 1727–1749.

Wiederman, M. W. (1993). Evolved gender differences in mate preferences: Evidence from personal advertisements. Ethology and Sociobiology, 14, 331–351.

Wiederman, M. W. (1997). Pretending orgasm during sexual intercourse: Correlates in a sample of young adult women. Journal of Sex and Marital Therapy, 23, 131–139.

Wilcox, A. J., Weinberg, C. R., & Baird, D. D. (1995). Timing of sexual intercourse in relation to ovulation. Effects on the probability of conception, survival of the pregnancy, and sex of the baby. The New England Journal of Medicine, 333, 1517–1521.

Wilke, M. (1998). Condom ads will debut along with Stern show: LifeStyles buys time in late-night program via CBS-owned stations. Advertising Age, 69, 8.

Williams, G., Abbou, C. C., Amar, E. T., et al. (1998). Efficacy and safety of transurethral aprostadil therapy in men with erectile dysfunction. MUSE study group. British Journal of Urology, 81, 889–894.

Williams, T. R., O' Sullivan, M., Snodgrass, S. E., & Love, N. (1995). Psychosocial issues in breast cancer. Postgraduate Medicine, 98, 97–99, 103–104, 107–108, 110.

Williamson, G. M., & Walters, A. S. (1996). Perceived impact of limb amputation on sexual activity: A study of adult amputees. Journal of Sex Research, 33, 221–230.

Wills, T. A., & DePaulo, B. M. (1991). Interpersonal analysis of the help-seeking process. In C. R. Snyder & D. R. Rorsyth (Eds.), Handbook of social and clinical psychology (pp. 350–375). New York: Pergamon.

Wilson, H. C., Kiefhaber, S. H., & Gravel, V. (1991). Two studies of menstrual synchrony: Negative results. Psychoneuroendocrinology, 16, 353–359.

Wilson, S. M., & Medora, N. P. (1990). Gender comparisons of college students' attitudes toward sexual behavior. Adolescence, 25, 615–627.

Wincze, J. P., & Carey, M. P. (1991). Sexual dysfunction: A guide for assessment and treatment. New York: Guilford Press.

Wingo, P. A., Tong, T., & Bolden, F. (1995). Cancer statistics. CA-A Cancer Journal for Clinicians, 45, 8–30.

Winick, C. (1992). Substances of use and abuse and sexual behavior. In J. H. Lowinson, P. Ruiz, R. B. Millman, & J. G. Langrod (Eds.), Substance abuse. A comprehensive handbook (pp. 722–732). Baltimore: Williams & Wilkins.

Winn, R. L., & Newton, N. (1982). Sexuality in aging: A study of 106 cultures. Archives of Sexual Behavior, 11, 283–298.

Wise, C. M. (1995). Gonococcal arthritis in an era of increasing penicillin resistance: Presentations and outcomes in 41 recent cases (1985–1991). The Journal of the American Medical Association, 273, 902.

Witt, D. K. (1998). Yohimbine for erectile dysfunction. The Journal of Family Practice, 46, 282–283.

Wolfe, J., Sharkansky, E. J., Read, J. P., Dawson, R., Martin, J. A., & Ouimette, P. C. (1998). Sexual harassment and assault as predictors of PTSD symptomatology among U. S. female Persian gulf war military personnel. Journal of Interpersonal Violence, 13, 40–57.

Wolfe, L. (1981). The Cosmo report. New York: Arbor House.

Wolner-Hanssen, P., Eschenbach, D. A., Paavonen, J., Stevens, C. E., Kiviat, N. B., Critchlow, C., DeRouen, T., Koutsky, L., & Holmes, K. K. (1990). Association between vaginal douching and acute pelvic inflammatory disease. Journal of the American Medical Association, 263, 1936–1941.

Woods, N. F. (1984). Human sexuality in health and illness (3rd ed.). St. Louis: Mosby.

World Health Organization Task Force on the Prevention and Management of Infertility. (1995). Tubal infertility: Serologic relationship to past chlamydial and gonococcal infection. Sexually Transmitted Diseases, 22, 71–77.

World Health Organization. (1987). Barrier contraceptives and spermicides: Their role in family planning care. Geneva, Switzerland.

Wright, L. K. (1991). The impact of Alzheimer's disease on the marital relationship. Gerontologist, 31, 224–237.

Wroe, M. (1996, November). Anglican bishop champions gay interests. London Observer Service @London. [online].

Wylie, K. R. (1997). Treatment outcome of brief couple therapy in psychogenic male erectile disorder. Archives of Sexual Behavior, 26, 527–545.

Wyman, M. A., & Snyder, M. (1997). Attitudes toward "gays in the military": A functional perspective. Journal of Applied Social Psychology, 27, 306–329.

Yao, M., & Tulandi, T. (1997). Current status of surgical and nonsurgical management of ectopic pregnancy. Fertility and Sterility, 67, 421–433.

Yarnall, K. S., Michener, J. L., Broadhead, W. E., & Tse, C-K, J. (1993). Increasing compliance with mammography recommendations: Health assessment forms. Journal of Family Practice, 36, 59–64.

Yescavage, K. (1999). Teaching women a lesson. Sexually aggressive and sexually nonaggressive men's perceptions of acquaintance and date rape. Violence Against Women, 5, 796–812.

Ying, Y. (1992). Life satisfaction among San Francisco Chinese-Americans. Social Indicators Research, 26, 1–22.

Youn, G. (1996). Sexual activities and attitudes of adolescent Koreans. Archives of Sexual Behavior, 25, 629–643.

Young, C. H. (1982). Sexual implications of stoma surgery. Clinics in Gastroenterology, 11, 383–391.

Young, M. (1980). Attitudes and behavior of college students relative to oral-genital sexuality. Archives of Sexual Behavior, 9, 61–67.

Zacks, R. (1994). History laid bare. New York: Harper Collins.

Zelnick, M., Kantner, J., & Ford, D. (1981). Sex and pregnancy in adolescence. Beverly Hills, CA: Sage.

Ziff, S. F. (1981). The sexual concerns of the adolescent woman with cerebral palsy. Issues in Health Care of Women, 3, 55–63.

Zigler, E. (1995). Can we "cure" mild mental retardation among individuals in the lower socioeconomic stratum. American Journal of Public Health, 85, 302–304

Zilbergeld, B. (1992). The new male sexuality. New York: Bantam Books.

Zoldbrod, A. P. (1998). Sex smart: How your childhood shaped your sexual life and what to do about it. Oakland, CA: New Harbinger.

Zubin, L. S., Hirsch, M. B., & Emmerson, M. R. (1989). When urban adolescents choose abortion: Effects on education, psychological status, and subsequent pregnancy. Family Planning Perspectives, 21, 248–255.

Zulkifli, S. N., Low, W. Y., & Yusof, K. (1995). Sexual activities of Malaysian adolescents. Medical Journal of Malaysia, 50, 4–10.

Zumoff, B. (1998). Does postmenopausal estrogen administration increase the risk of breast cancer? Contributions of animal, biochemical, and clinical investigative studies to a resolution of the controversy. Proceedings of the Society for Experimental Biology and Medicine, 217, 30–37.

PHOTO AND ART CREDIT LIST

Photo for "Dear Dr. Ruth" provided by Steve Friedman. For the following figures, the artwork was drawn using photographs created by Michal Heron Photography, NYC and Stephen Ogilvy Photography, NYC. Figures 8-9 through 8-24, 9-11, 9-12, 10-12A and B, 15-2A and B, 15-3, 15-5, 15-6A, 15-8, 15-11A and B, 16-6 and 16-10.

1-1   © FPG International
1-2   Courtesy of SanfordCourtesy Lopater
1-3A   © CORBIS
1-3B   © Jeffrey L. Rotman/CORBIS
1-4A   © Steve Chenn/CORBIS
1-4B   © CORBIS
1-5   © James H. Pickerell/Image Works
1-6A   © Vittoriano Rastelli/CORBIS
1-6B   © Richard T. Nowitz/CORBIS
1-6C   © John Garrett/CORBIS
1-6D   © Earl & Nazima Kowall/CORBIS
1-7A   © CORBIS
1-7B   Photo Lennar Nilsson/Albert Bonniers Förlag AB, A CHILD IS BORN, Dell Publishing Company
1-8   © AP/Wide World Photos
1-9   Courtesy of W. G. Carpenter, Phoenix, Maryland.
1-10   © AP/Wide World Photos
1-11A   Courtesy of Wyeth-Ayerst Pharmaceuticals.
1-11B   Burke & Triolo/Artville
1-11C   Courtesy of LDS Consumer Products.
1-12   © Chronis Jons/Stone
1-13   Courtesy of Sanford Lopater
1-14   © AP/Wide World Photos
1-15   © Richard AEF.Kirsch/The Image Bank
1-16   Courtesy of the Commonwealth of Virginia Division of Forensic Science.

2-1   © Alinari/Art Resource, NY
2-2   © Michael Nicholson/CORBIS
2-3A   Belvoir Castle, Leicestershire, UK/ Bridgeman Art Library
2-3B   Alinari/Art Resource, NY
2-3C   Borromeo/Art Resource, NY
2-4A   Scala/Art Resource, NY
2-4B   Scala/Art Resource, NY
2-5   Erich Lessing/Art Resource, NY
2-6   © CORBIS
2-7   Illustration by Spencer Phippen.
2-8   Scala/Art Resource, NY
2-9   © Dave Bartruff/PictureQuest, GA
2-10   © Bettmann/CORBIS
2-11   © PACHA/CORBIS
2-12   The Pierpont Morgan Library/Art Resource, NY
2-13   © Underwood & Underwood/CORBIS
2-14   © Hulton-Deusch Collection/CORBIS
2-15A   Courtesy of gayhistory.com. Reproduced from an original housed at the Archiv und Bibliothek des Schwulen Museums. Berlin.
2-15B   © Hulton-Deusch Collection/CORBIS
2-15C   © Bettmann/CORBIS
2-16   © Hulton-Deusch Collection/CORBIS
2-17   Courtesy of gayhistory.com. Reproduced from an original housed at the Archiv für Sexualwissenschaft, Berlin.
2-18   © Bettmann/CORBIS
2-19   © Bettmann/CORBIS

3-1   © Steve Mason/Photodisc
3-2   Photo Lennar Nilsson/Albert Bonniers Förlag AB, A CHILD IS BORN, Dell Publishing Company
3-3   From Bear M, Connors B, and Pardiso M. Neuroscience: Exploring the Brain, 2nd ed. Baltimore: Lippincott Williams & Wilkins, 2000.
3-4A   From Sadler TW. Langman's Medical Embryology, 7th ed. Baltimore: Williams & Wilkins, 1995.
3-4B   From Sadler TW. Langman's Medical Embryology, 7th ed. Baltimore: Williams & Wilkins, 1995.
3-5   From Sadler TW. Langman's Medical Embryology, 7th ed. Baltimore: Williams & Wilkins, 1995.
3-6   Courtesy of David A. Hatch, M.D.
3-7   From Sadler TW. Langman's Medical Embryology, 7th ed. Baltimore: Williams & Wilkins, 1995.
3-8   © James Marshall/CORBIS
3-9   Courtesy of Chippendales®
3-10   © AP/Wide World Photos
3-11   © CORBIS
3-12   © Peter Menzel/PictureQuest, GA
3-13   © George Hall/CORBIS
3-14   © AP/Wide World Photos
3-15   Courtesy of Dr. Leah C. Schaefer and Dr. Reneè Richards.
3-16A   David Rini, MFA, The Fine Art of Illustration, Baltimore, MD
3-16B   From Georgiade NG, Reifkohl R and Levine LS. Georgiade Plastic, Maxillofacial and Reconstructive Surgery, 3rd ed. Baltimore: Williams & Wilkins, 1997.
3-17A   David Rini, MFA, The Fine Art of Illustration, Baltimore, MD
3-17B   From Georgiade NG, Reifkohl R and Levine LS. Georgiade Plastic, Maxillofacial and Reconstructive Surgery, 3rd ed. Baltimore: Williams & Wilkins, 1996.
3-18   Courtesy of Carter-Wallace, Inc. Photo by Michal Heron, NYC/Stephen Ogilvy, NYC.
3-19   Courtesy of Carter-Wallace, Inc. Photo by Michael Zeppetello.
3-20   © The Purcell Team/CORBIS
3-21   © Bettmann/CORBIS
3-22   © Reuters NewMedia Inc./CORBIS
3-23   © Photofest
3-24   © Michael S. Yamashita/CORBIS
3-25   © Photofest

4-1   Michal Heron, NYC/Stephen Ogilvy, NYC
4-2   Michal Heron, NYC/Stephen Ogilvy, NYC
4-3   Michal Heron, NYC/Stephen Ogilvy, NYC
4-4   David Rini, MFA, The Fine Art of Illustration, Baltimore, MD
4-5   David Rini, MFA, The Fine Art of Illustration, Baltimore, MD
4-6   Davis G, Ellis J, Hibbert M, Perez RP, Zimbelman E. Female Circumcision: The Prevalence and Nature of the Ritual in Eritea. Military Medicine. 1999;164:11-16.
4-7   David Rini, MFA, The Fine Art of Illustration, Baltimore, MD
4-8   David Rini, MFA, The Fine Art of Illustration, Baltimore, MD
4-9   From Das Lexikon der Gesundheit. Munich: Urban & Volgel Verlag, 1996. Art by Jonathan Dimes, Parkton, MD
4-10   Michael Kress-Russick, Madison, WI
4-11   From Gartner LP and Hiatt JL. Color Atlas of Histlogy, 3rd ed. Baltimore: Lippincott Williams & Wilkins, 2000.
4-12   From Cormack DH. Essential Histology. Philadelphia: Lippincott-Raven, 1993.
4-13   From Das Lexikon der Gesundheit. Munich: Urban & Schwarzenberg Verlag, 1996. Art by Jonathan Dimes, Parkton, MD.
4-14   Michael Kress-Russick, Madison, WI
4-15   Michal Heron, NYC/Stephen Ogilvy, NYC
4-16   David Rini, MFA, The Fine Art of Illustration, Baltimore, MD
4-17   Courtesy of McGhan Medical Corporation.
4-18   Michal Heron, NYC/Stephen Ogilvy, NYC
4-19A   Giraudon/Art Resource, NY
4-19B   Erich Lessing/Art Resource, NY
4-20   David Rini, MFA, The Fine Art of Illustration, Baltimore, MD
4-21   From Das Lexikon der Gesundheit. Munich: Urban & Schwarzenberg Verlag, 1996. Art by Jonathan Dimes, Parkton, MD.
4-22   Michal Heron, NYC/Stephen Ogilvy, NYC
4-23   David Rini, MFA, The Fine Art of Illustration, Baltimore, MD
4-24   Courtesy of Singapore Medical Journal.
4-25   From Das Lexikon der Gesundheit. Munich: Urban & Schwarzenberg Verlag, 1996. Art by Jonathan Dimes, Parkton, MD.
4-25   From Eroschenko VP. di Fiore's Atlas of Histology with Functional Correlations, 8th ed. Baltimore: Williams & Wilkins, 1995.
4-26   Copyright by Dr. R. G. Kessel and Dr. R. H. Kardon, Tissues and Organs: A Text-Atlas of Scanning Electron Microscopy, 1979, W.H. Freeman, all rights reserved.
4-27   From Gartner LP and Hiatt JL. Color Atlas of Histlogy, 3rd ed. Baltimore: Lippincott Williams & Wilkins, 2000.
4-28   Copyright by Dr. R. G. Kessel and Dr. R. H. Kardon, Tissues and Organs: A Text-Atlas of Scanning Electron Microscopy, 1979, W.H. Freeman, all rights reserved.
4-29   From Das Lexikon der Gesundheit. Munich: Urban & Schwarzenberg Verlag, 1996. Art by Jonathan Dimes, Parkton, MD.
4-30   Michael Kress-Russick, Madison, WI

5-1ABC From Edge V and Miller M. Women's Health Care. St. Louis: Mosby, 1994.
5-2A   From Bates. Bates' Guide to Physical Examination and History Taking, 7th ed. Baltimore: Lippincott Williams & Wilkins, 1999.
5-2B   From Edge V and Miller M. Women's Health Care. St. Louis: Mosby, 1994.
5-3   Larry Ward, Salt Lake City, UT. From Fuller J and Schaller-Ayers J. Health Assessment: A Nursing Approach, 2nd ed. Philadelphia: J.B. Lippincott Company, 1994.
5-4   Michal Heron, NYC/Stephen Ogilvy, NYC
5-5   Michal Heron, NYC/Stephen Ogilvy, NYC
5-6A   From Brant WE and Helms CA. Fundamentals of Diagnostic Radiology, 2nd ed. Baltimore: Lippincott Williams & Wilkins, 1998.
5-6B   From Daffner RH. Clinical Radiology: The Essentials, 2nd ed. Baltimore: Lippincott Williams & Wilkins, 1998.
5-7   © Keith Brofsky/Photodisc
5-8AB   From Georgiade NG, Reifkohl R and Levine LS. Georgiade Plastic, Maxillofacial and Reconstructive Surgery, 3rd ed. Baltimore: Williams & Wilkins, 1997.
5-9   © Bettmann/CORBIS
5-10   © SIU Biomed com /Custom Medical Stock Photo
5-11   From Bates. Bates' Guide to Physical Examination and History Taking, 7th ed. Baltimore: Lippincott Williams & Wilkins, 1999.

5-12   From Cormack DH. Essential Histology. Philadelphia: Lippincott-Raven, 1993.

5-13   © Rawlins/Custom Medical Stock Photo

5-14   Michael Kress-Russick, Madison, WI

5-15A   © AP/Wide World Photos

5-15B   © Neal Preston/CORBIS

5-16   Michal Heron, NYC/Stephen Ogilvy, NYC

5-17   From Das Lexikon der Gesundheit. Munich: Urban & Schwarzenberg Verlag, 1996. Art by Jonathan Dimes, Parkton, MD.

5-18   Michael Kress-Russick, Madison, WI

5-19   Michael Kress-Russick, Madison, WI

5-20   From Brant WE and Helms CA. Fundamentals of Diagnostic Radiology, 2nd ed. Baltimore: Lippincott Williams & Wilkins, 1998.

6-1AB   © Photofest

6-2   © CORBIS

6-3   Maggie Heinzel-Neel/Artville

6-4AB   Courtesy of Behavioral Technology, Inc., Salt Lake City, UT.

6-5   From Bear M, Connors B, and Pardiso M. Neuroscience: Exploring the Brain, 2nd ed. Baltimore: Lippincott Williams & Wilkins, 2000.

6-6   From Bear M, Connors B, and Pardiso M. Neuroscience: Exploring the Brain, 2nd ed. Baltimore: Lippincott Williams & Wilkins, 2000.

6-7   From Bear M, Connors B, and Pardiso M. Neuroscience: Exploring the Brain, 2nd ed. Baltimore: Lippincott Williams & Wilkins, 2000.

6-8   From McArdle WD, Katch FI, and Katch VL. Exercise Physiology, 5th ed. Baltimore: Lippincott Williams & Wilkins, 2001.

6-9   Michael Kress-Russick, Madison, WI

6-10A-E   David Rini, MFA, The Fine Art of Illustration, Baltimore, MD

6-11   David Rini, MFA, The Fine Art of Illustration, Baltimore, MD

6-12   Michael Kress-Russick, Madison, WI

6-13   © Jack Hollingsworth/CORBIS

6-14   © Annie Griffiths Belt/CORBIS

6-15   © Jeff Greenberg/Image Works

6-16   Michal Heron, NYC/Stephen Ogilvy, NYC

6-17   Mary Anna Barratt, Parkton, MD

7-1   Mary Anna Barratt, Parkton, MD

7-2   Michael Kress-Russick, Madison, WI

7-3   © David Turnley/CORBIS

7-4   © Bettmann/CORBIS

7-5   Michael Kress-Russick, Madison, WI

7-6   Michael Kress-Russick, Madison, WI

7-7   From THE PROPHET by Kahlil Gibran,
(narrative)   Copyright 1923 by Kahlil Gibran and renewed 1951 by Administrators C T A of Kahlil Gibran Estate and Mary G Gibran. Used by permission of Alfred A. Knopf, a division of Random House, Inc. and Gibran National C

7-7   © E.O. Hoppé/CORBIS

7-8   © Photodisc

7-9   © Bettmann/CORBIS

7-10   © Bettmann/CORBIS

7-11   © CORBIS

7-12   Courtesy of Richard and Margaret Dimes, Winthrop, MA.

7-13   © Richard Hamilton Smith/CORBIS

7-14   © Ed Eckstein/CORBIS

7-15   © Worldwide Marriage Encounter, used with permission

7-16A   © Joseph Sohm; ChromoSohm Inc./CORBIS

7-16B   © Kit Kittle/CORBIS

7-16C   © CORBIS

7-17A   © AP/Wide World Photos

7-17B   © Robbie Jack/CORBIS

7-18A   © R.W. Jones/CORBIS

7-18B   © Chandra Clarke/CORBIS

7-19   Mary Anna Barratt, Parkton, MD

7-20   Carla Golembe/Artville

7-21   Reprinted with special permission of King Features Syndicate.

8-1   Eiji Miyazawa/ Black Star

8-2   Michael Kress-Russick, Madison, WI

8-3   © Jim Sugar Photography/CORBIS

8-4   Encyclical Letter of John Paul II, the Splendor of Truth (Veritatis Splendor), Copyright ©, 1993, Daughters of St. Paul. Used with permission of Pauline Books & Media.

8-5   Gustave Doré (French, 1832-1883) The Neophyte (First experience of the Monastery), c. 1866-68 Oil on canvas, 57-3/3 x 107-1/2 inches CHRYSLER MUSEUM OF ART, NORFOLK, VA, Gift of Walter P. Chrysler, Jr. 71.2061

8-6   © Bettmann/CORBIS

8-7   © Suzanne Arms/Image Works

8-8   © Mark Antman/Image Works

8-9   Art by David Rini, MFA, The Fine Art of Illustration, Baltimore, MD

8-10   Art by David Rini, MFA, The Fine Art of Illustration, Baltimore, MD

8-11   Art by David Rini, MFA, The Fine Art of Illustration, Baltimore, MD

8-12   Art by David Rini, MFA, The Fine Art of Illustration, Baltimore, MD

8-13   Art by David Rini, MFA, The Fine Art of Illustration, Baltimore, MD

8-14   Art by David Rini, MFA, The Fine Art of Illustration, Baltimore, MD

8-15   Art by David Rini, MFA, The Fine Art of Illustration, Baltimore, MD

8-16   Art by David Rini, MFA, The Fine Art of Illustration, Baltimore, MD

8-17   Art by David Rini, MFA, The Fine Art of Illustration, Baltimore, MD

8-18   Art by David Rini, MFA, The Fine Art of Illustration, Baltimore, MD

8-19   Art by David Rini, MFA, The Fine Art of Illustration, Baltimore, MD

8-20   Art by David Rini, MFA, The Fine Art of Illustration, Baltimore, MD

8-21   Art by David Rini, MFA, The Fine Art of Illustration, Baltimore, MD

8-22   Art by David Rini, MFA, The Fine Art of Illustration, Baltimore, MD

8-23   Art by David Rini, MFA, The Fine Art of Illustration, Baltimore, MD

8-24   Art by David Rini, MFA, The Fine Art of Illustration, Baltimore, MD

9-1   Courtesy of the Hungarian National Museum of Historical Photographic Archives.

9-2   © Mimmo Jodice/CORBIS

9-3   Courtesy of gayhistory.com. Reproduced from an original housed at the Archiv für Sexualwissenschaft, Berlin.

9-5   From Bear M, Connors B, and Pardiso M. Neuroscience: Exploring the Brain, 2nd ed. Baltimore: Lippincott Williams & Wilkins, 2000.

9-6   Illustration by Spencer Phippen.

9-7A   From Pilliterri A. Maternal & Child Health Nursing: Care of the Childbearing & Childrearing Family, 3rd ed. Philadelphia: Lippincott Williams & Wilkins, 1999. Courtesy of Janet Weber.

9-7B   © B. Proud

9-8   Maggie Heinzel-Neel/Artville

9-9   © B. Busco/The Image Bank

9-10   Keith Brofsky/Artville

9-11   Art by David Rini, MFA, The Fine Art of Illustration, Baltimore, MD

9-12   Art by David Rini, MFA, The Fine Art of Illustration, Baltimore, MD

9-13A   © 1998, The Washington Post Reprinted with permission. Art by Michael Kress-Russick, Madison, WI.

9-13B   © AP/Wide World Photos

9-13C   © AP/Wide World Photos

9.14   © AP/Wide World Photos

9-15   © AP/Wide World Photos

9-16   © AP/Wide World Photos

9-17   Mary Anna Barratt, Parkton, MD

9-18   Courtesy of St. Cloud Times.

9-19   © AP/Wide World Photos

T9-1   Michael Kress-Russick, Madison, WI

10-1   Courtesy of University of Chicago, photo by Matthew Gil son.

10-2A   Britt Matson/Artville

10-2B   © CORBIS

10-3   © SW Productions/Photodisc

10-4   From Bates. Bates' Guide to Physical Examination and History Taking, 7th ed. Baltimore: Lippincott Williams & Wilkins, 1999.

10-5   From Das Lexikon der Gesundheit. Munich: Urban & Schwarzenberg Verlag, 1996.

10-6   © Petit Format/Nestle/Science Source/Photo Researchers

10-7   © Copyright of Genetics & IVF Institute

10-8   Michael Kress-Russick, Madison, WI

10-9   Michael Kress-Russick, Madison, WI

10-10   © Photospin

10-11ABC   Michael Kress-Russick, Madison, WI

10-12A   Art by David Rini, MFA, The Fine Art of Illustration, Baltimore, MD

10-12B   Art by David Rini, MFA, The Fine Art of Illustration, Baltimore, MD

10-13   Photography Michal Heron, NYC/Stephen Ogilvy, NYC. Courtesy of Warner-Lambert, a Pfizer Company.

10-14   Neil O. Hardy, Westport, CT. From Stedman's Medical Dictionary, 27th ed. Baltimore: Lippincott Williams & Wilkins, 2000.

10-15   Neil O. Hardy, Westport, CT. From Stedman's Medical Dictionary, 27th ed. Baltimore: Lippincott Williams & Wilkins, 2000.

10-16   © Petit Format/Nestle/Science Source/Photo Researchers

10-17   Photo Lennar Nilsson/Albert Bonniers Förlag AB, A CHILD IS BORN, Dell Publishing Company

10-18A-D   From Daffner RH. Clinical Radiology: The Essentials, 2nd ed. Baltimore: Lippincott Williams & Wilkins, 1998.

10-19A-C   From Pilliterri A. Maternal & Child Health Nursing: Care of the Childbearing & Childrearing Family, 3rd ed. Philadelphia: Lippincott Williams & Wilkins, 1999. Photos by John Gallagher, with permission of University of Pennsylvania Medical Center, Philadelphia.

10-20   © Caroline Brown, RNC, MS, Ded

10-21   © Layne Kennedy/CORBIS

10-22   Courtesy of the Birthing Center at St. Luke's-Roosevelt Hospital Center in New York City.

10-23   Courtesy of Howard McClamrock, MD, Maryland Women's Center and University of Maryland Medicine.

10-24   Michael Kress-Russick, Madison, WI

10-25   Courtesy of RIMOS s.r.i.-ITALY.

10-26   © Rawlins/Custom Medical Stock Photo

10-27   From Das Lexikon der Gesundheit. Munich: Urban & Schwarzenberg Verlag, 1996. Art by Jonathan Dimes, Parkton, MD

10-28   By Jonathan Dimes, Parkton, MD. Adapted from IVF and GIFT: A Guide to Assisted Reproductive Technologies. Birmingham: American Society for Reproductive Medicine, 1995.

10-29   Courtesy of Procrea Biosciences, Montreal Canada. www.procrea.com

10-30   Michael Kress-Russick, Madison, WI

11-1   Michael Kress-Russick, Madison, WI

11-2   History of Contraception Museum, Janssen-Ortho, Inc., Toronto, Canada.

11-3A   © Bettmann / CORBIS

11-3B   Courtesy of Dr. Roy Greep of the Worcester Foundation for Experimental Biology.

11-3C   © PictureQuest

11-4   © Michael S. Yamashita/CORBIS

11-5   Courtesy of Wyeth-Ayerst Pharmaceuticals.

11-6   Courtesy of Wyeth-Ayerst Pharmaceuticals.

11-7   Courtesy of Carter-Wallace, Inc., BLAIREX and Ortho-McNeil. Photo by Michal Heron, NYC/Stephen Ogilvy, NYC.

INDEX

Page numbers in italics denote figures; those followed by a "t" denote tables.

A